# HEALTH PROMOTION
Throughout the Life Span

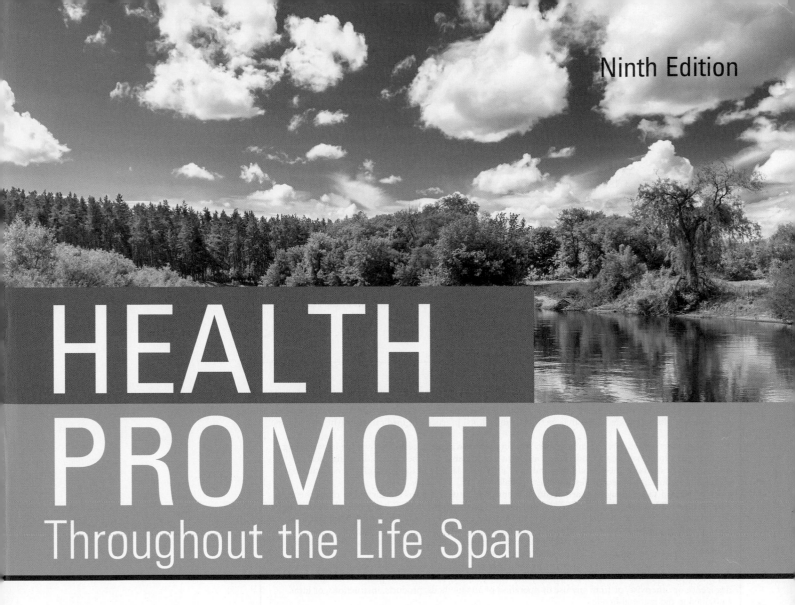

Ninth Edition

# HEALTH PROMOTION
## Throughout the Life Span

**CAROLE LIUM EDELMAN**, MSN, GCNS-BC, CMC
Private Practice
Professional Geriatric Care Management
Westport, Connecticut

**ELIZABETH CONNELLY KUDZMA**, DNSc, MPH, WHNP-BC, CNL
Professor
Director of MSN Program
School of Nursing
Curry College
Milton, Massachusetts

**ELSEVIER**

# ELSEVIER

3251 Riverport Lane
St. Louis, Missouri 63043

*Senior Content Strategist:* Jamie L. Blum
*Content Development Specialist:* Charlene Ketchum
*Publishing Services Manager:* Jeffrey Patterson
*Senior Project Manager:* Mary Pohlman
*Design Direction:* Margaret Reid

Printed in China.

Last digit is the print number:   9   8   7   6   5   4   3   2   1

To our wonderful families, friends, students, and colleagues —
that they promote health in themselves and others.

# CONTRIBUTORS

Kevin K. Chui, PT, DPT, PhD, GCS,
  OCS, CEEAA, FAAOMPT
Director and Professor
School of Physical Therapy
College of Health Professions
Pacific University
Hillsboro, Oregon

Kristi Coker, PhD, RN
Director of Nursing for Children's Hospital
Greenville Health System
Greenville, South Carolina

Donna DelloIacono, NP, PhD, CNL
Nurse Practitioner
Weiner Center for Preoperative Evaluation
Brigham and Woman's Hospital
Boston, Massachusetts

Susan Ann Denninger, PT, DPT, PCS
Physical Therapist
Kidnetics
Greenville Health System
Greenville, South Carolina

Christine Sorrell Dinkins, PhD
Associate Professor of Philosophy
Wofford College
Spartanburg, South Carolina

Susan A. Heady, PhD, RN
Professor
Webster University
St. Louis, Missouri

Rosanna F. Hess, BSN, MA, MSN,
  DNP, RN
Research Associate
Research for Health, Inc.
Cuyahoga Falls, Ohio

June Andrews Horowitz, PhD, RN,
  PMH, CNS-BC, FAAN
Associate Dean for Graduate Programs &
  Research and Professor
College of Nursing
University of Massachusetts
Dartmouth, Massachusetts

Susan Rowen James, PhD, RN
Professor Emeritus
School of Nursing
Curry College
Milton, Massachusetts

Debora Elizabeth Kirsch, RN, MS,
  CNS, PhDc
Retired Faculty
College of Nursing
SUNY Upstate Medical University
Syracuse, New York

Carolyn Cable Kleman, PhDc, MHA,
  BSN, RN
Doctoral Candidate
Kent State University
Kent, Ohio

Myrtle McCulloch, EdD, MS, RDN
Assistant Professor, Nutrition
School of Nursing and Health Studies
Georgetown University
Washington, DC

Staci McIntosh, MS, RD
Assistant Professor
Department of Nutrition and Integrative
  Physiology
University of Utah
Salt Lake City, Utah

Maureen Murphy, PhD, MSN, MEd,
  RN, CNM
Professor
School of Nursing
Curry College
Milton, Massachusetts

Anne Rath Rentfro, PhD, RN
Retired Professor
The University of Texas at Brownsville
Brownsville, Texas

Susan Scott Ricci, ARNP, MSN,
  MEd., CNE
Nursing Faculty
University of Central Florida
Orlando, Florida

Ratchneewan Ross, PhD, RN, FAAN
Cone Health Distinguished Professor
Chair, Department of Family and
  Community Nursing
School of Nursing
University of North Carolina at
  Greensboro
Greensboro, North Carolina

Leslie Kennard Scott, PhD, APRN,
  PPCNP-BC, CDE, MLDE
Associate Professor
Pediatric Nurse Practitioner BSN-DNP
  Programs Coordinator
College of Nursing
University of Kentucky
Lexington, Kentucky

Jeanne M. Sorrell, PhD, RN, FAAN
Contributing Faculty
Richard W. Riley College of Education and
  Leadership
Walden University
Minneapolis, Minnesota

Frank Tudini, PT, DSc, OCS, COMT,
  FAAOMPT
Professor
Sacred Heart University
Fairfield, Connecticut

Diane Marie Welsh, DNP, RN, CNE
Dean, School of Nursing
Regis College
Weston, Massachussetts

Sheng-Che Yen, PT, PhD
Assistant Professor
Department of Physical Therapy,
  Movement and Rehabilitation Sciences
Northeastern University
Boston, Massachusetts

## EVOLVE ASSET CONTRIBUTOR

Lois E. Brenneman, MSN, FNP
Family Nurse Practitioner and Adjunct
  Faculty
Fairleigh Dickinson University
Teaneck, New Jersey

# REVIEWERS

**Angeline Bushy, PhD, RN, FAAN**
Professor and Bert Fish Endowed Chair
College of Nursing
University of Central Florida
Orlando, Florida

**Margaret-Ann Carno, PhD, MBA, CPNP, D ABSM**
Assistant Professor of Clinical Nursing and Pediatrics
School of Nursing
University of Rochester
Rochester, New York

**Pamela N. Clarke, RN, MPH, PhD, FAAN**
Professor and Director of the Center for Community Health and
    Economic Development
Fay W. Whitney School of Nursing
University of Wyoming
Laramie, Wyoming

**Kim Clevenger, EdD, MSN, RN, BC**
Associate Professor of Nursing
Department of Nursing
Morehead State University
Morehead, Kentucky

**Donna DelloIacono, NP, PhD, CNL**
Nurse Practitioner
Weiner Center for Preoperative Evaluation
Brigham and Woman's Hospital
Boston, Massachusetts

**Maureen Murphy, PhD, MSN, MEd, RN, CNM**
Professor
School of Nursing
Curry College
Milton, Massachusetts

# PREVIOUS CONTRIBUTORS

Gary P. Austin, PT, PhD, OCS, FAAOMPT

Kathleen Blais, EdD, RN

Jennifer Elizabeth Brunton, PhD

Tawna Cooksey-James, PhD, RN, CNE

Dee Coover, PhD, RN

Michael Fortin, PT, DPT

Philip A. Greiner, DNSc, RN

Suzy Harrington, DNP, RN, MCHES

Yi-Hui Lee, PhD, MBA, MSN, BSN

Brian Pecchia, PT, DPT, ATC

Roseanne M. Prunty, DPT

Jeffrey R. Ross, BFA, MA, MAT

Ali Salman, MD, PhD, ND

Toni M. Tucker, MA, RD

## PURPOSE OF THE BOOK

The case for promoting and protecting health, and preventing disease and injury, was established by many accomplishments in the 20th century and continued into the 21st century. Americans and global populations are taking better care of themselves; public concerns about physical fitness, good nutrition, and avoidance of health hazards such as smoking have become adopted in the lifestyles of global citizens. Encouraging positive health changes has been a major effort of individuals, the government, health professionals, and society in general. In the United States, public and private attempts to improve the health status of individuals and groups traditionally have focused on reducing communicable diseases and health hazards. Concerns continue about how to deliver the best practices to improve access to and reduce costs of health services and to improve the overall quality of life for all people. Americans increasingly recognized that the health of each individual is influenced by the health environments of all individuals worldwide.

Throughout the history of the United States, the public health community has assessed the health of Americans. In 1789, the Reverend Edward Wigglesworth developed the first American mortality tables through his study in New England. Population statistics gathered in England and America, including those of Florence Nightingale, proved that useful data could change health outcomes. The *Report of a General Plan for the Promotion of Public and Personal Health* was completed by Lemuel Shattuck in 1880. *Healthy People, The Surgeon General's Report on Health Promotion and Disease Prevention,* was first published in 1979, and was followed by *Healthy People 2000: National Health Promotion and Disease Prevention Objectives,* which listed three goals:

- Increase the span of healthy life for Americans.
- Reduce health disparities among Americans.
- Achieve access to preventive services for all Americans.

These original documents were followed by *Healthy People 2010* and *2020*.

Health-promotion advances require a better understanding of the environment, health risks, behaviors, and intervention measures. *Healthy People 2010* identified important determinants of health status, which included:

- Individual behavior
- Biology and genetics
- Physical environment
- Social environment
- Health services

Outcome measures designed to assist individual and group efforts to change and improve behavior in these areas can lead to decreases in morbidity and mortality.

Professionals who undertake health-promotion strategies also need to understand the basics of health protection and disease and injury prevention. Health protection is directed at population groups of all ages and involves adherence to standards, outcomes, infectious disease control, and governmental regulation and enforcement. The focus of these activities is on reducing exposure to various sources of hazards, including those related to air, water, foods, drugs, motor vehicles, and other physical agents.

Health care providers present individuals, families, and communities with disease- and injury-prevention services, which include immunizations, screenings, health education, and counseling. To implement prevention strategies effectively, it is essential to develop activities targeted to and tailored for all age groups in various settings including schools, industries, the home, the health care delivery system, the larger community, and the world. *Healthy People 2010* addressed these health problems by establishing goals and objectives for the first decade of the new millennium. The vision for *Healthy People 2010* was "Healthy people in healthy communities" because, as nursing has long recognized, the health of each individual is inseparable from the health of families, communities, nations, and the world. Health is significantly affected by the environment in which each individual lives, works, travels, and plays. Dimensions of the environment are not only physical but also psychosocial and spiritual; including the behaviors, attitudes, and beliefs of each individual. Specific objectives in 28 focus areas supported 2 major goals:

- Increase quality and years of healthy life.
- Eliminate health disparities.

Released in 2010, *Healthy People 2020* reflects the earlier assessments of major risks to health, changing public health priorities, and emerging issues related to our nation's health preparedness and prevention. The following vision was established: A society in which all people live long healthy lives.

The mission within this vision is improving health through strengthening policy. *Healthy People 2020* will:

- Identify nationwide health improvement priorities.
- Increase public awareness and understanding of the determinants of health, disease, and disability and the opportunities for progress.
- Provide measurable objectives and goals that can be used at the national, state, and local levels.
- Engage multiple sectors to take action that are driven by the best available evidence and knowledge.
- Identify critical research and data collection needs.

The overarching goals for *Healthy People 2020* continue the tradition of earlier *Healthy People* initiatives of advocating for improvements in the health of every person in our country. They address the environmental factors and place particular emphasis on the determinants of health:

- Eliminate preventable disease, disability, injury, and premature death.
- Achieve health equity, eliminate disparities, and improve the health of all groups.
- Create social and physical environments that promote good health for all.
- Promote healthy development and healthy behaviors across every stage of life.

The databases within *Healthy People* continue to indicate targets and assessments of health status and risk for evaluations and future planning, not only for health policymakers and health care providers but also for individuals, families, and communities at the local, regional, national, and global levels. (Subscribe to the *Healthy People* listserv for the latest information and to receive e-mail notices of related news, events, and publications at http://healthypeople.gov/hp2020.)

The information in this edition of *Health Promotion Throughout the Life Span* includes these and other data and guidelines for health promotion, health protection, preventive services, and surveillance data systems, including those to the US Preventive Services Task Force (www.ahrq.gov/clinic/cps) and the Guide to Community Preventive Services (www.thecommunityguide.org).

## APPROACH AND ORGANIZATION

This edition presents health data with related theories and skills that are needed to understand and practice when providing care. This book focuses on primary prevention intervention; its three main components are: (1) health promotion, (2) specific health protection, and (3) prevention of specific diseases. Health promotion is the intervention designed to improve health, such as providing adequate nutrition, a healthy environment, and ongoing health education. Specific protection and prevention strategies, such as massive immunizations, periodic examinations, and safety features in the workplace, are the interventions used to protect against illness.

In addition to primary prevention, this book discusses secondary prevention interventions, focusing specifically on screening and education. Such programs include blood pressure, cholesterol, and diabetes screening and referral (the acute components of secondary prevention are generally not addressed in this book).

This text is presented in five parts, each forming the basis for the next.

Unit 1, *Foundations for Health Promotion,* describes the foundational concepts of promoting and protecting health, and preventing diseases and injuries, including diagnostic, therapeutic, and ethical decision-making.

Unit 2, *Assessment for Health Promotion,* focuses on individuals, families, and communities and the factors affecting their health. The functional health pattern assessments developed by Gordon serve as the organizing framework for assessing the health of individuals, families, and communities.

Unit 3, *Interventions for Health Promotion,* discusses theories, methodologies, and case studies of nursing interventions, including screening, health-education counseling, stress management, and crisis intervention.

Unit 4, *Application of Health Promotion,* also uses Gordon's functional health patterns, emphasizing developmental, cultural, ethnic, and environmental variables in assessing the developing person. The intent is to address the health concerns of all Americans regardless of gender, race, age, or sexual orientation. Although most human development theories discussed are primarily based on the research of male subjects, newer theories based on female subjects are included. The

hope is to describe human development that more accurately reflects the complexity of human experiences throughout the life span.

Unit 5, *Emerging Global Health Issues,* presents a single chapter that discusses changing population groups and their health needs as well as related implications for research and practice in the 21st century. Throughout the text, research abstracts have been added to highlight the science of nursing practice and to demonstrate to the reader the relationship among research, practice, and outcomes.

Throughout these units, the evolving health care professions and the changing health care systems, including future challenges and initiatives for health promotion, are described. Emphasis is placed on the current concerns of reducing health care costs while increasing life expectancy and improving the quality of life for all Americans. This promotes the reader's immediate interest in thoughts about the content of the chapters.

### Key Features

- A full-color design, including color photos, is implemented throughout for better accessibility of content and visual enhancement.
- Each chapter starts with a list of objectives to help focus the reader and emphasize the content the reader should acquire through reading the book.
- Key Terms including quality and safety terms are listed at the front to acquaint readers with the important terminology of the chapter.
- Each chapter's narrative begins with a Think About It section, the presentation of a clinical issue or scenario that relates to the topic of the chapter, followed by critical thinking questions. This promotes the reader's immediate interest in and thought about the chapter.
- Research for Evidence-Based Practice boxes provide brief synopses on current health-promotion research studies that demonstrate the links between research, theory, and practice.
- Diversity Awareness boxes offer cultural perspectives on various aspects of health promotion.
- Quality and Safety boxes provide information regarding specific scenarios to improve health.
- Genomics boxes explore current genetic issues, controversies, and dilemmas with respect to health promotion, providing an opportunity for critical analysis of care issues.
- Innovative Practice boxes highlight inventive and resourceful projects, programs, and research studies that draw upon new ways of implementing health promotion.
- *Healthy People 2020* boxes present a list of selected objectives that are relevant to each chapter's topic.
- The Case Study highlights a real-life clinical situation relevant to the chapter topic.
- The Care Plan relates to the Case Study with the standardized sections of Defining Characteristics, Related Factors, Expected Outcomes, and Interventions, and details nursing diagnoses relevant to health-promotion activities and the related interventions.
- Study Questions are located on the book's website to offer additional review and self-study practice.

## New Features

1. An increased focus on genomics reflects increasing scientific evidence supporting the health benefits of using genetic tests and family health history to guide public health interventions.
2. The latest information about The Patient Protection and Affordable Care Act is included.
3. Expanded discussion of QSEN competencies related to health promotion.
4. Guidelines and recommendations from the latest Guide to Clinical Preventive Services, issued by the US Preventive Services Task Force, is included as appropriate.
5. Updated photos bring a fresh look and feel to the text.

## Evolve Resources

The expanded website for this book provides materials for both students and faculty, and is accessible at http://evolve.elsevier.com/Edelman/.

### For Students

- Study Questions: Multiple choice NCLEX® examination format

### For Instructors

- TEACH for Nurses, including Nursing Curriculum Standards, Teaching Activities, and Case Studies
- Image Collection, with all images from the book
- Lecture Slides, in PowerPoint
- Test Bank, 700 questions in NCLEX® examination format

The current trend to emphasize the developing health of people mandates that health care professionals understand the many issues that surround individuals, families, national and world communities in social, work, and family settings, including biological, inherited, cognitive, psychological, environmental, and sociocultural factors that can put their health at risk. Most important is that they develop interventions to promote health by understanding the diverse roles these factors play in the person's beliefs and health practices, particularly in the areas of disease and injury prevention, protection, and health promotion. Achieving such effectiveness requires collaboration with other health care providers and the integration of practice and policy while developing interventions and considering the ethical issues within individual, family, and both national and world communities' responsibilities for health.

**Carole Lium Edelman**
**Elizabeth Connelly Kudzma**

# ACKNOWLEDGMENTS

We had the good fortune of receiving much assistance and support from many friends, relatives, and associates. Our colleagues read chapters, gave valuable advice and criticism, helped clarify concepts, and provided case examples.

We also acknowledge the contributions of all the authors. In developing this text, they gave the project their total commitment and support. Their professional competence aided greatly in the development of the final draft of the manuscript. The editors worked and learned from each other during the planning and development of this book; throughout the entire process, close contact prevailed. Elizabeth Kudzma, a long-standing contributor, is the co-editor of this edition. She has added much knowledge and perspective to the ninth edition.

Many thanks to the Elsevier editorial and production team: Charlene Ketchum, Jamie Blum, Mary Pohlman, and Jeffrey Patterson. We appreciate and thank them for their ongoing help and support. It is a true pleasure working with them.

I am fortunate to have faith in the Lord, who gives courage and strength to face life's difficulties in a positive manner. My children, John and Megan Gillespie, Tom and Heather Gillespie, and Deirdre O'Brien, and my grandchildren, Ryan, Caroline, Meredith, and Colleen, bring joy to me as a mother and grandmother. Their patience and love are truly appreciated. Fredric Edelman provides much encouragement and support. Both my brother and sister in law, John and Marilyn Lium, are inspirational to me and a reminder every day that health in life is precious.

**Carole Lium Edelman**

As a contributor from the first edition to the present, I thank Carole Edelman for inviting me to become a co-editor of this ninth edition. The insights and clinical experiences of Curry College faculty colleagues and students are continuing sources of enrichment. Thanks also to my family, including my sister and brother (Mary and Mark), daughter Katherine, and especially to my husband Daniel, who provided support, discussion, and insight throughout this project.

**Elizabeth Connelly Kudzma**

# CONTENTS

# Health Defined: Health Promotion, Protection, and Prevention

*Ratchneewan Ross and Carolyn Cable Kleman*

## OBJECTIVES

*After completing this chapter, the reader will be able to:*

- Analyze concepts and models of *health* as used historically and as used in this textbook.
- Evaluate the consistency of *Healthy People 2020* goals with various concepts of health.
- Analyze the progress made in this nation from the original Healthy People document to the foci in *Healthy People 2020*.
- Differentiate between health, illness, disease, disability, and premature death.

- Compare the four levels of prevention (primordial, primary, secondary, and tertiary) with the levels of service provision available across the life span.
- Critique the role of research and evidence as well as the nurse's role in health education and research for the promotion and protection of health for individuals and populations.

## KEY TERMS

Adaptive model of health
Applied research
Asset planning
Clinical model of health
Community-based care
Cultural competence
Disease
Ecological model of health
Empathy
Epidemiology
Ethnocentrism
Eudaimonistic

Eudaimonistic model of health
Evidence-based practice
Functional health
Health
Health disparities
Health promotion
Health-related quality of life (HRQoL)
*Healthy People 2020*
High-level wellness
Illness
Interprofessional practice
Levels of prevention

Person-centered care
Qualitative studies
Quality of life
Quantitative studies
Racism
Role performance model of health
Social determinants of health
Specific protection
Well-being
Wellness
Wellness-illness continuum

**Health** is a core concept in society. This concept is modified with qualifiers such as *excellent, good, fair,* or *poor,* on the basis of a variety of factors. These factors may include age, sex, race or ethnic heritage, comparison group, current health or physical condition, past conditions, social or economic situation, geographical location, or the demands of various roles in society. In addition, there is growing evidence that larger societal and environmental concerns determine health outcomes. This chapter will discuss health as a concept and related concepts such as wellness, illness, disease, disability, and functioning. These concepts are frequently embedded in theories, such as theories of health behavior (Pender et al., 2015) or health planning (Issel, 2014). Some motivating factors behind the move to disease prevention and health promotion in society will be examined with an introduction to *Healthy People 2020,* the federal government's health objectives for the nation. The implementation of these concepts as nursing actions will also be addressed from ideal and pragmatic standpoints. Research and evidence supporting these concepts, and recommendations for further research, will be presented.

Nurses understand the pivotal role they play in promoting health and preventing disease, the important role of research in the knowledge of what is "healthy," and the central role of **epidemiology** (the study of health and disease in society) and public health theories in the everyday practice of nursing.

## EXPLORING CONCEPTS OF HEALTH

Dr. Margaret Newman (2003), a nursing theorist, states that definitions of health in the nursing literature can be classified broadly within two major paradigms. The first paradigm is the **wellness-illness continuum,** a dichotomized portrayal of health and illness ranging from high-level wellness at the positive end to depletion of health at the negative end. **High-level wellness** is further conceptualized as a sense of **well-being,** life satisfaction, and **quality of life.** Movement toward the negative end of the continuum includes adaptation to disease and disability through various levels of functional ability. The wellness-illness conceptualization was the focus of early research and is consistent with some of the categories Smith (1983) identified in her philosophical analysis of health. Research based on this paradigm conforms primarily to scientific methods that seek to control contextual effects, provide the basis for causal explanations, and predict future outcomes (see, Kaplow and Reed, 2008).

The second paradigm characterizes health as a perspective developmental phenomenon of unitary patterning of the person-environment. The developmental perspective of health has been present in the nursing literature since 1970, but it was not identified clearly with health until the late 1970s and early 1980s. It has been conceptualized as expanding consciousness, pattern or meaning recognition, personal transformation, and, tentatively, self-actualization. This shift toward a developmental perspective has had clear implications for the way in which health is conceptualized (Newman, 2003). Although not endorsing the developmental perspective to the extent of Rogers (1970) and Reed (1983), Pender and colleagues (2015) and Allen and Warner (2002) state that health is an outcome of ongoing patterns of person and environment interactions throughout the life span. Research within this paradigm seeks to address the dynamic whole of the health experience through behavioral and social mechanisms over time. Health can be better understood if each person is seen as a part of a complex, interconnected biological and social system.

The **ecological model of health** (Institute of Medicine, 2003) is a comprehensive developmental approach, and is useful for promoting health at individual, family, community, and societal levels. This model was updated in 2008 (and the 2010 report adding quality of life) with an emphasis on the **social determinants of health**—those factors in society that have an influence on health and the options available to people to improve or maintain their health. (These models are also reviewed in Richard et al., 2011.) In this way, the ecological model of health is more compatible with Smith's descriptions of health as adaptation and eudemonia (self-actualization). The social determinants of health also form the basis for *Healthy People 2020* (US Department of Health and Human Services [USDHHS], Office of Disease Prevention and Health Promotion, 2011). Each of these ideas will be examined in more detail throughout this chapter.

People involved in health promotion must consider the meaning of health for themselves and for others. Recognizing differences in the meaning of health can clarify outcomes and expectations in health promotion and enhance the quality of health care. Because health is used to describe a number of entities, including a philosophy of care (health promotion and health maintenance), a system (health care delivery system), practices (evidence-based health practices), behaviors (personal health behaviors), costs (health care costs), and insurance (uninsured health care), the reason that confusion continues regarding the use of the term "health" becomes clear. People's use of the term "health," and its incorporation into these various entities, has also changed over time.

Americans born before 1940 experienced the greatest changes in how health is defined. Because infectious diseases claimed the lives of many children and young adults at that time, health was viewed as the absence of disease. The physician in independent practice was the primary provider of health care services, with services provided in the private office. The federal government was only beginning to establish its role in working with states to address public health and welfare issues (Barr et al., 2003).

As the national economy expanded during and after World War II in the 1940s and 1950s, the idea of role performance became a focus in industrial research and entered the health care lexicon. Health became linked to a person's ability to fulfill a role in society. Increasingly, the physician was asked to complete physical examination forms for school, work, military, and insurance purposes, while physician practice became linked more directly to hospital-based services. The federal government expanded its role through funding for hospital expansion and establishment of the new Department of Health, Education, and Welfare, currently the Department of Health and Human Services (Barr et al., 2003). It was recognized that a person might recover from a disease yet be unable to fulfill family or work roles because of residual changes from the illness episode. Concepts of disability and rehabilitation entered the health care arena. The work or school environment was viewed as a possible contributor to health, illness, disability, and death.

From the 1960s to the present, there have been incredible changes in the health care delivery system while federal and state governments attempted to control spending and health care costs escalated (Barr et al., 2003). Primary care providers, including nurse practitioners and other advanced practice nurses, now attempt to involve individuals and their families in the delivery of person-centered care, and teaching individuals about individual responsibilities and lifestyle choices has become an important part of their job. Health care became an interdisciplinary endeavor even while managed care companies limited the health-promotion options available under insurance plans. During this time the idea of adaptation had an important influence on the way Americans view health. Increasingly health became linked to individuals' reactions to the environment rather than being viewed as a fixed state. Adaptation fit well with the self-help movement during the 1970s and with the progressive growth in knowledge from research of disease prevention and health promotion at the individual level.

Emphasis is being placed on the quality of a person's life as a component of health (USDHHS, Public Health Service, 2000; USDHHS, Office of Disease Prevention and Health Promotion, 2011). Research on self-rated health (Cano et al., 2003; Idler & Benyamini, 1997) and self-rated function (Greiner et al., 1999) indicates that there are multiple factors contributing to a person's perception of his or her health, sometimes referred to as functional health (Gordon, 2016) or health-related quality of life (HRQoL) (Andresen et al., 2003; USDHHS, Office of Disease Prevention and Health Promotion, 2011). Multiple tools are available for measuring quality of life, including a general measure established by the World Health Organization (2004)

(World Health Organization Quality of Life, WHOQOL-BREF) and the McGill Quality of Life Questionnaire (Cohen et al., 1997) for use at the end of life (Box 1-1: Quality and Safety Scenario).

## Models of Health

Throughout history, society has entertained a variety of concepts of health (David, 2000). Smith (1983) describes four distinct models of health in her classic work.

### Clinical Model

In the clinical model, health is defined by the absence of signs and symptoms of disease and illness is defined by the presence of signs and symptoms of disease. People who use this model may not seek preventive health services or they may wait until they are very ill to seek care. The clinical model is the conventional model of the discipline of medicine.

### Role Performance Model

The role performance model of health defines health in terms of individuals' ability to perform social roles. Role performance includes work, family, and social roles, with performance based on societal expectations. Illness would be the failure to perform roles at the level of others in society. This model is the basis for occupational health evaluations, school physical examinations, and physician-excused absences. The idea of the "sick role," which excuses people from performing their social functions, is a vital component of the role performance model. It is argued that the sick role is still relevant in health care today (Burnham, 2012; Davis et al., 2011).

### Adaptive Model

In the adaptive model of health, people's ability to adjust positively to social, mental, and physiological change is the measure of their health. Illness occurs when the person fails to adapt or becomes maladaptive to these changes. As the concept of adaptation has entered other aspects of American culture, this model of health has become more accepted. For example, spirituality can be useful in adapting to a decreased level of functioning in older adults (Haley et al., 2001).

### Eudaimonistic Model

In the eudaimonistic model, exuberant well-being indicates optimal health. This model emphasizes the interactions between physical, social, psychological, and spiritual aspects of life and the environment that contribute to goal attainment and create meaning. Illness is reflected by a denervation or languishing, a lack of involvement with life. Although these ideas may appear to be new when compared with the clinical model of health, aspects of the eudaimonistic model predate the clinical model of health. This model is also more congruent with integrative modes of therapy (National Institutes of Health, National Center for Complementary and Alternative Medicine, 2011), which are used increasingly by people of all ages in the United States and the rest of the world. In this eudaimonistic model, a person dying of cancer may still be healthy if that person is finding meaning in life at this stage of development.

## ✅ BOX 1-1    QUALITY AND SAFETY SCENARIO

### *Fall Prevention in the Home*

Falls in the home are a common yet preventable source of both fatal and nonfatal injuries. In 2012, the Centers for Disease Control and Prevention reported in its *Morbidity and Mortality Weekly Report* QuickStats section that older adults aged 75 years or older had the most nonfatal injury falls in which health care providers were consulted because of the injury. These data, from the 2010 National Health Interview Survey, indicate that 12% of this older adult population experience a fall significant enough to seek health care.

There are specific factors that contribute to fall risk, including changes to the person attributable to age, medication use, and environmental hazards. Nurses are in key roles to work with older adults to assess fall risks and help them gain control over this aspect of their health. The National Center for Injury Prevention and Control at the Centers for Disease Control and Prevention provides guidelines for fall prevention in older adults at http://www.cdc.gov/ncipc/pub-res/toolkit/checklistforsafety.htm.

Risk factors attributable to the aging process include visual, hearing, and functional limitations. Although pets have proven to be a benefit for older adults by providing companionship and comfort, they can also scamper underfoot or the older adult may trip over the pet because the pet is not seen or heard. Loss of night vision and depth perception can also contribute to falls when lighting is poor or when a person is moving from room to room. Older adults should be encouraged to always wear prescribed vision and hearing aids when moving about the house or apartment. Loss of upper and lower body strength can also contribute to fall risk. Lower body strength is needed to lift the legs and feet high enough to navigate stairs and changes in texture of flooring. Upper body strength allows the use of supports when a person is moving about. Watch the person maneuver about the living space and note the use of furniture, walls, and other objects for support.

Medications can contribute to disequilibrium. A careful review of currently used medications, both prescribed and over-the-counter medications, can help identify medications that could possibly contribute to fall risks. Environmental risks include clutter, too much furniture for the room, placement of items in typical walkways, lighting problems, needed repairs to flooring and walls, and the need for supports such as grab bars and railings. Again, watching the person navigate through the home is helpful in recognizing potential trip hazards and areas where additional supports are needed. Adequate hydration is another consideration, especially if the person is taking medications that contribute to dehydration without regular fluid replacement or if the temperature of the home and environment is too high.

Health outcomes for the person can be significant. Falls can cause minor injury and embarrassment, but they can also cause life-threatening injuries such as fractures and head injuries. If a fall has occurred, it is helpful to do a root cause analysis to determine those factors that contributed to the fall. Ask permission before attempting to make any alteration to the home, because items and their placement may have sentimental importance to the person. Address medication changes with the person, pharmacist, and/or primary care provider. Some medication habits may be hard for the person to change.

The nursing implications of fall risk are many and varied. Assessment skills must be practiced in a variety of settings so that the nurse is vigilant for potential hazards and individual factors that might precipitate a fall. Older adults should be routinely observed performing their daily routines to identify visual, hearing, and functional decline. Also, if a person reports a fall, that report should trigger a more extensive evaluation of that individual because falls may be indicative of future fall risk.

Falls are a frequent but preventable occurrence, especially for older adults. Falls also contribute millions of dollars each year to the cost of health care as a result of personal injury and disability. That is why fall prevention is a key feature of quality and safety education for nurses.

**Questions**

- Can you identify at least four items in your own environment that may contribute to your fall risk?
- How would you structure an interview with an older adult to determine the presence of fall risks in that person's home?
- What evidence and arguments would you use to encourage an older adult to modify the home environment to decrease the risk of a fall?

Sources: Adams, P. F., Martinez, M. E., Vickerie, J. L., & Kirzinger, W. K. (2010). Summary health statistics for the U.S. population: National Health Interview Survey, 2010. *Vital and Health Statistics 2011*, *10*(251), 1–118; Centers for Disease Control and Prevention. (2012). QuickStats: Rate of nonfatal, medically consulted fall injury episodes, by age group. *Morbidity Mortality Weekly Report*, *61*(4), 81.

These ideas of health provide a basis for how people view health and disease and how they view the roles of nurses, physicians, and other health care providers. For example, in the clinical model of health, a person may expect to see a health care provider only when there are obvious signs of illness. Personal responsibility for health may not be a motivating factor for this individual because the provider is responsible for dealing with the health problem and returning the person to health. Therefore attempts to teach health-promoting activities may not be effective with this person. On the other hand, those who adopt a eudaimonistic model of health may find that practitioners working under a clinical model do not address their more comprehensive health needs. They may instead seek out a practitioner of alternative medicine or the counsel of a priest, rabbi, or minister to complement the services of the more traditional health provider.

### Wellness-Illness Continuum

The wellness-illness continuum, as stated earlier, is a dichotomous depiction of the relationship between the concepts of health and illness. In this paradigm, wellness is a positive state in which incremental increases in health can be made beyond the midpoint (Figure 1-1). These increases involve improved physical and mental health states. The opposite end of the continuum is illness, with the possibility of incremental decreases in health beyond the midpoint. This depiction of the relationship of wellness and illness fits well with the conceptual and clinical model of health (McMahon & Fleury, 2012).

### High-Level Wellness

From a dichotomous representation of health and illness as opposites, Dunn (1961) developed a health-illness continuum that assessed a person not only in terms of his or her relative health compared with that of others but also in terms of the favorability of the person's environment for health and wellness (see Figure 1-1). Adding this second dimension to the health-illness continuum created a matrix in which a favorable environment allows high-level wellness to occur and an unfavorable environment allows low-level wellness to exist.

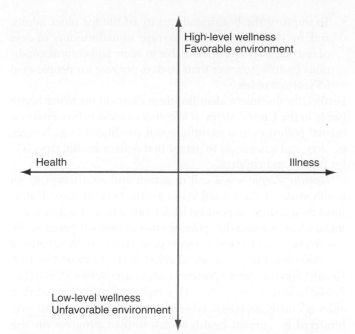

High-level wellness
Favorable environment

Health                                          Illness

Low-level wellness
Unfavorable environment

**FIGURE 1-1** Wellness-illness continuum with high-level wellness added. Moving from the center to the right demonstrates movement toward illness. Moving from the center to the left demonstrates movement toward health. Moving above the line demonstrates movement toward increasing wellness. Moving below the line demonstrates movement toward decreasing wellness. (Modified from US Department of Health and Human Services, Public Health Service, (1982); McMahon, S., & Fleury, J. (2012). Wellness in older adults: A concept analysis. *Nursing Forum, 47*(1), 39–51.)

With this addition, it became possible to combine the clinical model of health with models based on social and environmental parameters. The concept demonstrates that a person can have a terminal disease and be emotionally prepared for death, while acting as a support for other people and achieving high-level wellness. High-level wellness involves progression toward a higher level of functioning, an open-ended and ever-expanding future with its challenge of fuller potential and the integration of the whole being (Ardell, 2007). This definition of high-level wellness contains ideas similar to those in the eudaimonistic model of health. Additionally, high-level wellness emphasizes the interrelationship between the environment and the ability to achieve health on both a personal and a societal level.

## Health Ecology

An evolving view of health recognizes the interconnection between people and their physical and social environments. Newman (2003) expressed this interconnection within a developmental framework, and the work of Gordon (2016) applies this interconnection to functional health patterns as presented in subsequent chapters. Health from an ecological perspective is multidimensional, extending from the individual into the surrounding community, and including the context within which the person functions. It incorporates a systems approach within which the actions of one portion of the system affect the functioning of

the system as a whole (Institute of Medicine, 2003, 2010). This view of health expands on high-level wellness by recognizing that there are social and environmental factors that can enhance or limit health and healthy behaviors. For example, most people can benefit from physical activity such as walking, and people are more likely to walk in areas where there are sidewalks or walking paths and where they feel safe. Nurses can encourage people to walk but may also need to advocate safe areas for people to walk and work with others to plan for people-friendly community development.

## Functioning

One of the defining characteristics of life is the ability to function. Functional health can be characterized as being present or absent, having high-level or low-level wellness, and being influenced by neighborhood and society. Functioning is integral to health. There are physical, mental, and social levels of function, and these are reflected in terms of performance and social expectations. Function can also be viewed from an ecological perspective, as in the example of walking used previously. Loss of function may be a sign or symptom of a disease. For example, sudden loss of the ability to move an arm or leg may indicate a stroke. The inability to leave the house may indicate overwhelming fear. In both cases the loss of function is a sign of disease, a state of ill health. Loss of function is a good indicator that the person may need nursing intervention. Research in older adults indicates that decline in physical function is a sentinel event and may indicate the future loss of physical function and death (Boltz et al., 2012; Greiner et al., 1996).

## HEALTH

Health, as defined in this text, is a state of physical, mental, spiritual, and social functioning that realizes a person's potential and is experienced within a developmental context. Although health is, in part, an individual's responsibility, health also requires collective action to ensure a society and an environment in which people can act responsibly to support health. The culture and beliefs of people can also influence health action. This definition is consistent with the World Health Organization (WHO) definition of health as the state of complete physical, mental, and social well-being and not merely the absence of disease and infirmity (World Health Organization, 2004), but moves beyond this definition to encompass spiritual, developmental, and environmental aspects over time. The physical aspect includes one's genetic makeup, which when combined with the other aspects influences one's longevity. This broader definition is applicable across the life span, as well as in situations where illness may be a chronic state. For example, in this broader definition of health, a person with diabetes may be considered healthy if he or she is able to adapt to his or her illness and live a meaningful, spiritually satisfying life. Health is considered to be part of the metaparadigm for nursing (Fawcett & Garity, 2009), which includes the four components of person, health, environment, and nursing. As can be seen in the discussion thus far, health can be viewed in a variety of ways.

## ILLNESS, DISEASE, AND HEALTH

It is easy to think of health or wellness as the lack of disease and to consider "illness" and "disease" as interchangeable terms. However, "health" and "disease" are not simply antonyms and "disease" and "illness" are not synonyms. Disease literally means "without ease." Disease may be defined as the failure of a person's adaptive mechanisms to counteract stimuli and stresses adequately, resulting in functional or structural disturbances. This definition is an ecological concept of disease, which uses multiple factors to determine the cause of disease rather than describing a single cause. This multifactorial approach increases the chances of discovering multiple points of intervention to improve health.

Illness is composed of the subjective experience of the individual and the physical manifestation of disease (Hollingsworth & Didelot, 2005). Both are social constructs in which people are in an imbalanced, unsustainable relationship with their environment and are failing in their ability to survive and create a higher quality of life. Illness can be described as a response characterized by a mismatch between a person's needs and the resources available to meet those needs. Additionally, illness signals to individuals and populations that the present balance is not working. Within this definition, illness has psychological, spiritual, and social components. A person can have a disease without feeling ill (e.g., asymptomatic hypertension). A person can also feel ill without having a diagnosable disease (e.g., as a result of stress). Our understanding of disease and illness within society, overlaid with our understanding of the natural history of each disease, creates a basis for promoting health.

## PLANNING FOR HEALTH

Public health has always had the prevention of disease in society as its focus. However, during the past 30 years, the promotion of health and individual responsibility moved to the forefront within public health, becoming a driving force in health care reform.

A key milestone in promoting health was the advent of Healthy People (US Department of Health, Education, and Welfare, Public Health Service, 1979), the first Surgeon General's report on health promotion and disease prevention issued in the later years of President Carter's administration. This document identified five national health goals addressing the reduction of death in adults and children and the reduction of sick days in older adults.

- To continue to improve infant health, and, by 1990, to reduce infant mortality by at least 35%, to fewer than 9 deaths per 1000 live births.
- To improve child health, foster optimal childhood development, and, by 1990, reduce deaths among children aged 1 to 14 years by at least 20%, to fewer than 34 deaths per 100,000 children.
- To improve the health and health habits of adolescents and young adults, and, by 1990, to reduce deaths among people aged 15 to 24 years by at least 20%, to fewer than 93 deaths per 100,000 people.
- To improve the health of adults, and, by 1990, to reduce deaths among people aged 25 to 64 years by at least 25%, to fewer than 400 deaths per 100,000 people.
- To improve the health and quality of life for older adults, and, by 1990, to reduce the average annual number of days of restricted activity attributable to acute and chronic conditions by 20%, to fewer than 30 days per year for people aged 65 years or older.

Further, the document identified three causes of the major health issues in the United States as allowing careless habits, environmental pollution, and harmful social conditions (e.g., hunger, poverty, and ignorance) to persist that destroy health, especially for infants and children.

*Healthy People* was a call to action and an attempt to set health goals for the United States for the next 10 years. Unfortunately, a change in political leadership, a lack of political and social willpower, and the spiraling costs of hospital-based health care intervened. The need to report progress toward these national objectives led a larger, renewed effort in the form of *The 1990 Health Objectives for the Nation: A Midcourse Review* (USDHHS, Public Health Service, 1986). This midcourse review noted that, although many goals were achievable, the unachieved goals were hindered by current health status, limited progress on risk reduction, difficulties in data collection, and a lack of public awareness.

*Healthy People 2000* (USDHHS, Public Health Service, 1990) and *Healthy People 2000 Midcourse Review and 1995 Revisions* (USDHHS, Public Health Service, 1996) were landmark documents in that a consortium of people representing national organizations worked with US Public Health Service officials to create a more global approach to health. Additionally, a management-by-objectives approach was used to address each problem area. These two documents became the blueprints for each state as funding for federal programs became linked to meeting these national health objectives. While the objectives became more widely implemented, methods for collecting data became formalized, and the data flowed back into the system to form the revisions set in 1995. The core of these health objectives remained: that is, prevention of illness and disease was the foundation for health. *Healthy People 2000* established three broad goals:

- Increase the span of healthy life.
- Reduce health disparities.
- Create access to preventive services for all.

Additionally, the work included 22 specific areas for achievement, with objectives in each area based on age, health disparities, and health needs. By 1995, progress was made on 70% of the objectives. However, for 30% of the objectives, movement toward the goals was in the wrong direction, had experienced no change, or could not be determined because of a lack of data.

*Healthy People 2010* (USDHHS, Public Health Service, 2000) introduced two overarching goals:

- Increase quality and years of healthy life.
- Eliminate health disparities.

The first goal addressed the issues of longevity and quality of life. Both longevity and quality of life address the concern that people are living longer but frequently with numerous chronic health problems that interfere with the quality of their lives. However, quality of life is also an issue for people who are unable to achieve a long life. Combining these two ideas placed an emphasis on both longevity and quality of life as areas that need improvement.

The second goal, eliminating health disparities, addressed the continuing problems of access to care; differences in treatment based on race, gender, and ability to pay; and related issues such as urban versus rural health, insurance coverage, Medicare and Medicaid reimbursement for care, and satisfaction with service delivery.

From these goals, the *Final Report of the Commission on Social Determinants of Health* (Commission on Social Determinants of Health, 2008) was completed with the 733 objectives (of the original 969 objectives) for which tracking data were available. A total of 23% of these objectives were met, with another 48% moving toward their targets, representing positive responses on 71% of the objectives. However, 5% of the objectives demonstrated no change from the baseline, and 24% of the objectives moved in a negative direction from the target. For example, look at Focus Area 19: Nutrition and Overweight. Of 22 objectives, none were met, 2 moved toward the target, 3 demonstrated no change, and 15 moved away from the target. These findings are consistent with the epidemic of overweight and obesity in the United States and reflect the continuing influence of factors in our society that contribute to inactivity and weight gain (Fryar et al., 2014).

## HEALTHY PEOPLE 2020

### Goals

For *Healthy People 2020* (USDHHS, Office of Disease Prevention and Health Promotion, 2011), there are four overarching goals:
- Attain high quality, longer lives free of preventable disease, disability, injury, and premature death.
- Achieve health equity, eliminate disparities, and improve the health of all groups.
- Create social and physical environments that promote good health for all.
- Promote quality of life, healthy development, and healthy behaviors across all life stages.

These four goals established the territory in which health promotion and disease prevention efforts occur. Research in a variety of areas has clearly indicated that health disparities are directly and indirectly linked to longevity and quality-of-life issues (Barr, 2014). For example, the American Cancer Society reports that black men die of prostate cancer more frequently than any other racial or ethnic group, with their death rate almost 2.4 times higher than that of white men (American Cancer Society, 2016) (Box 1-2: Diversity Awareness).

The *Healthy People 2020* focus areas include adolescent health; blood disorders and blood safety; dementias, including Alzheimer disease; early and middle childhood; genomics; global health; health care–associated infections; health-related quality of life and well-being; lesbian, gay, bisexual, and transgender health; older adults; preparedness; sleep health; and social determinants of health. These focus areas are an expansion on previous areas and incorporate recent evidence more directly in each area.

The detailed objectives can be found at https://www.healthypeople.gov/2020/topics-objectives. These focus areas span age categories from conception to death and incorporate

---

### BOX 1-2   DIVERSITY AWARENESS

#### Influence of Personal Cultural Values on Health Care Delivery

Culture influences every aspect of human life, including beliefs, values, and customs regarding lifestyle and health care. As health care providers, nurses need to be aware of their own beliefs, values, and customs and how these ideas translate into behavior. It is easy to assume that an individual's own perspective is correct and shared by others. This is especially true when one is working with other health care providers who share the same culture. This concept is referred to as **ethnocentrism** and can lead to a devaluing of the beliefs, values, and customs of others, known as **racism**. Although it is impossible for any person to ignore the cultural influences on their lives, nurses and other health care providers have a special obligation to be aware of their own social and cultural biases. Our focus as nurses must be on the cultural influences in the daily lives of individuals through the development of **cultural competence** and cultural humility. The ability to view other people's situations from their perspective is known as **empathy**. Diversity awareness will continue to challenge providers to lifelong learning about the people for whom they provide care as the racial and ethnic mix in society changes.

---

prevention, access, treatment, and follow-up at the individual, family, provider, work site, and community levels. The 42 topical areas lead to specific objectives for each topical area. One example is used here for illustration.

*Objective PA-2.1. Increase the proportion of adults who engage in aerobic physical activity of at least moderate intensity for at least 150 minutes/week, or 75 minutes/week of vigorous intensity, or an equivalent combination.* This objective directly addresses each of the overarching goals, either directly or indirectly. Physical activity can contribute to the maintenance or improvement in mobility, which improves the quality of life and prevents disability. It is something in which most people can participate. It enhances positive mental health through stress reduction and physical fitness, which contribute to the development of healthy behaviors. However, it takes social action and awareness to address the need for social and physical environments that support physical activity across the life span.

Access to health care to obtain a complete physical examination before starting to exercise and the quality of the work or neighborhood environment available for exercise can contribute to success or failure of this objective. This objective is related to other objectives such as nutrition, obesity, and stroke prevention (Box 1-3: Innovative Practice).

Additionally, current knowledge of physical activity and specific populations was considered when the *Healthy People 2020* objectives were being created. Women, low-income populations, black and Hispanic people, people with disabilities, and those older than 75 years exercise less than do white men with moderate-to-high incomes (USDHHS, National Institutes of Health, National Heart, Lung, and Blood Institute, 2012). These health disparities can influence the number of people in these groups who develop high cholesterol levels or high blood pressure, which further increases their risk of heart disease and stroke. Although this objective addresses adults, other objectives address the need for beginning exercise activities at an early age and encouraging young adults to be actively engaged in exercise. How might this

### BOX 1-3 INNOVATIVE PRACTICE

*Process for Assessing, Evaluating, and Treating Overweight and Obesity in Adults*

Overweight and obesity are major concerns in public health because they contribute to other health problems such as high cholesterol level, high blood pressure, diabetes mellitus, heart disease, functional limitations, and disability. As part of the National Heart, Lung, and Blood Institute's (2000) obesity education initiative, titled Aim for a Healthy Weight, nurses have an important role to play in health education related to obesity prevention and control. More complete information and guidelines updated in 2012 can be obtained from http://www.nhlbi.nih.gov/health/public/heart/obesity/lose_wt/index.htm.

**Make the Most of the Individual's Visit and Set an Effective Tone for Communication:** Nurses ask individuals about their weight history, weight-related health risks, and desire to lose weight. The approaches used need to be respectful of a person's lifestyle, habits, and cultural influences. Discussions need to be nonjudgmental and goal directed.

**Assess the Individual's Motivation/Readiness to Lose Weight:** Nurses explain body mass index and why it is the preferred method of determining overweight and obesity in adults. Individuals need to understand the methods of data collection and measurement of height and weight, as well as waist circumference, risk factors, and comorbidities. Nurses develop skill in determining readiness and motivation to lose weight in their patients.

**Build a Partnership With an Individual:** Nurses work with individuals to determine what each person is willing to do to achieve a lower weight. This approach includes knowing the best practices in weight management and weight loss. Fad diets, dietary supplements, and weight loss pills may be inappropriate for most people, and formal weight loss programs may be too expensive for low- and moderate-income families. Use recommended diets that restrict caloric intake, set activity goals with your patients, encourage the person to keep a weekly food and activity diary, and provide information on diet and activity. Be sure to record individual goals and the treatment plan, including a health-education plan. Nurses are knowledgeable about current treatment options and their success. Holistic approaches are needed because food behaviors are influenced by many factors. Listen to individuals' stories about food and its role in their lives. Therapies should fit the individual's goals and lead to lifestyle change.

### BOX 1-4 HEALTHY PEOPLE 2020

*The 13 Focus Areas*

- Adolescent health
- Blood disorders and blood safety
- Dementias, including Alzheimer disease
- Early and middle childhood
- Genomics
- Global health
- Health care–associated infections
- Health-related quality of life and well-being
- Lesbian, gay, bisexual, and transgender health
- Older adults
- Preparedness
- Sleep health
- Social determinants of health

From US Department of Health and Human Services, Public Health Service. (2010). *Healthy People 2020.* https://www.healthypeople.gov.

100%. In 2011, 77.3% of people had a usual primary care provider, the baseline rate was 76.3% (2007), and the goal is 83.9%. Social determinants of health are represented by the leading health indicator of students who graduate with a regular diploma 4 years after starting 9th grade. There has been an overall increase from 79% (2010–11) to 81%, although there are dramatic differences in graduation rates according to race and ethnicity. Improving the health-related quality of life and well-being of adults is considered by measurement of the proportion of adults who self-report good or better physical and mental health. Men report good or better physical health at a rate of 82.5%, with women trailing at a rate of 75.4%, and 81.1% of men report good or better mental health compared with 77.3% of women. Education is related to good or better health. The more educated one is, the higher the level of reported good or better health (USDHHS, 2014).

Health care providers need to be responsible for offering health promotion, providing preventive health services, and monitoring behaviors. Unfortunately, many of the financial incentives for providers are to perform tasks and procedures rather than to counsel and help individuals choose between various behaviors. The Patient Protection and Affordable Care Act (US Congress, 2010) now requires primary care providers to provide free wellness services to older adults and others, and to provide person-centered care. Providers need to take the time to discuss behaviors that may improve the quality of life and extend the number of years of life. For example, the addictive nature of tobacco and its effect on the development and course of a variety of chronic health conditions are now well recognized. Providers should be asking every person if they use tobacco and should be providing them with ways to quit smoking, including economic and social incentives.

Providers also need to look for partnership in the community through which they can better serve the needs of individuals. *Healthy People 2020* emphasizes that person-centered care is essential to health promotion. One approach to person-centered care to build partnerships is the use of community nursing centers

objective be adjusted to the needs of an older adult population? The target for this objective is that 47.9% of adults engage in aerobic physical activity of at least moderate intensity for at least 150 minutes per week, or vigorous intensity for 75 minutes per week, or an equivalent combination. This target represents a 10% increase over the 2008 baseline. This approach emphasizes personal responsibility but now includes society's role in addressing the social and physical environments within which those choices are made (USDHHS, National Institutes of Health, National Heart, Lung, and Blood Institute, 2012).

The latest *Healthy People 2020* progress update on the goals of increasing access to health care services, addressing social determinants of health, and increasing the health-related quality of health for people indicates small improvements (Box 1-4).

The two leading health indicators for access to health care services of persons with medical insurance (<65 years old) and persons with a usual primary care provider showed little or no detectable change (USDHHS, 2014). The latest figure for the improvement in the rate of persons with medical insurance was 83.1% (2012), the baseline rate was 83% (2008), and the goal is

**BOX 1-5   HEALTHY PEOPLE 2020**

*Selected National Health Promotion and
Disease Prevention Objectives for Nutrition and
Weight Status*

- Increase the proportion of adults who are at a healthy weight.
- Reduce the proportion of adults who are obese.
- Reduce the proportion of children and adolescents who are considered obese.
- (Developmental) Prevent inappropriate weight gain in youth and adults.
- Increase the contribution of fruits to the diets of the population aged 2 years or older.
- Increase the variety and contribution of vegetables to the diets of the population aged 2 years or older.
- Increase the contribution of whole grains to the diets of the population aged 2 years or older.
- Reduce consumption of calories from solid fats and added sugars in the population aged 2 years or older.
- Reduce consumption of saturated fat in the population aged 2 years or older.
- Reduce consumption of sodium in the population aged 2 years or older.
- Increase consumption of calcium in the population aged 2 years or older.

From US Department of Health and Human Services, Public Health Service. (2010). *Healthy People 2020* objectives. https://www. healthypeople.gov.

as partnering organization (http://www.nncc.us/site/). The Health Promotion Center operated by Fairfield University School of Nursing in Fairfield, Connecticut, was one example. The nurses and nursing students who provided health education, screening, and referral services at the Health Promotion Center worked with existing community organizations to better meet the health care needs of underserved people. The Health Promotion Center worked with senior housing and senior centers to provide comprehensive cardiovascular screenings and medication review. As an extension of this work, funding was secured for a program called Step Up to Health, a project to increase physical activity in this population through interactive planning and consumer ownership of the activities. The project was part of the National Blueprint Project supported by the Robert Wood Johnson Foundation (http://www.agingblueprint.org). The project engaged older adults in walking programs, line dancing, gardening, and low-impact exercise programs, including programs from the National Arthritis Foundation (http://www.arthritis.org/) (Box 1-5).

Another approach to partnerships is to have providers serve as active participants on community boards and advisory committees, which allows providers to become aware of the service needs in the community and the resources available to meet those needs.

Work sites and communities need to become partners in providing opportunities for people to lead healthy lives through flexible work schedules, work site wellness programs, accessibility of safe parks, and availability of exercise facilities. Converting empty lots into community gardens provides beautification of the area, an opportunity for exercise in caring for the garden, and a source of fresh vegetables. The availability of bike paths encourages physical activity.

Churches, temples, and mosques can be vital partners in meeting *Healthy People 2020* objectives. Faith communities can break economic, social, racial, and gender barriers, making them an excellent source for sharing information on health promotion and disease prevention. Parish nurses are becoming increasingly prevalent, and they incorporate *Healthy People 2020* objectives into their activities (International Parish Nurse Resource Center, 2012).

Public health officials at all levels are necessary partners in meeting *Healthy People 2020* objectives. As part of the core public health functions of assessment, policy development, and assurance, the US Public Health Service and all state, county, and local health departments need to collect data, make information available to the public, create policies that support *Healthy People 2020* objectives, and ensure that needed services are available from a competent workforce.

*Healthy People 2020* can form the basis for planning, service delivery, evaluation, and research in every aspect of the health care system. The nurse needs to be familiar with this document and its intent. Nurses should compare their practices with the objectives of *Healthy People 2020*. Additionally, the nurse needs to be aware of the research and practice changes that occur as a result of the work toward these objectives.

## LEVELS OF PREVENTION

Prevention, in a narrow sense, means averting the development of disease. In a broad sense, prevention consists of all measures that limit disease progression. Leavell and Clark (1965) defined three levels of prevention: primary, secondary, and tertiary (Figure 1-2). Although the levels of prevention are related to the natural history of disease, they can be used to prevent disease and provide nurses with starting points for making effective, positive changes in the health status of the persons for whom they provide care. Primordial prevention, the earliest form of prevention, has been added as a type of prevention that reflects policy-level intervention aimed at affecting health before at-risk lifestyle behaviors are chosen or become habit. Within the four levels of prevention, there are five steps. These steps include health promotion and specific protection (primordial and primary prevention); early diagnosis, prompt treatment, and disability limitation (secondary prevention); and restoration and rehabilitation (tertiary prevention).

Some confusion exists in the interpretation of these concepts; therefore a consistent understanding of primordial, primary, secondary, and tertiary prevention is essential. The levels of prevention operate on a continuum but may overlap in practice. The nurse must clearly understand the goals of each level to intervene effectively in keeping people healthy.

### Primordial Prevention

"Primordial" refers to the timeframe *before* a risk factor develops and *before* disease occurs. Primordial prevention can begin as early as childhood or even prenatally and is closely linked to the determinants of health and the environment in which one lives (Salama, n.d.). Determinants of health include income, education, literacy, employment, working conditions, social and physical

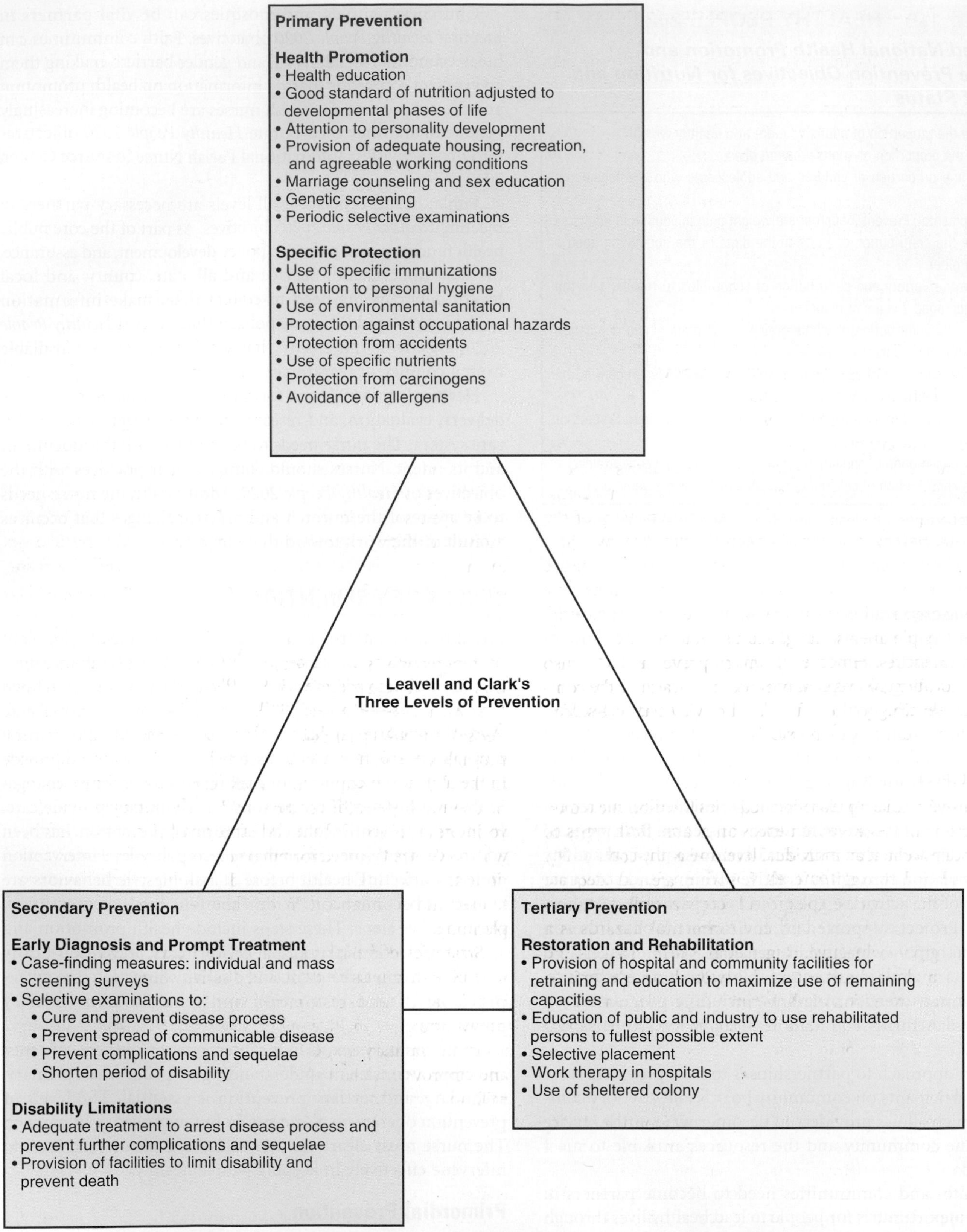

**Primary Prevention**

**Health Promotion**
- Health education
- Good standard of nutrition adjusted to developmental phases of life
- Attention to personality development
- Provision of adequate housing, recreation, and agreeable working conditions
- Marriage counseling and sex education
- Genetic screening
- Periodic selective examinations

**Specific Protection**
- Use of specific immunizations
- Attention to personal hygiene
- Use of environmental sanitation
- Protection against occupational hazards
- Protection from accidents
- Use of specific nutrients
- Protection from carcinogens
- Avoidance of allergens

**Leavell and Clark's
Three Levels of Prevention**

**Secondary Prevention**

**Early Diagnosis and Prompt Treatment**
- Case-finding measures: individual and mass screening surveys
- Selective examinations to:
  - Cure and prevent disease process
  - Prevent spread of communicable disease
  - Prevent complications and sequelae
  - Shorten period of disability

**Disability Limitations**
- Adequate treatment to arrest disease process and prevent further complications and sequelae
- Provision of facilities to limit disability and prevent death

**Tertiary Prevention**

**Restoration and Rehabilitation**
- Provision of hospital and community facilities for retraining and education to maximize use of remaining capacities
- Education of public and industry to use rehabilitated persons to fullest possible extent
- Selective placement
- Work therapy in hospitals
- Use of sheltered colony

**FIGURE 1-2** The three levels of prevention developed by Leavell and Clark. (Modified from Leavell, H., & Clark, A. E. (1965). *Preventive medicine for doctors in the community.* New York: McGraw-Hill; Ali, A., & Katz, D.L. (2015). Disease prevention and health promotion: How integrative medicine fits. *American Journal of Preventive Medicine, 49*(5), S230–S240.)

environment, health practices, genetic makeup, health services, gender, and culture (Association of Faculties of Medicine of Canada, n.d.). Primordial interventions are aimed at determinants of health. For example, if the social environment one grows up in discourages exercise or encourages eating high-fat food, that environment could be targeted for primordial prevention. Healthy eating and activity school-based programs, reduction of sodium in the food supply, and creation of safe places to ride bikes and walk are examples of primordial prevention (Weintraub et al., 2011). Most health-promoting primordial prevention occurs at the national, state, and community levels.

## Primary Prevention

Primary prevention precedes disease or dysfunction. However, primary prevention is therapeutic in that it includes health as beneficial to well-being, it uses therapeutic treatments, and, as a process or behavior toward enhancing health, it involves symptom identification when stress reduction techniques are being taught. Primary prevention intervention includes health promotion, such as health education about risk factors for heart disease, and specific protection, such as immunization against hepatitis B. Its purpose is to decrease the vulnerability of the individual or population to disease or dysfunction. Interventions at this level encourage individuals and groups to become more aware of the means of improving health and the actions they can take at the primary preventive health level and the optimal health level. People are also taught to use appropriate primary preventive measures. However, primary prevention can also include advocating policies that promote the health of the community and electing public officials who will enact legislation that protects the health of the public.

## Health Protection

Primordial and primary prevention activities focus on the reduction of threats and negative influences on health. Both types of prevention can occur at an individual level and at the community, state, national, and even global levels. Ensuring safe and adequate food, water, and medical therapies for all people as well as protecting them against workplace and environmental hazards is a regional and global objective. Ruger et al. (2015) suggest the formation of a global health fund that would unite efforts to ensure adequate protection of all the world's people concerning AIDS, tuberculosis, and malaria in recognition of the global responsibility for social protection.

## Health Promotion

The definitions of health promotion differ. O'Donnell (1987) has defined health promotion as "the science and art of helping people change their lifestyle to move toward a state of optimal health." Kreuter and Devore (1980) proposed a more complex definition in an article commissioned by the US Public Health Service. They stated that health promotion is "the process of advocating health to enhance the probability that personal (individual, family, and community), private (professional and business), and public (federal, state, and local government) support of positive health practices will become a societal norm."

*The theoretical basis of health promotion.* The theoretical underpinnings for health promotion have evolved since the early 1980s. Most of these theories are behaviorally based, derived from the social sciences, and extensively researched. These theories include the theory of reasoned action by Ajzen and Fishbein (1980), theories of behavior by Bandura (1976, 1999, 2004), the health belief model by Rosenstock (Champion & Skinner, 2008), Pender's health-promotion model (Pender et al., 2015), and stages of change theories by Prochaska (Prochaska et al., 2004). Internet searches on each of these theories will provide numerous websites where more detailed information is available.

*The social nature of health promotion.* Health promotion goes beyond providing information. It is also proactive decision-making at all levels of society as reflected in the *Healthy People 2020* objectives. Health promotion holds the best promise for lower-cost methods of limiting the constant increase in health care costs and for empowering people to be responsible for the aspects of their lives that can enhance well-being. Based on the need for health-promotion activities within the health care system, efforts must be made to identify the multiple determinants of health, determine relevant health-promotion strategies, and delineate issues relevant to social justice and access to care. Individuals, families, and communities must be active participants in this process so that the actions taken are socially relevant, economically feasible, and supportive of changes at the individual level.

*The active and passive nature of health promotion.* Health-promotion efforts, unlike those efforts directed at specific protection from certain diseases, focus on maintaining or improving the general health of individuals, families, and communities. These activities are conducted at the public level (e.g., government programs promoting adequate housing or reducing pollutants in the air), at the community level (e.g., Habitat for Humanity or community health centers), and at the personal level (e.g., voting to offer low-income housing or to elect public officials who recognize the need for public oversight). Nursing interventions are actions directed toward developing people's resources to maintain or enhance their well-being—a form of assets-based planning.

Strategies of health promotion that involve the individual may be either passive or active. Passive strategies involve the individual as an inactive participant or recipient. Examples of passive strategies include public health efforts to maintain clean water and sanitary sewage systems to decrease infectious diseases and improve health, and efforts to introduce vitamin D in all milk to ensure that children will not be at high risk of rickets when living in areas where sunlight is scarce. These passive strategies must be used to promote the health of the public when individual participation might be low but the benefit to society is high.

Active strategies depend on the individual becoming personally involved in adopting a proposed program of health promotion. Two examples of lifestyle change are performing daily exercise as part of a physical fitness plan and adopting a stress-management program as part of daily living. A combination of active and passive strategies is best for making an individual or society healthier. This text is concerned almost entirely with active strategies and the nurse's role in these strategies. Some passive strategies are presented but they are presented with the implicit belief that each individual must take responsibility for improving health. It is undeniable that passive strategies also have a valuable role, but they must be used within a context of encouraging and teaching individuals to assume more responsibility for their health.

*An application of theory to the practice of health promotion.* The transtheoretical model (TTM) is an excellent example and can be applied to this case study. TTM incorporates stages of change (readiness to take action), decisional balance (benefits to and detractors from changing a behavior), self-efficacy (personal confidence in making a change), and processes of change (cognitive, affective, and behavioral activities facilitating change). The bases of TTM are the stages of change; six stages that people spiral through on a path toward making and sustaining a behavioral change to promote health. These stages are:

| | |
|---|---|
| Precontemplative | Not considering change |
| Contemplative | Aware of but not considering change soon |
| Preparation | Planning to act soon |
| Action | Has begun to make behavioral change (recent) |
| Maintenance | Continued commitment to behavior (long-term) |
| Relapse | Reverted to old behavior |

Each stage offers opportunities for the nurse to provide information and support behavioral change. Encouraging people and suggesting changes to their environment that support behavioral change can increase individuals' self-efficacy and their chances of maintaining a change. This model also recognizes that people need multiple opportunities to make behavioral change before achieving success and that relapse should be expected (Prochaska et al., 2004).

Although health promotion would seem to be a practical and effective mode of health care, the major portion of health care delivery is geared toward responding to acute and chronic disease. Preventing or delaying the onset of chronic disease and adding new dimensions to the quality of life are not as easy because they take time to implement and evaluate and require personal action. These actions are more closely associated with everyday living and the lifestyles adopted by individuals, families, communities, and nations. Habits such as eating, resting, exercising, and handling anxieties appear to be transmitted from parent to child and from social group to social group as part of a cultural, not a genetic, heritage. These activities may be taught in subtle ways but they influence behavior and have as much of an influence on health as does genetic inheritance. Although the public may not appreciate the causal relationships between behavior and health, they should be apparent to health professionals. Arguably, the concept of risk is the most basic of all health concepts, because health promotion and disease protection are based on this concept.

Health-promotion strategies have the potential of enhancing the quality of life from birth to death. For example, good nutrition is adjusted to various developmental phases in life to account for rapid growth and development in infancy and early childhood,

physiological changes associated with adolescence, extra demands during pregnancy, and the many changes occurring in older adults. Good nutrition is known to enhance the immune system, enabling individuals to fight infections that could lead to disabling illnesses. Other individual activities are adapted to the person's needs for optimal personality development at all ages. As seen in Unit 4, much can be done on a personal or group basis, through counseling and properly directed parent education, to provide the environmental requirements for the proper personality development of children. Community participation is also an important factor in promoting individual, family, and group health (see Chapters 6–8).

Personal health promotion is usually provided through health education (see Chapter 10). An important function of nurses, physicians, and allied health professionals, health education is principally concerned with eliciting useful changes in human behavior on the basis of current research. The goal is to inculcate a sense of responsibility in individuals for their own health and a shared sense of responsibility for avoiding injury to the health of others. For example, encouraging child-rearing practices that foster normal growth and development (personal, social, and physical) addresses both the individual parent and the needs of society. Health education nurtures health-promoting habits, values, and attitudes that must be learned through practice. These must be reinforced through systematic instruction in hygiene, bodily function, physical fitness, and use of leisure time. Another goal is to understand the appropriate use of health services. For example, a semiannual visit to a dentist may teach a child better oral health habits and to visit the dentist regularly, although this is not the primary purpose of the visit. Parents, teachers, and caregivers play a vital role in health education. In addition to teaching individuals, nurses need to develop skills in group teaching and in providing education within community organizations.

Available research clearly shows an increase in longevity, a decrease in mortality and morbidity, and an improvement in the quality of life for individuals who have been involved in health-promotion activities such as physical activity and avoidance of smoking (Crimmins et al., 2011). It must be emphasized that health promotion requires lifestyle change. Once a lifestyle change has been adopted, vigilance is needed to ensure that the lifestyle change is maintained and modified to fit developmental and environmental changes.

Empirical data linking risk factors, health-promotion activities, and outcomes are sufficient to drive the development of the *Healthy People 2020* objectives and to be incorporated into quality improvement measures in managed care. One of the challenges posed in *Healthy People 2020* is the development of measurable outcome objectives that are based on more realistic economic models.

Health promotion is an important concept for nursing because it embodies many other concepts that nursing is concerned with today. As stated earlier, much of the nursing role is involved with health teaching. Standard 5B of *Nursing: Scope and Standards of Practice* (American Nurses Association [ANA], 2015b) includes a full section on the practice implementation of health teaching and health promotion. Nurses are expected to demonstrate professional role competence throughout their careers. Health education is clearly an important nursing role.

## Specific Protection

This aspect of primary prevention focuses on protecting people from injury and disease, for example, by providing immunizations and reducing exposure to occupational hazards, carcinogens, and other environmental health risks. These hazards and risks include not only protection of adults from work-related injuries (e.g., back injuries in nurses, dismemberment in machinists, exposure to chemicals used in boat repair or exposure to inhaled sawdust by carpenters) but also protection of infants and children from potential carcinogens (e.g., exposure of children to diesel emissions, damage to a fetus caused by radiation).

Primary prevention interventions are considered health protection when they emphasize shielding or defending the body (or the public) from specific causes of injury or disease. Implementing nursing interventions that prevent a specific health problem may seem easier than promoting well-being among individuals, groups, or communities because the variables are delineated more clearly in prevention than in promotion and the potential influences are less diverse.

*Examples.* Two examples may help demonstrate these differences. Immunization against influenza is quite popular and has become a regular activity for people at risk each fall. Nurses can participate in this specific protection role by giving the influenza injections in clinics and offices. Another example is the creation of nut-free schools to protect hypersensitive children from life-threatening allergic reactions to peanuts and nut products. Such initiatives have largely been the result of grassroots parent organizations working with formal community organizations to adopt policies that protect the health of these children. Nurses may be involved in the parent organizations or the school or public health boards that review the proposed policies. Additionally, nurses must be able to address the need to protect specific portions of the population at risk.

## Secondary Prevention

Although primary prevention measures have decreased the hazards of chronic diseases such as cardiovascular disease, conditions that preclude a healthy quality of life are still prevalent. Secondary prevention ranges from providing screening activities and treating early stages of disease to limiting disability by averting or delaying the consequences of advanced disease.

Screening is secondary prevention because the principal goal is to identify individuals in an early, detectable stage of the disease process. However, screening provides an excellent opportunity to offer health teaching as a primary preventive measure. Screening activities now play an important role in the control of diseases such as heart disease, stroke, and colorectal cancer. Additionally, screening activities provide early diagnosis and treatment of nutritional, behavioral, and other related problems. Nurses play an important role in screening activities because they provide clinical expertise and educationally sound health information during the screening process.

Delayed recognition of disease results in the need to limit future disability in late secondary prevention. Limiting disability is a vital role for nursing because preventive measures are primarily therapeutic and are aimed at arresting the disease and preventing further complications. The paradox here is that health education and disease prevention activities seem similar to those used in primary prevention, but are applied to a person or population with an existing disease. Modifications to the teaching plan must be made on the basis of the individual's current health status and ability to modify behavior.

## Tertiary Prevention

Tertiary prevention occurs when a defect or disability is permanent and irreversible. The process involves minimizing the effects of disease and disability by surveillance and maintenance activities aimed at preventing complications and deterioration. Tertiary prevention focuses on rehabilitation to help people attain and retain an optimal level of functioning regardless of their disabling condition. The objective is to return the affected individual to a useful place in society, maximize remaining capacities, or both. The responsibility of the nurse is to ensure that persons with disabilities receive services that enable them to live and work according to the resources that are still available to them. When a person has a stroke, rehabilitating this individual to the highest level of functioning and teaching lifestyle changes to prevent future strokes are examples of tertiary prevention.

## THE NURSE'S ROLE

Evolving demands are placed on the nurse and the nursing profession as a result of changes in society. Emphasis is shifting from acute, hospital-based care to preventive, **community-based care**, which is provided in nontraditional health care settings in the community. This demand for community-based services, with the home as a major community setting for care, is closely related to the changing demographics of the United States. While the home and community become the existing sites for care, nurses must assume more blended roles, with a knowledge base that prepares them to practice across settings using **evidence-based practice**. Within these roles, nurses assume a more active involvement in the prevention of disease and the promotion of health. Nurses can be more independent in their practice and place a greater emphasis on promoting and maximizing health, and more than ever nurses are accountable morally, ethically, and legally for their professional behavior.

## Nursing Roles in Health Promotion and Protection

Although nurses often work with people on a one-to-one basis, they seldom work in isolation. Within today's health care system, nurses collaborate with other nurses, physicians, social workers, nutritionists, psychologists, therapists, individuals, and community groups. In this **interprofessional practice**, nurses play a variety of roles.

### Advocate

As advocates nurses help individuals obtain what they are entitled to receive through the health care system, try to make the system more responsive to individual and community needs, and help people develop the skills to advocate for themselves. In the role of an advocate, the nurse strives to ensure that all persons receive high-quality, appropriate, safe, and cost-effective care. The nurse may spend a great deal of time identifying and coordinating resources for complex cases.

## Care Manager

The nurse acts as a care manager to prevent duplication of services, maintain quality and safety, and reduce costs. Information gathered from reliable data sources enables the care manager to help individuals avoid care that is unproven, ineffective, or unsafe. Reliable sources of information on best practices, evidence-based practices, and standard protocols are available from Internet sites sponsored by the federal government (e.g., https://www.nih.gov; https://www.cdc.gov), specialty organizations (e.g., http://www.arthritis.org; http://www.nursingworld.org; http://www.aginglifecare.org), and private foundations (e.g., http://www.rwjf.org; http://www.johnahartford.org). Successful care management depends on a collaborative relationship among the care manager, other nurses and physicians, the individual and his or her family, the insurance provider, and other care providers who work with the person. The wishes of the individual and the family need to be clear to the care manager as part of person-centered care provision. Facilitating communication among parties is one of the care manager's most important functions.

## Consultant

Nurses may provide knowledge about health promotion and disease prevention to individuals and groups as a consultant. Some nurses have specialized areas of expertise or advanced practice, such as in gerontology, women's health, or community/ public health, and they are equipped to provide information as consultants in these areas of specialization (ANA, 2015b). A gerontological nurse specialist might be on a community planning board offering advice about what types of health-promotion activities should be considered in planning a new senior housing development. All nurses need to develop consultation skills that can be integrated into practice and allow the individual nurse to take advantage of opportunities to provide support on an individual level or for future development at the organizational level (Norwood, 2003).

## Deliverer of Services

The core role of the nurse is the delivery of direct services such as health education, influenza vaccinations, and counseling in health promotion. Visible, direct delivery of nursing care is the foundation for the public image of nursing. The public demands that nurses be knowledgeable and competent in their delivery of services. This role is clearly expressed in *Nursing's Social Policy Statement* (ANA, 2010) and in the *Code of Ethics for Nurses with Interpretive Statements* (ANA, 2015a).

## Educator

Health practices in the United States are derived from the theory that health components such as good nutrition, industrial and highway safety, immunization, and specific drug therapy should be within the grasp of the total population. Even with its rich resources, society falls far short of attaining the goal of maximal health for all. The problem is not a lack of knowledge, but rather the lack of application; therefore it is incumbent on nurses to be excellent health educators. To teach effectively, the nurse must know essential facts about how people learn and the teaching-learning process (see Chapter 10).

In addition to their storehouse of scientific knowledge, nurses who are committed to their teaching role know that individuals are unique in their response to efforts to change their behavior. Teaching may range from a chance remark by the nurse, based on a perception of desirable individual behavior, to structurally planned teaching according to individual needs. Selection of the methods most likely to succeed involves the establishment of teacher-learner goals. Health promotion and protection rely heavily on the individual's ability to use appropriate knowledge. Health education is one of the primary prevention techniques available to avoid the major causes of disability and death today and is a critical role for nurses.

## Healer

The role of healer requires the nurse to help individuals integrate and balance the various parts of their lives (McKivergin, 2009). Healing resides in the ability to glimpse or intuit the "interior" of an individual, to sense and identify what is important to that other person, and to incorporate the specific insight into a care plan that helps that person develop his or her own capacity to heal. It requires a mindful blending of science and subjectivity (Benner et al., 2010; Siegel, 2007). Nurses have a special ability to help people heal. The art of nursing is the extraordinary ability to manage a broad array of information to create something meaningful, sensible, and whole (see Chapter 14).

## Researcher

In today's health care environment, nurses are constantly striving to understand and interpret research findings that will enhance the quality and value of individual care. To provide optimal health care, nurses need to use evidence-based findings as their foundation for clinical decision-making. When nurses or other clinicians use research findings and the best evidence possible to make decisions, the outcome is termed evidence-based practice. Evidence-based practice is defined as the conscientious, explicit, and judicious use of current best evidence in making decisions about the care of individuals. The practice of evidence-based nursing means integrating individual clinical expertise with the best available external clinical evidence from systematic research (ANA, 2015b).

The National Institute of Nursing Research (NINR) serves as the focal point in developing research themes for the future of the profession. NINR supports research to establish a scientific base for the care of individuals throughout the life span; from the management of individuals during illness and recovery to the reduction of the risks of disease and disability. The five "investment" themes NINR has identified are to enhance health promotion and disease prevention; to improve quality of life through symptom management; to improve palliative and end-of-life care; to enhance innovation in science and nurse practice; and to encourage a new generation of nurse scientists (NINR,

2011). Notice how the *Healthy People 2020* objectives match many of these themes.

Evidence-based practice involves searching for the best evidence with which to answer clinical research questions. Research evidence can be gathered from quantitative studies that describe situations, correlate different variables related to care, or test causal relationships between variables related to care (levels I to IV). Such studies become incorporated into screening and treatment standards such as those from the US Preventive Services Task Force (2014). Research evidence can also be gathered from qualitative studies that describe phenomena or define the historical nature, cultural relevance, or philosophical basis of aspects of nursing care (levels V to VII). Applied research is done to directly affect clinical practice (Burns & Grove, 2014). Sackett and colleagues (1996) stressed the use of the best evidence available to answer clinical questions and explore the next best evidence when appropriate. The next best evidence may include the individual clinical judgment that nurses acquire through clinical experience and clinical practice and other qualitative approaches to research.

Nurses need to recognize that research is important as a basis for their practice and that they need to participate in the research process. For example, both home health nurses and nurses in long-term care facilities are required to collect extensive data on the cognitive and physical functioning of individuals through the Outcome and Assessment Information Set (OASIS) and Minimum Data Set (MDS) assessment tools. These data are used as part of the quality improvement process to indicate areas for improvement in care, thereby contributing to nursing protocols. Nurses in hospital settings are asked to participate in research as part of the Magnet Hospital designation process.

Chapters 16 to 24 contain specific health-promotion research studies. Time should be taken to review these studies and explore the relationship between behavior and disease, to identify which population groups are at risk, and to discover what types of health-promotion programs work and why they work. Through knowledge of research, nurses can strengthen their confidence in making daily decisions about quality care (Box 1-6: Research for Evidence-Based Practice).

## IMPROVING PROSPECTS FOR HEALTH

### Population Effects

Cultural and socioeconomic changes within the population unequivocally influence lay concepts of health and health promotion. Currently there are areas of the United States where the Hispanic population is larger than any other population group. By the 2050, it is predicted that the majority of people in the United States will not be of white European descent (US Census Bureau, 2010a). Taken together as a portent for future health-promotion strategies, these predictions about the population indicate that current knowledge of and approaches to health promotion may not meet the needs of the future US population (see Chapter 2).

In addition to changes in the ethnic and racial distribution within the population, the projected changes in age distribution will affect health-promotion practice. Considerable growth is

---

### BOX 1-6 RESEARCH FOR EVIDENCE-BASED PRACTICE

#### Preventing Functional Decline in Hospitalized Older Adults

The ability to function independently is important throughout life, but especially as one ages. Although some loss of independence in physical functioning may be expected over time, hospitalization should not contribute to physical function loss. Current practice in most hospitals is to limit a person's mobility and independence in activities of daily living. At times these limitations are imposed to prevent falls or other events for the benefit of the individual. But at other times limitations are imposed for the convenience of the staff or to decrease the risk of liability.

Older adults are at risk of losing their functional abilities if the hospitalization-imposed limitations interfere with their normal level of activity. A prolonged hospitalization and rehabilitation period can lead to deconditioning, where the person loses muscle mass, strength, and range of motion as a result of a decrease in his or her activity. Research has demonstrated that such declines can further limit the activities of daily living for these older adults (Graf, 2006).

Evidence is now available to improve the quality of hospital and long-term care of older adults. Actions include establishing functional baseline data through geriatric assessments at the time of admission and at other set times during the stay; using protocols to improve self-care, nutrition, sleep quality, and cognition; minimizing the adverse events that may further influence loss of physical function; and improving the hospital environment to better serve an older adult population (Kleinpell et al., 2008). It is still the nurse caring for the individual person who is most likely to see the need for applying this evidence to improve the care of the hospitalized older adult.

From Graf, C. (2006). Functional decline in hospitalized older adults. *American Journal of Nursing, 106,* 58–67; Kleinpell, R., Fletcher, K., & Jennings, B. (2008). Reducing functional decline in hospitalized elderly. In R.G. Hughes (Ed.), *Patient safety and quality: An evidence-based handbook for nurses.* Rockville, MD: Agency for Healthcare Research and Quality. http://www.ncbi.nlm.nih.gov/books/NBK2629/?report=printable.

---

expected in the proportion of the population that is aged 25 years or older. For example, the post–World War II baby boom will increase the number of people in the 65 years and older age group between 2010 and 2030 (US Census Bureau, 2010b). Although there was a drop in births after 1960, this decrease has been offset by an increase in immigration, both legal and illegal. More restrictive immigration rules related to homeland security have limited legal immigration since 2002 (US Department of Homeland Security, 2016). Analysis of these population trends and projections helps health professionals determine changing needs. Additionally, analysis of the social and economic environment is necessary for the development of social policy concerning health.

## SHIFTING PROBLEMS

The provision of personal health services must be influenced by current information regarding environmental health. Environmental pollution is a complex and increasingly hazardous problem. Diseases related to industry and technology, including asthma and trauma, have become important threats to health.

The physical and psychological stresses of a rapidly changing and fast-paced society present daily problems, such as psychosocial and spiritual poor health habits. Posttraumatic stress disorder is becoming a more common diagnosis. Obesity, partly attributed to a lack of exercise and increasing food portion size, is a growing health issue. The ingestion of potentially toxic, nonnutritious, high-fat foods is another contributing factor (see Chapter 11). The abuse of tobacco, drugs, and alcohol also negatively affects health.

The emphasis on treating disease through the application of complex technology not only is costly but also contributes minimally to the improvement of health. An orientation toward illness clearly focuses on the effects rather than the causes of disease.

A substantial change in wellness patterns is occurring. Infectious and acute diseases were the major causes of death in the early part of the 20th century, whereas chronic conditions, heart disease, cerebrovascular accident (stroke), and cancer are the major causes today. An emphasis on the diagnosis and treatment of disease, which were highly successful in the past, is not the answer for today's needs, which are closely related to and affected by the individual's biochemical functioning, genetics, environment, and personal choices (Box 1-7). The Patient Protection and Affordable Care Act (US Congress, 2010) was enacted to begin the process of paying for health promotion by providing insurance coverage for more people and by covering preventive health services.

## MOVING TOWARD SOLUTIONS

Solutions are neither simple nor easy, but they can be focused in two major directions: individual involvement and government involvement. The first direction concentrates on actions of the individual, especially actions related to lifestyle choices across the life span. The learning and the inherent changes that are involved require the adoption of a new set of skills by people who will need the assistance of nurses to make those changes. Approximately one-fifth of the population of the United States is faced with the problem of getting the basic necessities of food and shelter. The other four-fifths, whose basic needs are met, must overcome problems resulting from affluence (USDHHS, Office of Disease Prevention and Health Promotion, 2011).

Motivational factors play a large role in influencing attitudinal change. As discussed in Chapter 10, programs for health promotion and health education are only part of the answer. Financial incentives for prevention may be another motivating factor, and health advocacy by professionals in the health field is critical. Additionally, private and public action at all levels is needed to reduce social and environmental health hazards. Toxic agents in the environment such as particles from diesel emissions and social conditions such as school overcrowding can present health hazards that may not be detected for years; therefore it is necessary for individuals and the government to play a role.

Legislation and financing that relate to primary prevention are discussed in Chapter 3. Government activity, in the form of legislation, is currently increasing in this area. For example, increasing the activity time in schools, mandating seat belt use, and implementing taxes on gasoline use are specific areas for governmental intervention. Health ecology and planning are

### BOX 1-7   GENOMICS

Genetic research is primarily concerned with discovering, detecting, and treating illnesses related to specific abnormal genetic sequences (Khoury, 2011). Genomics, as a research focus, involves the study of all human genes, which are collectively called the human genome. The study and practice of genomics is concerned with how genes express themselves and how they interact with each other and the environment to encourage or discourage disease (Allen et al., 2014). Genomic interests range from an individual level to a population-based level similar to health-promoting activities. Genomics at an individual level is concerned with an individual's risks related to that person's genomic profile and environmental stimuli. At the population level, genomics is concerned with large-scale patterns of genomic risk and how that plays out in the public arena. Therefore population-based public health genomics is involved with policy development, prioritizing useful genomic information, and ensuring that genomic information is discovered and used ethically and responsibly (Khoury, 2011).

Lifestyle, environment, and genetics and the interaction between the three are determining factors of disease. Currently the focus of much intervention is on the lifestyle and environmental contributors to disease. Because we are just beginning to look at the genomic components of disease and how they interact with lifestyle and environment, the current scientific discussion revolves around the ethical implications of private and public genomic interventions. Current debate surrounding population genomics focuses on the public's "right not to know" (Allen et al., 2014). Genomic information can be used to formulate public health information and initiatives. There are potential social justice ramifications in sharing large-scale genomic information which may accentuate discrimination and worsen stigma. If the information is too complex or difficult to comprehend, it may demotivate people from making needed positive changes. For example, if there is a health behavior that is linked to a particular genomic profile, knowing that could help those who do not have the genomic profile become motivated to change their behavior, whereas people with the genetic profile might become demotivated to change their behavior. Because it is a combination of factors that cause disease, just because a person has the genetic profile does not mean it is an absolute that the person will get the disease, so sharing this information incautiously may be a disservice to public health as opposed to a service. Careful consideration of the risks and benefits of sharing public genomic-related information is essential.

From Allen, C., Senecal, K., & Avard, D. (2014). Defining the scope of public engagement: Examining the "right not to know" in public health genomics. *Public Health Genomics, 42*(1), 11-18; Khoury, M. J. (2011). Public health genomics: The end of the beginning. *Genetics in Medicine, 13*(3), 206-209.

important areas for government involvement in the future. The redirection of the existing health care delivery system, putting more emphasis on primary prevention, is probably the most difficult and the most far-reaching goal; however, an emphasis on a wellness system is necessary to improve the health of the US population.

## TYING IT ALL TOGETHER USING THE NURSING PROCESS

### Problem Identification

How many problems are present in Frank's situation? The answer depends on who is asked the question and his or her position in relation to Frank. Each point of view focuses on different aspects of Frank's life. His physician, using a clinical model of

## CASE STUDY

### Health Assessment: Frank Thompson and Family

Frank Thompson's large brick home is located off a sparsely traveled country road. A few yards away stands the uninhabited shack where Frank was born during World War II.

Frank was raised knowing the odds that he faced as a poor tenant farmer. He helped his father, Ben, with their small tobacco and corn crops. They were unaware that the hazardous chemicals in the pesticides they used would later affect Ben's life. As his father often reminded him, Frank had to do better than others in school so he would not be doomed to the tenant farmer's life. However, Frank's school attendance was erratic because it was interrupted by the frequent demand of tending field crops. Thin and often tired, Frank had recurrent infections. The school nurse helped the Thompson family obtain the necessary medication for Frank's initial infection, but the family was never able to afford the penicillin that was necessary to prevent recurrent infections.

Inspired by the early work of Martin Luther King, Jr., Frank was intent on helping at home and building something better for his future. Frank managed to more than compensate for his lost time at school. He passed his college entrance examinations and was awarded one of the new equal opportunity grants, which offered him a choice of attending any of the Ivy League schools in the Northeast. Instead, he chose the prestigious Southern University and eventually earned a master of business administration degree. He married Sada, his longtime girlfriend, and the two planned their future.

With a good job in a large local sales firm, Frank built his house and started a family. He moved from being a salesman to being a division head and often traveled to regional meetings, sometimes accompanied by Sada and their three children. Frank's dream of sharing his success with his family included using part of his earnings to help his brothers and sisters with their education.

This new way of life meant Frank had little time for relaxation and frequently had to attend business luncheons and career-promoting social events. Frank kept late hours and worked long weekends. Good food, drinks, and cigarettes helped Frank relax before and after important business and social encounters; these softened the edges of hard bargaining and were status symbols.

Not surprisingly, Frank gained weight. He had a persistent cough, which was probably a result of the smoking habit that developed during the early years of his career. Frank's physician, whom Frank visited regularly at the corporation's health maintenance organization, said Frank's blood pressure and serum lipid levels were both higher than normal and that he had chronic bronchitis. The physician urged Frank to take the actions that Frank already recognized: reduce smoking, drinking, and intake of saturated fats and calories; get more exercise; and find ways to relax. However, Frank's life was too busy for exercise. He had to work harder because he was promoted in his company, but he also had to appear relaxed, which was an essential characteristic for a prospective vice president. To meet these goals, Frank tended to drink and smoke more. He also refused to take medication for problems he could not see. Without the outward signs of disease, Frank believed he was out of shape but generally healthy. Then Sada noted that his chance for promotion might actually improve if he lost some weight; therefore Frank registered for a physical fitness program for executives that he could attend on Sunday mornings and before work during the week. At his first workout, the classic sharp pain gripped his chest and Frank had a massive heart attack.

Weeks later, Frank was convalescing at home after being released from the university's coronary care facility. He was lucky to survive the heart attack and he was also fortunate to have most of the health care services covered by his medical insurance plan; in addition, 80% of his earnings were protected by the company's disability pension. (Most people in the United States do not have this protection.)

However, Frank's dreams of promotion were shattered. For many months he could go to the office only two or three times a week at most, simply to deal with routine matters. He could not travel, for business or otherwise, for a long time. He was also skeptical about his cardiac rehabilitation program because his heart attack happened during exercise.

**Reflective Questions:**
- As a nurse, how would you explain to Frank that his heart attack was not caused by his exercise?
- How might a family approach to diet and exercise work with this family, given its structure and background?
- Are there negative behaviors in your life that you see as status symbols?

health, might say that Frank has coronary heart disease with an acute myocardial infarction, hypertension, hyperlipidemia, chronic bronchitis, and obesity. But Frank's problems also represent a failure to meet several of the *Healthy People 2020* objectives on a personal level. His nurse can add that he has paid little attention to his lifestyle, even after changes were recommended. He continues to overeat, drink too much, smoke, not exercise, and live a stressful life. Frank's employer sees a man who has potential but who is now too disabled to take on new responsibilities and perhaps unable to continue performing his previous duties. Frank's children might feel that he can no longer take them on trips or play with them. His wife, Sada, knows that their plans for educating their children, and for travel and enjoyment, might suffer. The human resource personnel who manage Frank's health insurance and pension programs would say that he has an expensive disease, and the state health planner would point out that Frank's problem is only one of a growing number of disabling illnesses that result from preventable causes. A reviewer for *Healthy People 2020* might see Frank as part of the aggregated data on heart disease, indicating a continuing increase in the incidence of heart disease among black non-Hispanic men.

To Frank, his health problems are multidimensional. His initial fear of dying, pain, dependence, and frustration decreased as he began to feel better, but Frank is haunted by his realization that he might never be able to achieve his dreams for himself and his family. Although theoretically in his prime, Frank suddenly sees himself as far older than his years, both in body and in social achievement. He believes he has reached his limit and that he will never again have the freedom to choose his future. He and his family needed to evaluate their situation and make alternative plans based on asset planning. A care plan has been developed based on the situation of Frank and his family. (See the care plan at the end of this chapter.)

## Planning Interventions

Rather than emphasizing the chronic health issues and related problems, the nurse can begin with asset planning within the family. **Asset planning** is a planning approach that, given the realities of the present, helps focus the family members and their providers on the building blocks for their future. It focuses on the assets or strengths of the individual, the family, and the community, applying those assets to improve or maintain the current level of functioning.

Frank's physician and nurse can begin with the fact that Frank survived his first myocardial infarction. The coronary damage resulting from this event becomes the baseline for determining future change in the lives of Frank and his family. Earlier, Frank's physician had taken a broader time perspective when he advised Frank to reduce his cigarette smoking, which was contributing to both his bronchitis and his hypertension, and to change his high-fat diet and sedentary habits, which contributed to his weight problem and his high blood pressure. These lifestyle changes now become tools for Frank's recovery and for change within his family. His cardiac event also becomes a risk factor for heart disease in the lives of his children.

Looking at the immediate future, Frank's employer saw the effect of the event on Frank's position within the company. Frank would have a long recovery that could be successful if he adhered to his cardiac rehabilitation program. Asset planning at this level means examining how to move Frank back into his work role without further jeopardizing his health. Frank and Sada also need to examine if he could continue in this position, given its potential effect on his health.

Frank and his family used a broader perspective than the medical personnel or the corporation. They knew that to achieve the family's economic and educational goals and still spend time together they had to make decisions that would ultimately affect Frank's health. Similar to many Americans, they had been willing to live with Frank's job pressures and stressful lifestyle caused by the economy. The family members were aware of their impoverished roots and had no wish to return to them. However, they also recognized that the strength of their family, their ability to work together to achieve goals, and their faith were assets that could be used for support.

Frank's social network of friends, relatives, and church members became an additional asset. They helped the family through the difficult initial weeks at home by delivering meals, taking care of the yard work and laundry, and providing companionship so Sada could shop and have time alone. As Frank recovered, they would provide support for the social and lifestyle changes that Frank and his family needed to make.

The nurse-led cardiovascular rehabilitation group played a vital role in Frank's recovery. As the physician continued to monitor Frank's cardiac status, the nurse began the long process of working with Frank to modify his habits. He had stopped smoking while in the hospital, but with more free time than usual, he was craving to smoke again. Using an asset planning approach and Gordon's (2016) functional health patterns, the nurse identified the changes that Frank needed to make to decrease the risk of a second heart attack. A plan was developed to help Frank begin to take control of his life through behavior changes. These changes included relaxation techniques, diet modification, smoking cessation, and mild chair exercises. The support of the family was enlisted to reinforce the changes Frank was willing to make, because social support and environmental changes are shown to enhance personal decision-making. His employer was contacted and agreed to a plan enabling Frank to work from home using a computer while the workplace became smoke-free.

Frank became an asset to the workplace, serving as a spokesperson for the benefits of lifestyle change. He was enlisted to talk with other employees about stress management, exercise, weight reduction, and smoking cessation based on his personal experiences.

Health planners and public health officials used the broadest perspective in asset planning by viewing Frank as an example of a person whose potential shifted as a result of a preventable, disabling illness. The planners looked to public and private community patterns and policies that increase healthful habits and living conditions. Work schedules and work load; stress and safety in work environments; affirmative action programs for jobs and wages; availability of public transportation systems, recreational facilities, and economically accessible housing; farm price subsidies for food and tobacco crops that affect buying patterns; excise taxes and regulation of health-damaging drugs such as alcohol and nicotine were all taken into consideration (Grzywacz & Fuqua, 2000). The asset planning approach emphasized the positive actions that could be made at the personal, employment, community, and societal levels to minimize the effects of Frank's illness and related diseases, thereby addressing all levels of the ecological model of health.

## What Was the Actual Cause of Frank's Problem?

It is not possible to separate one cause from another because heart disease is a multifactorial disease. In Frank's case the sources of illness were found in the many interrelationships in his life. Attempting to treat or change each factor as a separate entity can have only a limited effect on the improvement of overall health. Frank's health problems were numerous. In addition to a poor diet, weight gain, lack of exercise, and smoking, his hyperlipidemia, an adaptive biological response to the pressures in his life, further debilitated him. It eventually led to clogged coronary vessels, and his responses became maladaptive. His hypertension, resulting from his diet and time-constrained lifestyle, complicated by the buildup of plaque secondary to hyperlipidemia, was also a biological attempt to adjust to a situation that contributed to an imbalance between his personal resources and the demands of his family and the economic world. Frank's smoking was a psychosocial means to help him relieve some of the emotional pressures. It may have served this short-term purpose, but only at a silently rising cost to his health. Cigarette use by persons who have hypertension or high serum cholesterol levels multiplies their risk of coronary heart disease (Izzo & Black, 2008).

## Evaluation of the Situation

The health status of an individual or population depends on a sustainable balance of the complex responses between physiological, psychological, and social and environmental factors. Health was initially conceived as a biological state, with genetic endowment as the starting point. However, health involves psychological and social aspects and is interpreted within the context of the immediate environment.

The interconnections between biophysical, psychological, and environmental causes and consequences did not end with Frank's heart attack. His heart attack was only the most dramatic sign that health-damaging responses outweighed health-promoting ones. The "tip of the iceberg" analogy is frequently used to illustrate the importance of identifying individuals with subclinical symptoms. High blood lipid levels, high blood pressure, obesity, smoking, and persistent worrying were no less important than the infarction in shaping the status of Frank's health. Repairing the damage to Frank's heart without changing his lifestyle, habits, and work environment would only buy a brief amount of time before further damage would occur.

The infarction and resulting disability also permanently reshaped Frank's environment. After a few months of working full-time, Frank realized that he needed to find a less stressful job. He recognized that his sales administration skills were an asset and began interviewing in the nonprofit sector. Ultimately, he landed a job at half his previous salary, but with excellent benefits and a flexible work environment. His reduced income meant that his children's educational opportunities were more limited than they were before his heart attack, but his family responded by seeking tuition support from community organizations. Frank found that his contacts in both the corporate and the nonprofit sectors increased his value to his new employer. Frank's entire life, internal and external, had changed. He had learned to adapt to his health problems and had developed a more **eudaimonistic** approach to health and life.

Frank's situation illustrates how causes and effects in life and health tend to merge into constant, inseparable interconnections between individuals and their worlds. A person's health status is a reflection of a web of relationships that characterize that person's life. Health is not an achievement or a prize but a high-quality interaction between a person's inner and outer worlds that provides the capacity to respond to the demands of the biological, psychological, and environmental systems of these worlds.

Which of the *Healthy People 2020* focus areas listed in Box 1-4 apply to the promotion of Frank's health?

Clearly, the area of heart disease and stroke is most applicable. The *Healthy People 2020* website (https://www.healthypeople.gov/2020/default) has a number of objectives that relate directly to the prevention of heart disease, hypertension, and hyperlipidemia, including objectives that relate to treatment options and training the public to recognize and respond to nutrition and weight (Box 1-5: *Healthy People 2020*). From the information about Frank and his experience, determine what his children should be taught on the basis of the *Healthy People 2020* objectives in this focus area.

## ◎ CARE PLAN

### Health Assessment: Frank Thompson and Family

*NURSING DIAGNOSIS: Risk of ineffective coping as a result of change in role performance and self-esteem

**Defining Characteristics**
- Inability to complete tasks
- Lack of focus on needs
- Feelings of inadequacy
- Inability to make decisions
- Sense of being overwhelmed
- Rest and sleep disturbance
- Frequent stress-related headaches
- Emotional fragility
- Assessment of situations does not match assessments of others

**Related Factors**
- Unexpected life changes
- Diagnosis of chronic disease
- Stressful life events
- Unsure of family supports
- Unrealistic expectations of self
- Unpredictable future
- Need to reassess abilities
- Insecure job status

**Expected Outcomes**
- The person will develop realistic expectations of capabilities on the basis of rehabilitation potential.
- The nurse and person will set mutually agreeable milestones for resuming functions.
- The person will develop a revitalized sense of self.
- The person and family will use available resources to examine social and role shifts that affect the family.
- The person and spouse will express to each other their hopes and fears about the future.

**Interventions**
- Listen to the concerns of the person and spouse regarding job, social, family, and medical concerns.
- Counsel the individual and spouse about realistic goals and expectations of cardiac rehabilitation.
- Assist the individual in setting realistic and reachable short-term goals.
- Assist the individual in developing more effective problem-solving skills.
- Provide support and positive feedback as short-term goals are met.
- Explore available community services that match the goals of the family.
- Facilitate family access to needed services through advocacy and supportive guidance.
- Supervise and teach about the use of prescribed and other medications.
- Coordinate communications between providers, employers, and other organizations to meet coping needs of the individual and his or her family.

## SUMMARY

The ways individuals define health and health problems are important because definitions influence attempts to improve health and care delivery. In the case study, Frank Thompson's health was affected by obvious, immediate, and personal factors, such as his diet and employment pressures. Nevertheless, his problems had their roots in the social and economic conditions of his parents; in his own early history of illness, education, and work; and in his and his family's hopes and aspirations. His physician defined Frank's problem in immediate biomedical terms. Public health planners, who saw Frank's problem on a longer-term population basis, sought policy solutions to the problem of preventing cardiovascular disease.

The view taken in this text is that a broad and longer-term perspective of health is the best guide to promoting health more effectively, even as nurses deal with individual problems on a daily basis. Health is a sustainable balance between internal and external forces. Health allows people to move through life free from the constraints of illness and promotes healing.

Illness represents an imbalance that human choices (intertwined social, political, spiritual, professional, and personal choices) create. In the United States, communities may still have time to reduce the onslaught of chronic disability and shift the direction, slow the pace, and humanize the scope of economic and social life.

Shifting directions in today's health care patterns may be possible only when nurses and other health professionals do what is expected of them as leaders in the care of health: to work with others through open processes; to provide leadership in finding the vision and the path; and to inform, educate, and reeducate themselves, their colleagues, the media, and the general public using research findings and evidence-based practice methods.

The responsibility of nurses as health professionals today is to see the health problem in new ways and help others to do the same. Responsibility means developing new roles and examining the problem through others' viewpoints, including those of individuals, the public, other professionals, and other nations. Responsibility also means evaluating the social and individual consequences, the long-term and short-term effects, and the public and private interests that are involved when one is deciding on the set of tools to use in the care of health.

## ⓔ EVOLVE CHAPTER FEATURES

http://evolve.elsevier.com/Edelman/
• Study Questions

## REFERENCES

Ajzen, A., & Fishbein, M. (1980). *Understanding attitudes and predicting social behavior.* Upper Saddle River, NJ: Prentice Hall.

Allen, F. M., & Warner, M. (2002). A developmental model of health and nursing. *Journal of Family Nursing, 8*(2), 96–135.

American Cancer Society. (2016). *Cancer facts and figures for African Americans 2016-2018.* Atlanta, GA: American Cancer Society.

American Nurses Association (ANA). (2010). *Nursing's social policy statement.* Washington, DC: ANA Publications.

American Nurses Association (ANA). (2015a). *Code of ethics for nurses with interpretive statements.* Washington, DC: ANA Publications.

American Nurses Association (ANA). (2015b). *Nursing: Scope and standards of practice.* Washington, DC: ANA Publications.

Andresen, E. M., et al. (2003). Retest reliability of surveillance questions on health related quality of life. *Journal of Epidemiology and Community Health, 57*(5), 339–343.

Ardell, D. B. (2007). What is wellness? http://www.seekwellness.com/wellness/what_is_wellness.htm.

Association of Faculties of Medicine of Canada. (n.d.). AFMC primer on population health. http://phprimer.afmc.ca/Part1-TheoryThinkingAboutHealth.

Bandura, A. (1976). *Social learning theory.* Upper Saddle River, NJ: Prentice Hall.

Bandura, A. (1999). *Self-efficacy: The exercise of control.* New York: W.H. Freeman.

Bandura, A. (2004). Health promotion by social cognitive means. *Health Education Behavior, 31*(2), 143–164.

Barr, D. A. (2014). *Health disparities in the United States: Social class, race, ethnicity & health.* Baltimore: Johns Hopkins University Press.

Barr, D., Lee, P., & Benjamin, A. (2003). Health care and health policy in a changing world. In H. Wallace (Ed.), *Health and welfare for families in the 21st century* (2nd ed.). Boston: Jones & Bartlett.

Benner, P., et al. (2010). *Educating nurses: A call for radical transformation.* San Francisco: Jossey-Bass.

Boltz, M., Resnick, B., & Galik, E. (2012). Interventions to prevent functional decline in acute care settings. In M. Boltz, E. Capezuti, et al. (Eds.), *Evidence-based geriatric nursing protocols for best practice* (pp. 104–121). New York: Springer.

Burnham, J. C. (2012). The death of the sick role. *Social History of Medicine, 25*(4), 761–776.

Burns, N., & Grove, S. K. (2014). *Understanding nursing research* (6th ed.). Philadelphia: Saunders.

Cano, A., et al. (2003). Family support, self-rated health, and psychological distress. *Primary Care Companion Journal of Clinical Psychiatry, 5,* 111–117.

Champion, V. L., & Skinner, C. S. (2008). The health belief model. In K. Glanz, B. Rimer, & K. Viswanath (Eds.), *Health behavior and health education: Theory, research and practice* (4rd ed.). San Francisco: Jossey-Bass.

Cohen, S. R., et al. (1997). Validity of the McGill Quality of Life Questionnaire in the palliative care setting. A multi-center Canadian study demonstrating the importance of the existential domain. *Palliative Medicine, 11,* 3–20.

Commission on Social Determinants of Health. (2008). *Closing the gap in a generation: Health equity through action on the social determinants of health. Final report of the Commission on Social Determinants of Health.* Geneva: World Health Organization.

Crimmins, E. M., Preston, S. H., & Cohen, B. (2011). Explaining divergent levels of longevity in high-income countries. http://www8.nationalacademies.org/onpinews/newsitem.aspx?RecordID=13089.

David, R. (2000). Keynote address: Leadership for innovation in health care. In Ford Foundation, John F. Kennedy School of Government, Summary of Proceedings, Local Innovations in Health Care Conference, Cambridge, MA, June 28-30, 2000.

Davis, M. A., Weeks, W. B., & Coulter, I. D. (2011). A proposed conceptual model for studying the use of complementary and alternative medicine. *Alternative Therapies in Health and Medicine, 17*(5), 32–36.

Dunn, H. (1961). *High-level wellness.* Arlington, VA: R.W. Beatty.

Fawcett, J., & Garity, J. (2009). *Evaluating research for evidence-based nursing practice.* Philadelphia: F.A. Davis.

Fryar, C. D., Carroll, M. D., & Ogden, C. D. (2014). Prevalence of overweight, obesity, and extreme obesity among adults: United States, 1960–1962 through 2011–2012. http://www.cdc.gov/nchs/data/hestat/obesity_adult_11_12/obesity_adult_11_12.pdf.

Gordon, M. (2016). *Manual of nursing diagnosis* (13th ed.). Sudbury, MA: Jones & Bartlett.

Greiner, P., Snowdon, D., & Greiner, L. (1996). The relationship of self-rated function and self-rated health to concurrent functional ability, functional decline, and mortality: Findings from the Nun Study. *The Journal of Gerontology. Series B, Psychological Sciences and Social Sciences, S51*(5), S234–S241.

Greiner, P., Snowdon, D., & Greiner, L. (1999). Self-rated function, self-rated health, and postmortem evidence of brain infarcts: Findings from the Nun Study. *The Journal of Gerontology. Series B, Psychological Sciences and Social Sciences, 54*(4), S219–S222.

Grzywacz, J., & Fuqua, J. (2000). The social ecology of health: Leverage points and linkages. *Behavioral Medicine, 26*(3), 101–115.

Haley, K., Koenig, H., & Bruchett, B. (2001). Relationship between private religious activity and physical functioning in older adults. *Journal of Religion and Health, 40*(2), 302–312.

Hollingsworth, L., & Didelot, M. (2005). Illness: The redefinition of self and relationships. Paper presented at the 4th Global Conference—Making Sense of: Health, Illness, and Disease Mansfield College, Oxford.

Idler, E., & Benyamini, Y. (1997). Self-rated health and mortality: A review of twenty-seven community studies. *Journal of Health and Social Behavior, 38*(1), 21–37.

Institute of Medicine. (2003). *The future of the public's health in the 21st century.* Washington, DC: National Academies Press.

Institute of Medicine. (2010). The future of nursing: Leading change, advancing health. http://iom.edu/Reports/2010/ThefutureofNursing-Leading-Change-Advancing-Health.aspx.

International Parish Nurse Resource Center. (2012). Resource catalog. http://www.parishnurses.org/.

Issel, L. M. (2014). *Health program planning and evaluation: A practical, systematic approach for community health* (3rd ed.). Sudbury, MA: Jones & Bartlett.

Izzo, J., & Black, H. (2008). *Hypertension primer* (3rd ed.). Philadelphia: Lippincott Williams & Wilkins.

Kaplow, R., & Reed, K. (2008). The AACN synergy model for patient care: A nursing model as a force of magnetism. *Nursing Economics, 26*(1), 17–25.

Kreuter, M., & Devore, R. (1980). Update: Reinforcing the case for health promotion. *Family & Community Health, 10,* 106.

Leavell, H., & Clark, A. E. (1965). *Preventive medicine for the doctor in his community.* New York: McGraw-Hill.

McKivergin, M. (2009). The nurse as an instrument of healing. In B. Dossey & L. Keegan (Eds.), *Holistic nursing: A handbook for practice* (5th ed., pp. 721–728). Sudbury, MA: Jones & Bartlett.

McMahon, S., & Fleury, J. (2012). Wellness in older adults: A concept analysis. *Nursing Forum, 47*(1), 39–51. doi:10.1111/nuf.2012.47.issue-1/issuetoc.

National Heart, Lung, and Blood Institute. (2000). Obesity education initiative. The practical guide: Identification, evaluation, and treatment of overweight and obesity in adults. NIH publication no. 00-4084. Bethesda, MD: US Government Printing Office.

National Institutes of Health, National Center for Complementary and Alternative Medicine. (2011). What is CAM? http://nccam.nih.gov/health/whatiscam/.

National Institute of Nursing Research (NINR). (2011). NINR strategic plan. http://www.ninr.nih.gov/NR/rdonlyres/8BE21801-0C52-44C2-9EEA-142483657FB1/0/NINR_StratPlan_F2_508.pdf.

Newman, M. (2003). A world of no boundaries. *ANS. Advances in Nursing Science, 26*(4), 240–245.

Norwood, S. (2003). *Nursing consultation: A framework for working with communities* (2nd ed.). Upper Saddle River, NJ: Prentice Hall.

O'Donnell, M. (1987). Definition of health promotion. *American Journal of Health Promotion, 1*(1), 4–5.

Pender, N. J., Murdaugh, C. L., & Parsons, M. A. (2015). *Health promotion in nursing practice* (6th ed.). Upper Saddle River, NJ: Prentice Hall.

Prochaska, J., Gill, P., & Hall, S. (2004). Treatment of tobacco use in an inpatient psychiatric setting. *Psychiatric Services, 55,* 1265–1270.

Reed, P. G. (1983). Implications of the life span developmental framework for well-being in adulthood and aging. *ANS. Advances in Nursing Science, 6*(1), 18–25.

Richard, L., Gauvin, L., & Raine, K. (2011). Ecological models revisited: Their uses and evolution in health promotion over two decades. *Annual Review of Public Health, 32,* 307–326.

Rogers, M. (1970). *An introduction to the theoretical basis of nursing.* Philadelphia: F.A. Davis.

Ruger, J. P., et al. (2015). From conceptual pluralism to practical agreement on policy: Global responsibility for global health. *BMC International Health and Human Rights, 15*(30), doi:10.1186/s12914-015-0065-8.

Sackett, D., et al. (1996). Evidence based medicine: What it is and what it isn't. *British Medical Journal, 312,* 71–72.

Salama, R. (n.d.). Concepts of prevention and control. http://www.pitt.edu/~super7/32011-33001/32311.ppt.

Siegel, D. (2007). *The mindful brain: Reflection and attunement in the cultivation of well-being.* New York: W.W. Norton & Co.

Smith, J. A. (1983). *The idea of health: Implications for the nursing profession.* New York: Columbia University Teachers College Press.

US Census Bureau. (2010a). The Hispanic population: 2010. C2010BR-04. http://www.census.gov/prod/cen2010/briefs/c2010br-04.pdf.

US Census Bureau. (2010b). The older population: 2010. C2010BR-09. http://www.census.gov/prod/cen2010/briefs/c2010br-09.pdf.

US Congress. (2010). Patient Protection and Affordable Care Act ("PPACA"; Public Law 111–148). http://www.healthcare.gov/law/full/index.html.

US Department of Health and Human Services. (2014). Healthy People 2020. http://www.healthypeople.gov/.

US Department of Health and Human Services, National Institutes of Health, National Heart, Lung, and Blood Institute. (2012). Obesity education initiative. http://www.nhlbi.nih.gov/health/public/heart/obesity/lose_wt/index.htm.

US Department of Health and Human Services, Office of Disease Prevention and Health Promotion. (2011). Healthy People 2020. Washington, DC. http://www.healthypeople.gov/2020/.

US Department of Health and Human Services, Public Health Service. (1986). *The 1990 health objectives for the nation: A midcourse review*. Washington, DC: US Government Printing Office, US Department of Health and Human Services.

US Department of Health and Human Services, Public Health Service. (1990). *Healthy People 2000: The Surgeon General's report on health promotion and disease prevention*. US Department of Health and Human Services publication no. 7955071. Washington, DC: US Government Printing Office.

US Department of Health and Human Services, Public Health Service. (1996). *Healthy People 2000 midcourse review and 1995 revisions*. Boston: Jones & Bartlett.

US Department of Health and Human Services, Public Health Service. (2000). *Healthy People 2010 (conference edition, in two volumes)*. Washington, DC: US Government Printing Office.

US Department of Health, Education, and Welfare, Public Health Service. (1979). *Healthy People*. Washington, DC: US Government Printing Office, US Department of Health and Human Services.

US Department of Homeland Security. (2016). Enforce and administer our immigration laws. https://www.dhs.gov/administer-immigration-laws.

US Preventive Services Task Force. (2014). Guide to clinical preventive services, 2014. http://www.uspreventiveservicestaskforce.org/Announcements/News/Item/uspstf-releases-2014-guide-to-clinical-preventive-services.

Weintraub, W. S., et al. (2011). Value of primordial and primary prevention for cardiovascular disease. A policy statement from the American Heart Association. *Circulation, 124*, 967–990.

World Health Organization. (2004). The World Health Organization Quality of Life *(WHOQOL)-BREF*. http://www.who.int/substance_abuse/research_tools/en/english_whoqol.pdf.

# 2

# Emerging Populations and Health

*Kevin K. Chui, Frank Tudini, and Sheng-Che Yen*

## OBJECTIVES

*After completing this chapter, the reader will be able to:*

- Differentiate among ethnicity, ethnic group, race, and minority group.
- Describe demographic data relative to emerging populations:
  - Arab Americans
  - Asian Americans/Pacific Islanders
  - Black/African Americans
  - Latino/Hispanic Americans
  - Native Americans
  - Homeless persons
- Describe health concerns and issues of emerging populations.
- Discuss selected cultural factors that may have an impact on the health and well-being of emerging populations.
- Contrast the folk healing system with the professional care system.
- Explain strategies for health care professionals to meet the needs of emerging populations.
- Describe initiatives to address the health care concerns of emerging populations.

## KEY TERMS

Chi
Complementary and alternative
  medicine (CAM)
Cultural competency
Culture
Emerging populations
Ethnic group
Ethnicity
Ethnocentric perspective

Female genital mutilation (FGM)
Folk healing system
Health disparities
Health equity
Homelessness
Hot and cold concept of disease
Jing
Minority group
Nurse care systems

Professional care systems
Race
Taoism
Transcultural nursing
Value orientations
Values
Yang
Yin

## HEALTH DISPARITIES AND HEALTH EQUALITY

Many magnitudes of disparity, particularly in health, exist within the United States and across countries (World Health Organization, 2015). There has been a growing awareness that racial and ethnic minority groups experienced poorer health compared with the general population in the United States. Various factors such as race or ethnicity, sex, age, disability, and socioeconomic status contribute to an individual's capability to attain good health, which is a function of one's ability to receive quality care and have access to health care (Agency for Healthcare Research and Quality, 2011). *Healthy People 2020* (http://www.healthypeople.gov) endeavors to improve the health of all groups (Hansen, 2011).

Health disparities is an umbrella term that includes disparities in health and in health care. It was defined by *Healthy People 2020* as "a particular type of health difference that is closely linked with social, economic, and/or environmental disadvantage," and "health disparities adversely affect groups of people who have systematically experienced greater obstacles to health based on their racial or ethnic group; religion; socioeconomic status; gender; age; mental health; cognitive, sensory, or physical disability; sexual orientation or gender identity; geographic location; or other characteristics historically linked to discrimination or exclusion" (US Department of Health and Human Services, Centers for Disease Control and Prevention, 2011). Health disparities represent a lack of efficiency within the health care system and account for unnecessary costs for and

## ? THINK ABOUT IT

### *A New Brand of Outreach for Chemically Dependent Homeless People With HIV/AIDS*

- Access to health care services is often a major barrier for people who are considered underserved by the health care system. Community outreach programs have shown some success in reaching persons with different types of health problems. However, outreach programs for certain marginalized populations have not always been successful in their efforts to reach the "hard to reach."
- A new approach in outreach programs for chemically dependent homeless people with HIV/AIDS is harm reduction. This approach "acknowledges the reality that drug use is a part of life. Rather than condemn or condone, harm-reduction practitioners seek to work collaboratively with the client."
- Harm reduction as a part of outreach programs:
  - Aims to build on the ability of individuals to make decisions about their own lives.
  - Views drug use along a spectrum, ranging from heavy use to abstinence.
  - Honors self-determination and individual dignity.
  - Functions as an alternative model of treatment that reinforces a hierarchical physician-patient relationship.
- Practitioners who view harm reduction as an essential component of outreach:
  - See their patients as experts of their lives and their addiction.
  - Consider the structural factors that influence adoption of healthy lifestyles.

- Facilitate an egalitarian relationship between the patient and the provider.
- Consider all the multiple pressures affecting patient functioning in all spheres of life.

With these premises and beliefs, an outreach program explored the service utilization of chemically dependent persons with HIV/AIDS. The study's purpose was to investigate whether hard-to-reach participants, lodged through a harm-reduction program at single-room occupancy hotels, access health services at the same level as those who report at the agency's drop-in center. Data indicate that low-threshold harm-reduction outreach did increase access to health services by reducing barriers to services.

The researcher concluded that this component of outreach is a "valuable intervention for increasing utilization among this highly marginalized group." Will this philosophy of outreach be effective in helping persons with chronic illnesses such as diabetes, hypertension, or obesity, to name just a few? Something to think about!

More comprehensive information on the harm-reduction approach for chemically dependent individuals with HIV/AIDS is available online at http://www.aids.org/topics/harm-reduction-and-hiv/.

From Shepard, B. (2007). Harm reduction outreach services and engagement of chemically-dependent homeless people living with HIV/AIDS: An analysis of service utilization data to evaluate program theory. *Einstein Journal of Biology and Medicine, 23*, 26–32.

---

diminish the quality of life of persons seeking care (Hansen, 2011).

Health equity is the accomplishment of the highest level of health for all people. Attaining health equity requires valuing everyone equally with focused and ongoing societal efforts to deal with preventable inequalities, historical and contemporary injustices, and the elimination of health and health care disparities (US Department of Health and Human Services, Centers for Disease Control and Prevention, 2011).

Although the diversity of the American population is one of the best assets for this country, one of the greatest challenges is reducing the disparity in health status of America's racial and ethnic minorities and other health disparity populations. The US Department of Health and Human Services (US Department of Health and Human Services, 2015) and the Institute of Medicine (2008) have well documented that racial and ethnic minorities, compared with whites, have less access to health care, receive lower-quality health care, and have higher rates of illness, injury, and premature death. A review of *Health, United States, 2014: With Special Feature on Adults Aged 55–64* (National Center for Health Statistics, 2015) will help one to understand the magnitude of the problem. For example, black or African-American men and women aged 20 years or older have much higher rates of hypertension and uncontrolled high blood pressure than white men and women. The issue of racial and ethnic health disparities has become one of the most urgent problems to plague the US health care system.

Efforts to eliminate disparities and achieve health equity have focused primarily on diseases or illnesses and on health care

services. However, the absence of disease does not automatically equate to good health. An individual's ability to achieve good health could be affected because of race or ethnicity, gender, sexual identity, age, disability, socioeconomic status, and geographical location.

## EMERGING POPULATIONS IN THE UNITED STATES

Currently, emerging populations include ethnic minorities and persons who are homeless. Ethnic minority populations could include Asian Americans/Pacific Islanders (AAPIs), black/African Americans (BAAs), Latino/Hispanic Americans (LHAs), Native Americans, and Arab Americans (Box 2-1: *Healthy People 2020*). The increasing population of immigrants has been a significant contributor to the presence of increasing numbers of major ethnic groups in the United States. Between 2000 and 2013 the immigrant population in the United States increased by 10.2 million (Migration Policy Institute, 2015). The US immigrant population accounted for about 11.1% of the total US population in 2000 and 13.1% in 2013 (Migration Policy Institute, 2015). From 1960 to 2013, more than 41 million people legally immigrated to the United States with the 10 most common countries of origin being (in rank order) Mexico, China, India, Philippines, Vietnam, El Salvador, Cuba, Korea, Dominican Republic, and Guatemala (Migration Policy Institute, 2015). In addition, there are approximately 11 million unauthorized immigrants in the United States, with Mexicans representing the majority (56%, or approximately 6 million) (Rosenblum & Soto, 2015). One

**Selected National Health Promotion and Disease Prevention Objectives for Emerging Populations**

- Increase the number of people with health insurance to 100% (baseline, 83.2% [lower in ethnic minorities] of people younger than 65 years covered by health insurance in 2008).
- Increase the proportion of people who have a specific source of ongoing care to 89.4% (baseline, 81.3% in 2008).
- Reduce the overall cancer death rate. Target of 161.4 deaths per 100,000 of the population (baseline, 179.3 deaths per 100,000 of the population in 2007).
- Prevent diabetes. Target of 7.2 new cases per 1000 per year, ages 18 to 84 years (baseline, eight new cases in past 12 months, as reported in 2006-2008) Increase the proportion of people with diabetes who receive formal diabetes education. Target of 62.5% (baseline, 56.8% of people with diabetes received formal education in 2008.)
- Reduce coronary heart disease deaths. Target of 103.4 deaths per 100,000 (baseline, 129.2 coronary artery disease deaths per 100,000 in 2007).
- Reduce AIDS among adolescents and adults. Target of 12.4 new cases per 100,000 (baseline, 13.8 cases of AIDS, aged 13 years or older in 2007).
- Increase the number of population-based data systems used to monitor data on (or for) lesbian, gay, and bisexual populations. Target of 12 data systems used to monitor data (baseline, 6 data systems used to monitor data in 2008).

From US Department of Health and Human Services. (2012). *Healthy People 2020* (Vol. 1). Washington, DC: US Government Printing Office. Also see developing data and goals for *Healthy People 2020* at http://www.healthypeople.gov.

in three Americans in the United States identifies as African American, American Indian/Alaska Native (AIAN), Asian, Native Hawaiian/Pacific Islander, Hispanic/Latino, or multiracial. It was estimated that this number is expected to increase to one in two Americans by 2050 (Kaiser Family Foundation, 2008). The increasing populations of ethnic groups are one of many factors producing disparities in health status and access to the health care system in the United States. The disparities in the health care system may cause increases of social costs attributable to the lost productivity or use of health care services among the ethnic minority populations.

## ETHNICITY, ETHNIC GROUP, MINORITY GROUP, AND RACE

Race and ethnicity categories in the United States are defined by the Office of Management and Budget, with the latest set based on a 1997 revision of a 1977 standard (Humes et al., 2011). The minimal race categories for collecting data on race and ethnicity are black/African American (BAA), American Indian/Alaska Native (AIAN), Asian, Native Hawaiian and other Pacific Islander, and white; and the minimal ethnicity categories are Hispanic/Latino and non-Hispanic/Latino origin (Humes et al., 2011).

Race and ethnicity are different but somewhat alike. Race is associated with power and indexes the history or ongoing imposition of one group's authority above another. Ethnicity focuses on differences in meanings, values, and ways of living (practices) (Markus, 2008). Race has been defined as "a dynamic set of

historically derived and institutionalized ideas and practices that: sorts people into ethnic groups according to perceived physical and behavioral human characteristics; associates differential value, power, and privilege with these characteristics and establishes a social status ranking among the different groups; and emerges (1) when groups are perceived to pose a threat (political, economic, or cultural) to each other's worldview or way of life; and/or (2) to justify the denigration and exploitation (past, current, or future) of, and prejudice toward, other groups" (Markus, 2008). A definition provided for ethnicity is that "ethnicity is a dynamic set of historically derived and institutionalized ideas and practices that allows people to identify or to be identified with groupings of people on the basis of presumed (and usually claimed) commonalities including language, history, nation or region of origin, customs, ways of being, religion, names, physical appearance, and/or genealogy or ancestry; can be a source of meaning, action, and identity; and confers a sense of belonging, pride, and motivation" (Markus, 2008).

A minority group consists of people who are living within a society in which they are usually disadvantaged in relation to power, control of their own lives, and wealth (Hammond & Cheney, 2009). For example, poverty rates for Native Americans and Alaskan Natives (27.0%) and blacks or African Americans (25.8%) are much higher than the overall poverty rate (14.3%) and that of whites (11.6%) and Asians (11.7%) (McCartney et al., 2013). In the 2010 US Census, just one-third of the US population reported their race and ethnicity as something other than non-Hispanic white alone, and this group was referred to as the "minority" population for the report (Humes et al., 2011). The minority population in the United States increased from 86.9 million to 111.9 million between 2000 and 2010, representing a growth of 29% during the decade (Humes et al., 2011).

## CULTURE, VALUES, AND VALUE ORIENTATION

Ethnicity is evidenced in customs that reflect the socialization and cultural patterns of the group. Culture, as an element of ethnicity, refers to integrated patterns of human behavior that include the language, thoughts, communications, actions, customs, beliefs, values, and institutions of racial, ethnic, religious, or social groups (Office of Minority Health, 2016a). It is "shaped by values, beliefs, norms, and practices that are shared by members of the same cultural group" (Giger, 2013).

Values are beliefs about the worth of something and serve as standards that influence behavior and thinking. Cultural values "are unique, individual expressions of a particular culture that have been accepted as appropriate over time. They guide actions and decision-making that facilitate self-worth and self-esteem" (Giger, 2013). Cultural values are integral to the manner in which individuals will employ health behaviors, maintain their health, how they will seek care for themselves and others, and where they are likely to go to receive care (Boyle, 2016).

Value orientations, learned and shared through the socialization process, reflect the personality type of a particular society. The dominant value orientations are shared by the majority of the group. Kluckhohn's model (1953) of value orientations

## ⊕ BOX 2-2   DIVERSITY AWARENESS

### Female Genital Mutilation: Taboo or Tradition

Some practices of individuals or groups are deeply rooted in beliefs connected to culture. These practices are considered unhealthy and/or unsafe in other cultures who do not share the same beliefs. This is the case for **female genital mutilation (FGM)**. What is the likelihood of health care providers having an encounter with circumcised women? It is probably high because "although the incidence of FGM in women is worldwide, rough estimates range from 114–130 million women" (Little, 2003). The increasing migration of circumcised women to the United States and the fact that "female circumcision has been practiced in the US since the 19th century" (Webber & Schonfeld, 2003) increase the probability of these women's presence in health care settings. In countries that legally prohibit FGM, parents often feign a holiday or vacation to the native country, where they have the young daughter circumcised.

Female circumcision and female genital mutilation have unknown origins. However, it is believed that the practice can be traced "in Africa as far back as the 5th century B.C. and has taken place in ancient Egypt, ancient Rome, Arabia, and Tsarist Russia" (Little, 2003). There are four types of FGM:

- Type 1, also known as clitoridectomy, is the excision of the clitoral prepuce and may also involve the excision of all or part of the clitoris.
- Type 2 is the excision of the clitoris and may also involve the excision of all or part of the labia minora.
- Type 3, also known as infibulation, involves excision of part or all of the external genitalia and the stitching or narrowing of the vaginal opening.
- Type 4 refers to all other genital procedures (Momoh, 2004).

It is a myth that FGM is advocated by specific individuals in cultures or societies that advocate and support this practice. Leval et al. (2004) analyzed the ways Swedish midwives discussed sexuality in circumcised African women. Their encounters with spouses in maternity wards dispelled the myth that men are the power holders. They were described as "always tender, caring, power shares, or even subordinates in the relationship." Support for this myth buster is seen in societies where adult women advocate and support the practice as an affirmation of their roles and high regard for their bodies (Little, 2003). Parents of young girls support the practice as an assurance of economic security for their daughters (Gruenbaum, 2005). In some societies, powerful women leaders who are feared and respected promote this practice (Little, 2003).

There are many explanations for female circumcision. Gruenbaum (2005) offers a comprehensive discussion of these. Her analysis to approaches for proposed changes in the practice or its elimination through the passage of laws is extremely enlightening and provides a deep understanding of the complexities of FGM. There are cultural reasons for this practice, including providing health benefits, preserving virginity before marriage, serving as a rite of passage, and providing economic security for women as well as for the people performing such acts (Berg et al., 2009; Gruenbaum, 2005; Little, 2003). Cultural beliefs about sexuality and sexual responses are also a factor (Leval et al., 2004).

FGM has many complications. The immediate ones include hemorrhage, infections, abscesses, and urinary difficulties such as retention and straining. Long-term complications include difficulty voiding, urinary and reproductive tract infections, and incontinence. Other complications are infertility, painful intercourse, keloids, introital and vaginal stenosis, dermoid cysts, and pain. For the circumcised woman during labor, there is obstructed labor, fetal distress, perineal tears, perineal wound infection, and postpartum hemorrhage and sepsis. Obermeyer (2005) contends that complications or consequences of FGM are poorly documented because of many methodological issues, including the quality of the data collected. Valid research on female circumcision is a fertile ground. Obermeyer's (2005) review of studies on FGM is an excellent resource for interested researchers.

What are the care implications for nurses? Midwives and nurses whose area of practice is women's health are more likely to have experiences with circumcised women. "It is essential that midwives recognize the cultural complexities of FGM and show sensitivity when caring and supporting women with FGM during pregnancy, labour, and the postnatal period" (Momoh, 2004). Identification can start by asking questions such as the following: "Have you been closed?" "Did you have the cut or operation as a child?" Referrals to a specialist would facilitate discussion of legal issues and possible reversal of the procedure (infibulation). Procedures to reverse infibulation during labor might be performed. Other invasive procedures need to be avoided to eliminate possible sources of pain and stress.

Following delivery, before reinfibulation or restitching is done, the health care provider needs to consider the laws governing the practice of FGM. The mother and the baby, if female, are cared for with a view toward the future of the baby.

The information presented is but a very small representation of the continuing interests and work of people from diverse backgrounds. One powerful statement made by these scientists and caregivers is that whatever is done to eliminate FGM, "the cultural integrity of the people" (Little, 2003) must be preserved. Readers are strongly urged to read the cited references for a fuller understanding of FGM.

Sources Berg, R. C., Denison, E., Lewin, S., & Odgaard-Jensen, J. (2009). International initiative for impact evaluation: Interventions to reduce the prevalence of female genital mutilation/cutting in African countries. http://www.ieimpact.org/admin/pdfs_synthetic/011%20protocol.pdf; Gruenbaum, E. (2005). Socio-cultural dynamics of female genital cutting: Research, findings, gaps, and directions. *Culture Health Sexuality, 7*(5), 420–441; Leval, A., Widmar, C., Tishelman, C., & Ahlberg, B. M. (2004). The encounters that rupture the myth: Contradictions in midwives' descriptions and explanations of circumcised women's sexuality. *Health Care for Women International, 25,* 743–760; Little, C. M. (2003). Female genital circumcision: Medical and cultural considerations. *Journal of Cultural Diversity, 10*(1), 30–34; Momoh, C. (2004). Attitudes to female genital mutilation. *British Journal of Midwifery, 12*(10), 631–638; Obermeyer, C. M. (2005). The consequences of female circumcision for health and sexuality: An update on the evidence. *Culture Health Sexuality, 7*(5), 443–461; Webber, S., & Schonfeld, T. (2003). Cutting history, cutting culture: Female circumcision in the United States. *American Journal of Bioethics, 3*(2), 65–66.

incorporates themes regarding basic human nature, the relationship of human beings to nature, human beings' time orientation, valued personality type, and relationships between human beings.

Ethnic groups have their unique beliefs and attitudes about health and health care services (Box 2-2: Diversity Awareness). Incongruent beliefs and attitudes about health and health care services among ethnic groups versus the rest of the population, particularly health care providers, are major barriers in improving the health status of ethnic group members. Health care providers need to become responsive to the cultural values of different peoples and to realize how this cultural understanding could augment effective and humanistic care delivery. Knowledge and culturally competent practices are essential for nurses to function effectively in rapidly changing multicultural societies to provide quality and safe care to all.

## CULTURAL COMPETENCY

Culture may have an impact on people's health, healing, wellness belief systems, perceived causes of illness and disease, behaviors of seeking health care, and attitudes toward health care providers. Culture may also influence the delivery of health care services by the providers, who use their own limited set of values to view the world.

Every culture has diverse illustrative models of illness and belief systems regarding health and healing. These models and wellness belief systems include views about the pathophysiology of diseases, the cause and the onset of symptoms, the natural history of illnesses, and the appropriate treatments for various health issues.

Cultural competency is one of the major elements in eliminating health disparities; it starts with an honest desire to disregard personal biases and to treat every person with respect. Cultural competence is a broad concept used to describe interventions to improve quality and access to health care for minorities (Truong et al., 2014) and a dynamic process that requires lifelong learning (Moore et al., 2010). Although the number of racial and ethnic populations is growing in the United States, it has produced a challenge to the system of health care delivery services. Health care providers and persons seeking care bring their individual cultures and health beliefs and values to the health care experience. Hence understanding the cultural underpinning of care is a challenging task because of the complexity and interaction between the person seeking care and the health care provider's cultural beliefs (Salman et al., 2007). In addition, providing health care services that are respectful of and responsive to diverse individuals' health beliefs, practices, and cultural needs is believed to contribute to fewer negative health outcomes (Management Sciences for Health, n.d.; Office of Minority Health, 2016a).

It is very important for health care providers to be aware of how persons interpret their health issues or illnesses and to be capable of providing culturally competent care. Simply recognizing and accepting cultural diversity is insufficient to attain cultural competency in health care. Culturally competent health care professionals should be able to consistently and thoroughly recognize and understand the differences in their culture and the culture of others; to respect others' values, beliefs, and expectations; to understand the disease-specific epidemiology and treatment efficacy of different population groups; and to adjust the approach of delivering care to meet each person's needs and expectations (Management Sciences for Health, n.d.). Cultural competency is usually reflected in a health care provider's attitude and his or her communication style.

Douglas and colleagues (2014) discuss universally applicable guidelines for achieving culturally competent care. Their guidelines include knowledge of culture; education and training in culturally competent care; critical reflection; cross-cultural communication; culturally competent practice; cultural competence in health care systems and organizations; patient advocacy and empowerment; a multicultural workforce; cross-cultural leadership; and evidence-based practice and research. For each guideline they discuss strategies and provide implementation examples for caregivers and health care organizations' leaders/managers.

Truong and colleagues (2014) conducted a systematic review of reviews on the effectiveness of interventions to improve cultural competence in health care. Nineteen reviews were included that examined a variety of health care contexts (i.e., a variety of minority populations, diseases, health care settings and professionals, and interventions). In this systematic review, three main types of outcomes were reported: patient-related outcomes, provider-related outcomes, and health service access and utilization outcomes. Most of the reviews reported moderate-level evidence for improvements in provider-related outcomes and health service access and utilization outcomes. Some, but weaker, evidence was reported for patient-related outcomes. Unfortunately, many of the self-reported measures, such as patient- and provider-related outcomes, used tools that were not validated.

Recently researchers have established and tested the Cultural Competence Health Practitioner Assessment (CCHPA-67), which purports to determine levels of cultural and linguistic competence (Haywood et al., 2014). The 67-item questionnaire has three domains; —knowledge, adapting practice, and promoting health—and has sound clinometric properties, including reliability and validity. CCHPA-67 can be used to examine the effectiveness of interventions to increase cultural and linguistic competence of health care practitioners and the association between their level of competence and health care outcomes.

## FOLK HEALING AND NURSING CARE SYSTEMS

Within its cultural and/or ethnic customs and traditions, each group has a healing system that incorporates the beliefs and practices deemed essential in maintaining and restoring health. Three components of the healing systems of people were defined: self-care, nurse care systems, and folk healing systems (Andrews, 2016). Nurse care is characterized by specialized education; advanced knowledge, skills, and abilities; responsibility; and expectation of remuneration of services provided (Andrews, 2016). A folk healing system embodies the beliefs, values, and treatment approaches of a particular cultural group that are products of cultural development. Folk health practices are seen in a variety of settings, including community groups, kinship groups, private homes, and healers' shrines. Unlicensed practitioners such as lay midwives, bone setters, and herbalists are part of the folk sector, as are religious practitioners such as spiritualists, Christian Scientists, and scientologists.

The choice of a health care system differs among ethnic groups and among individuals within the same group. Ethnic individuals' preference for their folk healing systems is motivated by their familiarity with the folk healer, who usually speaks the same language and is knowledgeable about the beliefs, customs, and traditions of the ethnic group. Easy access and the individual's ability to pay for the healer's services are real advantages when compared with the difficulty of getting appointments, the long waits, and the unfamiliar institutional settings in the professional care system. Despite ongoing developments in treatments provided by professional care systems, many folk healing practices maintain their popularity today. When folk healing practices are not effective, the individual may, as a last resort, turn to the professional care system. Through a culturally sensitive assessment process, nurses can determine which specific folk remedies individuals are using and whether their continued use would interfere with the prescribed medical regimen. Andrews and

Boyle (2016) and Giger (2013) have developed transcultural assessment guides, such as the Andrews & Boyle Transcultural Nursing Assessment Guide, that nurses can use when working with ethnically diverse individuals. Nurses must avoid an ethnocentric perspective when working with ethnic groups. An ethnocentric perspective, which views other ways as inferior, unnatural, or even barbaric, can serve as a major obstacle in establishing and maintaining good working relationships with consumers of health care services.

Ethnic groups will continue to use folk remedies and healing. Therefore nurses need to appreciate the many positive aspects of folk systems. A caring, holistic approach that incorporates family and support systems and considers the individual's viewpoint is one of the more positive aspects of folk systems. This approach is receiving recognition by the professional care system. A blend of both systems would optimize health care for ethnic Americans.

## ARAB AMERICANS

Arab Americans came to the United States in three immigration waves. The first wave of immigrants, who came between the late 1800s and World War I, were mostly from Greater Syria. The second wave came after the close of World War II and included many Muslims and refugees displaced by the 1948 Palestine War. The last wave occurred in the 1960s and consisted of many professionals, entrepreneurs, and skilled and semiskilled laborers (Abraham, 2014; Stussy, 2000).

The 2000 US Census was a milestone survey because for the first time it recognized Arab Americans as a separate ethnic group. Anyone from the following countries was considered to be of Arab ancestry: Algeria, Bahrain, Egypt, United Arab Emirates, Iraq, Jordan, Kuwait, Lebanon, Libya, Morocco, Oman, Palestine, Qatar, Saudi Arabia, Syria, Tunisia, and Yemen. The number of Arab Americans grew from approximately 850,000 in 1990 to approximately 1.2 million in 2000.

From 2006 to 2010, the American Community Survey 5-year estimates indicated that approximately 1.5 million people (0.5% of the total population) living in the United States has Arab ancestry (Asi & Beaulieu, 2013). On the basis of the 2010 US Census, there are approximately 1.7 million Arab Americans.

The six largest groups (in rank order) of Arab Americans are the Lebanese, Egyptians, Syrians, Iraqi, Palestinians, and Moroccans (US Census Bureau, 2016) Arab Americans live in all 50 states, but one-third of them live in California, Michigan, and New York. About 94% of Arab Americans live in metropolitan areas. The top five metropolitan areas of Arab American concentration are Los Angeles, Detroit, New York City/New Jersey, Chicago, and Washington, DC. One of the largest groups of Arab Americans live in Dearborn, Michigan (Arab American Institute Foundation, 2011). Three major religions represented among Arab Americans are Christianity, Judaism, and Islam (Arab American Institute Foundation, 2011). More than 45% of Arab Americans have a bachelor's degree or higher, compared with 28% of Americans at large. About 18% of Arab Americans have a postgraduate degree, which is nearly twice the American average (10%). Other statistical data and information on Arab Americans

---

### BOX 2-3   GENOMICS

A recent review on obesity-linked diabetes in the Arab world discusses a growing of evidence to support a genetically based association between obesity and diabetes in Arab populations. In addition to diet, physical activity levels (including social cultural barriers for women), and decreased level of awareness regarding the complication of obesity, there are genetic implications. Several studies on Arab populations have reported variations in the ADIPOQ gene that may affect the risk of type 2 diabetes, the risk of insulin sensitivity in obese diabetic individuals, and correlate with body weight, waist circumference, body mass index, and percentage of total body fat.

From Abuyassin, B., & Laher, I. (2015). Obesity-linked diabetes in the Arab world: A review. *Eastern Mediterranean Health Journal, 21*(6): 420-439.

---

can be found at the website of the Arab American Institute (http://www.aaiusa.org/).

## Health Care Issues of Arab Americans

There is limited health-related information and a scarcity of scholarship about Arab Americans. Similar to other ethnicities, Arab Americans have chronic health problems such as diabetes and coronary artery disease. Several factors place Arab Americans at high risk of developing adult-onset diabetes and cardiovascular disease, including obesity, age, gender, and low employment rates (Box 2-3: Genomics). Tailakh and colleagues (2012) examined the prevalence, awareness, treatment, and control of hypertension among Arab Americans by using a cross-sectional design. The prevalence of hypertension was high, with 36.5% of the sample having hypertension and 39.7% being pre-hypertensive. Of those with hypertension, only 67.4% were aware of their condition and only 52.2% were taking antihypertensive medication. Other significant findings included a higher prevalence in males than in females and a higher body mass index (BMI) in those with hypertension compared with normotensive participants. The study concluded that hypertension is a major health problem among Arab Americans and that prevention and treatment strategies are urgently needed for this population.

Another health concern is mental health and the role of acculturation in Arab Americans. Aprahamian and colleagues (2011) looked at the concept of mental health and the degree of acculturation and the implications for mental health counselors of Arab American individuals. They reported that age at migration, length of stay in the United States, religion, and discrimination experiences were significant predictors of mental health. Mental health counselors need to be aware of and consider these factors when helping Arab American individuals. Many Arab Americans seek their immediate and extended family, community, and traditional values and cultural practices for help during a health crisis. Consequently, given the unique nature of mental illness, many Arab Americans do not receive professional mental health attention when needed.

A health issue on the rise among Arab American adolescents is tobacco consumption, which is considered to be a major risk factor for many health problems affecting the respiratory and cardiovascular systems. Tobacco can be consumed in many ways; however, tobacco chewing, cigarette smoking, and use of a shisha (water pipe) are the three major methods used to consume tobacco products. Arabs, both men and women, have long traditions of using a water pipe and smoking cigarettes with their friends and families and at other social gatherings. Weglicki and colleagues (2008) reported that the percentage of Arab American youth smoking cigarettes was lower than that of non–Arab American youth. However, water pipe smoking was seen more often in Arab American youth when compared with non–Arab American youth. Tobacco use has been linked to a higher rate of chronic health problems such as heart disease, hypertension, and diabetes among Arab Americans than among non–Middle Eastern whites (Jamil et al., 2008). Current water pipe use has been better predicted by Arab ethnicity and a lower educational level. In another study on water pipe use, researchers examined nicotine dependence and barriers to cessation in Arab Americans who self-identified themselves as smokers (El-Shahawy & Haddad, 2015). Participants were divided into two groups, those who smoked cigarettes exclusively and those who were dual smokers (i.e., smoked cigarettes and used a water pipe). Dual smokers smoked significantly more cigarettes per day and had significantly higher scores for nicotine dependence and barriers to cessation (including addiction and external barriers). The water pipe seems to increase the addictive properties of cigarettes and increase barriers to cessation in this population of Arab Americans.

Access to culturally suitable and current care is essential given that the Arab American population suffers from a wide spectrum of diseases. Many barriers exist that prevent Arab Americans from using professional care services. Discrimination of Muslims or "Islamophobia" since 9-11 has further contributed to physical and mental health disparities in the United States and the United Kingdom (Liard et al., 2007). Additional barriers include religious beliefs and practices, cultural norms relating to modesty, family values of upholding the family's reputation, gender issues such as preference for a same-sex health provider, use of folk remedies, and stresses of assimilation and acculturation such as lack of English skills (Figure 2-1). There are also barriers related to the health providers, including a lack of culturally competent services and the possession of attitudes such as stereotyping and discrimination (Williams et al., 2008).

## Selected Health-Related Cultural Aspects

Arabs value the family and the ties it maintains; therefore the extended family, a clan, and a tribe are common kinship groups. Customs center on hospitality around food, family, and friends (Andrews, 2016). Arab American families are, on average, larger than non–Arab American families and smaller than families in Arab countries. According to the American Community Survey (Asi & Beaulieu, 2013), the average size of an Arab American household was 2.93 people, compared with the national average of 2.59 people. Yemeni averaged more than four people per household, and Palestinian, Jordanian, and Iraqi averaged more than three people per household. Traditionally, more children meant more pride and economic contributors for the family. The cost of having large families in the United States, however, and adaptation to American customs seem to encourage smaller families. Religion plays an important part in Arab culture, and there are dietary rules and prescribed rituals for praying and

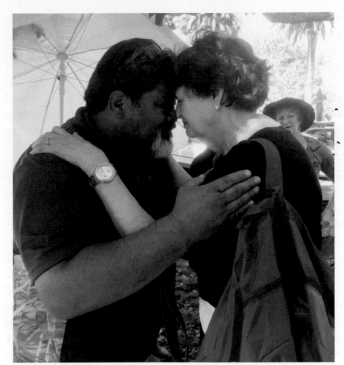

**FIGURE 2-1** One cultural norm of the Maori in New Zealand is to say goodbye by rubbing noses.

washing (Ehrmin, 2016). In addition, Arab Americans are present oriented and view the future as uncertain (Ehrmin, 2016).

## ASIAN AMERICANS/PACIFIC ISLANDERS

Asian Americans/Pacific Islanders (AAPIs) represent people from many different countries, so their origins, cultures, lifestyles, and religions are diverse, and they speak more than 100 languages and dialects (Africa & Carrasco, 2011). The six most common countries of origin are (in rank order) China, Philippines, India, Vietnam, Korea, and Japan. The number of AAPIs (alone or in combination) in the United States is about 17.3 million on the basis of 2010 US Census data, which represents an increase of 5.4 million since 2000 (Hoeffel et al., 2012).

Beginning in 1997, the Asian or Pacific Islander racial category was separated into two categories (one being Asian and the other being Native Hawaiian and other Pacific Islander) by the Office of Management and Budget directive (US Census Bureau, 2016.) "Asian" refers to a person having origins in any of the original peoples of the Far East, Southeast Asia, or the Indian subcontinent (Humes et al., 2011). According to the 2010 US Census, the estimated number of US residents of Asian descent corresponded to 5.6% of the total US population. Between the 2000 census and the 2010 census, Asian American and Pacific Islanders were the fastest growing (46% of growth) ethnic minority in the United States. In 2009 Chinese Americans were the largest Asian group, and following Spanish, Chinese was the most widely spoken non-English language in the United States. Most AAPIs live in metropolitan areas; California (5.6 million, or 14.9% of its population) is the state with the largest Asian population, followed by New York (1.6 million, or 8.2%) and Texas (1.1 million, or

4.4%) (Hoeffel et al., 2012). In Hawaii, 57% (or 781,000) of the total population are Asians. New Jersey also has a large concentration of AAPIs, where they represent 9.0% (or 795,000) of the total population.

AAPIs are often referred to as a "model minority"; this stereotype is frequently accepted because most AAPIs are viewed as being successful, resilient, hardworking, intelligent, and healthy. Education is highly valued in the AAPI communities. According to the reports from the US Census (Ryan & Bauman, 2016; US Census Bureau 2015a), Asian Americans have the highest percentage of college graduates of any racial or ethnic group. About 54% of Asian Americans have a bachelor's degree or higher level of education, compared with 32.5% of the total population in the United States. Approximately 17.2% of Asian Americans reported having no health insurance coverage in 2009. Native Hawaiians or Pacific Islanders refers to people having Hawaii, Guam, Samoa, or other Pacific Islands as origins (Humes et al., 2011). According to the 2010 US Census, Native Hawaiians and other Pacific Islanders formed the largest proportion of the total population in Hawaii. Among those who identified themselves as Native Hawaiian and other Pacific Islander, the poverty rate was 19%, and 20.7% of adults aged 25 years or older had a bachelor's degree or higher. Approximately 14.1% of Native Hawaiians and other Pacific Islanders were reported as being without health insurance (DeNavas-Walt, et al., 2013) A look at the status of AAPIs as a group reveals that they are doing relatively well in the United States. For instance, the median family income is higher than the national median income for all households. Their poverty level is lower than that of other ethnic groups (US Census Bureau, 2015a).

## Health Care Issues of Asian Americans/Pacific Islanders

Health care issues of AAPIs are relative to their ethnicity, religion, and status as immigrants. Some Asian American immigrants have carried diseases from their home countries, and they may now experience new diseases because of their new lifestyle and living conditions. However, AAPIs are more likely to be healthier than whites and other ethnic groups. Asian American women have the highest life expectancy (85.8 years) among all ethnic groups in the United States (Centers for Disease Control and Prevention, 2015). However, Asian Americans are challenged with various factors that threaten their health. Some negative causes are associated with infrequent medical visits as a result of language/cultural barriers, lack of health insurance, and fear of transportation (Centers for Disease Control and Prevention, 2015; Office of Minority Health, 2016b). Asians had the highest rate of health care–associated infections when compared with other races and ethnicities admitted to hospitals for cardiovascular disease, pneumonia, and major surgery (Bakullari et al., 2014). The researchers discuss how language barriers between patients and providers may serve as a possible explanation for their findings.

In general, AAPIs have health problems similar to those of the US population as a whole. Cancer, heart disease, stroke, unintentional injuries, and diabetes are the top five leading causes of death among AAPIs (US Department of Health and Human Services, 2010). A high BMI in Asian Americans was associated with an increased risk of total death at a rate similar to that for whites and black Americans in the United States (Park et al., 2014). Asian Americans also have a high prevalence of and risk factors for chronic obstructive pulmonary disease, hepatitis B, HIV/AIDS, smoking, tuberculosis, and liver disease (Office of Minority Health, 2016c). AAPI women were 30% less likely than non-Hispanic white women to have breast cancer (Office of Minority Health, 2016c). AAPI women are less likely to die of breast cancer, and death rates are lower compared with those for the other ethnic groups. However, AAPIs are three times more likely than non-Hispanic whites to have stomach cancer. Asian/Pacific Islander men are 40% less likely than white men to have prostate cancer, but they are twice as likely to have stomach cancer. In general, AAPIs have lower rates of being overweight and having hypertension and are less likely to be current cigarette users compared with white adults. By the end of 2009, AAPI cases accounted for approximately 1% of the total HIV/AIDS population in the United States (Centers for Disease Control and Prevention, 2014). Although the numbers of infected people are low compared with the numbers in the other groups in the United States, the increased rates of HIV/AIDS infections among AAPIs from 2006 through 2009 have raised concerns about this population (Centers for Disease Control and Prevention, 2014). Native Hawaiians/Pacific Islanders have a higher prevalence of substance abuse, depression, and delinquency when compared with Asian Americans (Wu & Blazer, 2015). Given the differences in substance abuse, mental health status, and other cultural, language, and socioeconomic characteristics, the researchers advise separating Native Hawaiians/Pacific Islanders and Asian Americans when topics that may inform health policy are being studied.

Disparities in the health status of AAPIs are primarily a result of subcultures within the larger group. There are many divergent and segregated cultures within AAPIs; however, all ethnic populations of AAPIs are currently often classified and viewed as an unvarying group. About two-thirds of AAPIs are foreign-born, whereas nearly 38% of Asian Americans do not speak English fluently (Ponce et al., 2009). The classification and cultural barriers (such as language) limit public awareness and restrain effective and culturally appropriate disease prevention for subgroups of the AAPI population. However, few studies have focused on AAPIs, and even fewer researchers have examined the subgroups, and this often creates a generalized and inaccurate picture of the experience and needs of AAPIs in the United States. The heterogeneity of subgroups among AAPIs and their relatively small representation in the US population make it challenging to have sufficient and representative samples from the AAPIs. Information about health status among the different subgroups of AAPIs is extremely limited; more studies are needed to fully understand their health issues.

## Selected Health-Related Cultural Aspects

AAPIs share many traditional values. A comprehensive description of traditional values in several Asian groups indicates commonalities and differences (Andrews & Boyle, 2016; D'Avanzo & Geissler, 2008).

The family is the most important social institution for AAPIs (Kavanaugh, 2008). The extended family has significant influence on Asian Americans. Although family dynamics and structure differ in the different AAPI subgroups, the family is often the major source of functional and psychological support for AAPIs. Usually, the interests and honor of the family are more important than those of individual family members. Older family members are usually respected and have authority that is often unquestioned. For instance, among Filipinos, calling older people by their first names is a sign of disrespect. Male friends of one's parents or grandparents are addressed as "tito" (uncle) followed by the first name. For female friends it is "tita" (aunt). These terms, denoting respect, have been substituted for Filipino terms that do not have English translations.

In the culture of Asian Americans, the oldest male family member is often the decision maker and spokesperson. Maintaining harmony is an important value in Asian cultures, and avoiding conflict and direct confrontation is strongly emphasized. Authorities and professionals are usually respected in the Asian American communities. Mostly, physicians and their recommendations are powerful and highly respected and valued. However, as a result of respect for authorities, AAPIs may avoid showing their disagreements with the recommendations of health care professionals. The health care providers need to recognize that lack of disagreement with recommended treatments or therapies does not mean that the Asian American patient and family agree with or will abide by the treatment recommendations.

The rates of psychological distress in AAPIs are similar to those in the general US population; however, AAPIs have a tendency to be the least likely to seek mental health services among all ethnicities. A variety of factors related to cultural values, such as stigma, cultural impact of shame, and language barriers, may contribute to their low utilization of mental health services (Africa & Carrasco, 2011). Asian cultures consider that the behavior of the individual reflects on the family; therefore mental illness or any behavior that indicates lack of self-control is viewed as producing shame and guilt in the family. Consequently, Asian Americans may be reluctant to discuss symptoms of mental illness or depression. Suicide was reported as the ninth leading cause of death among Asian Americans, compared with the tenth leading cause of death for white Americans; among all US women older than 65 years, Asian American women have the highest suicide rate (Office of Minority Health, 2016d).

In addition to reduced access to mental health care, the culture and values of AAPIs are associated with other health problems and risk factors that threaten health and act as barriers to accessing health care. For example, sexually related issues are taboo topics and considered a private matter that should not be discussed with anyone other than the spouse. Women may feel it is embarrassing to discuss sex, to visit physician clinics for sexually related health issues, or to receive some forms of physical examinations (e.g., Papanicolaou test). Such fears may have prohibited the willingness of AAPIs to access health care services and prevented health care providers from approaching this population for interventions. For example, the taboo topic of sexual issues was identified as one of the key barriers that makes it difficult for health care providers to approach Chinese American youths for HIV/AIDS prevention (Lee et al., 2012).

A different, but perhaps related, issue is barriers to health research participation by AAPIs (George et al., 2014). The most common barriers reported by AAPIs were mistrust, competing demands, unintended outcomes, lack of access to information, and stigma. Participants had concerns about signing the informed consent form (mistrust), which may have been related to language barriers and the lack of translated materials (lack of access to information).

Many people find the task of parenthood in a new country difficult because some of their cultural values conflict with the mainstream cultural values; for example, passivity to avoid conflict versus assertiveness. Exposure of children to different cultures in schools and in their neighborhood facilitates their adoption of other cultural beliefs and attitudes in their socialization. Additionally, the employment of immigrant women outside the home has exposed their children to other caretakers. Grandparents are often the caretakers of young grandchildren. Filipino American grandparents view their roles as part of their family responsibility (Kataoka-Yahiro et al., 2004).

Asian folk medicine and philosophies have a strong Chinese influence as a result of early Chinese migration throughout Asia. Therefore the folk medicines of Filipinos, Japanese, Koreans, and Southeast Asians are all imbued with Chinese principles. Taoism was the philosophical and theoretical foundation of Chinese medicine. The "Tao" is rooted in the idea of balancing natural processes and forces (such as yin and yang) and is closely related to Asians' activities of daily living, including traditional health practices such as acupuncture, holistic medicine, herbalism, meditation, and martial arts. According to Tao doctrine, humans are microcosms within the universe. Achieving harmony between the two is essential because the energies of both intertwine. Yin and yang are the two forces that keep innate energy, called chi, and sexual energy, called jing, in balance. Yin is feminine, negative, dark, and cold; yang is masculine, positive, light, and warm. An imbalance in energy can be caused, for instance, by yielding to strong emotions or eating an improper diet. In their interactions, humans and the universe are both susceptible to the elements of earth, fire, water, metal, and wood (Andrews, 2016; Ehrmin, 2016).

Asian folk medicine uses a wide variety of herbs for healing purposes, including roots, leaves, seeds, tree bark, and parts of flowers. Some aspects of Asian folk medicine have gained popularity within the professional care system. In general, the use or nonuse of healing traditions seems to be consistent with how closely Asians identify with their heritage (Tashiro, 2006). Of these, the best known is acupuncture (Andrews, 2016). Similar alternative treatment modalities that are slowly gaining wide acceptance include meditation, therapeutic touch, massage, imagery, relaxation, and bipolarity. Box 2-4: Research for Evidence-Based Practice discusses the use of complementary and alternative medicine (CAM) in the United States.

## LATINO/HISPANIC AMERICANS

The terms Hispanic and Latino are used interchangeably because the Office of Management and Budget demands federal agencies to use a "Hispanic or Latino" category to identify individuals

## BOX 2-4 RESEARCH FOR EVIDENCE-BASED PRACTICE

### Use of Complementary and Alternative Medicine in the United States

The National Center for Complementary and Alternative Medicine (2011) defines complementary and alternative medicine (CAM) as a set of varied medical and health care practices, systems, and products that are not usually considered part of conventional medicine. Medicine is practiced by holders of doctor of medicine or doctor of osteopathic medicine degrees and by their allied health professionals such as physical therapists, psychologists, and registered nurses. Conventional medicine is also called Western or allopathic medicine and is practiced by doctors of medicine and doctors of osteopathic medicine. Doctors of osteopathic medicine are fully licensed physicians. They provide a full range of services, from prescribing drugs to performing surgery, and use a "whole person" approach to health care. They focus special attention on the musculoskeletal system, a system of bones and muscles that makes up about two-thirds of the body's mass. They may use osteopathic manipulative treatment, a system of manual therapy, to treat mechanical strains affecting all aspects of the anatomy, relieve pain, and improve physiological function. Acupuncture, biofeedback, relaxation, music therapy, massage, art, music, and dance therapy are some examples of CAM. Western medicine, supported by improved knowledge and advances in technology, has been successful in addressing numerous illnesses. However, there remains a cadre of chronic illnesses and conditions that do not respond well to allopathic treatment. People who do not experience relief from chronic conditions often resort to CAM. However, the boundaries between CAM and conventional medicine are not fixed, and several CAM practices (e.g., acupuncture and music therapy) have been becoming more widely accepted.

A national survey found that about 38% of Americans use CAM, a group of diverse medical and health care systems, practices, and products that are not presently considered to be part of conventional medicine. Complementary medicine is used together with conventional medicine, and alternative medicine is used in place of conventional medicine (National Center for Complementary and Alternative Medicine, 2011). Another study used a comparative analysis of data from the 2002 and 2007 National Health Interview Survey of the civilian noninstitutionalized US population to investigate recent trends in CAM (Su & Li, 2011). The findings of this study suggest that CAM use has increased significantly in the United States. This increase was more obvious among non-Hispanic whites than among racial and ethnic minorities. The non-Hispanic white Americans had the highest prevalence rate of using at least one CAM therapy in the period from 2002 to 2007, followed by Asian Americans, black Americans, and Hispanics. This study also revealed that the use of CAM becomes more probable when there is limited access to conventional care. This study also pointed out that the increasing cost of conventional medical care has resulted in increasingly limited access to medical care and is a contributing factor to the rising prevalence of CAM use.

The dynamic interplay of many factors that serve as barriers for many ethnic groups to access traditional health care and the person's own cultural beliefs warrant a close look at how CAM can greatly augment health care services. This study revealed a growing prevalence of CAM use in the United States; however, the growth in CAM use was not equally distributed across racial and ethnic groups in the United States. The increasing prevalence and the increasing gap in CAM use across racial and ethnic groups highlight the critical need for assessing the health consequences of CAM therapies. There is limited information about the efficacy and the possible side effects associated with the use of any specific CAM therapy and its interactive effects with conventional medicine. More studies are needed to provide information about which CAM therapies can be used as an alternative or supplement to conventional medical care.

Sources National Center for Complementary and Alternative Medicine. (2011). What is complementary and alternative medicine? http://nccam.nih.gov/health/whatiscam#definingcam; Su, D., & Li, L. (2011). Trends in the use of complementary and alternative medicine in the United States: 2002-2007. *Journal of Health Care for the Poor and Underserved, 22*, 295–309.

from specific national origin. The Office of Management and Budget definition of Hispanic or Latino origin "refers to a person of Cuban, Mexican, Puerto Rican, South or Central American, or other Spanish culture or origin regardless of race." The largest Hispanic American subgroups are Mexicans, Puerto Ricans, and Cubans. Most Hispanics live in Texas, New York, Florida, and California (Office of Minority Health, 2016e). There are eight states in the United States with Hispanic populations greater than 1 million: Arizona, California, Colorado, Florida, Illinois, New Jersey, New York, and Texas.

Data from the 2010 US Census showed that the 50.5 million Latino/Hispanic people of the United States accounted for 16.3% of the total US population, making this population the nation's largest ethnic or racial minority (US Census Bureau, 2015b). There are 25 states in which Hispanics are the largest minority group. A 43% increase in the Hispanic population between 2000 and 2010 makes Hispanics the fastest-growing minority group in the United States after Asians (Humes et al., 2011). It was estimated that the Hispanic population of the United States will grow to 132.8 million or 30% of the nation's population, by 2050 (US Census Bureau, 2015b). The large size of the Hispanic population makes Mexico the only country that has a larger Hispanic population than the United States, and 64.3% of people of Hispanic descent in the United States were from Mexico (US Census Bureau, 2015b). About 76% of Hispanics aged 5 years

and older speak Spanish at home, and more than half of these Spanish speakers speak English "very well" (US Census Bureau, 2015b). The poverty rate among Hispanics increased from 23.2% in 2008 to 25.3% in 2009, and the percentage of Hispanics who lacked health insurance also increased from 30.7% in 2008 to 32.4% in 2009. Among the Hispanic population aged 25 years and older, 14% of them had a bachelor's degree or higher level of education in 2010.

## Health Issues of Latino/Hispanic Americans

Hispanic Americans' health is often associated with factors such as language/cultural barriers, lack of access to preventive care, and lack of health insurance. Latino/Hispanic Americans (LHAs) have many health issues complicated by multiple cultural, economic, political, and social factors. Hispanics are the highest uninsured racial or ethnic group in the United States (US Census Bureau, 2015b).

The leading causes of illness and death among Hispanics include heart disease, cancer, HIV/AIDS, stroke, and diabetes. Hispanic men and women have higher incidence and mortality rates for stomach cancer (US Department of Health and Human Services, Centers for Disease Control and Prevention, 2012a). Mexican American adults are almost twice as likely as non-Hispanic whites to have diabetes and 1.5 times as likely to die of this disease (US Department of Health and Human

Services, Centers for Disease Control and Prevention, 2012b). Although cardiovascular disease (US Department of Health and Human Services, 2011) and cancer are the first and second leading causes of morbidity and death among LHAs, their incidence in the general population is higher (US Department of Health and Human Services, Centers for Disease Control and Prevention, 2012a). Hispanic women were less likely to have had a mammogram within the past 2 years; however, they were slightly more likely to have had a Papanicolaou test during the past 3 years when compared with non-Hispanic white women (US Department of Health and Human Services, Centers for Disease Control and Prevention, 2012a). In addition, Hispanic adults aged 50 years and older were 34% less likely than non-Hispanic whites to report having undergone colonoscopy, sigmoidoscopy, or proctoscopy (Agency for Healthcare Research and Quality, 2015). Hispanic adults living in the United States generally have lower rates of prostate and breast cancer as compared with non-Hispanic White adults (US Department of Health and Human Services, Centers for Disease Control and Prevention, 2012a).

Some other health conditions and risk factors that significantly affect Hispanics include asthma, chronic obstructive pulmonary disease, HIV/AIDS, obesity, suicide, and liver disease. LHAs had the second-largest numbers of people with HIV/AIDS in 2014 (Centers for Disease Control and Prevention, 2014).

The difficulties experienced by LHAs in receiving appropriate health care services are comparable to those of the poor and other ethnic minorities. Other barriers include the lack of racial and ethnic diversity in the leadership and workforce of the health care system, lack of interpreter services for Spanish-speaking people, and lack of or inadequate culturally appropriate health care resources. Many Hispanic Americans may not readily seek care because they have continued reliance on their folk system of healing. Their preference for this is logical given their lack of health insurance and perceived difficulties negotiating the health care system because of language and other sociocultural barriers.

### Selected Health-Related Cultural Aspects

Each subgroup of the LHA population has distinct cultural beliefs and customs. However, a common heritage determines similar values and beliefs. For instance, the two most important aspects of all Hispanic cultures are the emphasis on the family and the emphasis on religion. For older Hispanic Americans, the family is an important component of good health. The family is the most important source of support; therefore the needs of the family as a whole supersede the needs of the individual. During times of illness and crisis, the family is there for the individual. Older family members and other relatives are accorded courtesy and respect and are often consulted on important matters (Andrews, 2016).

LHAs' dependence on spiritual strength to aid them in illness and dying is evident in their use of prayer. LHAs attribute the origins of disease and illness to spiritual or natural punishments, hot and cold imbalances, magic, dislocation of internal organs, natural diseases, and emotional and mental issues. The hot and cold concept of disease was derived from the Hippocratic theory of disease. Illness occurs when there is an imbalance. This concept of hot and cold guides Hispanics when they categorize illnesses and select appropriate treatments. For example, an elevated body temperature is managed by giving the person a cool drink to lower the temperature. For a person who has a cold, drinking warm fluids would be considered therapeutic (Chong, 2002).

LHAs attribute illness and disease to many supernatural and psychological causes. The evil eye, or the *mal de ojo*, is an example. Fright, or *susto*, and hysteria, or *ataque de nervios*, are caused by strong emotions, crises, and traumatic experiences (Chong, 2002). LHAs still resort to many home remedies and consult folk healers, including the curandero, spiritualist, *yerbero*, and *sabador*. Curanderos use a variety of folk remedies, including prayers, rituals, herbs, and the laying on of hands. Spiritualists use medals, amulets, and prayers to affect a cure. The *yerbero* is knowledgeable in the use of herbs, whereas the *sabador* is an expert in massage and manipulation of bones and muscles (Andrews, 2016). Other Hispanic Americans, such as Cubans, practice *Santeria*. People who are ill may seek the advice of a "godfather" who is a member of the *Santeria*. Wearing white clothes for a year, performing rituals, and following dietary restrictions are involved in bringing forth a cure to an illness (D'Avanzo & Geissler, 2008).

Folk remedies are used in combination with professional care approaches. The individual's belief in the folk remedy can have positive effects on the person's well-being. Therefore professional care personnel need to find ways to blend the two systems to the optimal benefit of LHAs and their families.

## BLACK/AFRICAN AMERICANS

"Black or African American" (BAA) refers to people having origins in any of the black racial groups of Africa (Humes et al., 2011) and the terms "Black" and "Black or African American" are used interchangeably by the US Census Bureau (2015). According to the 2010 US Census, the 43.1 million people of the BAA population made up 13.6% of the total US population (US Census Bureau, 2016). Black Americans are the second-largest minority population, following the Hispanic/Latino population (US Census Bureau, 2015).

As one of the largest ethnic groups in the United States, BAAs are considered a minority group, a label originating from their slavery roots. Most of the black Americans in the United States are descendants of enslaved people brought from Africa (Waters et al., 2014). Therefore they continue, in many ways, to experience extreme segregation and exclusion from mainstream society, and discrimination by the majority group.

In 2014, most of the black Americans in the United States lived in the Southern states, with the largest black American populations found in the following states: Georgia (33%), Maryland (32%), North Carolina (23%), Virginia (21%), New York (19%), Florida (18%), Illinois (16%), Pennsylvania (13%), Texas (13%), and California (8%) (US Census Bureau, 2014, estimate). BAAs that lived outside the South have a tendency to be more concentrated in metropolitan areas. The places with the largest black American populations were New York, Chicago, and Detroit, with Michigan being the state with the greatest proportion of BAAs (Rastogi et al., 2011).

BAAs have made substantial progress in many areas in the past century. However, there are still inequities in many areas, such as in business, education, political participation, and leadership. The reports of the 2010 US Census indicated that the rate of living at the poverty level for Black Americans was almost three times that for non-Hispanic whites (Office of Minority Health, 2016f). Educationally, BAAs have made substantial gains; 18% of BAAs who were 25 years or older had a bachelor's degree or a higher degree in 2010 (US Census Bureau, 2016b). The states with the highest BAA educational attainment (a bachelor's degree or higher) include Maryland, Colorado, Oregon, California, Massachusetts, Washington, New Jersey, Arizona, Georgia, and New York, all of which exceed 20%.

## Health Issues of Black/African Americans

A complex set of social, economic, and environmental factors can be identified as contributors to the current health status of BAAs. However, poverty may be the most profound and pervasive determinant of health status. Individuals and families who are below the poverty level or lack adequate resources have limited access to health care services such as prenatal and maternal care, childhood immunizations, dental checkups, well-child care, and a wide range of other health-promoting and preventive services. In 2014 the poverty rate in this population was reported as 26.2%, up from 24.7% in 2004; 11.8% of this population was reported as being without health insurance in 2014, down from 15.9% in 2013 (Smith & Medalia, 2015).

Two indices of the effects of poverty can be seen in the high rates of infant mortality and maternal mortality. Despite changes in living conditions, advances in infection control, and improved standards in neonatal care, BAAs still experience high infant and maternal mortality rates. Between 2005 and 2008 the infant mortality rate (number of deaths among infants aged <1 year per 1000 live births) for BAAs was 12.67, which is 2.4 times higher than that of non-Hispanic whites (Centers for Disease Control and Prevention, 2013). BAAs have the second-highest percentage of women who lack prenatal care in the first trimester of pregnancy (Office of Minority Health, 2016g). Black Americans have lower life expectancies than other races at age 65 years. In 2013, life expectancy for black American males (72.3 years) and females (78.4 years) was lower than that for white males (76.7 years) and females (81.4 years) (National Center for Health Statistics, 2015).

Black American children living below the poverty level also experience numerous health problems, including malnutrition, anemia, and lead poisoning. These problems and the lack of immunizations combine to inhibit normal growth and development and affect school performance. Poverty-stricken families usually live in depressed socioeconomic areas where housing conditions are unsafe and unhygienic. Unsafe buildings and other environmental structures cause accidents and injuries among young children. Young children have fallen to their deaths from windows that were unprotected by metal railings. Older people have suffered falls and other injuries from poorly lit stairways and hallways. Other hazards include uncollected garbage and abandoned buildings that are used as dumpsites or as meeting places for a variety of illegal activities.

Black Americans are affected disproportionately by the leading causes of death in the United States, including cancer, HIV/AIDS, obesity, diabetes, heart disease, and hypertension. The cancer and mortality rates for BAAs are higher than those for white Americans. In 2013 the age-adjusted mortality rate for black Americans was higher than that for whites for heart disease, cerebrovascular disease, malignant neoplasms, influenza and pneumonia, diabetes, HIV, and homicide (National Center for Health Statistics, 2015). Black American women are 40% more likely to die of breast cancer, and they are 2.1 times more likely to die of stomach cancer (Office of Minority Health, 2016h). Although black Americans are only 13% of the US population, they accounted for 47% of HIV/AIDS cases in 2012 (National Center for Health Statistics, 2015). Black American males have eight times the AIDS rate of white males. Black American females have 20 times the AIDS rate of white females (Office of Minority Health, 2016i).

Severe high blood pressure is more common for black Americans in both men and women. Black American adults are 40% more likely to have high blood pressure but 10% less likely to have blood pressure under control than their non-Hispanic white counterparts, and Black Americans are 30% more likely to die of heart disease compared with non-Hispanic white men (Office of Minority Health, 2016j). BAA adults are 60% more likely to have a stroke and males are 60% more likely to die of a stroke (Office of Minority Health, 2016k).

Other health issues including obesity and its contributing factors are also receiving attention. BAAs are twice as likely as non-Hispanic whites to receive a diagnosis of diabetes, and they are more likely to experience complications from diabetes (Office of Minority Health, 2016l). In addition, individual poverty level and living in a poor neighborhood increased the odds of having diabetes (Gaskin et al., 2014). Higher rate of diabetes may also be related to higher obesity rates among black Americans. BAAs had the greatest prevalence of obesity compared with other races in the United States (Flegal et al., 2012; US Department of Health and Human Services, 2009).

## Selected Health-Related Cultural Aspects

Differences in cultural beliefs, attitudes, and practices exist between rural and urban black Americans; however, they share some basic cultural beliefs. Black American culture is centered on the family and religion. The family, the strongest institution, provides strong extended kinship bonds with grandparents, aunts, uncles, and cousins. The family is considered the strongest source of support, especially in times of crisis and illness (Gary et al., 2003). Family members and relatives are consulted before BAAs seek care elsewhere.

Religion and religious behavior are an integral part of the BAA community. The church is a significant support system for many black Americans; it serves many purposes beyond worship and formation, including serving as a place to meet where members can pass on news, take care of business, and find strength of purpose; providing direct social welfare services; acting as a stabilizing force in the community; facilitating citizenship training and community social action; serving as a transmitter of cultural history; providing the means for coping and surviving in a hostile world (McGadney-Douglass, 2000); and counseling and community mental health (Avent et al., 2015; Hankerson et al., 2012; Young et al., 2003).

Africa Americans believe in the healing power of prayer (Vaughn et al., 2009). Black Americans were found to pray more for health reasons (Su & Li, 2011). The BAA church and spirituality play an important role in health issues. For instance, prostate education for older men is received more favorably when done within the parish nursing approach (Lambert et al., 2002), and religious involvement was found to have a positive effect on health behaviors (Holt et al., 2014).

BAAs define health as a feeling of well-being and the ability to fulfill role expectations. Diseases can be caused by natural or spiritual forces (Ehrmin, 2016); therefore BAAs' approach to health care is guided by these beliefs. Family members, such as grandmothers, and community members are often consulted for traditional home remedies. Traditionally, roots, herbs, potions, oils, powders, rituals, and ceremonies are still used in many Southern communities. The use of healers is also common, including the old lady, who is knowledgeable about folk remedies and child care; the spiritualist, who assists with financial, personal, spiritual, or physical problems; and the voodoo priest or priestess, who is knowledgeable about herbs, signs, and omens (Andrews, 2016).

As noted with the folk health practices of Asian and Hispanic Americans, BAAs' folk healing beliefs and practices can augment the professional care system. Black Americans often find comfort in the support that their religious leader or traditional healer can give them. Health care providers must find an appropriate place for these nontraditional modalities when caring for BAAs.

## AMERICAN INDIANS/ALASKA NATIVES

American Indian or Alaska Native (AIAN) refers to people who have origins in North America and South America (including Central America) and who maintain tribal affiliation or community attachment (Humes et al., 2011). Native Americans lived in America for thousands of years before the arrival of Europeans. AIANs are the original people of the land now occupied mainly by the Europeans. Evidence shows that AIANs have lived in North America for more than 75,000 years (Josephy, 1991). Native Americans came to be known as Indians, a label given by Columbus when he encountered the native peoples in the West Indies, which he mistook for the East Indies. This label was then extended to all the native peoples of North America and South America, from the Arctic to Tierra del Fuego. Before 1492 there were an estimated 5 million Native Americans. Columbus's discovery brought colonization and settlement by various European groups (Snipp, 2000). Thus the ancestral lands of the Native Americans were usurped, and the people were forced to labor on farms and in mines. Thousands died of disease and hard labor or were killed in attempts to escape from slavery. Other events, such as the removal of the Southeastern tribes in 1830, the Navajos' Long March to Fort Sumner in 1864, and the massacre at Wounded Knee in 1890, caused the Native American population to dwindle to 250,000 by 1890 (Fixico et al., 2001).

In 2010, 5.2 million people in the United States were identified as AIAN (a 26.7% increase since 2000), about 1.7% of the total US population (US Census Bureau, 2014). Between 2000 and 2010 the population of AIANs increased in all 50 states. Native Americans are concentrated in California, Oklahoma, Arizona,

Texas, New York, New Mexico, Washington, North Carolina, Florida, and Michigan (Norris et al., 2012). The states with the five highest percentage distributions of AIANs are California (13.9%), Oklahoma (9.2%), Arizona (6.8%), Texas (6.0%), and New York (4.2%). The cities with the highest number of AIANs in 2010, in rank order, were New York, Los Angeles, Phoenix, Oklahoma City, Anchorage, Tulsa, Albuquerque, Chicago, Houston, and San Antonio. The cities with the highest percentage of AIANs in 2010, in rank order, were Anchorage, Tula, Norma, Oklahoma City, Billings, Albuquerque, Green Bay, Tacoma, Tempe, and Tucson.

Of the total Native American population, 22% live on reservations or other trust lands and about 60% live in metropolitan areas (Office of Minority Health, 2016m). There are 565 federally recognized AIAN tribes and more than 100 state-recognized tribes (Office of Minority Health, 2016m). The Cherokees make up the largest tribe (Ogunwole, 2006).

The Native American percentages for higher education degrees are low in proportion to their total number. Among AIANs who are 25 years or older, 13% obtained a bachelor's degree or higher (US Census Bureau, 2014). Native Americans are making some progress in all levels of college education. However, low continuing educational attainment and low income levels combined with higher rates of poverty are socioeconomic issues that affect the health and the quality of life of this population. Native Americans experience the many negative situations that confront poor people both on the reservations and in the larger society.

### Health Care Issues of Native Americans

Many of the health problems of Native Americans can be linked directly to the social and economic conditions described here. These conditions predispose Native Americans to illnesses and health problems that afflict the poor. Some of these problems have been discussed for BAAs. Although Native Americans have responded well to prevention and treatment of infectious diseases, other health problems are closely linked with poverty and harmful lifestyle practices (Office of Minority Health, 2016m).

Cultural barriers, geographical isolation, inadequate sewage disposal, and low income are factors that prevent AIANs from receiving quality medical care. Some of the leading diseases and causes of death among AIANs are heart disease, cancer, unintentional injuries (accidents), diabetes, and stroke. A study examining trends in cancer mortality and incidence from 1999 to 2009 found less progress in cancer control for AIAN populations compared with white populations (White et al., 2014). American Indians/Alaska Natives also have a high prevalence of and risk factors for mental health and suicide, substance abuse, sudden infant death syndrome, teenage pregnancy, liver disease, and hepatitis (Office of Minority Health, 2016n). A study examining health behaviors and risk factors among AIANs from 2000 to 2010 found a higher prevalence of tobacco use, obesity, and no leisure-time physical activity (Cobb et al., 2014). In addition, AIANs had a lower prevalence of five or more servings per day of fruits and vegetables, cancer screening, and seat belt use.

AIANs have an infant death rate 1.5 times higher than the rate for non-Hispanic white Americans (Office of Minority Health, 2016o). Native American adults are 2.1 times more likely than white adults to have diabetes (Office of Minority Health, 2016p). Wong et al. (2014) found significantly higher infant, neonatal, and postneonatal death rates and average annual death rates for AIANs when compared with whites in almost all of the regions examined. Similar findings were also reported for pediatric death rates. They ranked the leading causes of infant, neonatal, post-neonatal, and pediatric deaths, most of which are potentially preventable. AIANs also have disproportionately high rates of death from unintentional injuries and suicide (Office of Minority Health, 2016m).

Many mental health problems also confront Native Americans. Difficult life situations and stresses of daily life contribute to an array of problems, including feelings of hopelessness, desperation, family dissolution, and substance abuse, specifically alcohol. The three most common lifetime diagnoses in the Native American population are alcohol dependence, posttraumatic stress disorder, and major depressive episode (Beals et al., 2005). Native American adults are twice as likely as white adults to have hepatic cancer and more likely to be obese. Their AIDS rates are 40% higher than those of non-Hispanic whites (Centers for Disease Control and Prevention, 2014).

The health problems of Native Americans are complicated by difficult access to health care. Poor health and limited health care options among urban AIAN populations have been well documented in many studies. Since 1972, the Indian Health Service (IHS), a government agency in the US Department of Health and Human Services, has stated a series of initiatives to fund health-related activities in off-reservation settings that make health care services accessible to urban AIANs. Federally recognized tribes are provided with health and educational assistance through the IHS (Office of Minority Health, 2016m). Approximately 1.9 million AIANs receive a health service delivery system operated by the IHS. About 36% of the IHS service area population resides in non-Indian areas, and 600,000 are served in urban clinics (Office of Minority Health, 2016m). Even though the IHS attempts to provide comprehensive, high-quality health care services to AIANs, the quality of care and access to health services need to be improved.

## Selected Health-Related Cultural Aspects

Native Americans are generally present oriented: they emphasize events that are occurring now rather than events that will happen later. They take one day at a time, and in times of illness they cope by hoping for improvements the next day (Ehrmin, 2016). Native Americans also value cooperation rather than competition. Sharing of resources, even among the poor, is an important component of this cultural value. Family and spiritual beliefs are important for Native Americans. Native Americans place great value on their families and relatives. Three or more generations form an extended kinship system, which is enlarged by the membership of nonrelatives, who are included through various religious ceremonies (Boyle, 2016).

Despite the great diversity in Native American groups in their beliefs and practices concerning health, illness, and healing, they share a common philosophical base. Native Americans believe that optimal health exists only when a person lives in a condition with balance and harmony in the inner and outer domains of life (Grandbois, 2005). The Earth is seen as a living entity that should be treated with respect; failure to do so harms the body. Instead of viewing illness as changes in a person's physiological state, Native Americans view it as an imbalance between the person and natural forces (Boyle, 2016; Grandbois, 2005). Native Americans believe that a person's sickness can be traced directly to that person having committed a violation against natural and spiritual laws; an individual can also inherit such a violation. The violation causes the person to have an imbalance that causes illnesses mentally, physically, emotionally, and spiritually.

Many AIANs proudly express spirituality, traditional medicinal practices, and cultural ceremonies in their lives. AIANs frequently seek traditional practitioners, who are medicine women or men known as shamans and are believed to have hypnotic powers, the gift of mind-reading, and expertise in concocting drugs, medicine, and poisons, and who carry out rituals and healing ceremonies that are believed to restore the sense of balance, harmony, and unity that the acute or traumatic event has caused (Grandbois, 2005).

# THE EMERGING RURAL AND URBAN POPULATIONS: HOMELESS PERSONS

## Homelessness: A Continuing Saga

Homelessness is a complex social and economic problem that continues to persist and grow. Many services and programs have been developed to address the issue, yet homelessness remains a significant problem. Homelessness could be defined as a lack of fixed, regular, and adequate nighttime residence resulting from extreme poverty and/or unsafe or unstable living environments (National Alliance to End Homelessness, 2012a; National Association for the Education of Homeless Children and Youth, 2016; National Coalition for the Homeless, 2009). In many studies, homeless people were counted as individuals who are in shelters or on the streets (National Coalition for the Homeless, 2009). However, homelessness is considered a temporary situation, not a permanent condition. Instead of the number of "homeless people," it has been suggested that the number of "people who experience homelessness over time" is a more appropriate measure of the magnitude of homelessness (National Coalition for the Homeless, 2009). Fortunately, homelessness declined by 9% and long-term homelessness declined by 7% from 2007 to 2013 (Henry et al., 2013).

It was estimated that about 3.5 million people (1.35 million of them children) are likely to experience homelessness in a given year (National Coalition for the Homeless, 2009). On a given night in January of 2013, 610,042 people were homeless, of which 23% were children younger than 18 years, 10% were aged 18 to 24 years, and 67% were 25 years or older (Henry et al., 2013). It was estimated that 42% of the homeless population are Black American, 39% are white, 13% are Hispanic, 4% are Native American, and 2% are Asian (National Coalition for the Homeless, 2009). The following five states account for more than half of the homeless population: California (22%), New York (13%), Florida (8%), Texas (5%), and Massachusetts (3%) (Henry et al., 2013). Between 2007 and 2013, New York, Massachusetts, Missouri, District of Columbia, and Ohio had the

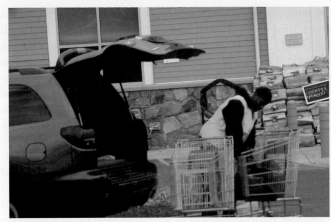

**FIGURE 2-2** A homeless man works at a day labor job to earn some money.

largest increases in the number of homeless people (Henry et al., 2013). During the same time period, California, Michigan, Texas, Washington, and New Jersey had the largest decreases in the number of homeless people.

## Why Families and People Become Homeless

Both structural and personal factors alone or in combination lead to lack of resources to secure and/or maintain housing. An increasing shortage of affordable rental housing and a simultaneous raise in poverty are two trends largely responsible for the growth of homelessness in the past 20 to 25 years (National Coalition for the Homeless, 2009a). Between 2005 and 2007, the number of repeated homeless individuals in the United States declined by 28% because of an increase in permanent supportive housing in the country. Recently, foreclosure has been a factor closely related to the increased number of people who experience homelessness in the United States (National Coalition for the Homeless, 2009b). Factors such as poverty, eroding work opportunities, a decline in public assistance, and lack of affordable housing are also significantly contributing to homelessness (National Coalition for the Homeless, 2009b) (Figure 2-2). Within the context of poverty and the lack of affordable housing, other additional major factors, such as lack of affordable health care, domestic violence, mental illness, and addiction disorders, can also contribute to homelessness (National Coalition for the Homeless, 2009b). In a study by Thompson et al. (2013), poverty, alcohol-use disorder (only), drug-use disorder (only), and both alcohol-use disorder and drug-use disorder were all significant predictors of first-time homelessness. In a systematic review of risk factors for homelessness among US veterans, substance abuse and mental illness were the two strongest and most consistent risk factors, followed by income-related factors (Tsai & Rosenheck, 2015).

## Health Issues of Homeless People and Families

Poor health is both an effect and a cause of homelessness. Homelessness and health care are closely interlinked. A serious health problem could force a person who does not have adequate health insurance to choose between paying bills for health care or paying rent for a place to live. The National Health Care for

the Homeless Council (NHCHC) reported that half of all personal bankruptcies in the United States are caused by health problems (National Coalition for the Homeless, 2009c).

Homelessness is associated with various behavioral, social, and environmental risks that expose individuals to many diseases. People experiencing homelessness usually have complex health problems. The lives of homeless persons and families are constant battles for daily survival. Homeless persons experience exposure to extremes in temperatures, unsanitary living conditions, crowded shelters, poor nutrition, and unsafe situations, wherever they live. They experience the same situations relative to health care; poor access because of lack of health insurance and inadequate resources to travel to health facilities.

As a result of poor living conditions and limited access to health care, homeless people are at a higher risk of being exposed to disease, violence, unsanitary conditions, malnutrition, stress, and addictive substances. The rates of serious illnesses and injuries among homeless people are three to six times the rates seen among the rest of the population (NHCHC, 2016a). This complex mixture of severe physical and/or psychiatric illness, substance abuse, and social problems is frequently found in homeless people (NHCHC, 2016b). Many diseases, including heart disease, cancer, liver disease, kidney disease, skin infections, HIV/AIDS, pneumonia, and tuberculosis, are common among the homeless population (National Coalition for the Homeless, 2009c). Compared with housed respondents, homeless patients were significantly more likely to be substance abusers (e.g., current smoker, binge drinking, high risk of alcohol and drug dependence, and any injection drug use), have a worse health status, experience food insufficiency, have chronic conditions (e.g., obstructive lung disease, liver and kidney conditions), experience two or more chronic conditions, and have mental health issues (e.g., psychological distress, depression, anxiety, panic disorder) (Lebrun-Harris et al., 2013). In addition, homeless patients surveyed were twice as likely to have unmet medical care needs and twice as likely to have visited the emergency department in the past year compared with housed respondents.

HIV/AIDS and homelessness are intricately associated. The homeless population has a higher prevalence of HIV/AIDS infections than the general population in the United States. It was estimated that 3.4% of homeless people were HIV positive in 2006, compared with 0.4% of adults and youths in the general population (National Coalition for the Homeless, 2009d). The conditions of homelessness may increase an individual's risk of becoming infected with HIV. Having substance abuse disorders and sharing or reusing needles to intravenously inject drugs greatly increases homeless peoples' risks of being infected with HIV. The homeless environment (such as limited privacy and communal sleeping and bathing at shelters) is not conducive to stable sexual relationships and makes it more likely for the homeless person to engage in risky sexual behaviors, therefore increasing the likelihood of contracting HIV (National Coalition for the Homeless, 2009d). Psychosocial distresses are not only associated with many mental health problems in homeless people but also influence behaviors that could affect the progression of HIV/AIDS (National Coalition for the Homeless, 2009d). Limited access to medical care severely prevents homeless people from receiving adequate HIV/AIDS treatment as well as education concerning HIV/AIDS prevention and risk reduction (National Coalition for the Homeless, 2009d). The homeless condition may also make adherence to HIV treatment regimens challenging for homeless patients and their caregivers (National Coalition for the Homeless, 2009d). In a study of HIV-infected drug users, homelessness and frequent heroin use were negatively associated with antiretroviral therapy adherence (Palepu et al., 2011). In addition, methadone maintenance was positively associated with antiretroviral therapy adherences, which speaks of the importance of improving housing status and methadone maintenance to increase adherence and thus survival in this population. To provide comprehensive services such as health education, HIV testing, case management, and mental health services, basic health care is needed for homeless people with HIV/AIDS.

Stress, depression, and other mental health problems are also common in homeless people. People who are homeless experience extreme stress on a daily basis. Multiple stresses of living in shelters and on the streets, physical problems, lack of resources, psychosocial issues such as shame and stigma, and feelings of hopelessness and despair often tax the homeless person's ability to cope. The homeless are also more likely to have gambling disorders (Shaffer et al., 2002). About half of people experiencing homelessness have mental health issues. Although only 6% of the general American population are severely mentally ill, about 25% of homeless people in the United States have serious mental illness, including chronic depression, bipolar disorder, and schizophrenia (National Alliance to End Homelessness, 2012b; National Coalition for the Homeless, 2009e). Homeless people are also more likely to have cognitive impairment (Depp et al., 2015), which further complicates their mental health.

The prevalence of substance abuse among homeless people is much higher than that among the general population (National Coalition for the Homeless, 2009f). It is estimated that more than half of all people experiencing homelessness have substance abuse disorders (United States Interagency Council on Homelessness, 2016). Substance abuse is both a leading cause and a consequence of the continuance of homelessness among individuals. Substance abuse was reported as the single major cause of homelessness for single adults and as one of the top three causes of homelessness for families, and more than half of homeless people reported that drugs and/or alcohol was a major cause of their homelessness (National Coalition for the Homeless, 2009f). Substance abuse also often arises after individuals become homeless. Homeless people abuse substances in an attempt to obtain temporary relief from their problems and eventually rely on drugs and alcohol to cope with their daily struggles; however, the substance dependence only worsens their problems and makes it more difficult for them to escape their homeless status (National Coalition for the Homeless, 2009f). Substance abuse and drug abuse often co-occur with mental health problems among homeless people (Polcin, 2015). It is estimated that almost half of all persons experiencing homelessness have substance abuse disorders, and most of the homeless individuals with substance abuse disorders also have moderate to severe mental illness (United States Interagency Council on Homelessness, 2016). A survey

of homeless youth found that 22% reported current prescription drug misuse and 13% were currently injecting drugs (Al-Tayyib et al., 2014). Furthermore, those that reported prescription drug misuse in the prior 30 days were significantly more likely to also have injected drugs during that same period.

Most homeless people do not have health insurance or the ability to pay for needed health care, and many providers refuse to treat homeless people (NHCHC, 2016a). Even though federally funded health care services provide primary care for homeless people, the homeless individuals who are able to benefit from these services are far fewer than those who desperately need care (NHCHC, 2016b). Several barriers that prevent access to health care have been recognized. These barriers include lack of knowledge regarding where to receive treatment, lack of access to transportation, and lack of identification (National Coalition for the Homeless, 2009c). Widespread access to affordable, high-quality, and comprehensive health care is necessary to stop homelessness (National Coalition for the Homeless, 2009c). On March 23, 2010, President Obama signed the Affordable Care Act into law, establishing new directives to improve access to affordable health coverage for all Americans and to protect Americans from obnoxious practices of insurance companies (USDHHS, 2016). The law gives all Americans access to care by their choosing affordable health insurance that fits their needs; this law also attempts to control health care costs without jeopardizing the quality of care (US Department of Health and Human Services, Center for Disease Control and Prevention, 2012).

## Strategies to Address Homelessness

Homelessness has long been recognized as a multidimensional problem of modern-day society. The homeless situation is a problem not only of individuals but also of families, communities, and societies. This problem needs to be addressed as a dynamic and not a static phenomenon, because as societies continue to change and evolve, there will always be those who are excluded and suffer consequences. These are the risks that must be actively anticipated so that strategic planning can forestall any devastating and long-lasting effects.

Many initiatives to address the issues of homeless people are being implemented by the NHCHC, which works with people who have experienced homelessness, health care and service providers, and policymakers; provides advocacy, research, and training; and collaborates clinical resources to break the connection between poor health and homelessness (NHCHC, 2016b). For more information about services and projects initiated by the NHCHC or its partners, visit http://www.nhchc.org.

Resolving health problems and resolving homelessness are dependently interrelated. Many health problems are highly prevalent in people experiencing homelessness. Health conditions such as diabetes, HIV/AIDS, addiction, and mental illness require ongoing treatment. If people do not have a stable place to stay, treating their health conditions and their finding time for healing and recovery from health problems are almost impossible. Preventive care can also be difficult for homeless people to access because it is often unaffordable (National Alliance to End Homelessness, 2012a). To end homelessness, mental and physical health conditions should be considered when effective, efficient strategies are being designed, and permanent stable housing together with supportive services is needed (National Alliance to End Homelessness, 2012b; NHCHC, 2016a). Fitzpatrick-Lewis et al. (2011) summarize recommendations for interventions for the homeless with concurrent mental illness and who are substance abuser and for the homeless with HIV. The Health Care for the Homeless Clinicians' Network has created clinical practice guidelines for the care of homeless patients. The recommended guidelines are available at http://www.nhchc.org/wp-content/uploads/2011/09/General-Recommendations-for-Homeless-Patients.pdf.

Research and practice have shown that permanent supportive housing works because housing is an essential part of treatment (National Coalition for the Homeless, 2009b). In addition to providing permanent supportive housing, strategies to assist homeless persons also include helping them gain access to the health care system and benefits, working with the community to obtain services and resources, educating homeless persons about their health, and educating health care personnel about homeless persons. Communities need to continue their in-kind work with homeless persons. Many schools and houses of religious worship have worked with local governments in extending support to the homeless. Food, clothing, night shelter, and short-term socializing have been provided. Parishioners may donate their time preparing meals, preparing the shelter, and serving as chaperones during the night. Much work is still needed to reduce homelessness. The needs of the recently identified rural homeless must be addressed. Every citizen should be educated so each person can serve as an advocate, and neighborhood coalitions should be established to prevent an increase in the number of homeless persons and to support the return of the homeless person as a dignified, contributing member of society. Health care providers must continue to seek effective ways to coordinate their efforts through the creation of comprehensive resource materials. Technology must be used at its maximal capability to facilitate assessment and monitoring. Preparation for health care for the homeless in both rural and urban settings should be strengthened as an essential part of the curriculums of the health care disciplines. Finally, more research regarding health care outcomes should be supported and data should be disseminated in a timely manner.

There is a greater degree of optimism today in dealing with the problems of homelessness. Individuals and communities are showing concern through increased involvement. Homelessness is everyone's problem, and people can ultimately effect the establishment of priorities to facilitate an improved quality of life. Increasing awareness and knowledge of the current status of homeless people will aid in understanding the problem and its ramifications. This understanding will serve as an excellent guide in providing input, taking necessary action, and making the final decision regarding the changes needed to make a healthy nation.

Health care professionals play a significant role in helping homeless persons. It is important for them to be capable of meeting the complex health needs of homeless people. Creative care planning is necessary for the homeless patient because standards of care may not be suitable for an individual who experiences homelessness and does not have a home where the basic requirements for self-care and recovery are available (Billings & Kowalski, 2008). Community health practitioners are also at the forefront of advocacy for the homeless as they work to effect changes and develop strategies to deal with the problems associated with the health status of homeless people.

## THE NATION'S RESPONSE TO THE HEALTH CHALLENGE

The National Institutes of Health has proclaimed health disparities as a major concern. It is putting significant effort into addressing and reducing health disparities involving cancer, diabetes, infant mortality, AIDS, cardiovascular illnesses, and many other diseases (Office of Minority Health, 2016a). In 2010 the US Congress stressed its commitment to health equity by elevating the National Center on Minority Health and Health Disparities to the National Institute on Minority Health and Health Disparities. In 2011 the US Department of Health and Human Services released two plans (The National Stakeholder Strategy for Achieving Health Equity and the HHS Action Plan to Reduce Racial and Ethnic Health Disparities) to reduce health disparities (Hansen, 2011). For more information regarding the two plans and the National Conference of State Legislatures, visit http://www.ncsl.org/.

### Healthy People 2020

*Healthy People 2020* outlines a comprehensive, nationwide health-promotion and disease-prevention agenda. This initiative is designed to serve as a road map for addressing and improving the health of all people in the United States. In the past 2 decades, one of Healthy People's primary goals has concentrated on disparities. In *Healthy People 2010,* the primary focus was not just as in *Healthy People 2000* to reduce health disparities among Americans, but also to eliminate health disparities. In *Healthy People 2020,* the goal has been expanded further: to achieve health equity, eliminate disparities, and improve the health of all groups (US Department of Health and Human Services, 2010). For more information about topics and objectives in *Healthy People 2020,* visit http://www.healthypeople.gov/.

### Office of Minority Health

The Office of Minority Health was created in 1986, and it was reauthorized by the Patient Protection and Affordable Care Act of 2010 (Office of Minority Health, 2016a). The Office of Minority Health has been working for more than 20 years to improve and protect the health of racial and ethnic minority populations through the development of health policies and programs that concentrate on eliminating health disparities. The Office of Minority Health is leading the charge to put into practice the HHS Action Plan to Reduce Racial and Ethnic Health Disparities at all levels of the Department of Health and Human Services and in the communities with whom it works.

In recent years, the Office of Minority Health started two initiatives (the National Partnership for Action to End Health Disparities and the Strategic Framework for Improving Racial and Ethnic Minority Health and Eliminating Racial and Ethnic Health Disparities) to guide its efforts toward eliminating health disparities in the United States. Both initiatives implemented a coordinated, systems-level approach that focused on eliminating health disparities and was contingent on science and knowledge to notify and continually improve policies and programs. The goals of the National Partnership for Action to End Health Disparities are to enhance awareness of the importance of health disparities and actions needed to improve health outcomes for racial and ethnic minority populations, strengthen and expand leadership for dealing with health disparities at all levels, improve health and health care outcomes for racial and ethnic minorities and underserved populations and communities, improve cultural and linguistic competency in delivering health services, and improve coordination and utilization of research and evaluation outcomes. The main purpose of the Strategic Framework for Improving Racial and Ethnic Minority Health and Eliminating Racial and Ethnic Health Disparities is to direct, organize, and coordinate the systematic planning, implementation, and evaluation of efforts that are targeted at improving racial and ethnic minority health and addressing racial and ethnic health disparities. For more information about trends in US public awareness of racial and ethnic health disparities, visit http://minorityhealth.hhs.gov/assets/pdf/checked/1/2010StudyBrief.pdf. Another initiative established by the Centers for Disease Control and Prevention is the Racial and Ethnic Approaches to Community Health, established in 2010. Its objective is to "eliminate disparities in health access and outcomes. These six health areas were selected for emphasis because they reflect areas of disparity that are known to affect multiple racial and ethnic minority groups at all life stages" (Office of Minority Health, 2016a). These areas include infant mortality; deficits in breast and cervical health promotion and disease prevention; and child and adult immunizations.

There are also minority health research initiatives sponsored by the National Institutes of Health, Centers for Disease Control and Prevention, and the Agency for Healthcare Research and Quality. Support for these initiatives and future ones must continue at all levels.

## NURSING'S RESPONSE TO EMERGING POPULATIONS AND HEALTH

The *Code of Ethics for Nurses* of the American Nurses Association (ANA) explicitly states the profession's commitment to provide service to people regardless of background or situation (ANA, 2016). Nurses have responsibilities to be aware of specific health needs and respond to illness in all populations. The ANA's Council on Cultural Diversity supports the work of nurses in their development of culturally competent care. The organization and its leadership, through the Ethnic-Minority Fellowship Program, have played an essential role in supporting the work and efforts of AAPIs, BAAs, LHAs, and Native Americans with graduate and doctoral work. Nurses continue to make many positive moves toward understanding culturally diverse populations. See the case study and care plan regarding Mr. and Mrs. Arahan, an older adult immigrant couple, at the end of this chapter, which propose nursing interventions to ensure their quality of life in

their later years. Nurses' awareness and understanding of transcultural issues have been facilitated by the works of leaders such as Leininger, Giger, Davidhizar, Andrews, and Boyle, to name just a few. In addition, wide dissemination of research findings has been made possible through the *Journal of Transcultural Nursing* and through annual conferences and other sponsored workshops. Additionally, nurses with advanced preparation have committed their time and energy to developing approaches and models for **transcultural nursing.**

Several nursing journals focus on cultural diversity, such as the *Journal of Cultural Diversity* and the *Journal of Multicultural Nursing and Health.* These journals and a variety of other publications are constantly increasing professionals' knowledge of health-related cultural issues. In addition, the *Minority Nurse Newsletter* provides excellent summaries of research studies, legislative updates affecting ethnic minorities, and relevant topics in education and practice. Ethnic nursing organizations are having an effect on greater cultural understanding through their dissemination of important works by clinicians, educators, and researchers (Box 2-5: Innovative Practice).

Major organizations such as the ANA, the National League for Nursing (Winland-Brown et al., 2015) publish culturally relevant materials to guide students, clinicians, and educators. Accrediting bodies for nursing education such as the Commission for Nursing Education Accreditation and the Commission on Collegiate Nursing Education support diversity with the inclusion of standards for maximizing diversity in the academic preparation of students pursuing bachelor's and master's degrees. Additionally, there is a cadre of nurses whose research on the cultural practices and beliefs of individuals and families gives professionals a sound base for improving practice and designing cost-effective and humanistic health care strategies. The quest to deliver culturally competent care has provided the impetus for nursing faculty to require transcultural courses in the nursing curriculum to facilitate awareness and understanding of cultural diversity. Transcultural nursing is an area of nursing study and practice that focuses on discovering and explaining cultural factors that influence the health, well-being, illness, or death of individuals or groups and seeks to provide culturally based appropriate care to people of diverse cultures (Leininger, 2001). Culture care diversity and universality theory (Leininger, 2002), developed by Madeleine Leininger, is a well-recognized theory used globally by many nurses, and it has significantly contributed to the establishment and advancement of transcultural nursing research knowledge and practice. It is essential for nurses to plan culturally tailored and competent care to mitigate health disparities and provide effective care in our rapidly changing multicultural societies, thereby delivering quality and safe care to all (Box 2-6: Quality and Safety Scenario).

Additionally, major textbooks focusing on specific clinical areas of practice devote material to health care issues of ethnic minorities. Other resources include a chapter or two on cultural diversity. In addition, discussion of specific health care problems and nursing care always includes cultural aspects. In the clinical setting, health care workers, through staff development and in-service programs, are provided with opportunities to learn and develop culturally sensitive care approaches.

## ✳ BOX 2-5   INNOVATIVE PRACTICE

### Spiritual Practices and Health

Spirituality and its relationship with health outcomes have been the focus of considerable interest in recent years (Como, 2007). Spirituality can be defined as an individual's sense of peace, purpose, and connection to others as well as the person's beliefs about the meaning of life. Many people believe that spirituality plays an important role in their lives (Gillum & Griffith, 2010; National Cancer Institute, 2012).

A growing amount of evidence reveals that spirituality and spiritual care play an important role in health and health care (Ehrlich, 2011). Considerable evidence has shown spiritual practices as an important and effective coping strategy and a common approach to dealing with health problems, particularly chronic diseases such as cardiovascular disease and cancer (Como, 2007; Medical University of South Carolina, 2012; National Cancer Institute, 2012). Spiritual practices are likely to improve coping skills and social support, promote feelings of optimism and hope, encourage healthy behavior, decrease feelings of depression and anxiety, and support a sense of relaxation (National Cancer Institute, 2012). Many studies have found that spiritual or religious beliefs and practices help patients with cancer as well as their caregivers to cope with the disease (National Cancer Institute, 2012). Studies also suggest that many patients would like health care providers to consider spirituality as a factor in their health care. It was reported that 94% of people admitted to the hospital agree that spiritual health is as important as physical health, and some studies show that health care providers' support of spiritual well-being helps improve patients' quality of life (National Cancer Institute, 2012).

A spiritual assessment may help health care providers understand how religious or spiritual beliefs will affect the way a patient copes with diseases and health problems. Few tools for assessing spiritual history and/or spiritual practices have been developed to help health care professionals consider patients' spiritual needs and/or plan appropriate spiritual interventions for their patients. A spiritual practices checklist (Quinn-Griffin et al., 2008) was developed to identify the religious or spiritual interventions used and the frequency of use of religious or spiritual interventions. The 12 items of the checklist include the most commonly used spiritual practices (e.g., prayer) and CAM interventions (e.g., meditation, yoga). Other examples of tools are the FAITH, the HOPE, and the FICA tools that help physicians assess patients' history of spirituality (Medical University of South Carolina, 2012). More information about the HOPE tool can be found at http://www.aafp.org/afp/2001/0101/p81.html?printable=afp.

It has been suggested by The Joint Commission that a spiritual assessment should be performed on every patient to identify patient's values, beliefs, and spiritual practices (Wesa & Culliton, 2004). Each person may have different spiritual needs, depending on cultural and religious traditions. For example, black Americans and Hispanic Americans were found to be more likely than European Americans to report prayer for health reasons (Gillum & Griffith, 2010). To better counsel and care for patients, health care providers should be aware of the common ethnic patients who may have more and special spiritual and religious needs and the common spiritual practices used by patients.

Sources Como, J. M. (2007). Spiritual practice: A literature review related to spiritual health and health outcomes. *Holistic Nursing Practice,* *21*(5), 224–236; Ehrlich, S. D. (2011). Spirituality. http://www.umm.edu/altmed/articles/spirituality-000360.htm; Gillum, F., & Griffith, D. M. (2010). Prayer and spiritual practices for health reasons among American adults: The role of race and ethnicity. *Journal of Religion and Health, 49*(3), 283–295; Medical University of South Carolina. (2012). Spirituality and cultural diversity. http://academicdepartments.musc.edu/family_medicine/Spirituality_and_Health/spiritualityculturaldiversity.htm; National Cancer Institute. (2012). Spirituality in cancer care (PDQ). http://www.cancer.gov/cancertopics/pdq/supportivecare/spirituality/HealthProfessional; Quinn-Griffin, M., Salman, A., Lee, Y., & Fitzpatrick, J. J. (2008). A beginning look at the spiritual practices of older adults. *Journal of Christian Nursing, 25*(2), 100–102; Wesa, K. M., & Culliton, P. (2004). Recommendations and guidelines regarding the preferred research protocol for investigating the impact of an optimal healing environment on patients with substance abuse. *Journal of Alternative and Complementary Medicine, 10*(1), 193–199.

## ✅ BOX 2-6   QUALITY AND SAFETY SCENARIO

### Immigrants and Health Care Providers

Mr. Jade and Madam Nora have four children: Nirman (6 months), Julia (18 months), Hady (4 years), and Jamella (6 years). Mr. Jade is an economist who immigrated to the United States from Iraq 4 years ago. The family has come to the well-baby clinic because Madam Nora has been concerned about Nirman; Nirman's skin appears paler than that of her siblings, and she is also not gaining weight. Mr. Jade gave a brief health history of Nirman's situation because his wife cannot express herself in English. "My wife believes that Nirman is not growing like the rest of our children. She breastfeeds her every 2 hours, but she is not eating." My wife is "upset that Nirman is not becoming bigger." The vital signs are as follows: pulse, 125 beats per minute; respirations, 22 breaths per minute; blood pressure, 100/70 mmHg; and rectal temperature, 99.4° F. Nirman's weight is 10 lb, 0 oz, and her length is 22 inches. Nirman appears pale. Madam Nora, aged 28 years, is wearing a headscarf covering her hair and a long dress. When Mr. Jade and Madam Nora are left alone, nurses can hear them arguing and raising their voices in a foreign language (Arabic), and Madam Nora appeared very upset. The medical history revealed a term baby female born by normal vaginal delivery with a normal birth weight. No history of vomiting, diarrhea, or

fever was reported. Pallor and jaundice were noted on physical examination. The family history revealed that both Mr. Jade and Madam Nora came from the same village and are Muslim and second-degree cousins. No genetic studies have been performed for the family members. Nirman's initial diagnosis is hemolytic anemia.

Nurses should consider the unique cultural background and family dynamics and functioning while providing care to this immigrant family to ensure safe and quality care. The family has an ineffective communication pattern and an inability to navigate through the complexity of the health care system. Madam Nora needs to communicate with health care providers through her husband, who, in turn, is not familiar with medical terminology. The fact that no genetic testing was performed among family members may be attributed to the unfamiliarity and complexity of the health care system in the United States as compared with the health services in their native country. It is important for nurses to have culturally competent skills and to identify cultural beliefs that may impact how immigrant patients may communicate with them. Hence effective approaches may be implemented to provide safe and quality care for this population and to mitigate health disparities.

## CASE STUDY

### *An Older Immigrant Couple: Mr. and Mrs. Arahan*

Mr. and Mrs. Arahan, an older couple in their 70s, have been living with their oldest daughter, her husband of 15 years, and their two children, aged 12 and 14 years. They all live in a middle-income neighborhood in a suburb of a metropolitan city. Mr. and Mrs. Arahan are both college educated and worked full-time while they were in their native country. In addition, Mr. Arahan, the only offspring of wealthy parents, inherited a substantial amount of money and real estate. Their daughter came to the United States as a registered nurse and met her husband, a drug company representative. The older couple moved to the United States when their daughter became a US citizen and petitioned for them as immigrants. Because the couple were facing retirement, they welcomed the opportunity to come to the United States.

The Arahans found life in the United States different from that in their home country, but their adjustment was not as difficult because both were healthy and spoke English fluently. Most of their time was spent taking care of their two grandchildren and the house. As the grandchildren grew older, the older couple found that they had more spare time. The daughter and her husband advanced in their careers and spent a great deal more time at their jobs. There were few family dinners during the week. On weekends, the daughter, her husband, and their children socialized with their own friends. The couple began to feel isolated and longed for a more active life.

Mr. and Mrs. Arahan began to think that perhaps they should return to their home country, where they still had relatives and friends. However, political and economic issues would have made it difficult for them to live there. Besides, they had become accustomed to the way of life in the United States with all the modern conveniences and abundance of goods that were difficult to obtain in their country. However, they also became concerned that they might not be able to tolerate the winter months and that minor health problems might worsen as they aged. They wondered who would take care of them if they became very frail and where they would live, knowing that their daughter had saved money only for their grandchildren's college education. They expressed their sentiments to their daughter, who became very concerned about how her parents were feeling.

This older couple had been attending church on a regular basis but had never been active in other church-related activities. The church bulletin announced the establishment of parish nursing with two retired registered nurses as volunteers. The couple attended the first opening of the parish clinic. Here, they met one of the registered nurses, who had a short discussion with them about the services offered. The registered nurse had spent a great deal of her working years as a community health nurse. She informed Mr. and Mrs. Arahan of her availability to help them resolve any health-related issues.

**Reflective Questions:**
- What strategies could be suggested for this older adult couple to enhance their quality of life?
- What community resources can they use?
- What can the daughter and her family do to address the feelings of isolation of the older couple?
- What health-promotion activities can ensure a healthy lifestyle for them?

## CARE PLAN

### *An Older Immigrant Couple: Mr. and Mrs. Arahan*

**\*NURSING DIAGNOSIS: Risk of continued feelings of isolation**

**Defining Characteristics**
- The couple no longer have a great deal of caretaking responsibilities.
- The daughter and her husband spend a great deal of time on their careers.
- Family dinners during the week are seldom.
- The daughter and her family socialize with their own friends.
- The older couple is thinking of returning to their native country.
- The couple is concerned about life in the United States with harsh winters and their minor health problems.
- The couple is concerned about their advancing years and future living arrangements.

**Related Factors**
- Transition from the native country to the United States.
- Differing religious, ethnic, and cultural backgrounds between the native country and the United States influence care decisions.
- Differing roles in family structures between the native country and the United States.
- Conflicting roles between the two generations.
- Limited opportunities for social support and assimilation for older immigrants to the United States.
- Health and health care needs, multiple and complex, for the elder population in the United States.

**Expected Outcomes**
The Arahans will:
- Join a senior citizen center for socialization and other activities.

- Volunteer at a nearby hospital or school several mornings or afternoons per week.
- Work with their daughter and her family to plan at least one family meal per week.
- Pursue some neglected hobbies.
- Get involved in a church group or in a civic organization.
- Begin a discussion on future alternate living arrangements.
- Make periodic visits to the native country to see relatives and friends.

**Interventions**
- Encourage the couple to have open discussions about their concerns with their daughter and her family.
- Support them in their choice of meaningful activities such as joining the senior center and volunteering.
- Provide information on resources for future living arrangements in the United States.
- Develop a plan for health monitoring on a regular basis.
- Provide a list of organizations that address issues and concerns of older adults such as the American Association of Retired Persons (AARP).
- Utilize their experience and expertise (if any) in managing the parish nursing clinic.
- Initiate an older support group in the parish with the Arahans as the first members.

The Arahans' situation is a very common one in most immigrant groups. The interventions outlined would need to consider the cultural traditions, personal preferences, health status, motivation level, physical ability, and resources of the couple to ensure positive outcomes and goal achievement.

## SUMMARY

This century will continue to be a time of great challenges as the population of the United States continues to be a nation of diverse peoples. The nation and its people have repeatedly overcome devastations by both nature and humankind itself. As citizens, emerging populations share similar concerns about life, including health, an acceptable standard of living, and quality of life. An array of cultural, economic, educational, social, and political barriers are being eroded at the local, national, and global levels to ensure the health and well-being of the people of the United States. The government, public and private industries, health care professions, and all individuals can work together to reduce health disparities and ensure a healthy nation for future generations.

## ⓔ EVOLVE CHAPTER FEATURES

http://evolve.elsevier.com/Edelman/
- Study Questions

## REFERENCES

Abraham, N. (2014). Arab Americans. In T. Riggs (Ed.), *Gale encyclopedia of multicultural America* (Vol. 1). New York: Gale.

Africa, J., & Carrasco, M. (2011). Asian-American and Pacific Islander mental health. http://www.nami.org/Template.cfm?Section=Multicultural_Support1&Template=/ContentManagement/ContentDisplay.cfm&ContentID=115281.

Agency for Healthcare Research and Quality. (2011). National healthcare disparities report. http://www.ahrq.gov/qual/qrdr11/index.html.

Agency for Healthcare Research and Quality. (2015). *National healthcare quality and disparities report. AHRQ publication no. 15-0007*. Rockville, MD: Agency for Healthcare Research and Quality.

Al-Tayyib, A. A., et al. (2014). Association between prescription drug misuse and injection among runaway and homeless youth. *Drug and Alcohol Dependence, 1*(134), 1–7.

American Nurse Association. (2016). Code of Ethics for Nurses. http://nursingworld.org/codeofethics.

Andrews, M. M. (2016). The influence of cultural health belief systems on health care practices. In M. M. Andrews & J. S. Boyle (Eds.), *Transcultural concepts in nursing care* (7th ed.). Philadelphia: Lippincott Williams & Wilkins.

Andrews, M. M., & Boyle, J. S. (2016). Andrews/Boyle transcultural nursing assessment guide for individuals and families. In M. M. Andrews & J. S. Boyle (Eds.), *Transcultural concepts in nursing care* (7th ed., Vol. Appendix A). Philadelphia: Lippincott Williams & Wilkins.

Aprahamian, M., et al. (2011). The relationship between acculturation and mental health of Arab Americans. *Journal of Mental Health Counseling, 33*(1), 80–92.

Arab American Institute Foundation. (2011). Quick facts about Arab Americans. http://www.aaiusa.org/demographics-old.

Asi, M., & Beaulieu, D. (2013). Arab Households in the United States: 2006–2010 American Community Survey Briefs. US Department of Commerce, Economics and Statistics Administration.

Avent, J. R., & Cashwell, C. S. (2015). The black church: theology and implications for counseling African Americans. *The Professional Counselor, 5*(1), 81–90.

Bakullari, A., et al. (2014). Racial and ethnic disparities in healthcare-associated infections in the United States, 2009-2011. *Infection Control and Hospital Epidemiology, 35*(S3), S10–S16.

Beals, J., et al. (2005). Prevalence of mental disorders and utilization of mental health services in two American Indian reservation populations: Mental health disparities in a national context. *American Journal of Psychiatry, 162*, 1723–1732.

Billings, D. M., & Kowalski, K. (2008). Teaching tips. Increasing competency in the care of homeless patients. *Journal of Continuing Education in Nursing, 39*(4), 153–154.

Boyle, J. S. (2016). Culture, family, and community. In M. M. Andrews & J. S. Boyle (Eds.), *Transcultural concepts in nursing care* (7th ed., pp. 317–358). Philadelphia: Lippincott Williams & Wilkins.

Centers for Disease Control and Prevention. (2013). CDC Health Disparities and Inequalities Report—United States, 2013. *Morbidity and Mortality Weekly Report, 62*(Suppl 3), 1–189.

Centers for Disease Control and Prevention. (2014). HIV surveillance report, 2014. http://www.cdc.gov/hiv/pdf/library/reports/surveillance/cdc-hiv-surveillance-report-us.pdf.

Centers for Disease Control and Prevention. (2015). Asian/Pacific American heritage month. http://www.cdc.gov/Features/AAPIHeritageMonth/.

Chong, N. (2002). *The Latino patient: A cultural guide for health care providers*. Yarmouth, ME: Intercultural Press.

Cobb, N., Epsey, D., & King, J. (2014). Health behaviors and risk factors among American Indians and Alaska natives, 2000-2010. *American Journal of Public Health, 104*(S3), S481–S489.

D'Avanzo, C. E., & Geissler, E. M. (Eds.). (2008). *Mosby's pocket guide to cultural health assessment* (4th ed.). St. Louis: Mosby.

DeNavas-Walt, C., Proctor, B. D., & Smith, J. C. (2013). *U. S. Census Bureau: Income, poverty, and health insurance coverage in the United States: 2012*. Washington, DC: US Government Printing Office.

Depp, C. A., et al. (2015). A quantitative review of cognitive functioning in homeless adults. *The Journal of Nervous and Mental Disease, 203*(2), 126–131.

Douglas, M. K., et al. (2014). Guidelines for implementing culturally competent nursing care. *Journal of Transcultural Nursing, 1–13*.

Ehrmin, J. T. (2016). Transcultural perspectiveness in mental health nursing. In M. M. Andrews & J. S. Boyle (Eds.), *Transcultural concepts in nursing care* (7th ed., pp. 272–316). Philadelphia: Wolter Kluwer Health: Lippincott Williams & Wilkins.

El-Shahawy, O., & Haddad, L. (2015). Correlation between nicotine dependence and barriers to cessation between exclusive cigarette smokers and dual (water pipe) smokers among Arab Americans. *Substance Abuse and Rehabilitation, 6*, 25–32.

Fitzpatrick-Lewis, D., et al. (2011). Effectiveness of interventions to improve the health and housing status of homeless people: a rapid systematic review. *BMC Public Health, 11*(638), 1–14.

Fixico, D., Kolata, A. L., & Neely, S. (2001). American Indian. In *The world book encyclopedia* (Vol. 10, pp. 136–185). Chicago: World Books.

Flegal, K. M., et al. (2012). Prevalence of obesity and trends in the distribution of body mass index among U.S. adults, 1999-2010. *Journal of the American Medical Association, 307*(5), 491–497.

Gary, F. A., Yarandi, H. N., & Scruggs, F. C. (2003). Suicide among African Americans: Reflections and a call to action. *Issues in Mental Health Nursing, 24*(3), 353–375.

Gaskin, D. J., et al. (2014). Disparities in diabetes: The nexus of race, poverty, and place. *American Journal of Public Health, 104,* 2147–2155.

George, S., Duran, N., & Norris, K. (2014). A systematic review of barriers and facilitators to minority research participation among African Americans, Latinos, Asian Americans and Pacific Islanders. *American Journal of Public Health, 104*(2), e16–e61.

Giger, J. N. (2013). Introduction. In J. Giger (Ed.), *Transcultural nursing: Assessment and interventions* (6th ed., pp. 2–18). St. Louis: Elsevier.

Grandbois, D. (2005). Stigma of mental illness among American Indian and Alaska Native nations: Historical and contemporary perspectives. *Issues in Mental Health Nursing, 26,* 1001–1024.

Hammond, R. J., & Cheney, P. (2009). Intro to sociology: Glossary of terms. http://freebooks.uvu.edu/SOC1010/index.php/glossary -of-terms.html.

Hankerson, S. H., & Weissman, M. M. (2012). Church-based health programs for mental disorders among African Americans: a review. *Psychiatric Services, 63*(3), 243–249.

Hansen, M. (2011). Strategies to eliminate health disparities. http:// www.ncsl.org/issues-research/health/strategies-to-eliminate-health -disparities.aspx.

Haywood, S. H., et al. (2014). Psychometric evaluation of a cultural competency assessment instrument for health professionals. *Medical Care, 52*(2), e7–e15.

Henry, M., Cortes, A., & Morris, S. (2013). The 2013 annual homeless assessment report to Congress. US Department of Housing and Urban Development.

Hoeffel, E. M., et al. (2012). The Asian population: 2010. 2010 Census Briefs. C2010BR-11.

Holt, C. L., et al. (2014). Positive self-perceptions as a mediator of religious involvement and health behaviors in a national sample of African Americans. *Journal of Behavioral Medicine, 37*(1), 102–112.

Humes, K. R., Jones, N. A., & Ramirez, R. R. (2011). Overview of race and Hispanic origin: 2010. http://www.census.gov/prod/ cen2010/briefs/c2010br-02.pdf.

Institute of Medicine. (2008). Challenges and successes in reducing health disparities. Workshop summary. http://www.iom.edu/ Reports/2008/Challenges-and-Successes-in-Reducing-He alth-Disparities-Workshop-Summary.aspx.

Jamil, H., et al. (2008). Comparison of personal characteristics, tobacco use, and health states in Chaldean, Arab American, and non-Middle Eastern white adults. *Journal of Immigration and Minor Health, 11*(4), 310–317.

Josephy, A. M. (1991). *The Indian heritage of America.* Boston: Houghton Mifflin.

Kaiser Family Foundation. (2008). Eliminating racial/ethnic disparities in health care: What are the options? http://kff.org/ disparities-policy/issue-brief/eliminating-racialethnic-disparit ies-in-health-care-what/.

Kataoka-Yahiro, M., Ceria, C., & Yoder, M. (2004). Grandparent caregiving role in Filipino American families. *Journal of Cultural Diversity, 11*(3), 110–117.

Kavanaugh, R. R. (2008). Transcultural perspectiveness in mental health nursing. In M. M. Andrews & J. S. Boyle (Eds.), *Transcultural concepts in nursing care* (5th ed., pp. 226–259). Philadelphia: Wolter Kluwer Health: Lippincott Williams & Wilkins.

Kluckhohn, C. (1953). Dominant and variant value orientations. In C. Kluckhohn, H. A. Murray, & D. A. Schneider (Eds.), *Personality in nature, society, and culture* (2nd ed.). New York: Alfred A. Knopf.

Lambert, S., et al. (2002). A comparative study of prostate screening, health beliefs, and practices between African American men and Caucasian men. *ABNF Journal, 13*(3), 61–63.

Lebrun-Harris, L. A., et al. (2013). Health status and health care experiences among homeless patients in federally supported health centers: Findings from the 2009 patient survey. *Health Services Research, 48*(3), 992–1017.

Lee, Y.-H., Salman, A., & Wang, F. (2012). Recruiting Chinese-American adolescents to HIV/AIDS related research: A lesson learned from a cross-sectional study. *Applied Nursing Research, 25*(1), 40–46.

Leininger, M. (2001). The theory of culture care diversity and universality. In M. M. Leininger (Ed.), *Culture care diversity and universality: A theory of nursing* (2nd ed., pp. 5–68). Boston: Jones & Bartlett.

Leininger, M. (2002). Culture care theory: A major contribution to advance transcultural nursing knowledge and practices. *Journal of Transcultural Nursing, 13*(3), 189–192.

Liard, D. L., et al. (2007). Muslim patients and health disparities in the UK and the US. *Archives of Disease Childhood, 92,* 922–926.

Management Sciences for Health. (n.d.). The providers guide to quality and culture: Health disparities. http://erc.msh.org/mainpage.cfm?file =7.1.0.htm&module=provider&language=English.

Markus, H. R. (2008). Pride, prejudice, and ambivalence: Toward a unified theory of race and ethnicity. *American Psychologist, 63,* 651–670.

McCartney, S., Bishaw, A., & Fontenot, K. (2013). Poverty rates for selected detailed race and Hispanic groups by state and place: 2007-2011. US Department of Commerce.

McGadney-Douglass, B. F. (2000). The black church response to the mental health needs of the elderly. In S. L. Logan & E. M. Freeman (Eds.), *Health care in the black community: Empowerment, knowledge, skills, and collectivism* (pp. 199–214). New York: Haworth Press.

Migration Policy Institute. (2015). Number of immigrants and immigrants as percentage of the U.S. Population, 1850 to 2013. http://www.migrationpolicy.org/programs/migration-data.

Moore, M. L., Moos, M. K., & Callister, L. C. (2010). *Cultural competence: An essential journal for perinatal nurses.* White Plains, NY: March of Dimes Foundation.

National Alliance to End Homelessness. (2012a). Federal policy brief: Changes in the HUD definition of "homeless." http:// www.endhomelessness.org/content/article/detail/3006.

National Alliance to End Homelessness. (2012b). Mental/physical health. http://www.endhomelessness.org/blog/c/ mentalphysicalhealth.

National Association for the Education of Homeless Children and Youth. (2016). Facts about homeless education. http:// www.naehcy.org/educational-resources/early-childhood.

National Center for Health Statistics. (2015). *Health, United States, 2014: With special feature on adults aged 55–64.* Hyattsville, MD: National Center for Health Statistics.

National Coalition for the Homeless. (2009). Who is homeless? http://nationalhomeless.org/factsheets/Whois.pdf.

National Coalition for the Homeless. (2009a). Why are people homeless? http://www.nationalhomeless.org/factsheets/ why.html.

National Coalition for the Homeless. (2009b). Strategies of state mental health agencies to prevent and end homelessness. http:// www.endhomelessness.org/content/article/detail/2592.

National Coalition for the Homeless. (2009c). Health care and homelessness. http://www.nationalhomeless.org/factsheets/health.html.

National Coalition for the Homeless. (2009d). HIV/AIDS and homelessness. http://www.nationalhomeless.org/factsheets/hiv.html.

National Coalition for the Homeless. (2009e). Mental illness and homelessness. http://www.nationalhomeless.org/factsheets/Mental_Illness.html.

National Coalition for the Homeless. (2009f). Substance abuse and homelessness. http://www.nationalhomeless.org/factsheets/addiction.html.

National Health Care for the Homeless Council (NHCHC). (2016a). What is the relationship between health, housing, and homelessness? https://www.nhchc.org/faq/relationship-health-housing-homelessness/.

National Health Care for the Homeless Council (NHCHC). (2016b). About the council. http://www.nhchc.org/about/mission/.

Norris, T., Vines, P. L., & Hoeffel, E. M. (2012). The American Indian and Alaskan Native Population: 2010. US Census Bureau. http://www.census.gov/prod/cen2010/briefs/c2010br-10.pdf.

Office of Minority Health. (2016a). About the Office of Minority Health. http://minorityhealth.hhs.gov/omh/browse.aspx?lvl=1&lvlid=1.

Office of Minority Health. (2016b). Native Hawaiians and Pacific Islanders profile. http://minorityhealth.hhs.gov/omh/browse.aspx?lvl=3&lvlid=65.

Office of Minority Health. (2016c). Asian American profile. http://minorityhealth.hhs.gov/omh/browse.aspx?lvl=3&lvlid=63.

Office of Minority Health. (2016d). Asian American mental health. https://minorityhealth.hhs.gov/omh/browse.aspx?lvl=4&lvlid=54.

Office of Minority Health. (2016e). Hispanic/Latino profile. http://minorityhealth.hhs.gov/omh/browse.aspx?lvl=3&lvlid=64.

Office of Minority Health. (2016f). Black/African Americans profile. https://minorityhealth.hhs.gov/omh/browse.aspx?lvl=3&lvlid=61.

Office of Minority Health. (2016g). Infant mortality and African Americans. http://minorityhealth.hhs.gov/omh/browse.aspx?lvl=4&lvlid=23.

Office of Minority Health. (2016h). Cancer and African Americans. https://minorityhealth.hhs.gov/omh/browse.aspx?lvl=4&lvlid=16.

Office of Minority Health. (2016i). HIV/AIDS and African Americans. http://minorityhealth.hhs.gov/omh/browse.aspx?lvl=4&lvlid=21.

Office of Minority Health. (2016j). Heart disease and African Americans. http://minorityhealth.hhs.gov/omh/browse.aspx?lvl=4&lvlid=19.

Office of Minority Health. (2016k). Stroke and African Americans. http://minorityhealth.hhs.gov/omh/browse.aspx?lvl=4&lvlid=28.

Office of Minority Health. (2016l). Diabetes and African Americans. http://minorityhealth.hhs.gov/omh/browse.aspx?lvl=4&lvlID=18.

Office of Minority Health. (2016m). American Indian/Alaska Native profile. http://minorityhealth.hhs.gov/omh/browse.aspx?lvl=3&lvlid=62.

Office of Minority Health. (2016n). Mental health and American Indians/Alaska Natives. https://minorityhealth.hhs.gov/omh/browse.aspx?lvl=4&lvlid=39.

Office of Minority Health. (2016o). Infant mortality and American Indians/Alaska Natives. https://minorityhealth.hhs.gov/omh/browse.aspx?lvl=4&lvlid=38.

Office of Minority Health. (2016p). Diabetes and American Indians/Alaska Natives. http://minorityhealth.hhs.gov/omh/browse.aspx?lvl=4&lvlID=33.

Ogunwole, S. U. (2006). We the people: American Indians and Alaska Natives in the United States. Washington, DC: US Census Bureau.

Palepu, A., et al. (2011). Homelessness and adherence to antiretroviral therapy among a cohort of HIV-infected injection drug users. Journal of Urban Health, 88(3), 545–555.

Park, Y., et al. (2014). Body mass index and risk of death in Asian Americans. American Journal of Public Health, 104(3), 520–525.

Polcin, D. L. (2015). Co-occurring substance abuse and mental health problems among homeless persons: Suggestions for research and practice. Journal of Social Distress and the Homeless, 25(1), 1–10.

Ponce, N., et al. (2009). The state of Asian American, Native Hawaiian and Pacific Islander health in California report. http://www.healthpolicy.ucla.edu/pubs/Publication.aspx?pubID=32.

Rastogi, S., et al. (2011). 2010 Census brief: The black population 2010. http://www.census.gov/prod/cen2010/briefs/c2010br-06.pdf.

Rosenblum, M. R., & Soto, A. G. R. (2015). An analysis of unauthorized immigrants in the United States by country and region of birth. Washington, DC: Migration Policy Institute.

Ryan, C. L., & Bauman, K. (2016). U. S. Census Bureau, Educational attainment in the United States: 2015. Washington, DC: US Government Printing Office.

Salman, A., et al. (2007). Cultural competence among staff nurses who participated in a family-centered geriatric care program. Journal of Nurses Staff Development, 23(3), 103–111.

Shaffer, H. J., Freed, C. F., & Healea, D. (2002). Gambling disorders among homeless persons with substance use disorders seeking treatment at a community center. Psychiatric Services, 53(9), 1112–1117.

Smith, J. C., & Medalia, C. (2015). U.S. Census Bureau, current population reports, P60-253, health insurance coverage in the United States: 2014. Washington, DC: US Government Printing Office.

Snipp, C. M. (2000). Selected demographic characteristics of Indians. In E. R. Rhoades (Ed.), American Indian health (pp. 41–57). Baltimore, MD: Johns Hopkins University Press.

Stussy, S. A. (2000). Arab Americans. In C. J. Moose & R. Wilder (Eds.), Racial and ethnic relations in America (Vol. 1, pp. 102–107). Pasadena, CA: Salem Press.

Su, D., & Li, L. (2011). Trends in the use of complementary and alternative medicine in the United States: 2002-2007. Journal of Health Care for the Poor and Underserved, 22, 295–309.

Tailakh, A., et al. (2012). Prevalence, awareness, treatment and control of hypertension among Arab Americans. Journal of Cardiovascular Nursing, 28(4), 1–9.

Tashiro, C. J. (2006). Identity and health in the narratives of older mixed ancestry Asian Americans. Journal of Cultural Diversity, 13(1), 41–49.

Thompson, R. G., et al. (2013). Substance abuse disorders and poverty as prospective predictors of first-time homelessness in the United States. American Journal of Public Health, 103(S2), S282–S288.

Truong, M., Paradies, Y., & Priest, N. (2014). Interventions to improve cultural competency in healthcare: A systematic review of reviews. BMC Health Services Research, 14(99), 1–17.

Tsai, J., & Rosenheck, R. A. (2015). Risk factors for homeless among US veterans. Epidemiologic Reviews, 1-19.

United States Interagency Council on Homelessness. (2016). People experiencing chronic homelessness. https://www.usich.gov/goals/chronic.

US Census Bureau. (2014). American Indian and Alaska Native heritage month: 2014. https://www.census.gov/newsroom/facts-for-features/2014/cb14-ff26.html.

US Census Bureau. (2015a). Asian/Pacific American heritage month: May 2015. https://www.census.gov/newsroom/facts-for-features/2015/cb15-ff07.html.

US Census Bureau. (2015b). Hispanic heritage month: 2015. https://www.census.gov/newsroom/facts-for-features/2015/cb15-ff18.html.

US Census Bureau. (2016a). http://www.census.gov/en.html.

US Census Bureau. (2016b). Black (African-American) history month: February 2016. https://www.census.gov/newsroom/facts-for-features/2016/cb16-ff01.html.

US Department of Health and Human Services. (2009). Differences in prevalence of obesity among black, white, and Hispanic adults—United States, 2006-2008. *Morbidity and Mortality Weekly Report, 58*(27), 740–744.

US Department of Health and Human Services. (2010). About Healthy People: Foundation health measures: Disparities. http://www.healthypeople.gov/2020/about/DisparitiesAbout.aspx.

US Department of Health and Human Services. (2015). Health, United States, 2015: With special feature on racial and ethnic health disparities. http://www.cdc.gov/nchs/hus/index.htm.

US Department of Health and Human Services. (2016). Health care: Facts & features: Key features of the Affordable Care Act. http://www.hhs.gov/healthcare/facts-and-features/key-features-of-aca/index.html.

US Department of Health and Human Services, Centers for Disease Control and Prevention. (2011). National vital statistics reports. http://www.cdc.gov/nchs/products/nvsr.htm.

US Department of Health and Human Services Centers for Disease Control and Prevention. (2012a). Health United States 2011: With special feature on socioeconomic status and health. http://www.cdc.gov/nchs/data/hus/hus11.pdf.

US Department of Health and Human Services Centers for Disease Control and Prevention. (2012b). Summary health statistics for U.S. adults: National Health Interview Survey 2010. http://www.cdc.gov/nchs/data/series/sr_10/sr10_252.pdf.

United States Interagency Council on Homelessness. (2016). https://www.usich.gov/.

Vaughn, L. M., Jacquez, F., & Baker, R. C. (2009). Cultural health attributions, beliefs, and practices: Effects on healthcare and medical education. *Open Medical Education Journal, 2*, 64–74.

Waters, M. C., Kasinitz, P., & Asad, A. L. (2014). Immigrants and African Americans. *The Annual Review of Sociology, 40*, 369–390.

Weglicki, L. S., et al. (2008). Comparison of cigarette and water-pipe smoking by Arab and non-Arab-American youth. *American Journal of Preventive Medicine, 35*(4), 334–339.

White, M. C., et al. (2014). Disparities in cancer mortality and incidence among American Indians and Alaska natives in the United States. *American Journal of Public Health, 104*(S3), S377–S387.

Williams, D. R., Neighbors, H. W., & Jackson, J. S. (2008). Racial/ethnic discrimination and health: Findings from community studies. *American Journal of Public Health, 98*(9 Suppl.), S29–S37.

Winland-Brown, J., Lachman, V. D., & Swanson, E. O. (2015). The new 'Code of Ethics for Nurses With Interpretive Statements' (2015): Practical clinical application, part I. *Medsurg Nursing, 24*(4), 268–271.

Wong, C. A., et al. (2014). American Indian and Alaska native infant and pediatric mortality, United States, 1999-2009. *American Journal of Public Health, 104*(S3), S320–S328.

World Health Organization (WHO). (2015). *Monitoring health inequality*. Geneva: World Health Organization.

Wu, L.-T., & Blazer, D. G. (2015). Substance use disorders and co-morbidities among Asian Americans and native Hawaiians/pacific islanders. *Psychological Medicine, 45*, 481–494.

Young, J. L., Griffith, E. E., & Williams, D. R. (2003). The integral role of pastoral counseling by African-American clergy in community mental health. *Psychiatric Services, 54*(5), 688–692.

# 3

# Health Policy and the Delivery System

*Debora Elizabeth Kirsch*

*Debora Elizabeth Kirsch*

## OBJECTIVES

*After completing this chapter, the reader will be able to:*

- Examine key developments in the history of health care that influenced the philosophical basis of American health care and separated preventive measures from curative measures.
- Differentiate between private and public sector functions and responsibilities in the delivery of health care.
- Describe the mechanisms by which health care in the United States is financed in both the private sector and the public sectors.

- Analyze the influence of health legislation on the health care delivery system.
- Differentiate between the purposes, benefits, and limitations of Medicare, Medicaid, and other government-sponsored programs in achieving health equity.
- Compare and contrast the health care delivery systems of the United States and other countries.
- Discuss the major provisions of the Patient Protection and Affordable Care Act of 2010 and its impact on improving population health.

## KEY TERMS

Accountable care organizations (ACOs)
Advanced practice nurses (APNs)
Advocate
Affordable Care Act (ACA)
Concierge care
Fee-for-service
Gatekeeper
Health insurance exchange

Health maintenance organizations (HMOs)
Health savings accounts (HSAs)
High-deductible health insurance plans (HDHPs)
Hospitalist
Indemnity insurance plans
Independent practice associations (IPAs)

Insurance
Managed care
Marketplace
Medicaid
Medicare
Nursing centers
Point-of-service (POS)
Preferred provider organizations (PPOs)
Primary care provider (PCP)

### ❓ THINK ABOUT IT

#### *The Federal Health Care Reform Law*

The passage of the health care federal reform law called the Patient Protection and Affordable Care Act ignited the national conversation on the expanding role of government in health care. Within the many provisions of the law, a federal government mandate now requires most American citizens to have health insurance coverage or face financial penalties. Although health insurance coverage is an essential element in promoting the health of an individual, questions remain on how best to serve the health care needs of all Americans.

- Will the provisions of the law solve the problems of access to affordable quality health care for all citizens?
- With a greater proportion of the population now mandated to have health insurance, will the overall health of the population be improved?
- How will the law curtail rising health care costs and issues of quality and safety?
- Why is the American health care system the most costly in the world?

The health care delivery system in the United States is a complex, multilayered entity that has the capacity to provide the newest technological treatments and implement the most advanced health care in the world. Research findings have sparked the development of international gold standards for practicing evidence-based medical and nursing care. The market-driven, multipayer, heavily private system is distinct from any other health care delivery system in the world, employing almost 12 million health care workers, practitioners, and health care support occupation workers in 2014, to serve more than 322 million people. The US Bureau of Labor Statistics reports the projection of 14 of the 20 fastest growing occupations between 2012 and 2022 are health care related (US Department of Labor, 2014). Of the 800 occupations the Bureau of Labor Statistics reports on, registered nurses constitute the largest number of professionals, with more than 2.7 million jobs, with an above-average salary of $69,790. A projected growth of more than 526,000 registered nurse jobs over the 2012 to 2022 period is predicted because of an increased emphasis on preventable care, the aging baby boomer population, and increased rates of diabetes, obesity, and other chronic conditions (US Department of Labor, 2015a,b). The American health care system is massive but so is the cost. The rising cost of health care is consuming a growing percentage of the nation's gross domestic product (GDP). The Centers for Medicare & Medicaid Services (CMS) reported in 2014 that national health expenditures consumed 17.4% of the nation's GDP (i.e., more than $3.0 trillion), which equates to $9255 per person, the highest dollar amount per capita of all industrialized countries. Projected health spending for 2014 to 2024 is expected to grow at 5.8% per year, resulting in a rise to 19.6% in the nation's GDP by 2024 (CMS, 2015a). The rising cost of health insurance premiums (and other related costs such as higher copays and deductibles) is a growing burden to working American families and employers.

Despite the vast economic resources devoted to financing the health care system, unequal access to care exists, especially among vulnerable populations. Although the availability and provision of health insurance is an important factor in health equity, vulnerable populations face additional obstacles, leading to health disparities across the nation. Health disparities (a particular type of health difference that is closely linked with social, economic, and/or environmental disadvantage) adversely affect groups of individuals especially vulnerable populations. The vision of *Healthy People 2020* is a society in which all people live long healthy lives. One of the overarching goals of *Healthy People 2020* is the attainment of the highest level of health for all people. The *Healthy People 2020* framework provides structure and guidance, identifying specific areas where action must be taken and targets met so as to achieve the goals by 2020 (US Department of Health and Human Services [USDHHS], 2015a). Federal and state governments, to improve the health of the population, enact health care reform policies and laws. In the past, health care reform consisted of incremental steps, mainly targeted at the poor and older adult populations to improve health (Medicare and Medicaid); however, with escalating health care costs, rising numbers of uninsured Americans, and concern for improvement in the quality and safety of care, a more substantive reform effort was taken. The new health care federal reform law called the Patient Protection and **Affordable Care Act (ACA)** was signed into law on March 23, 2010. The federal law requires the largest change in the financing of the American health care system since public Medicare and Medicaid programs were enacted in the 1960s. The law was designed to expand coverage, control cost, and improve the delivery of health care (Kaiser Family Foundation [KFF], 2013). A core component of the ACA is to reduce the number of uninsured individuals by expansion of the Medicaid program so that more individuals meet the expanded enrollment criteria and the establishment of marketplace subsidies for moderate-income individuals to assist with health care premium costs. Implementation of the law is occurring in increments, with full enactment of the ACA slated by 2018. The law is designed to address the issues of affordability, accessibility, and financing of health care, with focused efforts on meeting the needs of vulnerable populations. Implementation of the various provisions

of the ACA has required substantial changes in public insurance programs, private health insurance market regulations, and other components of the health care system. Because of lack of bipartisan support for the original ACA, and continued bipartisan disagreements over many of the provisions, a change in the political landscape of the Senate or House of Representatives in Washington or future actions filed in the court system may result in repeal of the law, dismantling of portions of the law, or additional amendments to some of the current and future provisions. For example, one of the first contested provisions of the ACA was the requirement for most United States citizens and legal residents to have health insurance or pay a federal tax penalty beginning in 2014. The Supreme Court in June of 2012 ruled in favor of the constitutionality of this contested provision and upheld the requirement for the individual mandate. However, the court also ruled that states had the option of expanding (or not) their Medicaid programs. Expanding the Medicaid program in every state would have increased coverage to a greater number of lower-income adults. A family of three, for example, in 2014 with an income of $27,300 or less would have been eligible for Medicaid coverage if they were living in a state that had expanded its Medicaid program. To encourage individual states to expand Medicaid coverage, additional federal tax dollars are allotted to states that have expanded coverage (KFF, 2013).

The past several years have been challenging times for state governments to arrange the implementation of the many provisions of the ACA. For example, one provision allows individuals to purchase coverage through a public or private **health insurance exchange**. The health insurance **marketplace**, or Obama care exchange, is for individuals who do not have health insurance or employer qualifying health insurance, Medicare, Medicaid, the Children's Health Insurance Program (CHIP), or other source that provide qualifying health insurance. Many individuals who qualify for marketplace coverage health insurance are eligible for financial assistance for a premium tax credit (subsidies) based on expected income for 2017. Marketplace plans must cover mandated essential health benefits, which include ambulatory patient services; emergency services; hospitalization; pregnancy, maternity, and newborn care; mental health and substance abuse services; prescription drugs; laboratory services; preventive and wellness services and chronic disease management; pediatric services, which include oral and vision care; and preexisting conditions, including pregnancy and preventive care. Plans must also have birth control benefits, and some covered contraceptive methods. Adult vision and dental coverage are not required in the mandated essential packages, but some plans may offer these benefits, or separate dental plans may be available for a separate additional premium. Marketplace plans have deductibles, co-payments, and other out-of-pocket costs for most covered services with the exception of some preventive care. All health insurance plans must cover the mandated essential health benefits, but each plan is different, with some states opting to cover additional services (HealthCare.gov, n.d.). The process for selecting and applying to join a plan can be challenging for many individuals, especially for those with low literacy levels and/or limited health literacy. Despite greater health insurance coverage for many more individuals, issues for the newly insured include paying for monthly premiums (if applicable), knowing how to use plan benefits effectively, finding a provider, navigating the health care system, and paying additional out-of-pocket expenses of deductibles and copays. A key role of nurses is to help individuals and families overcome these barriers.

This chapter will analyze the health status of the nation compared with other countries, examine historical influences in the delivery of health care, and describe the structure and mechanisms to deliver public (Medicare and Medicaid) and private health care in the United States and select other countries, the financing of the health care system, and key federal legislation with emphasis on the provisions of the ACA of 2010, which will strive to improve teamwork and communication between all these system pieces. The greatest savings in health care expenditures could be realized if individuals engage in consistent health-promotion and disease-prevention practices and avoid costly consequences of acute and chronic disease. The ACA includes requirements for essential health benefits designed to promote health screenings and other preventative measures, hoping that savings will be realized from early detection, decreasing hospital admissions, and unnecessary hospital readmissions. Nurses need to keep abreast of the various provisions and amendments of the law to help individuals and families navigate the health care system and be politically active in influencing health policy as an advocate of social justice for individuals and families.

## THE HEALTH OF THE NATION

*Health, United States* is an annually published document prepared by the USDHHS; it reports the health status of the nation by tracking a variety of specific, measurable health indicators. This annual report serves several key functions, but the main goal is to inform policymakers, the President, and Congress of the trends in the nation's health to guide the development of sound health policy and allocate resources to maintain and improve the health of the nation's citizens. The 2014 report indicates the health of the nation improved in many areas between 2003 and 2013 as a result of substantial funding of public health programs, research, provision of health care, and initiatives to support consumer education. Emerging trends indicate success in the reduction of morbidity and mortality for many diseases, control of widespread infectious diseases through widespread vaccination programs, improvement in motor vehicle safety, smoking cessation measures, and reduction of cardiovascular-related deaths. Life expectancy has increased for both men and women, and maternal and infant mortality rates on average are declining in many geographical locations. Heart disease remains the number one cause of death for Americans, responsible for 24% of all deaths in 2013, followed by cancer at 23% of all deaths in the same year. Education regarding leading a healthy lifestyle, controlling hypertension, smoking cessation, using cholesterol-lowering medications, and participating in routine screening has contributed to better health for many Americans, but concern about sedentary lifestyle, rising obesity trends, and chronic disease is noted. Recent national smoking cessation interventions for individuals aged 18 years or older are demonstrating some effectiveness as the percentage

of individuals who smoke dropped to 17.8% in 2013, compared with 23.2% in 2000. The percentage of adults who engage in aerobic exercise and muscle strengthening increased to 20.4% in 2013 (15.1% in 2000), but other health risk factors remain problematic, with 35.5% of adults older than 20 years reported as obese between 2009 and 2012, which is an increase from 30.5% for 1999 to 2002. The report cites the prevalence of childhood obesity as a growing concern—between 2009 and 2012, 10.2% of children aged 2 to 5 years, 17.9% of children aged 6 to 11 years, and 19.4% of adolescents aged 12 to 19 years were obese. As obesity trends often continue into adulthood, these children are at greater risk of developing diabetes, hypertension, and cardiovascular disease earlier in life and developing the sequelae of chronic disease in adulthood. Of noted concern is the rise in suicide and drug poisoning death rates in recent years. Suicide death rates rose 17% to 12.6 per 100,000 population and drug poisoning death rates involving opioid analgesics increased from 2.9 deaths per 100,000 population to 5.1 deaths per 100,000 population, with the highest rates among those aged 45 to 54 years (USDHHS, 2015a). Improvements in the nation's health have not been uniform, because factors affecting health equity include an individual's income, race, sex, ethnicity, education level, and geographical location (National Center for Health Statistics, 2014). In summary, the most effective intervention to decrease the growing cost of health care is to keep Americans healthy—preventing chronic diseases such as diabetes and heart disease with healthy eating, routine exercise patterns, and following recommended preventative measures with routine health screenings and early intervention if problems arise is needed.

### Healthy People 2020

As discussed in Chapter 1, on December 2, 2010, *Healthy People 2020* was launched, providing a 10-year agenda for improving the health of all Americans. The new overarching goals are listed in Box 3-1: *Healthy People 2020*.

One of the goals of *Healthy People 2000* was to reduce health disparities among Americans. Ten years later, Healthy People 2010's goal was to eliminate health disparities. The current 2020 goal is broader; to achieve health equity, eliminate disparities, and improve the health of all groups as measured by leading health indicators. Health disparities adversely affect groups of people who have systematically experienced greater obstacles to health on the basis of their race, color, or national origin;

---

♥ BOX 3-1  HEALTHY PEOPLE 2020

**Overarching Goals for Healthy People 2020**

- Attain high-quality, longer lives free of preventable disease, disability, injury, and premature death.
- Achieve health equity, eliminate disparities, and improve the health of all groups.
- Create social and physical environments that promote good health for all.
- Promote quality of life, healthy development, and healthy behaviors across all life stages.

Source HealthyPeople.gov. (2015). About healthy people. http://www.healthypeople.gov/2020/About-Healthy-People/.

ethnic group; religion; socioeconomic status; gender; age; mental health; cognitive, sensory, or physical or other disability; sexual orientation or gender identity; geographical location; or other characteristics historically linked to discrimination or exclusion (USDHHS, 2015b). Individuals and groups at risk of health disparity are considered vulnerable populations (KFF, 2010b). A more complete list of vulnerable populations can be found in Box 3-2: Vulnerable Populations. Public health nursing practice promotes and preserves the health of populations, looking at the community as a whole and its effect on the health of individuals, families, and groups. Community health nursing practice promotes, preserves, and maintains the health of populations through care provided to individuals, families, and groups and studies the effect of their health status on that of the community as a whole (Stanhope & Lancaster, 2012). A healthy thriving community is a community that is safe and inclusive and promotes a high quality of life and well-being, which can be measured by social networks, physical assets, economic opportunity, human development, and local institutions that sustain respect and support each of the dimensions (Community Health and Empowerment through Education and Research, 2015). *Healthy People 2020* supports the need for an effective public health infrastructure for planning, delivering,

---

### BOX 3-2  Vulnerable Populations

- Residents of rural areas
- Undocumented immigrants
- Low-income individuals and families
- Working poor
- Racial and ethnic minorities
- People with no health insurance coverage
- People with multiple chronic conditions
- People with language or cultural barriers
- The physically disabled or handicapped
- The terminally or mentally ill
- Persons with HIV/AIDS
- Alcohol or substance abusers
- Homeless individuals
- Individuals who do not speak English
- Individuals with communication difficulties
- Low education levels or illiteracy
- Anyone lacking health literacy

Sources Shi, L., & Stevens, G. (2010). *Vulnerable populations in the United States* (2nd ed.). San Francisco, CA: Jossey-Bass; Urban Institute. Health policy center vulnerable populations. http://urban.org/health_policy/vulnerable_populations/index.cfm.

---

and evaluating public health, with the key components being a capable and qualified workforce, up-to-date data and information systems, and public health agencies capable of assessing and responding to public health needs (Office of Disease Prevention and Health Promotion, 2015).

## Health Indicators of a Nation

Standard measures used to compare the health status of the population of one nation with another are actually death indicators. Although mortality-based indicators do not directly measure the health status of the living population, the data indirectly reflect the general health of a nation and are more readily available through government and world agencies. Table 3-1, International Comparisons of Core Health Indicators, compares the average life expectancy by gender as well as infant mortality rates of populations in select countries. According to Central Intelligence Agency (CIA) statistics (CIA, 2015), the life expectancy on average (both sexes combined) in the United States in 2015 was 79.68 years compared with 81.98 years in Sweden and 81.76 years in Canada. The life expectancy in Mexico was significantly lower at 75.65 years. In 1950, life expectancy in the United States for men was 56.2 years and for women was 65.5 years (Social Security Administration, n.d.), so much progress has been made in improving the health of the nation. Overall, life expectancy rates have risen sharply in the past 60 years in the United States and other industrialized countries, but in stark comparison, life expectancy in third world or poorer countries lags. For example, Afghanistan, a country with low levels of health care provisions, life expectancy today is on average 61.3 years. Compared with the United States, this gap is greater than 18 years, and life expectancy is less than life expectancies reported for women in the United States in 1950. During the preceding two decades, most nations have slowly increased life expectancy by 4 to 5 years (Table 3-2 for select countries). Although India, for example, is behind in life expectancy compared with other countries (average life expectancy in 2015 was 68.13 years), overall life expectancy has increased significantly in the last 2 decades (CIA, 2015).

Infant mortality rates (see Table 3-1) are one of the most important indicators of the health of a nation because they are associated with factors such as maternal health and access to health care. The US infant mortality rate (number of deaths in the first year of life) estimated in 2015 was reported as 5.87 (number of deaths of infants in the first year of life per 1000 live births), a dramatic improvement from 29.2 reported in 1950

---

### TABLE 3-1  International Comparisons of Core Health Indicator Estimates for 2015

|  | Afghanistan | Canada | France | Germany | Mexico | Sweden | United Kingdom | United States |
|---|---|---|---|---|---|---|---|---|
| Life expectancy at birth: males (years) | 60.5 | 79.15 | 78.65 | 78.26 | 72.88 | 80.09 | 78.37 | 77.32 |
| Life expectancy at birth: females (years) | 62.0 | 84.52 | 85.01 | 83.0 | 78.55 | 83.99 | 82.83 | 81.97 |
| Life expectancy at birth: both sexes (years) | 61.3 | 81.76 | 81.75 | 80.57 | 75.65 | 81.98 | 80.54 | 79.68 |
| Infant deaths per 1000 live births | 66.0 | 4.65 | 3.28 | 3.43 | 12.23 | 2.6 | 4.38 | 5.87 |

Data from the Central Intelligence Agency. (2015). The world fact book. http://www.cia.gov/library/publications/the-world-factbook/; World Bank. http://data:worldbank.org/indicator/SP.DYN.IMRT.IN.

TABLE 3-2 International Comparison of Life Expectancy Rates at Birth (in Years) Over Time for 1990, 2000, and 2013

| Location | Period | Male | Female | Both Sexes |
|---|---|---|---|---|
| Afghanistan | 2013 | 61 | 62 | 61 |
|  | 2000 | 42 | 42 | 42 |
|  | 1990 | 41 | 41 | 41 |
| Australia | 2013 | 80 | 85 | 83 |
|  | 2000 | 77 | 83 | 80 |
|  | 1990 | 74 | 80 | 77 |
| Canada | 2013 | 80 | 84 | 82 |
|  | 2000 | 77 | 82 | 79 |
|  | 1990 | 74 | 81 | 77 |
| China | 2013 | 74 | 77 | 75 |
|  | 2000 | 70 | 73 | 71 |
|  | 1990 | 67 | 71 | 69 |
| Denmark | 2013 | 78 | 82 | 80 |
|  | 2000 | 75 | 79 | 77 |
|  | 1990 | 72 | 78 | 75 |
| France | 2013 | 79 | 85 | 82 |
|  | 2000 | 75 | 83 | 79 |
|  | 1990 | 73 | 82 | 78 |
| India | 2013 | 65 | 68 | 66 |
|  | 2000 | 61 | 63 | 62 |
|  | 1990 | 57 | 58 | 58 |
| Mexico | 2013 | 73 | 78 | 75 |
|  | 2000 | 72 | 77 | 75 |
|  | 1990 | 68 | 75 | 71 |
| United Kingdom | 2013 | 79 | 83 | 81 |
|  | 2000 | 76 | 80 | 78 |
|  | 1990 | 73 | 79 | 76 |
| United States | 2013 | 76 | 81 | 79 |
|  | 2000 | 74 | 80 | 77 |
|  | 1990 | 72 | 79 | 75 |

Data from World Health Organization. Global health observatory data repository. http://apps.who.int/gho/data/view.main.680; World Health Rankings. Live longer life better. http://www.worldlifeexpectancy.com/country-health-profile/.

but higher than mortality rates in other developed nations (CIA, 2015). Mexico has an infant mortality rate of slightly more than 12, which is lower than that of other poor nations such as Ethiopia, which has an infant mortality rate of more than 53. Outliers for an extremely high infant mortality rate are Afghanistan, reporting 66.0, and Mali, reporting an estimate of more than 102 in 2015 (CIA, 2015) (Figure 3-1). The rationale of why the United States ranks less favorably in this health indicator than other industrialized nations is attributed to a number of factors. According to a working paper from the National Bureau of Economic Research (Chen et al., 2014), there is a lack of comparable microdata sets across countries that may account for about 40% of the difference in infant mortality rates between the United States and comparable countries because of the variability in the reporting of births near the threshold of fetal viability, so there are differences in how and what data are collected and used. This is also a factor in comparing neonatal mortality rates (infant deaths within the first 28 days of life) as countries may differ in reporting data based on gestational age and birth weight and survival. In the United States, low birth weight and congenital malformations were the two top reasons (38% of all infant deaths) in 2013 (CIA, 2015; Peterson Center on Healthcare & Kaiser Family Foundation Partnership, 2015; Mathews et al., 2015). Despite data collection and reporting variations, the United States overall has large disparities in health status by geographical areas, race, ethnicity groups, social class, and education levels. For example, infant mortality rates for black, non-Hispanic babies were more than twice those of white, non-Hispanic babies. According to 2013 figures (Figure 3-2), the infant mortality rate for white, non-Hispanic infants in the United States was 5.1, which is below the overall average for all races (6.0 years in 2013), but black, non-Hispanic babies had a disproportionately high rate of more than 10 infant deaths in the first year of life and American Indian/Alaska Natives had a rate of 7.6 deaths per 1000 live births in 2013 (Peterson Center on Healthcare & Kaiser Family Foundation Partnership, 2015). Preliminary data from the USDHHS reported similar infant mortality rates for 2013 (Table 3-3). Although the infant mortality rate from 2000 to 2013 in the United States improved by about 13%, there has been a persistent racial disparity in the United States, especially among black, non-Hispanic infants. The US infant mortality rate is higher than that of the other industrial nations presented in Table 3-1. A number of characteristics are reported with birth and infant death data sets that include in addition to race and ethnicity, infant mortality rates in which pregnancy care was started, smoking status during pregnancy, and education level of the mother. The lowest infant mortality rates are reported when a mother seeks prenatal care in the first trimester of pregnancy, is a nonsmoker during pregnancy, and has attained a bachelor's degree or higher (Table 3-4). Mothers who sought late or no prenatal care, smoked during pregnancy, or had less than a high school diploma had the greatest number of infant deaths. Large differences in infant death rates are readily apparent, as shown in Figure 3-3. The 2003 to 2005 the infant mortality rate of white mothers aged 20 years older with a college education was 4.2, whereas that of Asian women was even lower, at 3.8. These statistics are much more congruent with those of other industrialized countries. African American women with less than a high school education have the highest infant mortality rates, reported as 15.1. For most races and ethnicities, the higher a woman's educational achievement, the lower the overall infant mortality rate, as shown in Figure 3-1. In research terms this indicates a positive correlation between educational attainment of women and infant mortality rates. To improve health indicators and reduce health disparities of a population, interventions to promote educational attainment of women at least through high school need to occur as one strategy to decrease infant mortality rates. The mortality rate for infants of unmarried mothers (7.96) is 73% higher than that for infants of married mothers (4.60). Geographical variations also exist within the United States, with the highest percentage infant mortality rates reported in Mississippi at 9.6, Louisiana at 8.69, Alabama at 8.60 (compared with the national average of 5.96), and nine states reporting infant mortality rates of less than 5.0 (i.e., Massachusetts 4.18, Iowa 4.25, Vermont 4.35,

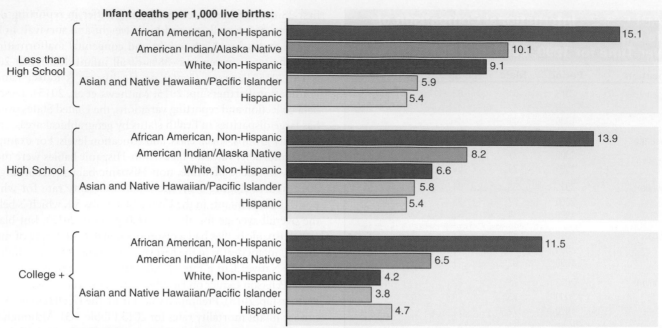

**Infant deaths per 1,000 live births:**

FIGURE 3-1 Infant mortality rates for mothers aged 20 years or older by race/ethnicity and education, 2003 to 2005. Data reported from 37 states, the District of Columbia, and New York City. (Data from the Centers for Disease Control and Prevention/National Center for Health Statistics, National Vital Statistics System, linked birth/infant death dataset. From *Health*, United States, 2008, Table 19.)

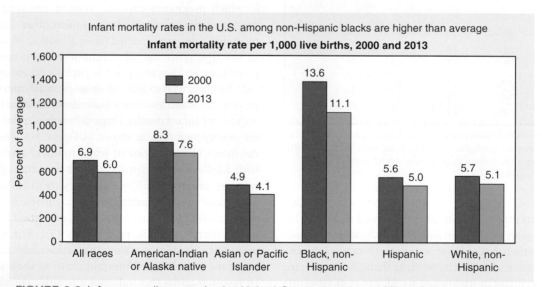

FIGURE 3-2 Infant mortality rates in the United States among non-Hispanic blacks are higher than average. (From National Vital Statistics System, National Center for Health Statistics, Centers for Disease Control and Prevention. Slide available from Kaiser Family Foundation. http://kff.org/Kaiser-slides/.)

California 4.76, Connecticut 4.79, New York 4.93) (Mathews et al., 2015). In summary, decreasing the nation's infant mortality rates will require community interventions to decrease teen pregnancy, promote educational attainment for all women to high school level or greater, and provide targeted interventions for specific racial groups and geographical areas.

## Historical Role of Women in Health Promotion

Nurses have a long tradition of involvement in health promotion, beginning with Florence Nightingale, the founder of modern nursing. While caring for wounded soldiers in a British camp outside Constantinople, Turkey, in 1854 during the Crimean

| TABLE 3-3 Infant Mortality Rate in the United States by Race/Ethnicity, 2013 | |
| --- | --- |
| Race/Ethnicity | Infant Deaths per 1000 Births[a] |
| Asian and Native Hawaiian/Pacific Islander | 4.07 |
| Hispanic | 5.0 |
| White, non-Hispanic | 5.06 |
| American Indian/Alaska Native | 7.61 |
| Black, non-Hispanic | 11.11 |
| All mothers | 5.96 |

[a]Births are categorized according to the race/ethnicity of the mother. Data from Department of Health and Human Services, Centers for Disease Control and Prevention, National Center for Health Statistics, Division of Vital Statistics. (2015). 2013 period linked birth/infant death data set. fdp://ftp.cdc.gov/pub/Health_Statistics/NCHS/Dataset_Documentation/DVS/periodlinked/LinkPE13Guide.pdf; Mathews, T. J., MacDorman, M. F., & Thoma, M. E. (2015). Infant mortality statistics from the 2013 period linked birth/infant death data set. *National Vital Statistics Reports, 64*(9), 1–30.

| TABLE 3-4 Infant Mortality Rates in 2007, by Trimester in Which Pregnancy Care was Started, Smoking Status During Pregnancy, and Education of Mother | |
| --- | --- |
| Characteristic | Rate |
| Prenatal care beginning in first trimester | 5.57 |
| Prenatal care beginning in second or third trimester | 6.3 |
| No prenatal care | 27.13 |
| Smoker during pregnancy | 10.41 |
| Nonsmoker during pregnancy | 6.1 |
| Educational attainment | |
| Less than high school diploma | 7.78 |
| High school diploma | 7.17 |
| Some college or technical school | 5.79 |
| Bachelor's degree or higher | 3.77 |

Data from Mathews, T. J., & MacDorman M. F. (2011). Infant mortality statistics from the 2007 period linked birth/infant death data set. *National Vital Statistics Reports, 59*(6):1–31.

War, she fought for hospital reform by crusading for nutritious food, cleanliness, and sanitation. She provided leadership for a group of nurses and comfort to the soldiers. Her careful recordings of care outcomes quantified needed reform in health promotion (University of Alabama at Birmingham, 2016). Later, Lillian Wald, appalled by the lack of medical care, ignorance, and living conditions of the poor in 1893, developed a settlement program in New York City that trained nurses, provided care to families, and developed education programs for the community. Wald, a leader in political activism, spearheaded organized public health in the direction of health promotion for families and communities (Henry Street Settlement, 2016). These pioneers and others set the stage for nurses' unique role in health promotion.

## A SAFER SYSTEM

The health care delivery system in the United States is experiencing significant changes sparked by health care reform and recommendations from large organizations involved in forming health policy. One of the large nonprofit organizations with seven divisions is the National Academies of Science, Engineering, and Medicine. One of the divisions, named the Institute of Medicine (IOM), conducts research from a systems approach to advise the nation's leaders in improving health. On March 15, 2016, the division that focuses on health and medicine (previously known as the IOM) was renamed the Health and Medicine Division (HMD). Several early IOM reports were instrumental in advising on the need to revise health policy to change the structure of health care delivery to deliver safer care. The 1999 IOM research report *To Err Is Human: Building a Safer Health System* (IOM, 1999) focused on prevention of medical errors, which account for approximately 98,000 deaths in hospitals each year. The startling findings concluded that the health care system, not bad practitioners, is the basic cause of

medical errors. In 2003 the IOM released another report, *Keeping Patients Safe: Transforming the Work Environment of Nurses* (IOM, 2003). This report shows that work environments in hospitals and nursing homes contribute to nurses' errors. Four main problem areas in nurses' work environments were identified: organizational management, workforce management, work design, and organizational culture. The researchers found that increased nurse staffing ratios, fewer nurses, mandatory overtime, inadequate continuing education, and lack of nurse involvement in decisions about client care create an environment that contributes to error-making. The data the IOM provided in this project support a direct link between nurse staffing and work environment with patient outcomes. Other efforts by the IOM to improve the health of the nation include the 2006 report *Preventing Medication Errors: Quality Chasm Series* (IOM, 2006). The report found in any given week, medication errors in prescribing or taking medication were not only common but also costly to the nation and recommended a comprehensive approach to decreasing the prevalence of medication errors by making changes in the health care system. A report released in January of 2012 discussed how standards of care can be defined as the level of health and medical care capable of being delivered when preparations are being made for public health emergencies such as pandemic influenza, large-scale earthquake, or any major disaster scenario in which the health system may be destroyed or stressed (IOM, 2012). The IOM has made recommendations in other areas promoting safety within the health care system. For example, in 2011 recommendations were made to improve transparency in the reporting of health information technology and promoting health literacy to encourage prevention and wellness, and in 2014 an IOM report, *Dying in America, Improving Quality and Honoring Individual Preferences Near the End of Life* (IOM, 2014) provided direction on improving end-of-life care for this vulnerable population. The IOM (now the HMD) has been productive in releasing hundreds of reports and

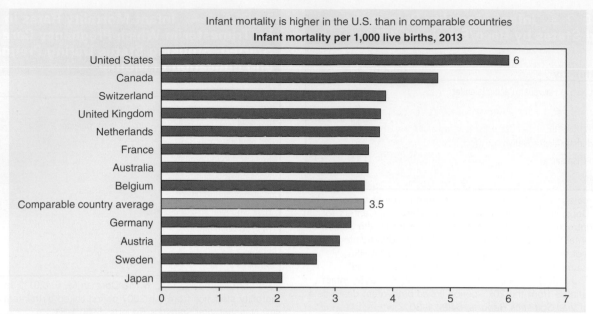

Infant mortality is higher in the U.S. than in comparable countries
**Infant mortality per 1,000 live births, 2013**

**FIGURE 3-3** Infant mortality is higher in the United States than in comparable countries. Infant deaths per 1,000 live births, 2013. Comparable countries are defined as those with above-median gross domestic product (GDP) and above-median GDP per capita in at least one of the past 10 years. In cases where 2013 data were unavailable, data from the last available year are used. (From OECD (2013). OECD health data: Health status: Health status indicators, OECD Health Statistics (database). doi:10.1787/data-00349-en; National Vital Statistics System, National Center for Health Statistics, Centers for Disease Control and Prevention. Slide from the Kaiser Family Foundation chart collection: How does infant mortality in the U.S. compare to other countries. Slide available from Kaiser Family Foundation. http://www.kff.org.)

workshop summaries of pressing concerns related to health and the health care system. New reports are generated each month by the HMD and can be found on the National Academy of Science website (see http://nationalacademics.org). Current topic areas include public health (367 reports), biomedical and health research (273 reports), quality and safety (222 reports), diseases (220 reports), health services, coverage, access (217 reports), and select populations and health disparities (163 reports). Other subject areas include food and nutrition, health care workforce, global health, veterans' health, mental health, education, aging, and women's health. The HMD in the first few weeks of April 2016 released six reports on topics as varied as vector-borne diseases, public health problems of hepatitis B and hepatitis C, and systems practices for the care of socially at risk populations, while in March 2016, ten reports were released pertaining to economics, protection of children, cancer care in low-resource areas, ovarian cancer, and Agent Orange updates and veterans. To provide safe, evidence-based care, nurses have a responsibility to be lifelong learners to stay abreast of new scientific findings and advocate health care policy changes that improve the health of the communities in which they practice and extend to the greater global population. Although health care is often equated with medical care, which focuses on the treatment of illness, this chapter presents the evolution and ongoing development of a broader concept of health based on the definition given in Chapter 1.

## GLOBAL HEALTH

The overriding objective of the World Health Organization (WHO) is to influence health opportunities and outcomes for all people so that they can attain the highest possible level of health. WHO recognizes the importance of families and health promotion, and has contributed to the family health policies of many nations by shaping global awareness for health promotion. The current agenda of WHO involves the following six goals: promoting development; fostering health security; strengthening health systems; harnessing research, information, and evidence; enhancing partnerships; and improving performance (WHO, n.d.a). Internationally, shrinking health care budgets have resulted in a variable level of achievement of these goals. In developing nations, such as those in Latin America and Africa, huge inequities in health care persist.

### Historical Perspectives

The complexities of the US health care system necessitate an understanding of the system as a whole before one can focus on the intermingled causative factors that have created a fragmented system of health care delivery. Many of today's problems have their roots in the decisions and directions of the past. It is not possible to identify and analyze current problems or to devise solutions without first exploring how the system developed. The relevance of the divergence between preventive and curative measures is apparent when the organization and financing of the delivery system are examined. The United States has established a system that uses two basic divisions of society to provide service: the public sector and the private sector. The merger of public health and welfare policies in the public sector is rooted in the Puritan ethic inherent in the historical development of the United States. The current focus on managed care as both an organizational strategy and a financing mechanism is highlighted in a discussion of how health care is delivered and financed.

## HISTORY OF HEALTH CARE

### Early Influences

Historical records of early civilizations (Egyptian, Indian, Chinese, Aztec, and Greek) show that ancient peoples were concerned with disease and practiced various methods of treatment. The earliest views of health can be seen as holistic in the sense that they emerged from an integrated worldview. Primitive peoples understood illness in mystical terms: sickness and cure theories were tied to the cosmic view of life, with natural and supernatural forces often inseparable. Most religions include a person's hygiene as part of their practice. For thousands of years, epidemics were viewed as divine judgments on human wickedness, with a gradual awareness that pestilence (any epidemic disease with a high death rate) has natural causes such as climate and other aspects of the physical environment. During the Middle Ages, infectious diseases in epidemic proportions (leprosy, bubonic plague, smallpox, and tuberculosis [TB]) were the leading causes of death. Clearly, health was viewed in terms of survival and absence of disease.

### Industrial Influences

The population of the Western world began to increase during the 1600s, when America was first being explored. The New World had many things to offer explorers. An adequate food supply made it possible for the population to live longer, and advances in transportation made distribution of food supplies and other goods and services possible. Manufacturing advances during the 18th century, through the invention of the flush toilet and cast iron pipe, made sanitary engineering possible, saving many lives by preventing diseases such as typhoid, paratyphoid, and gastroenteritis.

### Socioeconomic Influences

Although the Elizabethan poor laws (1601) in England provided a system of relief for the poor, which included infants, sick, and older people, and laborers in the workhouses, a new poor law was enacted in 1834 that was based on the harsher philosophy that regarded pauperism among able-bodied workers as a moral failing. If the worker did not earn a subsistence-level income, the attitude toward that worker was suspicious and punitive. These poor laws were the legal implementation of the Protestant work ethic that the Puritan forebears brought to the United States. According to this view, people are held directly accountable for their state in life, and health maintenance is the responsibility of the individual. The far-reaching implications of this ethic can be seen today in the organization, financing, and delivery of health services.

### Public Health Influences

Edwin Chadwick (1800–90) is known as the father of British and American public health. Chadwick established the English Board of Health, which emphasized environmental sanitation but excluded physicians outside times of crisis. Additionally, Chadwick was Secretary of the Poor Law Commission, which strove to improve the health of the masses for economic reasons. Chadwick's rationale was that disease among the poor was a major factor in their inability to support themselves. Therefore, governmental health and welfare policies have been joined in England since the 19th century.

Lemuel Shattuck, a leader of the public health movement, began the movement in the United States. He used the British system as the model, with public health services and welfare combined, despite the contradictory emphasis. Public health has focused on improving the health of the poor, whereas welfare has dictated subsistence at the minimal level. The influence of the Puritan ethic on the American health care system is apparent in the emphasis on the value of work and the attitude toward the poor. Today, health and welfare departments continue their contradictory approach to the poor.

### Scientific Influences

Until the 20th century, epidemics of infectious disease (plague, cholera, typhoid, smallpox, and influenza) were the most critical health problems and major causes of death and disability for Americans. Scientific advances during the 19th century by Louis Pasteur (germ theory), Robert Koch (origin of bacterial infection), Joseph Lister (antisepsis), and Paul Ehrlich (chemotherapy) expanded public health from its earlier concentration on sanitation to control of communicable diseases through a broad biological base. Public health became an important force in decreasing death rates and increasing life expectancy through the application of bacteriology. International environmental conditions were improved by the development of systems that safeguard water, milk, and food supplies; promote sanitary sewage disposal; and monitor the quality of urban housing.

Between 1936 and 1954 the discovery and use of sulfonamides and other antibiotics to treat bacterial infections reduced the death rate to its lowest point in history, with deaths caused by primary infections reduced to 4%, as compared with 33% only 50 years earlier (in 1886). The death rate did not change significantly between 1954 and the mid-1960s. Another decline in the death rate began after the mid-1960s and has continued (with the exception of a slight increase in 1995) with the control of many infectious diseases (Arias & Smith, 2003). As the life expectancy of the population increases, chronic diseases and comorbidities increase as well. Data from 2013 revealed heart disease, malignant neoplasm, chronic lower respiratory tract disease, unintentional injury, cerebrovascular disease, Alzheimer disease, diabetes, influenza and pneumonia, nephritis, and suicide in descending order are the top 10 leading causes of total death in the United States as reported by the Centers for Disease Control and Prevention (CDC, 2016).

Despite the progress in conquering infectious diseases, in vulnerable populations infections are once again among the top leading contributors to death in the United States. Influenza and pneumonia are the sixth leading cause of death for children aged 1 to 4 years, the seventh for children aged 5 to 9 years, and the eighth for children aged 10 to 14 years. Although not in the top 10 causes of death, some diseases that were thought to be under control, such as measles and TB, are resurfacing and new pathogens are emerging (CDC, 2016).

Some infectious diseases are difficult to eradicate from the population (e.g., TB). The most effective strategy for eliminating TB is to monitor those infected to ensure completion of treatment is by direct observed therapy, which requires the monitoring of a person's medication adherence for first-line drugs for 8 weeks and continuation of treatment for 4 to 7 months. Individuals who do not finish the prescribed medication regimen correctly are at risk of developing resistance to one or more first-line medications. Treatment of drug-resistant TB becomes more complicated and costly, and drug-resistant TB is difficult to eradicate. Resources are needed at local public health departments to provide monitoring and follow-up in this typically elusive TB-infected population. The National TB Surveillance System reports declining TB incidence on average, with 2013 data reporting the lowest number of TB cases in the United States since national reporting began in 1953. This is significant progress since TB cases peaked in 1992. In the United States in 2013, 65% of all TB cases and 90% of multiresistant cases occurred among people born in other countries. As reported by the CDC, in the United States in 2014 there were 2.96 TB cases per 100,000 persons. Foreign-born individuals in the United States had a 13 times higher rate (15.4 cases per 100,000 in 2014) than individuals born in the United States (1.2 cases per 100,000). The rates of TB in ethnic and racial populations differ as well in the United States. Native Hawaiians and other Pacific Islanders (16.9 TB cases per 100,000) and Asians (17.8 cases per 100,000) have the highest rates. Black or African Americans (5.1 cases per 100,000) and American Indians or Alaska Natives and Hispanics or Latinos both have the same rate of 5.0 cases per 100,000, whereas whites are reported to have the lowest rate at 0.6 cases per 100,000. To eliminate TB cases nationally will require adequate local community resources, targeted to groups at risk. Despite the relative low case rates in the United States, TB caused 555 deaths in 2013, up from 510 deaths in 2012 (CDC, 2015).

Globally, TB is the most common infectious disease and one of the world's deadliest diseases, with one-third of the world's population being infected. Major efforts have been put in place for TB prevention, screening, diagnosis, and treatment. WHO estimates 43 million lives were saved between 2000 and 2014 with targeted measures. Despite this progress, in 2014, 1.5 million people (1.1 million HIV positive and 0.4 million HIV negative) died of TB. This includes 140,000 children. TB is the leading cause of death in individuals with HIV. Targeted interventions have been distributed over wide regions of high disease–burdened countries because the risk of infection of the population is more widespread. Regions in Africa, for example, have 28% of the world's cases, with 281 cases for every 100,000 people. Indonesia was estimated to have 1 million new cases in 2014. WHO reported that in 2013, 9 million people around the world

became ill with TB. New strains of drug-resistant TB are now emerging that are resistant not only to isoniazid and rifampin, which are the most effective first-line TB treatment drugs, but also to second-line anti-TB drugs. TB remains an urgent public health problem, with more than 80% of the cases identified in 22 high-burden countries. Global interventions to reduce TB include targeted population- and age-specific interventions such as administration of the bacille Calmette-Guérin (BCG) vaccine to infants and small children in countries where TB is more common. The vaccine is given only if the child has negative TB skin test findings and cannot be separated from adults who are untreated or ineffectively treated for TB (CDC, 2015; WHO, 2015).

An effective, comprehensive public health system is imperative to enable the United States to respond to local, national, and global concerns. As new diseases emerge, older diseases reemerge (sometimes in drug-resistant forms), and natural and man-made disasters occur, a functioning public health system is warranted. The ACA calls for the establishment of a council within the USDHHS to be known as the National Prevention, Health Promotion, and Public Health Council, required to provide coordination and leadership at the federal level among all federal departments and agencies. The council is charged with obtaining input from relative stakeholders to develop a plan to improve the health status of Americans and reduce the incidence of preventable disease, disability, and illness, which will require the integration and coordination of many of the divisions of the USDHHS (Office of the Legislative Council, 2010). The CDC is the frontline agency for providing national health security and must remain vigilant in rapidly detecting and controlling disease outbreaks in the United States and abroad. The CDC's Emergency Operations Center is the command center for monitoring and coordinating emergency response to public health threats in the United States and worldwide, such as pandemic influenza, natural disasters, and terrorist attacks. Recent global outbreaks of the Hendra virus (1994); H5N1 bird flu (1997); Nipah virus (1999); severe acute respiratory syndrome–associated coronavirus (2003); monkey pox, mad cow disease, and avian flu (2006); H1N1 (2009); and Ebola (2014) pose challenges to global public health (CDC Foundation, 2012, 2016). According to the CDC, influenza pandemic occurs approximately three times a century, and in 1918 a severe influenza pandemic killed about 1% of those who contracted the influenza. When the bird flu virus H5N1 emerged in 1997, the CDC and others began tracking the novel form of influenza, fearing a potential pandemic. Because about 60% of individuals who contracted bird flu died, concern heightened when another influenza virus, H1N1, was first recognized in Mexico in 2009. The virus was identified as influenza A, H1N1, the same virus responsible for the 1918 Spanish influenza pandemic, which was responsible for 50 million deaths. Fearing another deadly pandemic, the CDC took quick actions and developed a vaccine that was distributed to as many Americans as possible, targeting infants, young adults, and pregnant women. Although the H1N1 flu outbreak of 2009 (known also as swine flu) killed 12,500 individuals, millions of Americans were protected against H1N1, preventing thousands of hospitalizations and deaths. The CDC remains on constant alert for new, deadly influenza viruses and other airborne diseases (CDC Foundation, 2012, 2016).

## Special Population Influences

The second goal of *Healthy People 2020*, as previously stated, is to achieve health equity, eliminate disparities, and improve the health of all groups. Vulnerable populations, especially those living in poverty, are at great risk of experiencing health disparities (USDHHS, Office of Minority Health, 2012). For many of these disadvantaged people, the issues of preventing disease and promoting good health are often secondary to the problems associated with everyday survival. Determinants of health in a population are related strongly to socioeconomic status and education level, with populations in the lower strata having worse outcomes. However, individual lifestyle behaviors, including dietary choices, level of physical activity, use of alcohol and tobacco, substance abuse, and risky sexual behavior, play a significant role in the health status of an individual. Access to health care for prevention, early detection, and treatment is paramount in diminishing health disparities, but programs promoting positive individual lifestyle behaviors are also needed (USDHHS, Office of Minority Health, 2012) (Box 3-3: Diversity Awareness).

## Political and Economic Influences

Political and economic considerations influence the health care system, and politics determines the decision makers who will negotiate a desired outcome. Economics defines the resources that are distributed and the manner in which they are distributed. The effect of economics and politics on the delivery of health care is illustrated by the situation in the United States following the Great Depression. Roosevelt's New Deal had an effect on health care, specifically in the passage of the Social Security Act in 1935, which authorized grants-in-aid to individual states to improve state and local public health programs. Funds were available for categorical assistance programs, with cash grants first given to needy blind and older individuals and later to disabled people. Medical care, through subsequent amendments, was an allowable budget item, but payments were often distributed for food, shelter, or other needs. Later, the Social Security Act resulted in the development of programs such as Medicaid and Medicare.

## Split Between Preventive and Curative Measures

The link between environmental health and personal medical care developed when sanitarians (people who work to maintain

---

🌐 **BOX 3-3  DIVERSITY AWARENESS**

### *Health and Human Services Action Plan to Reduce Racial and Ethnic Health Disparities*

**Community-Driven Approach to Reduce Health Disparities in the United States**

As a nation, health equity does not exist especially among racial and ethnic populations. Health disparities, as discussed in the report, are differences in health outcomes that are closely linked with social, economic, and environmental disadvantage, which are often driven by the social conditions in which individuals live, learn, work, and play. Marked differences in social determinants, such as poverty, low socioeconomic status, and lack of access to care, exist along racial and ethnic lines, leading to poor health outcomes. The economic burden between 2003 and 2006 attributable to health disparities was estimated to be $1.24 trillion. The major dimensions of racial and ethnic health disparities outlined are:

- Lack of insurance negatively affects the quality of health care received by minorities. One-third of the population consists of racial and ethnic minorities but constitutes more than half of the 50 million individuals without health insurance.
- Minorities are overrepresented among the 56 million people in the United States who have inadequate access to a primary care physician. Minority children are less likely than non-Hispanic white children to have a usual source of care.
- Racial and ethnic minorities often receive poorer quality of care and face more barriers in seeking care, including preventive care, acute treatment, and chronic disease management, than non-Hispanic whites.
- African Americans have higher hospitalization rates from influenza than other populations, and African American children are more than four times as likely to die of asthma as non-Hispanic white children. Higher obesity rates in the African American population contribute to the onset of diabetes, hypertension, and cardiovascular disease.

As the demographics of the United States continue to become more diverse, nurses need to be culturally competent as one strategy for eliminating racial and ethnic disparities. In the 2004 IOM report titled *In the Nation's Compelling Interest: Ensuring Diversity in Health Care Workforce*, diversity in the workforce was a key element of patient-centered care. Efforts to match the ethnic and racial composition of the health care workforce with the US population will contribute to addressing health disparities. Providers who speak a second language will also be needed because 24 million adults have limited English proficiency. Shortages of primary care providers in underserved areas significantly affect the health of ethnic and racial minorities. The primary care nurse practitioner is ideally suited to care for underserved populations in urban and rural areas. Additional funds from the ACA are funding Communities Putting Prevention to Work programs, which support statewide and community-based policy and environmental changes in nutrition, physical activity, tobacco control, and other factors that harm people's health. *Healthy People 2020* provides a comprehensive set of 10-year national goals and objectives with 42 topic areas and more than 600 evolving objectives. The leading health indicators outline high-priority health issues. One of the goals is to ensure that federal, state, tribal, and local health agencies have the necessary infrastructure to effectively provide essential public health services. A capable and qualified workforce, up-to-date data and information services, and public health agencies capable of assessing and responding to public health needs are three components necessary for an effective public health infrastructure (USDHHS, 2011). Nurses can play key roles as educators and providers of care in their communities to meet the needs of vulnerable populations and close the health disparity gap.

Sources US Department of Health and Human Services, Office of Minority Health. (2012). HHS action plan to reduce racial and ethnic health disparities. http://www.minorityhealth.hhs.gov/npa/templates/content.aspx; US Department of Health and Human Services (USDHHS). (2011). *Healthy People 2020*: Leading health indicators. http://www.healthypeople.gov/2020/LHI/data/.

a clean environment) realized that their efforts alone were not sufficient to prevent and cure the diseases of the population as a whole; improvement of personal health was also necessary. Early preventive services directed toward individuals originated in medical practice rather than public health but were limited to welfare medicine (caring for individuals through state programs). Community health centers that developed in America before World War I limited their scope to prevention and health education and, with the exception of some prenatal clinics, were generally located in poor neighborhoods. Delivery of preventive services developed separately from clinical medicine and became associated with public health. Most physicians, educated in hospitals, were interested in individuals for whom prevention had failed and whose illnesses brought them to the hospital ward.

Despite the separation of preventive and treatment services, the benefits of prevention were eventually incorporated into clinical medicine for individuals. Preventive and early detection measures became a part of pediatrics and obstetrics during the early part of the 20th century, when vaccines and vaginal cytology examinations became available and accepted. Later in the 20th century, internal medicine incorporated early detection of diseases such as diabetes, glaucoma, obesity, and hypertension. A shift to preventive medicine for the individual occurred, but the separate educational programs for public health and medicine still divided these areas. Not until the 1960s did the emphasis begin to turn from individual to societal values (Freyman, 1980).

This new emphasis on societal values parallels another evolution in the role of health in society. Greater governmental involvement in financing the health care delivery system has improved access to health care for many populations. Technological developments include computerized medical records, which should improve access to care through better communication with laboratories, primary care offices, hospitals, and care delivery agencies. The Patient Protection and Affordable Care Act (PPACA) of 2010, more commonly known as ACA, reformed certain aspects of the private health insurance industry and public health programs, increases coverage for individuals with preexisting conditions, and expands access to insurance for a projected 30 million more Americans (Office of the Legislative Council, 2010). This sweeping mandate extends a heavy layer of federal and state oversight, and since 2014 requires most Americans to obtain or purchase health insurance through a public or private plan, significantly diminishing the number of individuals who are uninsured.

## ORGANIZATION OF THE DELIVERY SYSTEM

The health care delivery system in the United States is a mammoth system composed of a network of public and private interrelated and in some cases overlapping components, designed to provide health care to the American people. The structure and financing of the health care delivery system is a system of multifaceted and complex interrelationship involving providers, consumers, and settings, with both the private sector and the public sector providing services. The public sector includes voluntary and nonprofit agencies, and official or governmental agencies. The

USDHHS is the principal federal regulatory agency whose mission is to enhance and protect the health and well-being of all Americans by providing effective health and human services and fostering advances in medicine, public health, and social services (USDHHS, n.d.b). Delivery of services is organized on three levels in both sectors: local, state, and national. Each of the three levels consists of private providers combined with official or voluntary public agencies. The nurse is often the professional who assists the health consumer to navigate throughout the complex delivery system; therefore a basic understanding of the system's organization is essential.

### Private Sector
#### Independent Practice

Traditionally, a person enters the health care delivery system by contracting directly with a health care provider for individual care on a fee-for-service basis. Free choice of the provider has been the hallmark of the American free-market system. However, more recently physicians and other health care providers have been working within managed health care organizations. Although private practice traditionally has been disease oriented, the current emphasis on primary care necessitates a much broader perspective. Primary care involves continual and comprehensive care that includes efforts to keep people as healthy as possible and to prevent disease.

Private care may be delivered in numerous settings, from inpatient (hospital or extended care facility) to outpatient (ambulatory) settings. Outpatient care is defined as any health care services that are not provided on the basis of an overnight stay in which room and board costs are incurred. Ambulatory settings include two major categories: care provided by owners and providers and care provided in service settings (Box 3-4). These categories overlap because many providers practice in their own offices and contract with one or more managed care organizations.

---

### BOX 3-4    Types of Ambulatory Care Settings

- *Owner provider:* Hospitals, community health agencies, managed care organizations, home health organizations, insurance agencies
- *Service settings:* Hospital-based clinics/centers, solo or group medical practices, ambulatory surgery and diagnostic procedure centers, telehealth service environments, university and community hospital clinics, military and settings within the Department of Veterans Affairs, nurse-managed clinics, managed care organizations, colleges and educational institutions, free-standing community facilities, care coordination organizations, walk-in clinics (some clinics are free clinics where patient-centered care can be provided for minimal or no fee—these types of clinics are an important safety net for vulnerable populations), urgent care centers, outpatient surgery centers, chemotherapy and radiation therapy centers, dialysis centers, neighborhood and community health centers, diagnostic and mobile imaging centers, occupational health centers, women's health clinics, wound care centers, fitness-wellness centers, health department clinics, nursing centers

Source American Academy of Ambulatory Care Nursing. (2011). *Definition of professional ambulatory care nursing report March 8, 2011.* Sudbury, MA: Jones & Bartlett.

Nursing centers are nurse-managed health centers, often situated in medically underserved rural and urban areas that primarily serve vulnerable populations in the provision of primary care to individuals and families. Nursing centers trace their origin to the Henry Street Settlement for the sick and poor of New York City, founded by Lillian Wald in 1893 and another visionary, Margaret Sanger, who opened the nation's first birth control clinic. The modern movement to establish nursing centers began in 1965 when the nurse practitioner role was created, which allowed nurses to provide primary care to individuals and families. Nursing centers (ambulatory care centers, family practice nursing centers, community nursing centers, and birthing centers) have provided high-quality nursing care from certified nurse midwives, nurse practitioners, and other advanced practice nurses (APNs). A number of nursing centers are academic nursing centers, established to provide nursing services to communities, learning experiences for students, and settings for faculty practice and research. The key components of a community nursing center include the following: a nurse as chief manager; a nursing staff that is accountable and responsible for care and professional practice; and nurses as the primary providers of care. Using a multidisciplinary collaboration framework, nurses have the opportunity to provide comprehensive primary care services, including a focus on wellness and health promotion, public health programs, and targeted interventions for populations with special needs. The Institute for Nursing Centers is a network of organizations whose focus is to promote and enhance the work of nursing centers by providing educational programs as well as a national repository of data for nurse-managed health centers funded by the W.K. Kellogg Foundation. Members of the Institute for Nursing Centers also provide mentoring and consultation to support colleagues in developing and advancing nursing centers (Institute for Nursing Centers, n.d.). The ACA specifically addresses nurse-managed health centers, describing them as a nurse practice arrangement managed by APNs who provide primary or wellness services to underserved or vulnerable populations.

Advanced practice nurses (APNs), an umbrella term for master's or doctoral prepared nurses who practice in the roles of nurse practitioners, clinical nurse specialists, nurse midwives, or nurse anesthetists, are well suited to provide cost-effective, quality care to individuals and their families, as well as to serve economically disadvantaged and vulnerable populations. APNs not only have specialized clinical knowledge and skills at the master's or doctoral level but also have pursued an advanced curriculum that includes research and theoretical foundations to determine best practices, evaluate health policy issues, and understand the intricacies of the health care system and financial management. Nurse practitioners play a key role within the health care system and often care for vulnerable populations in rural areas and inner cities, as well as practice in primary, acute, and long-term care settings.

## Move to Managed Care

Before the 1990s the traditional means for paying for health care was with indemnity insurance plans. A person would choose a physician or care provider and receive care, and the provider would either bill the individual's insurance company or be paid on a fee-for-service basis. Each separate service generated a professional fee, and the provider would receive payments directly from the insurance plan; alternatively, the individual would pay the provider, file an insurance claim for each covered expense, and receive reimbursement. The provider had autonomy to treat the person without oversight from the insurance company. In a traditional fee-for-service insurance system, there are no incentives to constrain cost and care (Barr, 2011). In an effort to control costs, managed care began to regulate the use of health care. Physicians or physician groups contracted with an insurance company for a negotiated fee-for-service, usually at a discounted rate. Today, managed care plans include a network of individual providers or physician groups, and individuals who choose to seek care from health care providers within their network usually have full coverage with or without a copayment. Individuals who choose health care providers outside the managed care network may not be covered, may be covered for a lesser amount, and or may have additional copayment costs, and thus face greater out-of-pocket expenses. Within the network, a person has a primary care provider who serves as a gatekeeper and is the foundation of the managed care concept in controlling health care costs within the organization. The primary care provider may be a physician, a physician assistant, or an APN. Physician primary care providers are usually general or family practitioners, but they may also be internists, pediatricians, or obstetrician-gynecologists. Physician assistants are educated and prepared to work under the direct supervision of physicians, whereas APNs who serve as primary care providers are typically nurse practitioners or certified nurse midwives. The term "gatekeeper" is a common managed care term, and the primary care provider has the role to coordinate and oversee an individual's care. The principal force behind the growth of managed care is the belief that health care costs can be controlled by managing the way in which health care is delivered and costs can be controlled because providers of care must be careful to provide only care that is absolutely necessary. Managed care plans are arranged agreements with a group of physicians, hospitals, and other health care providers to provide care at a certain cost (Barr, 2011). The gatekeeper concept is designed to manage the individual's use of resources, to reduce self-referral to specialists, and to protect the individual from unnecessary procedures and overtreatment (Shi & Singh, 2013). Decreasing hospital admission rates, readmittance to acute care, and costly procedures as well as limiting an individual's ability to self-refer to specialists is designed to achieve successful containment of health care costs. An oversupply of physician specialists has occurred in some areas, and a lack of primary care providers occurs in many rural areas; thus nurse practitioners are well suited to provide primary care. Providers of specialty care typically earn higher salaries than primary care providers, making career selection in a specialty area more attractive. Box 3-5 provides a glossary of key terms used in managed care.

## Health Maintenance Organizations

Health maintenance organizations (HMOs) deliver comprehensive health maintenance and treatment services to a group of enrolled individuals who prepay a fixed fee. The HMO accepts

## BOX 3-5   A Glossary of Managed Care Terms

*Access to health care:* The degree to which individuals are inhibited or facilitated in their ability to gain entry to and to receive care and services from the health care system.

*Beneficiary:* Any person, either a subscriber or a dependent, eligible for service under a health plan.

*Benefits:* The dollar amount available for the cost of covered medical services.

*Blue Cross/Blue Shield:* A combined medical plan offered through a worker's place of employment that combines both hospital and physician coverage.

*Capitation:* A fixed amount of payment per individual, per year, regardless of the volume or cost of the services each client requires.

*Copayments:* A fixed dollar payment that is made by the individual to the provider at the time of service.

*Cost sharing:* Provision of an insurance policy that requires the insured to pay some portion of the covered expenses (does not refer to or include the cost of the premium).

*Deductible:* A fixed dollar amount that the individual must pay before reimbursement begins.

*Gatekeeper:* A physician or advanced practice nurse who provides primary care and who makes referrals for emergency services or specialty care.

*Health care policy:* Decisions, usually developed by government policymakers, for determining present and future objectives pertaining to the health care system.

*Health maintenance organization (HMO):* A prepaid health plan delivering comprehensive care to members through designated providers, having a fixed monthly payment for health care services, and requiring members to be in a plan for a specified period.

*Indemnity:* Monies paid by an insurer to a provider, in a predetermined amount in the event of a covered loss by a beneficiary.

*Independent practice association (IPA):* An organization that physicians in private practice can join so that the organization can represent them in the negotiation of managed care contracts.

*Managed care:* A health care plan that integrates the financing and delivery of health care services by using arrangements with selected health care providers to provide services for covered individuals. Plans are generally financed by capitation fees. There are significant financial incentives for members of the plan to use the health care providers associated with the plan.

*Out-of-pocket expenditures:* The portion of medical expenses an individual is responsible for paying includes all health care goods and services, co-insurance fees, deductibles, and any amounts not covered as part of a health insurance plan (premiums paid for health insurance are counted as health insurance).

*Point-of-service (POS) plan:* A plan that contains elements of both HMOs and PPOs. They resemble HMOs for in-network services in that they both require copayments and a primary care physician. Services received outside the network are usually reimbursed on a fee-for-service basis

*Preferred provider organization (PPO):* A health plan generally consisting of hospital and physician providers. The PPO provides health care services to plan members usually at discounted rates in return for expedited claims payment.

*Primary care:* Basic health care that emphasizes general health needs rather than specialized care.

*Primary care provider:* A physician or APN who provides basic and routine health care services usually in an office or clinic.

*Reimbursement:* Payment of services. Payment of providers by a third-party insurer or government health program for health care services.

*Self-insured plan:* Plan offered by employers and other groups that directly assume the major cost of health insurance for their employees or members.

*Third-party payer:* In health care finance, this is an insurance carrier, Medicare, and Medicaid or their government-contracted intermediary, managed-care organization, or health plan that pays for hospital or medical bills instead of the individual.

*Underinsured:* Refers to people who have some type of health insurance, such as catastrophic care, but not enough insurance to cover all their health care costs.

*Uninsured:* Individuals or groups with no or inadequate health insurance coverage.

*Utilization review:* Evaluation of the necessity, appropriateness, and efficiency of the use of health care services, procedures, and facilities.

Source US National Library of Medicine, National Institutes of Health. Health economics information resources: A self-study course. http://www.nlm.nih.gov/nichsr/edu/healthecon/glossary.html.

responsibility for the organization, financing, and delivery of health care services for all enrolled members. Several HMO models have evolved. The traditional HMO structure was a group or staff model, in which the HMO owns the hospital and employs a group of physicians and some specialty services to provide care to its members. Salaried providers generally spent all of their time serving members of the HMO, with no financial incentive to provide more care. An example is Kaiser Permanente Health Care System, which also has its own hospitals. A capitation method of payment is used in which a service provider receives a fixed amount per person (the capitation rate) and in turn agrees to provide all necessary care to each enrolled member. The employer pays a monthly or annual rate directly to the HMO. The individual may also have out-of-pocket expenses such as copayments. Staff models were described as *closed panel,* because employed physicians provided care only for members of the HMO. A community physician (physician or health care provider outside the HMO) could not care for a member of the HMO without prearrangement or authorization by the HMO. In an HMO plan, individuals pay low out-of-pocket expenses

but must see a primary care provider first to be referred to a specialist. In a group-model HMO, the organization operates a health plan but contracts with groups of physicians and hospitals to provide care. The medical group receives a share of the capitation rate received by the HMO, and the group agrees to provide all necessary physician services for the member. The physician can be paid by salary or on a fee-for-service basis. An independent practice association (IPA) HMO will be discussed later. For all types of HMOs, a fixed amount of money is available each year for health care, based on the capitation fee and the number of members enrolled (Barr, 2011). Medicare enrollees since the 1970s have been offered the option of enrolling in fee-for-service or HMO plans. An earlier health reform law, the Medicare Modernization Act of 2003, renamed the program to include Medicare Advantage plans.

### Medicare Advantage Plans

Medicare Advantage plans are private health plans that are offered as an alternative to the traditional Medicare program and are available to 99% of Medicare beneficiaries. Those who enroll in a Medicare Advantage plan pay for the Part B premium (less any rebate if offered by the Medicare Advantage plan) and may pay an additional monthly Medicare Advantage plan premium for benefits and prescription drug coverage. The selected Medicare Advantage plan receives federal payments from Medicare for each enrollee. In 2015, 17 million Medicare beneficiaries were enrolled in 1 of more than 2000 plans offered that differ nationwide. Two-thirds of Medicare Advantage plans are HMOs. The KFF reports that the average beneficiary is able to choose from among 19 plans, with those living in metropolitan areas having a greater number of plans to choose from than those living in nonmetropolitan areas as the number of firms offering plans differs by location. Most Medicare Advantage plans (87% of plans in 2016) offer prescription drug coverage (MA-PD). Medicare beneficiaries who enroll in Medicare Advantage plans often have extra benefits such as vision, hearing, dental, and wellness plans when compared with those in the traditional Medicare program. In 2015 the average monthly premium for a Medicare Advantage plan HMO in 2015 was $39, for regional preferred provider organizations (PPOs) was $75.00, and for local PPOs was $79.00. Some Medicare Advantage plans have no additional monthly premium other than Medicare Part B premium and are called "zero premium plans." It is projected that approximately 80% of all Medicare beneficiaries will have access to some type of a zero-premium plan by the year 2016 which limits some out-of-pocket expenses as reported by the KFF. Members in the traditional Medicare program have no out-of-pocket limits under Medicare Part A and Part B, and thus have unlimited financial liability. Those who enroll in a Medicare Advantage plan have out-of-pocket expenses for services covered in Part A and Part B limited to no more than $6700 for services received from in-network providers. The out-of-pocket expense amount listed does not include expenses for prescription drugs or extra benefits not covered by the plan. The quality of a Medicare Advantage plan is rated at the contract level by a star system (one to five) with one star representing a poor rating, three stars representing an average rating, and five stars representing excellent performance. The CMS has assigned a star rating since 2012, and plans with high ratings receive higher rebate amounts. For example, plans rated with four or more stars receive 5% bonuses. Bonus percentages are doubled in some counties. Medicare members must select and enroll in a plan during the open enrollment period, but if a plan is rated five star, beneficiaries can enroll in those plans year round (KFF, 2015b). Selecting a Medicare Advantage plan that best fits the needs of an individual can be very confusing, especially since plan benefits change from year to year and the health care needs of an individual may change as well.

## Independent Practice Associations

Independent practice associations (IPAs) are organizations composed of independent physicians in solo or group practices who provide health care services to members of an HMO in their private offices, eliminating the expense of the staff model HMO, which furnished and owned the facility in which care was provided. The HMO for a fee-for-service or a prepaid price can purchase hospital care and specialty services not within the IPA. Physicians in an IPA contract may be restricted to caring only for members enrolled in the IPA, but some contracts may allow providers to care for nonmembers as well. Other variations of the staff model and IPAs exist. In a group practice model, an HMO contracts with all physicians and specialists needed by the HMO enrollees, but physicians remain independent. Some contracts are exclusive, requiring physicians to restrict care to members of an individual HMO, and other variations allow physicians to care for members outside the HMO. In a network model, HMOs contract with individual physicians and with physician groups for both primary and specialty services. The HMO maintains control over fee arrangements (Barr, 2011).

## Accountable Care Organizations

Accountable care organizations (ACOs) are key components in the ACA. ACOs in structure will be similar to traditional HMOs that are responsible for the quality and cost of care delivered to a defined population. An organization, either public or private, would be created that has a group of primary care physicians, providers, specialists, and hospitalist to provide health care in a local area. Physicians would accept the responsibility for the quality of care provided and the overall costs of delivering care to a defined population of individuals (Kovner & Knickman, 2015). In the ACA, ACOs will become an important part of Medicare reform. An ACO that serves a person in the Medicare system will be required to be composed of physicians, specialists, and hospitals that manage the health needs of a minimum number of Medicare beneficiaries for a specified period. ACOs will have financial incentives in place to encourage providers to keep health care costs low by not ordering unnecessary tests and procedures, and by focusing on prevention and treatment of individuals with chronic disease out of the hospital. Performance and savings benchmarks would be in place with a financial reward system as well as penalties.

## Concierge Medical Practices (Retainer Medicine)

According to an Accountability Office (2005) report to congressional committees and Concierge Medicine Today, concierge care is a newer model for providing primary care in a medical practice in which physicians charge individuals a membership fee averaging $1500 to $5500 per year in return for enhanced health care services or amenities. Approximately 12,000 physicians operate concierge-type practices, and 80% of concierge physicians accept insurance, whereas others are cash only. Amenities most often include same-day or next-day appointments for nonurgent care, 24-hour telephone/e-mail access to the physician, and routine periodic preventive examinations. Some concierge physicians do not accept insurance, but others report billing a person's health insurance for covered services and Medicare. Individuals electing to join a concierge practice are encouraged to have health care insurance for services used outside the practice, such as specialty care, complex diagnostics, and hospitalization. Although there is wide variation in the amenities offered, no–waiting time office visits, 24-hour access to physicians via cell phones and e-mail, same-day office appointments, and even the possibility of a house call serve as attractive incentives for individuals and families. Some medical issues can be handled digitally, with patient assessments made by phone images and e-mails, avoiding the need for an office visit. Physicians who provide concierge care typically care for fewer people (600 or fewer, compared with an average load of 2500 plus), allowing physicians more time to spend with each person and to provide expanded preventive services and practice amenities that are not available in a traditional practice. Concierge physicians typically treats 6 to 10 individuals per day, and according to Concierge Medicine Today's physician compensation report for 2014, earn on average the same salary as physicians in traditional medical offices. Fifty-seven percent of concierge physicians earn $300,000 or more and 23% earn $200,000 to $300,000 annually (Concierge Medicine Today, n.d.). Physician salaries are predominately derived from membership fees, and for those that except insurance, from insurance companies. The average profile of an individual in a concierge practice is upper middle class (household earnings $125,000 to $250,000 annually), and aged 50 years or older, although individuals and families with lower incomes may select concierge care for the convenience of high-quality holistic care. The number of concierge medical care practices is growing slowly, and they are not available in all areas, but there are those who oppose a model of care that favors the affluent receiving high-quality care. The shortages of primary care providers in traditional practices limits access to primary care at a time when the ACA has increased the number of insured individuals and families. If a physician leaves a traditional practice setting and begins a concierge practice, previous patients must find a new provider, which is problematic in areas where there is a shortage of providers. Physicians who choose concierge practice over traditional primary care offices report more time off, less paperwork, need for fewer office staff, and overall higher professional satisfaction as they are able to spend more time with patients. Additional time allows personalized service and the ability to provide holistic care. In turn, cost savings may be realized with a reduction in chronic disease or complications of disease, reduction in the need for emergency department visits, and reduction in the need for hospitalization and specialty visits (Concierge Medicine Today, n.d.).

## Hospitalist Movement

Responding to the same impetus that spurred managed care in outpatient settings, hospitalist programs—supported by HMOs, hospitals, and medical groups—were formed to control hospital costs without compromising quality or satisfaction with client care. Hospitalists are physicians or APNs whose professional focus is managing the comprehensive care of the hospitalized individual, providing direct inpatient primary, critical, and consultative care 24 hours a day. Hospitalists engage in clinical care, teaching, research, and leadership in the field of hospital medicine and meeting the needs of hospitalized patients with acute and chronic complex diseases. Hospitalists enhance the quality and safety of care of a patient within the hospital setting and the safe transitioning of care from the acute care hospital setting to post–acute care facilities or home. Studies have found that hospitals with a hospitalist model program have improved both the quality and the safety of care, with reduced lengths of stay, readmission rates, mortality rates, and complication rates, with efficient use of hospital and health care resources (Society of Hospital Medicine, n.d.).

## Point-of-Service Plans

Point-of-service (POS) plans evolved in response to concern about restrictions of consumer choice in selecting providers and services. POS plans allow members, for an additional fee and higher copayment, to use providers outside the individual HMO network. Members can choose to pay for this enhanced POS or stay within the HMO network for reduced copayments. If the individual receives care from a physician or hospital not within the list of providers or hospitals, the person pays a substantial portion of the cost of care, usually as out-of-pocket expenses.

## High-Deductible Health Insurance Plans

High-deductible health insurance plans (HDHPs) are structured similarly to traditional managed care plans and fee-for-service plans but have a very high annual out-of-pocket deductibles of $1000 or greater for individual coverage. A growing number of employers are offering these types of plans, and for those individuals who are generally healthy, the low monthly premium is an attractive option compared with the cost of other types of employer insurance plans. Plans usually have a set annual out-of-pocket limit. Attached to these plans, an employer can offer health savings accounts (HSAs) or savings options. Typically, an employer will make quarterly or annual deposits into the individual's health savings account, and the employee can elect to have additional funds withheld on a pretax basis to be deposited into the account, up to the annual Internal Revenue Service maximum. Individuals can withdraw money from the account at any age for health-related expenditures. The remaining money in the fund can be withdrawn at retirement without penalty. Most high-deductible health insurance plans are paired with in-network providers for additional savings. Some plans allow preventive services (e.g., adult physical examinations, cancer screenings, mammograms, routine gynecological visits, and well-child care) for no charge if an in-network provider is used. Office visits for sickness, laboratory tests, emergency and urgent care, and hospitalizations are covered all or in part after the deductible has been met. Because the annual out-of-pocket expenses are high, until the deductible has been met, individuals may decide to delay or not seek health care.

## Preferred Provider Organizations

Preferred provider organizations (PPOs) are a type of managed care plan in the private sector that has a preselected list of providers who have agreed to provide health services for those individuals enrolled in the plan. Contracted providers in the PPO agree to deliver services to members for a fee-for-service prenegotiated rate, which is usually discounted. To control costs, members must receive care exclusively from providers within the PPO or incur additional costs if a provider outside the PPO is used. Individuals are typically required to pay a copayment each time services are given. If an individual chooses to see a provider outside the PPO, he or she will pay additional costs. To control costs, the provider must receive preauthorization from the PPO for a member to be hospitalized or for some procedures or tests, and second opinions are usually required before major procedures or surgical operations are performed.

The KFF conducts an annual survey that reveals the distribution of the health plan type for individuals enrolled in employer health plans. Some employers, often those that are large, offer a variety of health plans to their employees. The distribution of health plan enrollment for covered workers reveals that 52% of workers have been enrolled in employer PPO plans, 24% of covered workers are enrolled in a high-deductible health insurance plan with a savings option, 14% are enrolled in an HMO, and 10% are enrolled in a POS plan, with 1% in a conventional or indemnity plan. POS plans were more popular among small firms, and PPOs were more popular for covered workers at large firms (KFF, 2015b).

## Public Sector

The public sector contains official and voluntary public health agencies operating at the local, state, federal, and international levels. Before 1900, public health was concerned with problems related to environmental risks and infectious diseases. After the 1900s the public health agenda expanded to address the needs of children and mothers. By midcentury, treating chronic disease had also been added to the agenda. As the century progressed, public health issues came to include substance abuse, mental illness, teenage pregnancy, long-term care, epidemics of violence and/or HIV/AIDS, and most recently bioterrorism and disaster preparedness (Nies & McEwen, 2014).

### Source of Power

The US Constitution is based on the sharing of sovereign power between federal and state governments. The powers of the federal government in relation to health are not delineated specifically in the US Constitution; they are derived from its authority to tax and to spend for the general welfare and from powers delegated to it by the states. The state governor or legislature usually appoints a health commissioner or secretary of health, who directs the health agency (usually the public health department) to protect citizens from communicable diseases and environmental hazards from waste, water, and food (Nies & McEwen, 2014). State health authority is based also on the Tenth Amendment, which reserves for the states, or for the people, those powers not delegated to the federal government by the US Constitution. The states then use their powers to create local governments and delegate authority to them in health matters. The US Public Health Service falls within the larger USDHHS. Box 3-6 lists the federal Public Health Service agencies within the USDHHS.

### Influence of Political Philosophy

The prevailing political philosophy regarding societal health needs affects the relationship among federal, state, and local governments. Although the federal government gained power to promote health and welfare in the early 20th century by the passage of the Sixteenth Amendment (giving it the authority to levy federal taxes), states retained sovereign power because the resources were distributed at the state and local levels. Beginning in the 1930s, however, New Deal philosophy began to displace power from the state and local governments to the federal government. Passage of the Hill-Burton Act of 1946 and establishment of what is now known as the CDC increased the federal

**BOX 3-6  The Department of Health and Human Services**

*The Federal Public Health Service Agencies*

Agency for Healthcare Research and Quality: Federal agency whose mission is to improve the quality, safety, efficiency, and effectiveness of health care for all Americans. Supports research with grants and funding.

*Centers for Disease Control and Prevention (CDC):* Working with states, it provides a system of health surveillance to monitor and prevent outbreaks of disease.

*Centers for Medicare & Medicaid Services (CMS):* Federal agency that runs the Medicare program and works with states to run the Medicaid program.

*Children's Health Insurance Program (CHIP) (Title XIX and Title XXI):* CHIP is a joint federal and state program that provides insurance for families who do not have health insurance and are not eligible for Medicaid.

*Food and Drug Administration (FDA):* Federal agency responsible for protecting the public, which includes ensuring foods are safe, wholesome, sanitary, and properly labeled; guaranteeing human and veterinary drugs, vaccines, and other biological products and medical devices intended for human use are safe and effective; protecting the public from electronic product radiation; ensuring cosmetics and dietary supplements are safe and properly labeled; and regulating tobacco products.

*Health Resources and Services Administration:* Primary federal agency for improving access to health care services for people who are uninsured, or medically vulnerable.

*Indian Health Service:* Responsible for providing federal health services to American Indians and Alaska Natives (approximately 1.9 million individuals) who belong to 556 federally recognized tribes in 35 states.

*National Institutes of Health (NIH):* Provides leadership and direction to programs designed to improve the health of the nation by conducting and supporting research. NIH funds basic, clinical, and translational biomedical and behavior research.

*Office of the Inspector General:* Office dedicated to combating fraud, waste, and abuse and to improving the efficiency of USDHHS programs. Provides oversight of Medicaid and Medicare, the CDC, the NIH, and the FDA

*Substance Abuse and Mental Health Services Administration:* Strengthens the nation's health care capacity to provide prevention, diagnosis, and treatment services for substance abuse and mental illness. Funds mental health and substance abuse prevention and treatment services

Source US Department of Health and Human Services Public Health Service Agencies Overview and Funding. October 13, 2015 CRS Report. http://www.FY2010-2016fas.org.

government's power over state and local affairs. The trend toward increased federal government involvement continued during the Kennedy-Johnson era, when the government focused on societal needs and health care to an unprecedented degree. During the Nixon-Ford era, the trend began to reverse as a New Federalism movement called for less federal encroachment into states' responsibilities and greater state and local responsibility. Clearly, the federal government's role varies according to political philosophy.

During the 1980s the Reagan administration supported free-market competition among insurance plans, physicians, and hospitals to offer the best possible services with the lowest price. Reagan was adamant in his opposition to adopting national health insurance legislation for what he labeled "socialized medicine." Reagan's procompetition policies supported a decrease in federal responsibility for health care, preferring to give states power by providing block grants and control at the state level.

During the Bush administration (1989–1993), incremental steps occurred in moving new legislation toward health care reform with a system of checks and balances in place so that no single political party controlled the White House, Senate, and House of Representatives. To avoid increasing taxes, President Bush proposed a system of tax deductions or tax credits to reduce the cost of private health insurance for families not covered by Medicaid or Medicare. Bush proposed the creation of large networks of small businesses to purchase group health insurance for their employees, voluntary measures to reduce insurance paperwork, encouragement of enrollment in HMOs, and legislation to reduce medical malpractice suits. Because of an economic recession, many workers employed by small businesses did not have employer health insurance plans, and these measures would have assisted in covering working families. However, congressional Democrats refused to support the proposed reform because it did not include an expansion of federal power with a plan for universal coverage or control over the growing cost of insurance premiums.

In 1993 the Clinton administration proposed the Health Security Act to achieve universal health care coverage in the United States by mandating that all employers provide health insurance for their employees and by giving small businesses and unemployed Americans subsidies with which to purchase insurance. The plan met severe opposition from the insurance industry and the business community. Mass media advertisements by these stakeholders questioned whether or not HMOs would provide choice and access to health care services. Large segments of the American public, especially the 80% who had employer-based private health insurance, began to fear being forced into HMOs, which would diminish their choice of, access to, and quality of health care. The cost of a socialized, universal health care coverage system was estimated to reach trillion-dollar levels. The act was defeated in Congress, and a time of political caution followed, stalling any further movement toward universal health care. Small incremental health reform was passed such as the portability of health care coverage in 1996 (Health Insurance Portability and Accountability Act [HIPAA]), allowing persons to access health care throughout the United States, and the focus shifted to balancing the federal budget. Other incremental legislation included the passage of the Balanced Budget Act of 1997, which made significant reforms in Medicare, as well as the formation of a new public insurance program—the CHIP. CHIP is a partnership between the federal and state governments to provide health insurance to uninsured children whose families earn too much to qualify for Medicaid but are unable to afford private insurance coverage. Each state operates its own CHIP, and some states have renamed the program; for example, Georgia's program is called Peachcare and New Mexico named its program Mexikids. The federal funding of CHIP, however, requires the program to be renewed every few years. On April 16, 2015, President Obama signed into law H.R. 2, the Medicare Access and CHIP Reauthorization Act of 2015, which extends CHIP for 2 more years. In 2013, 8.1 million children were enrolled in CHIP.

Another major expansion in the role of the federal government occurred in 2003, when Congress passed the Medicare Prescription Drug Act Part D, and in 2007 when legislation was signed to continue funding CHIP programs. The biggest expansion of federal oversight since Medicare and Medicaid from the 1960s came when the ACA was signed into law in March of 2010 (Box 3-7: Research for Evidence-Based Practice).

## Current Health Policy

On March 23, 2010, President Obama signed into law the ACA. The goals of the massive health care reform act were to dramatically reduce the number of uninsured Americans, pay for coverage without adding to the national debt, slow the rising cost of health care, and encourage a more efficient health care system (Kovner & Knickman, 2015). When first elected to office, President Obama pushed for health care reform and gained the support from a strong Democratic majority in both the House of Representatives and the Senate. Before it became law, bitter debates between Democratic and Republican members of the House of Representatives and the Senate occurred. Democratic control of the Senate and the House of Representatives allowed the bills to be quickly voted out of committee and introduced to the floors. In December 2009, the Senate bill passed with the partisan support of all Democrats. No Republican senators voted in favor of the bill. In March 2010 the bill came to a vote in the House of Representatives. This time there was bipartisan support against the bill, with 178 Republicans and 34 Democrats voting against it. The bill passed by seven votes (219 vs. 212), and 2 days later the health reform act of 2010 was signed into law, and an amended version was passed in May 2010 (Office of the Legislative Council, 2010). The 974-page document is long and complex, with many provisions and a timeline for incremental sections to be enacted, with most of the provisions taking place by 2014 (see http:// healthreform.kff.org/timeline.aspx for a timeline of detailed provisions by year). See Box 3-8 for a section-by-section title list of the ACA.

## Future Health Policy

Historically there has been a lack of consensus among the major political parties and stakeholders regarding health care reform. Since the ACA became law in March 2010, a number of states, individuals, and other organizations have filed actions in state and federal courts challenging the constitutionality of the law. The federal Supreme Court determined the constitutionality of the various provisions of this law in March 2012. Because the implementation of the law will occur over time (from 2010 to 2018), later provisions may also be met with legal opposition at the state and federal levels, which may result in amendments to the provisions. The timeline for implementation of the many provisions of the ACA began in 2010 under President Obama's term. Since full implementation was not slated to occur until 2018, and the Democrats lost federal political control with the November 2016 election, Republican control under the direction of President Trump will allow new opportunities to modify, amend, or repeal all or parts of the ACA. Since the executive branch of the federal government holds the power to change health care laws that state governments must then enact, substantial effort is needed in policy reform to prioritize both issues of access and cost containment. As future advances in science

## BOX 3-7   RESEARCH FOR EVIDENCE-BASED PRACTICE

### Connecting Eligible Immigrant Families to Health Coverage and Care: Key Lessons From Outreach and Enrollment Workers, October 2011

The 2014 provisions of the ACA significantly expand insurance coverage for low- and moderate-income families through an expansion in Medicaid eligibility and by making tax credits available to help individuals and families purchase insurance coverage through new health care exchanges. In 2010, 38 million immigrants resided in the United States, which was 12.5% of the population. Seventeen million were naturalized citizens, and 21 million were noncitizens. Noncitizens include both lawfully present and undocumented individuals. There are many more individuals who live in families with mixed immigration status, such as a US-born child with one or both parents being noncitizens. In 2009, it was estimated that 5.6 million children were living with at least one noncitizen parent. Most natural citizens have employer or private insurance coverage, whereas noncitizens are nearly three times as likely to be uninsured compared with US citizens. Since 1996, lawfully residing noncitizens have not been eligible to enroll in Medicaid and CHIP during the first 5 years of their legally residing in the United States. Some states eliminated or reduced the 5-year requirement to care for pregnant women and children. Undocumented immigrants are individuals who are not in the United States legally and are prohibited from enrolling in Medicaid or purchasing coverage through health exchanges. Individuals who enter any country illegally are typically not entitled to receive health care or other benefits provided to their citizens and legal residents.

In 2014, when the ACA provision takes effect to expand coverage to individuals with incomes up to 133% of the federal poverty level ($14,484 for an individual or $24,645 for a family of three in 2011), many more individuals will be eligible for Medicaid and individuals with incomes of up to 400% of the federal poverty level ($43,560 for individuals or $74,120 for a family of three in 2011) will be able to buy coverage through new health benefit exchanges using tax credits to help pay for the coverage. Lawfully residing immigrant families are expected to significantly benefit from the coverage expansion. To realize the benefit of the health reform law, enrolling immigrant families will be key and targeted outreach efforts will need to be employed. Immigrant families face numerous challenges in accessing needed care because of limited transportation options and language barriers. Immigrant families may also experience fear and confusion in navigating the health care system and being cared for by a primary care provider who may not have the capacity to provide culturally and linguistically appropriate services.

#### Methodology

To gain increased insight into barriers to coverage and care facing eligible immigrants, and to develop successful strategies to overcome these barriers, Health Outreach Partners and the Kaiser Commission on Medicaid and the Uninsured hosted focus group discussions with outreach and enrollment professionals who serve immigrant communities. Thirty-five professionals participated in one of four focus groups, with one focus group held in Florida, one focus group held in Washington, DC, and two focus groups held in California. With use of a structured interview guide, participants were asked questions concerning barriers to coverage, strategies they use to overcome these barriers, and perceptions of the potential impact of the coverage expansion on immigrant communities. Participants gave their consent for the interviews to be recorded and transcribed. Data were analyzed by qualitative software and supplemented with relevant research and data from a recent farm worker health outreach national needs assessment report. Participants were individuals who provide outreach and enrollment assistance in immigrant communities.

Successful strategies to overcome barriers to coverage and care were revealed, which included:

- use of trusted community organizations and individuals to provide outreach and enrollment assistance;
- providing direct one-on-one assistance from individuals with a shared background or experience;
- educating families about coverage options and the enrollment process;
- providing families with a list of required documents and identifying alternative options;
- offering both English and Spanish forms to document income;
- providing cards that families can present to request translation assistance;
- maintaining contact over time to assist families with renewal.

#### Recommendations and Conclusions

Addressing barriers that immigrant families face will require significant changes in processes and systems as well as a cultural shift among local eligibility offices that is focused on promoting coverage. The findings support the need both to provide outreach and enrollment assistance that meets the needs of immigrant families and to offer strengthening messages to dispel fears among the immigrant community.

Source Kaiser Family Foundation. (2011). *Connecting eligible immigrant families to health coverage and care: Key lessons from outreach and enrollment workers. Publication #8249.* Menlo Park, CA: The Henry J. Kaiser Family Foundation.

unfold, how resources are used to improve the quality and safety of patient-centered care will require ongoing adjustments in the provision and financing of health care (Box 3-9).

### Nursing's Role in Leading Change—2010 Recommendations of the Institute of Medicine

*Report on the future of nursing.* The Robert Wood Johnson Foundation and the IOM in 2008 launched a 2-year initiative to respond to the need to assess and transform the nursing profession. The IOM appointed the committee on the Robert Wood Johnson Foundation Initiative on the Future of Nursing and charged the committee with producing a report that would make recommendations for an action-oriented blueprint for nursing's future. The nursing workforce, composed of more than 3 million nurses, is the largest segment of the nation's health

care workforce. The IOM recognized that nurses play a key role in helping realize the objectives set forth in the 2010 ACA but a number of barriers exist that prevent nurses from being able to respond effectively to rapidly changing health care settings and an evolving health care system. The committee developed the following four key messages and seven recommendations (IOM, 2010):

- Nurses practice to the full extent of their education and training.
- Nurses achieve higher levels of education and training through an improved education system that promotes seamless academic progression.
- Nurses should be full partners, with physicians and other health care professionals, in redesigning health care in the United States.

## BOX 3-8    Sections of the Affordable Care ACT

**Title I**
Quality, Affordable Health Care for All Americans

**Title II**
The Role of Public Programs

**Title III**
Improving the Quality and Efficiency of Health Care

**Title IV**
Prevention of Chronic Disease and Improving Public Health

**Title V**
Health Care Workforce

**Title VI**
Transparency and Program Integrity

**Title VII**
Improving Access to Innovative Medical Therapies

**Title VIII**
Community Living Assistance Services and Supports Act (CLASS Act)

**Title IX**
Revenue Provisions

**Title X**
Reauthorization of the Indian Health Care Improvement Act

## BOX 3-9    Regulation of Quality and Safety of Medical Devices: Proposed Ban on the Use of Powdered Gloves

On May 28, 1976, the Federal Food, Drug, and Cosmetic Act became law, which authorized the United States Food and Drug Administration (FDA) to ban by regulation any device intended for human use on the basis of all available data if the device presented a "substantial deception" or an "unreasonable or substantial risk of illness or injury" which could not be, or has not been, corrected or eliminated by labeling or a change in labeling. The FDA protects the health of the public by monitoring reports of adverse events and other problems with medical devices. The FDA communicates safety concerns by alerting medical professionals and the public after analyzing the risks and benefits the devices poses to individuals. Information updates on recalls, current bans, and proposed bans can be found on the FDA website. On March 22, 2016, the FDA proposed a ban on powdered surgeon's gloves, powdered patient examination gloves, and absorbable powder for lubricating a surgeon's glove. Various types of powder have been added to gloves since the 1930s so wearers could don the gloves more easily. The proposed ban does not include powder intended for use on other medical devices or condoms. Before proposing the ban, the FDA reviewed the risks from the use of powder to both patients and users, including acute airway inflammation because of inhalation of the powder particles; hypersensitivity and allergic reactions; and risk of granuloma and adhesion formation to patients and care workers if internal tissue is exposed to powder. Once a ban is proposed, a period is allotted for comment before a final determination is made. As nonpowdered gloves are readily available and offer the same protection, the FDA expects if a powdered glove ban is implemented, reduction of adverse effects to both patients and health care workers will save $26.6 million to $29.3 million dollars annually. At that time, all unused powdered gloves will be required to be pulled from use and disposed of.

Sources US Department of Health and Human Services, Food and Drug Administration. http://www.fda.gov/MedicalDevices/Safety/default.htm; Federal Register. (2016). Banned Devices; proposal to ban powdered surgeon's gloves, powdered patient examination gloves, and absorbable powder for lubricating a surgeon's glove. https://www.federalregister.gov/articles/2016/03/22/2016-06360/banned-devices-proposal.

• Effective workforce planning and policy-making require better data collection and an improved information infrastructure.

For the IOM's report on the future of nursing recommendations, see Box 3-10: Innovative Practice. As discussed earlier, the IOM of the National Academies of Science, Engineering, and Medicine was renamed the Health and Medicine Division (HMD) in March 2016. The newly named division will expand the range of health matters analyzed to provide health policy advice to the nation's leaders (National Academies of Sciences, Engineering, and Medicine, 2016).

### Official Agencies

Official agencies are tax supported and therefore accountable to the citizens through elected or appointed officials or boards. The purpose and duties of official agencies are prescribed or mandated by law. This discussion is from the perspective of the individual gaining knowledge of or access to the health care system.

*Local level.* The health department of a town, city, county, township, or district is the local health unit and is usually the first line of access and health responsibility for the population that it serves. The mayor, the board of health, or some other executive governing body appoints the chief administrator, the health officer. The local health department's role and functions usually center on providing direct services to the public and depend on the state mandate and community resources. Local governments, but usually not health departments, have the responsibility to provide general health care services for the poor.

*State level.* Public health services are organized by each state, with wide variation from one state to another. The chief administrator is usually a state health officer or commissioner appointed by the governor. One agency, typically the state health department, performs the primary responsibilities in policy, planning, and coordination of programs and services for local units under its jurisdiction.

*Federal level.* The federal government assumes overall responsibility for the health protection of its citizens. Although all three branches of the government make health-related decisions, the major policy decisions are made by the president and the president's staff (executive branch) and by Congress (legislative branch). These two branches determine health policy. Once policy has been determined, other government agencies are responsible for oversight to ensure implementation.

## BOX 3-10  INNOVATIVE PRACTICE

### Institute of Medicine's October 5, 2010 Report on the Future of Nursing Recommendations

*Recommendation 1:* Remove scope-of-practice barriers. Advanced practice registered nurses should be able to practice to the full extent of their education and training.

*Recommendation 2:* Expand opportunities for nurses to lead and diffuse collaborative improvement efforts. Private and public funders, health care organizations, nursing education programs, and nursing associations should expand opportunities for nurses to lead and manage collaborative efforts with physicians and other members of the health care team to conduct research and to redesign and improve practice environments and health systems. These entities should also provide opportunities for nurses to diffuse successful practices.

*Recommendation 3:* Implement nurse residency programs. State boards of nursing, accrediting bodies, the federal government, and health care organizations should take actions to support nurses' completion of a transition-to-practice program (nurse residency) after they have completed a pre-licensure or advanced practice degree program or when they are transitioning into new clinical practice areas.

*Recommendation 4:* Increase the proportion of nurses with a baccalaureate degree to 80% by 2020. Academic nurse leaders across all schools of nursing should work together to increase the proportion of nurses with a baccalaureate degree from 50% to 80% by 2020. These leaders should partner with education accrediting bodies, private and public funders, and employers to ensure funding, monitor progress, and increase the diversity of students to create a workforce prepared to meet the demands of diverse populations across the life span.

*Recommendation 5:* Double the number of nurses with a doctorate by 2020.

*Recommendation 6:* Ensure that nurses engage in lifelong learning.

*Recommendation 7:* Prepare and enable nurses to lead change to advance health.

*Recommendation 8:* Build an infrastructure for the collection and analysis of interprofessional health care workforce data.

Source Institute of Medicine. (2010). The future of nursing: Leading change, advancing health. http://www.iom.edu/Reports/2010/The-Future-of-Nursing-Leading-Change-Advancing-Health.aspx.

The USDHHS, the main federal body concerned with the health of the nation, consists of a number of separate operating agencies (see Box 3-6). Under each of the federal public health service agencies listed there are numerous other departments. USDHHS agencies that relate directly to nursing include the Health Resources and Services Administration and the National Institutes of Health (NIH). The Bureau of Health Professions, within the Health Resources and Services Administration, contains a division of nursing, which is a source for nursing education and training grants. The National Institute of Nursing Research within the NIH funds nursing research, including health-promotion and illness-prevention studies.

**Chief nursing officer.** The chief nursing officer (CNO) serves in the US Public Health Service and leads the Commissioned Corps of the US Public Health Service (Corps) Nurse Professional Affairs. The CNO advises the Office of the Surgeon General and the USDHHS on the recruitment, assignment, deployment, retention, and career development of Corps nurse professionals. As the deputy associate administrator in the HIV/AIDS Bureau, Health Resources and Service Administration, the CEO manages funds for services for uninsured and underserved persons with HIV and training for professionals. The CEO also assists in managing funds for global HIV/AIDS programs. The current CNO, Rear Admiral Sylvia Trent-Adams, was appointed in November 2009 (US Public Health Nursing Services, n.d.).

**Federal emergency management agency.** The US Department of Homeland Security is another large branch of federal agencies with numerous offices, many of which have a connection with health care. Since 2003 the Federal Emergency Management Agency (FEMA) has been part of the US Department of Homeland Security. FEMA was established in 1979 by an executive order merging many separate disaster-related services into a single entity to assist states when a disaster overwhelms a state's capacity to respond. A disaster, as defined by FEMA, includes a hurricane, earthquake, tornado, flood, fire, hazardous spill, act of nature, or act of terrorism. The role of FEMA is to support citizens and first responders to build, sustain, and improve capacity to prepare for, protect against, respond to, recover from, and mitigate all hazards. Assistance is provided to individuals, communities, and states that are determined to be eligible. There are 10 regional FEMA offices located throughout the country, with headquarters in Washington, DC. In 2006 the Post-Katrina Emergency Management Reform Act created a "new FEMA" with an expanded mission and homeland security preparedness responsibilities in the areas of recovery, response, and logistics. The response directorate, for example, provides coordinated federal operational and logistical disaster response capability needed to save and sustain lives, minimize suffering, and protect property in a timely manner in communities overwhelmed by a disaster (US Department of Homeland Security, n.d.).

**Military health systems at the federal level.** The Military Health System (MHS) is a unique partnership of medical educators, medical researchers, health care providers, and support personnel who are prepared to respond anytime or anywhere with comprehensive medical capability to military operations, natural disasters, and humanitarian crises around the world and to ensure world-class health care is provided to all Department of Defense active duty members, retired US Military personnel, and their dependents.

The Department of Veterans Affairs (VA), an independent agency directly under the president, provides integrated health care services for veterans through the Department of Defense, which sponsors health care for military personnel on active duty. The VA uses an advanced computerized information system, which allows a person's medical record to be accessed in any VA site nationally, increasing efficiency in the provision of care. For active-duty service members and retirees of the seven uniformed services, their family members, survivors, and others who are registered in the defense enrollment eligibility reporting system, military health care is covered through the former Civilian Health and Medical Program of the VA. Following issues with delays in receiving medical care, the Veterans Choice Program went into effect in November 2014 and allows eligible veterans to receive care in their own community if their local VA medical facility is unable to schedule an appointment to be seen within a given time frame, or faces unusual or excessive burden in traveling to the nearest VA medical center based upon a number of given factors (VA, 2015). TRICARE is the health care program available to members of the National Guard and Reserves, retired members, and their families.

*Wounded warrior care.* When a soldier is severely injured, prolonged care and rehabilitation are often required before a decision can be made whether the soldier should remain on active duty. The MHS is responsible for providing clinical care to return service personnel to duty or to assist them in making the transition from MHS care to the VA health care system. Tremendous progress has been made in the rehabilitative care of injured combatants and coordination of MHS care with the VA health system.

*Americans with disabilities.* Starting in 1992, health care providers, both as employers and as providers of public services, were required to comply with requirements of the Americans with Disabilities Act of 1990. The act is considered the most sweeping civil rights legislation since the Civil Rights Act of 1964. The two parts that apply most directly to health care providers are the prohibition of employment discrimination and the requirements for provision of services to people with disabilities. An example of health care provider accommodation is to install wheelchair lifts in shuttle bus systems. Despite their need for health promotion and disease prevention, individuals with disabilities face numerous problems gaining access to health-promotion programs and preventive services. The barriers are financial, social, physical, and logistical (USDHHS, 2015c).

In 1990, President George H. W. Bush signed the Patient Self-Determination Act, which took effect in December 1991. This law was designed to increase individual involvement in decisions about life-sustaining treatment, ensuring that advance directives for health care are available to physicians at the time that medical decisions are being made and ensuring that individuals who have not prepared such documents are aware of their legal rights. As a condition of Medicare and Medicaid payment, the Patient Self-Determination Act requires health care facilities to comply with the law. The ACA has several provisions expanding the access requirements for services to people with disabilities.

*Federal health information privacy law.* Developed by the USDHHS as part of the Health Insurance Portability and Accountability Act of 1996, federal privacy standards were enacted by Congress requiring new safeguards to protect the security and confidentiality of health information, including paper, electronic, and oral communications. Health plans, pharmacies, physicians, nurses, and other health care providers must have a written privacy procedure, provide employee training on the Health Insurance Portability and Accountability Act, and designate a privacy officer to ensure procedures are followed. The privacy law permits disclosures without individual authorization to public health authorities authorized by law to collect and receive information for the purpose of preventing or controlling disease, injury, or disability (USDHHS, n.d.a).

*International level.* WHO, the United Nations' specialized agency for health as previously discussed, was established in 1948. WHO comprises members from more than 190 countries, and its core functions include giving worldwide guidance in the field of health; setting global standards for health; cooperating with governments in strengthening national health programs; and developing and transferring appropriate technology, information, and standards. The following is the six-point agenda of WHO: promoting development; fostering health security; strengthening health systems; harnessing research, information, and evidence; enhancing partnerships; and improving performance. In September 2015, a global plan of action for the next 15 years was developed with 17 Sustainable Development Goals and 169 targets. The new goals build upon what was not completed in the previous 15-year goals and seeks to meet the needs of the world's most disadvantaged people (women, children, poor), with the remaining overarching health goal of ensuring healthy lives and promoting well-being for all ages. Emerging challenges were recognized, such as noncommunicable diseases (diabetes and heart disease) and changing social and environmental factors, such as sanitation, pollution, urbanization, and climate change (WHO, n.d.b).

## Voluntary Agencies

The voluntary (not-for-profit) health movement, which began in 1882, stems from the goodwill and humanitarian concerns that are part of the nongovernmental, free enterprise heritage of the people of the United States. Nonprofit entities that maintain a tax-free status are often powerful forces in the health field, voluntary agencies, foundations, and professional associations. The tax-free status of these organizations is challenged at times on the basis of charge that some of them serve only a limited population. Voluntary agencies are influential in promoting health affairs and research agendas at the national policy level and often have significant influence on health legislation. Their prominent role was demonstrated by the American Cancer Society's early mass media announcements about the health hazards of smoking. An example of another voluntary agency is the Alzheimer's Association, which has local chapters that provide resources for families, including publications, services, respite for the caregiver, and support groups for individuals and families.

Philanthropic foundations provide valuable stimulation to the health field and operate under fewer constraints than do other sources in supporting research or training projects. Nurses interested in research or advanced clinical study that relates to the special interests of voluntary agencies or foundations may find grant monies available to support their work. For example, the John A. Hartford Foundation is a foundation established in 1929 and supports efforts to improve health care for older Americans. Recently, the trustees of this foundation awarded a $5 million, 5-year grant to create the John A. Hartford Foundation Institute for Geriatric Nursing at New York University, which promotes initiatives to improve care of older adults and training projects to prepare faculty to teach care of older adults in baccalaureate nursing programs. The institute has also raised the profile of geriatric nursing by creating nationally recognized awards for excellence in research and practice (John A. Hartford Foundation, 2012). Professional associations, organized at the national level with state and local branches, are powerful political forces. Nurses can support their professional organizations in influencing the direction of health policy through membership and active participation.

***The American Red Cross.*** The American Red Cross is a well-known volunteer-led humanitarian organization that is officially sanctioned by the federal government as a congressional charter, meaning it is not supervised by the government because it is not a governmental agency, but is recognized officially. Founded in 1881 by Clara Barton, the International Red Cross aids victims of war and natural disasters throughout the world. There are more than 700 local American Red Cross chapters in the United States, with more than 500,000 volunteers and 35,000 employees. The American Red Cross responds both to small local emergencies to help victims (such as in the case of a house fire) and to large natural disasters (such as hurricanes and earthquakes). The Red Cross is the largest supplier of blood and blood products in the United States, helps thousands of US service members separated from their families maintain communication, and offers communities a range of health and safety courses. The global network of national societies relies on public donations of money, time, and blood. Local Red Cross opportunities exist, including the donation of blood and assistance with blood drives and other volunteer activities (American Red Cross, n.d.).

## FINANCING HEALTH CARE

### Costs

The health care industry is the largest service industry in the United States today and the most powerful employer in the nation. The Bureau of Labor Statistics projects health care occupations will grow by 19% from 2014 to 2024, adding 2.3 million jobs (US Department of Labor, 2015b). National health expenditures in the United States were greater than those in any other country, with $3.2 trillion spent in 2015 (or $9990 per person), a marked increase from the $1.9 trillion spent in 2004. In 2015 health spending consumed 17.8% of the GDP and is projected to grow at an average rate of 5.8% per year from 2015 to 2025, and the health-share GDP is expected to rise to 20.1% by 2025. In 2014, the breakdown of national health spending was as follows: hospital expenditures $971.8 billion, Medicare spending in 2014 grew by 5.5% to $618.7 billion or 20% of the budget, Medicaid spending, which accounts for 16% of national health expenditures, grew by 11% to $495.8 billion, private health insurance spending was $991.0 billion or 33% of national health expenditures, out-of-pocket expenditures grew to $329.8 billion, or 11% of national health expenditures, physician and clinical service expenditures grew by 4.6% to $603.7 billion, and prescription drug spending increased by 12.2% to $297.7 billion. The trend in health care spending increases was projected to be 5.5% in 2015 and peak at 6.3% in 2020. In 2010 the per capita expenditure for health care (amount of money on average spent on each individual in the United States) was for the 65 years and older population $18,424, which is five times higher than the amount spent per child ($3628), and three times higher than the spending per working-age person ($6125), or on average $8402, per capita, the highest of all countries. Thirty-four percent of spending in 2010 was on older adults, who are the smallest group, or 13% of the population (CMS, 2015a, 2017). Canada, for example, which borders the United States, is reported to spend just more than $4000 per person, which is half of what the United States spends. Many other countries spend far less per capita, yet life expectancy is greater and infant mortality rates are lower. In addition to the United States spending more health care dollars per person than any other country, the rate of growth in per capita health expenditure in the United States is much steeper than that of other countries. The graphical representation in Figure 3-4 illustrates that in 1970 the per capita expenditure was $356, or 7% of GDP, and rapidly increased in each decade. The United States has outpaced all other countries and spends the most health care dollars per capita. Another measure of comparison is the amount of money a country devotes to health care in terms of GDP. Over time, the United States again outpaces the other nations in the percentage of GDP devoted to health care. In 2010, of the 305.2 million Americans, 49% had employer-based health insurance, 5% had private health insurance, 12% were enrolled in Medicare, 17% were enrolled in Medicaid, and 16% of the population were uninsured (Figure 3-5). A major focus of the ACA is aimed at reducing the number of uninsured Americans. These figures and expenditures, although numerous, introduce the topic of health care financing.

Health care analysts predict the accelerations in health care costs will continue, putting pressure on public and private payers to finance them. Factors driving costs include general inflation; health care cost inflation; application of new and more advanced technologies; growth in the proportion of older adults; government financing of health care services, including long-term care; growth of prescription drug use and costs; misdistribution of health care providers and services; expansion of medical technology and specialty medicine; and other costs associated with providing health care. For example, diagnostic and therapeutic techniques—including computer-aided technology and noninvasive imaging (such as magnetic resonance imaging), cardiac surgery, organ transplantation, joint replacements (particularly hips and knees)—enhance the capabilities of medicine while increasing costs.

A combination of the following factors results in hospitals having less time to offer prevention or health-promotion education to individuals: changes in hospital care and use of hospitalists, increased use of outpatient services, shorter inpatient stays, and increased time caring for chronic illness as opposed to acute illness. Moreover, workforce shortages, especially in nursing, increase the use of nonprofessional caregivers, and inadequate resources, reimbursement, and numbers of nurses may prevent health care professionals from offering the range of health promotion educational efforts requested in the *Healthy People 2020* objectives.

### Sources

Ultimately, the American people pay for all health care costs. Money is transferred from consumer to provider by various mechanisms. The major sources are the government (federal, state, and local monies collected by taxes), third-party payment (private insurance), independent plans, and out-of-pocket support, which totaled $3.2 trillion in 2015. The CMS provide statistics on the source of the nation's health care dollars and the manner in which they are spent. In 2014 (Figure 3-6) the largest percentage of the nation's health care dollars came from private health insurance (33%), and 11% of health care costs

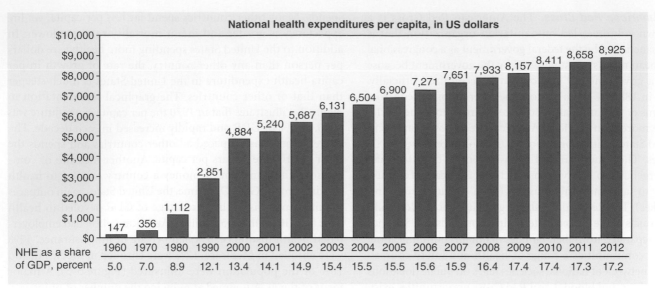

**FIGURE 3-4** National health expenditures per capita. *GDP*, Gross domestic product; *NHE*, national health expenditure. (From Kaiser Family Foundation calculations using national health expenditures data from Centers for Medicare and Medicaid Services, Office of the Actuary, National Health Statistics Group at http://cms.hhs.gov/NationalHealthExpendData/ [see national health expenditures by type of service and source of funds; file nhe12.zip]; GDP data from Bureau of Economic Analysis at http://bea.gov/national/index.htm#gdp [file gdplev.xlx]. Slide available from the Kaiser Family Foundation. http://kff.org/Kaiser-slides/.)

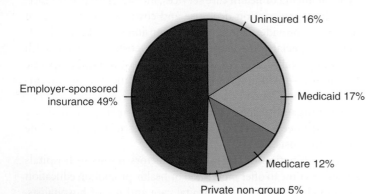

**FIGURE 3-5** Total expenditure on health care as a share of gross domestic product. Medicaid also includes other public programs: Children's Health Insurance Program, other state programs, military-related coverage. The numbers may not add up to 100% because of rounding. (From Health insurance coverage: KCMU/Urban Institute analysis of 2011 data from 2012 ASEC Supplement to the CPS. Health expenditures: KFF calculations using 2011 NHE data from CMS, Office of the Actuary. Found in Kaiser Commission on Medicaid and the Uninsured: Medicaid and its Role in State/Federal Budgets & Health Reform, April 2013. https://kaiserfamilyfoundation.files.wordpress.com/2013/04/8162-03.pdf.)

were out-of-pocket payments made by consumers. The cost of Medicare accounted for 20% of the health care dollars and federal, state, and local Medicaid costs accounted for 16%. In all, some form of health insurance funds 73% of the nation's health care. Figure 3-7 provides a similar schematic but displays where health care dollars are spent. Almost one-third (32%) of health care dollars are spent on hospital care, 20% on physicians and clinical services, 10% on prescription drugs, 5% on nursing care facilities

and continuing care retirement communities, 4% on dental care, 8% on administrative costs, and 14% on nonacute care. As discussed earlier, keeping Americans healthy and out of the hospital would save a tremendous amount of money.

## Employer Health Benefits

According to the employer health benefits survey's conducted by the KFF, the overall inflation rate of employer-sponsored health insurance for families has risen dramatically in the past decade. Between 1999 and 2015, health insurance premiums for individual and family coverage have risen significantly. The average employer-sponsored health insurance annual premium in 2015 was $6251 for individuals and $17,545 for family coverage. Since 1999 the average worker's contribution to family premiums has increased by 221%. The worker contribution for family coverage in 2001 was $1787 per year and in 2015 grew to $4955, whereas the employer contribution in 2001 was $7061 and jumped to $12,591 in 2015, for a total cost (does not include other costs associated with using the plan such as out-of-pocket expenses) of $17,545, making it difficult for both individuals and employers to pay for higher health care premiums (Figure 3-8). The cost for both single-coverage contributions of workers and employers in 2015 rose to $6251 (the employer contribution was $5179 and the individual worker's contribution was $1071). Again, this does not include the cost of using the benefits of the plan (KFF, 2015a). Most plans have additional out-of-pocket costs (co-payments) for use of the plan for office visits, laboratory testing, and other services, such as physical therapy. Almost all plans have some sort of prescription drug coverage but may limit coverage to certain medications (a formulary of what medications are covered or denied is usually part of a prescription plan). Some plans have a tiered list of medications with differing

**The nation's health dollar ($3.0 trillion), calendar year 2014, where it came from**

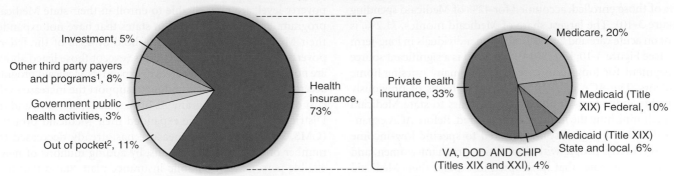

Investment, 5%

Other third party payers and programs[1], 8%

Government public health activities, 3%

Out of pocket[2], 11%

Health insurance, 73%

Private health insurance, 33%

Medicare, 20%

Medicaid (Title XIX) Federal, 10%

Medicaid (Title XIX) State and local, 6%

VA, DOD AND CHIP (Titles XIX and XXI), 4%

**FIGURE 3-6** Nation's health dollars ($3.0 trillion), calendar year 2014: where it comes from. The sum of the pieces may not equal 100% because of rounding. (From Centers for Medicare & Medicaid Services, Office of the Actuary, National Health Statistics Group. https://www.cms .gov/Research-Statistics-Data-and-Systems/Statistics-Trends-and-Reports/NationalHealthExpendData/ Downloads/PieChartSourcesExpenditures2014.pdf.)

**The nation's health dollar ($3.0 trillion), calendar year 2014, where it went**

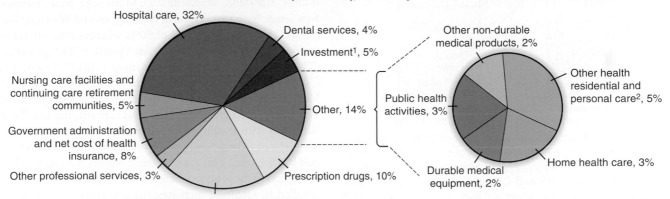

Hospital care, 32%

Dental services, 4%

Investment[1], 5%

Nursing care facilities and continuing care retirement communities, 5%

Government administration and net cost of health insurance, 8%

Other professional services, 3%

Other, 14%

Prescription drugs, 10%

Physician and clinical services, 20%

Other non-durable medical products, 2%

Public health activities, 3%

Other health residential and personal care[2], 5%

Home health care, 3%

Durable medical equipment, 2%

**FIGURE 3-7** Nation's health dollars ($3.0 trillion), calendar year 2014: where it went. The sum of the pieces may not equal 100% because of rounding. (From Centers for Medicare & Medicaid Services, Office of the Actuary, National Health Statistics Group. https://www.cms.gov/Research-Statistics-Data-and-Systems/Statistics-Trends-and-Reports/NationalHealthExpendData/Downloads/ PieChartSourcesExpenditures2014.pdf.)

**Average premiums increased by four percent between 2014 and 2015**

☐ Employer contribution
▨ Worker contribution

Single coverage:
2014: $6,025 ($4,944 / $1,081)
2015: 4% $6,251 ($5,179 / $1,071)

Family coverage:
2014: $16,834 ($12,011 / $4,823)
2015: 4% $17,545 ($12,591 / $4,955)

**FIGURE 3-8** Average annual health insurance premiums and worker contributions for family coverage, 2014 to 2015. (From Kaiser/HRET Survey of Employer-Sponsored Health Benefits, 2015. http://kff.org/report-section/ehbs-2015-section-one-cost-of-health-insurance.)

copayments. Generic medications (if available) generally have the least additional out-of-pocket cost and are listed in the lowest cost tier. Health care providers need to be aware of these variations between plans before prescribing medications, as out-of-pocket expenses may inhibit an individual from filling a prescription and following the prescribed medication plan.

Federal and state **Medicaid** spending showed an increasing pattern similar to that discussed earlier in this chapter, with Medicaid spending reported to be $5.3 billion in 1970, $207.0 billion in 2000, $309.0 billion in 2004, $366.5 billion in 2009, and $475.91 billion in 2014 (Figure 3-9). As a cost-savings mechanism, by 2000, 55.8% of Medicaid recipients were enrolled in some form of managed care plan. Although costly, the Medicaid program finances health care for low-income children, adults, seniors, and people with disabilities. Children comprise 48% of individuals in the program but account for only 21% of the spending of Medicaid dollars, adults account for 27% of individuals in the program and 15% of expenditures, and elderly people account for 9% of those enrolled and 21% of expenditures. The blind or disabled individuals in the program, representing only 15% of those enrolled, accounted for 42% of Medicaid spending (Figure 3-10). The largest share of Medicaid monies, 71.2%, is spent on acute care and 24.9% is spent on individuals in long-term care (see Figure 3-10; KFF, 2014). Medicaid is a significant source of payment for long-term care, covering many nursing home residents. The ACA of 2010 has added millions of previously ineligible individuals younger than 65 years to state Medicaid plans, diminishing the number of uninsured. Before ACA expansion, Medicaid eligibility was limited to specific low-income groups (elderly, people with disabilities, pregnant women, and children). For states that have opted to expand their Medicaid

programs, individuals, including adults below 133% of the federal poverty level, are now eligible to enroll in their state Medicaid program. Previously, and still in states that have not expanded their Medicaid program, the threshold of 45% of the federal poverty line was required and adults (except those listed above) are not eligible. A state that agrees to expand its Medicaid program accepts additional federal funding to support the increase in the cost of running the program. As of May 2015, 28 states and the District of Columbia have expanded their Medicaid program (CMS, 2015b). This one measure has already decreased the number of uninsured Americans, by adding millions of newly eligible persons to the public insurance plan. States that have not expanded their Medicaid plan continue to have higher numbers of uninsured.

Each state receives from the federal government a formula percentage of revenue to run a Medicaid program, leaving state budgets responsible for the remaining cost. Federal tax dollars must fund a minimum of 50% of a state's Medicaid cost. In 2014, 14 states—Alaska, California, Colorado, Connecticut, Illinois, Maryland, Massachusetts, Minnesota, New Hampshire, New Jersey, New York, Virginia, Washington, and Wyoming—were funded at the minimal level of 50%, whereas other states—for example, Mississippi (74.18%), West Virginia (72.62%), Kentucky (71.18%), Utah (70.99%), Arkansas (70.17%), and Idaho (70.23%)—received a much greater share of the cost of their Medicaid programs from the federal government (KFF, 2012). The greater the percentage of federal support, the less the state has to pay with state monies. For example, when a state receives only 50% of federal funding, the remaining 50% must be generated by state taxes. This is a tremendous burden on state residents. As the cost of the program increases and/or the number of persons enrolled in Medicaid increases, the taxpayers of the state must support the program, often through the raising of state, county, and local taxes. Because Medicaid is an entitlement program,

**Medicaid enrollees and expenditures, FFY 2209**

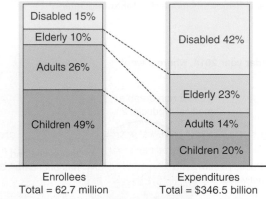

Enrollees
Total = 62.7 million

Expenditures
Total = $346.5 billion

**FIGURE 3-9** Medicaid enrollees and expenditures, fiscal year 2009. The sum of the pieces may not equal 100% because of rounding. (From KCMU/Urban Institute estimates based on federal FFY 2009 data from MSIS and CMS-64; 2012 MSIS FFY 2008 data were used for Pennsylvania, Utah, and Wisconsin, but adjusted to 2009 CMS-64. Slide available from the Kaiser Family Foundation. http://kff.org/Kaiser-slides/.)

**The majority of Medicaid expenditures are for acute care**

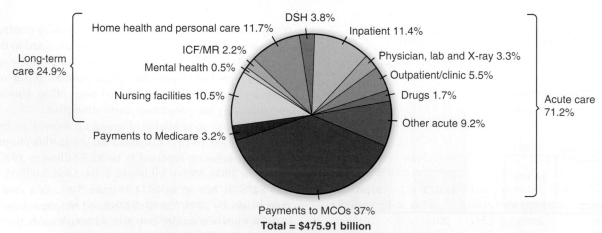

Total = $475.91 billion

**FIGURE 3-10** Most Medicaid expenditures are for acute care. By service, 2014. The total may not add up to 100% because of rounding. Excludes administrative spending, adjustments, and payments to the territories. (From Urban Institute estimates based on fiscal year 2014 data from CMS-64, prepared for the Kaiser Commission on Medicaid and the Uninsured. Slide available from the Kaiser Family Foundation. http://kff.org/Kaiser-slides/.)

any one individual who meets Medicaid's eligibility requirements is entitled to receive benefits; therefore there is no way to cap the Medicaid budget at the federal or state level under current law. Many states have more lenient eligibility requirements than those set by the federal government and offer more health services than are mandated. The ACA has addressed some of the disparities by mandating essential health benefits that all insurance plans must cover. The ACA has provisions to provide financial incentives for states that qualify, to provide enhanced services to Medicaid recipients by increasing their federal matching funds. One way states have cut costs in Medicaid programs is to decrease provider payment rates and limit services. These practices can jeopardize provider participation (providers willing to care for individuals enrolled in a Medicaid program) and limit access to care for Medicaid recipients. Decreasing eligibility requirements for individuals and families so they qualify for Medicaid coverage is part of the solution to reduce the number of uninsured by adding more lower-income individuals and families to the Medicaid program. Since more individuals will now qualify for Medicaid if the state expands its Medicaid programs, individual states need to enhance or develop efficient user-friendly systems to facilitate the enrollment process. Health care delivery systems in each state have needed to adjust to accommodate the increased number of Medicaid enrollees in the provision of safe and efficient quality care. The ACA has some provisions to increase payments for primary care services provided by primary care providers because Medicaid provider reimbursement rates for services provided are typically much lower than other sources of payment.

## Mechanisms

### Payment

Although some health care providers and other professionals in the private sector are paid on a fee-for-service basis, by third-party private insurance, or by public-supported insurance, most health workers, including nurses in institutional or community agencies and in the military, receive salaries or are paid by the hour regardless of the amount of care provided. Because nurses are salaried or paid by the hour, the separation of nursing costs from all other health-related costs is difficult. The cost of acute hospital nursing care is typically incorporated in the daily room and board charge in the acute care setting. Without documentation of specific nursing costs, validating the need for skilled nursing services is difficult.

In recent years, nurses and APNs have entered independent practice to provide direct services. The Bureau of Labor Statistics 2016 to 2017 report estimated in 2014 there were 170,400 jobs for APNs (122,050 nurse practitioners, 36,590 certified registered nurse anesthetists, and 5110 certified nurse midwives), with a projected need to increase the job numbers by 31% because of the effects of health care legislation, increased emphasis on preventive care, and need for health care of the aging population (US Department of Labor, 2015a).

Independent nursing practice may be viewed as a logical outgrowth of seeking higher levels of professionalism. The nurse practice acts of some states encourage nurses to use their knowledge more comprehensively than many agencies sanction. Although legislation in 1997 included the reimbursement of

APNs by Medicare, not all plans and provider groups include these nurses as primary care practitioners. Clearly, the nursing practice roles and prescriptive authority of APNs differ between states. Incremental steps have been taken to advance the APN role at both the federal level and the state level. Some states have passed laws for nurse practitioners to practice and prescribe medications without physician oversight. The IOM's 2010 report titled *The Future of Nursing: Leading Change, Advancing Health* supports nurses practicing to the full extent of their education and training.

Alternative forms of payment for APNs are salary and capitation. The salary system involves a set amount for services provided in a specified time frame. This system provides the employee with a fixed nursing income that is protected from changes in supply and demand, includes fringe benefits, and obviates fee collection problems. The salary system's flexibility makes it easier to fill unpopular jobs or jobs in underserved areas. The disadvantages of this system include a limit on income and constraints on schedules, vacations, and peer review. A nurse in a salaried position may not be able to earn overtime depending on the facility. Nurses who work beyond the scheduled hours are then uncompensated for additional time under a salary arrangement, which may lead to job dissatisfaction and burnout.

In the capitation system, such as in an HMO, each provider receives a flat annual fee for each participant regardless of how often services are used. Individuals who enroll in an HMO pay a fixed amount on a monthly basis whether or not they use the services; prepayment provides an incentive to provide efficient care. The objective is to keep people healthy to prevent costly services. Cost consciousness dictates that illness be treated as early as possible and in the most cost-effective setting. Capitation is simple to administer; no third-party insurance payments are present, and the HMO bears the risk of illness. Preventive primary care that avoids costly hospitalization keeps costs down, and the savings revert to the organization. On the negative side, individuals who make frequent or unnecessary visits to a provider in an HMO decrease the efficiency of the system.

### Cost Containment

The government's interest in hospital treatment cost containment was exemplified by the passage of the Social Security Amendments of 1983 (Public Law 98-21), which mandates the establishment by the Health Care Financing Administration of a prospective payment system for Medicare. This system stipulates that providers be paid at preset rates based on 470 diagnosis-related group categories used to classify the illness of each Medicare-insured person. Rates for each diagnosis were established according to regional and national amounts based on each hospital's urban and rural cost experience. The number of hospitals in the United States in 2012 was reported to be 5723, with more than 920,000 beds. In 2012 the average occupancy rate in hospitals was 65.2%. Large hospitals with 500 beds or more reported higher rates of occupancy, at 72.6%, whereas the smallest hospitals, those with 6 to 24 beds, had an occupancy rate of 30.8% (USDHHS, 2015b).

Another piece of legislation that targeted cost containment was the Balanced Budget Act of 1997, which also affected Medicare. This act reduced Medicare spending by limiting provider payments, increased options in the choice of managed care plans, and made medical savings accounts an option. As of 2007, medical savings accounts were linked to high-deductible Medicare Advantage plans (Medicare private health plans) and are currently available in some states. Medicare makes an annual deposit into an interest-bearing account on behalf of enrollees, who use the funds to pay for qualified health care expenses until they meet the deductible, at which point the plan will pay for all Medicare-covered services.

The Medicare Modernization Act of 2003 promotes private managed care plans to reduce the burden on the economy of Medicare entitlements. These HMO plans, called Medicare Advantage plans, discussed previously, typically have clients who are healthier than the average Medicare client. Older adults who are enrolled in these plans pay a monthly premium and are required to choose providers within the network. If care is provided outside the network of providers, individuals must usually pay out-of-pocket costs similar to those of other HMOs discussed earlier. This can be confusing to the older person because there are many Medicare Advantage plans to choose from and the person may not realize how a Medicare Advantage plan is different from traditional Medicare coverage. Provisions have been made for enrollees to change Medicare Advantage plans or to be disenrolled during specific time frames. Providers have been lobbying for increased reimbursement because Medicare dictates reimbursement fees based on a predetermined formula.

*Care management.* Care management began through public programs with nurses in public health departments, social workers in public welfare systems, and caseworkers in mental health departments. In care management, an experienced health care professional, such as a nurse, social worker, or gerontologist, helps determine the nursing care that is necessary, monitors that care, and arranges for individuals to receive care in the most cost-effective and most appropriate setting. Care managers are especially effective in meeting the needs of individuals recently discharged from the hospital, older adults, persons with medical conditions that are costly to treat (e.g., spinal cord injuries or persons with high-volume diseases such as chronic illnesses), persons with complex health and social needs, and other cases requiring multiple levels of care. The care manager must achieve a balance between cost and quality and must collaborate effectively with all providers involved, both inside and outside the health plan, and with the person's family to ensure appropriate quality care. Emphasis must be on health management across the continuum of health care services. As Medicaid and Medicare managed care systems continue to develop, demand for nurses to fill the care management role will continue to grow. In addition to working within organizations, care managers can have their own independent practices. Managed care organizations rely on care management to reduce inappropriate use of services, improve quality of care, and control costs (Nies & McEwen, 2014). Basic care management services are described in Box 3-11.

## Managed Care Issues

Managed care options will once again become more plentiful as states devise health care delivery systems to meet the ACA mandates. With a need to not only control costs but also to

---

### BOX 3-11    Care Management Services

- *Assessment:* Evaluating a person's physical, social, functional, psychological, financial, and spiritual needs, including the family within a specific environment
- *Care planning:* Setting goals and identifying specific services to meet individual and family needs, including how to allocate resources and refer to other resources
- *Geriatric care manager:* Manager who develops an individualized care plan for older adults with medical, functional, and cognitive conditions to receive care and services to remain at home, avoiding costly hospitalizations and emergency department visits when possible
- *Service coordination and referral:* Facilitating and coordinating access to needed providers
- *Care monitoring and periodic reassessments:* Evaluating progress, access to and use of services, and changes in needs

---

improve the functioning of the health care system to provide high-quality evidence-based care, new systems with groups of providers delivering care in more efficient ways must evolve. The use of technology has become a valuable resource for informing consumers and employers about health care issues and allowing them to search for and compare information on various types of health care plans. The Internet is also a tool nurses can use for their own continuing education needs, as well as to enhance others' education within a facility, public library, or home. Nurses can steer individuals toward appropriate websites for health-promotion and disease-oriented information (see the case study at end of this chapter). With the rapid expansion of scientific advances in health and medicine, it is not possible for the nurse to stay abreast of the growing body of research evidence without Internet assistance. Evidence-based practice is key in the provision of safe, quality nursing care. Registered nurses and APNs need to be able to obtain the best evidence, appraise the findings, and then apply them to practice with consideration of the culture and beliefs of the individual (Melnyk & Fineout-Overholt, 2014).

## Health Insurance

Positive elements of the health care system in the United States include excellent clinicians, health care facilities, and equipment—all of which are readily available to people with health insurance and adequate finances. The US system exhibits a high degree of technological change and innovation and excellent information, quality, and cost-accounting systems. Numerous studies have found that those who do not have health insurance are at risk of poorer health outcomes. The ACA has significantly decreased the number of those uninsured in states that have expanded their Medicaid programs and because most Americans are now required by federal law to purchase or obtain health insurance. A high number of uninsured individuals are disproportionately low-income persons and measures as discussed previously will increase the number of individuals in both private and public health plans. The plan does not address noncitizen foreign-born persons who have entered and are living in the United States illegally.

## Private Health Insurance

In the private sector, the following five types of organizations provide health care insurance:

- Traditional insurance companies (including the earliest insurer, Blue Cross, and Blue Shield, a nonprofit charitable organization) and for-profit commercial insurance companies
- PPOs acting as "brokers" between insurers and health care providers
- HMOs, which are independent prepayment plans
- POS plans, which combine features of classic HMOs with person choice characteristics of PPOs
- Self-insurance and self-funded plans, in which either the employer takes on the role of insurer or the enrollee sets up a trust account with tax savings.

Traditionally, private insurers charged employers or individuals annual premiums and provided services on a fee-for-service basis. Organized at the state and local levels, Blue Cross and Blue Shield generally complement each other, with Blue Cross reimbursing hospitals and Blue Shield covering physicians and other providers. After World War II, insurance companies began to provide health insurance plans in competition with Blue Cross and Blue Shield. Today, more than 800 commercial, profit-making insurance companies, such as Metropolitan Life and Aetna, offer policies that cover hospitalization and in-hospital or office-based physician care, and other major medical expenses. Much of the individual insurance sold today is supplementary, such as that designed to supplement Medicare, known as Medigap. These plans reimburse only deductibles and co-insurance payments associated with Medicare.

HMOs attempt to lower health care costs by emphasizing preventive rather than curative care, decreasing the progression and severity of some illnesses. Care is provided in outpatient settings when possible, and HMOs tend to use fewer services, with emphasis on the least costly means of providing a service.

POS plans enable enrollees to choose, at the POS, whether to use the plan's provider network or seek care from non-network providers. Typically, network providers are paid on a capitated or discounted fee basis, and non-network providers are paid on a fee-for-service basis.

Another change in the structure of the insurance industry is the growth of self-insured or self-funded plans. Self-insurance means that an employer (or union) assumes the claims risk of its insured employees, whereas self-funding refers to paying insurance claims from an established fund, such as a bank account or trust fund.

## Public Health Insurance and Assistance

*Medicare.* Medicare is a federal health insurance program that finances medical care for people older than 65 years, disabled individuals who are entitled to Social Security benefits, and people with end-stage renal disease requiring dialysis or a kidney transplant. The Medicare program, also known as Title XVIII of the Social Security Amendments, began in 1966 after decades of debate and is currently operated under the administrative oversight of the CMS. Medicare is an entitlement program, meaning individuals who contributed to Medicare through taxes are "entitled" to the benefits regardless of the amount of income and assets they have. The intent of Medicare was to protect older adults against the catastrophic financial debts often incurred in managing chronic illness and to assist in the payment of health care. In 1983 Medicare added hospice benefits for the last 6 months of life to cover services for the terminally ill. Hospice is based on a philosophy that views death as a normal part of the life cycle and emphasizes living the remainder of life as fully and comfortably as possible. Hospice care accounts for only a small amount of total Medicare expenditures. The total Medicare benefit payments in 2014 equaled $597 billion, accounting for 14% of the federal budget and 22% of the total national health spending in 2013. Twenty-six percent of Medicare expenditures went to Medicare Advantage plans, 23% went to hospital in patient services, 12% went to physician payments, 14% went to other payments (such as hospice, durable medical equipment, and Part B drugs), 11% went to outpatient prescription drugs, 3% went to home health, and 5% went to skilled nursing. There are four parts in the Medicare plan: Medicare Part A (hospital insurance), Medicare Part B (medical insurance), Medicare Part C (Medicare Advantage), and Medicare Part D (Medicare prescription drug coverage) (KFF, 2015c).

Medicare Part A is financed largely through a mandatory tax of 2.9% of earnings paid by employees and their employers (1.45% each) into the Hospital Insurance Trust Fund, which accounts for 87% of Part A's revenue. Individuals who earn more than $200,000 and $250,000 or more as a couple pay a higher payroll tax on earnings of 2.35%. Part A covers inpatient care in hospitals, skilled nursing facilities (not custodial or long-term care), home health services, and hospice care. For those individuals who have contributed to Medicare or whose spouse has contributed to Medicare for 10 years in Medicare-covered employment, there is no monthly premium for Part A. For those individuals who have not contributed for 10 years, premiums are pro-rated to the number of months (quarters of Medicare-covered employment), and in 2016 were up to $411 per month. The Part A benefits are subject to a deductible ($1288 deductible for each benefit period in 2016) and copayments, which differ depending on the number of days for each benefit period. For example, for days 1 to 60 there is zero co-insurance, for days 61 to 90 there is $322 co-insurance per day of each benefit period, and there are increased co-insurance rates for day 91 and beyond with defined limits (Medicare.gov, n.d.). Even if an individual does not pay a monthly premium for Part A, inpatient deductibles and co-insurance charges may be difficult for many older adults to manage as a result of fixed incomes.

Part B is supplementary voluntary medical insurance financed through a combination of general tax revenues (73%) and 25% of premiums paid by beneficiaries ($109.00 per month in 2016 with a $166 annual deductible). The Medicaid program pays the premium for low-income Medicaid beneficiaries. People with incomes $85,000 or higher or $170,000 for couples pay a higher income-related monthly Part B premium ranging from $152.78 to $349.13 per month in 2016. The ACA freezes the income thresholds for Part B through 2019. Beginning in 2020, income thresholds will be indexed to inflation and premiums are expected to grow. Part B covers physician visits, outpatient services, preventive services, and home health visits. Once the deductible has been met, individuals typically pay 20% of the Medicare-approved amount for most physician services, in-hospital physician services, outpatient therapy, and durable medical equipment (Medicare.gov, n.d.).

Part C refers to the Medicare Advantage program as previously discussed. Medicare Advantage programs such as HMOs and PPOs cover all of Part A and Part B, and typically Part D.

Part D is the voluntary, subsidized outpatient prescription drug benefit with additional subsidies available for low-income beneficiaries. Part D is financed through general revenues (74%), beneficiary premiums (15%), and state payments for dually eligible people (11%). The Part D benefit is offered through private plans that contract with Medicare. There are Medicare Advantage prescription plans and stand-alone prescription plans. The ACA includes a number of provisions that have enhanced benefits and gradually eliminated the Part D prescription drug coverage gap known as the donut hole. The Part D monthly premium differs by plan (KFF, 2014).

Individuals enrolled in both Medicare and Medicaid programs (duel) are considered vulnerable populations (older adults and poor), and Medicare premiums are subsidized. Medicare benefit payments accounted for 14% of the total federal spending in 2013 (Figure 3-11). The financial status of Medicare can be measured by the level of assets in the trust fund, compared with the level of benefit spending. If spending exceeds assets, the fund will become fully depleted. Each year the trustees predict the solvency of the trust fund (year in which funds will be fully depleted). In 2015, the trustees predicted the solvency of the Medicare Hospital Insurance Fund will be depleted in 2030 as the baby boom generation will reach Medicare eligibility and there will be a declining number of workers per beneficiary, resulting in a decrease in payroll tax contributions to the fund. The projected year to insolvency has varied, and the full impact of the ACA has not been fully realized. Future challenges include increased costs of health care services, increased costs of technology, and increased volume and use of services attributable to

population growth of older adults and increasing life expectancy. The number of older adults (65 years or older) and nonelderly disabled (younger than 65 years) who are enrolled in Medicare has increased steadily since 1966 (Figure 3-12), with 52 million in 2013. Neither Part A nor Part B of Medicare offers comprehensive coverage. Inherent in the program are deductibles, set amounts that the individual must pay for each type of service before Medicare begins to pay, and copayments, a percentage of charges paid by the individual. There are also limitations on the amount of coverage provided.

Out-of-pocket expenses do not include premium payments for Part B or for supplemental private health insurance, which can add significantly to out-of-pocket expenses. A comprehensive booklet available on-line or through the CMS details information on enrollment, costs, and services that are covered and not covered. With some exceptions, services not covered include acupuncture, chiropractic services (unless medically necessary to correct subluxation), and custodial care (activities of daily living such as help bathing, dressing, eating, getting in and out of bed). Other services that are not covered include most dental care such as cleanings, fillings, extractions, dentures, routine eye care, and spectacles for nondiabetic individuals, routine foot care for nondiabetic individuals (cutting or removal of corns, calluses, cutting of nails), hearing aids, long-term care (if only custodial care is needed), and health care while traveling outside the United States. Items not covered, especially custodial care, contribute significantly to out-of-pocket expenses. The main population at risk, the older adult, may have limited financial resources to seek preventive health services not covered. Some low-income enrollees may qualify for Medicaid services if income requirements are met, and others may have additional benefits through private insurance (Medicare.gov, n.d.).

In the Omnibus Budget Reconciliation Act of 1989, Medicare revised its payment scheme for physicians, assigning relative values to services on the basis of the time, skill, and intensity required to provide them, and a second limit was set on the amount that physicians could charge individuals above the amount that Medicare pays. This restriction was designed to limit growth of Medicare costs for physician payments.

The Balanced Budget Act of 1997, the Balanced Budget Refinement Act of 1999, and the Benefits Improvement and Protection Act of 2000 added services to the Medicare benefits package. These services include coverage for some screening tests, diabetes monitoring and diabetes self-management, and some immunizations.

The missing Medicare benefit causing great concern was the rising cost and lack of coverage for outpatient prescription drugs. On December 9, 2003, President George W. Bush signed into law the Medicare Prescription Drug, Improvement, and Modernization Act of 2003 (Public Law 108-173). This lengthy piece of legislation amended Title XVIII of the Social Security Amendments to provide a voluntary program for prescription drug coverage and to modernize the Medicare program. The Medicare prescription drug benefit Part D started on January 1, 2006, and covers some of the costs for prescription drugs. Different plans cover different drugs and require older adults to choose a plan that best meets their needs from a plethora of choices. Those

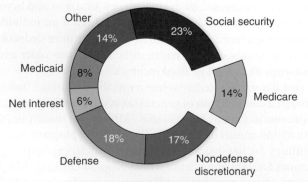

**Medicare spending is 14% of the federal budget**
**Total federal spending in 2013; $3.5 trillion**

Other 14%
Social security 23%
Medicaid 8%
Net interest 6%
Defense 18%
Nondefense discretionary 17%
Medicare 14%

**FIGURE 3-11** Medicare spending is 14% of the total federal spending, fiscal year 2013. All amounts are for fiscal year 2013. (From Congressional Budget Office, updated budget projections: 2014 to 2024, April 2014. Slide available from the Kaiser Family Foundation. http://kff.org/Kaiser-slides/.)

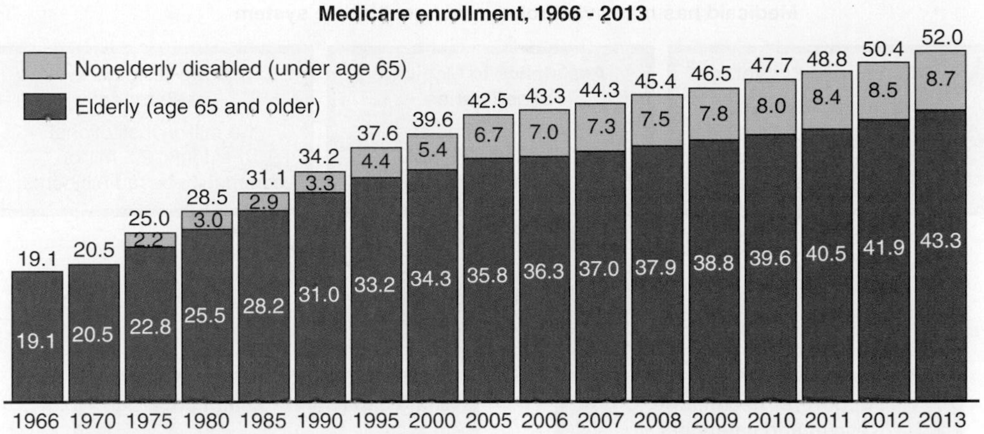

**Medicare enrollment, 1966 - 2013**

FIGURE 3-12 Medicare enrollment, 1966 to 2013. The numbers may not sum to the total because of rounding. People with disabilities younger than 65 years were not eligible for Medicare before 1972. (From Kaiser Family Foundation. Sources Centers for Medicare & Medicaid Services. Medicare enrollment: Hospital insurance and/or supplemental medical insurance programs for total, fee-for-service and managed care enrollees as of July 1, 2011: Selected calendar years 1966-2011; 2012-2013, HHS budget in brief, FY 2014. https://kaiserfamilyfoundation.files.wordpress.com/2013/06/july-2013-medicare-kaiser-slides.pptx.)

with low education or literacy levels, as well as debilitated older adults in long-term care facilities, may have difficulty selecting the best plan for their individual needs. The average monthly premium cost in 2016 is projected to be about $39.00 but may be higher in some plans and for those with higher incomes. The original Part D plan required the first $250 of prescription drug costs to be paid by the older adult each year. Medicare then pays 75% of the next $2000 worth of drugs on the plan's formulary. After that, there is a gap in coverage known as the "donut hole," where individuals pay 100% of drug costs until another $2850 has been spent out-of-pocket. At that point, Medicare will begin paying about 95% of the cost of covered drugs until the end of the calendar year. The ACA will gradually close the donut hole gap in prescription coverage (see http://www.cms.gov for the most up-to-date costs).

## Medicaid

Medicaid is an essential health insurance program available to certain low-income individuals and families who fit into an eligibility group that is recognized by federal and state law (Figure 3-13). Medicaid pays health care providers directly if they participate in the Medicaid program.

Medicaid is an assistance program, commonly referred to as welfare, managed jointly by the federal and state governments to provide partial or full payment of medical costs for individuals and families of any age who are too poor to pay for the care. Medicaid legislation, Title XIX of the Social Security Amendments, came into effect in 1967. The federal government provides funds to states on a cost-sharing basis, with 50% to almost 80% from the federal government and the remainder from the state, according to the per capita income of each state, to guarantee medical services to eligible Medicaid recipients.

Medicaid is an integral part of the health care system, providing health insurance coverage for 37% of all children, 51% of nonelderly people below the federal poverty level, and 64% of

nursing home residents (Figure 3-14). Medicaid serves as a safety net for low-income and high-need Americans.. Poverty guidelines are issued by the USDHHS to be used to determine financial eligibility for some federal programs. In 2015, the federal poverty level was $11,770 for individuals and $15,930 and for a family of two (USDHHS, n.d.b). The program will also support individuals and families with subsidies for insurance coverage in state-based health benefit exchanges. Individuals and families with income levels of 133% to 400% of poverty levels will be eligible to receive subsidies to assist in paying for health premiums. Previously, states established income eligibility requirements for their Medicaid program, and 47 states had income-eligibility levels for children in the Medicaid/CHIP program of 200%. Before the ACA, states could not cover nondisabled adults without children in a Medicaid program. As mentioned previously, the Supreme Court supported states' rights not to expand Medicaid eligibility. States that have not expanded Medicaid programs have higher numbers of uninsured people.

Additionally, Medicaid pays the Medicare premiums, deductibles, and co-insurance for certain low-income Medicare recipients. Medicaid plans are open-ended, meaning a state must admit into the program at any time all individuals who meet the criteria. A state is not allowed to cap the Medicaid budget for a particular fiscal year, thus making it difficult to determine exactly how much money needs to be appropriated.

States administer Medicaid under federal requirements and guidelines. The ACA mandates minimal essential health benefits, typically those that are offered in an employer's health plan must be offered, but states can provide enhanced benefits and offer a more comprehensive plan. Programs differed widely among states in terms of services covered. In summary, the ACA of 2010 includes a significant expansion of the Medicaid program, covering more of the uninsured and providing subsidies to help low-income individuals buy coverage through newly established health benefit exchanges.

**Medicaid has many vital roles in our health care system**

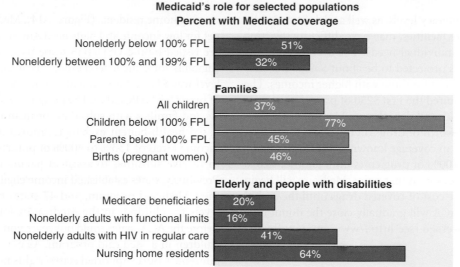

| Health insurance coverage | Assistance to Medicare beneficiaries | Long-term care assistance |
|---|---|---|
| 31 million children and 16 million low-income families; 16 million elderly and persons with disabilities | 9.4 million aged and disabled - 20% of beneficiaries | 1.6 million institutional residents; 2.8 million community-based residents |

**MEDICAID**

| Support for health care system and safety net | State capacity for health coverage |
|---|---|
| 16% of national health spending; 40% of long-term care services | Federal share can range from 50 - 83%. For FFY 2013, ranges from 50 - 73.4% |

**FIGURE 3-13** Medicaid has many vital roles in our health care system. *FFY,* Federal fiscal year. (From Kaiser Commission on Medicaid and the Uninsured. http://kaiserfamilyfoundation.files. wordpress.com/2013/03/medicaid-has-many-vital-roles-in-our-health-care-system-medicaid.png.)

**Medicaid's role for selected populations**
**Percent with Medicaid coverage**

Nonelderly below 100% FPL — 51%
Nonelderly between 100% and 199% FPL — 32%

**Families**

All children — 37%
Children below 100% FPL — 77%
Parents below 100% FPL — 45%
Births (pregnant women) — 46%

**Elderly and people with disabilities**

Medicare beneficiaries — 20%
Nonelderly adults with functional limits — 16%
Nonelderly adults with HIV in regular care — 41%
Nursing home residents — 64%

**FIGURE 3-14** Medicaid's role for selected populations. The federal poverty level (FPL) was $19,530 for a family of three in 2013. (From Kaiser Commission on Medicaid and the Uninsured [KCMU] and Urban Institute analysis of 2013 CPS/ASEC supplement; birth data-maternal and child health update, National Governors Association, 2012; Medicare data-Medicare Payment Advisory Commission, data book: Beneficiaries dually eligible for Medicare and Medicaid (January 2015), 2010 data; functional limitations-KCMU Analysis of 2012 NHIS data; nonelderly with HIV-2009 CDC MMP; nursing home residents-2012 OSCAR data. Slide available from the Kaiser Family Foundation. http://kff.org/Kaiser-slides/.)

The federal government, in the passage of the Deficit Reduction Act of 2005, made it harder for individuals to qualify for Medicaid nursing home benefits by increasing penalties on individuals who transferred assets for less than fair market value during the previous 5 years. Since long-term care is expensive, purchasing private long-term care insurance to cover nursing home care became an option in some states. Individuals who already have long-term care needs are not eligible, and the cost of the premium increases with an individual's age. For older persons, the cost of the premium makes long-term care insurance unaffordable.

Passage of the welfare reform bill in 1996 (Personal Responsibility and Work Opportunity Reconciliation Act of 1996, Public Law 104-193) revealed a significant philosophical shift in federal thinking about welfare assistance in the United States. For the first time, Medicaid was not linked directly to welfare programs. Ending a 61-year guarantee of federal aid, the Temporary Assistance for Needy Families program (formerly Aid to Families with Dependent Children) established by this legislation provides temporary financial aid with a 5-year lifetime limit. Legal immigrants who arrive in the United States after the passage of this bill must wait 5 years to become eligible for programs. The aim was to help parents become self-sufficient through welfare-to-work programs.

As part of the Balanced Budget Act of 1997, CHIP was enacted to provide health insurance coverage to children whose family's income is below 200% of the federal poverty level or whose family has an income 50% higher than the state's Medicaid eligibility threshold (CMS, n.d.). Some states had expanded their CHIP eligibility to include family coverage (see the previous discussion). The ACA has expanded Medicaid eligibility (see the previous discussion).

## Pharmaceutical Costs

The spiraling cost of prescription drugs continues to add to the complexity of providing adequate health care. Newer drugs cost more than the drugs they replace and contribute 50% of the increased cost. Increased use of prescription drugs adds to an increased cost per day of medications. Consumer demand sparked by drug advertisements, new indications for use, and increased consumer knowledge of available drugs has increased the demand for prescription medications. Increased drug cost is attributed to inflation, more days of therapy per user, greater number of drugs per user, cost of research and drug development (Box 3-12), and advertising costs. As discussed earlier, Part D of Medicare is the prescription drug component of the Medicare plan.

## The Uninsured: Who are They?

The number of uninsured Americans younger than 65 years was estimated to be 46 million in 2008 and rose as a result of the economic downturn and the growing cost of health plan

premiums (KFF, 2012). The 2010 ACA is expected to reduce the number of uninsured significantly with the expansion of Medicaid, subsidies to pay premiums in health insurance exchanges, a federal mandate requiring most legal citizens to enroll in an insurance plan or face tax penalties for noncompliance, and a provision allowing children to remain on their parents' employer family insurance until the age of 26 years (Figure 3-15). Previously, when children reached the age of 19 years and were not full-time college students, they were deleted from employer family insurance plans. Even with all the new options afforded by the ACA, a number of individuals will remain uninsured. Undocumented immigrants (those who are noncitizens and are living in the United States illegally) do not qualify for Medicaid or any other public insurance plan and are also exempt from paying the federal tax penalty. This population is extremely vulnerable because of language and cultural barriers and fear of being discovered as an illegal immigrant; therefore they typically do not seek health care. Provisions in current law require emergency care to be provided as well as care to be provided to pregnant women, regardless of alien status (KFF, 2010a). Another group of individuals are those who choose not to enroll in a qualified insurance plan and instead elect to pay the annual federal tax penalty. The ACA includes a federal tax penalty for individuals who do not obtain coverage beginning in 2014. The penalty increased every year for the next 3 years for any individual not exempted from the requirement who does not have coverage. For example, the per-adult penalty in 2014 was $95, rose to $325 in 2015, and rose to $695 in 2016. Exemptions from the federal penalty include undocumented immigrants, those whose incomes are below the minimum amount required to file federal income tax returns, those with incomes below 138% of the poverty level in states that have not expanded eligibility for Medicaid, and those who would have to pay more than 8.13% of household income for

---

### ⚕ BOX 3-12   GENOMICS

#### Genetics and Pharmacogenetics

The field of pharmacogenomics is rapidly expanding what is known about the influence of hereditary genetic attributes and how drugs respond in the body. A number of drugs have been found that affect certain ethnic groups and individuals in different ways. Individuals who metabolize a specific drug slowly (slow acetylators) will take longer to metabolize the drug into the active form and retain the active drug longer in the body. Slow or poor metabolizers may require a lower dose or a different choice of drug to avoid toxicity. Rapid metabolizers (fast acetylators) metabolize drugs quickly into the active form, which may then be metabolized more quickly into the inactive form, leading to therapeutic drug failure. Fast metabolizers may require no dosage adjustment or higher dosages for the dosage to be therapeutic. Other genetic variations in drug-metabolizing enzymes exist that significantly impact how a drug is metabolized. As the field of pharmacogenetics evolves, tools that determine genotyping of an individual may be used routinely to guide practitioners in the selection of therapeutic options. Optimal medication dosage and selection of drugs may personalize drug treatment regimens, preventing adverse effects and contributing to better patient outcomes. The financial and ethical decision-making aspects of the use of genotyping technology in medical decision-making will be issues to address in future health care legislation.

Source Woo, T., & Robinson, M. (2016). *Pharmacotherapeutics for advanced practice nurse prescribers* (4th ed.). Philadelphia: F.A. Davis.

---

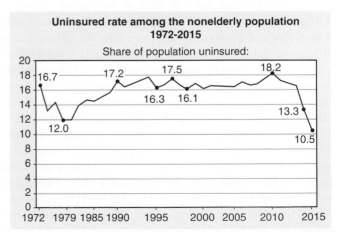

**Uninsured rate among the nonelderly population 1972-2015**

Share of population uninsured:

**FIGURE 3-15** Uninsured rate among the nonelderly population 1972 to 2015. The 2015 data are for the first and second quarters only. (From Centers for Disease Control and Prevention/National Center for Health Statistics, National Health Interview Survey, reported in http://www.cdc.gov/nchs/health_policy/trends_hc_1968_2011.htm#table01 and http://www.cdc.gov/nchs/data/nhis/earlyrelease/insur201511.pdf. Slide available from the Kaiser Family Foundation. http://kff.org/Kaiser-slides/.)

insurance. In 2016 the tax penalty was calculated to be the greater of the following two amounts: a flat dollar amount of $695 per adult and $347.50 per child, up to a maximum of $2085 for the family, or 2.5% of family income in excess of the 2015 income tax filing thresholds ($10,300 for a single person and $26,600 for a family). It is estimated that 7 million uninsured people are eligible for marketplace premium subsidies to assist with the cost of premiums. For about half who qualify, the cost of the lowest plan (a bronze plan) would have a zero premium cost. For others (an additional 3.5 million people) the cost of a bronze plan using their premium subsidy would be less than the penalty. However, although the cost of the premium for a bronze plan may be zero or reduced, which fulfills the ACA mandate, bronze plans typically have a higher copayment when used. The next level of insurance premiums, called silver premiums, may have a higher premium cost but significantly less copayment cost at the time of use. Health care providers and nurses need to stay abreast of all of these changes to help individuals and families navigate the complexities of the financial aspects of insurance. Once this portion of the law is fully enacted, it is expected that many more Americans will choose to obtain coverage as it will be less costly than paying the penalty. For some, the reality of the ACA insurance mandate will not be realized until federal tax returns are filed for 2016, in the early part of 2017 (KFF, 2016). Nurses and health care providers can assist individuals and families in both gaining coverage and selecting a plan that best suites their needs. Another group of individuals who may not have coverage are noncitizens who are legally traveling within the United States (business, education, tourism) unless they have purchased secondary travel insurance before entering the United States.

### Unauthorized Immigrants

The Pew Research Center (Gonzalez-Barrera & Krogstad, 2015) and the US Department of Homeland Security (2014) estimated the number of illegal aliens in 2014 in the United States was 11.3 million, or 3.5% of the nation's population. Almost 50% of unauthorized immigrants are from Mexico. Although it is difficult to determine exact numbers, in 2012, 8.1 million unauthorized immigrants were estimated to be working or looking for work. Some unauthorized immigrants entered the United States without valid documentation, whereas others arrived with valid visas but stayed past the visa expiration date. About 60% of unauthorized immigrants are located in six states: California, Texas, Florida, New York, Illinois, and New Jersey. Immigration reform remains a contested project with concern about both entry into the country and how to deal with unauthorized immigrants who are already living in the United States. In 2013, 662,483 individuals were apprehended: 438,421 individuals were removed and 178,371 individuals were returned. This is the lowest number of returned or removed individuals since 1972 (Gonzalez-Barrera & Krogstad, 2015). According to federal law, anyone entering an emergency department must be treated regardless of the ability to pay or immigration status. However, those individuals who are in the United States illegally may be reluctant to seek health care for fear of legal action, being removed, or being returned. This vulnerable population is not eligible to enroll in Medicare or Medicaid programs and have various unmet health care needs.

## HEALTH CARE SYSTEMS OF OTHER COUNTRIES

The United States spends the highest proportion of its GDP on health care of all industrialized countries (see Figure 3-4) with a reported GDP of 16% in 2008, 5.9% above the global average for the countries listed. The United States has the highest cost per capita (see Figure 3-2), reporting $7538 dollars were spent per person in 2008 compared with the next highest amount (Norway) at a little over $5000 and the lowest amount reported (Japan) at $2700. Figure 3-3 shows a graphical representation of the growth in health care expenditure per capita for different countries over time. The countries represented in Figures 3-2 and 3-3 all have some version of a universal health care plan and spend less money per capita. Life expectancy rates are higher and infant mortality rates are lower in these countries than in the United States. Although each country has a different type of health plan, all share many of the same problems of the US free-market system. As mentioned earlier, rising health care costs; issues of access and affordability; workforce shortages of health care providers; increased concern over medical errors, quality of care, and safety; changing demographic population trends; and escalating health care costs are some of the inherent issues faced by all nations in providing health care.

### Canadian Health Care System

The Canadian health care program, called Medicare, is a group of socialized health insurance plans that provide health coverage to all Canadian citizens regardless of medical history, personal income, or job status. The Canada Health Act, legislated at the federal level, determines what services must be provided, similarly to the Medicaid program in the United States, but provinces and territories may provide additional services not listed in the Canada Health Act. The Canada Health Act specifies basic services, including primary care and hospitalizations, leaving the individual province or territory responsible for the management, organization, and delivery of health services for its residents. The Canada Health Act does not include services such as physical therapy, dental coverage, corrective lenses, home care, or prescription medicines, but separate provinces can elect to provide enhancements. Some employers also offer private insurance plans to supplement the Canadian health care plan for services not offered, such as corrective lenses, medications, and home care. Every Canadian citizen has the same basic primary health insurance that is covered by the national health care plan. Each Canadian citizen applies for a provincial health card and, once it has been issued, the card provides access to a person's medical information and is used when the citizen visits a physician or health care provider, eliminating the need to fill out forms. Canadians pay for health care through a variety of federal and provincial taxes, just as US residents pay for Social Security and Medicare through payroll taxes. The federal government appropriates funds to the provinces and territories through cash and tax transfers. Because the government is the primary payer of medical bills, Canada's health care system is referred to as a single-payer arrangement. Some provinces gain additional funds through sales tax, lottery proceeds, and health premiums. Additional benefits differ among the provinces, but most provide prescription drugs to older adults and low-income clients. For Canadians with higher incomes and private supplemental insurance, private clinics are available that offer specialized services. The advantage of receiving care in a private clinic is reduced wait times for services. Private clinics offer specialized services not covered by the public health plan. Canadians covered by private health insurance typically have 80% of the costs covered at private clinics. Higher-income Canadians can pay out-of-pocket for care received at private clinics, which typically offer services with reduced wait times. For example, obtaining a magnetic resonance imaging scan in a hospital may require a waiting period of months, whereas a private clinic could offer the scan much earlier. Canadians with private health insurance and higher incomes have access to greater health care services and more expedient health care (Health Canada, 2016).

At one time, the Canadian system seemed to be an ideal model that the United States should adopt; however, increasing health care costs, access issues, delays in treatment, and workforce shortages of health care providers have caused political controversy and debate in Canada. Queuing refers to a system where a person is placed on a wait list before receiving certain types of tests or surgery, allowing a person who is in need of more immediate care to receive priority. If care needs are determined not to be life threatening, persons may need to wait for magnetic resonance imaging scans, heart bypass surgery, cataract removal, or hip replacement procedures for months because persons in urgent need of the procedures are higher on the list. Although all citizens receive the same level of public health care, private insurance allows a two-tiered system favoring Canadians with private health insurance or other financial resources to receive expedited care. If a person can pay out-of-pocket, he or she may elect to travel elsewhere (e.g., to the United States) to receive expedited care. A major shortage of physicians and nurses in Canada is due in part to lower reimbursement rates by the public health system as well as lower salaries, causing some health care providers to leave Canada and practice in other countries such as the United States. Over the years, the federal government has decreased contributions to the provinces and territories because of large federal budget deficits and limited fee increases to physicians for services. Regionalization of hospitals has caused access to care issues for those outside major cities. Expansion to offer better access to home care and community-based services is an emerging issue (Health Canada, 2016).

## SUMMARY

The nursing workforce, composed of more than 3 million nurses, is the largest segment of the nation's health care workforce, and nurses will be key players in moving forward the objectives set forth in the 2010 ACA and *Healthy People 2020*. To move these agendas forward, nurses need to understand the complexity of the health care system—the structures (federal, state, and local) and the financing mechanisms (public and private)—so

---

### CASE STUDY

#### Health Teaching: Using the Internet to Increase Health Literacy

Ella, age 34 years, has been married for 10 years to her husband Joe and recently moved to a new area with their two children, Billy, age 11 years, and Olivia, age 6 years. Joe just started a new position in a state agency and Ella plans to work 3 to 4 days a week as a home health aide. Joe completed a 2-year college degree, and Ella took a few college courses but never finished her degree. The family is new to a primary care clinic, and Ella asks the nurse for advice in choosing a health plan that will best meet the needs of her family. Ella and her husband would like to have a third child in the next year or so. Her husband Joe was given a folder at his new job with multiple health plans to choose from and asked Ella to "just pick one" because they are too complicated to understand. Joe considers himself healthy and active, although he has had recommendations in the past to lose 14 kilograms (30 lbs), is borderline hypertensive, and has slightly elevated blood lipid levels. He has a strong family history of coronary artery disease, and his father died of a myocardial infarction at the age of 65 years. Ella also struggles with her weight and often relies on fast food for quick dinners on the days she works. Their son Billy has attention-deficit–hyperactivity disorder and Olivia has asthma. Both children are above the recommended body mass index for their ages. The family has a home computer with Internet access, and Ella states she is "getting better at using it as her sixth grade son is learning computer literacy in school and is teaching Mom."

The nurse discusses the family's general health-promotion and health-protection needs and the special needs presented by the diseases that have been identified. She provides some resources for Ella to learn more about the health plans available to her and consumer-friendly health information websites.

#### Reflective Questions

- What additional information does the nurse need to assess this family's needs?
- What are the priority area teaching needs for this family?
- What community resources might be available to Ella and her family?
- What are some appropriate websites that Ella might find useful?

Before leaving, the nurse suggests the following:

- From the Agency for Healthcare Research and Quality, a federal government agency with health information for consumers on guidelines in choosing a health plan: http://www.ahrq.gov/consumer/insuranceqa/.
- From the US Department of Labor, a federal agency that provides information on health plans, benefits, and has many links: http://www.dol.gov/.
- For health care information on multiple topics:
  - Health Care Information: http://www.himss.org
  - WebMD: http://webmd.com/
  - Healthfinder: http://healthfinder.gov/
  - Mayo Clinic: http://www.mayoclinic.com/

---

interventions can be targeted to reduce health disparities, promote health equity, and elevate the level of health and wellness across the population. The IOM recognized a number of barriers exist that prevent nurses from being able to respond effectively to rapidly changing health care settings and an evolving health care system. Nurses need to be proactive in shaping policy that affects the health care system and need a working understanding of the complexity of the health care system to be able to educate individuals and families about health care resources, to coordinate services, and to influence health care policy at the local, state, and national levels. To accomplish this task, nurses need to become and remain well-informed citizens and health care consumer advocates.

A historical perspective and a description of the current health care delivery system in the United States provide a framework for the analysis of trends, values, and needs related to health. Awareness of global health indicators sets the stage for the nurse to then compare the health of the nation as a whole. The structure and financing of the health care system, both the public sector and the private sector, are complicated. The influence of recent health reform, the ACA of 2010, sparks an opportunity for nurses to be key players in engaging effectively to deliver high-quality evidence-based nursing care and move forward the agendas of *Healthy People 2020* and the IOM's *Future of Nursing: Leading Change, Advancing Health.*

## ⓔ EVOLVE CHAPTER FEATURES

http://evolve.elsevier.com/Edelman/
• Study Questions

## REFERENCES

Accountability Office. (2005). Physician services: Concierge care characteristics and considerations for Medicare. http://gao.gov/new.items/d05929.

American Red Cross. (n.d.). About us. http://www.redcross.org.

Arias, E., & Smith, B. (2003). Deaths: Preliminary data for 2001. *National Vital Statistics Reports, 51*(5), 1–44.

Barr, D. (2011). *Introduction to U.S. health policy: The organization, financing, and delivery of health care in America* (3rd ed.). Baltimore, MD: Johns Hopkins University Press.

CDC Foundation. (2012). How CDC saves lives by controlling REAL global disease outbreaks. http://www.cdcfoundation.org/content/how-cdc-saves-lives-controlling-real-global-disease-outbreaks.

CDC Foundation. (2016). Global disaster response fund. http://www.cdcfoundation.org/globaldisaste.

Centers for Disease Control and Prevention (CDC). (2015). Reported tuberculosis in the United States, 2014. U.S. Department of Health and Human Services, CDC, October 2015. http://www.cdc.gov/tb/statistics/reports/2014.

Centers for Disease Control and Prevention (CDC). (2016). 10 leading causes of death by age group, United States 2013. http://www.cdc.gov-injury-wisqars.pdf.

Centers for Medicare & Medicaid Services (CMS). (n.d.). State Children's Health Insurance Program (SCHIP) homepage. http://www.cms.gov/apps/firststep/content/schip-qas.html.

Centers for Medicare & Medicaid Services (CMS). (2015a). National health expenditure data: NHE projections 2014-2024-forecast summary fact sheets 7/28/15. http://www.cms.gov/Research-Statistics-Data-and-Systems/Statistics-Trends-and-Report.

Centers for Medicare & Medicaid Services (CMS). (2015b). In states that expand Medicaid, more low-income adults gain access to health coverage. http://www.cms.medicaid.gov.

Centers for Medicare & Medicaid Services (CMS). (2017). Historical national health expenditure fact sheet 2015. http://www.cms.gov.

Central Intelligence Agency (CIA). (2015). The world fact book. http://cia.gov/library/publications/the-world-factbook.

Chen, A., Oster, E., & Williams, H. (2014). Why is infant mortality higher in the U.S. than in Europe? NBER working paper no. 20525. http://www.nber.org.

Community Health and Empowerment Through Education and Research. (2015). About CHEER. http://communitycheer.org/about/.

Concierge Medicine Today. (n.d.). Concierge medicine today, 2014 stats, year-end data summary. http://www.conciergemedicinetoday.org.

Freyman, J. G. (1980). *The American health care system: Its genesis and trajectory*. Huntington, NY: Krieger.

Gonzalez-Barrera, A., & Krogstad, J. (2015). What we know about illegal immigration from Mexico. http://www.pewresearch.org/fact-tank/2015/11/20/what-we-know-about-illegal-immigration-from-mexico/.

Health Canada. (2016). Health Canada-a partner in health for all Canadians. http://www.hc-sc.gc.ca.

HealthCare.gov. (n.d.). Health benefits and coverage-what marketplace health insurance plans cover. http://www.healthcare.gov.

Henry Street Settlement. (2016). Lillian Wald. http://www.henrystreet.org/about/history/lillian-wald-html.

Institute for Nursing Centers. (n.d.). Home page. http://www.nursingcenters.org/.

Institute of Medicine (IOM). (1999). To err is human: Building a safer health system. http://www.iom.edu/Reports/1999/To-Err-is-Human-Building-A-Safer-Health-System.aspx.

Institute of Medicine (IOM). (2003). Keeping patients safe: Transforming the work environment of nurses. http://www.iom.edu/Reports/2003/Keeping-Patients-Safe-Transforming-the-Work-Environment-of-Nurses.aspx.

Institute of Medicine (IOM). (2006). Preventing medication errors: Quality chasm series. http://www.iom.edu/Reports/2006/Preventing-Medication-Errors-Quality-Chasm-Series.aspx.

Institute of Medicine (IOM). (2010). The future of nursing: Leading change, advancing health. http://www.iom.edu/Reports/2010/The-Future-of-Nursing-Leading-Change-Advancing-Health.aspx.

Institute of Medicine (IOM). (2012). Barriers to integrating crisis standards of care principles into international disaster response plans-workplace summary. http://www.iom.edu/Reports/2012/Barriers-to-Integrating-Crisis-Standards-of-Care-Principles-into-international.

Institute of Medicine (IOM). (2014). Dying in America, improving quality and honoring individual preferences near the end of life. http://www.iom.edu/2014/Dying-in-America.

John, A., & Hartford Foundation. (2012). About us. http://www.jhartfound.org/about_us.htm.

Kaiser Family Foundation (KFF). (2010a). *Health policy center: The uninsured*. Menlo Park, CA: Henry J. Kaiser Family Foundation. http://www.urban.org/health_policy/uninsured/index.cfm.

Kaiser Family Foundation (KFF). (2010b). Health policy center: Vulnerable populations. http://www.urban.org/health_policy/vulnerable_popuations/index.cfm.

Kaiser Family Foundation (KFF). (2012). Kaiser Commission on Medicaid and the uninsured. http://www./kff.org, Publication#8272–2.pdf.

Kaiser Family Foundation (KFF). (2013). Summary of the Affordable Care Act. http://www.kff.org/health-reform/fact-sheet/summary-of-the-affordable-care-act/.

Kaiser Family Foundation (KFF). (2014). Medicare at a glance. http://www.kaiserfamilyfoundation.files.wordpress.

Kaiser Family Foundation (KFF). (2015a). 2015 Employer health benefits survey: Summary of findings. http://www.kff.org.

Kaiser Family Foundation (KFF). (2015b). Medicare advantage 2016 data spotlight: Overview of plan changes (p 24). Issue brief, December 2015. http://www.kff.org.

Kaiser Family Foundation (KFF). (2015c). The facts on Medicare spending and financing (p 50). http:/www.kff.org.

Kaiser Family Foundation (KFF). (2016). The cost of the individual mandate penalty for the remaining uninsured December 2015 issue brief. http://www.kff.org.

Kovner, A., & Knickman, J. (2015). *Jonas & Kovner's health care delivery in the United States* (11th ed.). New York: Springer.

Mathews, T. J., MacDorman, M. F., & Thoma, M. E. (2015). Infant mortality statistics from the 2013 period linked birth/infant death data set. *National Vital Statistics Reports, 64*(9), 1–30.

Medicare.gov. (n.d.). Your Medicare coverage. http://www.medicare.gov.

Melnyk, B., & Fineout-Overholt, E. (2014). *Evidence-based practice in nursing and healthcare: A guide to best practice* (3rd ed.). Philadelphia: Lippincott Williams & Wilkins.

National Academies of Sciences, Engineering, and Medicine. (2016). About our division name. http://www.nationalacademies.org/hmd/About-HDM/Division-Name.

National Center for Health Statistics. (2014). *Health, United States, 2014 with special features on adults aged 55-64.* Hyattsville, MD: National Center for Health Statistics.

Nies, M., & McEwen, M. (2014). *Community/public health nursing: Promoting the health of populations* (6th ed.). St. Louis: Saunders.

Office of Disease Prevention and Health Promotion. (2015). About healthy people. http://www.healthypeople.gov/2020/About-Healthy-People/.

Office of the Legislative Council. (2010). Compilation of Patient Protection and Affordable Care Act as amended through May, 1, 2010. 111th Congress. PPACA Public Law 114–148.

Peterson Center on Healthcare & Kaiser Family Foundation Partnership. (2015). Peterson-Kaiser Health System Tracker. http://www.healthsystemtracker.org.

Shi, L., & Singh, D. (2013). *Essentials of the US health care system* (3rd ed.). Burlington, MA: Jones & Bartlett Learning.

Social Security Administration. (n.d.). History. http://www.ssa.gov/history/lifeexpect.html.

Society of Hospital Medicine. (n.d.). Definition of a hospitalist and hospital medicine. http://www.hospitalmedicine.org.

Stanhope, M., & Lancaster, J. (2012). *Public health nursing: Population-centered health care* (8th ed.). St. Louis: Mosby.

University of Alabama at Birmingham. (2016). The life of Florence Nightingale. Reynolds historic library. http://www.uab.edu.

US Department of Health and Human Services (USDHHS). (2012). Office of Minority Health. HHS action plan to reduce racial and ethnic health disparities. http://www.minorityhealth.hhs.gov/npa/templates/content.aspx.

US Department of Health and Human Services (USDHHS). (2015a). Healthy People 2020. http://www.healthypeople.gov/2020/Leading-Health-Indicators.

US Department of Health and Human Services (USDHHS). (2015b). *Health, United States, 2014 with special features on adults aged 55-64.* Hyattsville, MD: National Center for Health Statistics.

US Department of Health and Human Services (USDHHS). (2015c). Civil rights. http://www.hhs.gov/civil-rights/for-individuals/index.htm.

US Department of Health and Human Services (USDHHS). (n.d.a). Health information privacy. http://www.hhs.gov/ocr/privacy/hipaa/understanding/index.html.

US Department of Health and Human Services (USDHHS). (n.d.b). About HHS. http://www.hhs.gov.

US Department of Homeland Security. (2014) 2013 yearbook of immigration statistics. http://www.dhs.gov/sites/default/files/publications/0is_yb_2013_0.pdf.

US Department of Homeland Security. (n.d.). FEMA. http://www.fema.gov/Homepage.

US Department of Labor. (2014). Bureau of Labor Statistics: Occupational outlook handbook, fastest growing occupations. http://www.bls.gov/ooh/fastest-growing.htm.

US Department of Labor. (2015a). Bureau of Labor Statistics: Economic employment and wages summary—May 2014. http://www.bls.gov/news.release/ocwage.nr0.htm.

US Department of Labor. (2015b). The Bureau of Labor Statistics occupational outlook handbook 2016-2017. http://www.bls.gov.

US Public Health Nursing Services. (n.d.) Leadership. http://www.usphs.gov.

Veterans Administration (VA). (2015). In the news, VA makes changes to Veterans Choice Program. http://www.va.gov.

World Health Organization (WHO). (2015). *Global tuberculosis report 2015* (20th ed.). Geneva: World Health Organization.

World Health Organization (WHO). (n.d.a). MDGs: Progress made in health. http://www.who.int.

World Health Organization (WHO). (n.d.b) Global health observatory data repository. http://apps.who.int/gho/data/view.main.680.

# 4

# The Therapeutic Relationship

*June Andrews Horowitz*

The therapeutic relationship is the **milieu** (or context, setting) in which nursing care occurs. Nursing practice is shaped by the caregiver's ability to focus on the interests, concerns, and needs of the individual (Peplau, 1991; D'Antonio et al., 2014). Establishing a therapeutic relationship is critical to problem resolution. The nurse-person relationship comprises the key components of knowing each other, reciprocity, respect, and confidence (Errasti-Ibarrondo et al., 2015). Even in brief interactions, communicating a focus on and concern for the person is critical. A 56-year-old woman who experienced an unexpected myocardial infarction recalls that the clinician who made the most impact on her sat quietly at her bedside for a few moments and made eye contact to discuss what was most important about the woman's rehabilitation plan. What made this brief interaction memorable? It was the clinician's attention to the person who was experiencing the health crisis; it was the quiet pause from the acute care arena activity created by sitting, listening, and making eye contact: it was the clinician's focus on what was most important for the woman's recovery. Across delivery settings, the importance of the nurse-person relationship cannot be forgotten or minimized because of time constraints. As the example shared here illustrates, even episodic brief encounters can have profound effects as shown in this example. Moreover, in today's complex multicultural and global health care arena, nursing's concentration also extends beyond individuals to populations (Fawcett & Ellenbecker, 2015), yet the same critical elements of the relationship remain.

BOX 4-1  HEALTHY PEOPLE 2020

**Leading Health Indicators**
- Access to health services
- Clinical preventive services
- Environmental quality
- Injury and violence
- Maternal, infant, and child health
- Mental health
- Nutrition, physical activity, and obesity
- Oral health
- Reproductive and sexual health
- Social determinants
- Substance abuse
- Tobacco

**Priorities for Action**
- Adopt the 12 leading health indicators as personal and professional guides for choices about how to make health improvements.
- Encourage public health professionals and public officials to adopt the leading health indicators as the basis for public health priority setting and decision-making.
- Urge public and community health systems and our community leadership to use the leading health indicators as measures of local success for investments in health improvements.

Source US Department of Health and Human Services. (n.d.) *Healthy People 2020*. Leading health indicators. http://www.healthypeople.gov/2020/Leading-Health-Indicators.

BOX 4-2  **The Valuing Process**

**Choosing**
- Choosing freely
- Choosing from alternatives
- Choosing after careful consideration of potential outcomes of each alternative

**Prizing**
- Cherishing and being happy with personal beliefs and actions
- Affirming the choice in public, when appropriate

**Acting**
- Acting out the choice
- Repeatedly acting in some type of pattern

Particularly in health promotion, the nurse-person relationship is the context for care. Health promotion requires sensitivity to each person's goals and values; the individual's and the nurse's. Helping a person adopt health-promoting behaviors requires more than giving information. Health promotion also requires effective communication, which is why communication is a focus area of *Healthy People 2020* (US Department of Health and Human Services, 2010) and thus a priority for nursing practice. Successful health promotion involves interpersonal skills, personal insight, accountability, mutual respect, and a supportive working milieu. Essential to this interactional process are values clarification, communication, and the helping relationship. See Box 4-1: *Healthy People 2020* for the leading health indicators and priorities for action.

## VALUES CLARIFICATION

### Definition

Values are qualities, principles, attitudes, or beliefs about the inherent worth of an object, behavior, or idea that guide action by sanctioning certain actions and disavowing others. Values and beliefs are essential factors in design and implementation of nursing interventions. To serve the unique and diverse needs of individuals, it is imperative that nurses understand the importance of cultural differences by valuing, incorporating, and examining their own health-related values and beliefs and those of their health care organizations, for only then can they support the principle of respect for persons and the ideal of transcultural care (Beard et al., 2015). Cognitive values are those

a person ascribes to verbally and intellectually. Active values, in contrast, are those a person physically acts out. Judging the power of a given value by its ability to influence action is important. For example, a nurse may claim to value the worth of all people equally, but may treat individuals of various races differently and provide the most time and concern for those who are racially similar to the nurse. This cognitive value has little power to shape the nurse's behavior. If the nurse treated people of all races with equal respect, the value would also be active and have great power to motivate behavior.

Many forces shape values. Passed down from one generation to another, values color an individual's identity, goals, and sense of personal meaning. Values are embedded in the culture and taught within a family and social context, giving meaning to the life events and happenings outside the family's boundaries (Wright & Leahey, 2013). To engage in health promotion, the nurse must appreciate that values are culture bound and explore how culture, traditions, and practices in a multiethnic and multicultural society influence health-related values. Without this understanding, the nurse is likely to relate to individuals with a limited awareness of their assumptions and inadequate sensitivity to the uniqueness and perspective of the person, family, or community.

Values evolve; they are not static. Life events and social processes can spark a reappraisal of personal values. **Values clarification** is a method for discovering one's values and the importance of these values (Raths et al., 1978). Values clarification does not tell a person how to act, but it helps people recognize what values they hold and evaluate how those values influence their actions.

Box 4-2 outlines seven steps in the valuing process. The first three steps involve a cognitive process, the next two steps involve the affective or emotional domain, and the final steps involve behavior (Raths et al., 1978; Stuart, 2012). The nurse uses values clarification to examine personal values and their potential influence on nursing care, and to help people identify their values and reflect on their connection to health-related behaviors. Box 4-3 lists suggestions for putting values clarification into action. For a values clarification exercise, try following the steps outlined in Box 4-3 in regard to a personal value. Moreover, values clarification requires exploration of both overt and covert factors that affect our perceptions and actions. The process entails taking a

## BOX 4-3    Techniques for Assisting Individuals to Clarify Values

**Identify the Individual's Values**

"What is important to you?"

"Which of the following statements sounds most like the way you think?"

"What do you value most in life?"

**Use Reflection to Restate the Value and Make It Explicit**

"In what you've just told me, I hear that it is very important to you that…"

"I understand that you value…"

**Identify Value Conflicts or Conflicts Between Values and Actions**

"What connection does this value have to your current health or illness and to the healthy behaviors, interventions, or treatments needed to maintain or restore your health?"

"How does this particular value affect your behavior and health?"

"What are some ways that you might put your values into action?"

"Are your actions consistent with your values? If not, then what might you change?"

virtual flashlight to shine light on our past and current life experiences to examine the values that shape our attitudes and behavior.

Values clarification becomes a clinical aim when individuals' values lead to behaviors that conflict with the nurse's value of promoting health. For example, a nurse tells a childbirth education class consisting of pregnant women and their coaches that alcohol use poses serious risks to the fetus. After the class, one woman comments, "Do you really think that having a drink once in a while is bad for the baby? I'm sick of being told that I can't do things because of the baby." In this example, an apparent conflict in values between the nurse and the individual exists. Intervention is needed to examine how this woman's wish for freedom from restrictions clashes with her desire to have a healthy child. Nurses must consider their own values related to health promotion for the individual and the fetus and must weigh the importance of respecting individuals' rights to make decisions about their own health behaviors with potential risks to the fetus. Such value conflicts result in ethical dilemmas. Resolution rests on the nurse's ability to examine conflicting values and available evidence about possible outcomes when fashioning health-promotion interventions. Sharing the evidence to support the clinical recommendation also helps to reduce a judgmental message in the communication and opens communication for discussion about the strength of the evidence and its practical implications for health behaviors (Melnyk & Fineout-Overholt, 2011).

## Values and Therapeutic Use of Self

Therapeutic use of self is the application of one's cognitions, perceptions, and behaviors to create interpersonal encounters that promote health in another person, family, group, or community. Without self-awareness and clarification of values, therapeutic use of self is impaired. Self-concept and self-esteem are interrelated components of individuals' judgments and attitudes about themselves. Self-concept is a mental picture of the self; a composite view of personal characteristics, abilities, limitations, and aspirations. Self-esteem, the affective component of self-perception, refers to how individuals feel about the way that they see themselves. Internalized appraisals from others also influence self-concept and self-esteem.

Self-concept evolves throughout life. From birth, family experiences and parental identification mold the child's sense of identity. Self-esteem is learned from experience. To cultivate children's self-esteem and enable them to have a realistic perception of their strengths and weaknesses, parents should focus on positives, give feedback on abilities and limitations, and provide the child with a sense of belonging and realistic confidence. Positive, rewarding, anxiety-free interactions contribute to security, esteem, and positive self-view. Positive but realistic appraisals from significant others, especially the parents, help the young child to develop this healthy self-view. Parental resources—that is, social determinants of health (such as parental education, household income/zip code)—also have demonstrated positive effects on children's development (Sullivan, 1953; Walker et al., 2011).

The self does not develop solely in response to the reflected appraisals of others. Genetic endowment, experiential opportunities, and the individual's action shape self-concept. People can accept or reject the appraisals of others and modify their behavior. The ability to control actions and evaluate outcomes of interactions allows individuals to modify and alter their views of self. As such, the self is dynamic, changing through interaction with the outside world and in response to the various maturational and situational crises of life.

The ability to examine, reflect on, and evaluate the self is a uniquely human talent. Self-awareness involves interactions between the self and the external world and the symbolic connections created by the individual. The self includes an unconscious component that is only partially accessible and influences behavior. Self-awareness is influenced by the degree to which an individual has an accurate concept of all dimensions of the self.

The goal of high self-awareness is reached through three steps. The first step is listening to oneself and paying attention to emotions, thoughts, memories, reactions, and impulses. Frequently, people ignore their feelings and thoughts because they are anxious or because they are in a hurry to accomplish some other task. Without self-reflection, people act automatically and lose some of the meaning of living. To improve the ability of self-reflection, ask questions such as the following:

- What am I feeling now?
- What emotions have I experienced today and in the past day or so? What were my thoughts?
- What events led to these thoughts and feelings?
- What actions did I take? Did my behavior fit with my thoughts and feelings, or was there a lack of harmony?
- Was I aware of my reactions at the time that they occurred?
- How have I responded in clinical situations lately?
- How did I react in response to a particularly happy, sad, or difficult situation? In what way might I alter my actions now? What feelings and reactions did I experience while interacting with this individual?

The second step is listening to and learning from others. Feedback from others that conflicts with self-image can produce anxiety.

In response, the feedback is ignored or translated incorrectly to preserve self-image and reduce anxiety. However, this pattern of responding limits knowledge of the self and inhibits the ability to examine the appraisals of others, resulting in limited personal growth. Asking reflective questions enables the nurse to use feedback effectively. Helpful questions include "What feedback have I received today?" and "What is the other person trying to tell me now?" A person also can ask others directly for feedback. For example, a student nurse might ask another student how he or she comes across. The feedback might be used to alter aspects of behavior that are ineffective or problematic before the student nurse asks a faculty member for evaluative feedback. Using clinical supervision and consultation with colleagues provides needed opportunity for reflection on practice. How the nurse comes across to the individual, family, or community is crucial to successful health promotion, making self-awareness and sensitivity to feedback essential.

The third step is **self-disclosure**; sharing aspects of the self enriches interpersonal life. Through self-reflection/self-disclosure, people come to know themselves better because they have exposed their thoughts, actions, and feelings for examination with others. Self-disclosure is an indicator of a healthy personality and a strategy for developing one (Jourard, 1971; Stuart, 2012). Self-disclosure by one person tends to trigger self-disclosure by another in a reciprocal pattern of interaction. Therapeutic interactions characterized by reciprocity involve a mutual exchange—a pattern of communication between the nurse and an individual, not a one-way intervention from the nurse to the other person. Traditionally, clinicians have been wary of self-disclosure because it may cross a boundary from a professional to a personal relationship. Additionally, the nurse's self-disclosure might burden the individual and shift the focus of attention from the individual to the nurse. Although these guidelines are considered so as to prevent excessive or inappropriate self-disclosure, appreciation that self-disclosure occurs within all human interactions is needed. Baldor (2011) found that experienced psychiatric nurse practitioners and clinical nurse specialists identified appropriate self-revelation as an effective component of the therapeutic relationship. Self-disclosure was seen as effective when thoughtfully applied on the basis of the client's developmental stage, the length of the relationship, client need, and boundary strength. Effective self-disclosure was context dependent and related to relational skill of the experienced or expert nurse. Implications included participants' belief that self-disclosure by the clinician is unavoidable and that it can contribute to strengthening or weakening the therapeutic alliance. Thus evidence supports that nurses are not blank screens, robots, or technicians delivering care; individuals value nurses who engage in interactions as real people and who are willing to share information about themselves appropriately and thoughtfully. Seeking consultation from a colleague is helpful whenever a concern arises regarding the limits of appropriate self-disclosure.

**Practical reflection** (i.e., self-reflection) involves deliberating on one's own thoughts and recollections of events to understand them and to take needed corrective action. In reflection, thoughts are interpreted or analyzed. The process tends to be triggered by a seminal or meaningful event or situation, and the process

> **BOX 4-4  Components of the Self**
> - The *public self,* which is shown to others.
> - The *semipublic self,* which is seen by others but may be outside the individual's awareness.
> - The *private self,* which is known to the individual but is not revealed to others.
> - The *inner self,* which is the unconscious portion not known even to the individual because it has anxiety-provoking content.

results in increased understanding or awareness. These insights can then be used in the future when one is faced with a similar event or situation to implement a planned approach. Research outcomes show that self-reflection is associated with lowered practice stress and increased competence among nursing students (Pai, 2015). The process of practical reflection dovetails with steps toward self-awareness previously described and offers complementary helpful tips. First, the nurse recalls an incident when something went wrong. Then the nurse experiences the incident again by remembering images and by privately retelling events, statements, outcomes, and associated emotions. Next, the nurse interprets the story of communication that failed by examining expectations, ideals, goals, influences, personal actions, and others' actions that occurred during the event. The last step involves honest inspection of the nurse's own role in the story. Insights gained may be applied to prevent repetition of the problem and to plan future action (Box 4-4).

Why is it important for a nurse to clarify personal values and increase self-awareness? The nurse's values and self-understanding influence behavior. The self is the nurse's greatest tool: to use the self effectively, the nurse must be fully aware of how it functions. Thus reflection and self-awareness guide the nurse's practice framework. In addition, sensitivity to individuals' perspectives is required to build a collaborative partnership, the cornerstone of the nurse-person relationship. Helping individuals to explicate their values and direct their actions accordingly toward health-related goals embodies patient-centered care as defined by Quality and Safety Education for Nurses (QSEN, 2012): "Recognize the patient or designee as the source of control and full partner in providing compassionate and coordinated care based on respect for patient's preferences, values, and needs." In today's multicultural society, sensitivity to one's values as a health care provider and those of persons for whom we care becomes crucial to delivery of person-centered effective care (McCaffrey & McConnell, 2015).

## THE COMMUNICATION PROCESS

The **communication process** is the forum for all thought and relationships shared among people. In conjunction with the use of scientific and technological advances, communication is an essential tool for the nurse to engage in health-promotion interventions. Communication is the foundation for any professional relationship. Nurse-patient communication plays a vital role in the formation and development of the nurse-patient relationship. It is the glue that connects individuals' learning and satisfaction with care (D'Antonio et al., 2014; Tejero, 2011). Communication is an information exchange between individuals

## BOX 4-5   Use Strategies for Communicating Clearly/Enhance Health Literacy Capacity

- *Greet patients warmly:* Receive everyone with a welcoming smile, and maintain a friendly attitude throughout the visit.
- *Make eye contact:* Make appropriate eye contact throughout the interaction. Refer to Tool 10: Consider Culture, Customs and Beliefs for further guidance on eye contact and culture.
- *Listen carefully:* Try not to interrupt patients when they are talking. Pay attention, and be responsive to the issues they raise and the questions they ask.
- *Use plain, nonmedical language:* Don't use medical words. Use common words that you would use to explain medical information to your friends or family, such as stomach or belly instead of abdomen.
- *Use the patient's words:* Take note of what words the patient uses to describe his or her illness and use them in your conversation.
- *Slow down:* Speak clearly and at a moderate pace.
- *Limit and repeat content:* Prioritize what needs to be discussed, and limit information to three to five key points and repeat them.
- *Be specific and concrete:* Don't use vague and subjective terms that can be interpreted in different ways.
- *Show graphics:* Draw pictures, use illustrations, or demonstrate what you mean with three-dimensional models. All pictures and models should be simple, designed to demonstrate only the important concepts, without detailed anatomy.
- *Demonstrate how it's done.* Whether doing exercises or taking medicine, a demonstration of how to do something may be clearer than a verbal explanation.
- *Invite patient participation:* Encourage patients to ask questions and be involved in the conversation during visits and to be proactive in their health care.
- *Encourage questions:* Refer to Tool 14: Encourage Questions for guidance on how to encourage your patients to ask questions.
- *Apply teach-back:* Confirm patients understand what they need to know and do by asking them to teach-back important information, such as directions. Refer to Tool 5: Use the Teach-Back Method for more guidance on how to use the teach-back method.

Sources Agency for Healthcare Research and Quality. (2015). Communicate clearly: Tool #4. In *Health Literacy Universal Precautions Toolkit* (2nd ed.). Publication 15-0023-EF. Rockville, MD; Agency for Healthcare Research and Quality. http://www.ahrq.gov/professionals/quality-patient-safety/quality-resources/tools/literacy-toolkit/healthlittoolkit2-tool4.html.

through shared symbols and signs and commonly understood behavior (Ruesch & Bateson, 1987). This exchange involves all the modes of behavior that an individual uses, consciously or unconsciously, to affect another person. Communication includes the spoken and written word and nonverbal communication (gestures, facial expressions, movement, body messages or signals, and artistic symbols). Furthermore, communication errors between clinical providers and individuals or their proxies as well as ineffective communication among practitioners have been identified as a major source of personal and health care delivery safety problems (Box 4-5).

Increasingly, communication is electronic. **Telehealth**, mobile health (**mhealth**), or Internet health (**ihealth**)—the use of telecommunications and data technologies to deliver health care services, including assessment/diagnostic services, treatment, consultation, and health information across platforms—is rapidly growing as a communication/intervention system. Such electronic communication can encompass the spoken and written word, and nonverbal forms of communication. Using technology to engage individuals in clinical communications is already in place, with potential for future development, and brings its own challenges (Haskey et al., 2015). Issues of health literacy, as discussed later in this chapter, including access, technology competence, and sensory capacity (such as eyesight and hearing), influence the effectiveness of telehealth as a communication medium.

Thus clear communication is a major component of promoting an individual's, a family's, and a community's safety and quality care. Yet the format and interface differ from the modes of human communication available until the latter part of the 20th century and the 21st century, and changes will be exponential in the years to come. (For additional discussion, see Box 4-6: Innovative Practice.) Social determinants of health can play a crucial role in access to and the effectiveness of Internet-based health information and intervention delivery. Evaluation of Internet-based health education and intervention systems, including access, is a critical goal for translation of research to practice.

In nursing, communication is the cornerstone of a positive nurse-person relationship. Communication refers to a set of strategies and actions to enhance reciprocity, mutual understanding, and decision-making. Focusing the clinical discussion on the person's story rather than a version reformulated by the provider is essential to person-centered communication. Box 4-7 highlights strategies associated with person-centered communication based on evidence from the research literature.

Considerable evidence supports the effectiveness of these strategies. Research study results showed that nurses communicate effectively when they use a person-centered approach or nurse-person relational approach consisting of their being attentive, caring, accepting, empathetic, friendly, comfortable, calm, interested, sincere, and respectful (Doss et al., 2011; Tejero, 2011). Although these strategies sound simple and basic, such appraisals are noticeably absent in many instances and their presence is essential to quality nursing care (Box 4-8: Research for Evidence-Based Practice). Furthermore, research findings have indicated that nurses seek communication with individuals that supports openness and engagement of both the nurse and the person to form a bonding factor between them (Tejero, 2011).

## Function and Process

The following are core functions of communication:
- To obtain and send messages and to retain information.
- To use the information to arrive at new conclusions, to reconstruct the past, and to look forward to future events.
- To begin and to modify physiological processes.
- To influence others and outside events (Ruesch & Bateson, 1987).

Communication transmits information, both interpersonally and intrapersonally, and it provides the basis for action.

The process of communication consists of four components (Watzlawick et al., 1967). Nurses must be able to diagnose communication difficulties in any of these components. **Input** involves taking in information from outside the individual or group.

## BOX 4-6 INNOVATIVE PRACTICE

### Telehealth/mhealth/ihealth: Therapeutic Relationships in the Age of the Internet

Technological advances have produced rapid changes in communication. Automatic teller machines have replaced human tellers at banks for routine transactions. Voicemail rather than a receptionist routinely answers calls, and messages are recorded electronically. An electronic response to many calls directs the caller to a series of options that may not even include speaking to a person. E-mail, instant messaging, and "texting" are ubiquitous. Information in many areas is now available via access to a computer and an Internet connection. Wireless Internet (WiFi) access is increasingly used as a perk to lure customers to the local coffee spot and to ease passengers' irritation during long flight delays. Nurses use electronic records and communicate updated information via handheld devices.

In the past decade, we have witnessed exponential increases in computer penetration (Thielst, 2010). Such technology can improve work and expand capabilities. Who would prefer to use a traditional typewriter to prepare papers and documents after mastering a word-processing program? Yet many issues deserve examination as we move into the age of telehealth.

Telehealth or mhealth or ihealth—the use of telecommunications and data technologies to deliver health care services, including diagnostic services, treatment, consultation, and health information—is now omnipresent. Rather than replacing traditional care, telehealth is best understood as a complementary approach to long-distance care delivery, and faster and easily delivered contact. Telehealth has the potential to expand access to care, particularly for individuals receiving home care and those in remote areas, and to contain costs (Luptak et al., 2010). Moreover, the concept of telehealth also encompasses remote teaching, conferencing, and consulting (Ackerman et al., 2010).

Technological advances have produced benefits; however, technology can also reduce the need for direct interpersonal contact. Barriers to use include the need for financial investment to establish networks, inadequate reimbursement mechanisms, potential risks to confidentiality with electronic transmission, and licensure issues when care is transmitted across state lines. Challenges include conducting systematic evaluation of outcomes and cost-effectiveness, and ensuring that individuals' economic status and health literacy do not constrain access.

Perhaps the most important threat is that care can become impersonal when face-to-face contact is replaced by an electronic interface. Thus preserving core nursing values as electronic care systems are created, tested, and implemented is a crucial goal. Innovative practices to safeguard core professional values in the emerging age of telehealth include:

- The avoidance of a "one size fits all" approach through individualized or tailored algorithms and design features specific to the system's use. Moreover, clinician behaviors that facilitate a patient-centered style of communication include using open-ended questions, building partnerships, sharing decision-making and information, providing counseling, and using statements of concern, agreement, and approval. This style more successfully addresses individual needs and is associated with greater patient satisfaction, better psychosocial adjustment, and improved health outcomes. Adding opportunities for on-line questions and answers or an open electronic or telephone chat with a clinician can facilitate tailoring in this delivery approach. Text and/or e-mail prompts can also facilitate adherence to care. Also, providing user-friendly access, education/instruction, and tracking/monitoring use and problems are necessary ingredients for high user satisfaction (Young et al., 2011).
- The development and maintenance of therapeutic relationships by inviting exchanges between the nurse and the person; for example, by creating a series of layered screens that first introduce the nurse (visually and with a biography) and later invite exchanges, feedback, and sharing of experiences and stories from individuals.
- The fostering of individual autonomy by building components that encourage decision-making, problem-solving, and knowledge development that are timely and specific to the health problem and stage of treatment or management.
- The creation of flexible technology applications that work across a variety of platforms (e.g., computer, smartphone, tablet).

Consider the following questions about telehealth:

- What effects do technological changes have on the therapeutic relationship?
- Will face-to-face interaction become a rare occurrence? In the future, might therapeutic interactions occur primarily via technology, such as voicemail, the Internet, and video-recorded transmission? What advantages and disadvantages will appear with the increasing use of technology in nursing practice?
- What creative approaches may evolve using technology in therapeutic relationships?
- How can electronic communication systems be used in disaster preparedness to alert people at risk and direct actions to increase safety when a human-caused or natural disaster is suspected, imminent, or in progress?

Sources Ackerman, M. J., Burgess, L. P., Filart, R., Lee, I., & Poropatich, R. K. (2010). Developing next-generation telehealth tools and technologies: Patients, systems, and data perspectives. *Telemedicine and e-Health, 16*(1), 93–95; Agha, Z., Schapira, R., Laud, P., McNutt, G., & Roter, D. (2009). Patient satisfaction with physician-patient communication during telemedicine. *Telemedicine and e-Health, 15*(9), 830–839; Luptak, M., Dailey, N., Juretic, M., Rupper, R., Hill, R., Hicken, B., et al. (2010). The Care Coordination Home Telehealth (CCHT) rural demonstration project: A symptom-based approach for serving older veterans in remote geographical settings. *Rural and Remote Health, 10*(2), 1375; Thielst, C. (2010). At the crossroads: NRTRC white paper examines trends driving the convergence of telehealth, EHRs and HIE. *World Hospitals and Health Services, 46*(4), 17–23.

Once taken in, input must be transformed in some manner to be used. For example, symbols must be translated into words to transmit ideas. The flow and transformation of processed input refers to the way information is analyzed and stored within the individual, or the way it is transmitted from person to person within a human system (group or family) before communication with the external environment occurs. The outcome of information processing, **output**, involves further exchange with the environment or the other person. A new information exchange is triggered at this point in the cycle by the response called **feedback**, a monitoring system through which the person or group controls the internal and external responses to behavior

(output) and accommodates these responses appropriately. A feedback **loop** shows the dynamic nature of communication. Each piece of communication is both a stimulus designed to elicit a response and a response to a different stimulus.

When interpersonal communication is analyzed, two types of feedback can be identified: positive (encouraging change) and negative (encouraging homeostasis or no change). Parents' commands to a young child illustrate these types of feedback: positive, "Try that again; you almost had it," and negative, "Don't touch that; it's hot." The first statement shows the parent's attempt to encourage the child to continue new behavior; the second illustrates an effort to curtail undesired behavior. Rather than

---

**BOX 4-7    Strategies Associated With Person-Centered Communication**

- Permitting people to tell their stories in their own words and chronology.
- Using a conversational interviewing style.
- Being friendly through humor and social conversation, and nonverbal cues such as smiling.
- Eliciting people's views, perspectives, thoughts, wishes, goals, values, and expectations.
- Inquiring about the nature of the person's life.
- Attending to the person's needs.
- Avoiding overemphasis on technical aspects of care and tasks.
- Not being too busy to talk.

- Responding to cues concerning emotional issues and problems.
- Giving information about self-care and participation in decision-making.
- Developing mutual understanding.
- Creating collaborative health care plans.
- Showing empathy and concern for the individual's well-being.
- Connecting with individuals through humor, touch, and selective self-disclosure.
- Tuning in to individuals' preferences and style.
- Attending to and advocating individuals' needs.
- Maintaining confidentiality.

Sources Dziopa, F., & Ahern, K. (2009). What makes a quality therapeutic relationship in psychiatric/mental health nursing: A review of the research literature. *Internet Journal of Advanced Nursing Practice, 10*(1), 1–19; Bolster, D., & Manias, E. (2010). Person-centered interactions between nurses and patients during medication activities in an acute hospital setting: Qualitative observation and interview study. *International Journal of Nursing Studies, 47*(2), 154–165.

---

**BOX 4-8    RESEARCH FOR EVIDENCE-BASED PRACTICE**

### The Mediating Role of Nurse-Patient Dyad Bonding in Patient Satisfaction

**Study Overview**

Using a correlational path analytical research design, Tejero (2011) examined the direct and indirect relations of nurse characteristics and patient characteristics to patient satisfaction, as mediated by nurse-patient dyad bonding. A sample of 210 nurses and 210 patients from medical surgery, obstetrics, gynecology, otolaryngology, and ophthalmology units, the trauma ward, and medical intensive care units participated in the study. Characteristics of the nurses and patients were gathered through observation, interview, and medical record review. Instruments were used to measure nurse-patient bonding during observation and to measure patient satisfaction with nursing care in the interview. In addition, a checklist was used to collect information on patient complexity, vulnerability, and predictability as well as information on nurse clinical judgment and facilitation of learning.

**Results**

The results confirmed the importance of the nurse's role in the formation of a therapeutic dyadic relationship that results in patient satisfaction—a critical

part of quality outcomes in health care. Openness and engagement of nurses during interactions were significantly and positively correlated with patient satisfaction. Path analysis showed that nurse facilitation of learning was particularly important in mediating nurse-patient dyad bonding. Nurses' efforts to educate and provide information to patients displayed openness and engagement, which leads to openness and engagement from the patient. The manner, tone, and emotion of the nurse were also shown to affect patient satisfaction.

**Implications**

Formation of nurse-patient therapeutic dyadic relationships plays a major role in the quality of patients' experiences. Tejero (2011) stated that a key implication is that the nurse is the healthy individual in the dyad and clinical expert in the interaction, who is obligated to initiate and steer the dyadic relationship toward a therapeutic bond. The findings of this study showed that nurse facilitation of patient learning should be emphasized in practice and in teaching students so as to provide evidence-based practice and improve patient satisfaction.

Source Tejero, L. M. S. (2011). The mediating role of the nurse-patient dyad bonding in bringing about patient satisfaction. *Journal of Advanced Nursing, 68*(5), 994–1002.

---

meaning "good" or "bad," positive feedback and negative feedback refer to promotion of system change and stability, which is the process of balancing the direction and magnitude of change. Both types of feedback are needed, depending on the situation.

The situational context of communication is important. The context of communication is the setting's physical, psychosocial, and cultural dimensions. It includes the relationship between the sender and the receiver; their previous experiences, feelings, values, cultural norms, age, and developmental stage; and the physical location.

## Types of Communication

All human communication occurs in three forms: verbal, nonverbal, and metacommunication. Each affects the meaning and influences the interpretation of the message.

### Verbal Communication

Verbal communication is the transmission of messages using words, spoken or written. As symbols for ideas, words impart

meaning defined by a specific language. Communicating with language is a critical ability.

People who are deaf or hard of hearing often use sign language to communicate. Signs, similarly to spoken or written words, are used consistently to represent a particular meaning. Words may also be spelled out through finger spelling in a manner parallel to written communication. Braille assists blind and visually challenged people to read. Touch is used to interpret markings that represent letters and words. Sign language and braille blend aspects of verbal and nonverbal communication, but both forms of communication transmit meaning through a consistent language system.

Verbal communication with people who speak a different language poses a challenge. As societies become increasingly multicultural, assistance from specially trained interpreters is essential for the provision of culturally competent care. Confidentiality issues, the complexity of health information, and the need to validate understandings and reach mutual decisions make it inappropriate to use untrained personnel or relatives to interpret what is meant simply because they are available.

The importance of language development is apparent in its three functions: informing the person of others' thoughts and feelings; stimulating the receiver of a message by triggering a response; and serving a descriptive function by imparting information and sharing observations, ideas, inferences, and memories (Watzlawick et al., 1967). The ability of verbal communication to fulfill these functions is influenced by many factors, including the communicator's social class, culture, age, milieu, and ability to receive and interpret messages.

## Nonverbal Communication

Nonverbal communication or language encompasses all messages that are not spoken or written. The channels of nonverbal communication are the five senses. Movement, facial and eye expressions, gestures, touch, appearance, and vocalization or paralanguage all constitute nonverbal modes of communication (Blondis & Jackson, 1982). Although all communication has the potential of being misunderstood, nonverbal communication is particularly subject to misunderstanding because it does not always reflect the sender's conscious intent and is highly influenced by culture. Nonverbal messages also tend to be nebulous, without specific beginnings and endings.

Body motion or kinetic behavior includes facial expression (or facies), eye movements, body movements, gestures, and posture (Blondis & Jackson, 1982). When observing facial expression, the nurse notices the affect or emotion that is communicated. Does the person appear happy or sad; alert, distracted, or sleepy; contented, agitated, angry, or anxious? The degree of emotion expressed should also be noted. Does the person's face express what generally is considered an excessive degree of feeling for the situation, too little, or none at all? Eyes, in conjunction with the movement of other facial muscles, move in ways that convey affect. Eye contact conveys messages of interest or trust; lack of eye contact can imply lack of interest or anxiety; constant eye contact can send a message of hostility.

All of these nonverbal messages are culturally and situationally bound. Nonverbal behavior, particularly facial and eye expressions, is contextual. For example, in certain circumstances and cultures, avoidance of direct eye contact between some people can be a sign of respect. Yet in other situations and cultures, it can be interpreted as indicative of disinterest, avoidance, or disrespect. Therefore interpretation requires a cultural lens.

Sign language combines features of both nonverbal and verbal communication. Sign language involves nonverbal communication because, although it uses symbols that are communicated through specific signs, these are enhanced by facial expressions and body postures. However, sign language shares many aspects of verbal communication. It has syntax and grammar, words may be spelled out, and a standard meaning is assigned to specific signs to create symbolic language, just as words share common definitions.

*Importance of nonverbal communication.* Nonverbal communication has great power to transmit information about another's thoughts and feelings; therefore careful observation is essential. Even silence can be very revealing. The significance of nonverbal communication is best captured by the axiom "actions speak louder than words." Nurses' nonverbal messages that communicate distance from the person, or signal an unfriendly or uncaring attitude, thwart development of a therapeutic relationship (Henry et al., 2011) and thereby render health-promotion efforts unproductive.

## Metacommunication

Besides verbal and nonverbal communication, a phenomenon called metacommunication refers to a message about the message. Watzlawick and colleagues (1967) described metacommunication as the impossibility of not communicating: that is, "one cannot not communicate." Persons transmit a message about what is being communicated even when words are not spoken." Metacommunication is the relationship aspect of communication. In a sense, metacommunication involves reading between the lines or going past the surface content of the message to glean nuances of meaning. When the content and the relationship aspects, or metacommunication aspects, of a message are incongruent, interpreting the communication accurately may be difficult, leaving the receiver uncomfortable and confused.

## Group Process

In group settings, a special type of metacommunication is called process. A basic principle of group theory states that all communication has content and process. Content is what is said; process is the relationship aspect of what is communicated. Group process occurs during every group encounter. Staff meetings and clinically oriented psychoeducation, therapy, and counseling groups always involve group process. For example, consider two individuals in a smoking cessation group who always support each other by agreeing with each other and offering comments or criticism to any group member who disagrees. Although this pairing between the individuals offers them some protection from anxiety that may result from self-examination and feedback, it isolates them and curtails feedback from others. Examination of this group process is an essential task. The nurse leader and participants can transform this problematic situation into a learning opportunity by identifying the pattern and pointing out the behavior after it has occurred frequently; helping the pair and other group members consider what needs are being met through this pattern; looking at each person's role in fostering this process (e.g., why other group members have failed to confront the pair); and discussing potential outcomes of changing the behavior. These steps can be applied in clinical situations when greater self-understanding is a goal.

## Effectiveness of Communication

Understanding what makes communication effective improves the nurse's ability to assess needs and to intervene successfully to promote individuals' health. Steps to functional communication include firmly stating the case, clarifying the message, seeking feedback, and being receptive to feedback when it is received. Implementing these steps to functional communication between nurses and individuals, and between nurses and other care providers, is essential to ensure patient safety and quality care (QSEN, 2012).

To state the case, the sender needs to make the content and the metacommunication congruent; when they conflict, the message is confusing. For example, a nurse is angry with a colleague for making statements to an administrator that undermined the nurse's plans for reconfiguring a health-promotion program in their agency. When the nurse had a chance to speak with this colleague, they exchanged pleasantries without mention of what the nurse thought about the colleague's statements to the administrator. When the colleague asked if something was bothering the nurse, the nurse responded that nothing was wrong. The colleague senses that the nurse's verbal and nonverbal communication did not match; in other words, the content of the message and the metacommunication were incongruent. The colleague was left feeling uneasy, and the nurse failed to express his or her thoughts or to take effective action to rectify the perceived problem with the colleague. To make the communication functional, the nurse needed to bring thoughts and feelings into awareness and reflect on the intended message. Once these steps have been accomplished, the message's content and metacommunication can be adjusted to match, and the nurse's communication is likely to be effective. This example typifies ineffective communications.

To clarify the message, the sender must give a complete message. Important features should be emphasized and specifics of any request must be stated, not assumed. The message's importance must also be indicated. To illustrate this, a woman mentions to her nurse that it is nearly June. The nurse responds that he has noticed how warm the weather is becoming. On the surface, this communication may seem functional until the intent of the woman's message is considered. She meant to imply that June is the 5-year anniversary of her remission from cancer, and she hoped that her nurse would somehow know that she wanted him to comment on the significance of this anniversary. To make this communication functional, the woman needed to expand the message (e.g., "My anniversary after cancer treatment is coming up") and then clarify her wish to hear a sensitive response from the nurse (e.g., "This anniversary marks the goal for you to be cancer-free." "What will you do to celebrate?"). Additionally, she needed to show how important the message was (e.g., "I'd really like to do something special to mark this date"). If the nurse had been attuned to the metacommunication in this exchange, he could have clarified this woman's intent and met her need for recognition and dialogue.

One technique for clarifying and qualifying messages is called the "I" statement. Use of "I" statements helps the sender state what he or she wants, feels, thinks, or plans (including likes and dislikes). For example, "I felt unimportant when you forgot to recognize this anniversary" is an "I" statement that the person could have used to communicate effectively. Soliciting such "I" messages is a therapeutic technique to be encouraged.

Questions can clarify and qualify messages, depending on the type of question asked. Open-ended questions tend to elicit descriptive responses rather than one-word answers. For example, the question "Tell me what you did for exercise this week" is likely to yield a more elaborate description of a health behavior from a person than the question "Did everything go okay with your exercise plan?" However, direct questions that seek a one-word answer are useful when a specific piece of information is sought. "Did you spend 15 minutes or more walking today?" may be a better approach than "What was your activity like today?" when it is important to discuss and promote minimal exercise requirements. Also, for individuals having trouble expressing more than the simplest thoughts, asking direct questions that call for brief replies can be helpful, such as "Did you eat breakfast?" This approach is particularly useful with people who are depressed, regressed, cognitively impaired, or unable to handle complex information or communication at a particular time, or when a specific yes/no response is needed.

Seeking feedback is another element of functional communication. Consensual validation, confirming that both the sender and the receiver understand the same information, calls for the use of the clarification skills just described. In family communication, the parent, as the sender, should model this behavior for children by asking the child, as the receiver, to explain his or her sense of the message and how to ask the sender for further explanation. For example, "I want you to clean your room" (message from parent) can be followed by "Tell me how you think you will do that" (validating that the child and the parent agree about what the task entails). This style of seeking validation can be adapted to nurse-nurse or nurse-interprofessional exchanges between colleagues and to therapeutic interactions, and is critical to effective clinical care (Institute of Medicine, 2010). Such confirmation in communication is also essential when health-promotion interventions are being provided. Without validating that the person understands the information and its importance, and that the person has a behavior plan to follow, health-promotion efforts are likely to fail. Moreover, failure to validate understanding is a significant risk to patient safety (QSEN, 2012).

Being open to feedback is also crucial. A "no questions" attitude blocks functional communication, whether in the home, classroom, or clinical setting. Children, students, individuals, and even other nurses may be afraid to question anyone in authority or may assume that the person should magically know what is intended or expected. For example, a person may avoid confronting a nurse who fails to explain the clinical plan and then communicates that the person should know how to follow through. Statements by the sender such as "Tell me what you think" and "What is your understanding of what I said?" are helpful in eliciting confirmation of understanding and feedback.

Receiving and sending messages involve many of the same processes. Evaluation of the intent of the message, both the content and the metacommunication, is the first step. The receiver frequently needs to seek clarification and validate understanding of the message for communication to be effective. Clarification of expectations, active exchange of information, power sharing, and negotiation will enhance the quality of nurse-person communication. The outcome is a nurse-person relationship based on trust and partnership (Doss et al., 2011), critical ingredients of patient-centered care (Institute of Medicine, 2010).

## Interprofessional Communication and Teamwork

Interprofessional communication and teamwork for care design and delivery involve cross-disciplinary education and practice approaches that are now widely promoted as essential to an effective health care system (Lyons et al., 2016; Thistlethwaite, 2012). However, instruments to help students and clinicians to hone their observations of teamwork behaviors have been lacking. The Jefferson Teamwork Observation Guide is an easy-to-use short tool, with evidence of reliability and face and predictive validity, for observation of teams in action to identify behaviors, including communications indicative of good teamwork (Lyons et al., 2016). The Jefferson Teamwork Observation Guide is a helpful instrument for nurses to use to recognize, observe, and then implement the behaviors that comprise good teamwork and communication.

## Factors in Effective Communication

### Listening

Effective listening, an important part of communication, is more than passively taking information. Effective listening is actively focusing attention on the message. Asking questions to explore what is meant helps the listener reach an accurate assessment of the message's meaning.

Many forms of nonverbal communication have been identified that, from a Western or European perspective, commonly convey that the person is listening. These nonverbal communications include direct gazing and eye contact, head nodding, orienting one's body to maintain interpersonal closeness, leaning forward, making facial expressions such as eyebrow animation and smiling, and using brief verbal statements that indicate interest, such as "Please go on" or "Tell me more about that…."

For behavior to communicate that the person is listening also depends on the context and intensity of the activities, and the cultural norms of each person. For example, leaning close to a person might be interpreted as intrusive. Yet the same behavior could be seen as a sign of support, depending on the context and perspective of those involved. Sensitivity to nuances in communication and validation of meaning can be particularly helpful strategies when the nurse and the person come from different cultural backgrounds.

Reciprocity, the patterning of similar activities within the same interval by two people, can help the nurse communicate a listening stance in an effective way. When the nurse matches nuances of the individual's type and style of behavior, the chances that the person will interpret the nurse's behavior as an indication of active listening are increased, and the likelihood of misinterpretation is reduced. Nurses can enhance the quality of their communication, even when encounters are brief, by attending to reciprocity in their interactions and by validating whether or not reciprocity is associated with shared interpretations of meaning.

Poor listening blocks the nurse's understanding of the person. The nurse's failure to listen may be caused by anxiety; focus on other demands; lack of experience, which leads to excessive talking by the nurse; preoccupation with personal thoughts; or lack of practice. The importance of focusing on the individual's needs and concerns through effective listening is a recurrent theme in research concerning therapeutic interaction (Doss et al., 2011; Shipley, 2010; Stuart, 2012) and a cornerstone of patient-centered and safe care (Institute of Medicine, 2010; QSEN, 2012).

### Flexibility

Flexibility is a balance between control and permissiveness. In "overcontrol," every message is monitored. In exaggerated permissiveness, anything can be communicated in any way. For communication to be functional, rules are needed about what is appropriate, without rigid prescriptions that inhibit meaningful interchange. For example, the guideline that nurses will not answer questions concerning intimate details of their lives sets an appropriate limit; however, this does not mean that nurses should refuse to answer any question about themselves.

### Silence

Silence between people is often uncomfortable for the nurse who is somewhat insecure about what should occur during a therapeutic encounter. However, silence can be beneficial when used carefully. When one is seeking a verbal response, silence can be perceived as a lack of interest. At other times, silence allows individuals to reflect on what is being discussed or experienced, lets them know that the nurse is willing to wait until they are ready to say more, or simply provides them with comfort and support. Each situation needs evaluation and sensitivity. Rather than asking a flurry of questions to break the silence, the nurse allows the person time to decide when to comment or should make brief comments that do not demand answers, such as "It can be helpful to take time to think about what we've been discussing." Also, comments such as "Try putting your thoughts or feelings into words" and "I am here when you are ready to talk" can help the person to share these thoughts or feelings when silence is blocking rather than improving the communication.

### Humor

Humor is part of being human; it relieves tension, reduces aggression, and creates a climate of sharing. Humor can block communication when it is used to avoid subjects that might be uncomfortable or when it excludes other people. Humor can also inflict emotional pain and communicate negative views or stereotypes about particular individuals or groups through teasing and jokes concerning race, ethnicity, culture, country of origin, occupation, age, sex, sexual activity, or other traits that stand out or are devalued. A direct response to the latent content or message in this type of humor is an effective way to curtail its use and minimize its effect. For example, a response that shows disapproval of the latent message such as "That kind of joke makes me very uncomfortable. I don't find it funny to describe [the specific group in question] that way, and I would like you to stop" will send a clear message and be likely successful in stopping the offensive communication. In contrast, for humor to be helpful the meaning of the humor must be understood and its purpose supportive to the individual. Clarification of the meaning should be used when there is doubt or concern.

### Touch

Touch is an interesting means of nonverbal communication for nurses, who often touch individuals while administering care. The nurse's concern can be expressed by a gentle or soothing application of touch. Nevertheless, in some instances touch is inappropriate. For example, in interactions with individuals who have trauma histories or acute psychiatric disturbances, touch might be misinterpreted. A woman who has been raped might interpret touch during an examination as an attack. Evaluation of the context and meaning of touch to the individual is based on knowledge of that person and interpretation of feedback. Informing the individual about the purpose of touching and asking for permission and feedback are useful techniques to avoid unintended distress or misinterpretation of touching in a clinical encounter.

## Space

Space between communicators varies according to the type of communication, the setting, and the culture. Hall (1973) researched proxemics, the use of space between communicators, and identified four zones of space commonly used in interaction in North America; these are presented in Box 4-9 and Figure 4-1. It is critically important for nurses to be sensitive to how spacial zones vary across cultures when caring for persons from diverse backgrounds.

Understanding the appropriate distance for a given type of interaction helps the nurse to make nonverbal and verbal communication congruent and to avoid violating spatial norms.

Awareness of cultural customs concerning distance is important in shaping communication and interpreting the behavior of others. When people from different cultures or groups communicate, there may be discomfort about the acceptable distance between them when speaking. Recognition of differences helps the nurse adjust the distance and interpret the meaning of this nonverbal communication.

---

### BOX 4-9 Zones of Space Common to Interaction in North America

1. *Intimate space:* up to 18 in (45.5 cm); used for high interpersonal sensory stimulation (see Figure 4-1A)
2. *Personal space:* 45.5 cm to 1.2 m (18 in to 4 ft); appropriate for close relationships in which touching may be involved and good visualization is desired (see Figure 4-1B)
3. *Social-consultative space:* 2.7 to 3.6 m (9 to 12 ft); less intimate and personal, requiring louder verbal communication (see Figure 4-1C)
4. *Public space:* 3.6 m (12 ft) or more; appropriately used for formal gatherings, such as giving speeches (see Figure 4-1D)

Source Hall, E. (1973). *The silent language.* Garden City, NY: Doubleday/Anchor Press.

---

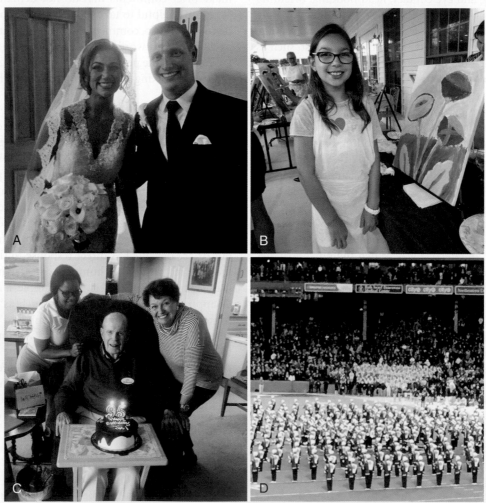

**FIGURE 4-1 A,** Intimate distance communication. **B,** Personal distance communication. **C,** Social-consultative distance communication. **D,** Public distance communication.

Many traits and components discussed in this chapter characterize functional communication. However, communication is a subtle and intricate process. Communication cannot be reduced to a set of parts and principles; its roles and nuances are far more complex and variable. Communicating by language and symbols is a special human ability. Healthy communication enables people to move from being alone to being together—clearly one of the crucial tasks of living. Effective communication is also the foundation for the helping relationship. Moreover, effective communication is essential to providing quality care and ensuring patient safety and well-being (QSEN, 2012).

## Health Literacy

Clear communication improves the quality of health care encounters. Health literacy, the capacity to read, comprehend, and follow through on health information, is a critical component of health promotion. Yet nearly 9 out of 10 adults encounter problems using everyday health information to make good decisions about health (Institute of Medicine, 2011). To combat low health literacy, nurses can encourage individuals to ask three essential questions at every health visit (National Patient Safety Foundation, n.d.; Speros, 2011):

- "What is my main problem?"
- "What do I need to do?"
- "Why is it important for me to do this?"

Nurses also promote health literacy by creating a safe and comfortable environment, sitting to establish eye contact rather than standing when communicating, using visual aids and models to illustrate conditions and procedures, and verifying understanding of care instructions by having individuals then teach the content; that is, using "teach-back" as a strategy (Speros, 2011). Resources are available to help nurses and other clinicians to increase individuals' understanding of health information across health literacy levels. The Agency for Healthcare Research and Quality (2015) *Health Literacy Universal Precautions Toolkit* provides easily accessible and highly useful resources to promote universal health precautions; that is, steps to take when clinicians assume that all persons may have some limitations in understanding health information and accessing health services. This toolkit provides evidence-based approaches for use from assessment to intervention. The toolkit suggests fundamental communication strategies to communicate clearly (see Box 4-5).

Three key factors regarding health literacy to consider are the educational level of the target audience or users; the reading/comprehension level for materials in on-line, verbal, or written format; and the native language of the target audience or users. A highly educated target audience generally has high health literacy because of strong command of the native language being used. Research evidence has shown that health information in use may be at a reading level above the comprehension level (i.e., at 9th grade level) of the users. The researchers recommended that quality be improved in materials and instruction, especially for those with low education/literacy skills (Ryan et al., 2014). Furthermore, nurses need to assess comprehension of all health information and instruction, particularly of complex medical/health information. Developing materials at the 5th or 6th grade reading level helps ensure that comprehension is very likely across wide ranges of the target audience. Word processing programs and on-line tools can evaluate the reading level of text. Published materials also are available to help in assessing and developing appropriate content (McKenna & Stahl, 2015). These available resources enable nurses easily to determine the reading level of all health and research materials, and to adjust the level by changing complex terms to more commonly used words with only one or two syllables and simplifying sentences to avoid complex construction with multiple phrases. Finally, adjusting word usage to avoid native colloquialisms will increase understanding among persons whose native language is not being used. Moreover, advocating the development and/or revision of existing materials to reach a 5th/6th grade reading level is an appropriate nursing mandate.

In the emerging age of telehealth, developing strategies for confirming understanding and individualizing methods of communicating health information is increasingly important (see Box 4-6: Innovative Practice). Health information and even access to appointments are steadily shifting from face-to-face interaction to access by telephone via voice prompts and Internet-based formats. Many factors involved in health literacy can impair individuals' ability to understand and respond to audio and/or visual commands. Consider the array of commands involved in the typical automated telephone system involved in ordering a prescription refill from a typical pharmacy. The individual must select from a list of options; next, multiple numbers must be keyed in that represent prescription numbers listed in small print from a prescription label and birthdays in appropriate format; finally, a variety of confirmations must be entered. Persons with auditory, visual, language comprehension, and/or cognitive limitations may not have adequate capacity to manage such common health care technologies. Therefore technology competence becomes another component of health literacy to be considered.

## THE HELPING OR THERAPEUTIC RELATIONSHIP

A helping or therapeutic relationship is a process through which one person promotes the development of another person by fostering the latter's maturation, adaptation, integration, openness, and ability to find meaning in the present situation (Peplau, 1969; D'Antonio et al., 2014). The therapeutic relationship emerges from purposeful encounters characterized by effective communication. In this relationship the nurse respects the individual's values, attends to concerns, and promotes positive change by encouraging self-expression, exploring behavior patterns and outcomes, and promoting self-help (Doss et al., 2011). The therapeutic relationship is the foundation of clinical nursing practice (D'Antonio et al., 2014)—the essential element of quality care with every individual in every situation (QSEN, 2012). Techniques, technology, interventions, and contexts differ, but the relational aspect of nursing practice produces a cohesive unity, allowing each nurse to see people holistically and as unique individuals. Although many components of the helping relationship are most germane to relationships that extend over time, the essentials of the helping relationship apply to even brief therapeutic encounters.

> ### BOX 4-10    Characteristics Associated With Therapeutic Effectiveness
>
> - Self-awareness and self-reflection
> - Openness
> - Self-confidence and strength
> - Genuineness
> - Concern for the individual
> - Respect for the individual
> - Knowledge
> - Ability to empathize
> - Sensitivity
> - Acceptance
> - Creativity
> - Ability to focus and confront

No perfect profile or personality of a helping person exists. However, certain traits can be nurtured without thwarting the nurse's unique personality. These characteristics enable the nurse to be an agent of therapeutic care (Peplau, 1963; Stuart, 2012). Box 4-10 lists characteristics associated with therapeutic effectiveness.

## Characteristics of the Therapeutic Relationship

No recipe is available for a successful therapeutic relationship. Techniques and concepts serve only as tools. As a nurse develops and evaluates a helping relationship, be it long term or brief in nature, the following guidelines may be useful.

### Purposeful Communication

Purposeful communication means that the nurse focuses communication toward a particular goal. Social chitchat, communication without a goal, should not make up the bulk of therapeutic interaction. This does not mean that the nurse should never discuss a social topic; nonetheless, there should be some purpose. For example, discussing the weather with a somewhat disoriented older adult individual serves the purpose of orienting that person to the environment. Discussing the Super Bowl with an avid football fan may provide valuable assessment data and engage the person in a current topic of social interest. Goals guide the nurse in focusing communication.

### Rapport

Rapport is a harmony and an affinity between people in a relationship. By using many of the traits listed for helping a person, the nurse can establish an atmosphere in which rapport can develop. To let the person know that his or her concerns interest the nurse and that working together may alleviate some of his or her difficulties and encourage growth, it is important to be genuine, open, and concerned.

### Trust

Trust is a necessary component of any helping relationship. Trust is the reliance on a person to carry out responsibilities and promises, based on a sense of safety, honesty, and reliability. Trust is an important component of partnership. The nurse promotes trust by modeling and structuring the relationship appropriately. The following strategies promote trust:

- Anticipating that the individual will do as promised.
- Clearly defining the relationship parameters and expectations, particularly the purpose and specifics of time, place, and anticipated behavior.
- Being consistent.
- Examining behaviors that interfere with trust.

### Empathy

Empathy is the ability to understand another's feelings without losing personal identity and perspective. Empathic nurses draw on emotions and experiences that enable them to place themselves in the other person's situation. While the person senses increasing understanding and acceptance from the nurse, the individual's distress decreases. Outcomes from research studies are building knowledge about the role that empathic nursing care plays in outcomes. Nurses learn behavioral approaches that enhance empathic relations with people through supervised experiential learning (Haskey et al., 2015). For example, nurses do not empathize by switching the focus of the interaction to themselves or by sympathizing (e.g., "I know exactly how you feel; that happened to me once"). Rather, they use clinical and personal experience to appreciate the individual's feelings and experiences: they try to imagine themselves in the person's situation. Using personal understanding based on some shared aspect of experience such as a loss while maintaining boundaries is the essence of empathy in the helping relationship. With empathic understanding, the nurse acknowledges the affective domain of personal experiences and uses this knowledge to appreciate the person's reactions. Empathy enables the listener to share human experiences as the basis for providing care.

### Goal Direction

A helping relationship is special in its goal-directed nature. Although most human relationships focus on mutual benefit, a helping relationship exists solely to meet some need or to promote the growth of the recipient. Although the nurse may benefit from the interaction, the relationship is centered on the recipient.

Goals are formulated as desired individual behaviors/outcomes. Short-term goals are likely to be achieved within 10 days to 2 weeks; all other goals are long term. All goals should be stated in measurable terms and should focus on a positive change or on the decrease of problematic behavior/health indicators. Ideally, a person works with the nurse to establish goals. However, some individuals, such as those who are seriously ill, depressed, psychotic, or cognitively impaired, may be unable to establish mutual goals. When an individual is unable to negotiate appropriate goals, the nurse establishes realistic goals and shares them to the degree possible with the person, who is free to participate or to reject efforts to reach these goals. In some circumstances when the care recipient is unable to collaborate regarding care decisions, then a family member or another designee/health care proxy may be the appropriate person for such communication.

### Ethics in Communicating and Relating

Ethical decision-making is closely linked with the goal-directed nature of helping relationships. Ethical issues are present in

## BOX 4-11   Guidelines for Ethical Interpersonal Communication

Ethical interpersonal communication involves:

- Being aware and open to changing concepts of self and others.
- Attending to role responsibilities; individual sacrifice, when it is required to make a "good" decision; and emotions, while guarding against letting emotions be the sole guide of our behavior.
- Sharing personal views candidly and clearly.
- Communicating information accurately, with minimal loss or distortion of intended meaning.
- Communicating verbal and nonverbal messages with congruent meanings.
- Sharing responsibility for the consequences among communicators.
- Recognizing the multicultural context of all communication.
- Respecting the dignity of every person.
- Avoiding coercion and use of power in communicating.
- Being sensitive to gender and cultural contexts of communication and interpretation.
- Building context for intercultural dialogue that is open with conditions of security and mutual respect.

- Eliminating any elements of your communication that denigrates, stereotypes, or devalues clients.
- Facilitating open and accurate communication among professional groups, professionals, staff and families, clinical care unit and department staffs or administrators, and clinical care facilities.

Unethical communication involves:

- Purposefully deceiving.
- Intentionally blocking communication—for example, changing subjects when the other person has not finished communicating, cutting a person off, or distracting others from the subject under discussion.
- Scapegoating or unnecessarily condemning others.
- Lying or deceiving that causes intentional or unintentional harm.
- Verbally "hitting below the belt" by taking advantage of another's vulnerability.
- Violating Health Insurance Portability and Accountability Act rules concerning protection of personal health information.

human interactions whenever behavior may affect others, whenever actions involve conscious choices of methods and ends, and whenever actions can be evaluated in reference to standards of right and wrong (Holmes, 2014). Guidelines that may be adapted as ethical standards for interpersonal communication are highlighted in Box 4-11.

Frequently the nurse may wish to set goals that the individual does not want to reach; the nurse must remember that the problem belongs to the person, as does the choice of care alternatives. The nurse assists the individual in decision-making, with the decision based on the individual's value system. However, the nurse should not take a laissez-faire approach and avoid assisting the person. The nurse's responsibility is to help the individual to examine values, identify conflicts, and prioritize goals and desired health care outcomes. Action follows from understanding values and the best available information. Both the individual and the nurse must bring interpreted facts and personally clarified values to the interaction to establish goals. Recognizing this interplay, the nurse must clarify personal values, subsequently respect the individual's rights, and act to support and protect the integrity of the person, family, group, or community.

Ethical communication also involves safeguarding protected health information. The individual's right to privacy motivated the passage of the Health Insurance Portability and Accountability Act in 1996. Individually identifiable health information is defined as (US Department of Health and Human Services, 2003):

*Information protected by law and includes demographic data, that relates to: the individual's past, present or future physical or mental health or condition, the provision of health care to the individual, or the past, present, or future payment for the provision of health care to the individual, and that identifies the individual or for which there is a reasonable basis to believe can be used to identify the individual. Individually identifiable health information includes many common identifiers (e.g., name, address, birth date, Social Security Number).*

Sharing personal health information (PIH) can be understood on the basis of "need to know" so as to care for the person. Stuart's (2012) concept of the circle of confidentiality provides a helpful guideline to nurses. "Within the circle, patient information may be shared. Those outside the circle require the patient's permission to receive information. Within the circle are treatment team members, staff supervisors, health care students and their faculty (only if they are working with the patient), and consultants who actually see the patient." Adhering to the rules concerning protection of identifiable health information is both an ethical and a legal requirement for the nurse.

## Therapeutic Techniques

Occasionally, clinicians who are novices in establishing helping relationships assume that they are bound to "say the wrong thing" and cause terrible damage to the person, or that they will learn some magical phrases and questions to create instant rapport. No nurse or other professional is so powerful that a "wrong word" will destroy the individual's self-concept or self-esteem. Even people with physical and emotional problems are resilient and have coped, at least to some degree, with a lifetime of stresses. Alternatively, no magical saying exists that the nurse can always plug into an interaction to communicate successfully. Although some techniques are often useful, they must be applied with purpose, skill, and attention to the individuality of each person and to the context of the interaction. The following techniques therefore should be viewed as guidelines, rather than prescriptions, for effective shaping of the therapeutic relationship.

### Focus on the Individual

The first step to therapeutic communication is focusing on the individual and the reason that the interaction is occurring. The nurse is not the focus; the person is. Although an overly business-like style fails to communicate concern and support, delving into one's own personal life to the extent that it diverts attention from the other person's concern is also problematic. Avoiding nurse-directed conversation can be difficult; a useful rule of

---

☑ BOX 4-12 **QUALITY AND SAFETY SCENARIO**

*Steps in Promoting Problem-Solving*

**Describe the Experience or Event of Concern**
*Helpful Verbal Nursing Strategies*
"Tell me what happened."
"Describe the experience to me."

**Analyze the Parts of the Experience and See the Relationships to Other Events**
*Helpful Verbal Nursing Strategies*
"What meaning does this have for you?"
"What pattern is there?"

**Formulate the Problem**
*Helpful Verbal Nursing Strategies*
"In what way is this problematic?"
"What do you want to see changed?"

**Validate the Formulation**
*Helpful Verbal Nursing Strategies*
"Do you mean...?"
"Let me tell you what I understand you to be saying."

**Use the Formulation to Identify Ways to Solve or Manage the Difficulty**
*Helpful Verbal Nursing Strategies*
"What would you do the next time?"
"In what way has your view changed?"
"What actions are needed to solve the problem that you've identified?"

**Try Out the Solutions, Judge the Outcomes, and Adjust the Plan Accordingly**
*Helpful Nursing Strategies*
Encourage application in new situations through role playing or through practice in appropriate settings; help the individual cycle through the preceding sequence as needed to evaluate the outcome and make adjustments to the plan.

Source Peplau, H. E. (1963). Process and concept of learning. In S. Burd, & M. Marshall (Eds.), *Some clinical approaches to psychiatric nursing* (pp. 333-336). New York: Macmillan.

---

thumb is to answer or respond to obvious questions and to switch the focus back to clinical concerns when other questions are asked. For example:

> *Individual* (looks at female nurse's wedding ring): "Are you married?"
> *Nurse:* "Yes, I am."
> *Individual:* "What does your husband do for a living?"
> *Nurse:* "Rather than get distracted by a discussion about me, let's get back to planning how you will manage at work."

Keeping focus on the person's concerns includes identifying the portion of the message that is clear and relevant to the purpose of the interaction, seeking validation, and helping the individual to clarify the rest of the message.

### Help the Individual to Describe and Clarify Content and Meaning

Too often the nurse rushes to offer an interpretation of the nature of the problem and quickly follows up by suggesting a solution. Solving problems efficiently makes the nurse feel effective, important, and powerful; however, the person's needs may not be met. A crucial step in using the therapeutic relationship effectively is to assist the individual to describe a particular experience or concern. Description is enhanced when the nurse prompts the person to clarify the description and interpret its meaning.

Use of who, what, where, and when questions helps the person to clarify and expand the content and meaning of what is communicated. Phrases such as "tell me," "go on," "describe to me," "explain it to me," and "give me an example" are also likely to elicit description of important content and to diminish distracting generalizations and abstractions. By seeking feedback, the nurse helps the individual to explain the meaning further. In clarifying the meaning, the nurse should avoid threatening, detective-like

questions. Questions that begin with "why" often increase the person's anxiety because they demand reasons, conclusions, analysis, or causes (Peplau, 1964). Reformulating questions to obtain descriptive data first and then helping the individual to analyze links among events, thoughts, feelings, actions, and outcomes is generally a more helpful approach.

A problem-solving approach by the nurse assists the person to describe and clarify the content and meaning of experience. Sequential steps help the individual to explain events, to change circumstances and responses that interfere with health, and to solve problems (D'Antonio et al., 2014; O'Toole & Welt, 1989; Peplau, 1963). This problem-solving approach can be adapted for use in health promotion to assist the person in problem-solving by working through the steps outlined in Box 4-12: Quality and Safety Scenario. These steps are a useful guideline for keeping the focus of concern on the individual and his or her definition of the problem. Rather than telling the person what is wrong and how to fix it, the nurse's primary goal is helping the person to describe the problem and formulate solutions in partnership. The cyclic nature of the process is illustrated in Figure 4-2.

### Use Reflection

Reflection is the restatement of what the individual has said in the same or different words. This technique can involve paraphrasing or summarizing the person's main point to indicate interest and to focus the discussion. Effective use of this approach does not include frequent, parrot-like repetition of the individual's statements. Instead, reflection is the selective paraphrasing or literal repetition of the person's words to underscore the importance of what has been said, to summarize a main concern or theme, or to elicit elaborated information. In addition, to verify understanding of health information, the nurse can ask the person

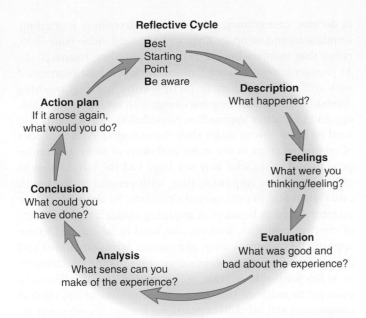

**Reflective Cycle**

**B**est
**S**tarting
**P**oint
**B**e aware

**Description**
What happened?

**Feelings**
What were you
thinking/feeling?

**Evaluation**
What was good and
bad about the experience?

**Analysis**
What sense can you
make of the experience?

**Conclusion**
What could you
have done?

**Action plan**
If it arose again,
what would you do?

**FIGURE 4-2** The process of reflection. The reflective process is illustrated here with entry at any point to examine events, associated thoughts and feelings, and analysis with a goal of understanding the events and one's reactions/actions as well as formulating a plan for responding effectively to similar events in the future.

to restate what has been communicated. Failure to confirm understanding interferes with desired clinical care outcomes. For example, Bolster and Manias (2010) identified failures in communication, including lack of comprehension of information from providers, as a barrier to consumers' participation in their care.

## Use Constructive Confrontation

Confronting an individual means that the nurse points out a specific behavior and then helps the person to examine the meaning or consequences of the behavior. For example:

> *Nurse:* "You missed your appointment for the consultation we had scheduled."
>
> *Individual:* "Oh, I didn't notice the date."
>
> *Nurse:* "You are usually very aware of time and appointments. What do you think was going on with you that you didn't notice the date this time?"

This type of confrontation is not an angry exchange but a purposeful way of helping the person examine personal actions and their meaning.

## Use Nouns and Pronouns Correctly

Some individuals have difficulty separating themselves from others or specifying the object or subject in their language. These individuals misuse pronouns by referring to we, us, they, she, he, him, and her, without clearly identifying the referent, and by making vague statements such as "They don't like me. They told me I was useless." Others may use general nouns, such as everyone, people, doctors, and nurses, to avoid clear communication about specific persons. The nurse can clarify the meaning

by asking, "Who are they?" or "Who is the person?" Additionally, the nurse must be careful to use separate pronouns when speaking of herself or himself and the individual, particularly when the person has disordered thinking. For example, when communicating with an individual who is confused or exhibits disordered or psychotic thinking, the nurse should say "you" and "I," rather than "us" or "we," to promote clear thinking and communication and to assist the individual to maintain personal boundaries (Peplau, 1963).

## Use Silence

Allowing a thoughtful silence at intervals helps the individual to talk at his or her own pace without pressure to perform for the nurse. Silence also permits time for reflection. Particularly helpful to the depressed or physically ill person, silence can reduce pressure and conserve energy. After several moments, the nurse can ask the person to share some thoughts. For example, "Try putting your thoughts into words," "Tell me what are you thinking or feeling now," or "I'll be here when you feel ready to talk."

## Motivational Interviewing

**Motivational interviewing (MI)** is a person-centered communication approach used widely in health care and life coaching to assist individuals to make behavioral changes regarding a wide variety of lifestyle and health issues (Barrett & Chang, 2016; Ostland et al., 2015). Key components of MI are:

- Engaging—involving the individual in talking about issues, worries, and desires, and to establish the basis for a trusting relationship.
- Focusing—narrowing the focus to habits or patterns that individuals wish to change.
- Evoking—eliciting motivation for change by increasing the sense of the importance of change, confidence, and readiness to change.
- Planning—developing practical steps that the individual wants to use to create the desired changes.

Nurses can seek training and use many available self-help and life coaching resources for health promotion (e.g., Hall, 2012). For example, *The Life Coach Workbook* (Raymond, 2014) is an example of a self-help book with useful tools that align nicely with MI that could be tailored to specific health care concerns. Such resources have high acceptability and can serve as helpful adjuncts to formal education and treatment/health-promotion guidance from nurses.

Current evidence supports the use of MI as an effective technique that can be taught to health professionals without advanced mental health training to promote desired behavioral change across health problems and settings. For training, use, and evaluation of MI implementation, nurses and other clinicians can use the Motivational Interviewing Skills in Health Care Encounters instrument, a reliable validated assessment tool to evaluate acquisition and use of specific MI skills and principles (Petrova et al., 2015).

## Barriers to Effective Communication

Barriers to effective communication can originate with the nurse, the individual, or both. The most obvious barrier is the nurse's failure to use the types of therapeutic techniques just described. Lack of knowledge or experience can limit the nurse's ability to assess the individual's needs and repertoire of skills. Supervision and study can help the nurse apply the steps of the nursing process by using effective intervention approaches.

Communication is also ineffective when some part of the communication-feedback loop breaks down. Failure to send a clear message, receive and interpret the message correctly, or provide useful feedback can interfere with communication. Diagnosing the source of the communication breakdown, taking steps to correct it, and using knowledge of the communication process and appropriate therapeutic techniques are the nurse's responsibility.

## Anxiety

When the nurse or individual is highly anxious during an interaction, perception is altered and the ability to communicate effectively is curtailed sharply. Defense mechanisms, such as denial, projection, and displacement, reduce anxiety but block understanding of the true meaning of an interaction. Severe anxiety and defense mechanisms distort reality and lead to disordered communication. To enhance interpersonal communication, the nurse identifies the feeling of anxiety and its source and uses anxiety-reducing interventions.

## Attitudes

Biases and stereotypes can limit the nurse's and the individual's ability to relate. When the difficulty is the individual's problem, the nurse can assist by examining those views that interfere with the person's relationships. When the problem is the nurse's, openness in the supervisory relationship to examine personal behavior is crucial. When the nurse fails to examine his or her attitudes toward the person, negativity may be communicated and perceptions of the interaction may be distorted.

## Gaps Between the Nurse and the Individual

Related to attitudinal barriers, differences in gender, age, socioeconomic background, ethnicity, race, religion, or language can block functional communication between the nurse and the individual. These factors can cause differences in perception and block mutual understanding. Newly licensed nurses have attributed communication problems to differences in language proficiency among nurses, including English as a second language, as well as to problems in understanding non–English-speaking individuals (Smith-Miller et al., 2010). To reduce such gaps, nurses can question unclear verbal or written communications, seek clarification or assistance from translators, and explore the ways in which perceptions may differ and meanings can be clarified (Box 4-13: Diversity Awareness and Chapter 2).

Moreover, generation gaps between faculty and student nurses can interfere with effective development of the interpersonal skills required for therapeutic nurse-person relationships (Bhana, 2014). Generation Y students, born from the early 1980s to the late 1990s, constitute a large cohort of current undergraduate/pre-licensure and graduate nursing students. Evidence from the literature demonstrates that this generation benefits from deconstruction pedagogies or interactive teaching strategies such as debates, case studies, role playing, storytelling, journaling, simulations and webpage links to audio and video page links, rather than more traditional didactic approaches (Bhana, 2014). As younger generations (e.g., millennials), who have been raised with technology at their fingertips, enter nursing, teaching approaches will require ongoing change with use of more technology and interactive approaches. Nonetheless, our students also need to learn how to adapt their technology-mediated modes of communication to the styles and skills of older generation persons and those who may not have had the same access to technology when communicating with persons in the health care system and in professional situations. So although faculty members need to be adept at engaging students with a variety of effective strategies, students also need to be coached to use appropriate communication approaches across situations and populations. For example, evidence supports the effectiveness of video feedback, another technological teaching/learning strategy, to enhance the quality of communication, clinical competence, and MI skills of practicing nurses (Noordman et al., 2014). Thus ongoing faculty development and testing of various teaching approaches to help students develop competence in therapeutic communication and relationships is crucial to nursing's future.

## Resistance

Resistance comprises all phenomena that inhibit the flow of thoughts, feelings, and memories in an interpersonal encounter and behaviors that interfere with therapeutic goals. Resistance arises from anxiety when a person feels threatened. To reduce this anxiety, the person implements resistant behavior to divert the focus, most often in the form of avoidance, such as being late, changing the subject, forgetting, blocking, or becoming angry.

Initially, the nurse should identify the behavior, whether it is the nurse's or the individual's behavior, and then attempt to interpret it in the context of the interaction. Exploration of possible threats in the relationship, goals, context, or a particular topic can lead to understanding the source of the resistance and finding the ability to handle these difficulties. Anxiety reduction is often a necessary step in dealing with resistant behavior.

## Transference and Countertransference or Distorting

Transference is reacting to another person in an exchange as though that person were someone from the past. Another term for this process is distorting. Transference, although a concept from the psychoanalytic/psychodynamic tradition in psychiatry and psychiatric nursing, retains relevance today. It is best understood as a process that distorts a current relationship or interaction on the basis of past learning, expectations, and/or relationships. Transference or distorting may involve a host of feelings that generally are classified as positive (love, affection, or regard) or negative (anger, dislike, or frustration). Typical transference reactions involve an important figure from the past such as a mother or father; however, at times transference may be more general to include all authority figures. Something about another person's characteristics, behavior, or position, in combination with individual dynamics and context, triggers this response.

## ⊕ BOX 4-13   DIVERSITY AWARENESS
### Multicultural Context of Communication

As health care providers, nurses might believe that they have expert knowledge about health promotion and the treatment of illness that will be beneficial to others. Therefore, it seems logical that nurses would select appropriate information to share with individuals to help them maintain health and manage illness or alterations in health status. However, consider the possible influences of cultural differences between the nurse and individual.

Much of the knowledge generated from nursing-related disciplines and the sciences is rooted in a Western perspective. Particularly in the United States, knowledge is developed and interpreted from the perspective of the dominant cultural group, a white, Anglo-Saxon, Christian point of view. When this perspective remains unexamined, alternative perspectives are ignored and invisible. Nurses who are members of the dominant cultural group may be well-intentioned, but ineffective, when they attempt to engage a person of a different cultural group in a relationship without questioning how culture influences interactions, interpretations of events and information, and beliefs and values concerning health and health care practices. Preconceived ideas about people based on some characteristic or group affiliation, such as racial or ethnic identity, religion, country of origin, gender, or sexual orientation, can interfere with nurses' abilities to relate to people as individuals. At the same time, a lack of knowledge of other cultural groups hampers nurses' understanding of the individual's point of view.

Guidelines for recognizing the multicultural context of communication in therapeutic relationships include the following:
- Make ethnocultural assessment a critical component of every clinical evaluation.
- Allow other people to define themselves.
- Ask the person, and the family as appropriate, about cultural health care practices and traditions.
- Respect cultural practices and traditions while providing opportunity for the person to voice preferences and make choices.
- Respect the language of others and do not assume superiority in language.
- Collaborate with trained translators and health promoters (people with the same ethnic or racial background as the individuals).
- Create intercultural open dialogue based on security and mutual respect.
- Avoid use of racist, sexist, ageist, and other forms of denigrating language.
- Do not perpetuate stereotypes in communication.

- Adapt communication to the uniqueness of the individual.
- Reject humor that degrades members on the basis of gender, race, ethnicity, religion, sexual orientation, country of origin, and so forth.
- Respect the rights of others to have different practices and customs.
- Do not allow injustice to continue through silence.
- Present information clearly to all people to help them make informed choices.
- Do not judge values, traditions, and practices on the basis of their similarity to or difference from personal values, traditions, and practices, but judge them on the basis of whether they facilitate human potential.

The following are some issues for the nurse to consider:
- When the nurse works with a person from a different cultural background, what are common barriers to establishing a therapeutic relationship?
- In learning about different cultural groups, is there a risk of creating new stereotypes that interfere with the ability to treat people as unique individuals?
- If the nurse has little or no knowledge about a person's culture, how can the nurse provide meaningful nursing care?
- Are the two previous questions contradictory? How can the nurse meet the different challenges that they imply?
- Research measurements typically are developed from the perspective of the dominant culture. If the nurse wishes to use a standardized instrument to measure clinical or research variables among members of different cultural groups, then what questions about the instrument should the nurse ask, and what problems might the nurse encounter? What would need to be done to determine whether or not an instrument truly measures the same phenomenon across different populations?
- Consider the possible influences of cultural differences between the nurse and the individual. Think of an example of two people from diverse cultural groups who developed a relationship. Examine how they got to know each other and what differences and similarities they uncovered. Did barriers to understanding each other exist? If so, how did they bridge these barriers? What did they learn about themselves? What did they learn about the ways that culture shapes perspective and interactions? Think about how a nurses can apply these insights to their relationships with people from cultural groups that differ from their own.
- How would a multicultural perspective change the practice?

People in a therapeutic relationship often develop strong transference feelings toward the helping professional, arising from the interaction's intensity and the care provider's authoritative or nurturing role. When transference or distorting reactions interfere with the current relationship (i.e., when reactions are out of proportion to the actual situation such as excessive anger in response to a nurse's suggestion), they require gentle probing by pointing out the reaction and asking about the associated thoughts and feelings, and possible past reactions in similar circumstances (e.g., responses to authority figures). To work with a person's transference reactions effectively, the nurse first helps the person to examine feelings and thoughts about the nurse with a nondefensive or reactive stance. Then the nurse assists the person to compare and contrast the nurse with people from the person's past to reduce distortions and comprehend the present reality to move forward effectively.

**Countertransference** is basically the same phenomenon and involves distorting, but it is experienced by the health care professional rather than the person. The nurse experiences many feelings toward the person; these feelings are not problematic, unless they remain unanalyzed and block the nurse's ability to work effectively with the individual. For example, if a nurse has strong feelings about the person and thinks that the person cannot possibly function after discharge without the nurse's aid, the nurse is likely to distort the person's abilities, encourage a childlike dependency, and interfere with the person's progress. This nurse needs to examine such personal feelings to understand their source. Once understood, countertransference reactions generally cease to interfere with the relationship. Consultation for supervision with an advanced practice psychiatric nurse or other mental health expert is recommended whenever transference or countertransference (i.e., distorting) reactions are persistent and problematic.

### Sensory Barriers

When the individual has sensory limitations, the nurse may need to use extra skill in communicating. Use of the other senses to send or receive messages should be attempted. Special help is often available from trained therapists and teachers; for example, many agencies have access to interpreters for deaf people, and visual aids may be useful. Nurses must be as creative as possible, learn from others who are skilled in alternative forms of communication, and make referrals as necessary. As technology evolves, new communication methods will continue to decrease these barriers. For example, voice recognition software programs assist persons with visual and motor challenges to communicate via text.

### Failure to Address Concerns or Needs

Failure to meet the individual's needs or to recognize the individual's concerns is the most serious barrier to effective interaction. This failure can arise from inadequate assessment, lack of knowledge, inability to separate the nurse's needs from the individual's needs, and confusion between friendship and a helping relationship, including unrecognized or unresolved sexual issues. To correct this problem, the nurse should recognize that a barrier to relating to the person exists. Using the supervisory process to determine the problem's source, the nurse should then take corrective action, such as obtaining more information or knowledge, performing a self-assessment with values clarification, and examining reactions, biases, and expectations. Nurses, particularly novice nurses and those transitioning to a new role (e.g., from staff nurse to nurse practitioner after graduate school), need to *demand* mentorship/clinical supervision that is not tied to performance evaluation. In other words, a supportive mentoring/supervisory relationship with a more senior nurse is a necessary ingredient in helping nurses to be effective. Cost-cutting efforts in today's health care system often neglect such needs. Yet consider the cost of a failed hire or ineffective relationships with care recipients. An argument for having professional support can be strong. Additionally, nurses can create their own cost-effective professional support systems by creating peer groups and/or engaging their own consultants with a peer group outside the work setting.

### Setting

The setting of a therapeutic interaction can affect the goals and the nature of the communication. The most important aspect of any setting is that the nurse and the individual are able to attend to each other. The nurse's attention to the person helps create this atmosphere. The nurse assesses the influence of factors such as lighting, noise, temperature, comfort, physical distance, and privacy; potentially disturbing factors can be altered or controlled within the limits of the setting. Occasionally the nurse has only minimal control over the setting, as in a busy clinic, health center, inpatient unit, emergency department, or the individual's home. Although far from the ideal of a quiet, pleasant, well-lit private office, these typical clinical settings can be used effectively by creating a sense of private space. Curtains can be drawn, doors shut, and two chairs pulled to a corner to shape an environment for interaction. When possible, however, nurses seek offices or rooms to establish privacy during significant communication or when imparting important or complex health information. Home settings can also be more comfortable for individuals than for nurses, yet also

can provide invaluable context when used. The nurse can also acknowledge verbally that some aspect of the environment, such as an interruption or noise, is bothersome. This strategy shows people that the nurse recognizes possible concentration difficulties and is sharing the environment with them.

### Stages

Therapeutic relationships follow sequential phases, which may overlap, differ in length, or involve issues that appear over time rather than in a set sequence. Orientation (introductory), working, and termination phases have been identified by researchers and clinicians (Canabrava, 2011; Stuart, 2012).

Originally these relationship stages were identified from clinical interactions that developed over a prolonged period. However, they can be observed in brief encounters that are effective; that is, interactions that meet individuals' needs rather than therapeutic interactions that have been reduced to little more than quick question-and-answer sessions. Whether the nurse is engaged in a long-term or short-term relationship with an individual, attention to the relationship stages is important. Brief therapeutic relationships will telescope the stages; therefore it is particularly important that the nurse focus on meeting the key demands of each relationship phase. It is important to note that individuals may move in and out of direct care episodes, while a therapeutic relationship can be maintained over a longer period. A relationship exists even when the nurse and the individual do not see each other for an extended period, and each encounter occurs within the trajectory of the relationship stages.

### Orientation or Introductory Phase

The orientation or introductory phase begins when the nurse and the individual meet. This meeting typically involves some feeling of anxiety; neither party knows what to expect. When the therapeutic relationship is primarily a counseling type of relationship, part of the nurse's role is to help structure the interaction by discussing several topics during the initial meeting and sometimes during the first few meetings. Box 4-14 lists topics appropriate to this phase. Discussion of these issues establishes a contract or pact and involves a mutual understanding of the parameters of the relationship and an agreement to work together.

The orientation stage is a critical juncture in any therapeutic relationship. Without successful transition through the orientation phase, no working alliance will exist and the treatment goals will remain unmet. Consistency, sensitive pacing of communication, active listening, conveying concern and warmth, and paying

---

**BOX 4-14   Key Topics of Discussion During the Orientation or Introductory Phase of the Therapeutic Relationship**

- What to call each other
- Purpose of meeting
- Location, time, and length of meetings
- Termination date or time for review of progress through follow-up
- Confidentiality (with whom clinical data will be shared)
- Any other limits related to the particular setting

attention to comfort and control help to establish a connection during the orientation phase. In contrast, inconsistency, unavailability, individual factors associated with trust, nurses' feelings about the other person, confrontation of delusions or strongly held views, and unrealistic expectations hamper relationships.

When the therapeutic relationship is not structured primarily as counseling with a specific number of sessions, the orientation phase may appear less distinct and the topics noted may seem irrelevant. In this case, the nurse can adapt the suggested topics to meet the specific situation. However, except in true emergencies, initial encounters should always include introductions by name, discussion of the purpose, and presentation of a plan for ongoing care or specific follow-up.

### Working Phase

The working phase of the therapeutic relationship emerges when the nurse and the individual collaborate as partners in promoting the person's health. The working phase may last for only a brief time to establish a treatment plan, may last for an established number of sessions, as in brief psychotherapy, or may extend over a longer period if the nurse is the primary care provider, care manager, or long-term caregiver in any setting or context for an individual or family. During the working phase, the relationship is the context through which change occur. Goals are set, and the nurse and the individual work mutually toward their accomplishment. Interventions are tailored to the specific situation and health needs of the person and the family. Solving problems, coping with stressors, and gaining insight are all part of the working phase. The nurse and the individual recognize each other's uniqueness and establish trust as the first step in establishing a working relationship.

Resistant behaviors may be observed during this phase while the nurse and the individual become closer and work on potentially anxiety-producing problems. The person may pull away through the use of defense mechanisms because change can be difficult. Overcoming the resistance becomes an important nursing task.

### Termination Phase

Termination marks the end of the relationship established in the therapeutic contract or negotiated in accordance with the limits of the contract. Ending a relationship can cause anxiety for both the individual and the nurse. Termination represents a loss; therefore it can trigger feelings of sadness, frustration, and anger. Termination in this case is the loss of a relationship and the loss of future involvement, with its attendant realistic expectations or fantasies. Termination also reawakens feelings of previously unresolved losses, such as a death or divorce.

Working through any feelings related to termination is an important part of clinical care. Some individuals require the nurse's assistance to experience the feelings of loss and to connect present reactions to past real or symbolic losses. Box 4-15 lists additional interventions for use during the termination phase.

Both the nurse and the individual can learn much during termination; the process directs both participants to examine problems and progress in the relationship, feelings, and reactions. The experience also helps the nurse and the individual gain

---

> ### BOX 4-15 Interventions for Use During the Termination Phase of the Therapeutic Relationship
>
> - Let the person know why the relationship is to be terminated.
> - Remind the person of the date and how many meetings or appointments are left.
> - Collaborate with other staff so that they are aware of how the person is reacting and any special needs that the person may have.
> - Help the person to identify sources of support and other people with whom a relationship is possible.
> - Review the gains and the remaining goals.
> - Discuss the pros and cons experienced during the relationship to help the person develop a realistic appraisal.
> - Make referrals for follow-up care as needed.

---

> ### BOX 4-16 Key Ingredients for a 15-Minute (or Shorter) Family Interview
>
> - Use manners to engage or reengage family members. Make an introduction by offering your name and role. Orient family members to the purpose of a brief family interview.
> - Assess significant areas of internal and external structure and function (obtain information from a genogram concerning basic family composition and external support data).
> - Ask family members three key questions.
> - Commend the family on one or two strengths.
> - Evaluate usefulness and conclude.

Source Wright, L. M., & Leahey, M. (2013). *Nurses and families: A guide to family assessment and intervention* (6th ed.). Philadelphia: F.A. Davis.

---

practice in ending relationships and in exploring reactions, which can be most helpful when future losses occur. Nonetheless, major gains can be accomplished with the deadline of termination. Options for follow-up or future treatment as the need determines also require exploration and planning.

### Brief Interactions

Time constraints in practice are unavoidable. Although challenging, brief therapeutic encounters can be meaningful and useful. Limited time is not a valid reason to avoid interviewing or interacting with individuals. Rather, nurses purposefully can structure brief interactions to achieve specific clinical outcomes (Wright & Leahey, 2013). Box 4-16 delineates key ingredients for a **15-minute** (or shorter) **interview** with a family.

These guidelines for brief interactions with families can be adapted for interviews with individuals. An effective 15-minute (or shorter) interview is feasible if nurses plan to introduce themselves, state the purpose of meeting, validate understanding with the person or the family, clarify parameters such as time, focus and listen, and elicit significant individual and family data. Most important, the goal of the interaction must be realistic and clearly defined. For example, the purpose may be to elicit a family's view of the problem for which the person has sought care or to prioritize problems to be treated. Even when time is limited, the interview is structured to provide an opportunity for the person or the family to engage in dialogue as an active participant in care, and the nurse's attention is completely focused on the individual.

Circumstances also can dictate the need for immediate and instructive communications that command specific actions. For example, during a crisis, directive, clear communication is paramount. Miller and McCurley (2011) demonstrated the importance of preparedness and communication strategies during disaster-related events. Planning in anticipation of human-caused and natural disasters is critical so as to have functional communications systems in place. Such systems increasingly will use various methods of telecommunication. After tragic events have

occurred, including shootings on college campuses, efforts to communicate more effectively are paramount. Universities, for example, have responded by instituting systems to communicate rapidly with a large campus community. Widely deployed strategies feature instant text messaging and e-mailing (see Box 4-6: Innovative Practice).

The following case study presents a detailed scenario of a home visit and questions related to how the nurse can develop a therapeutic relationship with the person. The care plan presents a plan of care for the person, including communication interventions.

## CASE STUDY

### A Health-Promotion Visit: Maria Sanchez-Smith

As part of a health-promotion visit for Maria Sanchez-Smith and Thomas, her 2-week-old infant, Jessica Wong, a registered nurse, planned to conduct an infant assessment, provide breastfeeding support, teach about normal infant development and care activities, and assess Mrs. Sanchez-Smith's adaptation to motherhood and her postpartum recovery status. Before the visit, Ms. Wong reviewed the clinical information she obtained during Mrs. Sanchez-Smith's hospitalization. Mrs. Sanchez-Smith is a 34-year-old Hispanic primiparous woman who delivered a 7-pound, 10-ounce healthy boy (Thomas) after a 12-hour labor. The labor had progressed well without complications. Mrs. Sanchez-Smith received epidural anesthesia at 6-cm dilatation, and the baby was delivered vaginally. Her husband, Mark Smith, provided labor support and was present for the delivery. After a 2-day hospital stay, Mrs. Sanchez-Smith was discharged. At discharge, the infant was breastfeeding, had normal newborn examination findings, and weighed 7 pounds, 5 ounces. Ms. Wong had been impressed by both parents' preparation for the birth. They had attended childbirth classes and read several books about infant development and parenting. Ms. Sanchez-Smith planned to take an 8-week maternity leave from her position as a lawyer in a large practice and had arranged for a child care provider to come to the family's home to take care of the infant beginning 2 weeks before the end of her maternity leave. Mr. Smith had not planned to take time off from his job because he had recently been promoted to a high-level managerial position in his company that required increased travel and time at work. He was able to postpone a business trip to be present at the delivery and had sent a plane ticket to his mother-in-law so she could come and stay at their home during the first week after Mrs. Sanchez-Smith and Thomas were discharged from the hospital.

During the visit, Ms. Wong first assessed the infant. She incorporated teaching concerning normal infant development and concluded that Thomas was a healthy 2-week-old infant who was feeding well. Thomas's circumcision was healing without complications and he had regained his birth weight.

When Ms. Wong asked how Ms. Sanchez-Smith was doing, Ms. Sanchez-Smith hesitated and then responded, "I'm not sure. I'm very glad that Thomas is doing well… but I worry sometimes that I'm not going to be able to do everything right for him. It's funny, but I've spent so many years getting an education and establishing my law career. It was hard work, but I managed to do well. Now a little infant overwhelms me. I don't know how I'll manage this." When Ms. Wong asked Ms. Sanchez-Smith to talk more about her concerns, Ms. Sanchez-Smith described how incompetent she felt while her mother was staying with her. "My mother could do everything so easily. I fumbled with every diaper. It felt like she criticized how I did things. When she told me about what she did when she had children, I felt pushed to do things 'her way' and not the way that I had planned. She even wanted to give him a bottle when I was trying so hard to get breastfeeding going. At least the doctor said Thomas had gained enough weight. Thomas' weight gain made me feel like I wasn't a total failure. I couldn't wait for her to go, but I fell apart after she left. I was alone. Mark is out of town until the weekend, and I couldn't get Thomas to stop crying yesterday. I thought I would

scream, so I put him down in his crib and I just sat there crying. What's wrong with me? I've never felt so out of control before. I want to be a good mother, but I feel like I can't give any more right now."

In response to Ms. Wong's follow-up questions about mental status, Mrs. Sanchez-Smith described frequently feeling irritated and sad, crying a few times over the previous several days, having difficulty sleeping even when the baby was asleep, feeling fatigued, and being worried about how she would be able to go back to work in only a few weeks. Ms. Wong also inquired about the family's cultural, ethnic, and religious backgrounds. Mrs. Sanchez-Smith responded, "Interesting that you should ask. That's actually another issue right now. I'm from New Mexico and my family is Hispanic and Catholic, but I'm not a practicing Catholic now. You might guess that I'm Latina from my hyphenated name. I added my maiden name to Smith when I got married to honor my family. Mark is Protestant, but not really religious. His family comes from New Jersey. They are very nice and were supportive when we got married. We were lucky that our families accepted us together. I have to admit, though, that we didn't really figure out what we would do about raising the baby. Mark thinks that we'd be hypocrites to have a Catholic christening. Plus, my mother told me that I'd be selfish to go back to work so soon. Can you help me? I feel like I'm going out of my mind and I don't know what to do."

This case study raises a variety of clinical concerns. As the nurse in this encounter, Ms. Wong could begin by considering the following questions.

**Reflective Questions:**

- What are my feelings as I listen to her story and her distress? Am I aware of how my values and expectations affect my interaction with this person? How can I establish a therapeutic relationship to support Ms. Sanchez-Smith during this stressful period?
- What is the significance of the distress symptoms that Ms. Sanchez-Smith reported? Given that the period during which many women experience postpartum blues has passed, what is the most appropriate action for referral to obtain a thorough mental status examination for postpartum depression?
- Who is the most appropriate health care provider to evaluate her for postpartum depression, and treat her if it is confirmed? How can I facilitate getting her the care she needs, and can I remain available to her? How can I assist Ms. Sanchez-Smith to meet the infant's developmental needs during this stressful period?
- In what ways do family dynamics, values, and expectations related to differing cultural and religious heritages contribute to the problems described? What can I do to explore these issues further? What strengths can be harnessed? Are there clergy who could be engaged for pastoral counseling? How can I engage support systems to ameliorate rather than exacerbate the difficulties? What can be done to engage both Mr. Smith and Ms. Sanchez-Smith in a therapeutic relationship to focus on the couple and parenting concerns, and to involve both partners in treatment strategies?

## CARE PLAN

### Transition to Parenthood: Maria Sanchez-Smith

*NURSING DIAGNOSIS: Risk of impaired parenting related to stress involved in transition to parenthood

#### Defining Characteristics

- Feeling overwhelmed with responsibilities of new parenthood
- Insecurity about tasks of infant care
- Crying
- Sadness
- Feeling out of control
- Difficulty sleeping even when the baby is asleep
- Worry about going back to work soon

#### Related Factors

- Transition from high career achievement to new role as mother.
- Differing religious, ethnic, and cultural backgrounds of the two parents and extended families.
- Confusion and lack of decisions about religious and cultural traditions to follow for their infant.
- Conflicting expectations of extended families, particularly from Ms. Sanchez-Smith's mother.
- Job pressures on Mr. Smith to travel and be away from home.
- Unanticipated social isolation for Ms. Sanchez-Smith during this postpartum period.
- Limited social support (particularly from the husband because of work-associated travel).

#### Expected Outcomes

- Competent mothering and infant care are displayed.
- Ms. Sanchez-Smith describes her feelings, concerns, and needs.
- Indicators of postpartum depression are evaluated, and referral for follow-up is made for positive findings.
- Social supports are engaged.
- Ms. Sanchez-Smith and Mr. Smith successfully negotiate immediate decisions about religious and cultural practice concerning their baby and agree to use counseling services to work out decisions concerning their child's upbringing and involvement of the extended family.

#### Interventions

- Health information is provided about normal newborn and postpartum adjustment.
- Infant care information is provided on the basis of Ms. Sanchez-Smith's needs.
- Expectations about postpartum adjustment and parenthood are elicited.
- Health information about postpartum depression is provided regarding prevalence and common symptoms.
- Personal and family histories are obtained, with a focus on mental health.
- Postpartum depression is evaluated with use of interview questions and an assessment measure, such as the Edinburgh Postnatal Depression Scale (Cox et al., 1987) or the Postpartum Depression Screening Scale (Beck & Gable, 2001).
- If symptom levels suggest postpartum depression, a referral for mental health evaluation is made. If there are any signs of safety risk to self or others, immediate protective action (e.g., emergency mental health evaluation) is taken.
- Sources of social support are solicited, and specific plans are made to use available support, such as the husband, friends, and hired infant care providers.
- Conflicts and areas of shared values, plans, goals for raising the baby are explored.
- Pros and cons of options for raising the baby are examined in relation to religious, ethnic, and cultural considerations.
- A follow-up plan is made to reassess symptoms of postpartum depression and to discuss ongoing concerns about how to raise the baby with Mrs. Sanchez-Smith and Mr. Smith.
- Referral is made to local support and psychoeducational programs for interfaith couples.

*NANDA Nursing Diagnoses—Herdman T. H. & Kamitsuru, S. (Eds.). Nursing Diagnoses - Definitions and Classification 2015-2017. Copyright © 2014, 1994-2014 NANDA International. Used by arrangement with John Wiley & Sons Limited. In order to make safe and effective judgments using the NANDA-I nursing diagnoses it is essential that nurses refer to the definitions and defining characteristics of the diagnoses listed in this work.

## SUMMARY

Relating to persons has many challenges and rewards for nurses. Although some aspects of this work are predictable, each person and family is unique and provides a chance for the nurse to learn, grow, and help in new ways. This chapter has provided guidelines for developing therapeutic relationships, but these guidelines do not guarantee success or an easy job. The desire and skill of the individual nurse bring this information to life. The blend of the nurse's artistry, humanity, knowledge, skill, and ethics sparks concern and the ability to help another human being communicate effectively; essential components of the nurse-person relationship.

The therapeutic relationship is the primary arena for health promotion. Values clarification, communication, and the helping relationship are its core components. For nurses, applying this knowledge to their varied roles is essential to promoting health and providing quality care.

Rising use of technology and mounting pressures for cost-effective care are here to stay. In this climate, the importance of the therapeutic relationship is underscored (see Box 4-6: Innovative Practice). Without a relational context, the care dimension in health care is lost, and health promotion is reduced to standardized, recipe-like prescriptions. Effective health promotion directed to the needs of individuals, families, and communities requires reflection on the value of caring, effective communication, and a helping relationship.

## EVOLVE CHAPTER FEATURES

http://evolve.elsevier.com/Edelman/

- Study Questions

## REFERENCES

Ackerman, M. J., et al. (2010). Developing next-generation telehealth tools and technologies: Patients, systems, and data perspectives. *Telemedicine Journal and E-Health: The Official Journal of the American Telemedicine Association, 16*(1), 93–95.

Agency for Healthcare Research and Quality. (2015). *Health literacy universal precautions toolkit* (2nd ed.). Publication 15-0023-EF. Rockville, MD.

Baldor, K. R. (2011). *Nurse clinician self-disclosure: A qualitative study.* Amherst, MA: University of Massachusetts.

Barrett, K., & Chang, Y. P. (2016). Behavioral interventions targeting chronic pain, depression, and substance use disorder in primary care. *Journal of Nursing Scholarship, 48*(4), 345–353.

Beard, K. V., Gwanmesia, E., & Miranda-Diaz, G. (2015). Culturally competent care: Using the ESFT model in nursing. (2016). *The American Journal of Nursing, 115*(6), 58–62.

Beck, C. T., & Gable, R. K. (2001). *Postpartum depression screening scale.* Los Angeles: Western Psychological Services.

Bhana, V. M. (2014). Interpersonal skills development in Generation Y student nurses: A literature review. *Nurse Education Today, 34,* 1430–1434.

Blondis, M. N., & Jackson, B. E. (1982). *Nonverbal communication with patients: Back to the human touch* (2nd ed.). New York: John Wiley & Sons.

Bolster, D., & Manias, E. (2010). Person-centered interactions between nurses and patients during medication activities in an acute hospital setting: Qualitative observation and interview study. *International Journal of Nursing Studies, 47*(2), 154–165.

Canabrava, D. D. S. (2011). Nursing consultation of mental health supported by the interpersonal relations theory: Report of experience [in Portuguese]. *Ciência, Cuidado e Saúde, 10*(1), 150–156.

Cox, J. L., Holden, J. M., & Sagovsky, R. (1987). Detection of postnatal depression: Development of the 10-item Edinburgh Postnatal Depression Scale. *The British Journal of Psychiatry: The Journal of Mental Science, 150,* 782–786.

D'Antonio, P. D., et al. (2014). The future in the past: Hildegard Peplau and interpersonal relations in nursing. *Nursing Inquiry, 21,* 511–517.

Doss, S., DePascal, P., & Hadley, K. (2011). Patient-nurse partnerships. *Nephrology Nursing Journal: Journal of The American Nephrology Nurses' Association, 38*(2), 115–124.

Errasti-Ibarrondo, B., et al. (2015). Essential elements of the relationship between the nurse and the person with advanced and terminal cancer: A meta-ethnography. *Nursing Outlook, 63,* 255–268.

Fawcett, J., & Ellenbecker, C. H. (2015). A proposed conceptual model of nursing and population health. *Nursing Outlook, 63,* 288–298. doi:10.1016/j.outlook.2015.01.009.

Hall, E. (1973). *The silent language.* Garden City, NY: Doubleday/Anchor Press.

Hall, P. (2012). *How to be the pilot of your own life: Flying lessons.* Tucson, AZ: Through a Different Lens, LLC.

Haskey, N., et al. (2015). Improving the hospital experience: Technology at the bedside. *Canadian Journal of Dietetic Practice & Research, 76*(3).

Henry, S., et al. (2011). Association between nonverbal communication during clinical interactions and outcomes: A systematic review and meta-analysis. *Patient Education and Counseling, 86*(3), 297–315.

Holmes, P. (2014). Intercultural dialogue: Challenges to theory, practice and research. *Language and Intercultural Communication, 14,* 1–6.

Institute of Medicine. (2010). The future of nursing: Leading change, advancing health. http://www.nationalacademies.org/hmd/Reports/2010/The-Future-of-Nursing-Leading-Change-Advancing-Health.aspx.

Institute of Medicine. (2011). Innovations in health literacy: Workshop summary. https://www.nap.edu/catalog/13016/innovations-in-health-literacy-research-workshop-summary.

Jourard, S. (1971). *The transparent self* (rev. ed). New York: Van Nostrand Reinhold.

Lyons, K. J., et al. (2016). Jefferson Teamwork Observation Guide (JTOG): An instrument to observe teamwork behaviors. *Journal of Allied Health, 45,* 49–53c.

McCaffrey, G., & McConnell, S. (2015). Compassion: A critical review of peer-reviewed nursing literature. *Journal of Clinical Nursing, 24*(19-20), 3006–3015.

McKenna, M. C., & Stahl, K. D. (2015). *Assessment for reading instruction* (3rd ed.). New York: Guilford Press.

Melnyk, B. M., & Fineout-Overholt, E. (2011). *Evidence-based practice in nursing & health care: A guide to best practice* (2nd ed.). Philadelphia: Lippincott Williams & Wilkins.

Miller, C., & McCurley, M. C. (2011). Federal interagency communication strategies for addressing radiation emergencies and other public health crises. *Health Physics, 101*(5), 559–561.

National Patient Safety Foundation (n.d.) Ask me 3 good questions for your good health. https://www.npsf.org/askme3.

Noordman, J., van der Weijden, T., & Van Dulmen, S. (2014). Effects of video-feedback on the communication, clinical competence and motivational interviewing skills of practice nurses: A pre-test posttest control group study. *Journal of Advanced Nursing, 70,* 2275–2283.

Ostland, A. S., et al. (2015). Motivational interviewing: Experiences in primary care nurses trained in the method. *Nurse Education in Practice, 15,* 111–113.

O'Toole, A., & Welt, S. R. (1989). *Interpersonal theory in nursing practice.* New York: Springer.

Pai, H. C. (2015). The effect of a self-reflection and insight program on the nursing competence of nursing students: A longitudinal study. *Journal of Professional Nursing, 31*(5), 424–431. doi:10.1016/j.profnurs.2015.03.003.

Peplau, H. E. (1963). Process and concept of learning. In S. Burd & M. Marshall (Eds.), *Some clinical approaches to psychiatric nursing* (pp. 348–352). New York: Macmillan.

Peplau, H. E. (1964). *Basic principles of patient counseling* (2nd ed.). Philadelphia: Smith Kline and French Laboratories.

Peplau, H. E. (1969). Professional closeness: As a special kind of involvement with a patient, client, or family group. *Nursing Forum, 8*(4), 342–360.

Peplau, H. E. (1991). *Interpersonal relations in nursing.* New York: Springer.

Petrova, T., et al. (2015). Motivational interviewing skills in health care encounters (MISCHE): Development and psychometric testing of an assessment tool. *Research in Social & Administrative Pharmacy, 11*(5), 696–707.

Quality Safety and Education for Nurses (QSEN). (2012). Patient centered care. http://qsen.org/competencies/pre-licensure-ksas/#patient-centered_care.

Raths, L., Harmin, M., & Simon, S. (1978). *Values and teaching.* Columbus, OH: Charles E. Merrill.

Raymond, J. (2014). *The life coach workbook*. London: John Murray Learning.

Ruesch, J., & Bateson, G. (1987). *Communication: The social matrix of psychiatry*. New York: W.W. Norton.

Ryan, L., et al. (2014). Evaluation of printed health education materials for use by low-education families. *Journal of Nursing Scholarship*, 46(4), 218–228.

Shipley, S. (2010). Listening: A concept analysis. *Nursing Forum*, 45(2), 125–134.

Smith-Miller, C. A., et al. (2010). Leaving the comfort of the familiar: Fostering workplace cultural awareness through short-term global experiences. *Nursing Forum*, 45, 18–28.

Speros, C. (2011). Promoting health literacy: A nursing imperative. *The Nursing clinics of North America*, 46(3), 321–333.

Stuart, G. W. (2012). *Principles and practice of psychiatric nursing*. (10th ed.). St. Louis: Mosby.

Sullivan, H. S. (1953). *The interpersonal theory of psychiatry*. New York: W.W. Norton.

Tejero, L. M. S. (2011). The mediating role of the nurse-patient dyad bonding in bringing about patient satisfaction. *Journal of Advanced Nursing*, 68(5), 994–1002.

Thistlethwaite, J. (2012). Interprofessional education: A review of context, learning and the research agenda. *Medical Education*, 46, 58–70.

US Department of Health & Human Services. (2003). OCR privacy brief: Summary of the HIPAA privacy rule. http://www.hhs.gov/ocr/privacy/hipaa/understanding/summary/privacysummary.pdf.

US Department of Health and Human Services. (2010). *Healthy People 2020: Improving the health of Americans*. Washington, DC: U.S. Government Printing Office.

Walker, S. P., et al. (2011). Inequality in early childhood: Risk and protective factors for early child development. *Lancet*, 378(9799), 1325–1338. doi:10.1016/S0140-6736(11)60555-2.

Watzlawick, P., Beavin, J. H., & Jackson, D. D. (1967). *Pragmatics of human communication: A study of interactional patterns, pathologies and paradoxes*. New York: W.W. Norton.

Wright, L. M., & Leahey, M. (2013). *Nurses and families: A guide to family assessment and intervention* (6th ed.). Philadelphia: F.A. Davis.

Young, L. B., et al. (2011). Home telehealth: Patient satisfaction, program functions, and challenges for the care coordinator. *Journal of Gerontological Nursing*, 37(11), 38–46.

# 5

# Ethical Issues Related to Health Promotion

*Christine Sorrell Dinkins*

## OBJECTIVES

*After completing this chapter, the reader will be able to:*
- Discuss health promotion as a moral endeavor.
- Describe the relationship of health care ethics to health promotion.
- Analyze the relationship of various ethical theories to the nursing role in health promotion.
- Discuss the historical development and importance to nursing of the codes of ethics.
- Describe contemporary ethical issues in health promotion (e.g., issues related to genetics, genomics, culture, end-of-life decision-making).
- Analyze problems related to health promotion using an ethical decision-making framework.

## KEY TERMS

| | | |
|---|---|---|
| Advocacy | Feminist ethics | Normative theories |
| Applied ethics | Genomics | Paternalism |
| Autonomy | Genetics | Phenotype |
| Beliefs | Genetic counseling | Practical wisdom |
| Beneficence | Genotype | Preventive ethics |
| Civil liberties | Informed consent | Privacy Rule |
| Codes of ethics | Justice | Social justice |
| Confidentiality | Maleficence | Trust |
| Consequentialist | Metaethics | Utilitarian theories |
| Consent | Moral | Value theories |
| Descriptive theories | Moral agency | Veracity |
| Duty-based theories | Moral distress | Virtue ethics |
| Ethical dilemmas | Moral philosophy | |
| Ethical issues | Nonmaleficence | |

## THINK ABOUT IT

### Assisted Suicide or Emotional Support?

A nurse in a clinic is accountable for ongoing assessments of pain management. One of the long-term clients, Ana, has required increasing amounts of narcotics for her pain management over the last year. The nurse has known for more than a year that Ana's husband, Victor, has amyotrophic lateral sclerosis, or Lou Gehrig disease. Victor's disease adds a great deal of stress to both their lives, which has had a negative effect on Ana's physical health. The nurse assesses the emotional toll of Victor's illness as part of Ana's pain assessment. During one of these discussions, Ana asks the nurse how much of her narcotic medication her husband would need to take to end his life.

- What are the implications of providing someone, indirectly, with the means to commit suicide?
- What questions would you have for Ana at this point of the conversation?
- Imagine how she might respond. What would you say or do in response to her answers?
- Do you have any obligations to Victor?
- Do you think you should collaborate with Victor's physician?
- What is in Ana's best interests?
- Who or what are your resources?
- Do national nursing organizations have written guidelines about assisted suicide?
- What is the law in your state?
- What should you do?

# HEALTH PROMOTION AS A MORAL ENDEAVOR

The American Nurses Association (ANA) designated the year 2015 as "The Year of Ethics." A highlight of the year was a revision of the *Code of Ethics for Nurses with Interpretive Statements*, which was the first revision since 2001. The revised code provides a succinct statement of ethical values, obligations, and duties of nurses and describes nursing's understanding of its commitment to society. The code frames how nurses provide service to society through health-promotion interventions; this care can be seen as a moral endeavor. Nurses confront moral issues in the process of attempting to enhance the well-being of a society overall, as well as promoting and protecting health for individual members of a society. Health is considered a human good because it helps people to have a desirable quality of life and achieve life goals. At the level of the individual, health promotion involves providing services that help people achieve their potential.

To set a higher standard of health for all people, it is important to understand the contexts of people's lives. This understanding entails consideration of a variety of factors that can affect a person's health status, such as mental, physical, spiritual, environmental, cultural, social, and genetic factors. Viewing health promotion as a moral endeavor is consistent with the intent and goals of the US government's prevention agenda for the nation as presented in *Healthy People 2020* (see https://www.healthypeople.gov).

The following are the four overarching goals of *Healthy People 2020*:

- Attain high-quality, longer lives free of preventable disease, disability, injury, and premature death.
- Achieve health equity, eliminate disparities, and improve the health of all groups.
- Create social and physical environments that promote good health for all.
- Promote quality of life, healthy development, and healthy behaviors across all life stages.

The purpose of health-promotion efforts, as discussed throughout this book, is to ensure that people have access to the tools and strategies to live at the highest level of well-being possible. Health-promotion efforts address environmental obstacles to human health, such as pollution, marketing of harmful products, and economic disparities. Thus health promotion is not the province of a single discipline but requires collaboration of patients, health care providers, and institutions working together to create a nurturing environment for achieving health goals.

This chapter focuses on understanding the health professional's moral responsibilities toward individuals and society with regard to facilitating health and well-being, or the relief of suffering. Professional responsibilities are obligations incurred by disciplines that provide a service to society. For example, the *Code of Ethics for Nurses with Interpretive Statements* (ANA, 2015) states that nursing addresses the "protection, promotion, and restoration of health and well-being; the prevention of illness and injury; and the alleviation of suffering, in the care of individuals, families, groups, communities, and populations." This document, along with the ANA's "Nursing's Social Policy Statement" (ANA, 2010), describes the ethical responsibilities of US nurses (Boxes 5-1

---

## BOX 5-1  Code of Ethics for Nurses

- The nurse practices with compassion and respect for the inherent dignity, worth, and unique attributes of every person.
- The nurse's primary commitment is to the patient, whether an individual, family, group, community, or population.
- The nurse promotes, advocates, and protects the rights, health, and safety of the patient.
- The nurse has authority, accountability, and responsibility for nursing practice; makes decisions; and takes action consistent with the obligation to promote health and to provide optimal care.
- The nurse owes the same duties to self as to others, including the responsibility to promote health and safety, preserve wholeness of character and integrity, maintain competence, and continue personal and professional growth.
- The nurse, through individual and collective effort, establishes, maintains, and improves the ethical environment of the work setting and conditions of employment that are conducive to safe, quality health care.
- The nurse, in all roles and settings, advances the profession through research and scholarly inquiry, professional standards development, and the generation of both nursing and health policy.
- The nurse collaborates with other health professionals and the public to protect human rights, promote health diplomacy, and reduce health disparities.
- The profession of nursing, collectively through its professional organizations, must articulate nursing values, maintain the integrity of the profession, and integrate principles of social justice into nursing and health policy.

Sources American Nurses Association. (2015). *Code of ethics for nurses with interpretive statements*. Washington, DC: American Nurses Association; American Nurses Association. (2015). *Guide to the code of ethics for nurses: Interpretation and application*. Washington, DC: American Nurses Association.

---

and 5-2). The weblinks for this chapter include a link to the ANA's *Code of Ethics for Nurses with Interpretive Statements*. The International Council of Nurses (2012) also has a code of ethics, revised in 2012, which serves as a standard for nurses worldwide and is easily accessible via the Internet.

Ethical issues focused on health promotion are best viewed as a subset of health care ethics that, in turn, has its roots in moral philosophy and value theory. This chapter discusses factors that can affect health promotion across the life span in diverse health care settings. The development, scope, and limits of ethical theories and perspectives are explored in relation to problems in health promotion. A basic assumption in this chapter is that the anticipation and prevention of ethical problems is a critical component of ethical professional action. A variety of real and hypothetical cases are presented to illustrate how ethical issues relate to health promotion. Strategies to aid nurses in identifying, anticipating, and addressing ethical issues are provided throughout.

The terms *ethical* and *moral* are used interchangeably throughout the chapter. Even though the two concepts are sometimes characterized differently, they have the same root meanings. The term *ethics* is derived from the Greek word *ethos*, meaning customs, conduct, or character. The term *moral* is derived from the Latin word *mores* and originally referred to doing something from a custom or habit (Sproul, 2015).

BOX 5-2   **Nursing's Social Policy Statement**
*Excerpt: Knowledge Base for Nursing Practice*

The knowledge base for nursing practice includes nursing science, philosophy, and ethics.

Nurses partner with individuals, families, communities, and populations to address such issues as:

- Promotion of health and safety
- Care and self-care processes
- Physical, emotional, and spiritual comfort, discomfort, and pain
- Adaptation to physiological and pathophysiological processes
- Emotions related to experiences of birth, growth and development, health, illness, disease, and death
- Meanings ascribed to health and illness
- Decision-making and ability to make choices
- Relationships, role performance, and change processes within relationships
- Social policies and their effects on the health of individuals, families, and communities
- Health care systems and their relationships with access to and quality of health care
- The environment and the prevention of disease

Source American Nurses Association. (2010). *Nursing's social policy statement. The essence of the profession* (3rd ed.). Silver Spring, MD: American Nurses Association.

## HEALTH CARE ETHICS

### Origins of Applied Ethics in Moral Philosophy

The discipline underlying ethical practice, or applied ethics, is moral philosophy. Moral philosophy is concerned with discovering or proposing what is right or wrong, or good or bad, in human action toward other humans and other entities such as animals and the environment. Singer (1993) described the crucial questions of moral philosophy as "What ought I to do? How ought I to live?" Among the tasks of moral philosophy is that of formulating theories or frameworks to guide action. Using a moral theory to propose and implement appropriate actions in troubling situations guides the decision maker toward good actions and the avoidance of harmful actions.

The theories that emerge as a result of philosophical inquiry about good action are called value theories; they are concerned with either discovering what humans seem to value (descriptive theories) or proposing what they ought to value (normative theories) to achieve predetermined goals. Value theories are based on observations of human behavior over time and in a variety of settings. Descriptive theories do not tell us what actions we ought to take. They are not directives; they merely tell us how people act toward each other and their environments and what they seem to believe are good or moral actions. Normative theories, in contrast, are concerned with ensuring good actions.

### Types of Normative Ethical Theories

Normative ethical theories are reasoned explanations of the moral purpose of human interactions, or they are believed to be objective truths about good action (divinely given in the case of religious ethics). Actions that are in accord with the foundational principles of the theory are the type of right or good actions we should take given that we believe the principles (e.g., fairness and trust)

are valid. What is often called the golden rule is a classic example of a normative principle. The golden rule commits us to treating other people in the manner that we would wish to be treated, given similar circumstances. Normative theories permit judgments about the value of actions on the basis of the extent to which these actions are consistent with the assumptions of the theory. They are key to decision-making and relevant for health promotion but may be overlooked by policymakers.

### Consequentialist Theories

The foundational principle of John Stuart Mill's (2002/1861) theory of utilitarianism proposes that actions are good insofar as they aim at yielding the greatest amount of happiness or pleasure or causing the least amount of harm or pain to individuals and overall society. This theory is often formulated as the greatest good for the greatest number. Mill viewed pleasure as a complex concept, with qualitative as well as quantitative aspects. This perspective is consequentialist: it holds that the consequences or intended consequences of actions matter for determining moral worth. Therefore from the consequentialist perspective, any decision about intended actions or interventions must take into account all knowable potential consequences. Among the implications of this type of theory for nurses is the imperative that data gathering must be thorough and complete. Additionally, the professional is accountable for possessing the appropriate skills and knowledge to undertake actions that will promote good. The professional's decision can be evaluated as bad or good to the extent that actions are in accord with the theory: in the case of utilitarianism, "right actions" would be those that are directed toward promoting the greatest good or causing the least harm. The propositions of the theory direct what is needed for moral action or, stated another way, for doing the right thing.

### Duty-Based Theories

Other normative value theories are not as heavily weighted toward producing good consequences. For example, duty-based theories, such as the theory of Immanuel Kant (1724–1804) and those of various religions (Judaism, Christianity, Islam), depend more on adherence to duties than on good consequences. Individuals are viewed as having certain duties that cannot be circumvented, even if deliberately avoiding the duty would result in good outcomes. For religions, these rules are imparted in some way by a divine being.

For Kant, our capacity to reason is what guides moral action. Moral reasoning has been proposed as a model for health promotion (Buchanan, 2006). Kant based his theory on the idea that what separates us from other life forms is our ability to make rules for ourselves using reason. His main rule, whereby each of us can determine for ourselves a moral course of action, is the categorical imperative. It is called the categorical imperative because it applies in all situations (categorical) and is a binding command (imperative). The categorical imperative was framed in several different ways by Kant. One major formulation is as follows: "Act only according to that maxim whereby you can at the same time will that it should become a universal law" (Kant, 1993/1785).

Kant's theory is easier to understand through examples. Kant argued that making a false promise is always wrong even if on some occasions it might produce a good outcome. It is wrong because it is irrational and the promise breaker is making a moral exception for himself or herself. If everyone made a false promise when the immediate outcomes were likely to be positive, humans would lose their ability to trust promises, and this would make promises pointless and ineffective. Thus making a false promise is irrational (and therefore unethical) because one is making a promise while counting on everyone else to act differently so that promises do not cease to exist. This formulation could thus be stated alternatively as a question to ask oneself before acting: "If I do this act, am I making a moral exception for myself? Am I counting on others to act differently than I am right now?" If a person asked this question before sneaking onto a bus without paying the fare, the answer would be "yes I am making a moral exception for myself (and therefore should not do this)," because if everyone rode without paying the fare, the bus service could not run anymore!

Another formulation of Kant's categorical imperative is "Act in such a way that you treat humanity, whether in your own person or in the person of another, always at the same time as an end and never simply as a means" (Kant, 1993/1785). Kant calls us all to recognize every human being as a full human being with his or her own ends (i.e., life and goals). To treat someone merely as a means would be to use or ignore that person for one's own purposes. For example, it would be wrong to pretend to be friends with someone just so that person could help us study for a test. The various formulations of the categorical imperative will always lead to the same decision, so when we are deciding on an action, we can choose whichever formulation is easier (or more relevant) to apply in the situation.

## Character-Based Theories

Also referred to as virtue ethics, character-based approaches to ethics center on the individual agent making the decision. Aristotle (384–322 BCE) argued that being moral was a matter of habits and desires. If a person can learn to desire the right things, then he or she will do the right things. For Aristotle (1985/350 BCE), doing the right thing is all about who you are. If you are a moral person with good ethical thinking skills, you will do the right thing. So, in any given situation, I might ask myself, "What would a good person do in this situation?" or "If I do this, will I be the kind of person I would consider to be a good person?"

Aristotle says that habits help us be moral in two ways: First, they help us put our desires in order. By always acting honestly, for instance, one will begin to form a desire for honest acts, so the habit of acting honestly makes one develop a desire to be honest. Second, habits help us learn how to be moral. The more one acts courageously, for instance, the better one become at it. By forming a habit of acting courageous, one is more likely to be able to know what the courageous thing to do is in any given situation, and will be more able to make oneself do it.

The advantage of Aristotle's character ethics is that instead of hard and fast rules to follow, he offers general advice, and thus his ethics is easily applicable to all situations. The drawback comes from the same source though: without any hard and fast rules to follow, it can be hard to look to virtue ethics to determine the right thing to do. Habits can help us learn, in general, how

to be courageous, honest, temperate, kind, etc. Also necessary, though, is practical wisdom (phronesis in the original Greek). Aristotle's writings on ethics do not try to tell us what the right thing to do is in any situation. Instead, he describes the skills needed to figure out what to do in any situation. He takes this approach because he believes there is no one right way to act at all times. Any moral decision depends on the situation and the person making the decision.

## Limitations of Moral Theory

Keep in mind that moral theories arise out of a particular perspective or philosophy about the world. They are conceptualized as a result of this perspective and within a historical and political context. The philosophical approach that evaluates value theories or ethical perspectives for their congruence and usefulness in human decision-making across environments is metaethics. Philosophers interested in metaethical questions investigate where our ethical principles come from and what they mean. Are they merely social inventions? Do they involve more than expressions of our individual emotions? Metaethics allows us to critique the adequacy of ethical approaches for application across a variety of practice settings and cultural environments. Other sorts of metaethical questions posed by moral philosophers include the following: Are there such things as absolute ethical truths? If so, how do we go about discovering these? If not, what foundations should we use to guide our actions? What is a valid moral theory? Should human values be congruent across settings and cultures?

Religiously based moral theories depend on the idea that good actions are those that obey the laws of a supreme being. However, because the foundational tenets of religions do not consistently mirror each other, what constitutes a moral or morally neutral action from a Jewish perspective may well be morally prohibited from a Roman Catholic perspective. Moreover, even within a religion, the tenets of its different sects or branches may not always lead to the same conclusions about good actions. Nurses and other health care professionals need to recognize the influence of religion in persons' lives because their duty to provide safe, competent, compassionate, and ethical care extends to an accommodation of religious and cultural values and practices.

As a result of diverse religious and cultural values, there are divergent but strongly held views on what is the good for humans. Many contemporary philosophers have argued that there can be no single approach that permits the identification or resolution of all moral problems (Rachels & Rachels, 2011; Weston, 2010). Even the golden rule can be problematic from a cross-cultural perspective. For example, I might want to be treated as an autonomous being capable of making my own decisions, but a person from Thailand might be more used to family-centered decision-making. Treating my Thai friend as I would wish to be treated would be a mistake. An understanding of cultural beliefs is necessary for good action in such cases (Box 5-3: Diversity Awareness). Health care professionals wishing to engage in ethics respectful of diversity may be well served by "listening to the stories of those who are different, who may be unseen, marginalized, and excluded in our healthcare systems" (Sorrell & Dinkins, 2006). If we fail to listen to these stories, we are likely to be

## BOX 5-3 DIVERSITY AWARENESS

### Self-Reflection

The increasingly multicultural society, multiple languages spoken, and diverse set of values presents health care providers with complex assessment and planning problems. Nurses and other health professionals are charged with practicing "with compassion and respect for the inherent dignity, worth, and unique attributes of every person" (ANA, 2015, Provision 1). It is not possible to know details about every culture as well as the unique differences of each individual, family community, and group within each culture. There are strategies, however, that a health professional can use to ensure that an individual's unique values and particular needs are the focus of health-promotion interventions.

When a particular culture is part of your population base, opportunities should be pursued for learning individual differences in beliefs, values, and needs related to that culture. To facilitate your assessment, perhaps the most important undertaking is self-reflection. The following are self-reflection and other considerations for providing culturally sensitive care:

- Commitment to increasing knowledge and skill in sensitivity to cultural differences.
- Self-awareness and awareness of one's own biases, beliefs, and values. Ask yourself:
  - what values and biases you bring to the relationship
  - how your background has influenced your beliefs
  - what knowledge and experience you have to draw on
  - what values you think you share with the client (validate with the client)
  - how comfortable you are with who you are
  - what further information you need to facilitate culturally competent care
  - who or what is the best resource for further information
- Awareness of the validity of different beliefs and values.
- Attempts to understand the meaning behind client behavior.
- Increased knowledge of the beliefs and values of other cultures.
- Developing cultural skills through encounters with people from other cultures.

Source American Nurses Association. (2015). *Code of ethics for nurses with interpretive statements*. Washington, DC: American Nurses Association.

oblivious to the harm being done in health care through unwitting oppression of minorities or people from other cultures.

Additionally, **utilitarian theories** emerged out of a particular era and as a result of perceived injustices in societal arrangements in England during the turmoil of the industrial revolution. Utilitarians such as Jeremy Bentham (1748–1832) and John Stuart Mill (1806–1873) sought frameworks that would permit the rectification of unjust policy decisions and the vast economic inequities within their society. For this reason, such theories have a tendency to privilege the good of the group over the needs of individuals. In health promotion, seeking a balance between good for the group or community and good for the individual can be a particular challenge. Utilitarian theories, in particular, are in danger of favoring the group (the majority) over those who are in fewer numbers (the minority).

The most famous illustration of how our ethical decision-making might be determined by our culture and context comes from Plato (~427 to ~347 BCE). In Plato's *Republic* (1992/360 BCE), the character of Socrates describes a cave where prisoners have been shackled since birth, and thus the cave is the only reality they know. The prisoners face a cave wall on which they see shadows cast by the fire behind them, but they cannot turn their heads to see the fire and do not even know it is there. When one prisoner is freed, he journeys upward, first seeing the fire and eventually making it out into the wider world, lit by the light of the sun. Socrates says this prisoner's journey is the moral journey each of us must take. We must recognize that the morals we are taught may just be shadows of the true moral good (represented by the sun in the story).

Health practitioners today should be aware that they are likely most familiar and comfortable with the ideals and morals they have been raised with, and it is not always good to be limited by this perspective. As our society becomes increasingly complex, there are new and emergent ethical issues, such as protection of the environment, use of technology, allocation of scarce resources, and health care reform. Normative ethical theories give each of us means to think for ourselves and reflect on what we believe is right. It is not prudent to adopt one theory to guide actions in every situation related to health promotion. If a moral theory is applied unreflectively, it can lead to actions that are problematic for an individual or group. Health-promotion activities mandate not only a general understanding of the nature of the problem or potential problem but also knowledge of the values, beliefs, needs, and desires of the person or population being served. In addition, it is advisable that individuals look for an action or decision supported by more than one ethical theory—such confluence means that the action or decision will be morally right from multiple perspectives or contexts.

Specific principles derived from ethical theories have proved useful because they highlight salient aspects of complex problems and help to examine implications of different proposed courses of action. Selection of pertinent principles, however, depends both on the context of the problem and on the beliefs and values of the individual or group for which action is needed. For example, imagine a woman who seeks assistance in deciding whether to undergo genetic testing for the breast cancer gene *BRCA2* because several members of her immediate and antecedent families have received diagnoses of breast or associated cancers. She tells her nurse practitioner that she is not sure whether it would be beneficial to be tested. The nurse practitioner, in facilitating the woman's health-promotion efforts, understands that she must use clinical judgment to facilitate the woman's autonomous choice. Understanding the requirements of the principle of autonomy is important in helping the woman make her decision. It is not sufficient, however, to understand the meaning of autonomy and its limits; the nurse practitioner must also know something about the woman's life, values, beliefs, and relationships to provide her with the information and resources necessary for her decision. If the woman is screened and the results are positive for the gene, the woman not only must decide her next actions but also must consider the implications of the results (e.g., how the results affect her children or her decision to have children). Box 5-4: Genomics presents information on **genetic counseling**. Individual principles of importance to decision-making in health care settings are explored in this chapter. They, along with associated ethical considerations such as professional, feminist, and virtue ethics, underpin a framework of moral decision-making for health promotion that is presented at the end of this chapter.

## ⚠ BOX 5-4  GENOMICS
### Nurses as Genetic Educators, Researchers, and Counselors

Nurses have always been important advocates for health care literacy and education. Since the International Human Genome Sequencing Consortium completed the Human Genome Project in 2003, nurses have stepped forward to gain new competencies and assume new roles related to genetics and genomics. In assuming these roles, nurses face ethical, legal, and social implications with patients and community members. These ethical, legal, and social implications require a basic genomic health literacy, as well as an understanding of the expectations of the public. Research strongly suggests that people want to have their genetic sequencing results to better understand their health profile.

The rapidly increasing discoveries in genetic research challenge nurses to gain new competencies so as to be knowledgeable about the often difficult ethical situations related to these discoveries. **Genetics** involves the study of a single gene's function. **Genomics** represents a wider view to include all genes in a person, including interactions of the genes with themselves and also the environment (Huddleston, 2013; Lyon et al., 2011). Two other terms sound similar but have different meanings. **Genotype** refers to a set of genes in our DNA that is responsible for a particular trait. **Phenotype** is the physical expression of that trait, and is determined by interaction between the genotype and the environment. Genotype is an inherited trait; the entire genetic information about an organism is contained in a genotype. Examples of genotype are the genes responsible for eye and hair color and the sound of one's voice. Phenotype is what you see; it is the visible expression of the results of the genes combined with the environmental influence on one's appearance or behavior. Examples of phenotypes are the *visible* or *observable* characteristic of eye and hair color and the sound of one's voice.

These terms help nurses to understand how the integration of genomic and genetic factors into areas such as biobehavioral research provides new opportunities to understand problems that are difficult to define. For example, Lyon and colleagues (2011) noted that attempts to study fatigue have "been stymied by the lack of phenotypic clarity." These nurse researchers have studied genetic-genomic approaches that may increase the precision and clarity of the study of fatigue, thus enhancing understanding of mechanisms by which fatigue occurs in various health conditions as a patient symptom. Nurses are making important contributions through integration of genetic-genomic measures into biobehavioral research. This research may lead to better prediction of risk for medical problems, as well as identification of biological markers of symptom onset, progression, and resolution. More research is also needed in examining the relationship between individual genetic/genomic variations and outcomes of nursing interventions so that nurses can use genetic/genomic information to plan nursing interventions. There are potentially many nursing interventions that would be more effective if they were individually tailored to a person's genetic/genomic profile, rather than a "one size fits all" approach (Munro, 2015).

The ever-expanding discoveries in genomics challenge the nurse to be competent in genomic applications to nursing care and knowledgeable in the often difficult ethical issues that arise with these discoveries. There is a need for nurses to position themselves so as to attain advanced knowledge and skills related to their serving as specialized genetic counselors. For example, behavioral phenotypes have emerged as an area of specialist practice for nurses in the field of intellectual disability (Higgins & Duffy, 2006). Although many health care professionals have the skills to counsel individuals about genetic testing issues, especially in their fields of expertise, genetic counselors are an increasingly important resource and are aware of ethical issues to consider in genetic screening.

Genetic counselors are specially trained master's-prepared individuals. These professionals can obtain certification through the American Board of Genetic Counselors. Their professional society is the National Society of Genetic Counselors. Genetic counselors enter the field from a range of backgrounds including biology, genetics, nursing, psychology, public health, and social work.

The goals of the discipline are outlined in the society's *Code of Ethics* (National Society of Genetic Counselors, 2006). Genetic counselors provide counseling services that are nondirective to avoid coercion or persuasion. Although there is controversy about how directive or nondirective advice should be based on the ethical ideals of autonomy, counselors strive to be nondirective while at the same time tailoring information to fit the specific needs of persons. Because advances in embryo preimplantation genetic testing, as well as in utero fetal testing, permit screening of individuals for certain superior characteristics or the screening out of certain genetic diseases, the perceived need to distance the profession from this issue is understandable.

Ethical issues related to genetic counseling for screening purposes that apply both for genetic counselors and for other health care providers include the following:

- Understanding the wider context of genetic testing implications (privacy, discrimination, economics, health insurance denials, implications for family members, anxiety and apprehension, and eugenics [striving for perfection] and its associated implications for individuals and society).
- Assisting people to determine the risks and benefits of screening.
- Assisting people to prepare for their future needs.
- Assisting people with their procreative planning.
- Understanding how cultural differences impact counseling needs.
- Addressing societal issues related to genetic advances, including determining research priorities, justice issues, and discrimination of the genetically disadvantaged.

Sources Andrens, L. B., Mehlman, M. J., & Rothstein, M. A. (2002). *Genetics: Ethics, law, and policy*. St. Paul, MN, West Group/Thompson; Higgins, S., & Duffy, J. (2006). Behavioral phenotypes: An emerging specialist role for nurses. *British Journal of Nursing, 15*(21), 1176–1179; Huddleston, K., (2013). Ethics: The challenge of ethical, legal, and social implications (ELSI) in genomic nursing. *OJIN: The Online Journal of Issues in Nursing. 19*(1), 6; Lyon, D. E., McCain, N. L., Pickler, R. H., Munro, C., & Elswick, R. K. (2011). Advancing the biobehavioral research of fatigue with genetics and genomics. *Journal of Nursing Scholarship, 43*(3), 274–281; Munro, C. L. (2015). Individual genetic and genomic variation: A new opportunity for personalized nursing interventions. *Journal of Advanced Nursing, 71*(1), 35–41; National Society of Genetic Counselors. (2006). *Code of ethics*. http://nsgc.org/p/cm/ld/fid=12.

## Feminist Ethics and Caring
### Feminist Ethics

Feminist perspectives on ethics derive from the feminist movement's efforts to expose and rectify injustices to women and raise awareness of the dominance of patriarchy in many ethical approaches. The feminist movement perspectives also often include problems common to all oppressed groups. **Feminist ethics**, emerging as it has out of feminist thought and feminist philosophy, is not another ethical theory as such; rather it presents a viewpoint on moral problems in health care and other areas of life that have been historically neglected.

Feminist scholars have noted that traditional moral theories, and the principles derived from them, have been unable to adequately capture the nature and origins of health care problems. Feminist critics assert that moral decision-making must include an investigation of both hidden and overt power relationships implicit in ethical problems. Additionally, understand the contexts of situations and the interrelationships of those involved because human beings are not isolated individuals who may be viewed as totally independent of others. Thus hidden power imbalances in various relationships and situations are an important element in moral decision-making. Feminist ethics, then, contributes a perspective that is often missing from traditional ethical approaches and aims to change the way ethical problems are perceived and explored.

The characteristics of feminist ethics include (Green, 2012):

- An understanding that human beings are inseparable from their relationships with others; relationships are the core variable of care.
- A focus on care and responsibility within relationships, rather than rights, rules, and an abstract system of thought.
- A concern with the development of character and attitudes within the context of relationships.
- A concern for the rights and equality of all persons.

Thus feminist ethics allows a critique of the treatment of individuals in the contexts in which they live. This approach to ethics often focuses on imbalances of power along with oppression attributable to sex, sexual orientation, ethnicity, socioeconomics, politics, and other characteristics. For example, a feminist ethicist might point out that a punitive approach to perinatal substance abuse is not associated with improved outcomes for the fetus; in fact, the fetus may be at greater risk because the possibility of such punishment makes women fearful of accessing health services.

## The Ethics of Care

The feminist ethic of care is an important concept for health promotion because it focuses on the nature of nurse-person relationships and on the context of people's lives. This approach to care has found increasing acceptance in nursing as both a virtue of the nurse and a responsibility of practice in which treatment is offered on a common ground basis that will support people within their relationships. Carol Gilligan's (1982, 2013) research, among that of others, has been instrumental in the acceptance of the concept of care as informing ethics in nursing practice. Gilligan was a graduate student and then colleague of Lawrence Kohlberg, a developmental psychologist. The main focus of Kohlberg's (1981, 1984) body of work was the nature of moral character development, which was informed by Piaget's work on the stages of cognitive development in children. Kohlberg's stages of moral development were derived from longitudinal studies of young men. These moral reasoning studies were designed around the idea that an ability to apply conceptions of justice, rules, and principles to difficult situations denoted the highest achievable level of moral development. Gilligan challenged the reliance on only males in the study of moral reasoning and implemented studies of women's experiences, discovering that women had a moral orientation based on the caring and nurturing of others. In this framework used by women, interrelationships and contexts are critically important in understanding the complexities of a given situation (Paulsen, 2011).

The ethic of care calls for a knowledgeable and skillful health professional to assume responsibility for unique needs of an individual in all of his or her complexities. Benner and colleagues (2009) define care as "the alleviation of vulnerability; the promotion of growth and health; the facilitation of comfort, dignity or a good and peaceful death," noting that care is "the dominant ethic found in [nurses'] stories of everyday practice."

### Limits of the Ethic of Care

One problem with using care as an ethic of health-promotion practice has to do with the concern of moral predictability or certainty (Nelson, 1992), much like with Aristotle's virtue ethics. If the emphasis in ethics of care is on relationships and there are no criteria for right and wrong actions, how can one be assured of the morally correct action in a given situation? An answer to this question could be that a morally correct action emerges as a result of judgment based on prior knowledge, experience, and an engaged relationship with the person. Thus the process of the interaction, coupled with the character, knowledge, experience, and intent of the moral agent, is the crucial factor that achieves the moral good for an individual. A person's control of his or her own care is important. In a nursing setting the action is right if the nurse incorporates this person control into meeting the complex needs of the person being cared for.

When the solution to one person's problems affects others, however, the rightness of the action depends on more than the one-on-one caring relationship. The problem remains one of choosing between this person's needs and the needs of others who might be affected by the actions chosen. This problem is resistant to resolution via an ethic of care alone. The problem analysis framework described later combines the ethic of care with other considerations. Both an ethic of care and the principles derived from traditional moral theory may be needed for health promotion.

The purpose of ethical inquiry in health promotion is to gain clarity on actual or potential moral issues arising in the context of health-promotion endeavors and to understand what is expected of the health-promotion agent viewed as a moral agent. Ethical inquiry will not permit the resolution of all problems, because the environments in which health-promotion efforts are conceptualized are incredibly complex. It is impossible to foresee all possible consequences of action, but ethical reasoning can facilitate appropriate and in-depth data gathering, permit the uncovering of hidden agendas and interests, and focus on the most salient aspects of a particular problem, thus enhancing professional judgment.

## PROFESSIONAL RESPONSIBILITY

Professional judgment and ensuing actions are integral to the goal of providing a good for the population of concern. Thus health promotion is a moral endeavor requiring morally sensitive and knowledgeable agents. But what are the scopes and limits of a nurse's obligations to anticipate, identify, and address morally problematic issues related to the promotion and protection of health for individuals, groups, and society? How do nurses balance their duties to individuals with a duty to the society? How are individuals' freedoms (autonomy) balanced with the collective responsibilities owed to society and future generations?

## Accountability to Individuals and Society

### Professions

Although this section focuses on the nursing discipline's mandate to promote health, the discussion can also be applied to the responsibilities of other health professionals who assume health-promotion responsibilities. Nursing is a profession insofar as it provides a service to society and is self-governing, and its members are accountable for their actions (Grace, 2001). A significant consequence of professional status is that members can be held accountable for their practice formally by professional licensure boards. More importantly, they are morally accountable for practicing according to their discipline's implicit or explicit code of ethics. One important characteristic of professions, especially those that provide crucial services to society, is that they have codes of ethics that provide essential elements of their promises of service to society. Codes of ethics provide a normative framework for professional actions. A professional implicitly accepts these codes on acquiring membership in the discipline. Thus each professional should establish a personal perspective on ethical practice within the broad framework of professional codes (Corey et al., 2014).

### Trust

Service professions such as nursing, medicine, and teaching are in part defined by their relationships to those in need of services. This relationship is one of **trust**. The professional has the knowledge and skills to meet an individual's needs or the needs of a group. The potential recipients of services lack the knowledge or ability to anticipate or meet their own needs but trust that the professional will keep their best interests as the primary goal and will strive to meet their needs. For example, in the current health care environment in the United States, people may have trouble accessing a specialist provider because of their particular insurance coverage or the inability to afford health care insurance or to pay on their own.

Nurses are responsible not only for promoting health and healing but also for recognizing and addressing barriers to health-promotion activities. "Nursing's Social Policy Statement" (ANA, 2010) provides a detailed account of the nursing discipline's responsibilities, which describes the social contract between society and the nursing profession and emphasizes the nurse's responsibility to advocate changes when health care services are threatened.

### Codes of Ethics

Codes of ethics are examples of normative ethics in that they prescribe how members of a profession ought to act, given the goals and purposes of the profession related to individuals and society. The provisions of codes of ethics for nurses provide direction and expectations of ethical behavior. They represent the profession's promises to society. Although the public is not directly involved in the formulation of such codes and, indeed, is for the most part not even aware of their existence, the

profession is responsive to the evolving needs of a given society. It can be said that codes of ethics are the tentative end results of a discipline's political process in that they are not static but result from debate and discussion over time among the profession's scholars, leaders, and members.

The current *Code of Ethics for Nurses with Interpretive Statements* presents a central foundation to guide nurses in their decisions and conduct (Epstein & Turnerm, 2015). The code establishes an ethical standard that is nonnegotiable; that is, the goals and intent of the code may not be ignored, diluted, or downplayed by individuals or institutions employing nurses in the United States (ANA, 1994). The 2015 code "addresses individual as well as collective nursing intentions and actions; it requires each nurse to demonstrate ethical competence in professional life" (ANA, 2015).

Codes of ethics tend to offer guidelines not only about responsibilities for ensuring good care but also about responsibilities for recognizing and addressing barriers to service. The ANA's *Code of Ethics for Nurses with Interpretive Statements* proposes that "the nurse promotes, advocates for, and protects the rights, health, and safety of the patient" (ANA, 2015, Provision 3). These actions would require a nurse to anticipate future health needs and political activity when necessary to ensure health promotion.

## Advocacy

**Advocacy**, as an expectation of nurses, is strongly reinforced both in the *Code of Ethics for Nurses with Interpretive Statements* and in innumerable scholarly articles. However, advocacy is a controversial concept. The meaning of the term *advocacy* is derived from its use in law. In legal jurisprudence, advocacy is aggressive action taken on behalf of an individual, or perhaps a group viewed as an individual entity, to protect or secure that individual's or group's rights. The individual lawyer does not have an opposing obligation to attend to social justice issues. This attention to broader questions of justice is the responsibility of other areas of the justice system.

Nurses and other health care professionals have a responsibility to speak up on behalf of people whose rights have been compromised or endangered. This is part of the nurse's role because people may not recognize either what is needed to meet their needs or when the care they are receiving is substandard. However, that is not the end of their responsibilities. They must also consider that specific actions they undertake in the name of advocacy may pose problems for other people who are relying on them for health care services.

For example, Juanita Rimmer, a nurse case manager, is assisting Jim Bailey to apply for services in a rehabilitation facility because he has residual hemiparesis secondary to a cerebrovascular accident. There is a waiting list at the facility, but Juanita believes it is a priority for Jim to be treated there because he lives with his frail, elderly mother, who will not be able to assist him with his activities of daily living. Because Juanita represents other people who will also benefit from rehabilitation, her decision to be an advocate for Jim must be weighed against the needs of these other people. A moral responsibility associated with advocacy in health care settings is that the effect of actions on others is considered. When one is advocating extra attention or specialized care for a given person, an injustice may be rendered simultaneously to other people in the nurse's care. Thus professional advocacy requires a balancing of the health needs of the individual with the health needs of the population (Grace, 2001).

Advocacy is an ideal of health care professions that requires attention to vulnerable individuals and groups and to broader societal concerns. Moral agency on the part of the nurse requires action and motivation directed to some moral end that is enacted through relationships. Being aware of one's self in relation to others helps to establish the moral choice required to be an advocate for them. Understanding the interdependent nature of individual and social needs facilitates preventive and health-promotion actions on the part of nurses both locally and globally.

In the last decade there has been a shift in global consciousness in both ethics and nursing, in which nursing views ethics in a much broader sense than just direct care provided to individuals (Tschudin, 2010). It may encompass such issues as unequal care in communities composed of a large minority population or for undocumented patients. Advocacy may include political activity to address populations of concern. Preemptive and sociopolitical advocacy identifies and challenges the source of the ongoing problems. Nurses have moral obligations related to sociopolitical advocacy on behalf of their populations of concern. Juanita Rimmer's obligations include recognizing the problems caused by a chronic shortage of rehabilitation services. Her concerns include discovering the source of this problem and joining with others in an attempt to address it at this level. Strategies for solving seemingly intractable problems of health care include collaboration with specialty nursing, medical, or client advocacy groups, and communication of the issues in both professional and popular media.

Advocacy for health promotion is a concept with broad implications. It includes activities that are directed toward remedying socially based inequities or inadequacies in the health care delivery system. Advocacy can be viewed as an ethic of practice that includes all activities directed toward the person's good. Advocacy carries risks, in that addressing or facilitating the good for individuals or groups may pit nurses against their peers or against potential adversaries who do not share the same professional goals.

The nurse's role of advocacy requires that professional knowledge and judgment be applied to a variety of situations, from the relatively simple to the complex. The 2010 Institute of Medicine report "The Future of Nursing: Leading Change, Advancing Health" emphasized the need for advocacy in nurses through practicing to the fullest extent of their education and training and as full partners with physicians and other health care professionals in redesigning health in the United States (Institute of Medicine, 2010). This process requires several steps. First, potential or real problems need to be identified and analyzed, often in collaboration with others. Second, appropriate actions need to be formulated and their likely consequences considered. Third, obstacles to action should be recognized and addressed. Finally, actions are performed and evaluated. These basic steps

are evident whether the object of health care or health promotion is an individual, a group, or society.

## Problem-Solving: Issues, Dilemmas, Risks, and Moral Distress

The nature of health care environments makes it inevitable that difficult decisions will have to be made. However, many of the ethical problems encountered in health-promotion settings are issues rather than dilemmas. Daniel Chambliss (1996), a sociologist who studied nurses in acute care institutional settings, asserts that organizations such as hospitals often give rise to "practical problems, not individual dilemmas." These practical problems are nonetheless moral problems because they interfere with the goals of promoting health, well-being, or the relief of suffering. In both institutional and noninstitutional health care settings, obstacles to good care may be caused by health care system arrangements, interprofessional conflicts, and/or lack of resources. Dilemmas are ethical issues of a special sort. Ethical dilemmas are those situations in which a choice must be made between two undesirable options. Weston (2010) claims that true dilemmas are actually quite rare and that often additional, better options can be found by one changing the way the situation is examined.

The goals of health promotion require that both issues and dilemmas be recognized and addressed. Neglected issues can become dilemmas. Because nurses are at the front line of providing health care, they are often the first to observe an issue with quality of care or safety. Sometimes this concern may lead the nurse to assume the whistle-blower role—bringing the concern into the open in the hope of effecting change. Various studies have identified whistle-blowing as key in highlighting a need for health reform (Jackson et al., 2014). There is considerable evidence, however, that the whistle-blower may experience significant negative and harmful consequences, such as being victimized or ostracized by colleagues and administrators or losing employment (Jackson et al., 2014).

When a nurse is in danger of losing his or her position as a result of advocating better conditions, a balancing of foreseeable risks and benefits to the individual or group is required. The process of decision-making in this situation can lead to moral distress. Moral distress occurs when a nurse knows the ethically correct action to take but feels powerless to take that action (Epstein & Delgado, 2010). Nurses who are faced with ethical issues that seem to be irresolvable may experience guilt, frustration, and a sense of powerlessness, sometimes because they do not believe that they can adhere to their personal values. Moral distress can occur when the nurse's values and perceived obligations conflict with the needs and prevailing views of the work environment. The framework for making ethical decisions that is discussed later in this chapter includes considerations related to personal security along with preserving integrity.

## Preventive Ethics

Just as preventive health care activities aim to forestall health problems, the practice of preventive ethics aims to forestall ethical problems before they develop. Preventive ethics is an important requirement of health-promotion endeavors that includes individual action by the nurse, as well as social and political activism with other nurses or professional nursing organizations. Preventive ethics requires the health promoter to envision potential problems and institute actions that halt their development. For example, it is possible to extend a dying person's life for a very long time with use of available technology and medications. Although a competent person has the right to refuse treatment and this right is legally recognized as a result of the Patient Self-Determination Act (PSDA) of 1991, many people become incapacitated before they are able to make their wishes known. All states recognize and honor advance directives, but the legally recognized form differs from state to state (Box 5-5). It is important to think about the nurse's role in supporting individuals and their families in end-of-life decision-making. Much more work needs to be done engaging people in discussion and helping them plan for such eventualities while they are still well. Preventive ethics in this situation entails initiating communication with persons and families before a problem arises. This communication is often missing both in institutional and in primary care settings.

Preventive ethics using a feminist ethics perspective would encourage the addressing of institutional practices to provide more humanistic care and underlying social issues that lead people to overeat, smoke, or be inclined toward violence. For example, preventive ethics would require the investigation of why as a society we have trouble discussing death and dying, and why we find it so hard to have a peaceful or good death. Weston (2010) notes that much of the energy used on the polarized abortion debate could be more profitably put to use in determining why people who do not want to be pregnant nevertheless become pregnant. Weston suggests that it would be useful to reframe the question to ask "why pregnancy, or pregnancy at the wrong time, is so unacceptably burdensome for many women." We need to ask questions about lack of support, lack of education, poor or difficult-to-use birth control methods, resistance from spouses and lovers, lack of child care, and so on. One strategy for identifying potential ethical problems before they occur or worsen is to examine problematic cases for their antecedents. We should ask fundamental questions about societal arrangements and influences on health trends.

On a local level, nurses and other health promoters need to use clinical judgment in anticipating and forecasting problems before they arise. For example, unrecognized health illiteracy may affect an individual's understanding of his or her rights and entitlements. When a nurse observes that a person and that person's family do not understand either the information that has been given to them or the implications of following a given course of action, the nurse engages in preventive ethics by supplying that information and ensuring that the information is understood. The nurse acts to prevent negative consequences that can arise as a result of poorly understood information. Other examples of opportunities to use preventive ethics include focusing on smoking or childhood obesity. Many problems in health care occur as a result of poor communication or because information has been provided too late for reasoned decision-making (Box 5-6: Quality and Safety Scenario).

## ETHICAL PRINCIPLES IN HEALTH PROMOTION

Although the tenets of nursing's codes of ethics and standards of practice provide some guidance about the nature of practice and the manner in which services will be provided, they often leave some ambiguity about the best course of action in morally troubling situations. The use of principles derived from a variety of ethical theories, along with feminist insights or an ethic of care, helps to provide further guidance in decision-making in morally problematic health situations. Beauchamp and colleagues (2007) noted that ethical principles provide an important starting point for moral judgment and policy evaluation, but that principles alone are not enough. In other words, principles such as autonomy, beneficence, and justice often serve as helpful starting points in teasing out the tangled elements of complex issues, but taken alone they are usually insufficient for moral problem-solving in health care environments. One must decide which principles are important to consider in a given case or situation, and this requires an exploration of the case as discussed in the decision-making framework provided later in the chapter.

Additionally, tenets of the *Code of Ethics for Nurses with Interpretive Statements* and other ANA position statements provide guidance regarding what a nurse's moral responsibilities are in a particular type of situation. Certain tenets address the responsibilities of the nurse in improving the larger health care environment. These obligations include collaborating with others to "protect human rights, promote health diplomacy, and reduce health disparities" (ANA, 2015).

### Autonomy as Civil Liberty

In health-promotion settings and endeavors the concept of **autonomy** can be understood from two different perspectives. From the vantage point of public health, the extent of individual autonomy, or freedom of action, may be limited by the duty of protecting the health and safety of the society. From this perspective there is an age-old struggle between civil rights and public safety. Moral questions ask to what degree society is justified in regulating the health and safety of society at large. There is an inevitable tension associated with curtailing **civil liberties** in the name of safety or health. This tension arises from perceptions that, in most Western contexts, freedom of action is a prerequisite of human flourishing.

Currently there are many indirect threats to the health and safety of our society including, but by no means limited to, bioterrorism and the spread of HIV/AIDS and drug-resistant tuberculosis. Actions to resolve any of these threats have the potential to impinge on civil liberties; such actions might include, for instance, surveilling citizens or requiring disclosure of disease status. Advances in genetic knowledge present the possibility of discrimination from a variety of sources. It will be difficult to maintain individual privacy, and discrimination based on class or gene profile will be made easier.

The current managed care environment, although having a stronger focus on inculcating healthy behaviors, can impinge on civil liberties. The behavior-change approach has been criticized as too paternalistic, without sufficient regard for the individual's or the group's own perceptions of what is important;

## BOX 5-5    Preventive Ethics: Patient Self-Determination Act and Advance Directives

Advance care planning is a process in which patients, their families, and their health care providers discuss the patient's goals, values, and beliefs and document how these should be reflected in future health care choices. It often cannot be predicted whether and when individuals will lose the ability to make their wishes for treatment and care known. Advance care planning is a health-promotion endeavor that can enhance an individual's quality of life, especially while having chronic illness.

In the last 2 to 3 decades, great technological and therapeutic advances have been made, with the resulting ability to save the lives of people experiencing catastrophic illnesses and trauma. One effect of these advances, unfortunately, is that sometimes we are successful only in prolonging the dying process. Although it is now recognized that people have a right to refuse treatment to prolong life, critically ill people may lose their ability to articulate their wishes for treatment. Advance directives are a way for people to help ensure that when they become incapacitated, the care and treatment they receive matches their predetermined wishes. At their best, advance directives have the potential to ease the strain felt by loved ones as they strive to make the "right" treatment choices for a friend or relative. Advance directives also guide health professionals in their decision-making regarding the person in question.

### Types of Advance Directives

There are various forms of advance directives but the types typically recognized by state law in the United States are the living will and the durable power of attorney for health care. Living wills document patient preferences for life-sustaining treatments and resuscitation, whereas a durable power of attorney documents one's choice of a surrogate decision maker. A major limitation of the living will is that it may not be applicable to every decisional dilemma the patient will actually face. Therefore it is important to also designate a surrogate decision maker who can provide guidance to health care professionals in cases where patients are incapacitated and the living will does not apply.

The Patient Self-Determination Act (PSDA) of 1991, which was formulated in response to 2 decades of ambiguity and litigation involving right-to-die cases, represented an attempt to ensure that people's rights were honored. The PSDA required changes in public policy, public and professional education, institutional policy, and social awareness. The PSDA was intended to improve communication related to end-of-life care issues and preferences among individuals, health care providers, and proxy decision makers. It requires institutions that receive Medicare and Medicaid funds to:

- give written information on admission to all (not just the Medicare and Medicaid) persons about their rights under the law to make their own treatment decisions;
- inform people of their rights to complete state-allowed advance directives and provide written policies about those rights;
- document when a person has an advance directive;
- not discriminate or make care conditional on the presence or absence of an advance directive;
- provide staff education about advance directives and personal rights.

Although the PSDA has great potential, it serves its purpose only to the extent that it is taken seriously as a responsibility of a given institution. Institutions may fail to ensure that a qualified person is available to impart the information or to request personal preferences. It is important for those involved in health promotion to understand and address why people may be reluctant to make an advance directive and why institutions are not diligent in providing information and education. Recent studies suggest that the percentage of older Americans who complete advance directives before their death has increased dramatically from 20% to approximately 70% over slightly more than the past decade but it is important to explore why, even in the presence of the PSDA, some people do not have advance directives.

### Impediments to the Use of Advance Directives

- Discussions with health care providers about the implications of desired choices have been inadequate.
- People do not want to talk about future incapacity or death. They may have cultural prohibitions about discussing the possibility of serious illness or death.
- Past encounters with the health care system have led to distrust.
- People cannot predict accurately their future preferences and they know too little about what constitutes life support.
- People may change their minds about what they will accept.
- The health care proxy may turn out to be a poor choice or may cause conflicts among other family members or loved ones. The person or family may ask for something that is morally unacceptable.
- Treatments may be specified to which the provider has conscientious objections.
- Documentation may be lost, misplaced, or not accessible in an emergency.
- Written instructions are too vague and open to divergent interpretation to be useful guides.
- Even the most diligent proxy cannot always know what the person would have wanted in the absence of a detailed treatment directive.
- The proxy may make a treatment choice contrary to the person's directive.
- The proxy may make a decision with which the institution or physician disagrees.

### Positive Outcomes of Use of Advance Directives

In spite of impediments, research has shown that advanced care planning has resulted in the following positive outcomes:

- Higher rates of completion of advance directives.
- Increased likelihood that clinicians and families understand and comply with a patient's wishes.
- A reduction in hospitalization and intrusive treatments at the end of life.
- Increased utilization of hospice services.
- Increased likelihood that patients will die in their preferred place.

Sources Detering, K., & Silveira, M. J. (2015). Advance care planning and advance directives. *UpToDate.* http://www.uptodate.com/contents/advance-care-planning-and-advance-directives; The Holdings Group. (2012). *The failure of the living will.* http://www.theholdinggroup.org/the-failure-of-the-living-will-2/.

this may increase the risk of failed interventions. Prioritizing behavior change in health-promotion endeavors over the need to address underlying social concerns, such as poverty and other forms of disadvantage, may obscure a focus on the social determinants of health. Rather than focusing on behavior change, a focus on empowerment may help a person gain control over

social and economic factors that contribute to health problems (Tengland, 2016).

### Autonomy as Self-Determination

A second, related, sense of autonomy has to do with individual choice. Autonomy is the moral principle that underlies the concept

## BOX 5-6   QUALITY AND SAFETY SCENARIO

### Patient-Centered Care

Recognize the patient or designee as the source of control and full partner in providing compassionate and coordinated care based on respect for the patient's preferences, values, and needs (http://qsen.org).

#### How Is Health Literacy Related to Ensuring Autonomy in Decision-Making for Individuals?

Autonomy is an important ethical principle for health-promotion activities. To ensure autonomy in individual decision-making, it is important to assess the individual's health literacy skills. These skills relate to a person's ability to obtain, process, and act on basic health information. Think how difficult it would be for a person with low literacy skills to navigate today's complex health care system. Adequate health literacy is essential for accessing necessary health care services and for fostering effective decision-making.

In the process of implementing health-promotion activities, the nurse should first determine whether the person has adequate health literacy skills. This can be assessed with tools such as the Rapid Estimate of Adult Literacy in Medicine-Short Form (REALM-SF) or the Test of Functional Health Literacy in Adults (TOFHLA). It is important however, not to base an approach to health promotion solely on the results of one of these tools, which may not reveal the extent to which health recommendations may be misunderstood. The nurse should take the time to establish a rapport with the individual that includes fostering a sense of trust and openness for the person to ask important questions.

Unrecognized health literacy may interfere with individuals' rights to autonomy in decision-making because they may make a decision based on inaccurate information or may automatically accept the decision of the health care provider without deciding for themselves whether or not the decision is appropriate for their individual situation. Thus it is an ethical obligation of the nurse to make sure that effective communication is implemented. A public health approach founded on health promotion principles can provide a useful scaffold for assessing the health literacy of persons in the community. This can help to ensure that the person is in control and a full partner in health-promotion decisions that respect his or her preferences, values, and needs.

Source Guzys, D., Kenny, A., Dickson-Swift, V., & Threlkeld, G. (2015). A critical review of population health literacy assessment. *BMC Public Health, 15*, 215.

---

of informed consent to treatment, interventions, and health-promotion efforts. In Western societies it is probably the most powerful moral principle underlying the treatment of individuals. This principle asserts that people have the ability to reason, and a consequence of the ability to reason is the capacity to make choices. These choices concern both one's own behavior and how one should act toward others. Although the idea that our ability to reason constitutes the essence of being human originated with Aristotle, Kant (1993/1785) developed this idea in meticulous detail in his work *Grounding for the Metaphysics of Morals*. According to Kant, people are capable of conscious desires and goals and are free agents capable of making decisions and setting goals as guided by their own reason. This principle is a salient consideration in health care settings: it underpins the health provider and promoter-person relationship and the issue of informed consent. However, there is limited agreement about the scope, limits, and strength of this principle (Beauchamp &

Childress, 2008). When describing autonomy in the context of health or treatment choices, we should delineate what we mean by autonomy in the context of the problem under discussion. Feminist criticisms of an emphasis on autonomy highlight the problem that our choices necessarily affect others because we are contextual beings inseparable from our relationships with one another.

Respect for human autonomy guides us to permit individuals to make and learn from their own mistakes. Generally, respecting autonomy requires that we permit individuals to make their own decisions, even when these decisions seem to others to be ill-informed. There are exceptions to this rule. Exceptions include those situations in which there is a high risk of serious injury or death and when it cannot be determined whether the person's judgment is impaired. Thus we make exceptions to the rule of autonomy when we suspect that an individual is not able to reason adequately. A person's reasoning ability may be impaired by psychological or physical conditions, or it may be impaired as a result of incorrect or incomplete information.

In health-promotion activities, respect for autonomy requires that individuals be given the information they need to make choices. Choices can be considered autonomous only if certain criteria are met. The criteria that determine whether or not a person is actually capable of autonomous (voluntary) choice include cognitive maturity, possession of appropriate information to permit decision-making, intact mental capacities (the ability to reason logically), the absence of internal or external coercive influences, and the ability to appreciate the risks and benefits of alternative choices. Assessing all such criteria is quite a tall order. And in one sense it may be that nobody acts totally autonomously at any given time because of the influences of entrenched beliefs and values that are derived, for the most part, from our cultural and environmental backgrounds. We are never entirely escaped from Plato's cave. Some of these influences are under conscious control in the sense that we can recognize what values we hold and even revise them if they are dissonant with other values. However, some of these influences are not readily recognizable: they lie beneath the surface of consciousness and are hard to access even if we are willing to try. We all have blind spots; autonomy viewed as informed, uncoerced, and reasoned action is therefore an ideal. Many of us fall short of the ideal.

### Informed Consent

Informed consent to research, treatments, or health-promotion endeavors is a process of ensuring that a person has all of the appropriate information necessary to reach a decision about participation that facilitates autonomous action. Beauchamp and Childress (2008) note that informed consent occurs when a person with substantial understanding, and without substantial control by others, intentionally authorizes a professional to intervene on his or her behalf. The key phrase is "with substantial understanding." It is important to understand that even after a consent form has been signed, a person has the right to rescind consent in light of additional information and/or changed consequences.

The components of the consent process include determining the person's competency to consent. There must be no physical or mental impairments that hinder the person in question from understanding and processing information. For example, a person with pneumonia who is febrile and confused is probably not capable of making an informed decision until the fever has been reduced and the confusion has cleared. To be substantially informed, a person must be made aware of important details of the proposed intervention, including its nature, purpose, probability of success, and important risks, and must also understand what alternatives (if any) are available. Because this information must be tailored to meet the specific needs of an individual and such a task requires knowledge of the person, an ethic of care is important to understanding a person's unique needs. We can check understanding to a certain extent by asking the individual to articulate how the proposed intervention will facilitate his or her own values and goals. There must be no subtle or overt coercion by professionals or others. Finally, appropriate supports must be available to complete the proposed intervention.

Obtaining consent for any interventions, or for involvement in research, is best viewed as a process that entails ongoing assessment of the person's status and evaluation of needs for further information or support. People may not understand information well when they are in stressful situations or when the information is complex. Thus we should assess people for and validate understanding on an ongoing basis.

Ensure that all individuals, regardless of age, make informed choices. Although the life span increases in society, nurses must be aware of strategies for ensuring that older adults, who may be less able to advocate their own health needs, participate in the making of informed decisions. More research is needed on ethical problems that confront nurses in caring for older adults in the community.

Adolescence is a period of transition between the dependence and vulnerability of childhood and the autonomy of adulthood. Adolescents are generally considered capable of making decisions related to health-promotion activities, and health professionals have a duty to respect those decisions, provided that doing so does not produce harm to adolescents or others (Larcher, 2012). Most health-promotion activities do not require formal informed consent. However, it is important to integrate the underlying principles and supporting research related to informed consent to be sure that the selected health-promotion strategies fit individuals' beliefs and values. It is also important to recognize that complex social factors may contribute to adolescents' inability to make well-thought-out decisions (Box 5-7: Evidence-Based Practice).

## Exceptions to Autonomous Decision-Making

In some cases, proxy decision-making on behalf of the individual is required (Box 5-8). Proxy decision-making must take into account what is known about the person and must follow a path of action that is most likely to respect that individual's goals and values. Researchers have found that surrogate family members who need to serve as proxies in making decisions for loved ones, often at the end of life, find the decision-making overwhelming and extremely stressful (Sorrell, 2014). Most surrogate decision makers have had little preparation for making these choices and worry that they are not making the right decision. Nurses should

### BOX 5-7    EVIDENCE-BASED PRACTICE

#### Influences on Sexual Decision-Making of Late Adolescents

Violence has been identified by the World Health Organization as a major risk to the health and well-being of all young women. Sexual activity without clear consent is one aspect of violence against adolescents, who are still developing their values and beliefs about sexual activity and sexual norms. In a qualitative research study, Fantasia (2011) used a narrative inquiry approach to explore what influenced adolescents' decision-making related to sexual activity. The research question was: What are late adolescents' perceptions of factors that influenced their sexual decision-making? Ten female adolescents aged 18 years or older were interviewed. They were asked to respond to the question "Please tell me, in your own words, the story of your decisions to have sex." Each participant constructed her own story without influence from the researcher.

The findings showed that in the most of the sexual encounters of these adolescents, sexual consent was implied, with no consent clearly stated. The participants discussed how sexual activity eventually occurred, even when they did not want it, because of partners who used "pressure to always say yes." Inability to communicate readily with partners and the influence of alcohol were identified as contributing factors to the lack of clear consent. None of the participants expressed emotion or anger over what had occurred, and they did not label it as rape. There appeared to be an acceptance of this type of nonconsensual sexual activity.

The findings from the study provide evidence that adolescent decisions involving consent for sexual activity are complex and are influenced by a myriad of social factors. All individuals have a right to clearly refuse or consent to sexual activity; this is imperative for the promotion of physical, emotional, and sexual health and safety. Nurses and other health care professionals who work with adolescents need to carefully assess sexual behaviors and recognize that these young women are at risk of nonconsensual sexual activity. Sexual violence education should include information on negotiation and communication skills that will help adolescents mediate complicated interpersonal situations. Appropriate educational programs can help to empower young women through opportunities for increased knowledge and self-confidence.

Source Fantasia, H. C. (2011). Really not even a decision any more: Late adolescent narratives of implied sexual consent. *Journal of Forensic Nursing, 7*(3), 120–129.

support these surrogate decision makers as they struggle with making a decision. Iverson and colleagues (2014) described what helps and hampers surrogate decision-making (Box 5-9: Innovative Practice).

Certain populations are considered less than fully autonomous for a variety of reasons. People with Alzheimer disease or other physical or psychological disruptions or deficits that prevent adequate comprehension may require proxy decision makers. It is important not to assume, however, that all persons with Alzheimer disease are incapable of providing informed consent, because many persons in the early stages of the disease are capable of making decisions related to their care (Sorrell & Cangelosi, 2009). Incarcerated people are restricted in their choices and may be subject to subtle or not-so-subtle coercion. Children are considered less than fully autonomous because they are not developmentally mature. Additionally, in people with certain mental illnesses, such as psychoses or bipolar disorders, the capacity for decision-making may fluctuate. The President's Commission for the Study of Ethical Problems in Medicine and Biomedical and Behavioral Research (1982) was formed to study

## BOX 5-8  Proxy Decision-Making

Autonomy based: person's previously articulated desires
- Written
  - Living will, advance directive
  - Document details to various degrees what the person will or will not accept
- Substituted judgment
  - Individual appoints a proxy who is expected to honor previously expressed preferences
  - Informal (nonappointed significant other)

Best interests
- Surrogate chooses the actions that will give the highest overall benefit—may or may not be based on a person's previously expressed desires; a quality of life determination based when possible on knowledge about the person (Beauchamp & Childress, 2008)
- Best interests may trump the proxy's choice; doubt about the proxy's motives possible

Reasonable person standard
- Based on the answer to "What would a reasonable person want?"

Beauchamp, T. L., & Childress, J. F. (2008). *Principles of biomedical ethics* (6th ed.). New York: Oxford University Press.

## BOX 5-9  INNOVATIVE PRACTICE

### Surrogate Decision-Making

Most end-of-life health care decisions are made by surrogate decision makers who are under a great deal of stress over their seriously ill family member. Both surrogates and clinicians have various degrees of preparation, knowledge, abilities, or comfort in working effectively with another in making very difficult decisions for someone else.

Iverson and colleagues (2014) explored surrogate decision makers' challenges in making decisions related to the care of patients in critical care. They interviewed 34 designated surrogates of critically ill patients receiving care in two tertiary care institutions. Surrogates were asked to describe and reflect on their experiences of making health care decisions for others. They identified factors that added to the difficulty in decision-making:
- Stress associated with assuming a decision-making role for which they felt unprepared
- Uncertainty of patient outcomes
- Difficulty in communicating with multiple health care providers who would provide different information
- Insufficient knowledge of patients' wishes
- Conflict within the family
- Fatigue resulting from near constant vigilance in the intensive care unit

Social networks that provided access to family and/or friends were helpful in the decision-making process, as they provided surrogate decision makers with emotional and informational support. Nurses were the preferred resource for day-to-day communication and information gathering except when major decisions needed to be made. Most participants perceived that nurses offered compassionate communication and were able to disentangle information that was difficult to understand.

The findings of the study suggest areas where clinicians can intervene to facilitate the processes of surrogate decision-making. Stress can be minimized by improving communication between surrogate decision makers and health care providers. Nurses are uniquely poised to intervene to improve communication and reduce surrogates' decision-making anxiety.

Source Iverson, E., Celious, A., Kennedy, C. R., Shehane, E., Eastman, A., Warren, V., et al. (2014). Factors affecting stress experienced by surrogate decision makers for critically ill patients: Implications for nursing practice. *Intensive and Critical Care Nursing, 30*(2), 77–85.

health care decision-making and noted that the minimal capacities needed for competent decision-making are "(1) Possession of a set of values and goals; (2) the ability to communicate and to understand information, and (3) the ability to reason and deliberate about one's choice." These criteria are generally accepted as a basic minimum (Beauchamp & Childress, 2008). It can be seen from these criteria that some children would be able to understand the implications of a given course of treatment, and adults with cognitive impairments may be deemed competent to make certain decisions. Competency to make autonomous choices is not an all-or-nothing capacity. Competency determinations are, as a rule, made for a given decision or task. Thus a person may vacillate between competency and noncompetency, depending on either the task at hand (degree of difficulty) or the physical or psychological status during the period when a decision must be made.

When advocating decision-making for a cognitively impaired person, consider the risks and benefits of allowing the individual to make his or her own decision. The benefits in terms of self-esteem may well outweigh the risks of many choices. However, if the risk of injury is high and it is obvious that the person is not able to reason effectively, autonomous decision-making may not be feasible. In this case, nurses can collaborate with the individual, family members, and other health professionals to arrive at a decision that is best for the individual.

When children are involved, it is often the parent or guardian to whom we turn for permission to treat the child. Nevertheless, in pediatric settings it is incumbent on people involved in health-promotion endeavors or in research with minors to gain assent from the child in addition to consent from the parent or guardian (Driessnack & Gallo, 2011; Lambert & Glacken, 2011). The example of 5-year-old Julianna Snow illustrates how difficult these decisions can be. Julianna had an incurable neurodegenerative illness and decided that she would rather die at home instead of returning to the hospital for treatment that would likely lead to death or being sedated on a respirator with little quality of life. Julianna's parents honored this decision and Julianna died. Ethical questions were raised about whether a child of this age could/should be allowed to make an irreversible decision without the maturity to understand the consequences (Cohen, 2015).

For a child's assent to be meaningful, an assessment of the level of maturity and comprehension is required, and information must be provided in language and terms that are appropriate for the developmental level. Conversely, when there is conflict between the decision of the parent and that of the child, the health care provider has a duty to ensure that the parental choice is in the child's best interest. Where there is serious doubt, it may be necessary to involve the courts.

## Confidentiality

Autonomy is also the principle underlying **confidentiality**: One expression of autonomy is the ability to maintain privacy in one's life (Burkhardt & Nathaniel, 2013). People have the right to decide who can have access to information about them, thus limiting the negative use of personal information by others. In certain situations, the status of confidentiality between a person and others, such as clergy, is considered a privilege and as such is shielded from exposure by the legal system. In health care, confidentiality does not carry as strong a status as clergy-supplicant or lawyer-client privilege (Grace, 2004). There may be occasions when health care providers have a duty to warn others who are unknowingly endangered. This duty was highlighted by the landmark Tarasoff case. On October 27, 1969, Prosenjit Poddar killed Tatiana Tarasoff. Poddar was receiving psychiatric care during this period. He had informed his therapist 2 weeks earlier that he was going to kill a certain girl, easily identifiable as Tarasoff, on her return from Brazil. At the time his therapist tried to have him committed. The police detained Poddar briefly but decided he was rational, so they released him. No one warned Tatiana of the danger. The courts concluded that "once a therapist does in fact determine, or under applicable professional standards reasonably should have determined, that a person poses a serious danger of violence to others, he bears a duty to exercise reasonable care to protect the foreseeable victim of that danger" (Tarasoff v. Regents of University of California, 1976). The court recognized the difficulty of predicting the degree of danger and the importance of maintaining confidentiality but determined that when the risk is high, confidentiality should be breached.

Nurses must strive to keep the person's personal information confidential so as to enhance trust within the nurse-person relationship. Therefore in health care settings there are strong penalties against breaching confidentiality. In theory, the principle of confidentiality may be overridden only in situations in which extreme harm to self or others is imminent. In practice, this is difficult to enforce, because in medical settings many people have access to the person's information. Insurance companies demand access to information before payment for services is made. In outpatient settings, challenges for privacy may occur when personnel are personally acquainted with the individual. When health professionals are members of the community in which they practice, there may be confidentiality issues associated with the intimate nature of small communities. Nurses and other health-promotion professionals may find themselves being asked by friends and relatives of the person for details about that person's health status. It can be very difficult to respond diplomatically while maintaining the person's privacy. The ethical implications of these threats to confidentiality are many. Thus it is important for nurses to be aware of potential breaches of confidentiality and to advocate confidential treatment of information for those they serve.

## The Privacy Rule

The Privacy Rule (45 Code of Federal Regulations Part 160, 164 subparts A & E) was developed as a result of the Health Insurance Portability and Accountability Act (HIPAA). Its intent was to ensure that individuals' health information is properly protected, while allowing the flow of information needed to provide and promote high-quality care (including use of information about the person receiving care for research) and to protect the public's health and well-being. HIPAA was meant to protect the privacy of individually identifiable health information in the face of advances in electronic technology and to limit the ways in which

"health plans, pharmacies, hospitals, clinics, nursing homes and other covered entities (any provider that conducts or conveys information in electronic form, e.g., physicians, nurse practitioners)" can use medical information (US Department of Health and Human Services [USDHHS], n.d.). "Covered entities" means those covered by the Privacy Rule. The limitations on the use of medical information extend to any identifiable information, written, oral, or computerized. Although there are some legal guidelines about disclosure, nurses and others are responsible for using clinical judgment in deciding what level of detail to share. It is important to understand that the purpose of the rule is to protect individual rights while still facilitating important public health and epidemiological research. Health-promotion activities include empowering people to exercise these rights. The Privacy Rule ensures that individuals are given a copy of the privacy practices at a given institution. Additionally, under the rule individuals have the following rights:

- To access their own information.
- To limit who may receive their information.
- To request corrections for errors.
- To receive an accounting of how their information has been used.
- To request special confidential reporting of their information to them at a location of their choosing (this may be especially important for individuals at risk for intimate partner violence).
- To pursue complaints with the Department of Health and Human Services Office for Civil Rights.

A rule of thumb for health professionals related to sharing information with others is to disclose only as much information as is pertinent to the situation and is necessary to provide optimal care. A decision about disclosure of a person's information requires balancing of the risks of information sharing with the benefits of treatment. Although the Privacy Rule was meant to help safeguard people's rights, some commentators and researchers are finding the rule overly restrictive and worry that it might discourage important research, especially genetic research, with its far-reaching implications for individual privacy.

### Adolescents: Special Considerations of Confidentiality

Adolescents often present health professionals with very tricky confidentiality issues. As Bandman and Bandman (2001) note, "the adolescent is torn between wanting to challenge authority and to assert independence while still needing the help and support of effective parents. Normal developmental needs, along with the results of risk-taking behavior such as drug and alcohol experimentation and risky sexual activity, mean that teenagers can pose a health-promotion challenge. The task of health promotion is to maintain and facilitate the adolescent's emerging autonomy and confidentiality needs, while mediating between the peer and parental figures who feel that they have a right to information about the adolescent. It is easy to become caught in the tension between the anger and perceived duties of the parent and the defensiveness and vulnerability of the adolescent" (Bandman & Bandman, 2001).

Although federal and state laws, as well as ethical considerations, generally serve to protect the privacy and autonomy of adolescents, health promotion involves more than mere protection. It involves facilitating the adolescent's health. Thus the responsibilities include helping an adolescent to grasp his or her authentic options and rights, facilitating interaction between the adolescent and parents or guardians, maintaining trust, and preserving confidentiality.

On the other hand, clinical judgment (which includes ethical judgment) is important in determining risk. If the risk of preserving the adolescent's privacy is high, on the basis of all pertinent and available evidence such as the presence of sexual or physical abuse, then it may be necessary to report this information to appropriate authorities. Mandatory reporting laws exist. Such laws are important for the general protection of a society's citizens. However, there may be rare occasions when a judgment must be made about whether upholding the legal obligation would cause more harm than good. In such circumstances there are two separate considerations. First, one must decide whether the risk to professional standing and licensure of not following the legally required path is something that the professional is willing to assume. The second consideration involves assessing the potential benefits and risks to the person resulting from failure to report. There is no easy resolution for these types of problems. If the situation is not an emergency, it is prudent to solicit appropriate advice from a peer, a counselor, or an ethics expert or resource. In any case, it remains the professional's ethical responsibility to handle the given situation in a manner that preserves trust and provides ongoing support.

## Veracity

Veracity, or devotion to the truth, is another principle that supports health-promotion activities. People whose health is in question are to various degrees reliant on the person who possesses the knowledge and skills to bring these to bear on their behalf. The contemporary bioethics literature favors characteristics of "veracity, ...candor, honesty and truthfulness" (Beauchamp & Childress, 2008) as virtues to be nurtured in the development of health professionals. This represents a change from the paternalistic (the physician knows what is best) attitudes that prevailed early in the 20th century and up to the late 1960s.

Veracity in giving people information about their health care needs facilitates autonomous choice and enhances personal decision-making. Nurses may be tempted to withhold certain details when this is seen as serving the person's best interests or when family members demand it. It is sometimes difficult to determine how much and what types of information will best serve a person's needs. Knowledge of the person's beliefs, values, and lifestyle preferences is essential to the process of supplying adequate information to support autonomous decision-making. Withholding information or providing information that is misleading or incomprehensible in an attempt to influence someone to agree to a treatment or intervention conflicts with veracity. It may be tempting to avoid the longer route to resolving such problems (e.g., education, understanding people's motives).

Veracity has some cross-cultural implications, in that some cultures have not traditionally valued truth-telling in the case of terminal illness. Decision-making about whether or not to honor veracity in such cases must take into consideration what is known about the culture, the particular person, the strength of his or her personal and cultural beliefs, and whether there is evidence about what sorts of things the person would like to know. The absence of veracity may interfere with autonomous action. In the case of terminal illness, it may deprive the person of the ability to plan the remainder of his or her life.

At first glance, veracity appears an easy concept to incorporate into health-promotion interventions. It may sometimes be difficult, however, in health education endeavors aimed at changing patterns of behavior in society. Should health professionals just present the facts or should they attempt to persuade people? What are the limits of veracity? Is it permissible to exaggerate the dangers of certain behavior in the interests of the health of society? These questions cannot be answered within the confines of this chapter but are important to keep in mind when one is assessing the merits of proposed population-based interventions.

## Nonmaleficence

Related to autonomy is the principle of nonmaleficence, which enjoins people not to harm other people. In general society, this principle constrains people from autonomous actions that are likely to harm others. For instance, a 25-year-old is allowed to drink alcohol but not to drink and drive because the latter may harm others. In health care settings, this principle prohibits clinicians from harming those for whom they provide services. For health promotion, it means that when activities are being planned on an individual or societal level, possible harms must be minimized. It is often impossible to foresee all the risks of a given course of action, but professionals who engage in health-promotion endeavors are responsible for foreseeing predictable adverse consequences and taking these potential consequences into consideration. The responsibilities include addressing social or health care policies that are discovered to have unintended effects.

Carter and colleagues (2011) illustrate how a policy designed to address obesity through use of a mass-media program can have unintended negative health effects. They describe how the program *How Do You Measure Up?* can carry the message to people to trim waistlines and "turn their lives around." Although mass-media campaigns such as this one are targeted at the population level, they may also have a deeply personal and emotional effect on individuals, stigmatizing individuals who feel incapable of making changes in their lives to lose weight.

Teaching about self-esteem and fitness may help people live with obesity more healthfully. Employer incentive programs that differentiate among individuals on the basis of their success in changing behaviors such as smoking or weight loss also carry the possibility of discrimination when they provide financial benefits to the most successful individuals, in that some individuals face significantly greater difficulty than others in achieving desired outcomes (Madison et al., 2011). Well-designed employer incentive programs, however, can help individuals overcome barriers they face in trying to avoid disease and disability. Systematic evaluation of incentive programs will enhance understanding of how to design programs to prevent discrimination and maximize equity (Sorrell, 2015).

Unintentional harm is a possibility for actions designed to promote health. Risks can be minimized by anticipation of potential negative effects and implementation of measures to control them. Professionals are responsible for understanding the limits of their knowledge or the data to which they have access. A synthesis of reflection, critical thinking, and knowledge, along with an understanding of the details and context of a situation, is required before one embarks on a course of action aimed at facilitating a person's health or well-being. The overall discomfort encountered by the individual must be the minimum possible to achieve the primary good intended. In other words, the health care provider is accountable for his or her judgment and for providing interventions most likely to bring about the desired result. Thus more than just the intention not to do harm is required.

Nurses and other health professionals can do harm inadvertently through such behaviors as ignorance or incompetence, referral to a provider who is incompetent or inappropriate, or inadequate supervision or training of those under their supervision. However, the duty of nonmaleficence does not mean that nurses are always accountable for foreseeing the consequences of their actions. For example, a course of exercise may be designed for a person who has had a thorough physical examination, but during an exercise session the person faints and fractures his arm. Further testing reveals a previously undetected cardiac anomaly that is subsequently surgically corrected. This is not maleficence; the main objective of the agent was therapeutic, and the event was, if not totally unforeseeable, not identified on routine preexercise testing. In this kind of case, we tend to look at the principle behind the action rather than the consequences. The clinician's duty was upheld, even though initially bad consequences were the unintended result. Thus both deliberate harm and harm caused by indifferent or incompetent decision-making should be considered maleficent, but when a competent practitioner evaluates a problem thoroughly in its appropriate context and intervenes with therapeutic intent, and nonetheless there is a partially negative outcome, such action does not violate the concept of nonmaleficence.

## Beneficence

Beneficence is the quality or state of doing or producing good. As a moral principle, beneficence presents us with the duty to maximize the benefits of actions while minimizing harms. There are two related aspects of the moral principle of beneficence in health-promotion settings: actions taken to further the overall health or well-being of the society in general and actions taken to promote the good of a particular individual.

When society formulates rules designed to protect people against the negative effects of their own actions, these rules are considered beneficent. It is important to emphasize, however, that beneficence should be performed in accordance with the person's will or values, and with respect for the person's autonomy (Kangasniemi, 2010; Keane, 2010). Sometimes rules designed to protect people are described as paternalistic because they override a person's autonomy to disobey them. For example, motorcycle helmet laws are paternalistic, as are rules governing the use of therapeutic or so-called recreational drugs. Paternalism is often

justified by the assertion that the persons affected will be better off or protected from harm.

The principle of beneficence, when it overrides an individual's autonomous choice so as to serve that individual's interests, is appropriate when a person lacks the capacity to make personal decisions. Thus any of the factors discussed earlier that interfere with rational decision-making may require the health care provider to beneficently override the individual's decisions. Generally, though, beneficence permits interference only when the risks of the individual's proposed actions are high. This is because autonomy is such a powerful principle in Western societies that a decision to override an autonomous choice is not taken lightly. One may be justified in preventing a person from taking an overdose of sleeping pills or jumping off a cliff because the risks of not doing so are high and, importantly, if the person succeeds there is no possibility of future autonomous actions.

Beneficence, unlike nonmaleficence, is not necessarily a moral requirement of action on the part of societal members toward each other (Grace, 2004). Whether beneficence is viewed as a moral requirement of societal members in everyday life very much depends on philosophical beliefs and the ethical theory or perspective (if any) recognized by the person. Kant (1993/1785), for instance, distinguishes between perfect duties and imperfect duties. Perfect duties must be followed and tend to be defined in negative terms (e.g., "do not lie," "do not steal"); imperfect duties are ones we are called but not bound to follow (e.g., stopping to help someone who is looking for something lost on the sidewalk). An individual is not necessarily morally required to go out of his or her way to help someone unless the person is endangered and assistance would mitigate the danger. In that case, failing to offer assistance could be seen as violating the principle of nonmaleficence. Also, when an individual has responsibility for vulnerable others, such as when parents must use beneficence on behalf of their children, beneficence is required.

In contrast to ordinary members of society, nurses have duties of beneficence because their professional goals involve meeting health care needs and thus are aimed at providing good. For such reasons, beneficence is a moral expectation of nurses. Beneficence is often a difficult principle to use in health-promotion settings, however, because of the dual nature of health-promotion goals—health for individuals and health for communities. As noted earlier, there is often a tension between the two.

A paradox exists when we try to change unhealthy behaviors but do not address the underlying causes of those behaviors. For example, although smoking cessation programs assist some people to stop smoking, and restricting areas where people may smoke tends to persuade some people that it is becoming too inconvenient to continue, we also should address problems such as advertising campaigns that aim to gather new smoking recruits from among adolescents. Some advertising campaigns encourage adolescents to try flavored cigarettes through offering a variety of flavors and attractive packaging. But these tobacco cigarettes are addictive and dangerous. Education-based health-promotion programs without underlying societal changes are often doomed to fail. Thus following beneficence, health professionals have obligations to address deep-rooted social problems that jeopardize health or are associated with health disparities.

## Beneficence: Conflict With Autonomy

The principles of beneficence and autonomy sometimes conflict. For example, seat belt rules are ostensibly created to protect people from injury, but they take away autonomous choice. Beneficence may justify overriding the decision of a febrile, confused person who refuses to take her antibiotics for treatment of pneumonia. What is the clinician's responsibility? The duties of beneficence seem to mandate medicating her against her will, ensuring that the good of health is facilitated although violation of the principle of autonomy. The justification for this must include an assessment of her status related to her capacity for autonomous decision-making. Preserving the person's life so he or she can make autonomous decisions in the future may be required by beneficence. However, it can be argued that beneficence takes precedence over autonomy only in those cases in which the choice cannot be considered autonomous. First, there has to be evidence that a choice has been made. In this case the choice was between accepting antibiotic treatment versus not accepting antibiotic treatment. Second, the reasonableness (or rationality) of the decision has to be discerned. It must be ascertained whether the person really has grasped the implications of refusing treatment. The reasons given for the treatment refusal, then, should illuminate gaps in information delivery or processing. Finally, it must be determined whether there are any external or internal coercion factors impinging on the decision. Perhaps the person feels she cannot afford the medicine (external), or perhaps she has a mistrust of antibiotics because of a previous experience (internal). When a decision cannot be said to be informed, the principle of beneficence directs us to decide on treatment on the basis of the person's best interests.

## Justice

Justice is an ethical principle of major importance in health-promotion settings. There are various conceptions of justice, and the term is used in a variety of ways. For the purposes of this chapter the discussion is about social justice rather than criminal justice. Social justice includes formal or informal systems within a society that are concerned with disparities in socioeconomic conditions leading to poor health and fairness in the distribution of goods such as health, education, food, and shelter (Powers & Faden, 2008). Buchanan (2000) notes that the concept of justice has been central to human understandings of socially significant values for a long time. Justice in health care is a major commitment of nursing, and thus the discipline of nursing is becoming more focused on active engagement in social justice issues.

In democratic societies, the requirements of social justice generally include equitable distribution of the benefits and burdens of societal life. "Justice as fairness" reflects the ideas behind Rawls's (1971, 1999) *A Theory of Justice*. Rawls identifies two rules that he argues will result in a fair and just society. "First: each person is to have an equal right to the most extensive liberty compatible with a similar liberty for others. Second: social and economic inequalities are to be arranged such that they are both (a) reasonably expected to be to everyone's advantage, and (b) attached to positions and offices open to all" (Rawls, 1971). Rawls formulates these rules as a result of his hypothetical method for deciding how a society's institutions should be arranged to provide fairness. Rawls proposes that these rules of justice would emerge as a result of an average person's reasoning about what social arrangements that person would prefer if that reasoning were done from behind a "veil of ignorance"; that is, if the person did not know what his or her personal impediments, assets, or characteristics were going to be, such as intelligence, socioeconomic status, race, gender, or (dis)ability. Rawls's two rules aim to balance overall good for society with respect for individual rights, in some ways a balance of Mill's utilitarianism and Kant's focus on respect for persons. That is why inequalities must be open to all and must be to everyone's advantage. It is arguably fair for a judge to be paid more than a janitor because the judge's higher salary is to the advantage of all because it leads to competition and motivates the brightest citizens to enter the profession. However, to truly be a fair situation, part (b) of the second rule would also have to hold true—the pathway to becoming a judge must be open to all. Meeting part (b) would presumably require, at least, quality public education and financial support for college and law school.

Rawls's theory, although respected by ethicists, is subject to criticism on a variety of fronts. One significant criticism is that justice as fairness does not provide much guidance for some common social problems, such as abortion, welfare, and the righting of previous wrongs (e.g., affirmative action, the rights of native people), and ignores the problems of those without legal rights such as undocumented workers (Buchanan, 2000; MacIntyre, 2007). Dinkins (2011), however, suggests that the "veil of ignorance" thought experiment described by Rawls may increase empathy in daily practice because it helps us realize that when we step out from the veil into the workplace being envisioned, we could be anybody: a single mother without insurance unable to access health care for her children, an elderly woman with a hoarding disorder who lives surrounded by piles and piles of decaying garbage, or a person from any other vulnerable population in our society.

An emphasis on justice in health care settings is sometimes called the impartialist perspective in that it considers the needs of all who fall under its umbrella. For example, within the prison system, this view of justice would mandate access to care for prisoners in need. Thus it would not permit arbitrary obstacles to access (such as requiring good behavior or favors) that might be presented by prison officers or by other prisoners who wish to exert physical or psychological control. Justice would also require improved access to care for the poor and underprivileged, in terms of both receiving care and having access to transportation or local availability of services.

Although justice might require consideration of the special needs of a disadvantaged group, it does so impartially: that is, it does not distinguish among the particulars of individuals. Each member within the group has an equal right to whatever is proposed. In an economically and profit-driven health care system, injustices occur both at the local level and at the societal level. Because justice viewed as fairness is impartial about individual differences, that moral perspective considered alone is not a perfect tool with which to look at health care disparities and their causes.

Health disparities are a specific subset of health differences that are important for social justice because they evolve from intentional or unintentional discrimination or marginalization (Braveman et al., 2011). Nurses and other health professionals need to move beyond thinking about "doing no harm" to identifying and addressing adverse social influences on the health of underprivileged groups and the implications of their consequent poor health (Rogers & Kelly, 2011). The combination of justice, feminist concerns about power and oppression, and the acknowledged responsibilities of nurses to promote health permit a comprehensive view of problems associated with health protection and promotion. This view incorporates an ethical approach to problems both for society and for individuals within the society. Buchanan (2000) captures this necessary synthesis of perspectives well, noting "the mutually reinforcing relationships among justice, caring and responsibility" which will help nurses to "enable people to live well."

## STRATEGIES FOR ETHICAL DECISION-MAKING

### Locating the Source and Levels of Ethical Problems

Most health-promotion problems are moral or ethical issues in the sense that obstacles exist that prevent an individual from living life well or achieving personal goals related to health. Throughout this chapter, discussions of both the larger (societal) and the narrower (individual) perspectives have been emphasized and their relationships highlighted. Sometimes tensions between the two require mediation and may force the health promoter to decide which problem must be addressed first. For example, a nurse at a family practice clinic cares for a teenager who is morbidly obese. At the level of the individual, the nurse is charged with discovering the underlying causes of the obesity (e.g., physical, psychological, contextual) and designing strategies with the individual to help resolve the problem. However, the nurse has responsibilities also to address the issue at the more political level with interested others.

To address health-promotion issues effectively, professionals need to possess not only their particular disciplinary expertise and an understanding of ethical language, principles, and perspectives, but also a willingness to understand their own values and preconceptions about health and people. Understanding personal philosophy, biases, and values permits one to control for these in the sense of being aware of the influences they have in our interactions with others.

### Values Clarification and Reflection

Gaining confidence in moral decision-making is a slow process. The following are suggestions that will guide development related to recognizing and addressing ethical issues.

### Examine Beliefs and Values

Cultivate the habit of examining how your personal values and **beliefs** relate to the human condition, justice, and responsibility. Be willing to revise your beliefs in line with your professional

knowledge base, experiences, or current research findings. For example, how do beliefs that "people get what they deserve" correlate with what we know—for example, that those of lower socioeconomic status have lower levels of health and that poor health interferes with functioning and is associated with depression? How do our attitudes change when we try to place ourselves in the context of the other person's life?

This is not to say that maintaining personal integrity is not important—it is. Maintaining both personal and professional integrity is essential to good practice. Integrity has to do with a sense of wholeness of the self and consistency of actions with truly examined beliefs and values. "Nurses have both personal and professional identities that are integrated and that embrace the values of the profession, merging them with personal values" (ANA, 2015). The *Code of Ethics for Nurses with Interpretive Statements* validates the nurse's preservation of integrity in those situations in which he or she feels that personal integrity is compromised. It notes that "when a particular decision or action is morally objectionable to the nurse,… the nurse is justified in refusing to participate on moral grounds" (ANA, 2015). In contemplating refusal to provide care, however, the nurse should ensure that the decision is based on sound ethical principles, not simply on personal beliefs. When opting out of care involves risk to the individual, other arrangements must be made to safeguard individual care. Decisions not to participate in a situation cannot be made trivially because of the trust relationship and a nurse's moral accountability for actions. The threat to the nurse's integrity must be serious and the person's well-being must not be jeopardized by the nurse's absence. Other arrangements must be made for care of the person in such circumstances. The nurse who encounters repeated threats to integrity has a responsibility to consider changing the situation in some way. Change efforts may be directed toward institutional policy or may require that an alternative work environment be considered.

A true examination of beliefs and values requires a willingness to admit that they may not always be justifiable; they may be remnants from childhood indoctrination of various sorts. For example, one might believe that certain ethnic groups are inferior in some way, or that one should not question authority. An honest and ongoing examination of one's values and biases permits one to control for these beliefs when providing care to diverse persons. Being willing to examine one's beliefs and values—being willing to continue that upward journey out of Plato's cave—is thus a key part of personal and professional integrity.

### The Influence of Personal Beliefs and Values

In addition to examining beliefs and values, we should also think about the influence that these characteristics have on our practice. An understanding of how personal beliefs and values either are congruent or are liable to interfere with the task at hand is crucial to ethical problem-solving. In any given situation, the health professional must ask himself or herself, "What are my beliefs and biases in this situation? How are these likely to influence my actions?" For example, if the home health nurse believes his below-poverty-level, depressed, obese, diabetic patient who smokes is responsible for the poor healing of her leg ulcer, he may be less inclined to work with the person to discover and address the person's goals.

## Reflection on Practice

A third helpful strategy is to reflect on situations afterward to discover what worked, what did not work, and what could be done differently in the future. It is often helpful to interact with peers or other experts after particularly difficult situations to discover alternative perspectives or resources for the purposes of future problem-solving. You might ask a peer or mentor to ask you questions to help you think through why you made a particular decision. Or you might practice some reflective writing to help you think through your reasoning and consider whether you would act differently in the future (Dinkins, 2015).

## Decision-Making Considerations

Decision-making in health-promotion settings has inescapable moral components. As noted earlier, the nurse has a professional responsibility to further the good for individuals and society. Thus the careful exercise of experience, skill, and knowledge is warranted when one is trying to formulate the best course of action for a given individual or group, or in resolving societal health-promotion problems. This framework is offered as a way of ensuring clarity about a particular case or situation. Because of the diverse nature of health-promotion activities, no straightforward models of decision-making can realistically be applied in all situations. Additionally, decision-making is often an ongoing process, and revisions to plans may be required in light of new information. The following are important facets of decision-making but do not necessarily occur in the order given.

## Identify the Main Problem or Issue

What level of problem is this: social, group, or individual? If the location of the problem is societal, it will also impact individuals and groups, and a decision has to be made about the order of interventions. Try to determine the main ethical principle involved or whether it is a problem of conflicting principles. For example, after identification of the problem, you may determine that to provide benefit to the person, the person's autonomy must be overridden. Is this a social justice issue? Is it an autonomy issue? What factors led to the problem? Is there coercion or other power imbalance? If so, who has an interest in maintaining the power imbalance and who gains the most from the imbalance? These are the questions feminist ethics would ask.

## Determine on Whom the Resolution Will Have an Impact

Who has a stake in the issue and in how it will be resolved? Answering this question will permit a determination of whose input is crucial to the decision-making process. Who and what are important considerations (e.g., institutions, individuals, businesses, social policy)? Does this issue result from a failure to predict the consequences of certain social policies?

## Determine the Prevalent Values

What are the values held by all the different players? Are there value conflicts? The value conflicts might be individual versus social, as in the case of a person with tuberculosis who refuses to take his medicines, thus putting at risk members of his family or members of the community. Value conflicts might also be interpersonal among the health-promotion team or they might be personal versus professional. As a general rule, more weight is assigned to the values of the individual who is most likely to be affected by a decision. It is important to consider the influence of culture on values when the issue involves health promotion for culturally diverse groups. It is also important to involve people who can help explain the cultural beliefs, especially when language difficulties are present. A knowledgeable but neutral interpreter may be helpful when liaison between groups is needed.

## Identify Information Gaps

Reflect on whether the decision makers are confident about what they know and do not know, and what they may be overlooking. This determination is not always an easy task. Information may exist that has not yet reached our awareness, or we might fail to ask a question that would reveal important information. How can we be confident about the scope and limits of our knowledge? Clinical judgment is a good tool but is not foolproof. When doubts exist or the decision is likely to have serious or risky consequences, we need to involve knowledgeable others or try to determine the best places to gain missing information.

## Formulate Possible Courses of Action and Probable Consequences

Courses of action may involve further information gathering, brainstorming, and possibly collaboration with other experts or specialists. Although further data may be needed to resolve problems at the level of individuals or small groups, it is especially necessary to enlist additional help when the issue is one that requires political action to effect policy changes. It may be necessary to recruit community members and leaders or to enlist the political power of specialty groups. Finally, a determination must be made about which proposed courses of action will be the least harmful and the most beneficial. Remember not to look just to likely consequences, however. Consider possible actions from the framework of duty and character as well.

## Initiate the Selected Course of Action and Evaluate the Outcome

Does the actual outcome match the anticipated outcome? If not, what happened that was unexpected? Would this outcome have been foreseeable given more data? Would you do things differently in another similar situation given what you have learned? Does the problem need to be addressed at a different level (institutional or public policy)?

## Engage in Self-Reflection and Peer or Expert Group Reflection

What could you have done differently? Would consulting with others have altered your conception of the problem or your course of action? What insights can you or your peers glean from this that could be appropriate for similar situations in the future? How might continuing education opportunities help you or your peers more appropriately address similar problems in the future? Would an ethics resource (committee or consultant) be helpful in such situations? Could you use this case as a focused learning experience for your peers and collaborators?

## ETHICS OF HEALTH PROMOTION: CASES

Some cases of special relevance to health promotion are presented next. They are followed by questions that can be answered by individual readers, but they also provide a good starting point for group discussion. Try using the decision-making strategies suggested throughout the chapter as you explore these problems. It is anticipated that you will want more information than is provided. Deciding what extra information would be helpful is an important part of the exercise.

### Case 1: Addressing Health Care System Problems—Elissa Needs Help

Elissa is 38 years old. She recently moved 200 miles from her home to a small town (population 6000) and separated from her abusive husband to escape his continuing threats and to be near her childhood friend. She suffers from chronic, sometimes incapacitating, depression, for which she has received antidepressant medications and counseling, with temporary relief. She has been unable to work and has no private health insurance. She is eligible for the state's Medicaid program, however, and has recently discovered that Medicaid will cover her health care needs. Her friend refers her to the only primary care center in the area, where she is seen by Jill, one of the two nurse practitioners. As part of her evaluation, Jill discovers that Elissa was abused as a child and has very poor self-esteem. Elissa affirms that her childhood friend is very supportive. Jill believes that longer-term psychological counseling would benefit Elissa and facilitate her well-being, but she also knows that none of the counseling services within a 50-mile radius accepts Medicaid payment. Elissa has no transportation.

- What are Jill's options? What are her responsibilities?
- What actions might Jill pursue both on a local level and on a political level? What are her resources?
- What is the responsibility of the health-promotion disciplines in cases such as this?

### Case 2: She's My Client!—Lilly and "Jake" (a.k.a. Paul)

Shirley, a nurse practitioner, is at a conference when a physician colleague discusses a difficult case. One of his clients, "Jake," is HIV positive but refuses any treatment. The physician explains that Jake fears that his wife will discover and recognize the names of the medications, because he knows "these drug names are discussed on television all the time." Jake has not told his wife that he is HIV positive and has no intention of ever doing so. Jake firmly believes his condition is his private information and, for now, the couple use condoms for birth control. The physician is concerned that Jake will not tell his wife. The physician is presenting this case to colleagues to highlight the public awareness campaigns that, to some extent, have affected client privacy. He argues, "Listen to how they call out your name and the drugs at the pharmacy counter."

Shirley recognizes bits and pieces of information and comes to the painful realization that Jake is really Paul, and Paul is the husband of one of her clients, Lilly. Lilly has begun to discuss with Shirley that she wants to get pregnant soon. The town is too small for Shirley to be mistaken. Or is it?

- Is it ethical for the nurse practitioner to ask the physician if Jake is Paul?
- Is it ethical for Shirley to tell Lilly she suspects Paul is HIV positive?
- Should this information change how Shirley counsels Lilly about a pregnancy?
- What is in Lilly's best interests? Is Shirley also obligated to consider Paul's interests?
- What resources are available?

### Case 3: Don't Touch My Things! Ms. Smyth and Autonomy

Ms. Smyth, 78 years old, had lived in the same home for 30 years. Never married, she cared for her disabled mother for 15 years. After her mother died, she lived alone on a small pension. She appeared to be well groomed and appropriately dressed when she left her house.

Ms. Smyth was hospitalized for a bowel obstruction, and Joe, a community health nurse, made a follow-up visit after discharge to her home. When Joe arrived at the house, he was overcome with the smell of rotting garbage, urine, and feces. Five small dogs ran back and forth among piles of garbage and magazines, overturned furniture, and discarded appliances. There was no running water, and the bathroom was not functional. Joe told Ms. Smyth that her living conditions were unhealthy and that he would contact a community agency to help her clean her house. Ms. Smyth became very angry and said no one had the right to take her things away.

- Is it ethical for Joe to overrule Ms. Smyth's autonomy in decision-making?
- What action is in Ms. Smyth's best interests?
- What action is in the community's best interests?
- What ethical issues are involved in caring for a client with a hoarding disorder, such as that seen in Ms. Smyth's situation?

## SUMMARY

Health promotion is a vast and complex practice area; consequently, the associated ethical challenges are diverse and multileveled. This chapter has outlined the nature and purpose of health care ethics and related this framework to the responsibilities of health care providers in health-promotion interventions. Health promotion should be viewed as a moral undertaking of health care providers. After reading this chapter, students will have knowledge of some of the tools and language needed to explore ethical issues, discuss these issues with others, and address problematic issues at both the individual level and the societal level. Perhaps the most important factor to consider is that ethical problems manifesting themselves at the level of the individual almost always have their origins in the broader societal environment.

## CASE STUDY

### Genetic Screening Programs

A US company has been sequencing the DNA of 20 individuals. With the individuals' consent, the results will be made available to researchers. Each donor will be offered information about genetic variations that might indicate a higher-than-average likelihood of developing a life-threatening condition.

There are hopes that genetic screenings of large populations will change the practice of health care from a focus on treating diseases to preventing them. Some researchers predict the complete sequencing of each human genome will provide routine data to health care providers, much like the common measurements of blood pressure, pulse, temperature, and blood counts today. Other research data show, however, that better predictors of determining the risk of diabetes are asking people about their family history of diabetes, their weight, and their age rather than sequencing their DNA.

**Reflective Questions:**

Apply different concepts and theories of ethics in thinking about the following questions.

- What are some of the ethical issues of these DNA analyses?
- What are the responsibilities of health care professionals in the genetic screenings of a population?
- What additional components could a community health nurse add to the following plan of care for participants having their DNA sequenced?

Sources Beery, T. A., & Shooner, K. A. (2004). Family history: The first genetic screen. *Nurse Practitioner: American Journal of Primary Health Care, 29*(11), 14–25; Huddleston, K. (2013). Ethics: The challenge of ethical, legal, and social implications (ELSI) in genomic nursing. *OJIN: The Online Journal of Issues in Nursing. 19*(1), 6; Knome. The Human Genome Interpretation Company; Lashley, F. R. (2007). *Essentials of clinical genetics in nursing practice.* New York: Springer.

## ◎ CARE PLAN

### Genetic Screening Programs

The use of developments in genetics research, including genetic counseling, testing, and screening, as well as advanced therapeutic and reproduction choices, influences the health of both present and future generations throughout the world.

As previously addressed, health care professionals have many complex ethical responsibilities in the applications of genetic developments with local, national, and international communities, as well as with individuals and families.

In the following care plan, the community health nurse from the preceding case study addresses aspects of the ineffective management of genetic screenings in a community.

\*NURSING DIAGNOSIS: Ineffective community therapeutic regimen management

#### Definition

Pattern in which a community experiences (or is at risk of experiencing) difficulty integrating a genetic screening program for the prevention/treatment of illness and reduction of risk

#### Defining Characteristics

*Major:* Community verbalizes desire to manage the genetic screenings and treatment of illness and prevention of sequelae; community verbalizes difficulty with regulation and integration of prescribed regimens for genetic screening and treatment of illness and its effects or prevention of complications.

*Minor:* Knowledge of risk factors for illness (expected or unexpected) is accelerated.

#### Related Factors

**Treatment Related**

- Complexity of genetic screening and therapeutic regimen
- Complexity of health care
- Financial costs
  - Actual cost of procedure
  - Potential cost (e.g., loss of health insurance)
- Side effects
  - Expected (e.g., anxiety)
  - Unexpected (e.g., despair)

**Situation/Environment Related**

- Health and health care needs, multiple and complex, especially for vulnerable population (e.g., unborn children)
- Presence of known and unknown environmental (including occupational) health hazards
- Availability of community resources for screening for risk factors of diseases
  - Less expensive (e.g., family health histories and physical exams); more expensive (e.g., genetic screenings)
  - Overall needs and financial resources

#### Expected Outcomes

With the community health nurses' guidance, community members will:

- Evaluate the actual and potential (e.g., significant increases in birth rates) health problems and resources of the community.
- Identify community resources that are needed to promote health and prevent illness, including genetic screenings.
- Participate in program development as needed to improve the effectiveness of the therapeutic regimen management of genetic screening programs.

#### Interventions

- Complete a community assessment including:
  - Actual and potential health problems and needs
  - Actual and potential resources for health
- Develop an overall program plan for genetic screenings
- Develop a specific program for the genetic screening of an individual, perhaps including the following components:
  - Complete initial interview, individual and family histories, and physical examination with appropriate laboratory studies
  - Generally, discuss the genetic screenings and informed consent, focusing on the concerns of the individual and/or family
- Assess barriers to learning:
  - Physical condition
  - Sensory status (e.g., vision, hearing)
  - Intelligence, learning abilities/disabilities
  - Emotional state(s) (e.g., fears, guilt)
  - Stressors, concerns

*Continued*

## ◎ CARE PLAN—cont'd
### *Genetic Screening Programs*

- Provide information:
  - Explain needed knowledge and perhaps changes (e.g., lifestyle behaviors)
  - Discuss and add to individual's knowledge of the pros and cons of genetic screening
  - Identify influencing factors to decision-making about individual's genetic screening
- Perform screenings (e.g., depression, financial resources).

- Give time to integrate new information, perhaps having a second appointment to:
  - Readdress questions
  - Develop informed consent, including policies on privacy
- Perform actual genetic screening procedure.
- Explain results with genetic and reproductive counseling.
- Repeat and follow up as necessary.
- Compare the diagnostic criteria for Ineffective Therapeutic Regimen Management with other differential diagnoses potentially present in the case study.

*NANDA Nursing Diagnoses—Herdman T. H. & Kamitsuru, S. (Eds.). Nursing Diagnoses - Definitions and Classification 2015-2017. Copyright © 2014, 1994-2014 NANDA International. Used by arrangement with John Wiley & Sons Limited. In order to make safe and effective judgments using the NANDA-I nursing diagnoses it is essential that nurses refer to the definitions and defining characteristics of the diagnoses listed in this work.

## ⓔ EVOLVE CHAPTER FEATURES

http://evolve.elsevier.com/Edelman/
- Study Questions

## REFERENCES

American Nurses Association (ANA). (1994). *Position statement: The nonnegotiable nature of the ANA code for nurses with interpretive statements.* Washington, DC: American Nurses Association.

American Nurses Association (ANA). (2010). *Nursing's social policy statement* (3rd ed.). Silver Spring, MD: American Nurses Association.

American Nurses Association. (2015). *Code of ethics for nurses with interpretive statements.* Washington, DC: American Nurses Association.

Aristotle. (1985). *Nicomachean ethics* (trans. T. Irwin). Indianapolis: Hackett. (original work ~350 BCE).

Bandman, E. L., & Bandman, B. (2001). *Nursing ethics through the life span* (4th ed.). Upper Saddle River, NJ: Prentice Hall.

Beauchamp, T. L., & Childress, J. F. (2008). *Principles of biomedical ethics* (6th ed.). New York: Oxford University Press.

Beauchamp, T. L., et al. (2007). *Contemporary issues in bioethics* (7th ed.). Belmont, CA: Wadsworth.

Benner, P., Tanner, C. A., & Chesla, C. A. (2009). *Expertise in nursing practice: Caring, clinical judgment, and ethics* (2nd ed.). New York: Springer.

Braveman, P. A., et al. (2011). Heath disparities and health equity: The issue is justice. *American Journal of Public Health, 101*(Suppl. 1), S149–S155.

Buchanan, D. R. (2000). *An ethic for health promotion: Rethinking the sources of human well-being.* New York: Oxford University Press.

Buchanan, D. R. (2006). Moral reasoning as a model for health promotion. *Social Science & Medicine, 63*(10), 2715–2726.

Burkhardt, M. A., & Nathaniel, A. K. (2013). *Ethics and issues in contemporary nursing* (4th ed.). Albany, NY: Delmar.

Carter, S. M., et al. (2011). Evidence, ethics, and values: A framework for health promotion. *American Journal of Public Health, 101*(3), 465–472.

Chambliss, D. F. (1996). *Beyond caring: Hospitals, nurses, and the social organization of ethics.* Chicago: University of Chicago Press.

Cohen, E. (2015). Heaven over hospital. Parents honor dying child's request. CNN Health. http://www.cnn.com/2015/10/27/health/girl-chooses-heaven-over-hospital-part-2/.

Corey, G., et al. (2014). *Issues and ethics in the helping professions* (9th ed.). Belmont, CA: Brooks/Cole.

Dinkins, C. S. (2011). Beyond patient care: Practicing empathy in the workplace. *Online Journal of Issues in Nursing, 16*(2), http://www.nursingworld.org/MainMenuCategories/ANAMarketplace/ANAPeriodicals/OJIN/Columns/Ethics/Empathy-in-the-Workplace.html.

Dinkins, C. S. (2015). Socratic pedagogy: Teaching students to think like nurses. In J. M. Sorrell & P. R. Cangelosi (Eds.), *Expert clinician to novice nurse educator.* New York: Springer.

Driessnack, M., & Gallo, A. M. (2011). Stop, look, and listen. Revisiting the involvement of children and adolescents in genomic research. *Annual Review of Nursing Research, 29*(1), 133–149.

Epstein, E. G., & Delgado, S. (2010). Understanding and addressing moral distress. *Online Journal of Issues in Nursing, 15*(3), http://www.nursingworld.org/MainMenuCategories/EthicsStandards/Courage-and-Distress/Understanding-Moral-Distress.html.

Epstein, B., & Turner, M. (2015). The nursing code of ethics: Its value, its history. *Online Journal of Issues in Nursing, 20*(2), http://www.nursingworld.org/MainMenuCategories/ANAMarketplace/ANAPeriodicals/OJIN/TableofContents/Vol-20-2015/No2-May-2015/The-Nursing-Code-of-Ethics-Its-Value-Its-History.html.

Gilligan, C. (1982). *In a different voice: Psychological theory and women's development.* Cambridge, MA: Harvard University Press.

Gilligan, C. (2013). *Joining the resistance.* Malden, MA: Polity Press.

Grace, P. J. (2001). Professional advocacy: Widening the scope of accountability. *Nursing Philosophy, 2*(2), 151–162.

Grace, P. J. (2004). Ethics in the clinical encounter. In S. Chase (Ed.), *Clinical judgment and communication in the nurse practitioner practice.* Boston: Boston College, William F. Connell School of Nursing.

Green, B. (2012). Applying feminist ethics of care to nursing practice. *Journal of Nursing Care,* doi:10.4172/2167-1168.1000111.

Huddleston, K. (2013). Ethics: The challenge of ethical, legal, and social implications (ELSI) in genomic nursing. *OJIN: The Online Journal of Issues in Nursing.*, *19*(1).

Institute of Medicine. (2010). The future of nursing: Leading change, advancing health. http://iom.nationalacademies.org/Reports/2010/The-Future-of-Nursing-Leading-Change-Advancing-Health.aspx.

International Council of Nurses. (2012). The ICN code of ethics for nurses. Geneva: International Council of Nurses. http://www.icn.ch/who-we-are/code-of-ethics-for-nurses/.

Iverson, E., et al. (2014). Factors affecting stress experienced by surrogate decision makers for critically ill patients: *Implications for nursing practice. Intensive and Critical Care Nursing, 30*(2), 77–85.

Jackson, D., et al. (2014). Whistleblowing: An integrative literature review of data-based studies involving nurses. *Contemporary Nurse, 14*(2), 240–251.

Kangasniemi, M. (2010). Equality as a central concept of nursing ethics: A systematic literature review. *Scandinavian Journal of Caring Sciences, 24*, 824–832.D.

Kant, I. (1993). *Grounding for the metaphysics of morals* (3rd ed.) (trans. J. W. Ellington). Indianapolis: Hackett. (original work published 1785).

Keane, M. (2010). Ethics as individual health interventions. *The American Journal of Bioethics, 10*(3), 36–38.

Kohlberg, L. (1981). *The philosophy of moral development: Moral stages and the idea of justice. Essays on moral development* (Vol. 1). San Francisco: Harper & Row.

Kohlberg, L. (1984). *The psychology of moral development: The nature and validity of moral stages. Essays on moral development* (Vol. 2). San Francisco: Harper & Row.

Lambert, V., & Glacken, M. (2011). Engaging with children in research: Theoretical and practical implications of negotiating informed consent/assent. *Nursing Ethics, 18*(6), 781–801.

Larcher, V. (2012). Moving from dependence to autonomy: Adolescents' decisions regarding their own health care. http://www.hinnovic.org/dependence-to-autonomy-adolescents%E2%80%99-health-care/.

MacIntyre, A. (2007). *After virtue: A study in moral theory* (3rd ed.). Southbend, IN: Notre Dame University.

Madison, K. M., Volpp, K. G., & Halpern, S. D. (2011). The law, policy, and ethics of employers' use of financial incentives to improve health. *Journal of Law, Medicine & Ethics, 39*(3), 450–468.

Mill, J. S. (2002). *Utilitarianism* (2nd ed.). Indianapolis: Hackett. (originally published 1861).

Nelson, H. L. (1992). Against caring. *Journal of Clinical Ethics, 3*(1), 8–20.

Paulsen, J. E. (2011). Ethics of caring and professional roles. *Nursing Ethics, 18*(2), 201–208.

Plato. (1992). *Republic* (trans. C. D. C. Reeve). Indianapolis: Hackett. (original work ~360 BCE).

Powers, M., & Faden, R. (2008). *Social justice: The moral foundations of public health and health policy* (2nd ed.). New York: Oxford University Press.

President's Commission for the Study of Ethical Problems in Medicine and Biomedical and Behavioral Research (1982). *Compensating for research injuries: The ethical and legal implications of programs to redress injured subjects.* Washington, DC: US Government Printing Office.

Rachels, J., & Rachels, S. (2011). *The elements of moral philosophy* (7th ed.). New York: McGraw-Hill.

Rawls, J. (1971 and 1999). *A theory of justice.* Cambridge, MA: Harvard University.

Rogers, J., & Kelly, U. A. (2011). Feminist intersectionality: Bringing social justice to health disparities research. *Nursing Ethics, 18*(3), 397–407.

Singer, P. (1993). *A companion to ethics.* Cambridge, MA: Wiley-Blackwell.

Sorrell, J. M. (2014). Deciding for others: Surrogates struggling with health care decisions. *Journal of Psychosocial Nursing and Mental Health Services, 52*(7), 17–21.

Sorrell, J. M. (2015). Employer-sponsored wellness programs for nurses: The ethics of carrots and sticks. *OJIN: The Online Journal of Issues in Nursing, 20*(1), 8, doi:10.3912/OJIN.Vol20No01EthCol01.

Sorrell, J. M., & Cangelosi, P. R. (2009). Respecting vulnerability: Informed consent in persons with Alzheimer's disease. *Southern Online Journal of Nursing Research, 9*(4), http://www.resourcenter.net/images/snrs/files/sojnr_articles2/vol09num04art02.html.

Sorrell, J. M., & Dinkins, C. S. (2006). An ethics of diversity. Listening in thin places. In C. S. Dinkins & J. M. Sorrell (Eds.), *Listening to the whispers. Re-thinking ethics in healthcare* (pp. 310–314). Madison, WI: University of Wisconsin Press.

Sproul, R. C. (2015). The difference between ethics and morality. *Ligonier Ministries.* http://www.ligonier.org/blog/difference-between-ethics-and-morality/.

Tarasoff v. Regents of University of California (1976). California Supreme Court 131. *California Reporter, 14.*

Tengland, P. A. (2016). Behavior change or empowerment: On the ethics of health-promotion goals. *Health Care Analysis, 24*, 24–46.

Tschudin, V. (2010). Nursing ethics: The last decade. *Nursing Ethics, 17*(1), 127–131.

US Department of Health and Human Services. (n.d.). Health information privacy. https://www.hhs.gov/ocr/hipaa/.

Weston, A. (2010). *A practical companion to ethics* (4th ed.). New York: Oxford University Press.

# 6

# Health Promotion and the Individual

*Anne Rath Rentfro*

## OBJECTIVES

*After completing this chapter, the reader will be able to:*
- Define the framework of functional health patterns as described by Gordon (2016).
- Describe the use of the functional health pattern framework to assess individuals throughout the life span.
- Illustrate health patterns of the functional, potentially dysfunctional, and actually dysfunctional categories of behavior.
- Identify risk factors or etiological aspects of actual or potential dysfunctional health patterns to consider with nursing diagnoses.
- Discuss the planning, implementation, and evaluation of nursing interventions to promote the health of individuals.
- Develop specific health-promotion plans based on an assessment of individuals.

## KEY TERMS

Age-developmental focus
Culturally competent care
Cultural attunement
Expected outcomes

Functional focus
Functional health patterns
Health status
Individual-environmental focus

Nursing diagnosis
Nursing interventions
Pattern focus
Risk factors

---

 **THINK ABOUT IT**

### *Assessment of Alcohol Consumption*

*Women have different patterns of alcohol consumption and different thresholds for problem drinking than men. Instruments such as the CAGE questionnaire detect alcohol dependence and would not be a sensitive enough measure for some women, in particular pregnant women, who are less likely than men to be alcohol dependent. The T-ACE instrument provides a measure of alcohol intake patterns more appropriate for women than that derived from the CAGE test (considered* Cutting *down on drinking, been* Annoyed *by criticism of drinking, feeling* Guilty *about drinking, and using alcohol as an* Eye-opener*). The T-ACE test, developed for use with women, was the first validated screening tool for assessing drinking risk in pregnant women and continues to provide a highly sensitive tool for identifying risk drinking (Bax et al., 2015). Screening is a useful strategy in health-promotion assessment and intervention (see Chapter 9). A pattern of drinking is established with use of the following questions:*

**T**—*How many drinks does it* Take *to make you feel high?*

**A**—*Have you ever been* Annoyed *by people criticizing your drinking?*

**C**—*Have you ever felt you ought to* Cut *down your drinking?*

**E**—*Have you ever had a drink first thing in the morning (*Eye-opener*) to steady your nerves or get rid of a hangover?*

Scores are calculated as follows:
- A reply of more than two drinks to question T is considered a positive response and scores 2 points, and an affirmative answer to question A, C, or E scores 1 point respectively.
- A total score of 2 or more points on the T-ACE indicates evidence of risk drinking.

Why would a nurse tailor the assessments to individual characteristics of a population? How effectively would this screening tool identify alcohol problems in women other than the pregnant women within the population? Why?

In health-promotion practice, nurses assess patterns and use their assessment to facilitate individuals' maintenance of well-being or their progression toward wellness. Health and illness within this context reflect changing patterns of the life process. For example, generally when disorganization or ineffective coping produce fluctuations in patterns that eventually result in illness, a treatment plan is designed to alleviate the symptoms or eliminate the illness altogether. The strategies used in this assessment process focus on identifying abnormalities. Conversely, health promotion aims to maintain effective coping strategies to prevent illness in the first place, therefore requiring different approaches to assessment and planning. One foundational concept in health promotion is strength or asset assessment. Using patterns of strength, according to Newman's theory of health as expanding consciousness, nurses should redirect the individual toward more harmonious patterns of health promotion (Bateman & Merryfeather, 2014). In practice the framework of holistic nursing is congruent with Newman's theory. Holistic nursing provides central unifying themes that connect pattern recognition to person-environment relationships for health promotion throughout the lifespan. Holism emerges from each of the holistic nursing core values of philosophy, caring process, communication, attunement, healing, cultural diversity, education, research, self-reflection, and self-caring (Dossey et al., 2016).

In the United States, *Healthy People 2020*, the national health-promotion initiative, establishes national goals and provides a framework for prevention (US Department of Health and Human Services, 2015). *Healthy People 2020* publishes national health objectives that identify the most significant preventable threats to health. Communities use these objectives and associated indicators to evaluate progress toward the overall goals of attaining high-quality longer lives, decreasing health disparity, and creating environments that promote health and improve the quality of life for all (US Department of Health and Human Services, 2015). *Healthy People 2020* added the following topics that were not part of the *Healthy People 2010* initiative:

- Adolescent health
- Blood disorders and blood safety
- Dementias, including Alzheimer disease
- Early and middle childhood
- Genomics
- Global health
- Health care–associated infections
- Health-related quality of life and well-being
- Lesbian, gay, bisexual, and transgender health
- Older adults
- Preparedness
- Sleep health
- Social determinants of health

Most of these new topics concern primary prevention for individuals in some way. Selected examples of how the *Healthy People 2020* (USDHHS, 2015) objectives address these primary prevention areas for individuals are presented in Box 6-1: *Healthy People 2020*. Furthermore, this initiative maintains current data to be used to evaluate regional efforts toward the national goals and for the nation to progress to a healthier status.

**BOX 6-1   HEALTHY PEOPLE 2020**

***Selected Examples of National Health-Promotion and Disease-Prevention Objectives for Individuals From* Healthy People 2020**

- **H-1**   Increase the proportion of adolescents who have had a wellness checkup in the past 12 months
- **AH-3.1**   Increase the proportion of adolescents who have an adult in their lives with whom they can talk about serious problems
- **AOCBC-10**   Reduce the proportion of adults with osteoporosis
- **EMC-2**   Increase the proportion of parents who use positive parenting and communicate with their physicians or other health care professionals about positive parenting
- **SDOH-1**   Increase the proportion of children aged 0 to 17 years living with at least one parent employed year-round, full-time
- **NWS-13**   Reduce household food insecurity and in doing so reduce hunger
- **SH-2**   Reduce the rate of vehicular crashes per 100 million miles traveled that are due to drowsy driving
- **SH-3**   Increase the proportion of students in grades 9 through 12 who get sufficient sleep
- **SH-4**   Increase the proportion of adults who get sufficient sleep
- **BDBS-1**   (Developmental) Increase the proportion of persons with hemoglobinopathies who receive recommended vaccinations
- **BDBS-6**   (Developmental) Increase the proportion of children with sickle cell disease who receive penicillin prophylaxis from 4 months to 5 years of age
- **G-1**   Increase the proportion of women with a family history of breast and/or ovarian cancer who receive genetic counseling
- **G-2**   (Developmental) Increase the proportion of persons with newly diagnosed colorectal cancer who receive genetic testing to identify Lynch syndrome (or familial colorectal cancer syndromes)
- **IID-1**   Reduce, eliminate, or maintain elimination of cases of vaccine-preventable diseases
- **OA-2**   Increase the proportion of older adults who are up to date on a core set of clinical preventive services
- **AHS-1**   Increase the proportion of persons with health insurance

From US Department of Health and Human Services. (2015). *2020 topics and objectives.* http://www.healthypeople.gov/2020/topics-objectives.

Long before this current focus on health promotion with the *Healthy People* initiatives in the United States, nursing theorists, such as Newman, Rogers, and Pharris, posited that nurses care for well individuals, as well as those who are ill (Bateman & Merryfeather, 2014). The International Council of Nurses (2015) defines nursing as encompassing the "autonomous and collaborative care of individuals of all ages, families, groups and communities, sick or well and in all settings. Nursing includes the promotion of health, prevention of illness, and the care of ill, disabled and dying people. Advocacy, promotion of a safe environment, research, participation in shaping health policy and in client centered care, health systems management, and education are also key nursing roles." This broad definition provides a foundation for nursing globally using the nursing process: assessment, diagnosis, outcome criteria, process criteria (including planned interventions), implementation, and evaluation. The nursing process, in turn, establishes a useful framework for the health-promotion assessment of the individual.

Nurses typically use assessment strategies including health promotion that address interactions among an individual's biophysical, psychosocial, and spiritual states and patterns with the environment. When assessing for primary prevention, the techniques also include generalized health promotion and specific protection from disease, both of which fall within the scope of nursing practice. The active process of promoting health involves protection (immunizations, occupational safety, and environmental control) along with lifestyle, value, and belief system behaviors that enhance health.

With health promotion serving as the underlying theme, this chapter addresses nursing assessment of individuals. In most areas of health care, tertiary care and prevention of further disease provide the assessment focus (Hopkins & Rippon, 2015). This tertiary care–focused assessment identifies deficits, thus excluding assessment of overall general health and wellness. Most nursing diagnoses approved by NANDA International (formerly the North American Nursing Diagnosis Association) are problem oriented. The NANDA International definition of **nursing diagnosis** includes life processes, as well as actual or potential health problems. One way to address nursing diagnoses in well individuals is to focus on human developmental or maturational tasks. Most approved nursing diagnoses reflect a focus on deficit assessment and problem-solving; however, these diagnoses include many life processes that provide the broad base needed for nursing to address strength-based healthy responses or potential for healthy responses (Paans et al., 2013). Furthermore, concentrating on strengths in the health-promotion setting provides a foundation to help individuals move toward improved health. Nurses support and enhance the ability of healthy individuals to maintain or strengthen their health.

Current US health care systems continue to use deficit assessment rather than the asset-based approach that is more appropriate for health-promotion settings. Mental health, social work, and nursing, however, embrace an asset-based approach to assessment within the health-promotion context. From using infant competencies to plan care and person-centered approaches for care of people with mental health disorders, nurses incorporate asset-based assessment into their diagnostic process (de Moura Quintana et al., 2014; Hopkins & Rippon, 2015; Thomé et al., 2014). Although NANDA International has stated that there is a need for work in this area of asset-based assessment and wellness, published material for using wellness diagnoses appears infrequently. The NANDA International taxonomy, however, uses multiple dimensions of human response in the consideration of each diagnosis. These seven dimensions include the status of the diagnosis that considers whether the diagnosis is addressing wellness, risk, or an actual problem (Gordon, 2016). More work is necessary to develop and promote useful language for health-promotion and wellness diagnoses.

Gordon's (2016) framework, which uses a **functional health patterns** assessment, provides the foundation for the construction of the NANDA International nursing diagnosis nomenclature. As NANDA International continues to develop diagnoses for health promotion, Gordon's framework will most likely continue to provide the foundation for these diagnoses. This same framework is used throughout this chapter to demonstrate assessment

| TABLE 6-1 | Aspects of a Nursing Assessment |
|---|---|
| **Definition** | **Deliberate and Systematic Data Collection** |
| Components | Subjective data:<br>    Health history, including subjective reports and<br>        individual perceptions<br>Objective data:<br>    Observations of nurse<br>    Physical examination findings<br>    Information from health record<br>    Results of clinical testing |
| Function | Description of person's health status |
| Structure | Organization of interdependent parts describing health, function, or patterns of behavior that reflect the whole individual and environment |
| Process | Interview, observation, and examination |
| Format | Systematic but flexible; individualized to each person, nurse, and situation |
| Goal | Nursing diagnosis or problem identification<br>Identification of areas of strengths, limitations, alterations, responses to alterations and therapies, and risks |

approaches, as well as family and community assessment (see Chapters 7 and 8). In addition, this chapter presents components of the nursing process as they relate to health promotion of the individual.

## GORDON'S FUNCTIONAL HEALTH PATTERNS: ASSESSMENT OF THE INDIVIDUAL

Nursing assessment determines the **health status** of individuals. Table 6-1 demonstrates aspects of a complete nursing assessment. Assessment, in this case, refers to collection of data that culminates in problem identification or a diagnostic statement. Effective health assessment considers not only physiological parameters but also how the human being interacts with the whole environment. Behavior patterns, beliefs, perceptions, and values form the essential components of health assessment when nurses consider the maximal health potential of the individual. Pattern recognition supports our understanding of health of individuals and is reflected in nursing theories such as those initially developed by nursing theorists such as Newman (Bateman & Merryfeather, 2014).

Historically, conceptual models in nursing have used Gordon's health-related behaviors particularly in regard to formulating a framework to guide assessment. The current expansion of electronic documentation from acute care to ambulatory settings requires continued emphasis on the standardization of language. (Doenges et al., 2013). Gordon's 11 functional health patterns interact to depict an individual's lifestyle. Using this framework, nurses combine assessment skills with subjective and objective data to construct patterns reflective of lifestyles.

## Functional Health Pattern Framework

Holism and the totality of the person's interactions with the environment form the philosophical foundations of Gordon's functional health patterns. This foundation provides a context for collecting data that provide information about the entire person and most life processes. By examining functional patterns and interactions among patterns, nurses accurately determine and diagnose actual or potential problems, intervene more effectively, and facilitate movement toward outcomes to promote health and well-being (Gordon, 2016). In addition to providing a framework to assess individuals, families, and communities holistically, functional health patterns provide a strong focus for more effective **nursing interventions** and outcomes. This stronger focus provides a solid position from which nurses participate as decision makers in health care systems at organizational, community, national, and international levels.

### Definition

Functional health patterns view the individual as a whole being using interrelated behavioral areas. The typology of 11 patterns serves as a useful tool to collect and organize assessment data and to create a structure for validation and communication among health care providers. Each pattern described in Table 6-2 forms part of the biopsychosocial-spiritual expression of the whole person. Individual reports and nursing observations provide data to differentiate patterns. As a framework for assessment, functional health patterns provide an effective means for nurses to perceive and record complex interactions of individuals' biophysical state, psychological makeup, and environmental relationships.

### Characteristics

Functional health patterns are characterized by their focus. Gordon (2016) uses five areas of focus: pattern, individual-environmental, age-developmental, functional, and cultural.

**Pattern focus** implies that the nurse explores patterns or sequences of behavior over time. Gordon's term *behavior* encompasses all forms of human behavior, including biophysical, psychological, and sociological elements. Pattern recognition, a cognitive process, occurs during information collection. Cues are identified and clustered while information is being gathered. Patterns emerge that represent historical and current behavior. Quantitative patterns such as blood pressure are readily identified, and pattern recognition is facilitated when baseline data are available. As the nurse incorporates a broader range of data, patterns imbedded within other patterns begin to emerge. Blood pressure, for example, is a pattern within both the activity pattern and the exercise pattern. Individual baseline and subsequent readings may present a pattern within expected norms. Erratic blood pressure measurements indicate an absence of pattern. Functional health pattern categories provide structures to analyze factors within a category (blood pressure: activity pattern) and to search for causal explanations, usually outside the category (excessive sodium intake: nutritional pattern) (Gordon, 2016).

The **individual-environmental focus** of Gordon's framework (2016) refers to environmental influences occurring within many

### TABLE 6-2   Typology of 11 Functional Health Patterns

| Pattern | Description |
| --- | --- |
| Health perception–health management pattern | Individual's perceived health and well-being and how health is managed |
| Nutritional-metabolic pattern | Food and fluid consumption relative to metabolic needs and indicators of local nutrient supply |
| Elimination pattern | Excretory function (bowel, bladder, and skin) |
| Activity-exercise pattern | Exercise, activity, leisure, and recreation |
| Sleep-rest pattern | Sleep, rest, and relaxation |
| Cognitive-perceptual pattern | Sensory, perceptual, and cognitive patterns |
| Self-perception–self-concept pattern | Self-concept pattern and perceptions of self (body comfort, body image, and feeling state); self-conception and self-esteem |
| Roles-relationships pattern | Role engagements and relationships |
| Sexuality-reproductive pattern | Person's satisfaction and dissatisfaction with sexuality and reproduction |
| Coping-stress tolerance pattern | General coping pattern and effectiveness in stress tolerance |
| Values-beliefs pattern | Values, beliefs (including spiritual), or goals that guide choices or decisions |

Modified from Gordon, M. (2016). *Manual of nursing diagnosis* (13th ed.). Sudbury, MA: Jones & Bartlett.

of the patterns. For example, environmental influences in the functional health pattern include role relationships, family values, and societal mores. Personal preference, knowledge of food preparation, and ability to consume and retain food govern the individual's intake. Cultural and family habits, financial ability to secure food, and crop availability also influence food intake. Additionally, the person who secures, prepares, and serves the food controls the nutritional intake for the family. Individuals' internal and external environments influence the health patterns in multiple ways.

Each pattern also reflects a human growth and **age-developmental focus** (Gordon, 2016). As individuals fulfill developmental tasks, complexity increases. These tasks, however, provide learning opportunities for individuals to maintain and improve their health. Erikson's framework, which organizes specific health tasks for individuals to accomplish at each developmental phase of the life cycle, continues to serve as a framework to assess and plan care (Kramp, 2014). Erikson's eight stages provide the traditional developmental assessment nurses generally use to plan care (Table 6-3). Each stage presents a central task or crisis that must be resolved before healthy growth can continue (Erikson, 1963). Individuals develop their sense of autonomy in early childhood and struggle with the sense of shame and doubt. When this developmental level is achieved or

**TABLE 6-3 Relationship Between Selected Developmental Tasks and Wellness Tasks for Each Stage of the Life Cycle**

| Erikson's Eight Life Stages | Havighurst's Developmental Tasks | Examples of Minimal Wellness Tasks for Each Developmental Stage |
|---|---|---|
| 1. Infancy (trust vs. basic mistrust) | Learning to walk<br>Learning to take solid foods<br>Learning to talk<br>Learning to control elimination of body waste | Acquiring ability to perform psychomotor skills<br>Learning functional definition of health<br>Learning social and emotional responsiveness to others and to the physical environment |
| 2. Early childhood (autonomy vs. shame and doubt) | Learning gender difference and sexual modesty<br>Achieving physiological stability<br>Forming simple concepts of social-physical reality<br>Learning to relate emotionally to parents, siblings, and others<br>Learning to distinguish right from wrong and developing a conscience<br>Learning physical skills necessary for ordinary games | Learning about proper foods, exercise, and sleep<br>Learning dental hygiene<br>Learning injury prevention (safety belts and helmets, sunscreen, smoke detectors, poisons, firearms, and swimming)<br>Refining psychomotor and cognitive skills |
| 3. Late childhood (initiative vs. guilt) | Building wholesome attitudes toward self as a growing organism<br>Learning to get along with peers | Developing self-concept<br>Learning attitudes of competition and cooperation with others<br>Learning social, ethical, and moral differences and responsibilities |
| 4. Early adolescence (industry vs. inferiority) | Learning appropriate gender identity: masculine or feminine role<br>Developing fundamental skills in reading, writing, and calculating<br>Developing concepts necessary for everyday living<br>Developing conscience, morality, and scale of values<br>Achieving personal independence<br>Developing attitudes toward social groups and institutions | Learning that health is an important value<br>Learning self-regulation of physiological needs—sleep, rest, food, drink, and exercise<br>Learning risk taking and its consequences (injury prevention) |
| 5. Adolescence (identity vs. role confusion) | Achieving new and maturer relations with peers and both genders<br>Achieving gender identity<br>Accepting physique and using body effectively<br>Achieving emotional independence of parents and other adults<br>Achieving assurance of economic independence<br>Selecting and preparing for occupation<br>Preparing for marriage and family life<br>Developing intellectual skills and concepts necessary for civic competence<br>Desiring and achieving socially responsible behavior | Learning economic responsibility<br>Learning social responsibility for self and others (preventing pregnancy and sexually transmitted diseases)<br>Experiencing social, emotional, and ethical commitments to others<br>Accepting self and physical development<br>Reconciling discrepancies between personal health concepts and observed health behaviors of others (use of alcohol, drugs, tobacco, firearms, and violence)<br>Learning to cope with life events and problems (suicide prevention)<br>Considering life goals and career plans and acquiring necessary skills to reach goals<br>Learning importance of time to self and world |
| 6. Early adulthood (intimacy vs. isolation) | Selecting and learning to live with a mate<br>Starting a family; managing a home<br>Taking on civic responsibility | Committing to mate and family responsibilities<br>Selecting a career<br>Incorporating health habits into lifestyle |
| 7. Middle adulthood (generativity vs. stagnation) | Accepting and adjusting to physiological changes<br>Achieving adult social responsibility<br>Maintaining economic standard of living<br>Assisting adolescent children | Accepting aging of self and others<br>Coping with societal pressures<br>Recognizing importance of good health habits<br>Reassessing life goals periodically |

**TABLE 6-3   Relationship Between Selected Developmental Tasks and Wellness Tasks for Each Stage of the Life Cycle—cont'd**

| Erikson's Eight Life Stages | Havighurst's Developmental Tasks | Examples of Minimal Wellness Tasks for Each Developmental Stage |
|---|---|---|
| 8. Maturity (ego integrity vs. despair) | Adjusting to decreasing physical strength and health<br>Adjusting to retirement and reduced income<br>Adjusting to death of spouse/life partner<br>Establishing an explicit affiliation with own age group<br>Establishing satisfactory physical living arrangements | Becoming aware of risks to health and adjusting lifestyle and habits to cope with risks<br>Adjusting to loss of job, income, and family and friends through death<br>Redefining self-concept<br>Adjusting to changes in personal time and new physical environment<br>Adjusting previous health habits to current physical and mental capabilities |

Sources Erikson, E. H. (1998). *The life cycle completed.* New York: W.W. Norton; Hockenberry, M. J., & Wilson, D. (2015). *Wong's nursing care of infants and children* (10th ed.). St Louis: Mosby; Osborn, K. S., Wraa, C. E., Watson, A. S., & Holleran, R. S. (2013). *Medical-surgical nursing.* New York: Pearson Higher Education; US Department of Health and Human Services, & Centers for Disease Control and Prevention. (2015). *The guide to community preventive services: What works to promote health.* http://thecommunityguide.org/about/index.html; US Department of Health and Human Services. (2015). *2020 topics and objectives.* http://www.healthypeople.gov/2020/topics-objectives; and Public Health Service Task Force on Community Preventive Services. (2005). *What works to promote health?* Atlanta, GA: Centers for Disease Control and Prevention.

resolved, the child moves on to develop initiative during the next stage.

Both age and developmental stage continue to provide the foundation for contemporary assessment of individuals' health status. Developmental tasks begin at birth and continue until death. By considering current epidemiological data and recommended health behaviors, Gordon's (2016) framework continues to be useful today for health promotion throughout the life span. Therefore in Unit 4 Gordon's framework is used to explore developmental tasks and their related health behaviors for health promotion.

**Functional focus** refers to an individual's performance level. Other disciplines plan care using functional patterns, but assessment data differ among disciplines (Stallinga et al., 2014). Physical therapists and occupational therapists, for example, focus on physical ability to perform activities of daily living and rely on assessments of independent ability to perform personal activities of daily living to develop their plans. For physicians, genitourinary function refers to frequency or voiding patterns and characteristics of urine, such as color, odor, and laboratory analysis results. In addition to these factors of genitourinary function, nurses assess how the particular voiding pattern affects lifestyle, particularly how urinary frequency affects sleep patterns and the ability to perform activities such as shopping or socializing. Additional concerns might include the individual's ability to walk or climb stairs to the bathroom or to manage these activities safely at night. It has been suggested that all health disciplines should use the *International Classification of Functioning, Disability and Health.* Relying on this classification could promote transdisciplinary communication about functional patterns when used along with the NANDA International taxonomy (Stallinga et al., 2014).

Culture, age, and developmental and gender norms, considered during assessment, influence development of health patterns.

Leininger defines transcultural nursing concepts of cultural care, health, well-being, and illness patterns in different environmental contexts and under different living conditions (Gordon, 2016). **Culturally competent care** is delivered with knowledge of and sensitivity to cultural factors influencing health behavior. Complex cultural patterns transmitted from former generations contribute to individuals' health behavior. Culturally competent care respects the underlying personal and cultural reality of individuals. Given that one may never be fully competent in cultures other than one's own culture, the term **cultural attunement** may be more descriptive of the aim. Nurses provide more culturally attuned care when they use cultural norms, values, communication, and time patterns in reflective practice (Andrews & Boyle, 2015). The nurse and the individual interact, and the nurse reflects on the interaction and resumes interaction, making changes on the basis of the self-reflection. For example, when one is tuning a piano, the pitch from the piano and that from the tuning fork must match. The tuning continues until the two sounds resonate. When individuals and nurses experience emotional and physiological resonance surrounding individuals' sociocultural contexts, such as race, ethnicity, religion, and sexual orientation, they resonate and achieve attunement (Pandit et al., 2014).

The concept of attunement is particularly valuable when nurses are caring for people of multiple cultures, such as in an urban setting (Niño et al., 2016). Even when the individual and the nurse share ethnic or racial backgrounds, their particular heritage may be quite different. For example, many different ethnic groups speak Spanish from different countries or provinces within a country (Spain, Mexico, Puerto Rico, Cuba, Columbia, etc.) but may have different colloquialisms within their speech and different cultural values and norms. A Spanish-speaking nurse of Mexican heritage may not be culturally competent in caring for a client from Spain. Asian clients will also have diverse languages and cultural values. Cultural attunement may be useful in these kinds of settings.

Functional health patterns form a framework that centers on health and can account for cultural factors. Most nursing assessments use functional pattern assessment as a foundation to their practice. Although nursing theoretical and conceptual frameworks differ, the functional health pattern framework is relevant to most conceptual models. In fact, functional health patterns provide the structure used by NANDA International to support nursing diagnosis nomenclature. Nursing classification of interventions and outcome nomenclature also use Gordon's functional patterns as a foundation (Gordon, 2016). The advantages of a functional health pattern framework specific to the practice of nursing include the following:

- It provides consistent nursing language through collecting, organizing, presenting, and analyzing data to determine nursing diagnoses.
- It allows flexibility to tailor content for individuals and situations.
- It suits diverse practice areas (e.g., home, clinic, institution) for assessment of individuals (adult/children), families, or communities.
- It supports theoretical components of nursing service, education, and research by organizing clinical knowledge using nursing diagnoses, interventions, and outcomes.
- It incorporates medical science data while retaining the focus on nursing knowledge and practice.

## The Patterns

Each pattern reflects a biopsychosocial spiritual expression of the individual's lifestyle or life processes from the perspective of both the individual and the nurse. This expression reveals the following elements: a pattern or sequencing of behaviors; the role of the environment (physical surroundings, family, societal, and cultural influences); and developmental influences. The assessment of each pattern includes its status as functional (strengths/wellness), dysfunctional (actual), or potentially dysfunctional (risk), as well as an indication of the individual's level of satisfaction with the pattern (Gordon, 2016). Nurses continue assessing in more depth to generate an explanation for the problem, to determine remedial actions to take, and to understand the perceived effect of these actions from the individual's perspective. An important goal when assessing each pattern is to determine the individual's knowledge of health promotion, the ability of the individual to manage health-promoting activities, and the value that the individual ascribes to health promotion with use of an asset-based approach to identify wellness diagnoses. Each pattern is presented in this chapter, with details for nurses to use to assess individuals and determine health-promotion diagnoses using a functional health pattern framework along with a discussion of nursing implications for use of the patterns in health-promotion practice.

## Health Perception–Health Management Pattern

The health perception–health management pattern involves individuals' health status and health practices used to reach the current level of health or wellness with a focus on perceived health status and meaning of health (Gordon, 2016). When eliciting this information, nurses discover areas for further exploration under other functional health patterns. For example, if the individual reports shortness of breath when mowing the lawn, the nurse stores this information for later retrieval when he or she is assessing activity and exercise patterns or cognitive-perceptual patterns.

Health perception–health management patterns affect lifestyle and ability to function even when individuals do not perceive actual health problems, are unaware of necessary health promotion in the absence of problems, do not feel capable of managing their health, or believe activity on their part is useless to promote health. Health-promoting activities (e.g., adequate nutrition, activity and exercise, sleep and rest), routine professional examinations, self-examinations, immunizations, and safety precautions (e.g., auto safety restraints and locked medicine cabinets) provide this pattern's clues to maintain optimal quality of life.

Assessment objectives for health perception–health management consist in obtaining data about perceptions, management, and preventive health practices (Gordon, 2016). Exploring values identifies potential health hazards, such as lack of adherence to a prescribed medical or nursing regimen or ability to manage health effectively. In addition to these kinds of assessment cues, nurses identify unrealistic health and illness perceptions and expectations. The transtheoretical model consists of five stages that can be useful in assessing an individual's readiness to change (see Chapter 10). These stages—precontemplation, contemplation, planning/preparation, action, and maintenance—have been used widely in health-promotion programs for diverse populations and multiple age groups with topics ranging from prevention of injury to nutrition-education programs (Doenges et al., 2013).

Assessment includes the following parameters:
- Health and safety practices of the individual
- Previous patterns of adherence or compliance
- Use of the health care system
- Knowledge of health service availability
- Health-seeking behavior patterns
- Means to access health care (e.g., financial resources, health insurance, and transportation)

In addition to methods of health management, nurses explore health perceptions as individuals describe their current health status, past problems, and anticipation of future problems associated with health or health care. These findings reveal beliefs about health, perceived susceptibility, self-efficacy, and level of knowledge of health status, taking into account the influence of culture (Andrews & Boyle, 2015) (Box 6-2: Diversity Awareness). Health and illness perceptions significantly influence overall direction for care planning. Health beliefs, also discussed in the section Values-Beliefs Pattern, directly impact participation in care. Partnership with providers and attunement is also more likely to yield better attention to self-care, particularly in cultures that value collective responsibility. In addition, individuals from cultures valuing collectivism are more likely to engage in self-care measures when their cultural patterns and social support within families are considered (Paek et al., 2014).

## BOX 6-2 DIVERSITY AWARENESS

### Health Perspectives for Emerging Majority Groups in the United States

| Group | TRADITIONAL DEFINITIONS | | TRADITIONAL METHODS | |
| --- | --- | --- | --- | --- |
| | Health | Illness | Maintain/Protect Health | Restore Health |
| American Indian and Alaska Native population | Total harmony with nature. Survive extremely challenging situations | Price paid for past/future. Details specific to nations. Results from presence of evil spirits. Contagious/generalized symptoms. Human body considered as whole, with harmony between origins and superficial structures. Integration within context of environment | Maintain positive relationship with nature. Treat body with respect. Purification acts using water/herbal remedies and rituals | Removal of external causative factor by traditional healer after special ceremony to determine cause. Drumming |
| Asian population | Total physical and spiritual harmony with universe. For the majority, religious traditions pose variations on cultural values. Examples include respect for life moderation; basic relationships balance between evil and good | Human body considered as whole with harmony between organs and superficial structures. Integration of human body within context of environment. Imbalance of yin and yang | Body is gift from parents/ancestors; must be protected. Dietary practices. Formal daily exercise (tai chi). Amulets (Chinese) | Acupuncture applying poultices. Cupping. Bleeding. Massage. Herbal remedies. Other products. Use physicians. Women treat women. Use of immunizations. Important to keep body intact (Chinese). Amulets |
| African population | Process/energy force rather than a state. Consists of body/mind/spirit harmony with nature. Older adults held in high esteem | Harmony; illness attributed to demons and evil spirits. Pain as sign of illness; if no pain, then illness is gone | Dietary practices. Rest; clean environment. Laxatives/cod liver oil taken internally; sulfur and molasses on back. Protective material of various substances (copper/silver/dried flesh); prayer | Voodoo and magic. Care for the entire community. Prayer. Use of healers. Pictures—Catholic saints/relics. Sugar and turpentine herbs, minerals, oral preparations, including hot water and lemon garlic, flannel with camphorated oil |
| Hispanic population | Gift from God | Imbalance in body; punishment for wrongdoing. Imbalance between hot and cold/wet and dry (definitions differ). Dislocation of body parts. Magic or supernatural causes such as evil | Maintain equilibrium in universe through behavior, diet, and work | Prayer, dietary practices of hot/cold magic/religious rituals, artifacts. Frequently in Catholic and Pentecostal traditions such as offerings, confession, candles, laying on of hands. Folk holistic healers using herbs, prayer, massage, social rapport, spiritual healing |

There is wide diversity among racial and ethnic groups. Cultural beliefs and language may be quite different from one group to another within the same race or ethnicity. For more information about these concepts see Richeson, J. A., & Sommers, S. R. (2016). Toward a social psychology of race and race relations for the twenty-first century. *Annual Review of Psychology, 67,* 439–463.

It is also important to assess health management practices. In a study about the influence of past health management practices on future health management in posttraumatic brain injury patients, Ulfarsson and colleagues (2014) demonstrated that past health management practices such as use of sick time and employment status influenced their posttraumatic brain injury health management. This study provides some support for the belief that if adherence to a prescribed regimen has not occurred in the past, future adherence is also unlikely. Nurses aim to identify and remedy the causes of the discrepancies between provider recommendations and the individual's implementation of those recommendations. For example, an individual with high blood pressure who has failed to keep follow-up appointments, not taken medication as prescribed, and eaten foods with high sodium content should be assessed to determine whether this evident nonadherence results from a conflict within the value system of the individual (health beliefs); inaccurate information; misunderstanding; inadequate ability to learn, retain, or retrieve information (knowledge deficit); denial of illness (health perception); or inability to access care and/or resources. Variables such as financial resources, transportation difficulties, nutritional preferences, daily activities (individual and family patterns), ability to read written instructions (literacy or visual acuity), and ability to manipulate numbers (numeracy) may affect the individual's behaviors.

## Nutritional-Metabolic Pattern

Nutritional-metabolic patterns center on nutrient intake relative to metabolic need (Gordon, 2016). These patterns include individuals' descriptions of food and fluid consumption (history), as well as evidence of adequate nutrition (physical examination). Nurses explore individuals' satisfaction with current eating and drinking patterns, including restrictions, and their perceptions of problems associated with eating and drinking, growth and development, skin condition, and attunement and healing processes.

Intake and supply of nutrients to tissues and organs influence bodily functions and interact with lifestyle. Sufficient food and fluid intake provides energy for performance, which includes both internal physiological functioning and external body movements. Interruption in acquisition or retention of food or fluids offsets balance and significantly alters lifestyle. In addition to individuals' nutrition and metabolism, genetic variation, specific genetic abnormalities, environmental influences, and prenatal nutrition also govern growth rates (Levitsky, 2016).

Assessment within this pattern includes data about typical patterns of food and fluid consumption and adequacy of consumption patterns, along with perceived problems associated with nutritional intake. Nurses attend to cues to conditions of overweight, underweight, overhydration, dehydration, or difficulties in skin integrity, such as breakdown or delayed healing. Individuals may also be at risk of developing these problems. Conversely, this pattern may exhibit assets or strengths that can be used to support the health-promotion plan.

The parameters for assessment for this pattern fall into two broad categories of evaluation: nutrient intake and metabolic demand. Intake may be assessed with a 24-hour recall of food and fluid consumption; a listing of dietary restrictions, food allergies, vitamin supplements, and caffeine and alcohol ingestion (when not included in the medication history); and a schedule of eating and drinking patterns. Assessment includes screening individuals for problems associated with swallowing or chewing.

With identified problems, focused assessments include food preferences, feelings about present weight, and eating habits. Intake may be affected when individuals eat alone. Frequent dining out may indicate the need for further exploration within the nutrition area or other functional patterns. Fast food consumption may be the predominant source of nutrients. Consumption patterns may be deficient in essential vitamins or minerals. Food security may also be explored. Who purchases food? Is shopping preplanned with a grocery list? Are financial resources and food budgets adequate? Is food stored properly? Who prepares food? How is food prepared (fried, broiled, steamed, boiled, or baked)?

Metabolic demands differ from individual to individual and vary within the same individual during times of illness, stress, growth, high- or low-activity levels, healing, or recovery. Developmental and environmental conditions alter metabolic demands. Appetite and reported changes in weight, skin integrity, attunement, and general healing ability are explored during the interview or health history. Individuals may also report decreased tolerances for hot or cold weather.

Nurses' observations and perceptions play a vital role when they are assessing nutritional and metabolic patterns. Physical examination allows assessment of both the nutrient supply to the tissues and the metabolic needs of the individual. Objective findings serve as indicators to validate subjective reports concerning nutrient intake. Gross metabolic indicators include temperature, height, and weight. Physical examination focuses on skin, bony prominences, dentition, hair, and mucous membranes. Skin and mucous membranes, in particular, use nutrients rapidly and provide excellent indices of nutritional adequacy. Skin assessment includes assessment of color, temperature, and turgor, and evaluation of any skin lesions, areas of dryness, scaliness, rashes, pruritus, or edema. Mucous membranes are examined for color, integrity, moisture, and lesions. Dentition is evaluated for structure. Are teeth erupted at normal stages of development? Are teeth firmly implanted? Do dentures fit properly? Additionally, decay and evidence of oral hygiene are evaluated. Healing is assessed when there is evidence of injury. The assessment may also include laboratory information such as levels of fasting glucose, lipids, blood urea nitrogen, creatinine, calcium, and vitamin D.

Although problem identification occurs after assessment of all 11 functional health patterns, a problem in any one area serves as a clue to dysfunction in others. Assessment of one pattern facilitates synthesis and analysis of data collected in other functional health patterns. Nutrition and metabolism influence patterns of health management, elimination, activity, sleep, cognition, roles, and stress tolerance. The values-beliefs pattern may significantly alter all other functional patterns. Sociocultural values and ethnic backgrounds play a major role in the determination of eating patterns. Other areas to consider include eating habits, food preferences, and patterns of nutrient supply and demand across the life span. Raw fruits and vegetables may be fun "finger food" for the toddler, but the older adult, especially one with loose dentures or arthritis of the temporomandibular joint, may find these foods intolerable. Older adults may also find gastrointestinal intolerances that develop over time and were not present in their youth.

A nutritional pattern focus emphasizes educational needs. Assessment aims to demonstrate strengths in functional patterns along with disclosing dysfunctional or potentially dysfunctional patterns. Nutritional health-promotion activities present a strength that provides impetus for similar activities in the other patterns. For example, if balanced nutritional intake improves functional level, individuals may extend their health-promoting behaviors to stress reduction or other behaviors. Understanding food/fluid intake and balance of body requirements helps individuals adjust caloric intake as growth slows to prevent overweight problems during the adult years.

## Elimination Pattern

Elimination patterns include those related to bowel, bladder, and skin function. Nurses determine regularity, quality, and quantity of stool through subjective reports about methods used to achieve regularity or control and any pattern changes or perceived problems. Perspiration quantity and quality determine excretory skin function (Gordon, 2016).

Elimination pattern significance differs from individual to individual. Many people view elimination patterns as a measure of health and as a sensitive indicator of proper nutrition and stress level. Individuals' perceptions determine whether patterns become problematic or dysfunctional. Misconceptions about regularity exist, particularly of bowel function, and self-treatment commonly occurs to correct perceived problems.

Elimination pattern dysfunction affects interpersonal interactions (Brito-Brito et al., 2014). Lack of control affects body image (self-perception), activity level, socialization, and sleep patterns. Age, developmental levels, and cultural considerations direct the interview. Pediatric assessment includes toilet training methods, whereas adult assessment may focus on regularity and patterns of dysfunction. In addition to constipation, older adults may begin to develop urinary control problems. Women past childbearing years often develop urinary stress incontinence.

Assessment includes data about regularity and control of excreta (Gordon, 2016). Nurses investigate cues suggesting constipation patterns, diarrhea, or incontinence through focused assessment. Elimination pattern changes, pain, discomfort, and perceived problems receive attention. Data collection includes exploration of the individual's explanation of the problem, methods of self-treatment, and perceived results (Gordon, 2016).

The quantity, quality (color, odor, and consistency), frequency, and regularity of stool, urine, and perspiration determine the direction of further exploration. Nurses assess excretory mode, time patterns, and control. Encouraging discussion aims to reveal more detailed information about pattern changes, perceived problems, and elimination habits. Examination includes gross screening of specimens, noting the amount, consistency, color, and odor. Skin assessment includes careful observation and description of wound/fistula drainage.

Transition from nutrition to elimination pattern assessment can occur seamlessly. Fluid intake affects elimination. Dietary fiber affects bowel elimination patterns. Skin integrity heralds concerns about urinary incontinence, leading to additional discussion of elimination patterns. Direct questions about laxatives may be necessary because of the availability of over-the-counter treatments for constipation (Bardsley, 2015). Discrepancies between dietary intake and reported bowel regularity indicate the need for further questioning (Lee, 2015). Laxative dependency in the form of oral supplements, suppositories, or enemas may indicate knowledge deficits in the area of bowel elimination. Health education about normal bowel function, nutritional guidelines to assist the individual in elimination, or implementation of an exercise program may significantly reduce elimination pattern dysfunction. Although overuse of laxatives is generally considered a solution older adults use to cope with constipation, young adults with bulimia and anorexia should also be assessed for laxative overuse, abuse, and dependency (Elran-Barak et al., 2014). Furthermore, nurses should explore this issue with parents of children who struggle with constipation. These parents may rely on excess use of stimulant laxatives for the effected child, resulting in chronic laxative use.

Urinary frequency and urinary tract infection (UTI) require health education as well. Several approaches to prevention of UTIs in women have some evidence to support their use (Harvard Women's Health Watch, 2015). Drinking 8 ounces of cranberry juice a day for 6 months to a year, low-dose prophylactic antibiotics, vaginally administered estrogen to promote growth of lactobacilli in postmenopausal women, and probiotic vaginal suppositories containing lactobacilli for premenopausal women have each been shown to be effective in preventing UTI in some women. Presenting symptoms of UTI in both men and women include urinary urgency, urinary frequency, and nocturnal polyuria. Research indicates that prolonged time between urinations is linked to UTIs (Harvard Women's Health Watch, 2015; Nazarko, 2015). Evidence-based practice guides the nurse in establishing a more suitable elimination routine for the individual.

## Activity-Exercise Pattern

The activity-exercise pattern centers on activity level, exercise program, and leisure activities. Parameters to explore include movement capability, activity tolerance, self-care abilities, use of assistive devices, changes in pattern, satisfaction with activity and exercise patterns, and any perceived problems (Gordon, 2016). Limitations in movement capabilities or ability to perform activities of daily living significantly alter lifestyle and may affect every other functional health pattern. Mobility and independent functioning in self-care are almost universally valued. Childrearing practices demonstrate this value: parents boast about their infant who walks early, their toilet-trained toddler, and their preschooler who dresses without assistance.

Activity-exercise patterns provide effective indicators for commitment to health promotion and prevention (Figure 6-1). Exercise's impact on health status has been extensively documented with increased public awareness. Overweight and obesity, linked to sedentary lifestyle, has reached epidemic proportions worldwide. More than 1.9 billion adults (39%) are overweight, with 13% of the world's population designated as obese (World Health Organization, 2015). The World Health Organization also regards 42 million children younger than 5 years as either overweight or obese. The obesity epidemic extends from developing countries with undernourished populations to industrialized nations. Worldwide obesity prevalence has doubled since 1980 (World Health Organization, 2015). Modifiable habits such as tobacco use, poor nutrition, and sedentary lifestyle contribute to half of preventable deaths globally (National Research Council & Institute of Medicine, 2015). Assessments, plans, and interventions to prevent obesity have a major impact on global health and health promotion in the United States.

Activity-exercise patterns also indicate energy expenditure and activity tolerance levels. Movement directly affects activities of daily living, along with control of the immediate environment. The environment contributes to mobility as well. For example, individuals living alone in high-crime areas may limit their activity for fear of harm. Factors such as inclement weather, distance from public transportation, lack of outdoor spaces, and negotiating stairways with a cane can also influence decisions about activity (Gebel, 2015; Oreskovic et al., 2015). Environmental barriers significantly impair exercise activity patterns for individuals with neuromuscular or perceptual disturbances. Moreover, leisure

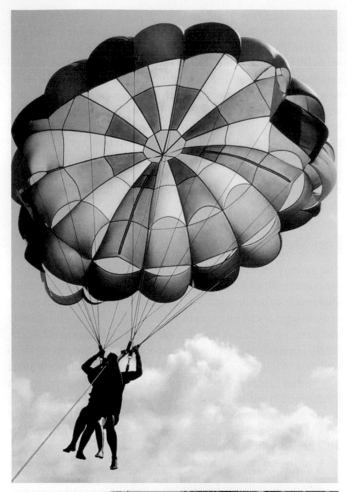

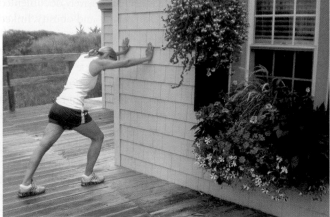

**FIGURE 6-1** Activity-exercise patterns provide effective indicators for commitment to health promotion and prevention.

activities provide clues to individuals' value systems (Sahlqvist et al., 2015). For example, work ethic, socioeconomic status, competitiveness, stage in career, and age influence how individuals perceive leisure and recreational activities.

The objective of assessment within the activity-exercise pattern is to determine the pattern of activities that require energy expenditure. The components reviewed are exercise, activity, leisure, and recreation (Gordon, 2016). The nurse seeks

clues to discover strengths and weaknesses within the pattern. Decreased energy levels, perceived problems, coping strategies, changes within the patterns, and associated explanations for these changes are all important clues that require further exploration. Generally, individuals with respiratory or cardiac disease warrant in-depth assessment, and focused assessment is indicated for individuals with neuromuscular, perceptual, or circulatory impairments.

The dimensions to be described and assessed within the activity-exercise pattern include daily activities, leisure activities, and exercise. Daily activities include occupation (position, hours of work or school, and amount of physical exercise versus cognitive or sedentary activities), self-care abilities (feeding, bathing, grooming, dressing, and toileting), and home-management routines (cooking, cleaning, shopping, laundry, and outdoor activities) (Gordon, 2016). Problems within any of these areas require explanation. Is it a problem of energy expenditure, mobility limitations, or decreased motivation caused by depression, grieving, or incongruent values?

Exercise parameters include the type, frequency, duration, and intensity of the individual's regular exercise. Nurses also assess the value the individual places on exercise as a part of determining their (i.e., the individual's) feelings about it. A 24-hour recall of the previous day's activities provides an initial picture of the pattern, whereas each major component addresses specific elements. Weekly logs provide follow-up assessment for suspected problems (Gordon, 2016). In addition to weekly logs, focused assessments include details about modes of transportation. Is a car used for transportation? If public transportation is used, how far away is the route? Are elevators or stairs used more often? Factors interfering with exercise or mobility include dyspnea, fatigue, muscle cramping, neuromuscular or perceptual deficits, chest pain, and angina. As with other patterns, feelings of satisfaction and perception of problems provide valuable indications of dysfunctional or potentially dysfunctional patterns.

Nurses evaluate subjective complaints, such as dyspnea, noting an individual's difficulty with breathing during the interview and physical examination. Examination includes objective circulatory, respiratory, and neuromuscular indicators. Assessment also includes skin color, skin temperature, apical heart rate, radial heart rate, and blood pressure, as well as respiratory rate, rhythm, depth of inspiration, and effort involved. Gait, posture, and balance are evaluated during ambulation. Muscle tone, strength, coordination, and range of motion provide useful clues to validate reports of activity and exercise. Assistive devices or prostheses are evaluated for proper use, proper fit, and degree of assistance or support provided.

Information obtained during the interview is linked closely to the examination findings. Examination alone may not disclose the invaluable subjective reports of early morning pain and joint stiffness. When appropriate, the nurse may ask the individual to climb stairs or perform self-care activities under observation to assess impairment. Direct observation validates assessment findings and is a valuable technique used by health care educators and home health nurses to evaluate adequate performance of self-care activities, such as dressing, cooking, and insulin administration. Various instruments have been designed to quantify the level of ability or disability. For some individuals, a metabolic activity index, in which each activity is measured according to kilocalories of energy expended per minute, helps to quantify assessment results and plan care.

Developmental norms have been established for infants and toddlers. Milestones such as sitting, crawling, walking, running, and hopping determine a child's development and should be screened in children with use of standardized screening instruments (Tonelli et al., 2016). Careful assessment of ability, limitations, and interests helps to guide the nurse in a more holistic assessment. Problem identification is reserved for the conclusion of the assessment after all 11 patterns have been constructed. Useful clues within a pattern lead into other pattern areas; however, premature closure of a topic during the examination is avoided. At this point, only tentative diagnoses are possible. Often explanations of problems lie in other functional health patterns. For example, when the individual expresses an inability to perform exercise on a routine basis, barriers may be discovered in another pattern. Barriers may be associated with knowledge deficit, the personal or family value system, overriding priorities, or low value placed on exercise. Is the inability to perform activities a result of general fatigue caused by inadequate or decreased sleep time associated with anxiety, nocturia, pain, or an infant waking every 3 hours for feeding? Are responsibilities associated with caring for several preschoolers and inadequate financial resources to secure a babysitter the cause? The assessment's purpose is to narrow the number of possible explanations.

## Sleep-Rest Pattern

Perhaps the single most important factor assessed in the sleep-rest pattern is the perception of adequacy of sleep and relaxation. Subjective reports of fatigue or energy levels provide some indication of the individual's satisfaction. People make assumptions about the roles that sleep and rest play in preparing the individual for required or desired daily activities. This pattern becomes extremely important when sleep and rest are perceived as insufficient. Sleep serves a restorative function in most individuals. Sleep deprivation studies provide vivid demonstrations of the need for different types of sleep: light, deep, dream, and rapid eye movement sleep. Again, problems within this pattern may cause problems in other patterns. A person who has difficulty with sleep may be tense and irritable, unable to tolerate stress, more prone to infectious processes, and incapable of making health-promoting relationships. Appetite alterations, elimination difficulties, and activity intolerance may occur (Luyster et al., 2015). Some degree of cognitive dysfunction generally occurs as well.

The objective when the nurse is assessing the sleep-rest pattern is to describe the effectiveness of the pattern from the individual's perspective (Gordon, 2016). Wide variation in sleep time (from 4 hours to more than 10 hours) does not necessarily affect functional performance; different individuals require different amounts of sleep. Difficulty experienced with sleep onset, sleep interruptions, and awakening are areas of assessment to consider. The nurse also evaluates disturbances such as dreaming and nightmares, sleepwalking, nocturnal enuresis, and penile tumescence. Counseling, institution of safety measures, or medical referral may be necessary. In addition to sleep, the nurse assesses rest and relaxation according to the individual's perceptions. Activities of the sedentary isolate type, such as reading or crocheting, may be relaxing for some individuals. Passive involvement, as with television viewing, may provide the only source of relaxation for the individual. Daily naps or relaxation exercises (meditation, yoga, or breathing exercises) may also be a part of this pattern.

Assessment parameters of the sleep dimension are divided into two parts: sleep quality and sleep quantity. Sleep quality includes the individual's perception of sleep adequacy, performance level, and physical and psychological state on awakening. Sleep quantity, in addition to focusing on the hours slept each day, is used to build a schedule of sleep times. The nurse assesses the individual for regularity of the time of retiring, time of awakening, and additional periods of sleep throughout the day. Sleep onset, the number of awakenings, and the reasons for awakening provide clues to problems. The dimensions of rest and relaxation include the parameters of the type, frequency or regularity, and duration. The perceived effectiveness of methods used to promote rest is also assessed.

When problems exist, focused assessment that evaluates efficiency of sleep compared with actual sleeping time is warranted. Individuals are conditioned to sleep under certain circumstances, and maintaining bedtime rituals is a distinct advantage in sleep promotion. A person who expects to sleep will usually sleep if such routines are maintained. Nurses assess schedule and routine changes associated with bedtime. When assessing bedtime routines, rituals along with other aids to sleep, such as natural aids (warm milk) or medications (prescription and nonprescription), should be explored. Physical examination includes general appearance, behavior, and performance changes. As with pain, sleep is a subjective experience. Comprehensive examination, which is beyond the scope of this chapter, may be performed, including polysomnography when indicated. Research indicates that subjective reporting of sleep quality and measures of sleep time closely approximate electroencephalographic findings.

Nursing care focuses on the need to identify evidence of sleep disturbances to design appropriate interventions before sleep deprivation occurs. Frequent awakenings do not necessarily imply sleep interruption. Many individuals awaken numerous times during the night but return to sleep within seconds. These awakenings occur in older adults, who generally spend most of the night in stages of light sleep. The normal developmental pattern of aging does not include deep sleep; therefore awakenings may not affect the sleep cycles. Older individuals, however, more often have trouble returning to sleep because they experience discomfort or anxiety. Biological rhythm and peak performance time may be helpful to the nurse when he or she is planning health education and return visits. Individuals commonly refer to themselves as morning people or night owls; therefore patterns of retiring and arising provide clues. Patterns of sleep and rest in conjunction with subjective reports of physical and mental well-being help determine appropriate interventions.

## Cognitive-Perceptual Pattern

Cognitive patterns include the ability of the individual to understand and follow directions, retain information, make decisions, solve problems, and use language appropriately. Auditory, visual, olfactory, gustatory, tactile, and kinesthetic sensations and perceptions determine perceptual and sensory patterns. Pain perception and tolerance are analyzed within this pattern area (Gordon, 2016). Capacity for independent functioning is considered a major role of thinking and perceiving. Compensation for cognitive-perceptual difficulties ensures safety. Health requires a balance between the individual and the environment. Decreased levels of cognition or perception require increased levels of environmental control. For example, mentally-impaired or sensory-impaired individuals may require sheltered work environments and supervised group living arrangements.

Interrelationships among the individual, the developmental stage, and the environment contribute to several patterns. For example, the behavior patterns of a 20-year-old high school "dropout" who works in a factory may differ from those of a 20-year-old second-year premedical student. Developmental stage plays a role in cognitive and perceptual abilities as well. Vision and hearing achieve full potential when children reach school age, with 20/30 vision considered normal in preschoolers. Developmental stage determines the ability to solve problems and conceptualize as described by the theorist Piaget (2003). As adults mature, visual acuity and the senses of hearing, touch, and even taste decline. Cognitive function must be evaluated within the context of the environment (Gordon, 2016). Environmental complexity results in different levels of functioning.

Assessing cognitive-perceptual patterns includes evaluating language capabilities, cognitive skills, and perception related to desired or required activities (Gordon, 2016). Nurses address clues indicating potential problems, particularly sensory deficits, sensory deprivation or overload, and ineffective pain management. Cognitive dysfunction may cause impaired reasoning, impaired judgment, or knowledge deficits related to health practices, as well as memory deficits.

Assessment parameters include hearing and vision test results. Changes in sensation or perception should be noted. In addition to decreased ability or acuity with regard to hearing, vision, smell, and taste, evaluation includes other perceptual disturbances, such as vertigo; increased or decreased sensitivity to heat, cold, or light touch; and visual or auditory hallucinations or illusions. Use and perceived effectiveness of assistive devices, such as hearing aids, eyeglasses, and contact lenses, is also noted.

Discomfort and pain are evaluated further. Useful tools that use pain scales have been designed to record and quantify changes in pain perception (Cunha Batalha et al., 2015). The location, type, degree, and duration of pain provide indicators of possible causes or sources. Relief measures to control pain and their effectiveness both provide data as well as a focus for health education. Attitudes toward pain should be considered. For example, someone may fear that medication is a sign of weakness or that it will result in a loss of independence. A pharmacological approach may be complemented with nonpharmacological strategies, such as heat or cold applications, distraction (music, reading, television), guided imagery, music therapy, and structured relaxation techniques (Cunha Batalha et al., 2015; Malcolm, 2015). For all individuals, exploring tolerance to pain is appropriate, using questions such as "Do you feel you are particularly sensitive to pain?" and "What level of pain is associated with your (cut, sprain, broken bone, or labor contractions)?"

Other areas of cognitive patterning to be explored include educational level, recent memory changes, ease or difficulty in learning, and preferred method of learning. Even when no problems are apparent or suspected, the nurse may assess these areas in more detail to determine areas of strength for use with health teaching plans.

Objective data are accumulated throughout the interview or assessment process. This data collection begins with the nurse's perception of the individual's general appearance: hygiene and grooming, proper use of clothing, neatness and appropriateness of dress, and indication that these are appropriate to the individual's developmental stage. Language and vocabulary use, the ability to convey an idea with words or with actions when speech is impaired or not yet developed, and grammatical correctness provide clues to cognitive functioning. Amplitude and quality of speech, affect and mood, as well as attention and concentration are all indicative of the individual's mental status. For many individuals, this information is sufficient to relay a sense of the level of understanding, memory, and mentation. Problem-solving abilities can usually be determined when the individual is asked to relate any perceived problems, provide an explanation of the problems and/or actions taken to solve the problems, and describe the results of the actions taken. Because this is a basic assessment in each functional health pattern, the nurse already has an idea of whether thought processes are logical, coherent, and relevant for this individual.

When problems within the cognitive realm do not surface, the information is recorded as part of the objective data or findings of the physical examination. The data to be noted include language; vocabulary; attention span; grasp of ideas; level of consciousness; orientation to person, place, and time; language spoken (whether primary or secondary); and behavior during the data collection process, including posture, facial expression, and general body movements.

When a problem is apparent or suspected based on age, hereditary factors, or inconsistencies in the assessment data, a focused assessment is essential. Coma scales or functional dementia scales may be appropriate. More commonly, a Folstein Mini–Mental Status Examination (MMSE) is performed to assess orientation, attention, calculation, language (ability to name objects, repeat abstract ideas, and follow commands), and recall (immediate, short-term, and long-term memory). Abilities to read, write, and copy designs can also be assessed (see Chapter 24). The examination of a sensory-perceptual pattern evaluates hearing, vision, and areas of pain at a screening level; comprehensive examinations are available and may be indicated. A full neurological assessment is warranted when specific sensory deficits are identified during the examination.

Although completing these assessment areas may seem overwhelming, the time required is generally less than that in most other pattern areas, perhaps because more information relevant to the cognitive-perceptual patterns becomes available as each pattern is assessed. Transition into the cognitive-perceptual pattern from other patterns may be facilitated by referring to a problem already described, with a question such as "Do you generally find it easy to solve problems effectively?" The self-perception pattern follows the cognitive pattern particularly well because mental status measures include feelings and perceptions of the individual regarding self. Mood, affect, and responses to the interviewer, such as eye contact, are indications of self-esteem. Cognitive-perceptual ability greatly influences the ability to function (self-care) or manipulate (activity and exercise) within the environment.

The placement of each of the patterns in a sequence suitable to each nurse, individual, or situation has been discussed. When the cognitive-perceptual pattern is dysfunctional, however, the individual is most likely unreliable as the historian; therefore it is wise to consider this pattern early in the assessment process. Approaching this pattern early saves valuable time and permits the identification of patterns that can be assessed more reliably.

Every person has experienced temporary memory lapses at one time or another. These events alone are not a sufficient basis for judgments. Sequencing of behaviors and clustering of appropriate signals (defining characteristics) are necessary to determine any nursing diagnosis. Equally important is the need to assess all pattern areas before data analysis and problem identification.

Cognitive and sensory ability data guide the nurse in planning care, which is especially apparent in health teaching. Formulation of health teaching plans ideally reflects each individual's preferred method of learning. The effective plan considers the individual's demonstrated developmental level; the ability to store information, retrieve information, and compensate for deficits; and also the neuromuscular and sensory levels necessary for skills development. An individually tailored plan contains mutually developed goals and short-term objectives. Although self-care might be an outcome for any person in whom diabetes mellitus has been newly diagnosed, the behaviors expected of an adult with diabetes will differ from those expected of a child.

## Self-Perception–Self-Concept Pattern

The self-perception–self-concept pattern encompasses the sense of each individual's personal identity, goals, emotional patterns, and feelings about the self. Self-image and sense of worth both stem from the individual's perception of personal appearance, competencies, and limitations, including the individual's self-perception and others' perceptions. The nurse assesses physical, verbal, and nonverbal cues (Gordon, 2016).

The significance of the sense of self to the whole person is best exemplified by personal experiences. Individuals who feel good about their self worth look and act differently from those who feel unable to accomplish anything worthwhile. Self-concept changes may affect patterns of eating, sleeping, and activity.

The individual's developmental level affects and is affected by this pattern. One of the tasks identified during the later phases of Erikson's developmental framework, described previously, is

building wholesome self-esteem. Delays in self-esteem and self-concept development affect progress toward subsequent tasks (Blakely-McClure & Ostrov, 2016) (see Table 6-3).

Family climate and relationship patterns provide the environmental impact that influences the self-concept pattern (see Chapter 7). People who are closely associated with the individual affect that person's self-esteem. Most people care about what others think of them; therefore the support of significant others affects the self-perception–self-concept pattern (Tranväg et al., 2015; Philips, 2015) (Figure 6-2).

The assessment objective in this pattern area is to describe each individual's patterns and beliefs about general self-worth and feeling states (Gordon, 2016). The nurse looks for clues that indicate identity confusion, altered body image, disturbances in self-esteem, and feelings of powerlessness. Nurses often identify anxiety, fear, and depression states that are responsive to nursing interventions (Webb et al., 2015).

The nurse notes the general appearance and effect of each individual, which may have been assessed as part of a formal mental status examination. Low self-esteem may be indicated by head and shoulder flexion, lack of eye contact, and mumbled or slurred speech. Anxiety or nervousness might be revealed through extraneous body movements such as foot shuffling or tapping, facial tension or grimace, rapid speech, voice quivering, twitches or tremors, and general restlessness or shifts in body position. Any of these indicators demands further exploration to determine underlying problems for each individual.

Self-concept influences each individual's interaction with others. In their study of 74 graduating college students, Wilt and colleagues (2016) linked meaning in life (MIL) to psychosocial functioning and self-concept at a time when the participants were embarking on a major life transition. The concept of MIL

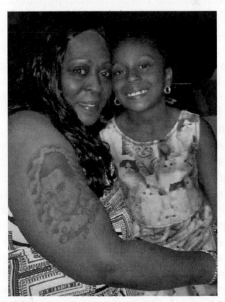

**FIGURE 6-2** Most people care about what others think of them; therefore the support of significant others, such as a grandmother supporting a student grandchild, affects their self-perception–self-concept pattern.

incorporates the belief that life is comprehensible and existence is important. Participants in this study who interacted with their family and friends had a higher level of MIL than those participants who experienced graduation and academic life without such interactions (Wilt et al., 2016).

Because the information in this pattern is personal, sharing the information may actually facilitate the process of goal setting and intervention planning when the nurse possesses strong communication skills and a caring attitude.

## Roles-Relationships Pattern

The roles-relationships pattern describes the position assumed and the associations engaged in by the individual that are connected to that position. The individual's perception is a major component of the assessment, and exploration of the pattern includes each individual's level of satisfaction with roles and relationships.

The need for relationships with other people is universal. Dossey and colleagues (2016) have identified basic needs for communication, fellowship, and love in high-level wellness. The ability to communicate with other people in a meaningful way greatly affects the whole person. The understanding of health as the harmonious balance between the individual and the environment indicates the major role that relationships with others play in health. Developmental hypotheses about readiness propose that attainment of each stage is required to progress to the next stage. For example, a person can become immersed in a relationship of genuine intimacy only after self-identity has stabilized. Developmental tasks that promote family development have also been identified similarly by Duvall and Miller as noted by Gilbert (2015) (see Chapter 7). The emphasis within these models is on the individual's relationships within the nuclear family.

The objective of the roles-relationships pattern assessment is to describe an individual's pattern of family and shared circumstances, with the associated responsibilities. The individual's perception of satisfaction with the established relationship contributes to this assessment. Loss, change, and threat produce the major problems within this pattern. Clues indicative of impaired verbal communication, social isolation, alterations in parenting, independence-dependence conflicts, dysfunctional grieving, and potential for violence are pertinent.

Assessment focuses on family, work, and community roles and relationships. Within the family, assessment parameters include the family structure, tasks performed, social support systems, and other dynamics, such as decision-making, power, authority, division of labor, and communication patterns. Parenting or marital difficulties and family violence issues are explored. The roles of student and employee are explored to determine specific occupation or position, along with work responsibilities and work environment. Parameters such as stress, safety, and health factors should be included (see the case study and the care plan at the end of this chapter). Financial concerns, job security, and retirement plans are elicited. Activity-rest patterns elicit information about time commitments, leisure activities, and physical exercise; therefore the assessment at this point addresses the impact of these factors on the roles-relationships pattern. Community roles and relationships indicate involvement within the neighborhood and other social groups, such as the level of socialization and the amount of social support available. Within all three components (family, work or school, and community) the individual is asked to describe the level of satisfaction with the roles and relationships.

Threat of change, actual change, and loss are areas to be explored further. In addition, family or work roles alone may not cause stress, but combining them may cause difficulties, as with the working mother or traveling husband and father.

Objective data for assessment within this pattern are usually unavailable unless the nurse makes a home visit or sees the individual in the company of significant others in some other capacity. Family interaction and communication patterns are noted whenever possible. Cognizant of meaningful relationships within the family, the nurse identifies potential problems, such as those that occur with the college student away from home, the individual who travels or moves frequently, and sole family survivors when older adults outlive their family members and friends (Gilbert, 2015). The relationships among the functional health patterns are clearly apparent in light of the developmental stages. Difficulties within the self-concept pattern and difficulties with relationships often appear together (Thomé et al., 2014). Relationships affect the whole person; therefore problems in the roles-relationships pattern may be exhibited in other areas, such as sleep, appetite, and sexuality.

## Sexuality-Reproductive Pattern

The sexuality-reproductive pattern describes the individual's sexual self-concept, sexual functioning, methods of intimacy, and reproductive areas. Data collection combines subjective information, nursing observations, and physical examination. Normal development and perceived satisfaction combine to provide the elements of this pattern (Gordon, 2016).

Sexuality is the behavioral expression of sexual identity. The importance of this pattern area to the individual's life and health is closely related to the self-perception and the relationships patterns. Body image, self-concept, and role and gender identity are linked to sexual identity. This concept of sexual self and the individual's relationships pattern indicate the level and the perceived satisfaction of sexual functioning. Sexual functioning involves, but is not limited to, sexual relations with a partner. Reproductive patterns are equally significant to this pattern assessment, the whole individual, and the family and community (see Chapters 7 and 8).

As discussed, individual development influences reproductive capacities; these include genotype, secondary sex characteristics, genital development, phenotype, ego integrity, and the family life-cycle stage (Gilbert, 2015). The environment also plays a part in expression of the sexuality-reproductive pattern. Cultural and family norms may contribute to the expression of sexuality and combine with other factors, such as the family's financial stability, to influence reproductive patterns (Sutherland et al., 2015). Norms within society may create issues in expressions of sexuality.

During the assessment process, nurses consider the continuum of sexual identity expression, including heterosexuality, bisexuality, and transgender, gay, or lesbian sexuality. The information gathered guides the health-promotion plan in those who inquire about their sexual identity. Cochran and colleagues (2016) indicate that sexual orientation influences the risk of death in their analysis of National Health and Nutrition Examination Survey data. Heterosexual participants ($n = 14,521$) were more likely to experience lower death risk than their nonheterosexual counterparts ($n = 1045$). These findings were consistent with the view that sexual orientation–related health disadvantages create this disparity in death risk. Nurses should remain informed about sexual orientation health disadvantages, such as mental distress, tobacco use, binge drinking, and lack of health insurance.

One objective of assessment in this pattern is to describe behavioral problems or difficulties (Gordon, 2016). Equally important is assessing the individual's knowledge of sexual functioning and preventive health practices, such as breast and testicular self-examination, Papanicolaou tests, effective contraceptive use, and avoidance of infection. Clues are evaluated for potential or actual sexual dysfunction.

The following parameters are assessed: sexual self-concept, which may be derived from information collected in the self-perception–self-concept and the roles-relationships patterns; sexual functioning, with the nurse noting evidence of some form of intimacy, the level of sexual activity or libido, and the effect of health or illness on sexual expression; and reproductive patterns, in which the nurse collects data pertinent to health-promotion factors, such as feelings related to aging, preventive practices, and knowledge of sexual functioning. For women, reproductive pattern assessment would also include information about menstruation, such as onset, duration, and frequency, date of last menstrual period, discomfort, and menopause, as well as information about reproductive stage, such as pregnancy history and birth control methods.

The level of satisfaction with sexual self-concept, sexual functioning, and reproduction is also explored. Difficulties such as ineffective or inappropriate sexual performance, discharges, infections, venereal disease, discomfort, and history of abuse are evaluated. Focused assessment to collect additional information is warranted with sexual dysfunction or trauma. Physical examination evaluates genital development and secondary sex characteristics. Signs of intimacy between partners, such as holding hands and hugging, are noted.

People may feel threatened by discussion of topics in this pattern; the depth of exploration is governed in part by the individual's wishes. Dialogue is encouraged but may be postponed until a firm and trusting relationship is established. A clear representation of the individual's knowledge and use of preventive practices facilitates planning for health promotion. Although sex education is usually associated with school programs, information and discussion about sexuality is just as important for adults of all ages. Sex education is a key element of parenthood classes. Improved understanding of sexuality and sexual function leads to discovery and increased satisfaction.

## Coping–Stress Tolerance Pattern

Gordon (2016) describes the coping–stress tolerance pattern as a depiction of general coping and the individual's ability to effectively manage stress. This pattern includes the individual's ability to process life crises and to resist disruptive factors that will influence self-integrity of ego, mode of conflict resolution, stress management, and accessibility to necessary resources (Box 6-3: Quality and Safety Scenario).

The ability to manage stress effectively in life is a learned behavior. Stress is a necessary part of life; without it there is no motivation to grow. Vulnerability to stress may be linked to individuals' coping strategies, such as avoidance behavior (Gorka et al., 2016). Stress is exacerbated by accumulation of minor irritations. Stress is inherent not in the event but in the individual's perception of that event. Whereas one individual may experience stress from missing a bus and can think only of being 10 minutes late, another will consider the same event an opportunity to spend 10 minutes reading the newspaper. This difference in perception may represent the different values used to identify sources of stress or it may represent coping strategies.

For purposes of assessing this pattern, coping, which is considered the individual behavioral response to stress, includes both problem-solving ability and use of defense mechanisms. Coping is viewed not as a single act but as a process incorporating many behaviors. The function of coping is to deal with the threat or emotional distress of an event. Coping effectiveness is assessed from the individual's perspective and from the nurse's observation of the individual's ability to function in the presence of actual or potential stressors in the environment.

The perception of stress and the ability to manage it depend on personal development, the amount of stress previously

---

### ☑ BOX 6-3 QUALITY AND SAFETY SCENARIO

Improving the quality of health promotion was explored in four primary health centers in Australia. These centers served Australian Indigenous people. The researchers aimed to describe the scope and quality of health-promotion activities and introduce health-promotion interventions. The findings suggest that quality-improvement projects can improve the delivery of evidence-based health promotion by engaging front-line health practitioners in redesign of systems. In addition to medical care, primary health centers that have health promotion as a core function should also deliver counseling, preventive medicine, health education and promotion, rehabilitative services, antenatal and postnatal care, and maternal and child care programs. Often organizational support for such core functions is inadequate. This study attempted to engage the centers in a systems approach to quality improvement to address the organizational components that hindered health-promotion delivery. The researchers used an iterative action research strategy to explore current practice, introduce best practices, and engage physicians, nurses, Aboriginal health workers, and administrative staff in the action plan to redesign health-promotion delivery systems within the four primary health centers.

From Percival, N., O'Donoghue, L., Lin, V., Tsey, K., & Bailie, R. S. (2016). Improving health promotion using quality improvement techniques in Australian Indigenous primary health care. *Frontiers in Public Health, 4*, 53.

experienced, the current level of stress within the environment, and the sources of social support. For example, an older adult may experience many stresses during life and manage them effectively, but now coping may no longer be possible because too many stressors are present, such as physical incapacitation, fixed income, fear of illness or injury, and lack of transportation (Bielderman et al., 2015; Boehm et al., 2015). In addition, this person may no longer have a social support system, which has been associated with promotion of health. Determining individuals' stress tolerance and past coping patterns becomes the objective of assessment for this functional pattern. Clues to difficulties in managing past and current stressors and changes in the effectiveness of a coping pattern help to determine personal coping capacity.

The following assessment parameters are included: the coping task, including the physical, psychological, and socioeconomic stimuli with which the individual must cope; coping style, or the tendency to use a specific style, such as approach oriented, avoidance oriented, or nonspecific; coping strategies, including specifics; and coping effectiveness. Coping strategy may be divided into information seeking, direct action (fight or flight), inhibition of action, or use of social support. Individual resources include the variety of coping mechanisms used by the individual, the flexibility of these mechanisms, and the health-promotion value associated with each of them. For example, in their study of problem-solving intervention with 166 stroke rehabilitation clients, Visser and colleagues (2016) report that their problem-solving intervention improved task-oriented coping and general health-related quality of life. However psychosocial health-related quality of life associated specifically with stroke in their sample did not seem to improve.

Stress tolerance patterns elicit the amount of stress effectively processed in the past. Use of anticipatory coping is assessed along with whether the individual knows how to cope, but does not cope (production deficit), or simply does not know how to cope (skill deficit). Other indicators of value within this pattern are discussed in the section Self-Perception–Self-Concept Pattern. Objective data of concern include physical signs of restlessness, irritability, and nervousness, such as increased heart rate, blood pressure, and perspiration. Evidence of coping ability and tolerance to stress are found in every other functional health pattern. Stress also affects the other patterns, thereby resulting in health problems such as insomnia, weight loss, and poor concentration (Dossey et al., 2016; Gordon, 2016).

Health can be promoted through early intervention to reduce stress. Coping patterns and stress tolerance in the past may uncover unhealthy coping behavior, such as smoking and alcohol consumption, that needs to be replaced by alternative coping strategies. Stress-reduction workshops would be helpful for most of the population because the future undoubtedly holds stressful events, some of which may be overwhelming without coping strategies. Box 6-4: Innovative Practice includes information about a unique company that offers stress-management interventions. Dossey and colleagues (2016) offer categories for stress management: social engineering strategies, such as time management or planned change; personality engineering strategies, such as assertiveness training or cognitive rehearsal; and altered states

---

## BOX 6-4 INNOVATIVE PRACTICE
### The Humor Potential Inc.

The Humor Potential, Inc., is a company that provides resources, products, and seminars for stress management with the use of humor. Company president Loretta LaRoche is a recognized expert on stress management, emphasizing the importance of balancing daily living experiences with humor. The Humor Potential offers seminars and lectures to health care professionals, schools, corporations, other organizations, and the general public. The company also produces television programs that have been televised nationally in the United States. One television program, *The Joy of Stress*, was nominated for a regional Emmy Award.

Books, prints, audiotapes and videotapes, and other products dealing with humor can be purchased from Loretta LaRoche's website. The collection consists of audiotapes and videotapes that have been developed for corporate meetings and training. An example is *Lighten Up!* This is a videotape and action guide that increases productivity by reducing stress. A catalog is available for e-mail, fax, phone, and mail orders.

**Contact information:**
The Humor Potential Inc.
Corporate Offices
50 Court Street
Plymouth, MA 02360
Website: www.lorettalaroche.com
Telephone: 800-99-TADAH (800-998-2324)

Based on data from the Humor Potential Inc. (http://www. lorettalaroche.com).

---

of consciousness, such as meditation or relaxation. Planning based on the assessment of all functional health patterns to help determine a coping pattern should include these kinds of strategies.

## Values-Beliefs Pattern

The values-beliefs pattern describes values, including the individual's spiritual values, beliefs, and goals. This pattern also includes perceptions of what is right, what is good, and conflicts that beliefs or values impart. Each of the 11 patterns addresses the value systems of individuals, their family, and society. Individual beliefs or values develop over time and govern life through personal experiences and family and societal influences (Boehm et al., 2015; Bielderman et al., 2015). The objective in assessing this pattern is to determine the basis for health-related decisions and actions (Gordon, 2016). Individuals engage in preventive health behavior when a threat to wellness or health status exists. Several other health belief models expand on this concept by including other motivations, such as personal values and environmental influences. Clues to conflict within the individual's value system or between the person's value system and that of the family or society are explored.

The dimensions of assessment include the individual's values, beliefs, or goals that guide choices or decisions that are related to health. The nurse collects information while exploring each pattern, while summarizing, clarifying, and securing additional information. Specifically, values and beliefs about self, relationships, and society are appraised. Individuals' beliefs, goals, and purposes of life are reviewed, along with any conflicts, perceived philosophies, and philosophies of the family, culture, and society. Sources of strength, such as a higher being or significant individual practices, are explored, including religious beliefs and preferences. Past goals and expectations are assessed through the individual's satisfaction. The nurse must identify the individual's goals and expectations concerning health, clarifying them to help the individual achieve them. To be effective, health-promotion interventions are based on the individual's value system and health beliefs (Dossey et al., 2016). The brevity of this discussion is not an indication of the importance that the values-beliefs pattern plays in the assessment of the individual. Individual values play a role in all the patterns.

## INDIVIDUAL HEALTH PROMOTION THROUGH THE NURSING PROCESS

The nursing process—the systematic approach to reduce or eliminate the individual's health problem—is accomplished in several steps, the first being the collection of necessary data. With the individual, the nurse analyzes the data, identifies a nursing diagnosis, projects outcomes, prescribes interventions, and evaluates effectiveness. Reassessment, reordering of priorities, new goal setting, and revising the plan continue as part of the process toward outcome attainment (Carpenito-Moyet, 2012).

### Collection and Analysis of Data

Assessment is a systematic technique for learning as much as possible about the individual. The main purpose in collecting data from a new individual is to see whether health problems exist and to identify the individual's health goals. Data collection includes biographical data, such as age, sex, and the purpose of the visit. This process is followed by assessment of the previously outlined 11 functional health patterns. Subjective reporting, nursing observations and perceptions, and the physical examination findings are assessed and recorded. The remaining discussion focuses on nursing diagnosis.

### Problem Identification

As the concept of problem identification evolved, most nurses have distinguished *nursing diagnosis* as the most useful label. Diagnosis is a careful examination and analysis of the facts to provide a basis for nursing intervention. Nursing diagnosis is the naming of individual, family, and community responses to actual or potential health problems or life processes (Gordon, 2016; NANDA International, 2011). Nursing diagnoses provide the basis for selection of nursing interventions to achieve outcomes for which the nurse is accountable (Gordon, 2016). Leadership from NANDA International has provided standardization of the descriptions of human responses that nurses manage. The most recent revision of this taxonomy has been approved for clinical testing and has been endorsed by the American Nurses Association (ANA) (NANDA International, 2011). Although Wang and colleagues (2015) describe issues associated with the use of the NANDA International taxonomy, such as inadequacy of terms to describe complex nursing care and nurses' reluctance to incorporate these diagnoses into their documentation language,

the NANDA International taxonomy remains the most widely used standardized language for nursing diagnoses.

Gordon (2016) proposes the accepted format of nursing diagnosis that lists the problem, cause, and signs and symptoms, or defining characteristics, for each diagnosis accepted for clinical testing. The NANDA International taxonomy uses a multiaxial framework for nursing diagnoses, including diagnostic concept (e.g., parenting), acuity (e.g., altered), unit of care (e.g., individual), developmental stage (e.g., adolescent), potentiality (e.g., at risk of), and descriptor, for creation of the diagnostic statement (NANDA International, 2011). Box 6-5: Research for Evidence-Based Practice discusses how this nursing classification system compares with a nonnursing system.

In discussions of problems, the meaning of the problem must be clearly defined and identified. The concept as used in this text refers to Gordon's (2016) proposition that a health problem is defined as a dysfunctional pattern and that nursing's major contribution to health care is in preventing and treating such a pattern. A pattern is dysfunctional when it represents a deviation from established norms or from the individual's previous condition or goals. (Normative behavior is further discussed in Unit 4.) A dysfunctional pattern is a problem when it generates therapeutic concern on the part of the individual, others, or the nurse and when it is amenable to nursing therapies.

As patterns are assessed, the nurse proposes several hypotheses regarding functional or dysfunctional labeling. At the completion

---

### BOX 6-5  RESEARCH FOR EVIDENCE-BASED PRACTICE

Evidence-based strategies should be used to promote individuals' health. Adolescent sexual health promotion efforts may be inaccessible and lack confidentiality. Multiple interrelated risks develop among adolescents, requiring multifaceted health-promotion strategies. Champion and colleagues (2016) aimed to explore these issues in their study exploring psychological distress, violence, and substance use among African American ($n = 94$) and Mexican American ($n = 465$) adolescent women with a history of risky sexual behavior. These adolescent women self-reported psychological distress, sexual risk behavior, sexually transmitted infection (STI), personal and friend/peer substance use, alcohol use, and violence. Substance-using friends, physical violence, and STI were highly associated with personal substance use in these adolescent women. Alcohol users were five times more likely than nonalcohol users to use other substances.

Adolescents in this study self-reported adverse sexual health outcomes, including initial and repeated unplanned pregnancies, HIV infection, and other STIs. Predictors of substance use in these women were ethnicity, friend substance use, physical violence history, STI history, and history of alcohol use. Nurses should consider social determinants, including demographic, educational, environmental, and behavioral components, in their assessment of specific adolescent populations such as ethnic minority females. The authors recommend that nurses integrate these complex health disparities into their health-promotion practice. They aim for their findings to guide health-promotion strategies in primary care settings for women experiencing multiple health disparities.

From Champion, J. D., Young, C., & Rew, L. (2016). Substantiating the need for primary care–based sexual health promotion interventions for ethnic minority adolescent women experiencing health disparities. *Journal of the American Association of Nurse Practitioners, 28*(9), 487–492.

of the assessment, conclusions must be drawn. The possibility exists that all patterns are functional, that some are functional, and that others are dysfunctional or potentially dysfunctional. Functional refers to wellness and optimal health. Dysfunctional patterns, indicating some health problems, may be present in the absence of disease; that is, nursing care may be needed for health promotion and health maintenance, not health restoration. The case history of Frank Thompson in Chapter 1 effectively illustrates the multiple nursing care needs of an individual who is not ill. In potentially dysfunctional patterns, sufficient evidence exists or enough **risk factors** are present to indicate that a pattern dysfunction will likely occur if interventions are not made. Early identification of potential problems is possible through systematic data collection and analysis.

## Contributing Etiological Factors

To plan care the nurse must first determine what has caused the actual or potential health problem: its contributing etiological factors. The etiological factors of most dysfunctional patterns lie within another pattern or patterns. Although cause is never an absolute within human sciences, the projection of outcomes or goals must be based on probable causes. Interventions then focus on mediating or resolving the probable causes. Most often, many factors are involved, and problems are said to relate to rather than be a result of these factors. Potential problems are not actual problems but risk states; therefore they have no specific cause and are identified when risk factors are present. Nursing intervention is directed toward risk reduction through education (classes or brochures) to improve nutrition, prevent accidents, and so forth. Risk estimate theory and potential health problems are developed further in Chapters 7 and 8 and Unit 4.

## Diagnostic Variables

The ability to arrive at an accurate diagnosis, even when comprehensive data are unavailable, is governed primarily by the nurse's clinical knowledge. Experience improves the effectiveness when nursing is performed as a scientific process. Nursing requires the gathering of information, interpreting it based on normative values, organizing and grouping information on the basis of healthy findings, identifying the problem, and then planning appropriate goals and interventions. Difficulties are encountered when there are no available norms that occur frequently in the psychosocial assessment components. Use of the 11 interdependent functional health patterns helps to solve these difficulties. By focusing on each of these areas, nurses find it easier to recognize whether a problem does or does not exist. Any change within the pattern may be a sign of dysfunction or an unhealthy but stabilized behavior. For example, a sign of dysfunction might be a 2-year-old child who is still not walking; developmental growth is a major factor in activity patterns of infants, toddlers, and children.

The use of physiological parameters clearly demonstrates the idea of a stabilized dysfunctional pattern, but equal attention must be given to psychological development. For instance, a 26-year-old man who lives with his mother and gives no indication of independent decision-making should be evaluated. It should be apparent that assessment information primarily comes from the initial contact with the individual and the database, which is generally the case in health-promotion activities. However, in any acute situation or emergency, quick assessment of the major problems is given high priority on a hierarchy-of-needs basis, and the full nursing assessment is postponed temporarily. For further understanding of the nursing diagnosis, the nurse is referred to those authors who discuss the development of diagnoses, the diagnostic process, and specific details of each accepted diagnosis (Carpenito-Moyet, 2012; Gordon, 2016; NANDA International, 2011).

## Planning the Care

In the nursing process, planning is the proposal of diagnosis-specific treatment to assist the individual toward the goal, or expected outcome, of optimal health. The individual's goals and the determined nursing diagnosis provide the basis for planning. Clear goals and diagnoses are critical to development of an effective plan of care. The nursing process identifies the following purposes of the planning phase: to assign priority to the problems diagnosed; to specify the behavioral outcomes or goals with the individual, including the expected time of achievement; to differentiate individual problems that can be resolved by nursing intervention, those that can be handled by the individual or family member, and those that should be handled with or referred to other members of the health team; to designate specific actions, the frequency of these actions, and the short-term, intermediate-term, and long-term results; and to list the individual's problems (nursing diagnosis) and nursing actions (frequency and **expected outcomes,** or goals) on the nursing care plan or blueprint for action (Carpenito-Moyet, 2012). This plan provides the direction for individual and nursing activities and is the guide for the evaluation. There are many research studies involving outcomes from which nurses can draw to increase the effectiveness of the care they provide.

## Implementing the Plan

Implementation consists of the actions necessary to fulfill the goals for optimal health; it is the enactment of the nursing care plan to elicit the behaviors described in the proposed individual outcome. The selection of a nursing intervention depends on several factors: the desired individual outcome, the characteristics of the nursing diagnosis, the research base associated with the intervention, the feasibility of implementing the intervention, the acceptability of the intervention to the individual, and the capability of the nurse (Carpenito-Moyet, 2012). A nursing interventions classification is being developed. As discussed in Unit 1, a critical component of effective communication is the accurate interpretation of the individual's information. This feedback process continues throughout all phases of the nursing process; the nurse continues to collect data to modify the plan as needed and does not blindly implement the care plan. As discussed in Unit 3, the most frequently used nursing interventions in health promotion are screening, education, counseling, and crisis intervention. All these interventions require strong communication abilities from the nurse. Checklists and screening instruments may be used to document nursing assessment and help to ensure transmission of reliable and quality information for client-centered care. Implementation requires transdisciplinary collaboration in the analysis and plan. Computerized data entry, information systems, and electronic medical records may facilitate communication; however, ongoing interaction with other health care providers is essential for collaboration.

## Evaluating the Plan

The process of analyzing changes experienced by the individual occurs in the evaluation phase of the nursing process, with the nurse examining the relationships between nursing actions and the individual's goal achievement. The nursing process emphasizes that evaluation is always considered in terms of how the individual responds to the plan of action (Osborn et al., 2013). As discussed, the nursing diagnosis (or health problems) and the goal (or expected outcome) guide the evaluation of the nursing care plan. Many variables influence outcomes: the interventions prescribed by the health care providers, the health care providers themselves, the environment in which the care is received, motivation, the individual's genetic structure, and the individual's significant others (Box 6-6: Genomics). The task for nursing is to define which outcomes are sensitive to nursing care so as to identify the expected and attainable results of nursing care for each individual (NANDA International, 2011). Families and clients are partners in the process of client-centered care (Spruce, 2015). Documentation of all components of the nursing process in the individual's health care record is then performed (Osborn et al., 2013).

---

### ⚕ BOX 6-6  GENOMICS

The *Healthy People 2020* genomics goal to improve health and prevent harm through valid and useful genomic tools in clinical and public health practices has two associated objectives, both of which are linked to health promotion assessment of the individual.

**G-1**  Increase the proportion of women with a family history of breast and/or ovarian cancer who receive genetic counseling

Women with a family history of breast and/or ovarian cancer face multiple decisions that encompass both a cognitive and an emotional component. Risk estimates, disease course, family/reproductive plans, potential interventions, and timelines should be discussed. Open dialogue should include numerical risk, past experiences with cancer and deaths in the family, whether the women has children, anxiety, depression, and general risk aversion. Treatment option discussion should include the types of breast cancers that develop in *BRCA1* and *BRCA2* carriers, the role of age at diagnosis, surgery, risk-reducing medications, surveillance, and surgical options (mastectomy and salpingo-oopherectomy). Information presented clearly with time and emotional support as decisions are made is essential. The efficacy of risk-reducing mastectomy has been supported in large-scale studies; however, the efficacy and side effects of salpingo-oopherectomy are less well established. Moreover, physical and psychosexual adverse effects may accompany these approaches. A genetic counselor who specializes in these disorders is the preferred provider to provide individualized care based on the specific gene mutation.

**G-2**  (Developmental) Increase the proportion of persons with newly diagnosed colorectal cancer who receive genetic testing to identify Lynch syndrome (or familial colorectal cancer syndromes)

Two to four percent of all colorectal cancers (CRCs) are associated with the autosomal dominant disorder Lynch syndrome. Additionally, individuals with Lynch syndrome have a 50% to 80% lifetime risk of developing CRC. The criteria (Amsterdam II) to determine which individuals should be screened for Lynch syndrome include:

- three biological relatives with CRC or another Lynch-associated cancer (endometrial, ovarian, upper urinary tract, small bowel) who are linked through a first-degree relative;
- at least two consecutive generations affected;
- one cancer diagnosis when younger than 50 years.

Individuals who meet the criteria but choose to forego genetic screening should receive aggressive surveillance with colonoscopy every 1 to 2 years starting at the age of 20 to 25 years. Failure to identify at-risk individuals is common, and aggressive screening is often not completed.

One potential barrier is provider lack of knowledge regarding recommended screening guidelines. Nurses who promote health should be aware of these screening criteria.

From Hartmann, L. C., & Lindor, N. M. (2016). The role of risk-reducing surgery in hereditary breast and ovarian cancer. *New England Journal of Medicine, 374*(5), 454-468; Patel, S. G., Ahnen, D. J., Kinney, A. Y., Horick, N., Finkelstein, D. M., Hill, D. A., et al. (2016). Knowledge and uptake of genetic counseling and colonoscopic screening among individuals at increased risk for Lynch syndrome and their endoscopists from the Family Health Promotion Project. *The American Journal of Gastroenterology, 111*(2), 285-293.

---

## CASE STUDY

### *Spiritual Distress: Cindy*

Cindy is a single 28-year-old woman. Cindy studies nursing and shares an apartment with two friends. She was having increasing difficulties with her course work and was placed on academic probation. Cindy became concerned about the effect of stress on her ability to finish her studies and on her future career. She grew increasingly nervous and began to ask, "Will I ever be okay?" and "Will I ever be able to finish school and function as a nurse?" Cindy expressed her fear of weakness and feelings of isolation, loneliness, helplessness, and loss of control. These feelings began to find expression in anger related to this major life disruption. She verbalized her anger at God for allowing this to happen to her. Her incapacity deprived her of her normal outlets for expressing and finding support for such concerns. Cindy was unable to participate in the practices of her faith, in which she had previously found strength in facing life's challenges. Her inability to concentrate and her growing feeling of lethargy added to her frustration. Expressing these fears and concerns was difficult for Cindy. The nurse, however, developed a trusting relationship with Cindy, permitting her to express her fears, anxieties, and concerns. Based on the nurse's assessment, the nursing diagnosis of spiritual distress was formulated.

#### Reflective Questions

- What differential diagnoses should the nurse consider?
- Describe other individuals you know who have experienced spiritual distress.

## ⊙ CARE PLAN

### *Spiritual Distress: Cindy*

**\*NURSING DIAGNOSIS: Spiritual distress related to a threat to well-being, loss of meaningful role, and separation from religious and family ties**

**Defining Characteristics**
- Experiences a disturbance in the belief system.
- Demonstrates discouragement or despair.
- Chooses not to practice religious rituals.
- Shows emotional detachment from self and others.
- Expresses concern, anger, resentment, and fear, related to a major life disruption.

**Related Factors**
- Threat to well-being from change in role as a student and fear of failure
- Loss of meaningful role as a student
- Separation from religious and family ties

**Expected Outcomes**
- Person will verbalize a greater sense of purpose, meaning, and hope.
- Person will express feelings of anger verbally and will discuss anger with another person.

**Interventions**
- Take time to be present and available to listen to the individual.
- Convey a nonjudgmental attitude.
- Encourage the individual to verbalize feelings.
- Pray with the individual as indicated.
- Engage the individual in values clarification.
- Encourage the individual to acknowledge feelings of anger and to acknowledge and name any other feelings experienced.
- Reassure the individual that it is acceptable to feel anger toward a supreme being.
- Encourage honest dialogue with a peer whom the individual trusts.
- Offer consultation with an appropriate spiritual advisor.
- Inform the individual of religious resources.

\*NANDA Nursing Diagnoses—Herdman, T. H. & Kamitsuru, S. (Eds.). Nursing Diagnoses—Definitions and Classification 2015–2017. Copyright © 2014, 1994–2014 NANDA International. Used by arrangement with John Wiley & Sons Limited. In order to make safe and effective judgments using the NANDA-I nursing diagnoses it is essential that nurses refer to the definitions and defining characteristics of the diagnoses listed in this work.

## SUMMARY

Data relevant to the health-promotion activities of the individual focus primarily on the assessment of the current health status so that the nurse can identify problem areas, or areas of dysfunction, within the individual's health and lifestyle pattern. This process is a fundamental first step and precedes all other components of the nursing process. Without a clear picture of the problem, nursing activities are fruitless. Gordon's (2016) functional health pattern framework provides guidance for the individual assessment. The focus of each pattern includes the age-developmental influences exerted, cultural and environmental roles played, functional ability displayed, and behavioral patterns specific to each individual. The interaction between internal mechanisms and the environment is assessed through these 11 functional health patterns. When assessing each pattern, the nurse must understand the pattern definition, the significance of the pattern to the whole individual, the developmental influences, the environmental role, the assessment objectives, the assessment parameters and indicators, and the nursing implications. Assessment is essential to all components of the nursing process in health promotion for the individual.

## ⓔ EVOLVE CHAPTER FEATURES

http://evolve.elsevier.com/Edelman/
- Study Questions

## REFERENCES

Andrews, M. M., & Boyle, J. S. (2015). *Transcultural concepts in nursing care* (7th ed.). New York: Wolters Kluwer.

Bardsley, A. (2015). Approaches to managing chronic constipation in older people within the community setting. *British Journal of Community Nursing, 20*(9), 444–450.

Bateman, G. C., & Merryfeather, L. (2014). Newman's theory of health as expanding consciousness: A personal evolution. *Nursing Science Quarterly, 27*(1), 57–61.

Bax, A. C., Geurtz, C. D., & Ballachova, T. N. (2015). Improving recognition of children affected by prenatal alcohol exposure: Detection of exposure in pediatric care. *Current Developmental Disorders Reports, 2*(3), 165–174.

Bielderman, A., et al. (2015). Understanding how older adults living in deprived neighbourhoods address aging issues. *British Journal of Community Nursing, 20*(8), 394–399.

Blakely-McClure, S. J., & Ostrov, J. M. (2016). Relational aggression, victimization and self-concept: Testing pathways from middle childhood to adolescence. *Journal of Youth and Adolescence, 45*(2), 376–390.

Boehm, J. K., et al. (2015). Unequally distributed psychological assets: Are there social disparities in optimism, life satisfaction and positive affect? *PLoS ONE, 10*(2), e0118066.

Brito-Brito, P. R., et al. (2014). Case study: Community nursing care plan for an elderly patient with urinary incontinence and social interaction problems after prostatectomy. *Journal of Nursing Knowledge, 25*(1), 62–65.

Carpenito-Moyet, L. J. (2012). *Nursing diagnosis: Application to clinical practice* (14th ed.). Philadelphia: Lippincott Williams & Wilkins.

Cochran, S. D., Bjorkenstam, C., & Mays, V. M. (2016). Sexual orientation and all-cause mortality among adults aged 18 to 59 years, 2001-2011. *American Journal of Public Health, 106*(5), 918–920. doi:10.2105/AJPH.2016.303052.

Cunha Batalha, L. M., et al. (2015). Pain assessment in children with cancer: A systematic review. *Revista De Enfermagem Referéncia,* (5), 119–127.

de Moura Quintana, J., et al. (2014). Use of the Classification of Functioning, Disability and Health for elderly care. *Revista De Enfermagem Referéncia*, 4(1), 141–148.

Doenges, M. E., Moorhouse, M. F., & Murr, A. C. (2013). *Nursing diagnosis manual: Planning, individualizing and documenting client care* (4th ed.). Philadelphia: F.A. Davis.

Dossey, B. M., Keegan, L., & Guzzetta, C. E. (2016). *Holistic nursing: A handbook for practice* (7th ed.). Boston: Jones & Bartlett.

Elran-Barak, R., et al. (2014). Eating patterns in youth with restricting and binge eating/purging type anorexia nervosa. *Journal of Eating Disorders*, 47(8), 878–883.

Erikson, E. H. (1963). *Childhood and society*. New York: Norton.

Gebel, K. (2015). Improving current practice in reviews of the built environment and physical activity. *Sports Medicine*, 45(3), 297.

Gilbert, P. (2015). When it hurts: Too young or too old. *The Journal of Nursing Care*, 4(228). doi:10.4172/2167-1168.1000228.

Gordon, M. (2016). *Manual of nursing diagnosis* (13th ed.). Sudbury, MA: Jones & Bartlett.

Gorka, A. X., LaBar, K. S., & Hariri, A. R. (2016). Variability in emotional responsiveness and coping style during active avoidance as a window onto psychological vulnerability to stress. *Physiology & Behavior*, 158, 90–99.

Harvard Women's Health Watch. (2015). When urinary tract infections keep coming back. *Harvard Women's Health Watch*, 23(1), 5.

Hopkins, T., & Rippon, S. (2015). *Head, hands and heart: Asset-based approaches in health care*. London: The Health Foundation.

International Council of Nurses. (2015). Definition of nursing. http://www.icn.ch/who-we-are/icn-definition-of-nursing/.

Kramp, G. (2014). Symbolic loss in American adolescents: Mourning in teenage cinema. *Journal of Religion & Health*, 53(2), 363–372.

Lee, A. (2015). Combating the causes of constipation. *Nursing & Residential Care*, 17(6), 327–331.

Levitsky, L. L. (2016). Nutrition and growth–a multitude of manifestations and room for further investigation. *Current Opinion in Endocrinology, Diabetes and Obesity*, 23(1), 48–50.

Luyster, F. S., et al. (2015). Screening and evaluation tools for sleep disorders in older adults. *Applied Nursing Research*, 28(4), 334–340.

Malcolm, C. (2015). Acute pain management in the older person. *Journal of Perioperative Practice*, 25(7/8), 134–139.

NANDA International (2011). *Nursing diagnoses: Definitions and classifications* (9th ed., pp. 2012–2014). Oxford: Wiley-Blackwell.

National Research Council, & Institute of Medicine (2015). *Measuring the risks and causes of premature death: Summary of workshops*. Washington, DC: The National Academies Press.

Nazarko, L. (2015). Solve the case: Urinary frequency and recurrent urinary tract symptoms. *Nurse Prescribing*, 13(9), 458–463.

Niño, A., Kissil, K., & Davey, M. P. (2016). Strategies used by foreign born family therapists to connect across cultural differences: A thematic analysis. *Journal of Marital and Family Therapy*, 42(1), 123–138.

Oreskovic, N. M., et al. (2015). Adolescents' use of the build environment for physical activity. *BMC Public Health*, 15(1), 1596–1603.

Osborn, K. S., et al. (2013). *Medical-surgical nursing* (2nd ed.). New York: Pearson Higher Education.

Paans, W., Müller-Staub, M., & Nieweg, R. (2013). The influence of the use of diagnostic resources on nurses' communication with simulated patients during admission interviews. *The Journal of Nursing Knowledge*, 24(2), 101–107.

Paek, H., Lee, H., & Hove, T. (2014). The role of collectivism orientation in differential normative mechanisms: A cross-national study of anti-smoking public service announcement effectiveness. *Asian Journal of Social Psychology*, 17(3), 173–183.

Pandit, M. L., et al. (2014). Practicing socio-cultural attunement: A study of couple therapists. *Contemporary Family Therapy*, 36(4), 518–528.

Philips, A. (2015). Diabetes and relationships: How couples manage diabetes. *Practice Nursing*, 26(6), 298–301.

Piaget, J. (2003). *The psychology of intelligence*. London: Taylor and Francis.

Sahlqvist, S., et al. (2015). Mechanisms underpinning use of new walking and cycling infrastructure in different contexts: Mixed-method analysis. *International Journal of Behavioral Nutrition and Physical Activity*, 12(24). doi:10.1186/s12966-015-0185-5.

Spruce, L. (2015). Back to basics: Patient and family engagement. *AORN Journal*, 102(1), 33–39.

Stallinga, H. A., et al. (2014). Functioning assessment vs. conventional medical assessment: A comparative study on health professionals' clinical decision-making and the fit with patient's own perspective of health. *Journal of Clinical Nursing*, 23(7-8), 1044–1054.

Sutherland, S. E., et al. (2015). Understanding the phenomenon of sexual desire discrepancy in couples. *Canadian Journal of Human Sexuality*, 24(2), 141–150.

Thomé, E. S., et al. (2014). Applicability of the NANDA International and Nursing Interventions Classification taxonomies to mental health nursing practice. *Journal of Nursing Knowledge*, 25(3), 168–172.

Tonelli, M., et al. (2016). Recommendations on screening for developmental delay. *Canadian Medical Association Journal*. doi:10.1503/cmaj.151437.

Tranväg, O., Petersen, K. A., & Näden, D. (2015). Relational interactions preserving dignity experience. *Nursing Ethics*, 22(5), 577–593.

Ulfarsson, T., et al. (2014). A history of unemployment or sick leave influences long-term functioning and health-related quality-of-life after severe traumatic brain injury. *Brain Injury*, 28(3), 328–335.

US Department of Health and Human Services (USDHHS). (2015). 2020 topics and objectives. http://www.healthypeople.gov/2020/topics-objectives.

Visser, M. M., et al. (2016). Problem-solving therapy during outpatient stroke rehabilitation improves coping and health-related quality of life randomized controlled trial. *Stroke; a Journal of Cerebral Circulation*, 47(1), 135–142.

Wang, N., Yu, P., & Hailey, D. (2015). The quality of paper-based versus electronic nursing care plan in Australian aged care homes: A documentation audit study. *International Journal of Medical Informatics*, 84(8), 561–569.

Webb, J. B., et al. (2015). Assessing positive body image: Contemporary approaches and future directions. *Body Image*, 4(6), 130–145.

Wilt, J., Bleidorn, W., & Revelle, W. (2016). Finding a life worth living: Meaning in life and graduation from college. *European Journal of Personality*, 30(2), 158–167.

World Health Organization. (2015). Global strategy on diet, physical activity, and health. http://www.who.int/mediacentre/factsheets/fs311/en/.

# 7

# Health Promotion and the Family

*Anne Rath Rentfro*

 **THINK ABOUT IT**

### Caring for Older Adults

*Adult family members, who may have health problems of their own, find themselves caring for their older adult parents as well as grandchildren. Increased life expectancies combined with increased age at the birth of the first child present adults with the caring for older parents along with young children (Suh, 2016). This population, known as the sandwich generation, is expected to become more prevalent in the coming years. An increasing number of parents of children older than 18 years provide financial support or care for grandchildren younger than 18 years along with caring for an older parent aged more than 65 years (Suh, 2016).*

- What are the implications of this growing situation for individuals? For families? For communities? For the nation?
- How will this trend affect individual lives personally and professionally?
- How does multigenerational caring affect family finances?

A family consists of a group of interacting individuals related by blood, marriage, cohabitation, or adoption who interdependently perform relevant functions by fulfilling expected roles. Relevant family functions include practices and values placed on health. Family health practices, whether effective or ineffective, encompass activities performed by individuals or families as a whole to promote health and prevent disease. How well families complete developmental tasks and how well families, including individuals within a family, generate health-promoting behaviors determine a family's potential for enhancement of family health practices.

How family members relate to one another influences their understanding of behavior, which is demonstrated in the family's structural, functional, communicational, and developmental patterns (Glover & Justis, 2015). Families provide the structure for many health-promotion practices; therefore family assessment informs health-promotion and disease-prevention planning. Within families, children and adults are nurtured, provided for, and taught about health values by word and by example. Family members first learn to make choices to promote health within the family structure (Table 7-1). Appreciating how families make decisions and encouraging family participation in all aspects of

## TABLE 7-1  Variety of Family Structures

| Configuration | Positions in Family |
|---|---|
| Single parent (separated, divorced, or widowed) | Mother or father, sons(s), daughter(s) |
| Unmarried single parent (never married) | Mother or father, sons(s), daughter(s) |
| Unmarried cohabiting couple | Two adults living together in a long-term relationship that resembles marriage |
| Unmarried parents | Two adults, sons(s), daughter(s) |
| Commune family | Mothers, fathers, adults, shared son(s), daughters(s) living together |
| Stepparents | Adults with son(s), daughter(s) from previous marriage |
| Adoptive family | Adults who provide a permanent home to son(s) and/or daughter(s) through a legal process |
| Family of choice | Adults with selected partners and family members |
| Married couple | Two cohabiting adults living in a recognized legal union |
| Same sex couple | Two persons of the same gender sharing an intimate, romantic, or sexual relationship |
| Married parents | Mother and father, son(s), daughter(s) |
| Nuclear family | Mother and father, son(s), daughter(s) |
| Gay, lesbian, transgender family | Adults and children living together with one or more members of the group who identifies as gay, lesbian, or transgender |
| Immigrant family | Adults and children living together with one or more members of the group who is foreign born |
| Biracial or multiracial family | Mother, father, adults, or children include two or more races |
| Transracial family | Mother, father, adults, or children include at least one member who is born of one race and decides to represent themselves as another race |
| Blended family | Mother, father, adults, or children represent members of from previous unions |
| Joint-custody family | Adults living with children who are legally awarded to both biological parents |
| Conditionally separate families | A family member is separated from the family but remains a significant member of the family (military service, incarceration, distant employment, hospitalization) |
| Extended family | Significant family members beyond the nuclear family that may include grandparents, aunts, uncles, and other adults who live nearby or in one household |
| Foster family | Adults, serving as state-certified caregivers, for children placed into a ward, group home, or private home |
| Grandparent(s) | Grandchildren, son(s) and/or daughter(s)<br>Grandmother and/or grandfather |

Modified from Brown, S. L., Manning, W. D., & Payne, K. K. (2016). Family structure and children's economic well-being: Incorporating same-sex cohabiting mother families. *Population Research and Policy Review, 35*(1), 1–21; Edwards, J. O. (2009). *The many kinds of family structures in our communities.* https://www.scoe.org/files/ccpc-family-structures.pdf.

care from acute care to health promotion helps families and individuals acquire new behaviors (Parkinson et al., 2016).

Families influence children's lifestyle choices. *Healthy People 2020* views families in the United States as a means of providing important opportunities for health promotion and disease prevention (US Department of Health and Human Services, 2015). Through family planning, parents assume the responsibility of caring for their children. Prenatal care and breastfeeding give infants a healthy start. Nutritious diets support physical growth and development. Children first observe and learn behaviors within their family. Patterns of nutrition, activity, oral hygiene, and coping develop at early ages, supported by the example of family members. Patterns of alcohol consumption and tobacco use are similarly established within families. Learning about human development fosters a healthy self-concept, including positive awareness of the family member's sexuality. Promoting self-esteem and reinforcing positive behaviors also strengthen the health of children. Primary care providers support positive behaviors by offering family members scientifically sound health-promotion and clinical preventive services, such as anticipatory guidance for developmental tasks, immunizations, screening for early detection, and appropriate counseling.

This chapter uses **family theory, systems theory, developmental theory**, and **risk-factor theory** to guide the nursing process with families. The 11 functional health patterns described in Chapter 6 establish the structure for interview questions during data collection. The analysis phase of the nursing process categorizes these data within stages of family development, and from the analysis, nursing diagnoses are formulated. **Family health status** is considered functional, potentially dysfunctional (potential problem), or dysfunctional (actual problem) (Gordon, 2016). The planning phase begins when family goals and objectives are stated. The family, the nurse, or another health professional facilitates implementation. Later in this chapter, four types of interventions for health promotion and disease prevention are discussed: increasing knowledge and skills; increasing strengths; decreasing exposure to risks; and decreasing susceptibility. Nurses assume various roles throughout the stages of family development, and these roles are also presented. Evaluation of a family plan considers outcomes that are specific, objective, and measurable and that rely on the family's subjective interpretation of concerns and probability of success, as well as that at the population level (Maurer & Smith, 2014).

## THE NURSING PROCESS AND THE FAMILY

The nursing process when promoting the health of families includes the family as a group and the interactions among family members. The National Center on Parent, Family, and Community Engagement (NCPFCE) views the entire family as the participant that guides assessment from a holistic framework (NCPFCE, 2015). Partnerships with families begin with an assessment (NCPFCE, 2015). The home is a natural environment for health-promotion encounters, although the process may occur in other settings as well. Different age groups (infants, children, and older adults) are likely to be present in the home. Nurses observe physical surroundings firsthand during home visits. For example, household safety hazards are observed directly. Nurses also monitor family unit rituals, roles, and interpersonal interactions. Generally the nurse contacts the family and establishes an appointment time for visiting the family. Including each family member in the visit provides a broad perspective. During visits, the nursing process develops mutually with families; it is not a treatment done for the family. Families collaborate with nursing in all phases of the process. Guidelines for home visits are presented in Box 7-1.

---

### BOX 7-1 Guidelines for Home Visits to Promote Health and Prevent Disease

**Planning the Visit**
- Make arrangements with the family.
- Study information regarding the family from agency records, referral forms, and other sources.
- Contact family and state the purpose of the visit.
- Obtain appropriate supplies and teaching aids for visits.

**Making the Visit**
- Offer an introduction and explain the purpose of the visit.
- Establish rapport.
- Show respect. Include all family members in the discussion.
- Identify the family's request for assistance.
- Understand the situation from the family's perspective.
- Identify appropriate activities for health promotion and disease prevention.
- Identify how the home visit is to be financed.
- Make a contract with the family that states specific goals and objectives that the family wants to reach.
- Think about safety before and during the visit.
- Identify and respond to health and home safety issues.
- Terminate the visit with specific instructions and information about the next visit: when it will occur, what will happen, who will be present, and what the family must accomplish before then.
- Carry through promptly on agreements made.
- Record notes promptly.

Modified from Alaska Parent Information and Resource Center. (n.d.). *Home visiting guidelines.* http://akpirc.org/wp-content/uploads/2011/04/Home-visiting.pdf; Vanderbilt Kennedy Center. (n.d.). *Home visits.* http://kc.vanderbilt.edu/kennedy_files/HomeVisitsTipsandResourcesJune2011.pdf.

---

Comprehensive family assessment provides the foundation to promote family health (NCPFCE, 2015). Several factors influence family assessment, such as nurses' perceptions about family constitution; theoretical knowledge; norms; standards; and communication abilities during visits. In addition to factors that pertain to the nurse, familial factors also influence assessments, such as family cooperation, mutual agreement to work toward goals, and family ability to recognize the relevance of health-promotion plans. Useful health-promotion family assessments involve listening to families, engaging in participatory dialogue, recognizing patterns, and assessing family potential for active, positive change (NCPFCE, 2015).

The assessment phase of the nursing process seeks and identifies information from the family about health-promotion and disease-prevention activities. To obtain this information, nurses follow family progress through developmental tasks and identify strengths in the family's ability to generate behaviors associated with disease prevention. The approaches considered in this chapter include the developmental framework, strength-based assessment, and the risk-factor estimate. Developmental phases for families as proposed by Duvall and Miller (Duvall, 1988; Duvall & Miller, 1985), strength-based assessment using a standardized tool (e.g. Canadian Family Assessment Tool) proposed by Wright and Leahy (2013), and risk-factor estimates delineated by *Healthy People 2020* can be used to guide nurses through the steps of the nursing process when they are working with families.

### The Nurse's Role

Nurses collaborate with families using a systems perspective to understand family interaction, family norms, family expectations, effectiveness of family communication, family decision-making, and family coping mechanisms. The nurse's role in health promotion and disease prevention includes the following tasks:

- Become aware of family attitudes and behaviors toward health promotion and disease prevention.
- Act as a role model for the family.
- Collaborate with the family to assess, improve, enhance, and evaluate family health practices.
- Assist the family in growth and development behaviors.
- Assist the family in identifying risk-taking behaviors.
- Assist the family in decision-making about lifestyle choices.
- Provide reinforcement for positive health-behavior practices.
- Provide health information to the family.
- Assist the family in learning behaviors to promote health and prevent disease.
- Assist the family in problem-solving and decision-making about health promotion.
- Serve as a liaison for referral or collaboration between community resources and the family.

Nurses use family theoretical frameworks to guide, observe, and classify situations. Nursing roles for families in various stages of development are presented in Table 7-2.

## FAMILY THEORIES AND FRAMEWORKS

Family theory stems from a variety of interrelated disciplines (Atkin et al., 2015). Family systems theory explains patterns of

## TABLE 7-2   Possible Nurse's Roles in Health Promotion and Disease Prevention Through Stages of Family Development

| Stage | Possible Nursing Role |
|---|---|
| Couple | Counselor on sexual and role adjustment<br>Teacher of and counselor on family planning<br>Teacher of parenting skills<br>Coordinator for genetic counseling<br>Facilitator in interpersonal relationships |
| Childbearing family | Monitor of prenatal care and referrer for problems of pregnancy<br>Counselor on prenatal nutrition<br>Counselor on prenatal maternal habits<br>Emotional support for amniocentesis<br>Counselor on breastfeeding<br>Coordinator with pediatric services<br>Supervisor of immunizations<br>Referrer to social services<br>Assistant in adjustment to prenatal role |
| Family with preschool or school-age children | Monitor of early childhood development; referrer when indicated<br>Teacher of first-aid and emergency measures<br>Coordinator with pediatric services<br>Counselor on nutrition and exercise<br>Teacher of dental hygiene<br>Counselor on environmental safety in home |
| Family with adolescents | Facilitator in interpersonal relationships<br>Teacher of risk factors to health<br>Teacher of problem-solving issues regarding alcohol, smoking, diet, and exercise<br>Facilitator of interpersonal skills with adolescents and parents<br>Direct supporter of, counselor on, or referrer to mental health resources<br>Counselor on family planning<br>Referrer for sexually transmittable disease |
| Family with young or middle-aged adults | Participant in community organizations involved in disease control<br>Teacher of problem-solving issues regarding lifestyle and habits<br>Participant in community organization involved in environmental control<br>Case finder in home and community<br>Screener for hypertension, Pap test, breast examination, mental health, and dental care<br>Counselor on menopausal transition |
| Family with older adults | Facilitator of interpersonal relationships among family members<br>Referral for work and social activity, nutritional programs, homemakers' services, and nursing home<br>Monitor of exercise, nutrition, preventive services, and medications<br>Supervisor of immunization<br>Counselor on safety in home<br>Counselor on bereavement |

Modified from Australian College of Nursing. (2015). *Community & primary health care nursing position statement.* https://www.acn.edu.au/sites/default/files/advocacy/Community_and_Primary_Health_Care_Postition_Statement.pdf.

living among the individuals who comprise family systems. In systems theory, behaviors and family members' responses influence patterns. Meanings and values provide the vital elements of motivation and energy for family systems. Every family has its unique culture, value structure, and history. Values provide a means for interpreting events and information, passing from one generation to the next. Values usually change slowly over time. Families process information and energy exchange with the environment through values. For example, holiday food traditions may be changed slightly by a daughter-in-law, whose own daughter may then adjust the traditional recipe within her own nuclear family.

System boundaries separate family systems from their environment and control information flow. This characteristic forms a family internal manager that influences and defines interactions and relationships with one another and with those outside the family system. The family forms a unified whole rather than the sum of its parts—an integrated system of interdependent functions, structures, and relationships. For example, one drug-dependent individual's health behavior influences the entire family unit.

Living systems are open systems. As living systems, families experience constant exchanges of energy and information with the environment. Change in one part or member of the family results in changes in the family as a whole. For example, loss of a family member through death changes roles and relationships among all family members. Change requires adaptation of every family member as roles and functions assume new meanings. Changes families make are incorporated into the system.

When the system is the family, issues can be clarified by family processes, communication interaction among family members, and family group values. In Bowen's family systems theory, birth order is considered an important determinant of behavior. In addition, family patterns of behavior differentiate one family from another (Vedanthan et al., 2016; Vess & Lara, 2016). When an individual family member expresses behaviors that differ from the learned family pattern, differentiation of self occurs. Interaction among family members and the transmission of these interaction patterns from one generation to the next provide the framework for the family systems approach (Rothenberg et al., 2016).

The framework for health promotion introduced by Pender and colleagues (2014) recognizes the family as the unit of assessment and intervention because families develop self-care and dependent-care competencies; foster resilience among family members; provide resources; and promote healthy individuation within cohesive family structures. Furthermore, because the family often provides the structure for implementation of health promotion, family assessment becomes an integral tool to foster health and healthy behaviors (Pender et al., 2014).

## THE FAMILY FROM A DEVELOPMENTAL PERSPECTIVE

Building on Erikson's (1998) theory of psychosocial development, Duvall and Miller (1985) identified stages of the family life cycle and critical family developmental tasks. Although Duvall's classification has been criticized for its middle class homogeneity and lack of diversity in family forms, this conceptual model helps to anticipate family events and has formed the basis for more contemporary developmental models (Duvall & Miller, 1985). Knowing a family's composition, interrelationships, and particular life cycle helps nurses predict the overall family pattern. Box 7-2 lists characteristics of healthy families. From Duvall's perspective, most families complete these basic family tasks. Each family performs these tasks in a unique expression of its personality. Progression through the stages occurs in a linear fashion; however, regression may occur and families may experience tasks in more than one stage at a time (Duvall & Miller, 1985). Specific tasks arise as growth responsibilities during family development. Failure to accomplish a developmental task leads to negative consequences. For example, intimate partner violence or child abuse or neglect may result in intervention by police, welfare, health department, or other agencies. Life cycle tasks build upon one another. Success at one stage is dependent on success at an earlier stage. Early failure may lead to developmental difficulties at later stages.

As families enter each new developmental stage, transition occurs. Families move through new stages as a result of events ranging from marriage (heterosexual, homosexual), gay and lesbian relationships, childbirth, single-led families, joint custody,

---

### BOX 7-2 Characteristics and Indicators of Healthy Families

Nurturing RELATIONSHIPS
- Maintains trust traditions and shares quality time.
- Communications are open and members listen to each other.

Establishing ROUTINES
- Maintains routines that promote health patterns of nutrition, hygiene, rest, physical activity, and sexuality.
- Maintains routines to promote safety and injury prevention; health protection; disease prevention; smoking and alcohol or substance abuse; and/or violence.
- Establishes patterns to promote mental health: interacting, communicating, and expressing affection, aggression, sexuality, and similar interactions.

Maintaining EXPECTATIONS
- Maintains morale and motivation, rewarding achievement, meeting personal and family crises, setting attainable goals, and developing family traditions, loyalties, and values.

ADAPTING to challenges
- Evolves during crises and respects each member of the group.
- Promotes strategies to make decisions about health and illness.

Connecting to COMMUNITY
- Family table time and conversation occur regularly.
- Members act as interactive caregivers across the life span to socialize children and adolescents, to participate in the community, and to support members as they age.

Modified from Search Institute. (2016). *Family strengths.* http://www.search-institute.org/research/family-strengths.

---

or remarried families; to adolescents maturing into young adults and leaving the home; to the aging years.

Each new developmental stage requires adaptation with new responsibilities. Concurrently, developmental stages provide opportunities for families to realize their potential. Nurses anticipate change through analysis of progress through each stage. Each new stage presents opportunities for health promotion and intervention. Family developmental stages, although reflective of traditional nuclear families and extended family networks, also apply to nontraditional family configurations (Coyne et al., 2016; Edwards, 2009). A family systems approach addresses the interaction of these multiple family configurations. For example, couples may marry and bring children from a previous marriage to a blended family that works toward achieving developmental tasks of couples along with family stages for the children. Both the couple and their children possess values and beliefs from the past that must integrate within the present union. Childless couples present developmental tasks that are different from those proposed for couples with children. One family conceptual model proposed by Vedanthan and colleagues (2016) illustrates the multiple connections among interdependence among family systems, shared environment, parenting style, caregiver perceptions, and genomics to promote cardiovascular health.

Nurses collect data to determine progress toward family developmental task attainment during the family assessment. Use of assessment tools that include gathering factors that strengthen and protect the family such as the Canadian Family Assessment Tool and the Family Development Matrix used in California provides more robust information (Harper Browne, 2014). These newer assessment tools focus on the assessment of family assets and social network resources that families currently use. These kinds of assessments intend to build on strengths at particular developmental stages to promote healthy family environments. Assessment of family developmental stages entails use of guidelines to analyze progress toward developmental tasks, family growth, and health-promotion needs.

## THE FAMILY FROM A STRUCTURAL-FUNCTIONAL PERSPECTIVE

Families consist of both structural and functional components. Family structure refers to family composition, including roles and relationships, whereas family function consists of processes within systems as information and energy exchange occurs between families and their environment.

## THE FAMILY FROM A RISK-FACTOR PERSPECTIVE

Family risk factors can be inferred from lifestyle; biological factors; environmental factors; social, psychological, cultural, and spiritual dimensions; and the health care system. As outlined in the Frank Thompson case study in Chapter 1, lifestyle habits such as overeating, drug dependency, high sugar and cholesterol intake, and smoking influence health outcomes. Biological risk factors may include the elements of genetic inheritance, congenital malformation, and mental retardation. To fully explore environmental risk factors that influence family function, nurses explore work pressures, peer pressure, stress, anxieties, tensions, and air, noise, or water pollution. Social and psychological dimensions such as crowding, isolation, or rapid and accelerated rates of change are areas to consider when nurses are assessing family risk factors. Cultural and spiritual aspects may include traditions of preventing illness such as daily prayer and meditation practices. Finally, health care system factors such as overuse, underuse, inappropriate use, or accessibility are considered in the family risk assessment.

To reduce risk factors, nurses help families focus on influencing health behaviors of their members. Society glamorizes many hazardous behaviors through advertising and mass media promotions that minimize negative health consequences. Families influence their members to weigh the consequences of risk-taking behavior. Awareness of risk factors may prompt families to reduce modifiable risk factors. Healthy behavior, including use of preventive health care services, is a significant area of family responsibility.

Traditionally, epidemiology has used levels and trends of mortality and morbidity rates as indirect evidence of health. Data such as infant mortality rates, stillbirth rates, and leading causes of death have long been used as indicators of collective community health. Healthy family functioning links the family life cycle stages with specific risk factors. Epidemiology often describes a disease association in terms of risk. Health risks can be physiological or psychological. Physiological risks arise from genetic background, whereas psychological risks include those related to low self-image. Risks also arise from environmental

considerations, including the physical environment and socio-economic condition (Freudenberg et al., 2011). Risk-factor theory considers families a pivotal part of the environment and also an important support system used to decrease health risks for individuals. As young family members mature developmentally and seek more independence from the family, peers may influence risk to compete with family values.

Risk estimates calculate differences between two groups: one with the risk factor and one without. The frequency of deaths, illnesses, or injuries with some specific risk factor compared with those for another group without the risk factor, or the population as a whole, determines the risk estimate. Some diseases (e.g., sickle cell anemia in Black-American families and Tay-Sachs disease in families of Ashkenazi Jewish descent) occur more frequently in certain families and can be identified by carrier screening (Azimi et al., 2016). Other recessive genetic disorders (e.g., cystic fibrosis and Gaucher disease) have decreased in incidence with prenatal carrier screening with genetic counseling in couples with suspect family histories (Azimi et al., 2016). Azimi and colleagues (2016) compared current strategies that target specific high-risk families to next-generation DNA sequencing (NGS) that provide high-level sensitivity and specificity for carrier screening. They developed a mathematical model to screen individuals for 14 recessive disorders commonly recommended for screening in targeted populations. The mathematical model provides support to transition from traditional lower-accuracy genotyping to more accurate NGS techniques focused on the most prevalent disorders (Azimi et al., 2016). Other diseases such as iron-deficiency anemia may not be attributed to a specific genetic background. The natural history of a chronic disease predisposes family members to greater risk, but specific causes may be difficult to identify. Well siblings, particularly adolescents, may be affected. Larsen (2016) describes nine phases that individuals and families may experience as they progress through chronic illness adaptation from the time before the disorder is recognized through a stable adjustment phase to the final relinquishment of life interest and activities.

The probabilities of risk change may also change depending on the family's activities in health promotion and disease prevention. Stages of family development are used to classify risk factors. Age-specific developmental stages, along with their associated age-specific health risks, are given in Table 7-3, which displays periods during which families become most sensitive to certain problems, with corresponding key times for health promotion and disease prevention. The risk behaviors highlighted include tobacco and alcohol use, faulty nutrition, overuse of medications, fast driving, stress, and relentless pressure to achieve. Habits learned in family settings help to develop individual lifestyle behaviors. In fact, 5 habits—nutrition, smoking, exercise, alcohol use, and stress—affect at least 7 of the 10 leading causes of death listed in *Healthy People 2020* (USDHHS, 2015). See Box 7-3: *Healthy People 2020* for selected objectives related to families.

## GORDON'S FUNCTIONAL HEALTH PATTERNS: ASSESSMENT OF THE FAMILY

Gordon's (2016) 11 functional health patterns help organize basic family assessment information. Patterns form the standardized

## TABLE 7-3   Family Stage: Specific Risk Factors and Related Health Problems

| Stage | Risk Factors | Health Problems |
|---|---|---|
| Beginning childbearing | Lack of knowledge of family planning<br>Adolescent marriage<br>Lack of knowledge concerning sexual and marital roles and adjustments<br>Low-birth-weight infant<br>Lack of prenatal care<br>Unmarried status<br>First pregnancy before age 16 years or after age 35 years<br>History of hypertension and infections during pregnancy<br>Rubella, syphilis, gonorrhea, and AIDS<br>Genetic factors<br>Lack of safety in home | Premature baby in family<br>Birth defects<br>Birth injuries<br>Accidents<br>Sudden infant death syndrome (SIDS)<br>Sterility<br>Pelvic inflammatory disease<br>Fetal alcohol syndrome<br>Mental retardation<br>Injuries<br>Birth defects<br>Underweight |
| Family with school-age children | Working parents with inappropriate use of resources for child care<br>Generational pattern of using social agencies as way of life<br>Multiple, closely spaced children<br>Low family self-esteem<br>Children used as scapegoats for parental frustration<br>Repeated infections, accidents, or hospitalizations<br>Parents immature, dependent, and unable to handle responsibility<br>Unrecognized or unattended health problems<br>Strong beliefs about physical punishment<br>Toxic substances unguarded in the home | Behavior disturbances<br>Speech and vision problems<br>Communicable diseases<br>Dental caries<br>School problems<br>Learning disabilities<br>Injuries<br>Chronic diseases<br>Homicide<br>Violence |
| Family with adolescents | Health disparities<br>Lifestyle and behavior patterns leading to chronic disease<br>Lack of problem-solving skills<br>Family values of aggressiveness, competition, rigidity, and inflexibility<br>Daredevil risk-taking attitudes<br>Conflicts between parents and children<br>Pressure to live up to family expectations | Violent deaths<br>Unwanted pregnancies<br>Sexually transmitted diseases |
| Family with middle-aged adults | Hypertension<br>Smoking<br>High cholesterol levels<br>Genetic predisposition<br>Use of oral contraceptives<br>Geographical area or occupation<br>Residence | Cardiovascular disease, principally coronary artery disease and cerebrovascular accident (stroke)<br>Diabetes<br>Accidents<br>Homicide<br>Abnormal fetus<br>Mental illness<br>Periodontal disease and loss of teeth |
| Family with older adults | Age<br>Drug interactions<br>Metabolic disorders<br>Pituitary malfunctions<br>Cushing syndrome<br>Hypercalcemia<br>Chronic illness<br>Retirement<br>Loss of spouse<br>Past environments and lifestyle<br>Lack of prevention for death | Mental confusion<br>Reduced vision<br>Hearing impairment<br>Hypertension<br>Acute illness<br>Infectious disease<br>Influenza<br>Pneumonia<br>Injuries such as burns and falls<br>Death without dignity |

Risks of poverty, abuse, neglect, substance abuse, poor nutrition, denial behavior, and socioeconomic status affect all ages. Depression, suicide, cancer, overweight, obesity, sedentary lifestyles, and respiratory distress syndrome affect most age groups. Therefore, these items have been excluded from the table.

Modified from US Department of Health and Human Services. (2015). *2020 topics and objectives.* http://www.healthypeople.gov/2020/ topics-objectives.

## ♥ BOX 7-3   HEALTHY PEOPLE 2020

### Selected Examples of National Health-Promotion and Disease-Prevention Objectives for Families

**BDBS-2**   (Developmental) Increase the proportion of persons with a diagnosis of hemoglobinopathies and their families who are referred for evaluation and treatment.

**BDBS-3**   (Developmental) Increase the proportion of persons with hemoglobinopathies who receive care in a patient/family-centered medical home.

**EMC 2.3**   Increase the proportion of parents who read to their young child.

**WS-13**   Reduce household food insecurity and in doing so reduce hunger.

**EH-15**   Increase the percentage of new single-family homes constructed with radon-reducing features, especially in high radon–potential areas.

**Family Planning Objectives**

**FP-1**   Increase the proportion of pregnancies that are intended.

**FP-2**   Reduce the proportion of females experiencing pregnancy despite use of a reversible contraceptive method.

**FP-3**   Increase the proportion of publicly funded family planning clinics that offer the full range of FDA-approved methods of contraception, including emergency contraception, on-site.

**FP-4**   (Developmental) Increase the proportion of health insurance plans that cover contraceptive supplies and services.

**FP-5**   Reduce the proportion of pregnancies conceived within 18 months of a previous birth.

**FP-6**   Increase the proportion of females or their partners at risk of unintended pregnancy who used contraception in the most recent sexual intercourse.

**FP-7**   Increase the proportion of sexually active persons who received reproductive health services.

**FP-8**   Reduce pregnancy rates among adolescent females.

**FP-9**   Increase the proportion of adolescents aged 17 years or younger who have never had sexual intercourse.

**FP-10**   Increase the proportion of sexually active persons aged 15 to 19 years who use condoms to both effectively prevent pregnancy and provide barrier protection against disease.

**FP-11**   Increase the proportion of sexually active persons aged 15 to 19 years who use condoms and hormonal or intrauterine contraception to both effectively prevent pregnancy and provide barrier protection against disease.

**FP-12**   Increase the proportion of adolescents who received formal instruction on reproductive health topics before they were 18 years old.

**FP-13**   Increase the proportion of adolescents who talked to a parent or guardian about reproductive health topics before they were 18 years old.

**FP-15**   Increase the proportion of females in need of publicly supported contraceptive services and supplies who receive those services and supplies.

**G-1**   Increase the proportion of women with a family history of breast and/or ovarian cancer who receive genetic counseling.

**DH-20**   Increase the proportion of children with disabilities, from birth through age 2 years, who receive early intervention services in home or community-based settings.

From US Department of Health and Human Services. (2015). *2020 topics and objectives.* http://www.healthypeople.gov/2020/topics-objectives.

format for family assessment using a systems approach with emphasis on developmental stages and risk factors. Assessment includes evaluation of dysfunctional patterns within families, with corresponding details in one or more of the other interdependent patterns (see Chapter 6).

The presence of risk factors predicts potential dysfunction. Developmental risk and risk arising from dysfunctional health patterns increase whole family risk (see Table 7-3). Gordon (2016) interprets risk states as potential problems. To formulate nursing diagnoses, nurses identify problems along with their associated and etiological factors. Influencing factors may precede or occur concurrently with the problem and are used to plan care. Interventions aim to modify influencing factors to promote positive change.

Family history begins with the health perception–health management pattern. Exploring issues within this pattern first provides an overview to help locate where problems exist in other patterns and to determine which problems require more thorough assessment. Interviewing from the family's perspective helps families define situations. The roles-relationships pattern defines family structure and function. The remaining nine patterns address lifestyle indicators.

## Health Perception–Health Management Pattern

Characteristics of family health perceptions, health management, and preventive practices emerge with assessment of the health perception–health management pattern. The National Survey of Children's Health (http://www.childhealthdata.org/) and other data sources contribute additional information to help identify health-promoting behaviors of families. Data collected in the Survey of Children's Health include information about the frequency of family meals; attendance at religious services; characteristics of parental relationship with children; parental coping abilities while parents are raising children; and methods for handling family disagreements. The intent of the survey is to provide a data source to explore research questions related to *Healthy People 2020* and the variables correlated with drug use. However, such data have also been associated with eating disorders and risk behaviors other than drug use. These assessment indicators also provide data to guide the remaining functional health pattern assessment. Patterns overlap, and findings in one pattern may encourage further assessment in another pattern. The following are some research questions that concern family health promotion:

- What are the chief concerns of parents and other adults in the household about their children's development, learning, and behavior?
- How do children's health status and the health practices (physical activity and smoking behavior) of the adults compare?
- What health-related behaviors, such as eating three meals a day at regular times, eating breakfast every day, exercising for a minimum of 2 or 3 days a week, sleeping for 7 to 8 hours each night, and abstaining from smoking, are practiced by the family?
- How safe are homes, schools, and neighborhoods from the perspective of the family?

Health practices differ from family to family. Families identify and perform health-maintenance activities based on their beliefs about health. Exploration during the assessment also includes the following areas:

- What is the family's philosophy of health? Does each family member hold similar beliefs? Do family members practice what they believe?
- In what negative behaviors or lifestyle practices, such as smoking, alcohol, and drug abuse, do the family engage?
- What chronic disease risk behaviors are exhibited within the family?
- Are risk factors present for infections, such as lack of immunization, lack of knowledge of transmittable diseases, and poor personal hygiene?
- Are risk factors for bodily injury, accidents, or substance abuse present in the home?
- Do older adult members know what medications they are taking and the reasons for their using them?
- Does the family discard outdated medications or those not used?
- What unattended health problems exist?
- Is there a history of repeated infections and hospitalization?
- Is the home understimulating or overstimulating?
- Where does the family obtain health and illness care?
- Is the family engaged in a dental program?
- How does the family describe previous experiences with nurses and other health care professionals?

## Nutritional-Metabolic Pattern

The nutritional-metabolic pattern depicts characteristics of the family's typical food and fluid consumption and metabolism (Gordon, 2016). Included in it are growth and development patterns, pregnancy-related nutritional patterns, and the family's eating patterns. Risk factors for obesity, diabetes, anorexia, and bulimia are identified.

Dietary habits, learned within the family context, involve behavioral patterns central to daily life. Keeping a diary of intake for a week is a useful strategy for assessing family food and fluid intake patterns. Assessment notes both meals shared with the whole family as well as additional consumption by individuals. Recent research provides evidence that family meal sharing is associated with healthier eating habits. For example, Utter and colleagues (2013) report that family meal sharing in their sample of New Zealand adolescents ($n = 9101$) was positively associated with higher well-being scores, lower depression scores, and fewer risk-taking behaviors. In a follow-up report of this same population, Utter and colleagues (2016) found the same positive associations with better nutritional indicators (fruit and vegetable intake), better mental health indicators (fewer depressive symptoms), and stronger family connections in adolescents who knew how to prepare food compared with those adolescents without the cooking abilities. However, the adolescents with cooking ability were more likely to have higher body mass index.

Exploration during nutrition pattern assessment includes the following areas:

- What kinds of foods are typically consumed?
- Who eats together at mealtimes?
- How is food viewed (reward/punishment)?
- Is there adequate storage and refrigeration?
- How is food purchased?
- How is food prepared?
- Who prepares food?

## Elimination Pattern

The elimination pattern describes characteristics of regularity and control of the family's excretory functions (Gordon, 2016). Bowel and bladder function and environmental factors such as waste disposal in the home, neighborhood, and community that influence family life are considered in this pattern.

Questions are phrased according to the age-specific developmental stage of the family. For example, when the nurse is attempting to determine whether there is a problem in the preschool stage, it would be appropriate to ask whether the child is being toilet trained. In families with adolescents, the nurse may ask how often individuals have bowel movements and whether there have been any changes from usual patterns. The nurse may ask older adult members whether they have any problems with constipation. Issues that particularly concern older adults include constipation, diarrhea, polyuria, and incontinence, as well as use of antacids and constipation-relieving agents and strategies. The nurse evaluates whether use of these strategies is appropriate or possibly contributing to poor health.

## Activity-Exercise Pattern

The activity-exercise pattern represents family characteristics that require energy expenditure (Gordon, 2016). The nurse reviews daily activities, exercise, and leisure activities. Families create settings for individual members to be physically active, sedentary, or apathetic toward physical activity. The quantity of sedentary activities such as television and video game screen time is explored.

Exploration during assessment of this pattern includes the following areas:

- How does the family exhibit its beliefs about regular exercise and physical fitness being necessary for good health?
- What types of daily activities include physical exercise and who does what with whom?
- What are the television viewing habits of children?
- How are other screen-viewing activities (computers, video games) incorporated into the daily routines?
- How often do children exercise?
- How are these activity and exercise factors related to children's health?
- What does the family do to have fun (Figure 7-1)?

## Sleep-Rest Pattern

Rest habits characterize the sleep-rest pattern (Gordon, 2016). Without the restorative function of sleep, individuals exhibit decreased performance, bad temper, and decreased stress tolerance, and may rely on alcohol or other chemicals to induce sleep. Regular, sufficient sleep patterns are linked to better mental status, including learning and decision-making. Most families have sleeping patterns, although in some families these patterns may

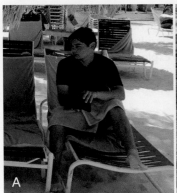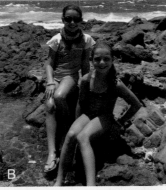

**FIGURE 7-1** Family outings can be **(A)** leisurely and restful or **(B)** adventurous and exciting.

not be readily apparent. It is important to elicit the data about sleep and rest from the family's perspective.

Assessment of the sleep-rest pattern includes the following:
- What are the usual sleeping habits of the family?
- How suitable are they to the age and health status of the family members?
- What are the usual hours established for sleeping?
- Who decides when and how children go to sleep?
- Do family members take naps or have other regular means of resting or relaxing?
- How early does the family rise? What are the patterns related to bedtime and rising?
- Do all family members have the same general sleep-rest pattern?
- Is there a family member with sleep disruption?

## Cognitive-Perceptual Pattern

The cognitive-perceptual pattern identifies characteristics of language, cognitive skills, and perception that influence desired or required family activities (Gordon, 2016). Specifically, this pattern concerns how families access information to make decisions, how concrete or abstract the thought processes are, and whether the decisions focus on present or future issues. Decision-making in families is associated with power in family functioning. Highly educated families usually have greater repertoires for problem-solving. Power and ability to solve problems are linked to leadership; family leaders must be acknowledged if nursing interventions are to be implemented.

Cognitive-perceptual pattern assessment includes the following:
- How does the family access and interpret information, especially about health (e.g., newspaper, books, computer, television, or radio)?
- What are the usual family reading patterns and strategies used for ongoing learning (e.g., continuing education programs)?
- What kinds of materials does the family read to the children?
- How does the family usually make decisions about health promotion and disease prevention?
- How do family members contribute to the decision-making process?
- How knowledgeable is the family about risk factors and developmental milestones?

- How are choices made regarding lifestyle?
- How knowledgeable are family members about correct information?
- How do family members acquire information?
- How accurate are the information sources used to make health-promotion choices?
- How do family members describe whether their health behavior is constructive or destructive?
- How do family members recognize signs and symptoms of deteriorating health?
- How do family members decide when medical attention is necessary?
- Who makes the decisions about when to seek health care?
- What factors contribute to delays from the time of onset to the time of treatment?
- How long do families wait before seeking care?
- What are some of the cues that signal to families that care is needed?
- How is professional care accessed?
- What type of health care is generally used health maintenance for immunizations (well-child care or emergency/urgent care facilities)?
- How are decisions made about the use of over-the-counter medications or the use of alternative or traditional health practices?

## Self-Perception–Self-Concept Pattern

The self-perception–self-concept pattern identifies characteristics that describe the family's self-worth and feeling states (Gordon, 2016). Rapport between the family members and the nurse facilitates disclosure. Families have perceptions and concepts about their image, their status in the community, and their competencies as a family unit. Families manifest these perceptions through shared aspirations, values, expectations, fears, successes, and failures. Relationships in families determine the amount of sharing that occurs. Situations affecting one member influence perceptions of the entire family group. How each member describes the family often gives clues to the family self-concept.

Exploration during assessment includes the following:
- How is this family similar to or different from other families?
- How does this family perceive itself to be similar to and different from other families?
- What special assets does each member contribute to the family?
- What changes would each member like to see occur in the family?
- What kinds of feelings do family members have for each other?
- Describe the general tone of feelings in the family. Is the tone indifferent, secretive, angry, or open?
- How does the family think it assimilates into the neighborhood and community?
- How does the family handle stress and crisis situations?
- How does the family experience changes in the way it feels about itself?
- How does the family describe the events that led to a change?

## Roles-Relationships Pattern

The roles-relationships pattern identifies characteristics of family roles and relationships (Gordon, 2016). Both structural and functional aspects of the family are assessed. Structural aspects of families include each member's name, age, sex, education, occupation, and role in the family. Traditionally, families have been described as nuclear and extended. The traditional nuclear family consists of husband, wife, and children, with an extended family that would include aunts, uncles, cousins, and grandparents. Today there are many varieties of nuclear and extended families. Edwards (2009) describes various contemporary family structures: traditional nuclear family, extended families, single-parent families, stepfamilies, cohabiting families, gay and lesbian families, grandparent-headed families, foster families, and fragmentary families. Traditional nuclear family structure has been influenced by societal changes, such as the women's movement, employment of mothers, divorce, and remarriage. Exploration of family origin and genetic heritage completes family identification data collection. Cultural practices in the home may or may not reflect the family's genetic heritage; therefore it is important to explore the diversity of cultural and ethnic practices during the family assessment (Andrews & Boyle, 2015).

The American Academy of Pediatrics regards the family as the most enduring link to health for children. For example, findings from the Early Childhood Longitudinal Study, Birth Cohort ($n = 5000$) maternal health behaviors at each phase of early development (9 months, 2 years, 4 years, 5 years) indicated the importance of the mother-child relationship in health promotion (Prickett & Augustine, 2016). The US Census Bureau (2014) released information in 2011 from the *Annual Report of Families and Living Arrangements*. The proportion of young adults aged 15 to 34 years living in their parents' homes increased from 14% in 2005 to 19% in 2011 and has extended beyond the economic recession. In regard to children aged 5 to 15 years, 69% live with both parents. Children living with only one parent are more likely to live with their mother. Grandparents live in 10% of the homes that have children younger than 18 years. The proportion of children with stay-at-home mothers decreased from 24% in 2007 to 23% in 2011. There is also an overall trend of increasing proportions of individuals living alone in their home, increasing from 13% in 1960 to 28% in 2011.

Schoon and colleagues (2012) suggest that children in the United Kingdom experiencing poverty for the first 5 years of life are at higher risk of impaired cognitive development than those who do not experience poverty. These data indicate the need to identify family structure for poverty-related factors to determine those families at risk and effectively intervene (see Figures 7-1, 7-2, and 7-3). Family structure and function influence family stability and pose a challenge to the nurse in health promotion and disease prevention.

Divorce and remarriage involve a complex transition that requires the disintegration of one family structure and reorganization to another (Hiyoshi et al., 2015). How parents cope during situational crises, as well as after the divorce, is a significant variable in long-term individual and family adjustment. See the case study at the end of this chapter for the presentation of a stepfamily situation. Developmental levels of children, individual temperaments of children, and quality of environmental support for children all contribute to family response to crises. For example, Feise and Bost (2016) explore how families' responses impact obesity risk in children. They link family system factors, such as family meal routines and distress during meals, with the biological risk of obesity.

A family resilience framework may be useful to promote strategies for prevention efforts aimed at strengthening families as they face life challenges. Masten and Monn (2015) describe an integrated method for understanding and promoting resilience in children and families. Family disruption has been associated with substance abuse and psychosocial maladjustment in adolescents and young adults. Family supports are associated with adherence, and substance abuse may decrease healthy social support systems. Moreover, both family dissolution and family disruption may be associated with substance abuse, alcohol consumption, and externalizing behaviors such as theft, property destruction, fighting, and assault (Masten & Monn, 2015). The current literature provides support for the importance of the roles-relationships patterns in the development of health-promoting behaviors (Gordon, 2016; Masten & Monn, 2015).

Family organization influences performance of health-promotion and disease-prevention functions. For example, a single parent without an extended family network may be in need of more community resources to help raise the children. A two-parent family living near its extended family may need less support to raise children, but family members may need to know about growth and developmental stages and immunization schedules. Individuals may experience a variety of family structures in one lifetime. A person may be part of a nuclear family as an infant, a single-parent family after the parents have divorced, a stepparent family after the mother or father has remarried, and an unmarried couple family when the person is one of two adults who share a household. The person brings the values and beliefs about health promotion and disease prevention that were practiced in previous unions to each new family configuration. Divergent values may result in conflicting expectations unless the new union forms a set of integrated values and beliefs. The current trend away from the nuclear family with the extended family may influence the general direction of the health care system and the strategies used to promote health with other family configurations.

Certain health-promotion issues are of particular concern to the nurse while he or she is assessing family health promotion and disease prevention. Violence is a health problem that threatens the integrity of all families. Alhusen and colleagues (2015) provide an overview of several studies reporting that the National Violent Death Reporting System lists a rate of 2.9 homicides per 100,000 live births. Often pregnancy-associated suicides involved intimate partner conflict attributable to the suicide, and almost half of the pregnancy-related homicides are related to family violence (Alhusen et al., 2015). According to Alhusen and colleagues (2015) these homicides outnumber the reported numbers of deaths from some of the common obstetrical causes. Furthermore, bullying contributes to violence issues that pertain to families. Bullying is addressed in *Healthy People 2020 Objectives* (USDHHS

2015). The measure used for this objective (IVP-35 Reduce bullying among adolescents) is the percentage of children bullied on school property during the 12 months before the survey (USDHHS, 2015). The midterm measure in 2013 (19.6%) was a 10% reduction since 2010 and moved toward the 2020 target of 17.9%. The role of the family dysfunction and support is linked to bullying behavior (Kann et al., 2013). Furthermore, bullying within families among siblings also occurs (Berry & Adams, 2016).

Family violence includes child abuse, spousal abuse, and elder abuse, with women being victimized more often during pregnancy. Death in pregnancy is often associated with domestic violence (Alhusen et al., 2015). Health promotion and violence prevention require a complex set of skills. Nurses use approaches to reduce violence-related injuries and deaths by acquiring the role of advocate and helping to eliminate victim blaming (Box 7-4: Research for Evidence-Based Practice). Explorations to assess families for health promotion and violence prevention may include the following:

- What formal positions and roles does each of the family members fulfill?
- What roles are considered acceptable and consistent within the family's expectations?
- What kind of flexibility in roles occurs when needed?
- What informal roles exist? Who plays informal roles and with what consistency?
- What purpose do the informal roles serve?
- How are the family social support networks associated with health and development?
- Who were the role models for the couples or single people as parents?
- Who were the role models for marital partners and what were their characteristics?
- How does the family manage daily living? How are the household tasks divided?
- How are problems handled? How are problems with children handled?

## BOX 7-4 RESEARCH FOR EVIDENCE-BASED PRACTICE

Twenty Latina women who had experienced domestic violence participated in this mixed-methods single subject design. Participant journaling and one-on-one interviews with research assistants were included in the design. Data were collected at multiple intervals during the 5-week training period for *promotoras* (community health workers).

These women were all born outside the United States. Average age of 36 years and 10.6 years of completed education, employment in the service industry characterized the sample. Quantitative measures, interviews, and journals revealed that the training increased leadership competency.

These findings provide support for recognizing the contribution of *promotoras* to community and public health. These types of development programs may also empower the *promotoras* to continue their community participation and model their engagement within their communities for other women.

From Serrata, J. V., Hernandez-Martinez, M., & Macias, R. L. (2016). Self-empowerment of immigrant Latina survivors of domestic violence: A promotora model of community leadership. *Hispanic Health Care International, 14*(1), 37–46.

- Who is employed outside the home?
- Who takes care of the children when both parents are employed outside the home?
- How does the family care for its ill members? How does it care for its older adult members?
- Are behaviors appropriate for family stages of development?
- Is decision-making allocated to the appropriate members?
- Does the family respond appropriately to its members' developmental needs?
- Is there fair distribution of tasks among family members?
- Is the family's emotional climate conducive to growth and development?
- Is there a connection between family and community crime?

In their study of 413 adolescents, Hardaway and colleagues (2016) provide evidence that family relationships protect adolescents from harm in violent communities. They report that interaction with the extended family and parental engagement act as resources for youth who are exposed to violence in their neighborhoods. These findings indicate that nurses working with families should encourage parents to maintain open communication within the family and that parents should enlist additional support from their extended family members as a larger network of positive influence for their children.

When this initial assessment reveals possible neglect, abuse, or violence, further assessment is warranted with a branched assessment that may include the following assessment parameters and questions:

- What cues are present to indicate chemical abuse?
- Who are the significant adult members of the household? (Determine the presence of a boyfriend/girlfriend.)

Nursing diagnoses and planning stem from a thorough assessment. High-quality evidence-based intervention is based on this systematic approach to assessment. For example, quality intervention for victims of intimate partner violence can be planned in advance to promote the safety and well-being of the victims (Box 7-5: Quality and Safety Scenario).

### Genogram

A **genogram**, or family diagram, represents the family on the basis of identification data that depict each member of the family with connections between the generations. This useful technique gathers data on at least three generations, including the current one; their parents, grandparents, aunts, uncles; and their children. The genogram explores clues within family histories contributing to health problems. Figure 7-2 depicts accepted genogram symbols, with a sample genogram of the fictional Graham family portrayed in Figure 7-3 (Stanhope & Lancaster, 2015). The Graham family genogram shows a variety of family structures, including changes resulting from marriage, divorce, death, and childbearing. This information highlights family health patterns to use for anticipatory health guidance; for example, in the case of the Graham family, hypertension, type 2 diabetes, cancer, and hypercholesterolemia. Family histories provide the unique perspective of family risk of inherited diseases as well as the family environmental contribution (Pender et al., 2014). Although *My Family Health Portrait* (https://familyhistory.hhs.gov/FHH/html/index.html)

**BOX 7-5  QUALITY AND SAFETY SCENARIO**

### Domestic Violence: Intimate Partner Violence

If the person is still in the relationship:

- Think of a safe place to go if an argument occurs—avoid rooms with no exits (bathroom) or rooms with weapons (kitchen).
- Think about and make a list of safe people to contact.
- Keep a cell phone with you at all times.
- Memorize all important numbers.
- Establish a "code word" or "sign" so that family, friends, teachers, or coworkers know when to call for help.
- Think about what to say to the partner if he/she becomes violent.
- Remind the individual that he/she has the right to live without fear and violence.

If the person has left the relationship:

- Change the phone number.
- Screen calls.
- Save and document all contacts, messages, injuries, or other incidents involving the batterer.
- Change locks, if the batterer has a key.
- Avoid staying alone.
- Plan how to get away if confronted by an abusive partner.
- If a meeting is necessary, have it in a public place.
- Vary the routine.
- Notify school and work contacts.
- Call a shelter.

If the individual is leaving the relationship or thinking of leaving, that person should take important papers and documents to facilitate application for benefits or take legal action. Important papers include Social Security cards and birth certificates for self and children, marriage license, leases or deeds, checkbook, charge cards, bank statements and charge account statements, insurance policies, proof of income (pay stubs or W-2s), and any documentation of past incidents of abuse (e.g., photos, police reports, medical records).

The National Coalition Against Domestic Violence provides information to health care providers, a network of shelters, and counseling programs, and operates a national hotline: 800-799-SAFE (7233); website: http://www.ncadv. org; address: One Broadway, Suite B210, Denver, CO 80203; phone: 303-839-1852; fax: 303-831-9251; telecommunication device (TTY): 303-839-1681; e-mail: mainoffice@ncadv.org.

Adapted from information on the National Coalition Against Domestic Violence. http://www.ncadv.org/.

takes a more traditional approach to family history, encouraging families to visit the website helps them explore their own family history. Resources for this continuously evolving topic of genomics can be found at the National Human Genome Research Institute (http://www.genome.gov/HealthProfessionals/), and on-line genetics education resources can be found at the National Institute of Health's National Genetics Research Institute at http://www.genome.gov/10000464. Box 7-6 explores how family assessment incorporates genomics.

### Ecomap

The ecomap, which is similar to the genogram, uses pictorial techniques to document family organizational patterns with visual clarity. A genogram is constructed for a family or household. It begins with a circle in the center of the page. Outside the circle, smaller circles are drawn and labeled with the names of

significant people, agencies, and institutions in the family's social environment. Lines are drawn from the family-household to each circle. Solid lines indicate strong relationships. Dotted lines reflect fragile or tenuous connections. Slashed lines signify stressful relationships. Arrows can be drawn parallel to the lines to indicate the direction for the energy flow or for resources (Stanhope & Lancaster, 2012). Figure 7-4 shows an ecomap for the fictional Graham family. Both the genogram and the ecomap provide useful information and can be incorporated into family systems assessment (O'Brien, 2014; Tramonti & Fanali, 2015). The ecomap helps to overcome the issues of the genogram encountered when one is assessing nontraditional families. The ecomap uses a functional rather than a structural approach to the assessment of family roles and function.

Health-promotion nursing relevance cannot be underestimated. Nurses who maintain competency position themselves to determine the most accurate risk profiles and family risk assessment.

## Sexuality-Reproductive Pattern

Sexuality is the expression of sexual identity. The sexuality-reproductive pattern describes sexuality fulfillment (Gordon, 2016), including behavioral patterns of reproduction. This pattern also includes perceptions of satisfaction or disturbances in sexuality, sexual relationships, reproduction (including contraception), and developmental changes throughout the life span, such as menarche and menopause. The sexuality-reproductive pattern addresses transmission of information within the family about sexuality, as well as sexuality for the couple, including their sexual relationship, perception of problems, manner in which problems are handled, and actions taken to solve problems (Gordon, 2016). Information transmission during childhood is an important area to explore to better understand how issues related to sexuality and gender identity are addressed within the family (Gordon, 2016).

Topics to explore during the assessment may include the following areas:

- How do the adults in the family communicate their needs to each other?
- How do family members commit to, love, and care for each other, as well as fulfill their obligations and responsibilities toward one another?
- How do the adults in the family view marriage, parenthood, and their relationship as lovers?
- How does the family address family planning and birth control?
- How do family members participate in the choice of family planning and contraceptives used?

When needed, complete pregnancy histories include sexual practices and partners, the number and ages of children, the number and outcome of pregnancies (including live births, miscarriages, spontaneous/therapeutic abortions), and the birth control methods used. Nurses also observe the comfort levels the adults demonstrate when discussing their own sexuality, or if an adult seems uninformed when discussing sexual subjects with children. Because of the impact that sexual relationships within the family have on children, exploring the variety of sexual

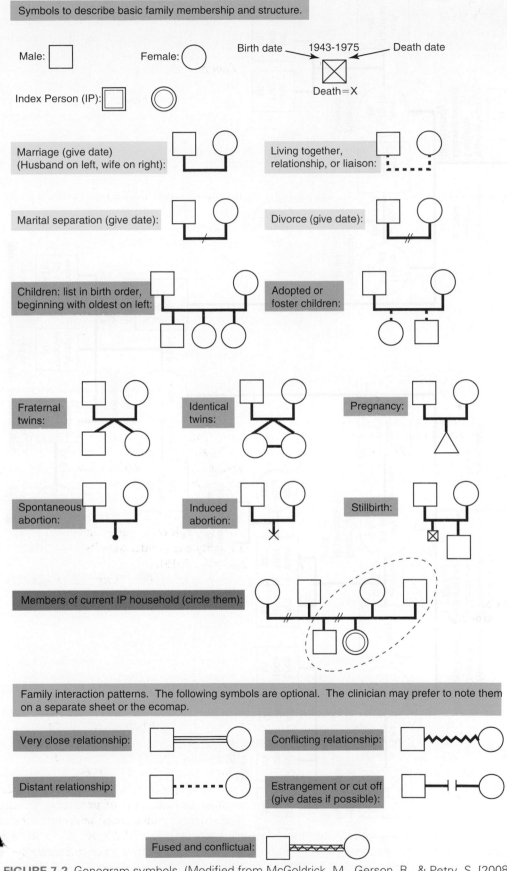

**FIGURE 7-2** Genogram symbols. (Modified from McGoldrick, M., Gerson, R., & Petry, S. [2008]. *Genograms: Assessment and intervention* [3rd ed.]. New York: Norton.)

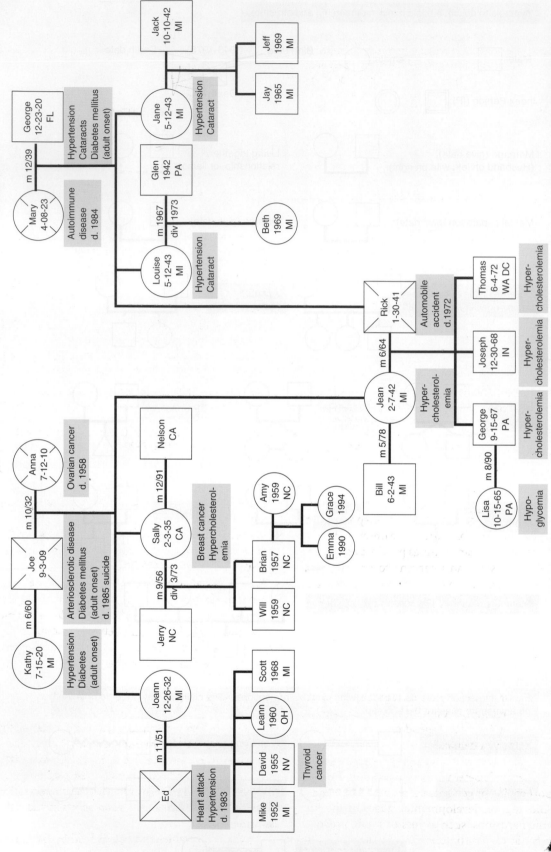

**FIGURE 7-3** Genogram of the Graham family. (From Stanhope, M., & Lancaster, J. [2015]. *Public health nursing: Population-centered health care in the community* [9th ed., p. 632]. St. Louis: Mosby.)

## BOX 7-6   Genomics and Family Assessment

Family assessment is the first line of assessment for genetic testing. Family assessment encompasses both genetic and environmental risks shared among family members. Family assessment provides the foundation for the complex process of genetic assessment, which includes nondirective genetic counseling to facilitate the balance of risk versus benefit (Wilson & Nicholls, 2015).

Thanksgiving Day, a day in the United States when families customarily gather, has been designated by the US government's Family History Initiative as Family History Day. Family History Day sets aside Thanksgiving Day as a time when family members can discuss their health history (https://www.genome.gov/17516481/). Multiple tools have now been designed to facilitate gathering and sharing information in preparation for use in an electronic health record (EHR) environment. The design of these tools is intended to improve quality, while decreasing disease burden and cost.

Evidence supports multiple genomic interventions that are derived from accurate family assessment. A number of conditions have been identified as tier 1 disorders. Tier 1 designation indicates that genomic and family health history synthesized studies support implementation of the evidence into practice. Currently the following disorders that rely on accurate family assessment are classified as tier 1:

### Breast/Ovarian Cancer
- Hereditary breast and ovarian cancer in women (see Box 6-6: Genomics)
  - *BRCA1* and *BRCA2* genes related
  - Deleterious mutation of the BRCA gene
- Chemoprevention of breast cancer

### Colorectal Cancer
- Newly diagnosed colorectal syndrome (test for Lynch syndrome; see Box 6-6: Genomics)
- Known Lynch syndrome in family
- Metastatic colorectal cancer (*KRAS* gene, cetuximab, panitumumab)
- Invasive colorectal cancer (carcinoembryonic antigen–related cell adhesion molecule 5)

### Cardiovascular Disease
- Familial hypercholesterolemia (DNA testing and low-density lipoprotein cholesterol concentration measurement)
- Cholesterol screening

### Other
- Osteoporosis screening in Women—parental history of hip fracture
- Hereditary hemochromatosis–family health history, especially siblings
- Newborn screening of 31 core conditions

Other tier 1 genomic applications, in addition to family assessment, could be used to reduce morbidity among affected people and their families (Douglas & Dotson, 2015).

Adding family health history to meaningful use standards for EHRs may also decrease the gaps between the evidence and how it is implemented in practice. Promoting the importance of family assessment through education and policy may facilitate identification of at-risk families (Kolor & Khoury, 2015).

From Douglas, M. P., & Dotson, W. D. (2015). Evidence matters in genomic medicine, round 2 from the Office of Public Health Genomics, Centers for Disease Control and Prevention. http://blogs.cdc.gov/genomics/2012/08/23/evidence-matters-in-genomic-medicine-round-2/; Kolor, K. & Khoury, M. J. (2015). Evidence matters in genomic medicine–round 3: Integrating family health history into preventive services. http://blogs.cdc.gov/genomics/2012/09/27/evidence-matters-in-genomic-medicine-round-3/; Wilson, B. J., & Nicholls, S. G. (2015). The Human Genome Project, and recent advances in personalized genomics. *Risk Management and Healthcare Policy*, (8)2, 9–20.

practices within heterosexual, homosexual, and bisexual relationships in the family is an important part of health-promotion assessment (Hockenberry & Wilson, 2015). The onset of the use of electronic health records in many settings provides an opportunity to systematically assess and intervene to provide best practices and eliminate disparities in these populations (Donald & Ehrenfeld, 2015).

## Coping–Stress Tolerance Pattern

The coping–stress tolerance pattern helps to depict the family's adaptation to both internal and external pressures (Gordon, 2016). On a daily basis, family members generate energy to face evolving needs. Society continually compels families to adapt to new situations. Survival and growth depend on coping mechanisms as families face external demands required to move from one developmental stage to the next. The family's ability to cope with everyday living demands determines family success. Family relationships support coping or generate more stress. Life events, such as divorce, moving, or developmental stages of the life cycle, and economic hardships, such as loss of a job, provoke stress and mobilize family coping strategies. Exploration of coping and stress tolerance includes the following assessment areas:
- How does the family cope with stressful life events?
- What experiences have family members had with chemical abuse?

- What strengths does the family have and use to counterbalance the stresses?
- What stressful family situations are experienced?
- How does the family view the association between stress and children's health and development?
- How does the family make appraisals of the situations, and are they realistic?
- Describe the family's resources. How do family members use knowledge or links to family networks or community resources?
- What kinds of dysfunctional adaptive strategies are used, such as chemical abuse or violence?

## Values-Beliefs Pattern

The values-beliefs pattern characterizes the family's perspective and attitudes about life meanings, values, beliefs, and spirituality and the way these issues affect behavior (Gordon, 2016). Assessment, diagnosis, and intervention are based on these attitudes. Assessment of this pattern enhances the interpretation of family behavior. Exploration of values and beliefs includes the following assessment areas:
- What are the values and beliefs held by the family?
- How flexible are rules?
- How do family members interact (calm, aggressive, competitive, or rigid)?
- How do family members view spirituality?

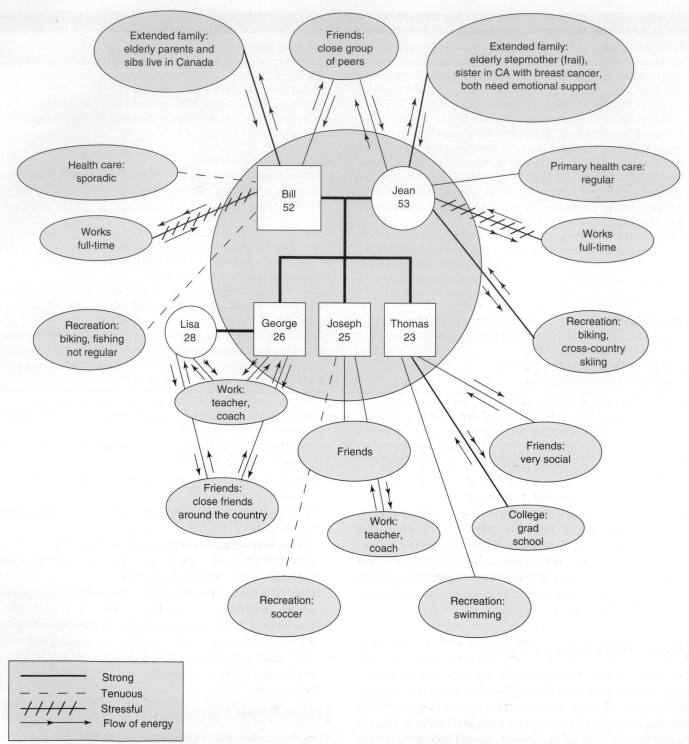

**FIGURE 7-4** Ecomap of the Graham family. (From Stanhope, M., & Lancaster, J. [2012]. *Public health nursing: Population-centered health care in the community* [8th ed., p. 636]. St. Louis: Mosby.)

- Describe the cultural or ethnic group with which the family identifies. What family practices are consistent with the norms of that ethnic group? How are the practices inconsistent with these norms?
- What are the family's traditions and practices?
- How do the significant cultural beliefs affect health or illness?
- Describe the role that religion plays in the family on a regular basis and during times of stress. How does the family rely on religious practices?
- How does the family perceive its competency during crisis?
- What are the family goals, and do members perceive that they are attaining these goals?
- How are value conflicts demonstrated within the family?
- How do identified family values affect the health status of the family?

Spirituality, defined as life purpose and connection with others, affects health. The metaphysical and transcendental phenomenon of spirituality, as well as the religious and nonreligious systems of belief within families, should be assessed (Denham et al., 2015). How well families communicate their unconditional love and forgiveness for injury or betrayal may contribute to physical symptoms within families. Clearly, spirituality and social skills promote health and prevent disease.

Data collected in the 11 functional patterns reveal ideas about family health-promotion and disease-prevention practices. Risks to healthy family functioning may be identified in each pattern. Risk factors may be found in more than one area. For example, passive smoke from one family member's cigarettes may be identified as an environmental risk factor in the home. However, the family's reaction to passive smoking determines the family members' perceived susceptibility, their perceived severity of the problem, and whether they will make a change in the environment to promote family health. The pattern indicates high risk if chronic asthma is described during the family history. In this situation, several other pattern areas support the finding. The nurse determines each risk behavior along with its effects on the others.

## ENVIRONMENTAL FACTORS

The environment also influences family health and well-being. The home, neighborhood, and community constitute the family environment. Assessment includes exploration of the following home environment areas (Figure 7-5):
- What type of dwelling is it (condominium, single dwelling, low-income apartment, or temporary shelter)?
- How has the family acquired the home (purchase, rental)?
- What is the condition of the home (interior/exterior: glass, trash, broken stairs, peeling paint, inadequate insulation, inadequate lighting on stairs, or broken fixtures)?
- Are the number and type of rooms adequate for the size of the family?
- How satisfactory are the furnishings to meet the needs of the family (enough chairs and beds, and a kitchen table)?
- How comfortable is the temperature (warm in winter and cool in summer, insulated)?
- How adequate is lighting for reading, sewing, and other activities?

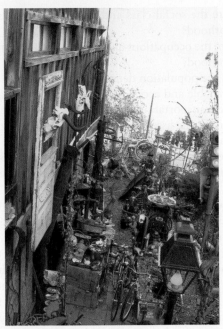

**FIGURE 7-5** Assessment of the home includes environmental assessment of the yard.

- How adequate is the water supply (sufficient/clean/fluoridated/polluted)?
- Does the family have access to a telephone, and are emergency numbers available?
- How safe are the kitchen sanitation and refrigeration capabilities?
- How adequate are the bathroom sanitation facilities, water supply, toilet, and towels and soap?
- Are the sleeping arrangements adequate for family members, considering age, sex, relationships, and spatial needs?
- How adequate is the plan for escape in an emergency (smoke detectors/escape route/plan inside the home)?
- What are the arrangements for and knowledge of first aid (directions posted for poisons, burns, lacerations, and other first-aid needs)?
- What signs of rats, mice, or cockroaches are present inside or outside the home?
- What are the family's impressions about the home? How do the family members describe the adequacy of their living space for privacy, their own interests, and status?
- How are chemicals stored in the home (out of reach of children)?
- How is safety ensured in the home? What safety issues are evident?

The areas to explore for neighborhood assessment are as follows:
- What is the condition of the dwellings and streets (maintenance/deterioration)?
- How and when is the garbage collected?
- What is the incidence of violent crime, burglaries, and automobile accidents?
- What kinds of industry are nearby and do they produce air pollution or toxic waste?

- What are the social class and ethnic characteristics of the neighborhood?
- What are the occupations and interests of the families in the neighborhood?
- What is the population density?
- How available and accessible is public transportation? Why is public transportation not used if it is available?

Exploration during assessment of the community includes the following areas:

- What resources, such as schools, church, transportation, shopping, and recreational facilities, are available for family use?
- How accessible are the health facilities, such as physician's office, clinic, hospital, gym, swimming pool, natural food store, and weight-reduction clinic?

By driving or walking around the area, the nurse can obtain neighborhood and community data. Other sources of information include the family, health professionals, teachers, business people, and others who work in the area. Official resources, such as the reports from the US Census Bureau (http://www.census.gov/) or statistics from the city or state health departments and libraries, are also helpful in describing a neighborhood and community.

## ANALYSIS AND NURSING DIAGNOSIS

### Analyzing Data

After completing the data collection, the nurse and the family analyze the data. Several approaches are used to analyze health data, including systems theory, developmental theory, and risk-estimate theory. A systems approach categorizes families as open or closed, with permeable or rigid boundaries determining both structural and functional components of family systems.

Developmental theory approaches families from the perspective of tasks and progression through cycles. Nurses analyze data to identify accomplishment of family life cycle stages and family tasks needed to function successfully. Family developmental needs are determined considering the wide variety of family structures and functions in society. Although most family models are based on nuclear family structures, additional family structures should be explored as indicated by current population trends (Brown et al., 2016; Coyne et al., 2016; Edwards, 2009). The stages of family development guide the baseline data analysis. Gaps, missing data, or conflicting information is identified and clarified.

### Couple Family

The first stage of family development begins when adults define themselves as a family regardless of the legal status. When individuals move from their family of origin to a new couple relationship, adaptation to role expectations of a partner becomes a developmental task for each individual. Establishing a mutually satisfying adult relationship that converges with the kinship network is one family developmental task. Adjustment for couples includes learning how to weave together two personalities, two life histories, and two aspirations of growth. Decisions in this stage include whether adults are gainfully employed, how money is managed, where they live, how they socialize with friends and

other family members, patterns of sexual activities, and whether the couple has decided to have children. Determining how to divide household tasks of cooking, washing, cleaning, and shopping occurs either consciously or subconsciously.

Developmental tasks that integrate health practices and habits into the couple's lifestyle require consideration during analysis. Health behavior constitutes particular actions to promote health and prevent disease. Examples of health-promotion and disease-prevention activities may include maintaining well-balanced rest, exercise, diet, and contraception; attending smoking-cessation classes; wearing seat belts; and directing activities toward self-actualization. Each individual brings values and beliefs to the relationship. Practices from the family of origin and values from personal experiences combine to form the adult beliefs of the individual. Achieving mutually satisfying relationships also depends on couples' conflict management. Strategies that stem from congruent value systems facilitate couple's adjustment. When couples use divergent strategies, problem-solving tends to be less effective.

### Childbearing Family

Decisions about adding children to the family commit couples to more complex long-term responsibility. Family development and primary health needs change to focus on additional members. To analyze the learning needs of couples with a pregnant member, nurses consider aspects of decisions and motivations involved with the pregnancy. With single-parent families (usually mothers) becoming increasingly common through divorce, death, adoption, or the choice to have a child out of wedlock, analysis of family function addresses these diverse family structures (Atkin et al., 2015; Coyne et al., 2016; Edwards, 2009).

Attitudes and practices in society regarding sexuality have influenced the incidence of sexually transmitted diseases, such as genital herpes, gonorrhea, and syphilis. Acquired immunodeficiency syndrome (AIDS), first described in 1981, poses a threat to the family and society, in addition to affected individuals. Human immunodeficiency virus (HIV) is transmitted through heterosexual, homosexual, or oral sexual intercourse, as well as through direct contact with infected blood, shared needles during intravenous drug use, and perinatal transfer from infected mothers to their infants. Prevention of HIV transmission requires abstinence from and modification of relevant behaviors.

Risk factors associated with sexuality include lack of knowledge of safe sexual practices, the reproductive system, and personal hygiene; lack of prenatal care; pregnancy before age 16 years; pregnancy after age 35 years; a history of hypertension or infection during pregnancy; and unplanned or unwanted pregnancy.

Risk factors for premature pregnancies and unsatisfying marriage consist of ignorance about, or values regarding, family planning; adolescent age; and sexuality and role adjustment problems. In unplanned pregnancies, adolescent parents put themselves and their developing child at risk. Lack of knowledge of prenatal care, childbirth, and childrearing practices compounds the risks for both the mother and the child. Parents who are unable to perform parenting roles risk an unsatisfying relationship and inappropriate developmental growth for this beginning stage

## 🌐 BOX 7-7   DIVERSITY AWARENESS

### Preconception Care

Preconception care is a significant health-promotion opportunity for the whole family. The importance of this care has been recognized by *Healthy People 2020,* the Institute of Medicine, and the Public Health Services Expert Panel on the Content of Prenatal Care.

One important area of preconception care is evaluating a couple's genetic history as documented on the standard family genogram. Further evaluation should be considered for couples who are related outside marriage or who have ethnic backgrounds such as Mediterranean, black, or Ashkenazi Jew, and for women older than 35 years or younger than 16 years who have preexisting medical conditions. Couples who have family histories of any of the following health problems should be referred for further genetic testing and counseling: cystic fibrosis, hemophilia, phenylketonuria, Tay-Sachs disease, thalassemia, sickle cell disease or trait, birth defects, or mental retardation.

Modified from Johnson, K. A., Floyd, R. L., Humphrey, J. R., Biermann, J., Moos, M. K., Drummon, M., et al. (2014). Action Plan for the National Initiative on Preconception Health and Health Care (PCHHC). A report of the PCHHC Steering Committee. http://www.cdc.gov/preconception/documents/ActionPlanNationalInitiativePCHHC2012-2014.pdf.

of the family life cycle. If couples decide to remain childless, learning needs include information about contraception.

The birth or adoption of a child begins a new family unit. Family members adjust to new roles as the unit expands in function and responsibility. As described more fully in the section Formulating Family Nursing Diagnoses, parents' history as a dyad and their experiences in other groups, particularly their families of origin, influence the development of the triad (Box 7-7: Diversity Awareness). Accommodating new members disrupts family equilibrium. As a group, families explore ways to meet each other's needs, to minimize differences, and work together. First-time parents often feel a lack of emotional support during the first several months of parenthood. Some, but not all, new parents have available family leave policies that may facilitate this transition. Without a family network or friends, the first days after the birth or adoption may be difficult. Parents may care for the child proficiently, but may need assistance to grow in the parenting role. If parents are both employed outside the home, they may encounter difficulty with the routines of baby care and being confined to the house more for child care. Anxiety about the adequacy of income may cause parents to increase their work hours to increase their income. Exhaustion for both parents is common from working full-time while providing child care as the infant develops. Single parents, usually mothers, carry these same burdens alone. Emotional support may be limited, particularly if one has not found satisfaction in parenthood. The families of origin or other support systems, such as self-help groups, neighbors, or friends, assist family members as they struggle to adapt to a new member. King and colleagues (2015) reported their findings from a US longitudinal study (Adolescent and Adult Health). Their structural equation modeling indicated that perceived family belonging for adolescents of stepfather families (*n* = 2085) was strongly associated with the perceived quality of parent relationships particularly with both the stepfather and

the birth mother. Nurses facilitate processes within families of origin, families of choice, or other support systems to promote health in the newly formed family unit.

Some parents thrive during the period when an infant needs almost constant care and nurturing. These parents find support in a network of family and friends. Couples who find satisfaction in parenthood seem to realize that parental influence begins at birth and is the single most important factor in the child's physical, emotional, and cognitive development. The parents' ability to assume responsibility depends on a complex array of factors: their own maturity; how they were nurtured as children; their conceptions about self, culture, social class, and religion; their relationship with each other; their values and philosophy of life; their perceptions of and experiences with children and other adults; and the life stresses they have experienced.

In analyzing the needs of childrearing families, nurses consider many factors, including providing for physical health, economic support, and nurturing actions that are vital to learning and social development of children. In analyzing couples' needs during this stage, nurses recognize the importance of interactions among the triad. Observing decision-making helps nurses determine family functioning, member roles, and effectiveness of family members. Risks associated with role relationships include working parents with insufficient resources for child care, abuse or neglect of children, multiple closely spaced children, low family self-esteem, children used as scapegoats for parental frustration, immature parents who are dependent and unable to handle responsibility, and strong beliefs about physical punishment or obedience.

### Family With Toddlers/Preschool Children

Families may have more than one child, each growing and developing at an individual pace. Preschool children place great demands on families. Families adjust to each new member with space and equipment for expansion. The needs and interests of preschool children influence home environments. Nurses assess the quality of the home environment for whether children have healthy amounts of stimulation-promoting opportunities. Safety balanced with exploration by the child results in health-promoting home environments. Rather than removing children from the kitchen or garden, finding ways to include them in a cooking or planting activity provides learning experiences. Other environmental influences affecting the child's rate and style of development include religious practices, ethnic background, education, and discipline techniques.

Evidence increasingly demonstrates the link between environment and health. Home environments that contain contaminated air, water, or food increase health risks. For example, lead poisoning, a preventable disease that continues to affect thousands of children, often results from lead paint and other factors in the home, such as water. Although restrictions exist in the United States to limit lead-based paint to exteriors, many homes have lead in the interior. Generally, lead in water is attributed to poor infrastructure in the home plumbing or the city. As a result, poorer neighborhoods are at higher risk of lead poisoning from their water source. For example, families in Flint, Michigan, experienced increased lead in the water coming into their homes when the local government changed their water source. Hanna-Attisha and colleagues (2016) reported the incidence of elevated blood lead levels within the city ($n = 1473$; before change 736; after change 737) increased from 2.4% to 4.9% ($p < 0.05$) after a water source change without a comparable change in blood lead levels outside the city ($n = 2202$; before change 1210; after change 992). The incidence of elevated blood lead levels was highest in neighborhoods with poor families. Both homes and automobiles are also considered possible sources of exposure to the poisonous agent carbon monoxide. Nurses also review data for home safety, including storage of dangerous materials, such as detergents, insecticides, and medications.

Health-promotion needs for young children include proper foods, adequate exercise and sleep, and dental hygiene. Parents teach children through modeling and use of positive reinforcement. Family developmental tasks include adjusting to fatigue resulting from parenting demands. Nurses explore alternatives to relieve parents. Parents need time for themselves, individually and as a couple (e.g., to exercise, socialize), while knowing their children are safe with a responsible person. Economic restraints may limit relaxation time away from the children. Sharing child care with friends and the family provides one source of support for new parents.

## Family With School-Age Children

A family with children in school may have reached its maximal size in numbers and interrelationships. The parents' major problem during this stage is the dichotomy between pursuing self-interests and finding fulfillment in producing the next generation. Family developmental tasks revolve around goals of reorganization to prepare for the expanding world of school-age children. School achievement becomes a critical task for socialization. Viewing social and educational goals from the perspective of family culture and parents' defined goals becomes particularly important during this developmental stage. For example, many opportunities for health education exist in schools, including influencing healthy beliefs and behaviors. However, school health programs focus on problems such as tobacco and substance abuse with messages aimed at problems and crises rather than healthy behaviors. Families influence health at home and in school both by teaching children ways to assess and manage risky situations and by describing the benefits to expect when healthy behaviors are practiced.

As children's activities broaden away from the home, another important developmental task for both the parent and the child becomes "letting go." Parents become involved in community groups such as the parent-teacher association, scout groups, sports teams, and other volunteer organizations. Encouraging children to join in family discussions to learn about their heritage can foster understanding of self within the family network (Figure 7-6). Children exposed to unsafe home environments are at risk of behavior disturbances, school problems, and learning disabilities. Parents who cannot manage their children in growth-promoting ways soon experience energy depletion and may turn to dysfunctional relief from parenting (e.g., drug and alcohol abuse).

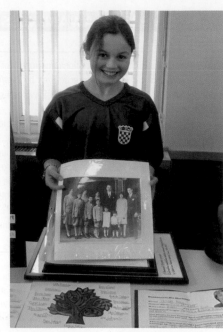

**FIGURE 7-6** School-age girl learns about her family heritage and presents this information through a school project.

## Family With Adolescents

Parents with adolescent children may experience a late pregnancy, resulting in care for an infant while other children in the family are in school. A new family member at this stage may be a source of joy or frustration for the family. The overall goal with adolescent members is to loosen family ties to allow greater responsibility and freedom in preparation for releasing young adults. Although each member of the family strives to achieve individual developmental tasks in the midst of social pressures, the family as a whole has tasks to accomplish. Strengthening the marital relationship to build a foundation for future family stages is a critical task during this time.

Open communication is often difficult during this stage, partly because of the differing developmental tasks of adolescents and adults. Adolescents seek their own identity, and adults attempt to facilitate adolescent decision-making processes. Choices about values and lifestyles may differ. Adolescents may challenge family values and standards. Although parents maintain some authority, adolescents tackle their own desires and needs. Adolescents want to do what their friends do, have their own cars, and make their own money to spend in ways that they see fit. Parents who give adolescent members opportunities to experience social, emotional, and ethical situations with others are providing learning opportunities to enhance their sense of autonomy and responsibility. As adolescents become mature and emancipated, families face balancing freedom with responsibility. Health problems in this age group include violent deaths, including suicide, injuries, and alcohol and drug abuse. Contributing risk factors involve lack of problem-solving skills, family values of aggressiveness and competition, socioeconomic factors, peer relationships, rigid and inflexible family values, daredevil risk-taking attitudes, and conflicts between parents and children. Environmental risk–related violent deaths and injuries are influenced by the highway system, automobile manufacturers, and the legislation of standards of safety. Families rely on public health officials and nurses' efforts as advocates to reduce environmental risks.

Families support adolescents in this stage of development by including them in decision-making and ensuring that they experience the positive and negative consequences of their choices. Family values of winning at all costs, aggressiveness, and competition may need to be explored during this period. Adolescents may discard these values if they are no longer applicable. Considerable change in adolescent values produces conflict and poses a threat to family cohesiveness. Families may place pressure on adolescents to conform to family values. In matters of life and death—for example, in regard to driving rules—parents must stay firm.

Families with adolescents experience identity crises for the adolescent, the adults, and the family as a whole. Adolescents move from childhood to adulthood while adults progress beyond parenthood. Adolescents struggle to find independent identities that remain connected to their family. Adults, in midlife, must resolve their own adolescent fantasies to move toward an identity for their remaining life.

## Family With Young Adults

Families with young adults act as a launching center when children begin to leave home. As children leave home, parents relinquish their parenting roles of many years to return to the marital dyad. The couple builds a new life together while maintaining relationships with aging parents, children, grandchildren, and in-laws. Couples focus on redefining relationships during this stage. As children develop, they no longer need a primary caregiver, often their mother, in the same way as during childhood. When mothers/caregivers devote years to raising children, their role and purpose within the family changes as children develop. Transition from a life with children as the priority to new or renewed interests (e.g., career, community service) may require assistance and support from the entire family. Careers at this stage may become more stable. Developmental tasks at this stage for the family's adults require focus on future prospects. In addition to individual changes occurring at this stage, families with young adults may experience other pressures. Aging parents and adult children may require financial or emotional support. Financial and emotional responsibilities to other family members hinder the couple's ability to focus on relationships during this developmental phase. Health-promoting activities to be focused on during this stage include coping with pressures of social roles and occupational responsibilities, maintaining health tasks to promote healthy aging, and reassessing life goals.

## Family With Middle-Aged Adults

Families consisting of only two members are able to enhance self-concept and support their relationship during middle age. Usually children have left home and adults experience a sense of freedom and well-being. Some relationships, by this stage, have reached a level of security, stability, and meeting each other's needs. Parenting pressures diminish, allowing parents to enjoy the accomplishments of their children and grandchildren. Couples

have acquired a network of friends. Long-time acquaintances seek participation from the couple in neighborhood rituals and events. Economic security and personal self-esteem may be at a peak.

In contrast, some relationships falter at this time. Departed children create a quiet house with less activity, known as the "empty nest." When individuals are unprepared for this stage, they might seek opportunities to enhance self-concept from outside of the family. With parenting roles now complete, adults may develop feelings of inadequacy or begin new relationships, start new families, or resort to substance abuse. In addition, this life phase may include becoming grandparents, parenting grandchildren, coping with the needs of middle-aged children, and caring for older adults (children, siblings, or parents).

Health tasks in this developmental stage require new awareness of susceptibility or vulnerability to health problems. Couples adjust their lifestyle and habits to cope with health risks. Losses promote health problems, and at this stage couples begin to cope with deaths among family and friends, along with declining income. If either member has developed physical or mental illness, the other adjusts to the resultant physical and mental impairments, redefining self-concept.

Middle-aged families face a host of risk factors leading to three prevalent causes of death: heart disease, cancer, and cerebrovascular accident (stroke). Family lifestyle may decrease risks by placing a high value on being physically active, refraining from smoking, maintaining adequate and sound nutritional habits, and consuming moderate amounts of alcohol. Lifestyle habits that are transmitted through role modeling have a greater influence on the younger members of the family than any verbal edict. Middle-aged members positively influence their health if they are able to choose environments low in water and air pollution and free from crippling stress factors such as excessive noise, traffic, and overcrowding. Family members can also apply pressure on key members of the community to decrease risks in the environment.

## Family With Older Adults

Retirement affects many aspects of life for couples and each individual in the family and their relationships with others. Besides decreased work hours, retirement also means reduction in income and fixed incomes for most people. Adjusting living standards to retirement income and being able to supplement this income with wage-earning activity is one task of the family with older adults. Other tasks during this stage include ensuring a safe and comfortable home environment, preparing for end of life, and adjusting to the loss of a spouse and finding meaning in the grief process (MacKinnon et al., 2016). In their qualitative pilot study, MacKinnon and colleagues (2016) reported that participants ($n = 12$) used group intervention (meaning-based group counseling) to establish effective coping strategies, adapt to their loss, and reframe life goals.

Health promotion aims to maintain functional ability, limit the effects of disabling conditions, and maintain quality of life. Older adults may fear becoming helpless, feeling useless, and being incapable of caring for themselves. When analyzing risk factors in the aging family, nurses look for the couple's ability

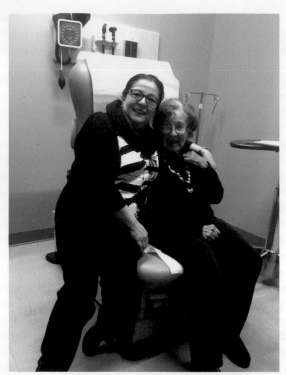

**FIGURE 7-7** As with all people, older adults hope for a state of well-being that allows them to function at their highest capacity physically. Medicare now has a yearly wellness visit for those older than 65 years.

to function well enough to carry out normal roles and responsibilities. As with all people, older adults hope for a state of well-being that will allow them to function at their highest capacity physically, psychologically, socially, and spiritually (Figure 7-7). Many older adults remain in their own homes, and most of these individuals are vigorous and completely independent. Assuming that most older adults prefer to remain in their own homes, assessment of the family for this age group should consider predictors of independence or those factors that indicate a need for institutionalized care such as assisted living, adult day care, or nursing homes. In their report of a longitudinal 22-year study of 1032 Finnish adults aged from 73.1 to 92.3 years (average age 83.5 years), Salminen and colleagues (2016) reported that falling several times a year, absence of nearby assistance, diminished cognitive function, and both high and low body mass index significantly increased the likelihood of institutionalization. These findings highlight the importance of assessing fall risk, social support networks, cognitive function, and body weight in families with older adults.

Ego integrity (the union of all previous phases of the life cycle) is the challenge in this stage and demands successful aging through continued activity. Having gone through the various stages of family development, the couple accepts what they have done as their own. At this time, they may need family or professional support to pursue other interests or maintain former activities to feel needed and useful.

The nurse and the family jointly analyze the information, comparing the family's data with documented norms of health promotion and disease prevention in older adults. Norms or expected values can be derived from the family's baseline information of 11 functional pattern areas, knowledge of growth and development for all age groups and the family as a whole, risk-factor estimates, and population norms. Population norms specify normal ranges for these groups. For example, age is associated with various risk factors; some disorders are so common that they are referred to as diseases of the older person. In certain diseases, such as lung cancer, there is a long period of exposure. Risk increases with cumulative exposure; therefore the incidence and prevalence of diseases increase with age.

*Sexuality.* Because of the popular perception that older adults are asexual, their sexual concerns may be disregarded (Salladay, 2016). The strength of sexual desire of the older women may be more influenced by age, education, and attitude than by biomedical factors.

General population norms for values, beliefs, self-perception, or role relationships may be less available than physical population norms. Cultural, ethnic, and religious factors contribute to values and beliefs about health. Family baseline information provides important comparative criteria for analysis. Family records provide useful information when available. The first contact assessment provides baseline information for subsequent comparison and evaluation of progress. Whether the family perceives situations to be problematic should also be considered in the analysis phase. Nurse and family perceptions about problems may differ.

## Formulating Family Nursing Diagnoses

Writing a **family nursing diagnosis** helps families promote health throughout the life cycle and prevents disease through decreasing risk-taking behaviors. Nurses derive diagnoses from assessed validated data. As a concise summary statement of a problem or potential problem, diagnoses provide direction for outcomes and interventions by identifying negative health states and factors to change to alleviate or prevent the problem (see Chapter 6). Describing health and validating potential or actual health problems with families facilitates cooperation. Assessment and negotiation continue until agreement occurs and a plan for resolution develops.

**Cultural competence** and respect for familial beliefs forms a foundation for the nursing process of assessing, determining nursing diagnoses, planning, intervening, and evaluating (see Chapter 2 for more detail). With changing trends in families and shifts in heritage within society, cultural competence and cultural attunement become priorities for family assessment and nurses. Pandit and colleagues (2014) define "socio-cultural attunement (SCA) as the ongoing process of experiencing clients' emotions around the intersection of socio-cultural contexts (i.e., gender, race, ethnicity, religion, sexual orientation, etc.)." Their definition of sociocultural attunement (SCA) was derived from a study that developed a working model of SCA in which 13 therapists and five couples participated in a total of 25 therapy sessions. Four cycles of qualitative analysis resulted in a working model for the SCA process. The process of SCA these researchers designed includes three recursive phases: the initial guiding lens, sociocultural interpretation, and client and therapist resonance (Pandit et al., 2014).

Cultural values, such as those connected to nutrition, influence most health-promotion practices. As globalization occurs, diversity will also expand, and competent care for indigenous populations and migrating populations will be needed (Andrews & Boyle, 2015). Cultural competence increases the efficacy of health promotion for all families, particularly families from within vulnerable populations (Andrews & Boyle, 2015).

## PLANNING WITH THE FAMILY

Intervention planning stems from complete assessment, analysis, and nursing diagnosis. The plan's purpose aims for behavioral change in families to promote health or prevent dysfunction. As in the assessment phase, family members play an active role in the planning process. Family responsibility for personal health status enhances the success of behavioral change outcomes. The planning process involves several steps, with the nurse and family identifying the following:

- Order of priority for problems or potential problems
- Items that can be handled by the nurse and the family and items that must be referred to others
- Actions and expected outcomes

The nursing plan provides direction for implementation and the framework for evaluation (see the care plan at the end of this chapter).

As mentioned, a family's health status can be diagnosed as functional, potentially dysfunctional, or dysfunctional. Functional family health status warrants verification by the nurse with a plan for periodic reevaluation that is formulated jointly. Plans to continue healthy living behaviors are reinforced. The nurse provides specific information requested by the family, such as immunization schedules, growth and development milestones, and recommended dietary allowances. In working with healthy families, the nurse controls the assessment and analysis phases of the nursing process. If the health status is judged functional, then planning health-education materials, scheduling periodic examinations, and providing accessibility of the nurse remain professional responsibilities. Implementation and evaluation of health-promotion activities become family responsibilities.

In health-promotion and disease-prevention settings, life-threatening situations rarely occur; however, when such situations do occur, they become the highest priority for intervention. For other identified potential or actual problems, the nurse relies on the family to decide which problem or potential problem to approach. After the ordering of priorities has been established, the family and nurse determine who will work on the problem. Problems or potential problems to be resolved by the nurse are identified separately from those requiring referral or family intervention. Problems for the family to handle or those the family is already addressing are considered strengths and are acknowledged and supported by the nurse. For example, when there is consistency among values and actions, physical fitness, weight management, and ability to cope with stress, the family is already taking informed and responsible action in these areas. The extent to which family members can provide their own health promotion and disease prevention will depend on their knowledge, skills, motivation, and orientation toward health.

Problems that need medical, legal, or social attention are referred to appropriate agencies. The nurse should have a directory of resources in the community when referrals are needed. Nursing intervention requires clearly stated actions that are purposeful, moral, capable of being accomplished, and adapted to the particular life situation, beliefs, and expectations of the family.

### Goals

Goals are statements describing desired outcomes. Family outcome statements include expected family behaviors, circumstances for exhibited behaviors, and criteria for determining performance. Health-promotion goals reflect a desire to function at a higher level of health and to grow beyond maintaining health or preventing disease.

## IMPLEMENTATION WITH THE FAMILY

The implementation phase is dynamic. As the nurse and family work together, new information is used to adapt and change the plan as necessary. Family nursing interventions aim to assist families in performing functions that members cannot perform for themselves. In health promotion and disease prevention, nurses assist families to improve their capacity to act on their own behalf. Ten studies were identified in a systematic review of the literature about family interventions (Deek et al., 2016). This review linked reduced readmission rates, emergency department visits, and anxiety levels and family-centered interventions. Evidence to support the use of family-centered interventions, including active learning strategies, transitional care, and appropriate follow-up in families with chronic conditions, was presented.

Families may know that they take risks by smoking, drinking, and engaging in a stressful lifestyle. As the nurse explains the rationale behind the proposed changes, families may choose to deny how they jeopardize their future health and continue their risk-taking behaviors. Factors that the nurse has not considered may cause the family's resistance. For example, families may have more pressing basic needs such as food, clothing, and housing. The Patient Protection and Affordable Care Act (2010) addressed some of these health care issues of the family by permitting parents to retain children on their health insurance plans until the age of 26 years, regardless of their marital status, living situations, or employment (unless in some cases where health insurance is an employee benefit). New insurance plans must cover preventive benefits such as well-child visits and immunizations without additional cost to the insured. Although the Patient Protection and Affordable Care Act (PL 111-148) became law on March 23, 2010, and was amended by the Health Care and Education Reconciliation Act of 2010 (PL 111-152), the statute was brought before the US Supreme Court beginning March 26, 2012, as unconstitutional, citing four major arguments (requiring the individual mandate, applying the Anti-Injunction Act, lacking a severability clause, and expanding Medicaid). The Supreme Court ruled in favor of the statute in June 2012.

Health promotion and disease prevention may not have been part of the family's life experiences, giving the nurse the educational task to try to change attitudes and values by expanding the options for families to consider health promotion. Four types of nursing interventions appear in health-promotion and disease-prevention planning: increasing knowledge and skills; increasing strengths; decreasing exposure; and decreasing susceptibility. Increasing knowledge and skills to improve family capacity for health-promotion and disease-prevention behavior may be the primary strategy. Use of this strategy helps families make informed choices about healthful lifestyle behaviors and to eliminate harmful environmental influences that affect health. Improved knowledge aims to create awareness as the nurse and family work together to uncover actual or potential problems. Nurses recognize particular families at risk and move toward motivating and supporting behavioral change in these families. Box 7-8: Innovative Practice presents an example of one program that provides education and support to people with cancer and their families.

**Family strengths** or forces that contribute to family unity and solidarity foster the development of inherent family potential (Carrascosa, 2015). These factors include:

---

### ☀ BOX 7-8 INNOVATIVE PRACTICE

#### *The Wellness Community and Gilda's Club*

The Wellness Community, which was founded in the 1982 by Dr. Harold Benjamin in California, has many local chapters throughout the United States. Comedian Gilda Radner attended the Wellness Community during her battle with ovarian cancer and shared her experiences in her book *It's Always Something*. After her death, Joel Siegel and Mandy Patinkin began Gilda's Club and opened the first club house in New York in 1991 with the support of her spouse Gene Wilder. These two organizations shared 45 years of offering free educational and support programs for people with cancer and their families on both coasts. Emphasis is placed on the family to acknowledge that no person with cancer makes the journey alone. Weekly support groups help family members support one another, explore new ways of coping with the stresses of cancer, and learn ways to become the most effective partners possible with their health care teams. These two organizations have now partnered to continue their vision with the Cancer Support Community to "ensure that all people impacted by cancer are empowered by knowledge and strengthened by action, and sustained by community."

These communities now offer a wide variety of workshops and programs (Gentle Strength and Stretch, Meditation and Guided Imagery, Nutrition Matters, Nutrition and the Immune System, Nutrition at Midlife: Preventing Heart Disease and Osteoporosis, tai chi, yoga, mindfulness, and feng shui). Social events are organized (comfort food potluck dinner, couples networking groups, singles networking group, family and friends networking group). Although chapters generally do not charge for their services, donations are appreciated and necessary to help serve the thousands of people with cancer and their families.

#### Contact Information:
Cancer Support Community
1050 17th Street, NW
Suite 500
Washington, DC 20036
Phone: 202-659-9709
Toll-free: 888-793-9355
Fax: 202-659-9301
E-mail: help@cancersupportcommunity.org
Website: http://cancersupportcommunity.org/default.aspx

---

- Physical, emotional, and spiritual factors
- Healthy childrearing practices and discipline
- Meaningful and clear communication
- Support, security, and encouragement
- Growth-producing relationships and experiences
- Responsible community relationships
- Growth with and through children
- Self-help and acceptance of help
- Flexibility in family functions and roles
- Mutual respect for individuality
- Crisis as a means for growth
- Family unity and loyalty and intrafamily cooperation
- Adaptability of family strengths

In recent years, a shift of family health care from an illness or problem and deficiency focus to a strength-based focus has occurred (Aston et al., 2015). Multiple models in nursing view families as systems and base their assessment and nursing process on strengths rather than deficits. These models of nursing provide the framework to assess and plan care using family strengths and resources (Carrascosa, 2015). Family members develop and maintain health-promoting behaviors by using commitment, appreciation, affection, positive communication, time together, a sense of spiritual well-being, and ability to cope with stress and crisis. Multiple assessment tools are available for nurses to use to generate discussion among family members about their strengths. Aston and colleagues (2015) describe the importance of corresponding nursing interventions to support and further develop the family dynamics of socialization, support, and nurturance.

Families with significant strengths may need to learn new, unfamiliar skills for mastering a specific technique, such as meditation, and to apply new tools for decision-making. These families rarely require ongoing supervision or support of sustained interventions aimed at changing their coping patterns, communication, or role behavior. They may be highly capable of seeking and using information. Assisting functional families may simply involve providing information in terms that can be understood and offering opportunities to ask questions and clarify information. Unit 3 contains individual chapters devoted to many of the strategies commonly used in health-promotion intervention, such as health teaching and counseling.

Decreasing exposure to risk factors may include enhancing parents' ability to assess and adjust their behavior to their child's temperament. Parents with limited literacy may need assistance to learn to respond constructively to their child's communication attempts. Health promotion includes teaching parents to avoid exposure to risks—for example, to use adequate restraints in automobiles, to protect their toddler from wandering into dangerous streets, and to supervise children to avoid falls and hazardous materials.

Although no substitute can be found for continuous supervision of a child, homes can be made safer if common hazards are moved out of children's reach. This effort includes storing all cleaning solutions and medications beyond children's reach; erecting barriers in front of exposed heaters, high windows, and stairways; keeping pots and pans turned inward on the stove;

fencing in a yard or a swimming pool; and teaching children to avoid dangerous areas. Becoming aware of peeling paint and toxic chemicals that parents might carry home from the job on their clothing can also protect the child.

Decreasing susceptibility means educating families about prevention principles. Families who realize how diseases are spread are better able to avoid transmission from person to person; through air, water, and food; and by insects and the rodents on which insects live. Health promotion includes emphasizing the role of personal hygiene and cleanliness to avoid infection. Families who know signs and symptoms that require medical attention and how to treat minor illnesses are better able to maintain healthy environments.

Pender and colleagues (2014) cite research that demonstrates how perceived susceptibility predicts preventive behavior. Perceived susceptibility is the family's estimated subjective probability that a specific health problem will be encountered. Family members' perceptions of health risks and their susceptibility to them will determine how they change their behavior. If the overweight family believes obesity is a threat to the health of the family, the family members are more likely to react positively to the changes suggested by the nurse than is a family who perceives no health threat. Nurses who introduce threat as a motivator to action are morally obligated to reduce the threat by meaningful and purposeful interventions. Table 7-2 lists various nursing roles used in the implementation stage.

## EVALUATION WITH THE FAMILY

The purpose of evaluation is to determine how the family has responded to the planned interventions and whether these interventions were successful. Goals and objectives that are stated in specific behavioral terms will make evaluation much easier than when they are given in general terms. The criteria used to evaluate interventions, such as weight change, increased lung capacity from an exercise program, and lower pulse rate as a result of relaxation exercises, are simple to measure. Other results of health promotion and disease prevention are not as easy to measure but must be considered in the evaluation step of the nursing process. When considering such factors as values, beliefs, self-perceptions, or role relationships, the nurse may base the evaluation on whether the family indicates that the interventions were successful. Additionally, the family's baseline data are used as comparative criteria in evaluation. The nurse reassesses the situation and compares the new information with that on the original assessment to determine whether change has occurred.

The following five measures of family functioning can be used to determine the effectiveness of interventions: changes in interaction patterns; effective communication; ability to express emotions; responsiveness to needs of members as individuals; and problem-solving ability. Using these measures, the nurse returns to the original assessment of the family's functioning and compares current observations with previous data. These characteristics of family functioning continue to provide a useful framework even today, when family structures are becoming more diverse and the nuclear family is becoming less prevalent (Brown et al., 2016; Coyne et al., 2016; Edwards, 2009).

When, during the planning phase of the nursing process, the nurse has identified the criteria (norms and standards) for the desired outcomes, these outcomes are the basis of evaluation. Data from the family that describe the behavior of family members relative to the desired outcomes determine whether the nursing care was successful. With the criteria stated, the goals and objectives outline how the family can demonstrate a successful outcome and the behavior change expected to result from nursing intervention. The more objective and measurable the desired outcome is, the more reliable the results of evaluation will be.

After the goals and objectives have been reached, the problem no longer exists. If evaluation shows the nursing actions did not achieve the goals or objectives, the nurse must review the nursing process to determine whether there were gaps in the assessment data, errors in analysis or nursing diagnosis, or alternative interventions that might have been considered. The nurse also needs to review the process with the family to determine whether the family members have contributed to outcome failure. Finally, the agency employing the nurse may be another factor; if intervention is costly or a shortage of staff exists, then health promotion and disease prevention may have low priority.

---

## CASE STUDY

### *Family Member With Alzheimer Disease: Mark and Jacqueline*

Mark and Jacqueline have been married for 30 years. They have grown children who live in another state. Jacqueline's mother has moved in with the couple because she has Alzheimer disease. Jacqueline is an only child and always promised her mother that she would care for her in her old age. Her mother is unaware of her surroundings and often calls out for her daughter Jackie when Jacqueline is in the room. Jacqueline reassures her mother that she is there to help, but to no avail. Jacqueline is unable to visit her children on holidays because she must attend to her mother's daily needs. She is reluctant to visit friends or even go out to a movie because of her mother's care needs or because she is too tired. Even though she has eliminated most leisure activities with Mark, Jacqueline goes to bed at night with many of her caregiving tasks unfinished. She tries to visit with her mother during the day, but her mother rejects any

contact with her daughter. Planning for the upcoming holidays seems impossible to Mark, because of his wife's inability to focus on anything except her mother's care. Jacqueline has difficulty sleeping at night and is unable to discuss plans even a few days in advance. She is unable to visit friends and is reluctant to have friends visit because of the unpredictable behavior of her mother and her need to attend to the daily care.

**Reflective Questions**
- How do you think this situation reflects Jacqueline's sense of role performance?
- How do you think that Jacqueline may be contributing to her own health?

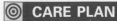

## CARE PLAN

### Family Member With Alzheimer Disease: Mark and Jacqueline

**\*NURSING DIAGNOSIS: Risk of ineffective role performance related to caring for a family member with Alzheimer disease**

**Defining Characteristics**
- Feeling exhausted
- Inability to complete tasks
- Feeling loss of usual or expected relationship with care receiver
- Increased stress or nervousness about the future
- Preoccupation with care routine
- Withdrawal from social contacts or change in leisure activities

**Related Factors**
- Illness severity of care receiver
- Increasing needs of care receiver
- Addiction or codependency of caregiver or care receiver
- Conflicting role demands
- Caregiver health impairment
- Unpredictable illness course or instability in the care receiver's health
- Psychological or cognitive problems in the care receiver
- Caregiver not developmentally ready for caregiving role
- Developmental delay or retardation of the care receiver or caregiver
- Marginal family adaptation or dysfunction before the caregiving situation began
- Marginal coping patterns of caregiver
- Providing direct, ongoing in-home care
- History of poor relationship between caregiver and care receiver
- Care receiver who exhibits deviant, bizarre behavior
- Incontinence in the care receiver

**Expected Outcomes**
- Caregiver distinguishes obligations that must be fulfilled from those that can be controlled or limited.

- In conjunction with the nurse, the caregiver develops a plan of care for the individual.
- Caregiver receives and accepts appropriate levels of support from family members, friends, and others.
- Caregiver describes help available from informal and formal support systems in the community and takes steps to obtain help.

**Interventions**
- Assess the level of the caregiver's stress.
- Assist the caregiver in developing a realistic plan of care, considering the care receiver's abilities and limitations; the plan will require modification as the person decompensates.
- Instruct the caregiver to encourage the person to participate, to the greatest extent possible, in social and self-care activities such as bathing, dressing, dining out with friends, and playing cards.
- Facilitate a family meeting to help the primary caregiver seek assistance from other family members.
- Support the caregiver and family members as they adjust to the degenerative nature of the disease; be aware that over time the stress associated with caring for the person increases.
- Identify community resources that may offer the caregiver relief from constant supervision of the individual (home health aides, respite care, and adult day care).
- Help the caregiver contact informal sources of support, such as church groups, extended family, and community volunteers.
- Encourage the caregiver to attend an Alzheimer disease support group.
- Refer the caregiver to the Alzheimer's Association.

\*NANDA Nursing Diagnoses—Herdman, T. H. & Kamitsuru, S. (Eds.). Nursing Diagnoses–Definitions and Classification 2015–2017. Copyright © 2014, 1994–2014 NANDA International. Used by arrangement with John Wiley & Sons Limited. In order to make safe and effective judgments using the NANDA-I nursing diagnoses it is essential that nurses refer to the definitions and defining characteristics of the diagnoses listed in this work.

## SUMMARY

Learning about health promotion and disease prevention begins at birth, with the family providing the stimulus for incorporating health in the value system of its members. From a systems perspective, the family has both structure and function; relevant functions include values and practices related to health. The effective execution of health-related functions involves the family's progression through its developmental tasks and its ability to generate low risk-producing behaviors associated with disease prevention.

Developmental and risk-estimate theories can be applied effectively to the nursing process with the family. The nurse uses functional patterns (an inherent part of both theories) to collect data for assessment. After organizing information on family life cycle stages for analysis with the family, the nurse writes the nursing diagnosis and plans, implements, and evaluates the interventions used to promote health and prevent disease in the family.

## EVOLVE CHAPTER FEATURES

http://evolve.elsevier.com/Edelman/
- Study Questions

## REFERENCES

Alhusen, J. L., Ray, E., et al. (2015). Intimate partner violence during pregnancy: Maternal and neonatal outcomes. *Journal of Women's Health, 24*(1), 100–106.

Andrews, M. M., & Boyle, J. S. (2015). *Transcultural concepts in nursing care* (7th ed.). New York: Wolters Kluwer.

Aston, M., Price, S., et al. (2015). The power of relationships exploring how public health nurses support mothers and families during postpartum home visits. *Journal of Family Nursing, 21*(1), 11–34.

Atkin, A. J., Corder, K., et al. (2015). Perceived family functioning and friendship quality: Cross-sectional associations with physical activity and sedentary behaviours. *International Journal of Behavior Nutrition and Physical Activity, 12*(1), 23.

Azimi, M., Schmaus, K., et al. (2016). Carrier screening by next generation sequencing: Health benefits and cost effectiveness. *Molecular Genetics & Genomic Medicine, 4*(3), 292–302.

Berry, K., & Adams, T. E. (2016). Family bullies. *Journal of Family Communication, 16*(1), 51–63.

Brown, S. L., Manning, W. D., & Payne, K. K. (2016). Family structure and children's economic well-being: Incorporating same-sex cohabiting mother families. *Population Research and Policy Review, 35*(1), 1–21.

Carrascosa, L. L. (2015). Ageing population and family support in Spain. *Journal of Comparative Family Studies, 46*(4), 499–516.

Coyne, E., et al. (2016). Understanding family assessment in the Australian context; what are adult oncology nursing practices? *Collegian (Royal College of Nursing, Australia)*, in press.

Deek, H., Hamilton, S., et al. (2016). Family-centered approaches to healthcare interventions in chronic diseases in adults: A quantitative systematic review. *Journal of Advanced Nursing, 72*(5), 968–979.

Denham, S., Eggenberger, S., et al. (2015). *Family-focused nursing care*. Philadelphia: F. A. Davis.

Donald, C., & Ehrenfeld, J. M. (2015). The opportunity for medical systems to reduce health disparities among lesbian, gay, bisexual, transgender and intersex patients. *Journal of Medical Systems, 39*(11), 1–7.

Duvall, E., & Miller, B. (1985). *Marriage and family development* (7th ed.). New York: Harper Collins.

Duvall, E. M. (1988). Family development's first forty years. *Family Relations, 37*, 127–134.

Edwards, J. O. (2009). The many kinds of family structures in our communities. https://www.scoe.org/files/ccpc-family-structures.pdf.

Erikson, E. H. (1998). *The life cycle completed*. New York: W. W. Norton.

Fiese, B. H., & Bost, K. K. (2016). Family ecologies and child risk for obesity: Focus on regulatory processes. *Family Relations, 65*(1), 94–107.

Freudenberg, N., Pastor, M., & Israel, B. (2011). Strengthening community capacity to participate in making decisions to reduce disproportionate environmental exposures. *American Journal of Public Health, 101*(Suppl. 1), S123–S130.

Glover, J. J., & Justis, L. M. (2015). Child maltreatment ethics and the identification and response to child abuse and neglect. In J. E. Korbin & R. R. Krugman (Eds.), *Child maltreatment: Contemporary issues in research and policy* (Vol. 4, pp. 157–171). Dordrecht, Netherlands: Springer.

Gordon, M. (2016). *Manual of nursing diagnosis* (13th ed.). Sudbury, MA: Jones & Bartlett.

Hanna-Attisha, M., LaChance, J., et al. (2016). Elevated blood lead levels in children associated with the Flint drinking water crisis: A spatial analysis of risk and public health response. *American Journal of Public Health, 106*(2), 283–290.

Hardaway, C. R., Sterrett-Hong, E., et al. (2016). Family resources as protective factors for low-income youth exposed to community violence. *Journal of Youth and Adolescence, 45*(7), 1309–1322.

Harper Browne, C. (2014). *The strengthening families approach and protective factors framework: Branching out and reaching deeper*. Washington, DC: Center for the Study of Social Policy. http://www.cssp.org/reform/strengtheningfamilies/2014/The-Strengthening-Families-Approach-and-Protective-Factors-Framework_Branching-Out-and-Reaching-Deeper.pdf.

Hiyoshi, A., Fall, K., et al. (2015). Remarriage after divorce and depression risk. *Social Science & Medicine, 141*(9), 109–114.

Hockenberry, M. J., & Wilson, D. (2015). *Wong's nursing care of infants and children* (10th ed.). St. Louis: Mosby.

Kann, L., Kinchen, S., et al. (2013). Youth risk behavior surveillance — United States. *Morbidity and Mortality Weekly Report, 63*(4), 1–172.

King, V., Boyd, L. M., & Thorsen, M. L. (2015). Adolescents' perceptions of family belonging in stepfamilies. *Journal of Marriage and Family, 77*(3), 761–774.

Larsen, P. D. (2016). *Lubkin's chronic illness: Impact and interventions* (9th ed.). Sudbury, MA: Jones & Bartlett.

MacKinnon, C. J., Smith, N. G., et al. (2016). A pilot study of meaning-based group counseling for bereavement. *OMEGA-Journal of Death and Dying, 72*(3), 210–233.

Masten, A. S., & Monn, A. R. (2015). Child and family resilience: A call for integrated science, practice, and professional training. *Family Relations, 64*(1), 5–21.

Maurer, F. A., & Smith, C. M. (2014). *Community/public health nursing practice: Health for families and populations* (5th ed.). St. Louis: Saunders.

National Center on Parent, Family, and Community Engagement (NCPFCE). (2015). PFCE research to practice series. http://eclkc.ohs.acf.hhs.gov/hslc/tta-system/family/rtp-series.html.

O'Brien, V. (2014). Responding to the call: A conceptual model for kinship care assessment. *Child & Family Social Work, 19*(3), 355–366.

Pandit, M. L., Chen-Feng, J., et al. (2014). Practicing socio-cultural attunement: A study of couple therapists. *Contemporary Family Therapy, 36*(4), 518–528.

Parkinson, J., Gallegos, D., & Russell-Bennett, R. (2016). Transforming beyond self: Fluidity of parent identity in family decision-making. *Journal of Business Research, 69*(1), 110–119.

Pender, N. J., Murdaugh, C. L., & Parsons, M. A. (2014). *Health promotion in nursing practice* (7th ed.). Upper Saddle River, NJ: Pearson.

Prickett, K. C., & Augustine, J. M. (2016). Maternal education and investments in children's health. *Journal of Marriage and Family, 78*(1), 7–25.

Rothenberg, W. A., Hussong, A. M., & Chassin, L. (2016). Intergenerational continuity in high-conflict family environments. *Development and Psychopathology, 28*(1), 293–308.

Salladay, S. A. (2016). Sex in the nursing home. *Journal of Christian Nursing, 33*(1), 13.

Salminen, M., Vire, J., et al. (2016). Predictors of institutionalization among home-dwelling older Finnish people: A 22-year follow-up study. *Aging Clinical and Experimental Research*, doi:10.1007/s40520-016-0530-9.

Schoon, I., Jones, E., et al. (2012). Family hardship, family instability, and cognitive development. *Journal of Epidemiology and Community Health, 66*, 716–722.

Stanhope, M., & Lancaster, J. (2012). *Public health nursing* (8th ed.). St. Louis: Mosby.

Stanhope, M., & Lancaster, J. (2015). *Public health nursing* (9th ed.). St. Louis: Mosby.

Suh, J. (2016). Measuring the "sandwich": Care for children and adults in the American Time Use Survey 2003–2012. *Journal of Family and Economic Issues, 37*, 197–211.

Tramonti, F., & Fanali, A. (2015). Toward an Integrative model for systemic therapy with individuals. *Journal of Family Psychotherapy, 26*(3), 178–189.

US Census Bureau. (2014). More young adults are living in their parents' home, Census Bureau reports. http://www.census.gov/newsroom/releases/archives/families_households/cb11-183.html.

US Department of Health and Human Services (USDHHS). (2015). 2020 topics and objectives. http://www.healthypeople.gov/2020/topics-objectives.

Utter, J., Denny, S., et al. (2016). Adolescent cooking abilities and behaviors: Associations with nutrition and emotional well-being. *Journal of Nutrition Education and Behavior, 48*(1), 35–41.

Utter, J., Denny, S., et al. (2013). Family meals and the well-being of adolescents. *Journal of Paediatrics and Child Health, 49,* 906–911.

Vedanthan, R., Bansilal, S., et al. (2016). Family-based approaches to cardiovascular health promotion. *Journal of the American College of Cardiology, 67*(14), 1725–1737.

Vess, L., & Lara, T. (2016). Career counseling and family therapy. An interview with Mark Savickas, PhD. *The Family Journal, 24*(1), 85–94.

Wright, L., & Leahey, M. M. (2013). *Nurses and families a guide to family assessment and intervention* (6th ed.). Philadelphia: F. A. Davis.

# 8

# Health Promotion and the Community

*Anne Rath Rentfro*

## OBJECTIVES

*After completing this chapter, the reader will be able to:*

- Describe the 11 functional health patterns and explain how they are used for data collection to assess communities.
- Evaluate community characteristics that indicate risk.
- Identify developmental aggregates of potential or actual dysfunctional health patterns.
- Explain methods of community data collection and sources of information.
- Describe a method of planned change for the community.
- Discuss the planning, implementation, and evaluation of nursing interventions in health promotion with communities.
- Develop a health-promotion plan based on community assessment (including resources), nursing diagnoses, and other contributing factors.

## KEY TERMS

| | | |
|---|---|---|
| Advocate | Community risk factors | Measurement data |
| Ambient | Demography | Observation data |
| Community | Developmental theory | Policy decision-making |
| Community diagnosis | Focus groups | Risk-factor theory |
| Community evaluation | Function of a community | Structure of a community |
| Community health promotion | Interview data | Systems theory |
| Community nursing intervention | Key informants | Windshield survey |
| Community outcomes | Lobbying | |
| Community pattern | Lobbyist | |

---

### ❓ THINK ABOUT IT

#### Teenagers: Drinking and Driving

*In a small rural community, seven teenagers have died in alcohol-related car accidents within the past 3 months. Alcohol and drug education is taught during the first year at the local high school, but driver's education classes are not offered because the school cannot afford the program. Parents within this community are extremely concerned.*

- What other information must be acquired before a diagnosis is made?
- What health-promotion ideas could be recommended based on the information provided?

In the last few decades, several social trends in the United States have increased public interest in health promotion and disease prevention. The *Healthy People 2020* initiative shifts the focus of health care from reactive to proactive with its emphasis on disease prevention and health promotion (US Department of Health and Human Services, 2015). By stating national health objectives as population-specific risks to good health, this venture guides community strategies to promote health, thereby reducing

disease risk factors. Box 8-1: *Healthy People 2020* highlights the emphasis this initiative takes in an environmental and community context.

Another social trend creating interest for health promotion is the changing population of the United States (see Chapter 2). As baby boomers entered older age beginning in 2011, the older population continues to expand and will grow more in the next 2 decades (Figure 8-1). The proportion of those older than 85 years has also increased by almost 5% (8.8% in 1980; 13.6% in 2010) as the US older population continues to age (West et al., 2014). These changes in the rates of the oldest-old contribute to a growing number of older people with disability in our communities (He & Larsen, 2014). Community assessment for health promotion will need to consider disability more thoroughly, because disability is currently viewed from a social model perspective (resulting from social and physical barriers). Older people also tend to have more chronic diseases and consume larger portions of health care resources than people in other age groups. This aging population will require more home services than previous generations because of increased life span and the

BOX 8-1    **HEALTHY PEOPLE 2020**

### Select Examples of National Health-Promotion and Disease-Prevention Goals and Objectives for Communities

The *Healthy People 2020* framework has expanded its focus to accentuate health-enhancing social and physical environments. Because the *Healthy People 2020* framework addresses health and health behaviors at multiple levels, almost all *Healthy People 2020* goals and objectives could be listed as examples of national health-promotion and disease-prevention objectives for communities. The following list consists of selected exemplars aimed specifically for aggregates and for health promotion rather than those that are individual level objectives with a tertiary care focus. When multiple objectives for one topic are pertinent to community assessment, the more general goal rather than specific objectives is listed.

| | |
|---|---|
| **AH-Goal** | Improve the healthy development, health, safety, and well-being of adolescents and young adults. |
| **AOCBC-11** | Reduce hip fractures among older adults. |
| **BC-13** | (Developmental) Decrease the prevalence of adults having high-impact chronic pain. |
| **BDBS-Goal** | Prevent illness and disability related to blood disorders and the use of blood products. |
| **C-15-18** | Increase the proportion of individuals who receive cancer screening and counseling. |
| **CKD-1** | Reduce the proportion of the US population with chronic kidney disease. |
| **DIA-2** | Reduce the proportion of preventable hospitalizations in adults aged 65 years or older with diagnosed Alzheimer disease and other dementias. |
| **D-16** | Increase prevention behaviors in persons at high risk of diabetes with prediabetes. |
| **DH-Goal** | Maximize health, prevent chronic disease, improve social and environmental living conditions, and promote full community participation, choice, health equity, and quality of life among individuals with disabilities of all ages. |
| **EMC-4** | Increase the proportion of elementary, middle, and senior high schools that require school health education. |
| **ECBP-Goal** | Increase the quality, availability, and effectiveness of educational and community-based programs designed to prevent disease and injury, improve health, and enhance quality of life. |
| **EH-Goal** | Humans interact with the environment constantly. These interactions affect quality of life, years of healthy life lived, and health disparities. The World Health Organization defines environment, as it relates to health, as "all the physical, chemical, and biological factors external to a person, and all the related behaviors." Environmental health consists in preventing or controlling disease, injury, and disability related to the interactions between people and their environment. |
| **FP-Goal** | Improve pregnancy planning and spacing, and prevent unintended pregnancy. |
| **GH-2** | Reduce the tuberculosis case rate for foreign-born persons living in the United States. |
| **HC/HIT-13** | Increase social marketing in health promotion and disease prevention. |
| **HRQOL/WB-1** | Increase the proportion of adults who self-report good or better physical and mental health. |
| **ENT-VSL-Goal** | Reduce the prevalence and severity of disorders of hearing and balance; smell and taste; and voice, speech, and language. |
| **HDS-Goal** | Improve cardiovascular health and quality of life through prevention, detection, and treatment of risk factors for heart attack and stroke; early identification and treatment of heart attacks and strokes; and prevention of repeat cardiovascular events. |
| **HIV-Goal** | Prevent HIV infection and its related illness and death. |
| **IID-1** | Increase immunization rates and reduce preventable infectious diseases. |
| **IVP-Goal** | Prevent unintentional injuries and violence, and reduce their consequences. |
| **LGBT-1** | Increase the number of population-based data systems used to monitor *Healthy People 2020* objectives that include in their core a standardized set of questions that identify lesbian, gay, bisexual, and transgender populations. |
| **MICH-Goal** | Improve the health and well-being of women, infants, children, and families. |
| **MPS-2.1** | (Developmental) Reduce the proportion of patients suffering from untreated pain due to a lack of access to pain treatment. |
| **MHMD-2, 12** | Reduce suicide attempts by adolescents and increase the proportion of homeless adults with mental health problems who receive mental health services. |
| **NWS-Goal** | Promote health and reduce chronic disease risk through the consumption of healthful diets and achievement and maintenance of healthy body weights. |
| **OSH-1-2** | Reduce nonfatal injuries and deaths and from work-related injuries. |
| **OA-1-3 & 12** | Increase the proportion of older adults who use the Welcome to Medicare benefit, have received current clinical preventive services, and report confidence in managing chronic conditions, and make information publicly available for older adults on the characteristics of victims, perpetrators, and cases of elder abuse, neglect, and exploitation. |
| **OH-8, 9 & 13** | Increase the proportion of low-income children and adolescents who received any preventive dental service during the past year and increase the proportion of school-based health centers with an oral health component and increase the proportion of the US population served by community water systems with optimally fluoridated water. |
| **PA-2, 3 & 15** | Increase the proportion of adults and adolescents who meet current federal physical activity guidelines for aerobic physical activity and for muscle-strengthening activity and increase legislative policies for the built environment that enhance access to and availability of physical activity opportunities. |
| **PHI-2** | (Developmental) Increase the proportion of tribal, state, and local public health personnel who receive continuing education consistent with the core competencies for public health professionals. |

BOX 8-1   **HEALTHY PEOPLE 2020—cont'd**

*Select Examples of National Health-Promotion and Disease-Prevention Goals and Objectives for Communities*

| | |
|---|---|
| **RD-7-8** | Increase the proportion of persons with current asthma who receive appropriate asthma care according to National Asthma Education and Prevention Program guidelines and increase the number comprehensive asthma surveillance systems for tracking asthma cases, illness, and disability. |
| **STD Goal** | Promote healthy sexual behaviors, strengthen community capacity, and increase access to quality services to prevent sexually transmitted diseases and their complications. |
| **SH Goal** | Increase public knowledge of how adequate sleep and treatment of sleep disorders improve health, productivity, wellness, quality of life, and safety on roads and in the workplace. |
| **SA-Goal** | Reduce substance abuse to protect the health, safety, and quality of life for all, especially children. |
| **TU-Goal** | Reduce illness, disability, and death related to tobacco use and secondhand smoke exposure. |
| **U-20** | Increase the number of states and the District of Columbia, territories, and tribes with sustainable and comprehensive evidence-based tobacco control programs. |
| **V-Goal** | Improve the visual health of the nation through prevention, early detection, timely treatment, and rehabilitation. |

From US Department of Health and Human Services. (2015). *2020 topics and objectives.* http://www.healthypeople.gov/2020/topics-objectives.

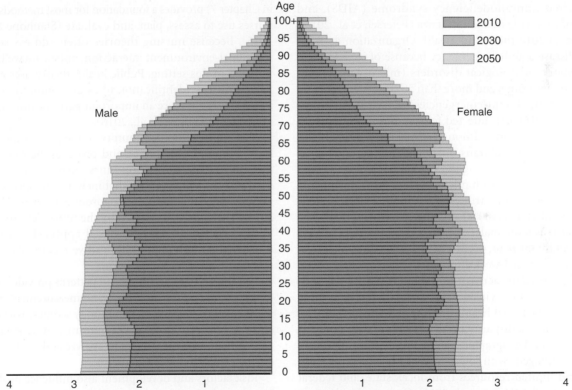

**FIGURE 8-1** Age and gender structure of the population for the United States: 2010, 2030, 2050. (From Ortman, J. M., & Guarneri, C. E. [2009]. *United States population projections: 2000 to 2050.* http://www.census.gov/population/projections/files/analytical-document09.pdf.)

concurrences of health problems (including altered levels of functioning).

The term **community** is used in various contexts with various meanings, depending on the frame of reference. Nursing generally adopts a broad sense of community that includes the concepts of groups of people that share social relationships, generally live within the same geographical location, and share common interests (Stanhope & Lancaster, 2015). A broad definition of community encompasses a wide variety of settings, such as school, workplace, and the international community.

Nurses in the nation's schools serve youth and provide access to community resources. Linking school nurses with communities can increase access to resources to improve health-promoting behaviors. *Healthy People 2020* addresses this issue: "ECBP-5: Increase the proportion of the Nation's elementary, middle, and senior high schools that have a full-time registered school nurse-to-student ratio of at least 1:750" (US Department of Health and Human Services, 2015). In 2006 the Health Indicators Warehouse (http://www.healthindicators.gov/) reported that 40.6% (confidence interval 35.3–45.9%) of US schools had the specified full-time registered nurse-to-student ratio (1:750). The 2012 evaluation of this indicator is not yet available.

People are integral to any concept of community; human beings give each community shape, character, and form. The diversity within a community and the diversity among various communities contribute to the health of that community. Individual health is reflected in each community through each person's contribution to its statistical rates and cultural and psychological makeup. Conversely, the context of the community is reflected in the individual through similar modes of expression (Pender et al., 2014).

This chapter focuses on the application of the nursing process to the community with independent, interdependent, and dependent nursing activities. Globalization has affected communities. Swift methods of travel and Internet communication impact community health (Petersen et al., 2016; Young et al., 2016). Communities globally are exposed to emerging infectious diseases such as Zika virus disease, Ebola fever, severe acute respiratory syndrome (SARS), human immunodeficiency virus (HIV)/acquired immunodeficiency syndrome (AIDS), and pandemics of tuberculosis and influenza (Petersen et al., 2016). For example, in 2016 the World Health Organization declared Zika virus disease a global emergency because of its associated serious newborn neurological disorders (microcephaly) and Guillain-Barré syndrome, and more than 50 countries reporting cases (http://www.who.int/emergencies/zika-virus/situation-report/28-april-2016/en/). Infected female mosquitos transmit most Zika virus infections. Although sexual intercourse, blood transfusions, and perinatal transmission have been proposed as alternative means of contracting the virus, among mothers who delivered infants ($n = 35$) with microcephaly, 74% remembered rashes in the first or second trimester (21 in the first trimester). Most infected individuals (80%) experience few symptoms. The symptoms, such as fever, malaise, rash, conjunctivitis, headache, and muscle and joint pain, occur about 1 week after the insect bite, then last for about 1 week after onset (Petersen et al., 2016).

Disparities in health across the world are associated with poverty, industrialization, violence, social disruption, education, food access, and maternal health. Even in developed countries with health resources, disparity occurs. Health may be different in urban versus rural geographical areas. Rural communities are doubly disadvantaged, with lower levels of health-promotion behaviors and limited resources from local, state, and federal public health agencies (Harris et al., 2016). Compared with urban Americans, rural people have increased levels of all the following: death from chronic obstructive pulmonary disease, suicide, and obesity (Harris et al., 2016). Furthermore, rural individuals (23%) are more likely to lack health insurance than their suburban counterparts (19%) (Harris et al., 2016; Meit et al., 2014).

Methods of data collection and sources of information about communities differ from individual sources. **Systems theory**, **developmental theory**, and **risk-factor theory** guide the nursing process. Developmental theory refers to a variety of explanations of phases of human development—physical, psychosocial, cognitive, and spiritual dimensions—based on descriptive research studies. Similarly, risk-factor theory identifies human characteristics and behaviors that increase the likelihood of the manifestation of health problems. Diverse communities require comprehensive assessment techniques that gather information about the unique characteristics of the population (e.g., cultural health practices or herbal remedies).

Gordon's (2016) functional health patterns provide the assessment framework for this chapter. Although other community assessment strategies exist, Gordon's (2016) patterns are useful to align community assessment findings with those of families and individuals to plan health promotion. An example of a data collection guide pattern is presented to facilitate the comprehension, synthesis, and application of **observation data**, **interview data**, **focus groups**, and **measurement data**. An example of data analysis, nursing diagnosis, planning, implementation, and evaluation follows, along with a description (Table 8-1).

## THE NURSING PROCESS AND THE COMMUNITY

Community nursing stems from a theoretical base that recognizes the impact of systems on health. General systems theory (described in Chapter 7) provides a foundation for most methods community nurses use to assess, plan, and evaluate (Stanhope & Lancaster, 2015). Because nursing theories often address self-care and individual-environment interaction, nurses are well prepared to function in this setting. Public health theory uses a population focus with risk identification to assess communities. Assessing aggregates is therefore an important part of community nursing assessment (Thomas et al., 2016).

The approach to community nursing assessment addresses each community as unique and provides the rationale for the assessment. The community nurse may use a comprehensive needs-assessment approach that includes all aspects of the community and is the traditional rigorous approach (Thomas et al., 2016). The approach selected by the nurse determines the data to be collected. In strength-based approaches and Gordon's functional pattern approach, positive factors play a consistent role in the information gathering.

Gordon's (2016) health-related patterns provide a useful guide to collect observation, interview, and measurement data. Health-related patterns depend on community settings, assessment focus, and the preference of each community. Assessing all pattern areas provides a basic data set to analyze and use for comparison during evaluation (see Chapter 6).

Risk factors and development also influence health patterns. For example, health concerns may occur in one pattern area, such as the increased age-related factor of teenage pregnancy (sexuality-reproductive pattern). Data from other areas may reveal that parental opposition (values-beliefs pattern) tends to restrict sex education and limit sex education in schools (coping–stress tolerance pattern). Attempting to restrict sex education or "ignoring" it in school and primary care may place the community at risk of unwanted pregnancy in its young people of childbearing age. Factors from several pattern areas may form clusters of risk for certain groups (see Chapter 6).

## THE NURSE'S ROLE

Community health nursing combines nursing practice and public health concepts to promote the health of populations without

## TABLE 8-1   Implementation of Community Health Plans With Objectives and Rationale

**Nursing Diagnosis:** Potential for increasing the incidence of fatal motor vehicle accidents in high school population related to alcohol use and driving.

**Goal:** North High School population will have reduced incidence (at least 20%) of fatal motor vehicle accidents related to alcohol use and abuse by December.

| Objective | Plans | Rationale |
|---|---|---|
| 1. Community will have access to information about incidence of fatal motor vehicle accidents and drunken driving arrests of its high school population for the past 5 yr by March | Interview local police about the incidence of fatal automobile accidents and substance abuse in the community. <br> Interview parents of deceased high school students, students, teachers, physicians, clergy, and emergency department personnel about the incidence of the problem and suggested measures for decreasing the incidence; suggest that interviews be broadcast over the high school radio station. <br> Have several people write to the community newspaper, commenting on the broadcast and the problem. | *Unfreezing:* For change to occur, the community has to become dissatisfied with the status quo and sense a need for change. <br> *Empiric-rational strategy:* People are rational; discussion of facts can result in support for change. <br> Important elements for preventing the problem include educating the public and having key community leaders discuss their views; concern lends credibility and is necessary for action. <br> People tend to listen to those with informal power. Keeping the issue before the community can raise consciousness. |
| 2. Community will take action to inform the population at risk about responsible drinking and driving by June | Suggest to the school principal and the school board the creation of a task force of community residents to plan a health program on individual responsibility and alcohol use in high school. <br> Conduct focus group discussions with the task force and develop collaborative group goals and strategies. <br> The task force should include teachers, students, parents, clergy, police, nurses, and physicians. The task force will examine ways to determine and teach content, integrate it into the curriculum, and recommend that community members, such as a nurse, be involved in teaching content. | *Changing:* Moving to a new level; community involvement will influence acceptability of changes. <br> Community residents like to be involved in decision-making. <br> It is important to establish trust and collaboration among community groups; this opens communication channels between adolescents and the health community. <br> Community involvement facilitates acceptance of change. |
| 3. Community will implement an educational program for its high school population related to use of alcohol and individual responsibility | Implement educational plans. | *Refreezing:* Moving to level of change brought about by community forces. <br> Educational strategies built around the concept of individual responsibility are essential elements in promoting health of young adults. |

limitation to any particular individual or group of individuals (Stanhope & Lancaster, 2015). Nursing concerns become the community's responses to existing and potential health-related problems, including such health-supporting responses as monitoring and teaching population groups. Nurses supply educational information to at-risk communities to develop health-oriented skills, attitudes, and related behavioral changes.

Community nurses also develop essential relationships aimed at accomplishing the community's health-related missions. Complex and dynamic communities, with their increasing public involvement in health and health policy, highlight the importance of human interactions inherent in nurses' responses to potential health problems, needs, and expectations. For example, active participation in environmental issues, such as decreasing control of toxic substances, provides an avenue for nurses to promote healthy environments by influencing policy.

In June 2015, the US Congress passed a bill to reform the Toxic Substances Control Act of 1976. The US Senate passed legislation in December 2015 that will move the bill to conference committee to be reconciled with the bill passed by Congress. Nurse opinion at this stage in the development of the new law

may influence legislators to construct a law that considers issues related to public health, such as preventing toxic toys from being imported and maintaining the states' influence over chemical regulation. According to Katie Huffling (2015), "Nurses have been instrumental in states like Maryland, Washington, New York, and Connecticut in pushing for laws to protect children and families from toxic chemicals. By taking away the rights of states to regulate these chemicals, dangerous chemicals are protected regulation for years before the federal government acts."

Concern about harmful effects of environmental contaminants includes decreased fertility in women, demasculinization of men exposed to plastics, and premature maturation of the reproductive tract with a trend toward earlier sexual maturation. Community nursing practice, therefore, requires a broad knowledge base derived from the natural, behavioral, and humanistic sciences with application of intellectual, interpersonal, and technical skills using the nursing process.

## Influencing Health Policy

The primary responsibility of the nurse is to the individual, family, group, or community served. A major portion of the nurse's role is to be an **advocate** not only for the individual but also for justice in health care delivery. Nurses need to be aware of issues that have an effect on the health of the American people and know how to influence necessary change.

Health and the environment are integrally connected; therefore nurses who engage in all planning aspects facilitate the health potential of those communities they serve. Involvement that includes attention to policy decisions and political action affects broader aspects of environmental, biophysical, and socioeconomic conditions of homes, schools, workplaces, communities, and health care delivery. For example, nurses could take active roles in how plastics impact population health (http://envirn.org/pg/groups/3755/environmental-health-scope-and-standards-of-practice), and in safeguarding natural resources. One organization, the Alliance of Nurses for Healthy Environments (ANHE), has created a website called the Knowledge Network (http://envirn.org/) to facilitate nurses' participation and competence in environmental health issues. In 2010 ANHE and the American Nurses Association (ANA) joined forces to develop the ANA's *Scope and Standards of Practice for Nurses* (Leffers et al., 2015). By virtue of their numbers, nurses, who constitute the largest group of health care providers in the United States, have tremendous potential to influence decision-making.

Participation in **policy decision-making** requires that nurses take a proactive stance to determine needs before a problem arises. Policy development and change occur on many levels, from within the nurse's agency or work group to the community, state, and national levels. At the institutional level, clinical decisions influence policy, as do management issues. The nurse examines the rationales underlying existing or planned policy and determines their current relevance. Nurses, by virtue of their education and experience, develop communication skills and apply change theory to influence policy.

Health-related decision-making often results from legislation at the local, state, or national level. Laws—rules enforced by a ruling authority by which society is governed—and regulations—agency or department rules developed to implement laws—define the services offered. Politics influence change and provide an arena for nursing to participle in shaping the future of health care. Political involvement may include voting, communicating with local representatives, supporting candidates, contributing time or financial support, and running for city, county, state, or national office. Voting, after nurses have become well informed on current issues and candidates, and serving on local and state committees are important ways for nurses to be actively involved.

In addition, knowing local representatives, informing them about health care issues, and advising them as to their constituents' needs are other ways nurses become involved. Legislators are influenced by the information that they receive and by the sources of that information. Nurses have a wealth of knowledge about health care. The process of seeking to influence legislators' views and votes is called **lobbying**. When an individual is employed to lobby, he or she is known as a **lobbyist** and is required to register as the representative of a special interest group. The ANA, located in Washington, DC, employs nurse lobbyists, as do many states. Individual nurses, however, can support colleagues who represent nursing's interests and who run for political office.

The ANA Nurses Strategic Action Team (N-STAT) network is an organized grassroots effort by nurses to help elect endorsed candidates and to inform legislators about policy issues of concern to nurses. When nurses join N-STAT, they receive alerts and updates detailing specific legislative issues. Financial contributions to Nurses for Political Action Coalition, the ANA's political arm, increase the power base of nurses. Membership of professional and community groups provides nurses with the collective voice to influence legislators.

Communicating with a legislator is essential and can be done by phone, writing a letter, personal visits, or e-mail correspondence. Legislators have staffs of experts in various areas, and each legislator is assigned to committees. To understand the legislative process, the nurse follows the progress of a bill. Thousands of bills are introduced at both the state level and the federal level and must be passed within 2 years or they will die by default. Once a bill has been introduced, it is referred to committee, and the committee chairperson determines which bills will be considered. Hearings are then held on the considered bills. When hearings have finished in committee, a bill is "reported out" at the federal level to the floor of the Senate or House of Representatives for a vote. Both the Senate and the House of Representatives must pass identical versions of the bill and, once passed by both chambers, it is forwarded to the President for signing. If signed, it is enacted into law (Bhushan, 2015). It is important for nurses to lobby, to inform legislators of new issues, and to give expert testimony on introduced bills. Nurses who are politically aware extend the collective nursing voice to its full potential.

Unfortunately, nursing's collective voice is rarely heard. Only about 20% of the entire nursing workforce are members of a collective professional organization (Woodward et al., 2015). Other health care professionals, such as members of the American Medical Association, have more united professional organizations with large memberships, providing a united voice and political clout that influences health care policy and law. Nurses have multiple professional organizations. With high membership dues, nurses likely join only a few groups and may gravitate toward their specialty organization. Without a single national organization with the majority of nurses as members, nursing's voice is diluted. When organizations promote an issue, the collective voice of the group rather than the voice of the individual sends a more powerful message to influence policymakers. Without a collective voice, nursing's influence on shaping health care policy is weakened.

To strengthen nursing's collective voice, the ANA has undergone significant reorganization with emphasis on increasing membership, by collaborating with its state constituent organizations, specialty organizations, and nonnursing health organizations. Engaging students in these strategies early in legislative processes will help to provide more well-informed practicing nurses. Well-informed, empowered professional nurses play significant roles in supporting legislative initiatives that promote and protect the health of the public. Other ways for nurses to be involved in policy change are to support candidates and run for office. Volunteering during campaigns to help a specific candidate or to encourage voter registration and voting are ways that nurses can influence policy. Many nurses now represent their local constituencies and have increasing visibility at the state and national levels. For example, five nurses currently serve in the United States 114th Congress (http://www.nursingworld.org/MainMenuCategories/Policy-Advocacy/Federal/Nurses-in-Congress).

Community nurses' roles include the interaction of independent, interdependent, and dependent functions. Independent functions include assessing, analyzing, diagnosing, planning, implementing, and evaluating communities for health promotion and health education. Interdependent functions include collaboration with community members and interdisciplinary teamwork functions that are crucial to effective community health. Dependent functions include implementing the therapeutic plans of team members.

Community health promotion includes all the following (US Department of Health and Human Services, 2015):

- Community participation, with representatives from multiple community sectors, including government, education, business, faith organizations, health care, media, voluntary agencies, and the public
- Assessment guided by a community-planning model to determine health problems, resources, perceptions, and priorities for action
- Targeted and measurable objectives to address health outcomes, risk factors, public awareness, services, and protection
- Comprehensive, multifaceted, culturally relevant interventions that have multiple targets for change
- Monitoring and evaluation of the objectives and strategies used

## METHODS OF DATA COLLECTION

Nurses obtain community assessment data through observation, interviews (including focus groups), and measurement. These three methods are used most frequently in various combinations to ensure the validity of the information. Obtaining data through observation—often referred to as the windshield survey approach to assessment—includes the use of the senses (sight, touch, hearing, smell, and taste) to determine community appearances. These appearances include the types and condition of residential dwellings and their people and also physical and biological characteristics, such as animal and plant life, temperature, transportation, sounds, and odors. Some communities have a characteristic "flavor." A community's physical characteristics influence health. What type of space is available? Children need space to run and play; young and middle-aged adults require space for recreation and exercise. What spatial barriers exist? Where is this space located in relation to traffic and schools? What does the air feel and smell like? What does the water taste like?

Community nurses obtain abundant subjective data by simply walking or riding around a community. Data obtained by observation provide important clues about the community, its actual or potential health problems, and its strengths. Technological advances such as the use of geographical information systems (GIS) enhance nurses' ability to assess communities. For example, Keddem and colleagues (2015) identified community vacant properties, illegal dumping, parks, tree canopy, aggravated assaults,

and theft to assess neighborhood irritants, neighborhood safety, walkability, pollen, and environmental allergens. The influence and intensity of these community features on asthma control was analyzed by use of GIS.

Analysis of observation data generates hypotheses to explore further with use of interview, focus group, and measurement data.

Interview data, the most common source of information from people, include verbal statements from community residents, key community officials, health care personnel, and various community agency staff. Key informants provide useful ways to learn how members perceive their community. Key community leaders often provide important information about community health concerns, necessary health resources, and community strengths, along with particular health beliefs and community health goals. Community residents provide useful information about their perceptions of health, health concerns, and needs, as well as their perceptions of the availability, accessibility, and acceptability of health services. Health agency personnel provide data about health resources, the population served, availability, and perceptions of concerns and needs. Developing a basic set of questions in advance enhances the relevance of interview data.

Community partners can be approached in groups to participate in assessment, planning, intervention, and evaluation (Andrews et al., 2012b; Frerichs et al., 2016). Community nurses who have expertise in building partnerships engage the community partnership model to conduct assessment, planning, the choosing of effective strategies, and evaluation (Stanhope & Lancaster, 2015). Andrews' research team uses this strategy for multiple community issues and health-promotion projects. The toolkit used for assessing partnership readiness is available on-line at http://academicdepartments.musc.edu/sctr/programs/community_engagement/Documents/SCTR%20CCHP%20Are%20We%20Ready%20Toolkit.pdf. Strategies initiated by engaged community members empower community partners and enhance the ability to transfer evidence-based strategies into their unique communities.

Measurement data use instruments to quantify data during information collection. Measurement data include population statistics, pollution indices, morbidity and mortality rates, census statistics, and epidemiological data. These data can be accessed by the Internet or locally in community libraries; health departments; environmental protection agencies; schools; police and fire departments; local health system agencies; and town, city, or state planning offices. Publicly supported agencies share their information, and community nurses readily use such data.

## SOURCES OF COMMUNITY INFORMATION

Census information available from http://www.census.gov, and also found in libraries and public agencies, is the most complete source for population information. Because the US Census is completed once every 10 years at the beginning of a decade, data for most communities become less accurate as the decade progresses. Community agencies and local planning commissions, project statistics, and developmental trends are how nurses understand population patterns and dynamics. Many communities and states also have databases available for public use.

Environmental measurement data can be obtained from the local branch of the US Environmental Protection Agency. Generally, local health departments monitor water, food, and sanitation systems. Nurses may be called on to facilitate safeguarding of natural resources protecting communities from industrial toxins. In areas that use well water, testing should be performed regularly. Community health nurses can participate in interventions to promote testing to assure the safety of water used in home. For example, Nova Scotia and areas across the northern United States risk exposure to arsenic that occurs naturally in the groundwater (Chappells et al., 2015). At-risk private well users should be testing their well water regularly. Community nurses in this setting could intervene using an integrated knowledge-to-action method. This method would include strategies including community outreach, home visits, and environmental home assessment planning. These strategies use community partnerships and home visits for informing the public and testing water in the private wells. Possible long-term public health initiatives for involvement of community health nurses include trainings that include awareness, testing, and treatment; low-cost or no-cost convenient testing stations; and mandatory regulated enforced testing at the point of property transfer or when new wells are constructed (Chappells et al., 2015).

Health departments along with school nurses and administrators provide school health information. Town, city, or county administrators provide information about land use, boundaries, housing conditions, utilities, and community services. Community newspapers supply information about community dynamics, health-related concerns, cultural activities, and community decision-making. The documentation techniques for community observation, interview, and measurement data are similar to those used for individuals and families. A triple-column format that separates the data obtained with each method facilitates recording.

## COMMUNITY FROM A SYSTEMS PERSPECTIVE

Systems theory provides an overall framework to connect and integrate community data. Systems consist of interrelated, interacting parts or components within boundaries that filter both the type and the rate of input and output (Frerichs et al., 2016). Similarly to how families form systems (see Chapter 7), communities viewed as systems have both structure and function. Assessment of communities includes exploration of aspects of the population within specific geographical areas.

### Structure

The structure of a community system or subsystem consists of a formal or informal arrangement of parts, including both animate and inanimate properties. Nursing, which operates within the context of the health system, can be considered within the context of community systems. Figure 8-2 shows the arrangement of a community system. The macrosystem includes societal ideologies, social norms, and culture, and shapes the larger part of the system that encompasses numerous subsystems, the exosystem, microsystem, and the individual (Joly, 2016). Communities' structural parts form the subsystems, each of which is in itself

a system. Health agencies, schools, fire departments, and governmental bodies are examples of structural parts. Joly (2016) places Bronfenbrenner's bioecological theory into a contemporary context. The subsystems, such as individuals, family, school, and community, lie within overarching macrosystems. These systems and subsystems interact and change over time within a social context. For example, development during adolescence and young adulthood influences the disparity found in social determinants that subsequently impact health (Joly, 2016). The arrangement and organization of a community, such as age distribution and types of health-promotion/protection programs, change over time. The parts fluctuate depending on environmental processes occurring locally and within the larger environment.

Community leadership provides direction for both health-promotion and health-protection activities; therefore community assessment includes exploration of various community systems as they relate to health. The practice of viewing community structure as a population (collection of people) and considering the arrangement of the community's health care parts (existing health services) plays an important role in the assessment process.

The study of populations is referred to as **demography**. A population is a group defined as an aggregate of people who share similar personal or environmental characteristics. Demography provides information about population characteristics—such as size and racial composition, along with the distribution of age, sex, marital status, nationality, language, religious affiliations, education, and occupation. Demographic data provide the basis for analysis and a means to identify groups who may have high risk of health concerns. Such information also provides direction for health strategies. For example, examination of the age distribution over several years reveals important population shifts with associated needs for additional health-promotion activities. The increasing numbers of individuals older than 65 years require changes in community health priorities that reflect this group's needs. Comparing population characteristics statistically enables nurses to make inferences about the community. Comparisons are made among three systems: the town, which is a part of the county; the county, which is a part of the larger system; and the state. Comparisons between affluent and poor communities, rural and urban communities, and diverse and homogeneous communities may provide important information for planning.

### Function

The **function of a community** refers to the process of dynamic change with adaptation in the system's parts and the ways that community systems and subsystems interact. Decision-making and allocation of health-promotion and health-protection resources are important considerations for community assessment. As health educators, nurses interact with communities to promote health. Community health promotion involves a complex array of responsibilities. Nurses act as advocates using proactive planning and collaboration with other disciplines and agencies. As a community liaison, the nurse establishes priorities for programming, matches resources with needs determined by a community needs assessment, empowers community members, and facilitates social, environmental, and political change. These multifaceted

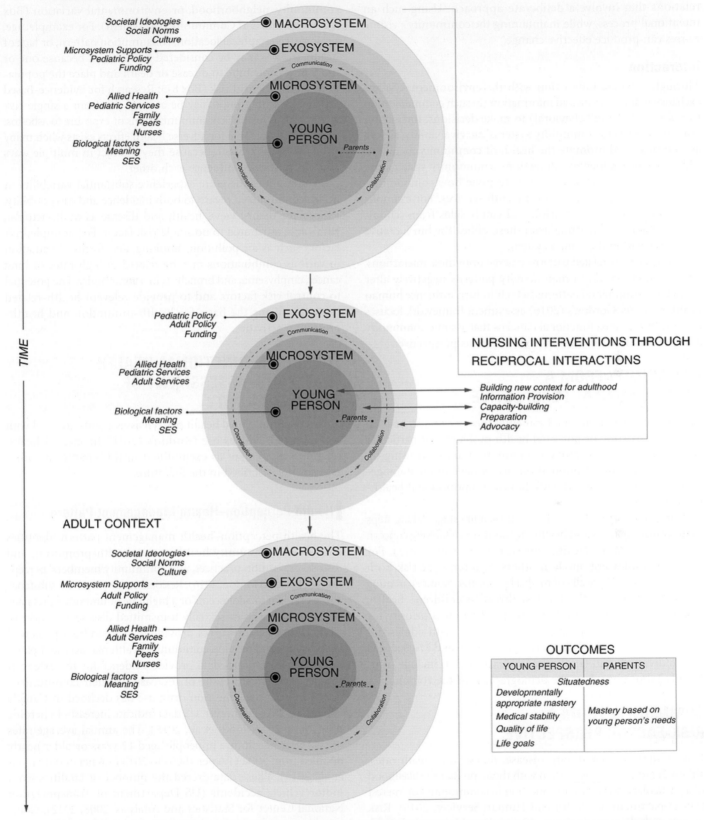

PEDIATRIC CONTEXT

*Societal Ideologies*
*Social Norms*
*Culture*
● MACROSYSTEM

*Microsystem Supports*
*Pediatric Policy*
*Funding*
● EXOSYSTEM

● MICROSYSTEM

*Allied Health*
*Pediatric Services*
*Family*
*Peers*
*Nurses*

*Biological factors*
*Meaning*
*SES*
● YOUNG
PERSON
*Communication*
*Parents*
*Coordination*
*Collaboration*

TIME

*Pediatric Policy*
*Adult Policy*
*Funding*
● EXOSYSTEM

*Allied Health*
*Pediatric Services*
*Adult Services*
● MICROSYSTEM

*Biological factors*
*Meaning*
*SES*
● YOUNG
PERSON
*Communication*
*Parents*
*Coordination*
*Collaboration*

NURSING INTERVENTIONS THROUGH
RECIPROCAL INTERACTIONS

Building new context for adulthood
Information Provision
Capacity-building
Preparation
Advocacy

ADULT CONTEXT

*Societal Ideologies*
*Social Norms*
*Culture*
● MACROSYSTEM

*Microsystem Supports*
*Adult Policy*
*Funding*
● EXOSYSTEM

*Allied Health*
*Adult Services*
*Family*
*Peers*
*Nurses*

*Biological factors*
*Meaning*
*SES*
● MICROSYSTEM

● YOUNG
PERSON
*Communication*
*Parents*
*Coordination*
*Collaboration*

OUTCOMES

| YOUNG PERSON | PARENTS |
|---|---|
| *Situatedness* | |
| Developmentally appropriate mastery | Mastery based on young person's needs |
| Medical stability | |
| Quality of life | |
| Life goals | |

Interacions within and berween the microsystem, exosystem and macrosystem can impact the achievement of transition outcomes. Interventions are depicted for context changes related to the movement between pediatric and adult services. Other contextual changes can occur in medical/biological factors or microsystem components, for example. Interventions start even before the context changes and continue over time until situatedness in th new context is achieved

**FIGURE 8-2** Community systems and subsystems model. *SES,* Socioeconomic status. (From Joly E. [2016]. Integrating transition theory and bioecological theory: A theoretical perspective for nurses supporting the transition to adulthood for young people with medical complexity. *Journal of Advanced Nursing, 72*[6], 1251–1262.)

functions require expertise in communication and interpersonal relations that involve a deliberate approach. Using such an intentional process, while maintaining the community's vision, nurses can produce effective change.

### Interaction

Through dynamic interaction with the environment, systems exchange matter, energy, and information (in such communication forms as verbal and behavioral) to make decisions. Interaction also contributes to community systems' survival ability, as well as to protect and promote the health of community members. Through environmental interactions, community systems use adaptation mechanisms. Nurses determine how communities apply these mechanisms toward health services. For example, policy that removes soft drink and candy sales from schools must consider lost revenue from these unhealthy but lucrative structures within the school system.

Various health-related patterns emerge from these interactions. For example, certain human-activity patterns negatively alter natural environmental patterns, which in turn influence human health patterns. Gordon's (2016) assessment framework focuses on 11 health-related functional patterns that assume community and environment interaction from a systems perspective.

## COMMUNITY FROM A DEVELOPMENTAL PERSPECTIVE

A framework based on developmental theory can also be used to identify existing or potential health problems for particular age groups in communities. Community nurses, focusing on the total community population, use a developmental, age-correlated approach to identify health-promotion and health-protection activities.

Nurses identify age-related risks at each life stage, taking steps to maximize wellness and health promotion as a lifelong concern (US Department of Health and Human Services, 2015). For example, adolescent single mothers of infants, at risk both emotionally and physically of medical problems, require parenting skills. Accidents are the greatest threat to children's health; therefore accident-prevention activities become a priority for communities with a young population and with adolescent mothers. Age-related risk factors (see Chapters 6 and 7) associated with individuals and families can be extended to include community groups based on the demographics of the community.

## COMMUNITY FROM A RISK-FACTOR PERSPECTIVE

Risk factors associated with disease, illness, and death rates, although not causally associated with them, predict the likelihood of a particular adverse health condition in communities of interest (US Department of Health and Human Services, 2015). Risk factors include a combination of demographic, psychological, physiological, and environmental characteristics (or they may include a single characteristic). The influence of various risk factors differs from person to person and from group to group because of genetic composition, geographical location, lifestyle patterns, resources, socioeconomic status, education level, and community, neighborhood, or environmental variation (Box 8-2: Genomics and Community Assessment). For example, age, sex, race, geographical location, consumption pattern, or lack of health services may be considered risk factors, because one or more may contribute to disease or death and place the population sharing them at risk (Box 8-3: Research for Evidence-Based Practice). Some groups may be at high risk from a single risk factor, such as insufficient immunizations or exposure to asbestos. A combined potential for adverse health effects exists when many risk factors are present, because they interact in multiple ways and synergistically influence each other.

Communities therefore experience substantial variability in health conditions in regard to both incidence and susceptibility. Risk-factor theory views health and disease as multifactorial, with cause attributed to no single risk factor. For example, risk factors such as air pollution, smoking, and forms of radiation in various combinations may be related to high rates of lung cancer, emphysema, and bronchitis in a community. The potential to control risk factors and to provide relevant health-related resources forms the basis for health-promotion and health-protection activities.

## GORDON'S FUNCTIONAL HEALTH PATTERNS: ASSESSMENT OF THE COMMUNITY

A variety of functional health pattern assessments are used with communities. Nurses use Gordon's (2016) functional health reference assessment as exemplified in this chapter or other assessments described in the literature.

### Health Perception–Health Management Pattern

The health perception–health management pattern identifies data about community health status, health-promotion and disease-prevention practices, and community members' perceptions of health (Gordon, 2016). Residents may perceive a substance abuse problem in adolescents or a high rate of unwanted pregnancies, breast cancer, or sexually transmitted disease as concerns. Community health nurses provide data to address perceived health issues and develop community health management plans. For example, national data provide evidence for the extent of the perceived health issue of increases in their community's injection drug use. Injection drug use has declined in Canada (Roy et al., 2016); however, US data indicate increases in heroine use (Jones, 2013; Jones et al., 2015). The annual average rates of past-year heroin use in people aged 12 years or older nearly doubled from 2002 (1.6 per 1000) to 2013 (2.6 per 1000) (Jones et al., 2015). These data exceed the number of fatalities from motor vehicle accidents (US Department of Transportation National Center for Statistics and Analysis, 2008, 2012). Community partners compare these data with local data to determine public health issues to pursue.

Valuable information can be elicited by nurses conducting focus group discussions and by interviewing key community members about their health concerns and issues. Mortality and

## BOX 8-2 GENOMICS

### Community Assessment

Combinations of genetic, individual, and environmental factors interact to affect the risk of and/or protection from many chronic disorders, such as diabetes, Alzheimer disease, cardiovascular disease, and depression. Genetic modifications at both the individual level and the community level impact these disorders. Moreover, these disorders modify genetic expression in both individuals and communities. Exchanges between the environment and genetics alter manifestations of these complex disorders. In contrast, manifestation of the disorder alters the environment and genetics. Community environment may influence mental health issues such as depression (Ware et al., 2016). Socioeconomic factors, chronic stressors (violence, unemployment, visual appeal), and community cohesion provide general measures in many studies.

In their study about predicting depressive symptoms, Ware and colleagues (2016) describe findings from studies linking community measures with genetic predictors of depression or depressive symptoms. The studies explored to provide support for their research included gene (serotonin transporter gene [5-HTT] promoter variant) interactions with the environment. The designs included only narrow individual-level samples or the wider county-level samples, rather than smaller less heterogeneous community samples. The findings from these few studies include gene interactions with environmental factors, such as a personal history of stressful life events, the proportion of individuals receiving public assistance (county level), county-level infant mortality rates, and county-level crime rates. These findings indicate that different risks of depression exist for different genotypes depending on their individual environment and their broader environment.

Use of phenotypic approaches to sample selection (depression symptoms) rather than diagnosed depression increases the sample size and extends the research to genome-wide/gene-region analysis rather than candidate gene analyses (Ware et al., 2016). Gene-region analysis explores the effects of genetic variability on phenotypic variability. Important genetic predictors have already been identified by analysis of genetic regions. Genetic predictors for numerous disorders have been identified after single nucleotide polymorphism (SNP) analysis revealed no statistically significant associations. Predictors for disorders such as bipolar disorder, coronary artery disease, hypertension, Parkinson disease, amyotrophic lateral sclerosis, Crohn disease, rheumatoid arthritis, type 1 and type 2 diabetes, and age-related eye disease arose from the analysis of gene regions rather than SNPs (Peng et al., 2010).

The Multi-Ethnic Study of Atherosclerosis, a longitudinal cohort study, included six sites participating in the National Institutes of Health (NIH) SNP Health Association Resource (SHARe) project (http://www.nhlbi.nih.gov/research/resources/genetics-genomics/share). Approximately 1 million SNPs were genotyped, and the use of programs available from the NIH increased the number of available SNPs to about 2.5 million markers.

Ware and colleagues (2016) provide evidence to support SNP interactions in gene region 9 neighborhood index score (G 9 NIS) of depressive symptoms within the neighborhood level. This significant neighborhood gene region involves regulatory function of depressive symptoms. The gene-expression foundation for regulation of depression may be established early in life, with changes in depressive symptoms later in life. Molecular-level adaptation and brain response to local stimuli may depend on G 9 NIS changes. These community-level interactions in the G 9 NIS region may interact to influence depressive symptoms.

This novel study explored the influence of gene-region interactions on depressive symptoms and supports the idea that community or neighborhood context may interact with genetic factors in shaping depressive symptoms. Replication in other samples is necessary before firm conclusions can be drawn.

From Peng, G., Luo, L., Siu, H., Zhu, Y., Hu, P., Hong, S., et al. (2010). Gene and pathway-based second-wave analysis of genome-wide association studies. *European Journal of Human Genetics, 18*(1), 111–117; Ware, E. B., Smith, J. A., Mukherjee, B., Lee, S., Kardia, S. L. R., & Diez-Roux, A. V. (2016). Applying novel methods for assessing individual and neighborhood-level social and psychosocial environment interactions with genetic factors in the prediction of depressive symptoms in the Multi-Ethnic Study of Atherosclerosis. *Behavior Genetics, 46*(1), 89–99.

## BOX 8-3 RESEARCH FOR EVIDENCE-BASED PRACTICE

### Associations Among Parent/Peer Relationships and Individual Characteristics of Children

Salzinger and colleagues (2011) use socioecological theory as a foundation to explore associations among parent/peer relationships and individual characteristics in their sample of 667 children. Three rounds of data were collected over 3 years. Each round consisted of a 45- to 90-minute interview with the guardian of the child. Instruments were used to measure internalization of problems (depression, anxiety), externalization of problems (aggressive behavior), exposure to community violence, exposure to family violence, attachment to parents, attachment to friends, delinquency of friends, self-reported competence, moral disengagement (justification for the use of aggression), household dysfunction, and mental health of guardians. The consent process explained that counseling services would be available and child abuse would be reported. Stepwise hierarchical linear regression was used to analyze the data. High exposure to violence was associated with little protection from normally protective factors (e.g., attachment to parents) compared with low exposure to violence. In the low exposure to violence setting, peer protective factors (e.g., friends) were effective. Less internalizing of problems was independently associated with individual competence. Externalizing problems was independently associated with variables from all domains, and exposure. Parent attachment and other protective factors were associated with decreased problems, whereas increased problems were associated with risk factors, such as a friend's delinquency.

In a meta-analysis of the research literature on peer attachment and youth internalizing problems, Gorrese (2016) reported that Salzinger and colleagues' (2011) research clearly delineated the links between the quality of peer attachment relationships and internalizing symptoms over time. Gorrese's (2016) meta-analysis provides additional evidence for the implementation of community violence reduction, health-promotion, and health-prevention programs that emphasize and promote protective factors with parents and peers. Initiating such programs may decrease adverse behavioral outcomes in adolescents.

From Gorrese, A. (2016). Peer attachment and youth internalizing problems: A meta-analysis. *Child & Youth Care Forum, 45*(2), 177–204; Salzinger, S., Feldman, R. S., Rosario, M., & Ng-Mak, D. S. (2011). Role of parent and peer relationships and individual characteristics in middle school children's behavioral outcomes in the face of community violence. *Journal of Research on Adolescence, 21*(2), 395–407.

morbidity statistics and other public health information sources provide measurement data (see Chapter 2).

## Nutritional-Metabolic Pattern

The nutritional-metabolic pattern identifies data relevant to community consumption habits as reflected in accessibility and availability of food stores and subsidized food programs for infants, children, and older adults. Community well-being, which depends on adequate dietary habits, food intake, and supply of nutrients, is influenced by culture, the presence or absence of kitchen facilities, and adequate plumbing.

Community assessment includes the collection of data by driving or walking through the community while using all five senses; it provides information about grocery stores, fast-food establishments, ethnic shopping facilities, and street corner vendors. Even affluent and developed countries contain areas without adequate access to food, or "food deserts," places where fresh food is not available. Income and food insecurity are highly correlated. Urban food insecurity (15% of city dwellers) in the US has grown with the growth in the urban poor population. As less than 2% of inhabitants still farm, movements to respond to food insecurity and access have evolved, promoting strategies such as backyard gardening, community gardening, community-supported agriculture, or local markets (Clendenning et al., 2016). Government programs, private soup kitchens, and food donations by houses of worship also provide information about nutritional patterns of communities.

## Elimination Pattern

The elimination pattern identifies environmental factors, including exposure to pollutants in the community through contaminated soil, water, and air, and the food chain. This pattern further classifies environmental factors into the two broad categories—physical and biological. Alterations in environmental processes threaten the health and integrity of communities, necessitating health-promotion and health-protection activities. For example, humans eliminate most endocrine-disrupting chemicals, pharmaceuticals, and personal care products into the environment (Noguera-Oviedo & Aga, 2016). Antibiotics and hormones from animals and fish also contaminate the environment. Groundwater, drinking water, surface water, and treatment plant effluents can be affected. Furthermore, some contaminants transform into contaminants that are more toxic than the original substance. For example, the antiviral acyclovir is excreted as a transformed product that is more toxic than the original drug (Schlüter-Vorberg et al., 2015).

Physical agents include geological, geographical, climatic, and meteorological aspects of the community. Certain population groups are particularly susceptible to acute respiratory disease and aggravated asthmatic episodes when the air quality is poor (Solomon et al., 2016). For example, when schools are located in high-pollution or high-traffic areas, children are exposed to polluted air. In addition, when home cooking devices pollute home air, families are exposed to polluted air (Pillarisetti et al., 2016). Use of solid fuel combustion such as wood or coal for cooking inside produces polluted home air. Community health nurses can use the Household Air Pollution Intervention Tool to plan interventions (Pillarisetti et al., 2016). Depending on resources, community collaborations, and partnerships, the community health nurse may use a variety of possible interventions to eliminate home air pollution from solid fuel cooking indoors. These interventions include simple chimney stoves with adequate exhaust, stoves with fan-assisted combustion, and/or clean fuel (Pillarisetti et al., 2016).

The geographical locations of communities, and major waterways, highways, or mountains located within communities, act as barriers to access to health facilities. Inaccessibility of health care services also hinders health in at-risk groups. Knowledge of climatic conditions provides clues to susceptibility to illness resulting from temperature or humidity in certain populations.

Biological agents include living things—such as plants, animals and their waste products, disease agents, microbial pathogens, and toxic substances—that can be hazardous to health. For example, Lyme disease, viral hepatitis, pneumonia, influenza, and the large number of diseases associated with childhood continue to be threats to community health. Observation, focus groups, and interviews with key community members reveal information concerning elimination patterns. The Environmental Protection Agency (http://www.epa.gov/) and the Centers for Disease Control and Prevention (http://www.cdc.gov/) provide excellent resources for community health nurses.

## Activity-Exercise Pattern

The activity-exercise pattern identifies physical activities and recreational options within communities. Science and technology have increasingly influenced productivity while simultaneously reducing or eliminating physical work. Consequently, physical activity no longer occurs during the work day for most community members, leaving leisure time as the only time for physical activity. Physiological evidence demonstrates that physical activity improves many biological measures associated with health and psychological functioning. Regular physical activity and musculoskeletal fitness are important for healthy, independent living as people grow older. Physical activity reduces the risk of many diseases, including obesity, heart disease, hypertension, cancer, osteoporosis, and diabetes mellitus.

Observation, focus groups, and interviews provide clues to a community's ability to provide cultural and recreational activities (Figure 8-3). Furthermore, noting whether the community has evidence of recreational facilities or is a "built community" with physical activity options (such as bike/walking trails), assessing transportation options, and observing community development that encourages walking should be included in the community assessment of the activity-exercise pattern.

## Sleep-Rest Pattern

The sleep-rest pattern identifies a community's rhythm of sleeping, resting, and relaxing. Some towns never close, with stores, traffic flow, and recreational facilities operating during both day and

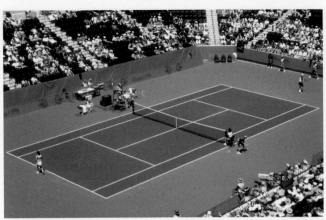

**FIGURE 8-3** The activity-exercise pattern identifies a community's physical activities and recreational options.

night hours. This ongoing activity produces unpleasant disturbances, such as unwanted noise that may be harmful to community well-being. Excessive noise from highways or airplanes produces physiological or psychological problems eliciting responses ranging from mild irritation to pain or permanent hearing loss. Although noise cannot be eliminated, efforts to minimize and control it are possible. Observation, focus groups, and interviews provide clues to this pattern.

## Cognitive-Perceptual Pattern

The cognitive-perceptual pattern identifies information about problem-solving and decision-making within communities. Systems depend on decision-making and resource allocation processes for survival. Communities require functional decision-making bodies to ensure adherence to rules and attainment of goals. Individual patterns and environmental patterns connect with important implications for community health. Community assessment includes appraisal of interaction with the environment, as in the participatory processes of community-based system dynamics. The effectiveness of the strategies used depends on a collaborative evolution and long-term commitment of the nurse in the community (Frerichs et al., 2016).

One strategy, bargaining, offers communities a plan to exchange resources for health service. For example, a community that owns a mammography machine but has no primary care facility might negotiate with another community to provide mammography for primary care services in return. Strategies using outside authority (legal bureaucratic methods) ensure compliance through rules and structures. In this case, states may mandate that communities maintain certain health standards. For example, a law may require all schoolchildren to be immunized against specific diseases before they enter public school. Cooperative strategies promote health when members share common goals (Andrews et al., 2012a). For example, community residents may unite to oppose a chemical landfill that is a health hazard.

Convincing people to comply because they hold some loyalty in the situation or relationship is another method that mobilizes communities. For example, community residents might expend a great deal of effort and money to retain a particular health clinic because of loyalty to the agency. Identifying decision-making patterns used by communities provides clues about health priorities and values, as well as matches and mismatches between existing circumstances, health goals, and planning strategies. Data can best be obtained by observation, focus groups, and interviews.

## Self-Perception–Self-Concept Pattern

The self-perception–self-concept pattern identifies self-worth and personal identity of communities. Characteristics such as image, status, and perceived competency with problem-solving indicate community self-concept. Housing conditions, buildings, and cleanliness reflect community image. School systems, crime rates, accidents, and opinions about whether the community is considered a good place to live suggest community perception of self-worth. Competency with social and political issues as well as community spirit creates positive self-evaluation. Community pride facilitates development of innovative health programs. Emotional tone (fear, depression, or positive emotional outlook) relates to findings in other pattern areas. For example, tensions in the cognitive-perceptual pattern (conflict between groups concerning health issues) may explain a general feeling of fear among the residents. Data are obtained through observation, focus groups, and interviews.

## Roles-Relationships Pattern

The roles-relationships pattern identifies communication styles along with formal and informal relationships. Of particular concern are roles and relationships affecting community ability to realize health potential. Patterns of crime, racial incidents, and social networks form indices of human relationships in communities. Publicizing health promotion becomes more effective when patterns of official communication are used. Health program success depends on support from prominent community members. Community members involved in health programs help identify other key community leaders. Use of media and other mass information programs improves communication, the flow of health information, and the number of community members reached. Interviews, television, the Internet, and newspapers are examples of ways to obtain and convey information.

## Sexuality-Reproductive Pattern

The sexuality-reproductive pattern identifies reproductive data of communities, which is reflected in live birth statistics, mothers' ages, ethnicity, and marital status. This information provides clues to the health-promotion needs of a particular community group. Premature infant rates, low-birth-weight infants, and abortion rates, as well as neonatal, infant, and maternal death rates reflect reproductive patterns of communities. Such information identifies at-risk groups on the basis of particular characteristics associated with these rates. Mismatches between existing health services, health education, and community health statistics also indicate health concerns. Availability of sex education in schools, the levels of spousal and child abuse, and the number of sex-related crimes also indicate health-promotion issues. Minutes of meetings, health records, statistical data, and public documents provide sources for these data.

## Coping–Stress Tolerance Pattern

The coping–stress tolerance pattern identifies the community's ability to cope or adapt. Communities respond to stress in different ways, some of which might threaten their integrity. Community responses reveal the group coping patterns. Communities develop abilities to exchange goods, services, goals, values, and ideals to survive and to promote community health. Community efforts to obtain goods from the environment, contain goods within the environment, retain goods within the community, and dispose of goods play significant roles in influencing health. Examples of resources that communities obtain from the environment to promote health include local, state, or federal funding; health services; health-related workforce personnel; new knowledge; and technological advances. Some communities obtain abundant health care services; however, primary services often remain inadequate or nonexistent. Lack of available health services, or lack of ability to obtain them, characterizes community health need. Examples of problems communities may attempt to control include sex-related crimes, diseases, substance abuse, industry, hazardous waste in the water supply, and noxious chemicals in the air.

Community coping patterns aim to retain certain health-protection services, such as immunization services for children and adequate health facilities. Coping efforts may also include strict zoning laws and housing codes or certain values such as sex education within the home. Expendable goods of communities include industrial and human wastes. Data can be obtained through minutes of meetings, public documents, health surveys, statistical data, and health records.

## Values-Beliefs Pattern

The values-beliefs pattern identifies the community values and beliefs. Such information provides clues for health-promotion and health-protection efforts valued by the community. Values underlie decisions about community health education and tax support for schools, hypertension screening for the public, disease-prevention programs, or well-child clinics. Traditions, norms, and cultural and ethnic groups share values and beliefs in communities. Data can be obtained through focus groups and through interviews with key community members and health-related personnel.

## ANALYSIS AND DIAGNOSIS WITH THE COMMUNITY

Analysis refers to data categorization and pattern determination. Data synthesis and organization occur to ascertain patterns of health activities and trends. An example of a clinical scenario about a particular community is presented in the case study and care plan at the end of this chapter. Decision-making and

### TABLE 8-2 Stages of Change

| Stages | Interventions |
|---|---|
| Precontemplation | Provide information (identify risk factors) <br> Raise doubts about current behaviors and future outcomes |
| Contemplation | Discuss risks of not changing <br> Discuss benefits of changing |
| Planning or preparation | Help plan phases of change <br> Help implement phases of change |
| Action | Help develop strategies to prevent relapse, emphasizing self-efficacy <br> Offer encouragement |
| Maintenance | Highlight past successes and future benefits |

Modified from Pender, N. J., Murdaugh, C. L., & Parsons, M. A. (2014). *Health promotion in nursing practice* (6th ed.). Upper Saddle River, NJ: Pearson.

judgment inherent in the nursing process become most important during the analysis and diagnostic phases. Table 8-2 presents an example of one way to organize community data using Prochaska's stages of change (Pender et al., 2014).

## Organization of Data

Charts, figures, and tables graphically display population distributions, morbidity and mortality data, or vital statistics to pinpoint significant community concerns with actual or potential health problems along with health-related responses to these concerns. Another valuable organizational technique—mapping—facilitates data analysis. For example, a series of maps gathered with use of technology such as GIS displays data that change over time. Analysis of several variables occurs simultaneously. Overlap of the locations of environmental hazards, densely populated areas, health-promotion services, and major highways becomes apparent. Poor environmental conditions; the distribution of illness, disease, and death rates; and accessibility of health-protection and health-promotion activities for the population appear at a glance with dotted scatter maps. Use of maps requires knowledge about the community's population base. Less-populated rural areas with fewer health facilities or fewer neonatal deaths in a community with fewer women of childbearing age are examples of how population statistics influence interpretation of mapping techniques. Use of theoretical frameworks for community health and Gordon's (2016) 11 pattern areas facilitates analysis of community data. Several guidelines, presented next, help community nurses analyze population data. Analysis often supports the need for further data collection.

## Guidelines for Data Analysis
### Check for Missing Data

The complexity, size, and number of community characteristics prohibit all possible facts about the health-related pattern areas being gathered; however, missing or insufficient data that indicate areas for further assessment should be identified. Additional assessment may determine specific approaches or a particular community diagnosis. Examples of missing data in community assessment include pollution indices, links between health resources and population groups, accessibility to resources, and morbidity statistics. Dates for census data used should be noted.

The nurse examines community data for incongruities and conflicting information. For example, a key community official might deny the existence of pollutants in the water supply, whereas newspaper reports of health department water analysis findings indicate otherwise. The nurse evaluates such inconsistencies before identifying existing or potential health concerns.

## Identify Patterns

Clues about a community pattern emerge from subjective and objective data gathered. During this stage, community nurses make decisions, begin to formulate diagnostic hypotheses (ideas and tentative judgments about possible health concerns), identify community groups that might be at risk, and establish probable causes or relationships. Ideas generated from this activity direct the search for additional clues in the data to confirm, reject, or revise hypotheses. Judgments about hypotheses continue to support patterns in the data.

To narrow the huge list of possible community health-promotion and health-protection concerns, community nurses formulate broad problem statements based on the health-related pattern areas (Gordon, 2016). For example, the community nurse differentiates among elimination problems (e.g., noxious chemicals), coping and stress-tolerance problems, and health perception–health management problems (e.g., high teenage mortality rate from motor vehicle accidents). Developing these general categories facilitates analysis.

## Apply Theories, Models, Norms, and Standards

Analysis of community data requires extensive knowledge of developmental, age-related risks, as well as theories and concepts of nursing, public health, and epidemiology. Such a broad foundation enables nurses to identify additional clues in health-related patterns that contribute to community nursing diagnoses and intervention. Developmental approaches form a basis to identify groups with potential health concerns. Age groups differ in susceptibility; therefore nurses examine community resources directed toward highly susceptible groups. For example, community data that show increases in the number of live births among older women indicate a need for health-promotion services for this group. If community data show increasing numbers of aging citizens, nurses explore the availability and accessibility of existing health services for this older group.

Analysis of data for common personal or environmental characteristics also occurs. For example, select groups may be at risk on the basis of a shared health concern, such as substance abuse, lack of immunizations, unsafe housing conditions, high exposure to asbestos or noxious chemicals, or inadequate health services. Shared characteristics, such as race or ethnicity, provide clues to susceptibility and the need for screening activities. For example, black populations warrant screening for hypertension. Additionally, if a fluoridated water supply is unavailable, additional intervention to prevent dental caries in children is justified. In addition, community literacy contributes to health-promotion

activity development methods used by nurses to establish educational programs. A low literacy level limits the ability to use all available resources.

Environmental information is readily available on the Internet. Databases and search engines provide useful information about environmental hazards and other environmental problems in communities. Prevention of disease worldwide depends on the dissemination of global environmental health information (US Department of Health and Human Services, 2015). Analysis of data relies on standards developed nationally or globally. For example, community data regarding air quality can be compared with state or national ambient air quality standards to determine health. In this context, the term ambient refers to outside air in a town, city, or other defined region. In the United States, air-monitoring stations are generally located in urban and rural areas within each state. One source for air quality information is the CHARTing Health Information for Texas, which is maintained by the University of Texas Health Science Center at Houston School of Public Health. The goal of this center is to serve as a resource in Texas for publicly available data to use for analysis and research. Data and links to other sites are continually monitored and updated (University of Texas Health Science Center at Houston, 2012). Current information about community resources enables more effective strategies to prevent risk factors and avoid health problems. Internet access facilitates identification of gaps in health-promotion and health-protection services.

## Identify Strengths and Health Concerns

Interpretation of community data occurs with regard to community concerns, community strengths, and feasibility studies. Community nurses make judgments and inferences about community health, community responses to health situations, and population needs. One approach assumes health concerns exist unless assessment data indicate otherwise (Gordon, 2016). Other systems of assessment base decisions on community strengths. With the problem-focused assessment of health concerns, nurses make diagnoses based on summarized data using the nursing process, which results in one or more of the following determinations:

- No problem exists, but providing health-promotion or health-protection services may address a potential health concern. For example, providing health education in a high school could offset a potential for increased sexually transmitted disease in the high school population.
- A problem exists but is recognized by community members or health-related professionals with effective strategies for problem-solving; for example, flu immunizations.
- A problem exists that the community recognizes, but resources are inadequate or the community has not responded. Assistance is needed; for example, highway traffic noise.
- A problem exists that the community recognizes but cannot cope with at this time, such as a lack of fluoridated water systems. Dentists, nurses, and nutritionists could be assigned to assist the community in resolving actual problems of dental caries.
- A problem or potential health concern exists that needs further study; for example, lack of sidewalks.

Use of strength-based approaches to assessment emphasizes strengths and integrates health-promotion and health-protection activities into a person's plans. For example, a community may have nutritional feeding programs for older adults, women, and children that are underutilized. Community members may not use them because communication is inadequate. Examples of community strengths and concerns are shown in Table 8-3.

### Identify Causes and Risk Factors

Data are examined for factors or characteristics that contribute to identified potential and existing health-related concerns. Nurses make inferences about population groups and identify risk factors. Identification of risk factors guides community nursing actions. Some risk factors signify immediate health concerns, such as a polluted water supply, whereas other risk factors indicate potential problems, such as lack of knowledge of childhood disease prevention. Nurses consider whether community risk factors can be altered, eliminated, or regulated through nursing actions. Nurses modify risk factors when possible by using strategies such as health education (Box 8-4: Diversity Awareness).

### Community Diagnosis

Community assessment, as previously described, culminates in nursing diagnoses. The following components are included in the community diagnosis process: community situations or states within a population or population group; data collection using some combination of observation, focus groups, interview, and measurement; a framework; existing or potential health concerns; risk factors related to health concerns; and potential solutions through nursing actions. Diagnoses form the basis for planning, implementing, and evaluating solutions to health concerns (Gordon, 2016). Box 8-5: Quality and Safety Scenario and Box 8-6: Innovative Practice provide an overview of how workplace violence contributes to quality and safety and how leaders might intervene to prevent or diffuse violence.

Community diagnoses and problem structuring facilitate communication among community health professionals, team members, and community members through the use of clear and concise nomenclature with development of diagnostic categories using both inductive and deductive reasoning specific to community nursing (Frerichs et al., 2016). Diagnoses may be written or stated according to the structural and functional aspects of a community.

Structural aspects include those related to the population, such as the demographic characteristics of groups with similar characteristics (preschool children, adolescents, or a high school population). Functional aspects include those related to the psychosocial, physiological, or spiritual health patterns, such as decision-making (cognitive-perceptual pattern) or communication links among health care resources (roles-relationships pattern). Functional health patterns guide data collection about health concerns and risk factors. Structural and functional aspects of the community provide a framework for diagnostic statements (see Chapter 6).

---

### TABLE 8-3　Examples of Community Strengths and Concerns

| Strengths | Concerns |
| --- | --- |
| Well-child clinic available | Unavailable |
| Feeding program accessible to older adults | Inaccessible |
| Sex education in schools acceptable | Unacceptable |
| Family planning services accessible | Inaccessible |
| Fluoridated water system | Nonfluoridated water system |
| Open communication | Dysfunctional communication |
| Interagency cooperation | Dysfunctional transactions |
| Adequate kitchen and plumbing facilities | Inadequate |
| High interest of key leaders in health promotion | Lack of interest |

---

### 🌐 BOX 8-4　DIVERSITY AWARENESS

#### Comparing Poverty Rates by Racial and Ethnic Categories

The United States uses the Current Population Survey to assess the labor force, but this survey also provides a broad-based database that includes demographic data facilitating comparison among groups (US Census Bureau, n.d.). According to the 2007–11 American Community Survey, the poverty rate (14.3%) increased by 2.3% from the level in 2007 (US Census Bureau, n.d.). Racial and ethnic disparities in poverty rates persist, with the highest rates for American Indians and Alaska Natives (27%). The next highest rates of poverty, listed in order from highest poverty rate to lowest, are for blacks or African Americans (25.8%), Native Hawaiians and other Pacific Islanders (17.6%), and the Asian population (Korean [15%], Vietnamese [14.7%], and Filipino [5.8%]). Among Hispanic subpopulations, the poverty rates ranged from a low of 16.2% for Cubans to a high of 26.3% for Dominicans. Non-Hispanic whites continue to maintain the lowest poverty rate among the racial ethnic data collected (9.9%).

Poverty experiences place these populations at risk for many health problems, such as developmental delay, asthma, and heart disease. Identifying harmful social determinants of health during community assessment facilitates health promotion for communities experiencing poverty (Chung et al., 2016). Assessment of the community should explore whether organizations exist to assist with food access, child health insurance options, employment opportunities, restraining orders, and securing safe housing. Access to health services, particularly mental health services, should also be included in assessment of impoverished communities. Furthermore, community members who remain informed about the unique resources available locally offer important information for planning care and referral to community-based programs.

Local health agencies, nonprofit groups, and community resource lists may provide additional information about resources available within the community. The community assessment gathers information about the issue encountered most frequently. Other issues may be less common, but because of their severity should be assessed, such as the incidence of child maltreatment.

From Chung, E. K., Siegel, B. S., Garg, A., Conroy, K., Gross, R. S., Long, D. A., et al. (2016). Screening for social determinants of health among children and families living in poverty: A guide for clinicians. *Current Problems in Pediatric and Adolescent Health Care, 45*(5), 135–153; US Census Bureau. (n.d.). Current population survey. http://www.census.gov/programs-surveys/cps.html.

## ✔ BOX 8-5 QUALITY AND SAFETY SCENARIO

### Workplace Violence

Targets for violent acts may be places where people work to support their families. Workplace violence was once considered isolated, unplanned incidents that fell under the jurisdiction of the federal Occupational Safety and Health Administration (OSHA). Currently, workplace violence prevention and preparation often also include external threats of terrorism. The following are some recommendations to minimize workplace violence:

- Encourage public awareness campaigns.
- Develop workplace policies and plans.
- Adopt a zero-tolerance workplace violence policy.
- Apply preventive law enforcement policies.
- Perform background checks on employees.
- Study government agencies that make workplace violence a priority.
- Provide proper training for employees, supervisors, and managers about warning signs of violent behavior.
- Encourage a workplace culture that facilitates health relationships, creative problem-solving, and voicing concerns while discouraging a hostile environment.
- Expect nonautocratic leadership styles.
- Prevent/minimize negative coworker behavior.
- Encourage social support (listening, recognition) for employees to succeed at their work.
- Implement strategies to minimize absenteeism, turnover, and low performance.
- Implement strategies to encourage participatory management.
- Ensure protection of the abused person when domestic violence or stalking occurs in the workplace.
- Develop and distribute clear and comprehensive legal and legislative guidelines.

- Evaluate programs and strategies after they have been implemented. Suggestions for approaches included the following strategies:
- Educational efforts should reflect cooperative efforts by government agencies, major corporations, unions, and advocacy groups, with OSHA acting as a facilitator and coordinator.
- Enact multidisciplinary no-threats/no-violence policies and prevention plans.
- Violence prevention training should occur regularly and include practicing the plan.
- The work space and policies should provide a physically secure work environment.
- Preventive measures should be established, including documenting incidents, planning antiviolence strategies, and conducting threat assessments.
- Systems should be developed for the monitoring of incidents of workplace violence.
- Resource lists should be maintained and include social service, mental health, legal, and other agencies that provide assistance.
- Training programs should extend community policing concepts to workplace violence. Government or private organizations should develop training materials for small employers. Employers should keep the abuser out of the workplace (e.g., screening telephone calls, making the victim's work space physically more secure, instructing security guards or receptionists).
- Employers should provide resources for emotional, financial, and legal counseling. Clear, comprehensive, and uniform legal guidelines should be distributed widely.
- Incentives for employers should be identified and instituted.

Modified from Cowie, A. K. (2016). Some predictors of workplace violence. *From Science to Practice: Organizational Psychology Bulletin, 2*(1), 13-14.

## ☀ BOX 8-6 INNOVATIVE PRACTICE

### Intervention Techniques to Prevent and Diffuse Workplace Violence

Lanza and colleagues (2016) reported their findings from a research study exploring the benefits of an innovative community intervention to prevent and diffuse workplace violence. The community meetings used a format (the violence-prevention community meeting) designed to minimize violence and promote nonviolent problem-solving and acting with civility. Their study included patients and staff on seven locked psychiatric units in the US Veterans Health Administration. During 21 weeks, each site had violence-prevention community meetings (VPCM) during the middle 7 weeks, with 7 weeks before the VPCM and 7 weeks after the VPCM. After the VPCM, aggression rates dropped. In addition to innovative strategies such as the VPCM, the following techniques may also be useful:

- Recognize warning signs, which include changes in mood, personal hardships, mental health issues (e.g., depression, anxiety), negative behavior (e.g., untrustworthy, lying, bad attitude), verbal threats, and history of violence.
- Do not limit at-risk behavior to a standard profile.
- Environments should be designed to detect signs of impending violence and to prevent violence with security cameras, key card access, administrative controls, and behavioral strategies.

- Reporting systems should be confidential and seamless.
- Stay calm; create a relaxed environment and speak calmly.
- Separate the individual from the group, if possible.
- Use nonthreatening body language; build trust and strengthen the relationship.
- Keep your verbal communication simple, clear, and direct; be open and honest.
- Reflect on the person's message to allow time for clarification, allow the person to verbalize, listen attentively, and stop what you are doing and give full attention.
- Ask for examples to help illustrate the points that are being made. Carefully define the problem, exploring it with open-ended questions.
- Silence allows the individual time to clarify thoughts.
- Monitor the tone, volume, rate, and rhythm of your speech.
- Seek opportunities for agreement.
- Be creative and open to new ideas.

From Lanza, M., Ridenour, M., Hendricks, S., Riordan, J., Zeiss, R., Schmidt, S., et al. (2016). The violence prevention community meeting: A multi-site study. *Archives of Psychiatric Nursing, 30*(3), 382–386.

## PLANNING WITH THE COMMUNITY

Community health planning begins with nursing diagnoses. Nurses design goals to resolve existing or potential health concerns. For example, high rates of childhood diseases in the community require goals aimed at decreasing rates. Identification of specific or potential health concerns with planned actions to achieve desired community outcomes provides the framework and data for community evaluation.

### Purposes

The following are major purposes of the planning phase:

- Prioritization of problems and identification of diagnoses through assessment
- Differentiation of problems resolved through nursing actions from those best resolved by others
- Identification of immediate, intermediate, and long-term goals, as well as behavioral objectives oriented to the community derived from the goals and specific actions to achieve objectives
- Formalization of a community nursing care plan (see the care plan at the end of this chapter) that includes written problems, actions, and expected behavioral outcomes

The planning phase culminates in a nursing plan that provides the framework for evaluation. Once developed, the plan is implemented. The costs associated with the delivery of health services and personnel, as well as the financial resources available, influence the priorities for implementation. Community values and the nurse's philosophy about people, health, the community, and nursing also influence implementation. High-priority issues often include infectious agents, sexually transmitted disease, alcohol and drug use, smoking, inadequate nutrition, inadequate infant and child care, high death rate from motor vehicle accidents, texting while driving, heroine overdose, and unwanted teenage pregnancies.

Community participation in health planning facilitates effective assignment of priorities. As health service recipients, community members strive for reasonably priced, high-quality services. Residents aim to acquire appropriate benefits for the needs and concerns of the population. Communication and the rationale for designating priorities help to resolve differences in opinion.

During the planning phase, nurses determine those problems most amenable to community nursing intervention, behavior implemented by the nurse to fulfill a health goal of the community. Community nurses differentiate problems nursing can resolve from those health concerns that could best be managed by community members, referred to health-related professionals, or handled with community support. Nurses refer problems related to the presence of rodents, poor sanitation conditions, or the absence of community recreational facilities to appropriate community leaders or agencies.

Community nurses focus on determining goals, developing measurable behavioral objectives, and designating actions to achieve expected outcomes. Nurses describe specific behaviors intended to reach projected outcomes. Evaluation includes appraisal of the effectiveness of nursing actions. Health planning emphasizes promoting and protecting population health; therefore problems, solutions, and actions are defined at the group level. Community nurses plan and implement health plans for groups, such as school-age children, and facilitate development of health-promotion services for all residents. Nurses frequently act as change agents by taking responsibility for influencing health patterns and behavior. Decisions about health interventions stem from community nurses' appreciation of human behavior and principles of planned change.

### Planned Change

Planned change results from efforts by individuals or groups, and involves fundamental shifts in behavior (Pender et al., 2014). Individuals act as agents of their own health conditions. Community health objectives often depend on active decisions by individuals to change their lifestyles (reducing alcohol consumption or quitting smoking). Efforts to influence and reinforce changes in community health behavior become the central focus of effective risk reduction programs (Brown et al., 2016).

Studies attempt to explain why some groups of people effectively participate in certain health programs or make lifestyle changes, whereas others do not. Early work by Rosenstock, who developed the health belief model, has evolved to models such as those by Pender and Prochaska used to explain and change health-promotion behaviors (Pender et al., 2014). These models identify critical concepts for understanding how individuals change their health behavior. Rosenstock's model includes the following four steps:

- Perceiving behavior as a health threat in terms of susceptibility and seriousness
- Believing the behavior is a threat to their personal health
- Taking action to adopt preventive health behaviors
- Reinforcing the new behavior

In Rosenstock's model, community members take a passive role at first, and then transition from passive to active between the second and third steps (belief to action). Ultimately, to improve community health through risk reduction programs, community members assume more responsibility for their own health, become more active in adopting healthy lifestyles, and monitor resources in the community to achieve healthy behaviors. In planning health-promotion activities, nurses consider effective strategies to motivate and support community transition from a passive to an active state.

Plans guide nursing actions. Nurses make additions and changes on the basis of community problems, resources, and problem resolution to maintain a viable plan. Table 8-1 provides one example of a community-oriented, health-promotion plan based on the goals recommended by the Surgeon General's report about health promotion and disease prevention. The report's general goal generates several specific objectives. Nursing diagnoses guide the direction of the objectives, including the risk factors to be addressed. Examples of various rationales in Table 8-1 show how nurses incorporate important concepts of planned change into community-based health-promotion plans.

Communicating plans to other health professionals, community members, and key officials remains an essential aspect of planning. Unification of care systems and linkages through shared data entry, computerized documentation, and electronic medical records contribute to more streamlined and transparent communication and collaboration. Local newspapers, local bulletins, and school correspondence to parents provide avenues to communicate with the community about health-promotion plans. Other community-based actions, such as those for nursing involvement in prevention of alcohol abuse in the community, can be used. The various plans have been categorized according to the health patterns to show that a community problem can be approached from multiple directions. Feasible plans that are well formulated facilitate implementation (US Department of Health and Human Services, 2015).

## IMPLEMENTATION WITH THE COMMUNITY

Implementation of the nursing process begins on the basis of the health-promotion and health-protection plans. In collaboration with community members or other health team members, the nurse tests feasibility and implements the plan. Involving key community members, in the assessment and planning process, is crucial for success. To ensure involvement, activities must be accessible. For example, schedule meetings in accessible areas, offer child care services, and provide light refreshments. Identify clearly what the community perceives as health-promotion needs. Maintain open communication—clear and correct information at regular intervals.

Intellectual, interpersonal, and technical skills of the community members facilitate the collaborative contribution. Community nurses often prepare community members with development of technical skills of community engagement and empowerment. Success also depends on the overcoming of expected resistance to change. Resistance to new health-promotion and health-protection activities, however, provides useful feedback to improve planning. People generally resist change to defend values that appear to be threatened by the change. Collaborating with communities initially facilitates change during the implementation phase. Table 8-4 lists factors that deter community participation. Informed nurses collaborate with community members throughout the process.

Community nurses implement health-promotion and health-protection plans in multiple community settings (schools, industry, public and private health agencies, and ambulatory care settings) where population groups experience relatively good health. Nursing centers provide nursing faculty, staff, and students with unique opportunities to assess health and plan, implement, and evaluate care (including holistic health promotion and primary health care) for individuals, families, and communities with unmet health care needs (Harvey et al., 2012). Community assessment includes observation of reciprocal interaction between the individual and his or her environment, which is similar to those techniques used for individual and family health promotion assessment (see Chapters 6 and 7 respectively). Community assessment also commonly uses factors related to self-efficacy and Bandura's social learning theory to explain relationships between human behavior and the environment. The complexity of health actions differs from one community to another. Community advisory boards play a critical role in community planning. As plans evolve, nurses learn more about the community and their own responses, strengths, limitations, and abilities to cope or adapt (Subica et al., 2016). Although implementation takes an action focus, it also includes assessment, planning, and evaluation activities to monitor actions taken to resolve, reduce, eliminate, or control the health concern.

## EVALUATION WITH THE COMMUNITY

During the evaluation phase of the process, community nurses learn whether planned actions achieved desired outcomes. Communities and nurses determine progression toward goal achievement through methods that expand collaborations (Frerichs et al., 2016). Nurses take overall responsibility for the process; however, collaborating with community members and health team members in the process produces the most valid results. For example, if implemented plans intend to reduce the incidence of fatal motor vehicle accidents, nurses guide the process to obtain community indicators and outcomes data, requisite community actions, and expected outcomes achieved from joint collaboration with community stakeholders.

Nursing plans, which include nursing diagnoses, expected outcomes, and interventions, provide the evaluation framework. With a community focus, goals and objectives define the evaluation, considering how the community responded to planned actions. For example, if childhood disease rate reduction is expected to result from certain nursing actions, community responses before the actions are compared with those after the actions. Comparison determines the level of effectiveness (complete, partially effective, or ineffective) of the nursing actions to achieve the goal.

Community nurses approach the dynamic process of evaluation in a purposeful, goal-directed manner (Stanhope & Lancaster, 2015; US Department of Health and Human Services, 2015). Determining the effectiveness of nursing actions evaluates the degree to which goals are achieved. The frequency of evaluation depends on the situations, changes expected, and objectives.

| TABLE 8-4   Potential Sources of Resistance to Health-Promotion Programs, With Agent Responses | |
| --- | --- |
| **Source of Resistance** | **Response** |
| Lack of communication about implementation of program | Communicate through community newsletter, newspapers, high school radio station, and posters |
| Misinformation regarding time and place of healthy activity | Disseminate valid information |
| Fear of unknown | Inform and encourage |
| Need for security | Clarify intentions and methods |
| No desired need to change behaviors | Demonstrate opportunity for change |
| Cultural or religious beliefs or vested interests threatened | Enlist key community leaders in planning change |
| Inaccessibility | Focus activities near the largest target population and in an area accessible by public transportation |

For example, an individual who is bleeding may need evaluation at frequent intervals, whereas behavioral changes in community groups occur slowly and require long-term evaluation methods. Evaluation intervals differ depending on immediate, intermediate, and long-range goals. The evaluation process continues until community goals are realized.

Evaluation results indicate the need for reassessment, revision, or modification of plans. Community nurses reassess situations, plan new approaches, and implement and evaluate revised plans, creating the continual cycle of the nursing process. Self-evaluation determines strengths and weaknesses as well as ways the nursing plan could have been more effective or efficient. The quality of community health-promotion and health-protection efforts depends on the professional qualities of those providing the services along with effective use of the nursing process.

Workable, cost-effective programs of community health promotion are needed. Nurses play an important role in providing evidence to support effective community health plans. Historically, documentation of effective health-promotion activities has been limited (Maurer & Smith, 2014; Pender et al., 2014). Effectiveness is determined through research studies that include analyses and outcomes evaluation of home-based and community-centered nursing interventions designed to meet the needs of high-risk families, geographical communities, and vulnerable populations. For example, in a study of 679 women eligible for the Special Supplemental Nutrition Program for Women, Infants and Children, health-promotion strategies of nutrition, physical activity, and social support were used to reduce the incidence of depressive symptoms (Surkan et al., 2012). Surkan and colleagues (2012) demonstrated that health-promotion interventions delivered through home visits and telephone calls reduced the incidence of depressive symptoms at 15 months postpartum among low-income, ethnically diverse women. Such evidence-based practice and research helps to garner support for community health-promotion programs. The *Healthy People 2020* objectives include examples of national and state partnerships establishing health objectives and sustaining the initiatives (US Department of Health and Human Services, 2015).

## CASE STUDY

### *Community Efforts to Decrease Adolescent Pregnancy Rates*

The community health nurse is facilitating a grassroots community group that is determined to decrease the adolescent pregnancy rate in the city. The community population hovers around 100,000. It is a community that lies on the Mexican border of the United States. The population is predominantly Mexican American, and there is a high poverty rate.

The schools offer health courses twice between seventh grade and twelfth grade. The only formal sex education provided occurs within the context of these two health courses. There is community opposition to increasing the amount of sex education in the curriculum. A community group that has researched the problem has decided to use a social marketing approach because of this community resistance.

Most of the materials reviewed do not address the cultural needs of the region. Many of the Spanish language materials use Spanish from countries other than Mexico. The situations posed in the audiovisual materials show people who the adolescents will perceive as different from themselves.

#### Reflective Questions
- How could the community group approach its goal to decrease the adolescent pregnancy rate in a manner that will be culturally competent?
- How might the community group approach this issue without the support of the school district?

## ◎ CARE PLAN

### *Community Efforts to Decrease Adolescent Pregnancy Rates*

**\*Nursing Diagnosis: Risk of ineffective community coping related to increased levels of teen pregnancy**

#### Defining Characteristics
- Absence of education or support for sexually active teenagers
- Absence of programs for pregnancy testing, counseling, or teaching young women to care for infants
- Absence of sex education in the home, school, and community
- Community conflicts over what to teach adolescent and preadolescent children about sex
- Failure of teenagers to perceive the long-term effects of having babies
- High incidence of infants who are born prematurely or with health problems
- High rate of teen pregnancy
- Lack of access to birth control pills or devices for teenagers
- Lack of community support for preventive sex education

#### Related Factors
- Community members' lack of knowledge about the causes of and contributing factors in teen pregnancy
- Inadequate community resources for preventing teen pregnancy
- Lack of adequate communication patterns and community cohesiveness regarding strategies to prevent teen pregnancy

#### Interventions
- Assess teenagers' knowledge of sex and sexuality to determine their educational needs.
- Work with schools to develop pregnancy-prevention programs that provide adolescents with information about the risks, problems, and complications of early pregnancy.
- Work closely with individual adolescents who are pregnant to assess their needs and provide care.
- Implement an outreach and health-promotion program to raise community members' awareness of the need to approach teen pregnancy as a community problem. Consider taking the following five steps:
  - Work with teachers, school psychologists, counselors, school nurses, students, and the parent-teacher association to determine the extent of the teen pregnancy problem.
  - Encourage local youth groups, churches, and social service organizations to feature presentations on pregnancy prevention at their meetings.
  - Contact representatives of local corporations to ask for funding for educational programs.

## ◎ CARE PLAN

### Community Efforts to Decrease Adolescent Pregnancy Rates—cont'd

- Help community members (school nurses, counselors, and teachers) recognize adolescent girls who need counseling regarding such issues as peer pressure to be sexually active and the long-term consequences of pregnancy. Remind community members of the importance of listening attentively and remaining nonjudgmental.
  - Provide education on birth control measures (including abstinence from sex) and make this information available at school.
- Establish clubs for adolescent girls in the community. The goal of these clubs is to foster self-esteem. During club meetings, members should have the opportunity to openly discuss difficult questions, such as why girls consider a baby a status symbol and how to respond to peer pressure to be sexually active. Increasing self-esteem has been found to be the most effective way to reduce teen pregnancy rates.
- Encourage adolescents to participate in peer support networks where they can openly discuss social and dating pressure and other issues related to teen pregnancy, to allow them an opportunity to express their feelings openly and obtain support from peers.
- Encourage community members to establish school-based clinics in which teens can have access to reproductive system models, pregnancy tests, and nonprescription birth control measures to support the teenagers who make the decision to protect themselves from unwanted pregnancies.
- Develop a list of referrals for teenagers, such as hospitals with human sexuality courses, charities that provide prenatal care and childbirth services, women's clinics, and Planned Parenthood, to compensate for restricted access to information in the adolescent's home or school.
- Encourage community members to implement an information campaign to educate adolescents, parents, and community members about the problems associated with teen pregnancy.
- Work with community members to evaluate the effectiveness of the teen pregnancy prevention program and assist in modifying it as needed to ensure its effectiveness and promote the program as a model for preventive health.
- Collect statistical data from the schools to analyze the teen pregnancy rates, to help evaluate the effectiveness of the prevention program.

**Expected Outcomes**
- Community members express awareness of the seriousness of the high adolescent pregnancy rate in their community.
- Community members express the need for a plan to reduce the prevalence of teen pregnancies.
- Community members develop and implement plans to prevent teen pregnancy.
- Community members evaluate the success of the plan in meeting goals and objectives.
- Community members continue to revise the plan to prevent teen pregnancy as necessary.

*NANDA Nursing Diagnoses—Herdman, T. H. & Kamitsuru, S. (Eds.). Nursing Diagnoses–Definitions and Classification 2015–2017. Copyright © 2014, 1994–2014 NANDA International. Used by arrangement with John Wiley & Sons Limited. In order to make safe and effective judgments using the NANDA-I nursing diagnoses it is essential that nurses refer to the definitions and defining characteristics of the diagnoses listed in this work.

## SUMMARY

Risk factors, injury, and disease are not inevitable events experienced equally among a community's members. Effective community nurses understand the dynamic and complex nature of communities (Figure 8-4). Nurses use various theoretical frameworks to assess health-related patterns, health concerns, and health action potential and to implement the nursing process within communities. Collection and analysis of community data identify susceptible subpopulations. Planning contributes to the development of effective and efficient health-promotion and health-protection services. The nursing process enhances the efficacy of planning activities.

Many communities experience obvious deficiencies in health services that warrant health planning action. Community nurses play a significant role in health planning directed toward reducing the risks associated with disease, premature death, and injury as well as health promotion among community members. Nurses use principles of planned change to increase community awareness of health, promote healthy behaviors, and encourage participation in preventive health services. The complexity differs from one community or geographical area to another. Community nurses connect health-promotion actions to specific community phenomena, providing scientific evidence to support nursing actions in the community.

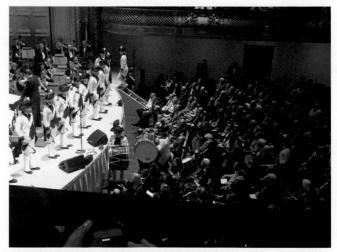

**FIGURE 8-4** Communities come together for the enjoyment of one of their traditional holidays. (From iStockphoto/Thinkstock.)

## ⓔ EVOLVE CHAPTER FEATURES

http://evolve.elsevier.com/Edelman/
- Study Questions

# REFERENCES

Andrews, J. O., Newman, S. D., et al. (2012a). Partnership readiness for community-based participatory research. *Health Education Research, 27*(4), 555–571.

Andrews, J. O., Tingen, M. S., et al. (2012b). Application of a CBPR framework to inform a multi-level tobacco cessation intervention in public housing neighborhoods. *American Journal of Community Psychology, 50*(1-2), 129–140.

Bhushan, B. (2015). Perspective: Science and technology policy–What is at stake and why should scientists participate? *Science and Public Policy, 42*(6), 887–900.

Brown, T. J., Todd, A., et al. (2016). Community pharmacy-delivered interventions for public health priorities: A systematic review of interventions for alcohol reduction, smoking cessation and weight management, including meta-analysis for smoking cessation. *BMJ Open, 6*(2), e009828.

Chappells, H., Campbell, N., et al. (2015). Understanding the translation of scientific knowledge about arsenic risk exposure among private well users. *Science of the Total Environment, 505*, 1259–1273.

Clendenning, J., Dressler, W. H., & Richards, C. (2016). Food justice or food sovereignty? Understanding the rise of urban food movements in the USA. *Agriculture and Human Values, 33*(1), 165–177.

Frerichs, L., Lich, K. H., et al. (2016). Integrating systems science and community-based participatory research to achieve health equity. *American Journal of Public Health, 106*(2), 215–222.

Gordon, M. (2016). *Manual of nursing diagnosis* (13th ed.). Sudbury, MA: Jones & Bartlett.

Harris, J. K., Beatty, K., et al. (2016). The double disparity facing rural local health departments. *Annual Review of Public Health, 37*(3), 167–184.

Harvey, S. T., Fisher, L. J., & Green, V. M. (2012). Evaluating the clinical efficacy of a primary care–focused, nurse-led, consultation liaison model for perinatal mental health. *International Journal of Mental Health Nursing, 21*(1), 75–81.

He, W., & Larsen, L. J. (2014). *Older Americans with a disability: 2008–2012. US Census Bureau, American Community Survey reports*. Washington, DC: US Government Printing Office. http://tilrc.org/assests/news/publications/older_americans_with_a_disability12_2014.pdf.

Huffling, K. (2015). Statement from the Alliance of Nurses for Healthy Environments on TSCA reform legislation in the Senate. Alliance of Nurses for Healthy Environments. http://envirn.org/pg/blog/read/86057/statement-from-the-alliance-of-nurses-for-healthy-environments-on-tsca-reform-legislation-in-the-senate.

Joly, E. (2016). Integrating transition theory and bioecological theory: A theoretical perspective for nurses supporting the transition to adulthood for young people with medical complexity. *Journal of Advanced Nursing, 72*(6), 1251–1262.

Jones, C. M. (2013). Heroin use and heroin use risk behaviors among nonmedical users of prescription opioid pain relievers–United States, 2002–2004 and 2008–2010. *Drug and Alcohol Dependence, 132*(1-2), 95–100.

Jones, C. M., Logan, J., et al. (2015). Vital signs: Demographic and substance use trends among heroin users—United States, 2002–2013. *Morbidity and Mortality Weekly Report, 64*(26), 719–725.

Keddem, S., Barg, F. K., et al. (2015). Mapping the urban asthma experience: Using qualitative GIS to understand contextual factors affecting asthma control. *Social Science and Medicine, 140*(8), 9–17.

Leffers, J. M., Smith, C. M., et al. (2015). Developing curriculum recommendations for environmental health in nursing. *Nurse Educator, 40*(3), 139–143.

Maurer, F. A., & Smith, C. M. (2014). *Community/public health nursing practice: Health for families and populations* (5th ed.). St. Louis: Saunders.

Meit, M., Knudson, A., et al. (2014). The 2014 update of the rural-urban chartbook. Rural Health Reform Policy Research Center. http://worh.org/sites/default/files/2014-rural-urban-chartbook.pdf.

Noguera-Oviedo, K., & Aga, D. S. (2016). Lessons learned from more than two decades of research on emerging contaminants in the environment. *Journal of Hazardous Materials, 316*, 242–251.

Pender, N. J., Murdaugh, C. L., & Parsons, M. A. (2014). *Health promotion in nursing practice* (7th ed.). Upper Saddle River, NJ: Pearson.

Petersen, E., Wilson, M. E., et al. (2016). Rapid spread of Zika virus in the Americas–implications for public health preparedness for mass gatherings at the 2016 Brazil Olympic Games. *International Journal of Infectious Diseases, 44*, 11–15.

Pillarisetti, A., Mehta, S., & Smith, K. R. (2016). HAPIT, the Household Air Pollution Intervention Tool, to evaluate the health benefits and cost-effectiveness of clean cooking interventions. In E. A. Thomas (Ed.), *Broken pumps and promises: Incentivizing impact in environmental health* (pp. 147–169). Cham, Switzerland: Springer International Publishing.

Roy, É., Arruda, N., et al. (2016). Epidemiology of injection drug use: New trends and prominent issues. *The Canadian Journal of Psychiatry, 61*(3), 136–144.

Schlüter-Vorberg, L., Prasse, C., et al. (2015). Toxification by transformation in conventional and advanced wastewater treatment: The antiviral drug acyclovir. *Environmental Science and Technology Letters, 2*(12), 342–346.

Solomon, G. M., Morello-Frosch, R., et al. (2016). Cumulative environmental impacts: Science and policy to protect communities. *Annual Review of Public Health, 37*(3), 83–96.

Stanhope, M., & Lancaster, J. (2015). *Public health nursing: Population-centered health care in the community* (9th ed.). St. Louis: Elsevier.

Subica, A. M., Grills, C. T., et al. (2016). Communities of color creating healthy environments to combat childhood obesity. *American Journal of Public Health, 106*(1), 79–86.

Surkan, P., Gottlieb, B., et al. (2012). Impact of a health promotion intervention on maternal depressive symptoms at 15 months postpartum. *Maternal and Child Health Journal, 16*(1), 139–148.

Thomas, S. J., Wallace, C., et al. (2016). Mixed-methods study to develop a patient complexity assessment instrument for district nurses. *Nurse Researcher, 23*(4), 9–13.

University of Texas Health Science Center at Houston. (2012). CHARTing health information for Texas. https://sph.uth.edu/charting/.

US Department of Health and Human Services. (2015). 2020 topics and objectives. http://www.healthypeople.gov/2020/topics-objectives.

US Department of Transportation National Center for Statistics and Analysis (2008). *Traffic safety facts. A compilation of motor vehicle crash data from the Fatality Analysis Reporting System and the General Estimates System*. Washington, DC: National Highway Traffic Safety Administration. http://www-nrd.nhtsa.dot.gov/Pubs/811162.PDF.

US Department of Transportation National Center for Statistics and Analysis (2012). *Traffic safety facts. A compilation of motor vehicle crash data from the Fatality Analysis Reporting System and the General Estimates System.* Washington, DC: National Highway Traffic Safety Administration. http://www-nrd.nhtsa.dot.gov/Pubs/812032.pdf.

West, L. A., Cole, S., et al. (2014). *US Census Bureau. 65+ in the United States: 2010* (pp. 23–212). Washington, DC: US Government Printing Office.

Woodward, B., Smart, D., & Benavides-Vaello, S. (2015). Modifiable factors that support political participation by nurses. *Journal of Professional Nursing, 32*(1), 54–61.

Young, S. K., Tabish, T. B., et al. (2016). Backcountry travel emergencies in Arctic Canada: A pilot study in public health surveillance. *International Journal of Environmental Research and Public Health, 13*(3), 276.

# 9

# Screening

*Elizabeth Connelly Kudzma*

### Screening Then and Today

In the 1920s, educators started to investigate the concepts of intelligence quotient, lower intelligence, and mental handicaps. Intelligence categories were separated numerically, and "cretin" became a medical term used to describe a lower level of intelligence. Neonatal hypothyroidism (cretinism) was more common in mountainous inland areas away from sea salt sources of iodine. It is very rare in the modern world because of the required screening of all infants at birth (blood tests measure levels of thyroid-stimulating hormone and thyroxine). Screening testing of mothers during pregnancy and of infants shortly after birth with dried blood spot (DBS) technology allows treatment and lifetime monitoring before the serious signs of thyroxine deficiency occur. This disorder and others (e.g., phenylketonuria [PKU]) are health screenings' modern success stories. Neonatal hypothyroidism has virtually disappeared in the developed world as a result of the screening of babies (target population) followed by appropriate treatment for affected individuals. However, the storage and research use of DBS technology raises significant controversy over lack of parental knowledge and consent for research activities; in some states privacy laws may inhibit retention of DBS samples without explicit parental knowledge (Botkin et al., 2013).

Very recently biotechnology companies have developed tests that aim to screen an individual's DNA for genes associated with diseases or population subgroups (Nickolich et al., 2016). DNA testing examines a person's genetic code to provide information about genealogy or ancestry that may be helpful in assessing a person's risk of disease. Personalized DNA testing kits are available to help consumers discover their risks of developing disorders (such as Alzheimer disease, diabetes, and breast cancer). An over-the-counter home test for human immunodeficiency virus (HIV) was approved by the Food and Drug Administration and was marketed to consumers in 2012. The availability of screening options that may be novel, but unproven, raises new questions about media information provided to the public, the politics involved (Lin & Gostin, 2016), and the reliability and validity of screening methods and associated necessary counseling.

- Why has the newborn period been identified as an important time to require screening tests?
- Each government regulates a list of mandated screening for newborns. Do you know what your government/state/ministry of health requires?
- The availability and feasibility of screening tests is constantly changing. How are new screening tests evaluated and added to the mandated requirements?
- What characteristics of screening tests have to be considered for neonates? What characteristics of screening tests have to be considered for individuals of any age?
- How is the margin of error further defined for screening tests/instruments?
- What aspects of screening program development should nurses participate in? Assessment, data analysis, implementation, evaluation of health outcomes?

*Evidence-based preventive services are effective in reducing death and disability, and are cost-effective or even cost-saving. Preventive services consist of screening tests, counseling, immunizations or medications used to prevent disease, detect health problems early, or provide people with the information they need to make good decisions about their health. While preventive services are traditionally delivered in clinical settings, some can be delivered within communities, work sites, schools, residential treatment centers, or homes (National Prevention Council, 2011, p. 18).*

Clinical and community preventive services are vital to health promotion and disease prevention. Identified as such, they have become one of the four strategic directions of the National Prevention Strategy (safe community environments, elimination of health disparities, clinical and preventive services, empowered people). Most adults are not up-to-date on the core set of clinical preventive services recommended at various ages, and the proportion of older adults who are current with their screening or are unwilling to be screened diminishes as more screening strategies are added (Bynum et al., 2012; Davis et al., 2012). Screening is an important component of clinical preventive services because it is a valuable tool for health care professionals to identify chronic conditions and risk factors before the condition becomes costly both in financial terms and for quality of life. This is particularly important as the health care paradigm shifts from medical and volume-based to a health-promotion and value-based model of care. Although health education about screening is categorized as part of the rubric of primary prevention, the actual process of screening is part of **secondary prevention.**

The primary goal of screening is to detect risk factors and a condition early, to prevent or treat it, and to deter its progression.

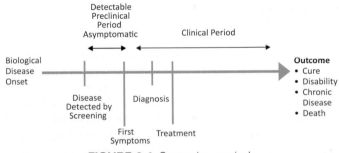

**FIGURE 9-1** Screening periods.

An important assumption underlying the use of screening is that detection early in the asymptomatic period allows treatment at a time when the eventual course of the disease can be altered significantly. Similarly, identifying risk factors assists in identifying the populations needing screening and focuses attention on needed behavior change before disease develops. Screening strategies are based on the principle that the selected disease is preceded by a period of **asymptomatic pathogenesis** or latency (disease development before symptoms first appear) when risk factors predisposing a person to the disease are building toward full manifestation of the disease (Figure 9-1). Screening takes advantage of the prepathogenic state and the early pathogenic state—identifying risks relating to disease in the earliest and most treatable stages.

Screening strategies are essential to the core of the health-promotion metaphor—the upstream/downstream narrative. When health care providers are so preoccupied with managing the acute care (ill/dying) of the drowning downstream, they have little time to focus on why individuals become ill and fall into the river upstream. Screening tests focus attention on going upstream to the source to better identify valid determinants of health status. Identification of valid health status measures involves accurate screening tests.

Administration of screening tests, some of which might be fairly simple and relatively inexpensive when compared with the burden of disease, provides value in improved quality of care and decreased health care costs. Screening is not generally a diagnostic measure, nor is it curative. It is a preliminary step to identify (upstream) individuals who need more diagnostic workup to prevent further development of the condition or disease and to ameliorate adverse disease outcomes. More importantly, it is a step toward empowering individuals to make more informed choices about their health and health behaviors. A second, but equally important, objective of screening is to reduce the costs of managing the disease by avoiding more intensive interventions required in later disease stages. A cost-conscious approach to health care mandates that health care professionals, at all levels, acquire a basic understanding of the screening process and its application. Unfortunately, upstream screening and the application of screening processes involves complicated decision-making, and is entangled with social policy, communication and media information, and personal choice.

## ADVANTAGES AND DISADVANTAGES OF SCREENING

### Advantages

Some screenings are very simple and performed at home (blood pressure, heart rate, weight, even currently oxygen saturation), and nurses are involved in promoting their use and educating people about their use. This chapter, however, will focus more on the efficacy and efficiency of clinical, procedural, and laboratory-based tests. Screening tests offer several advantages. Although some screening procedures are simple and relatively inexpensive, others are expensive and may not be cost-effective. The simplicity of some screening procedures decreases the time and cost of the health care personnel involved, especially when compared with the cost of treating the disease after symptoms appear, and enables less skilled technicians to administer the test.

A second advantage is the ability to apply the screening process to both individuals and larger populations. In an **individual screening** program, one person is tested by a health professional who has selected the individual as high risk (such as prior hypertension). The practitioner can make this decision independently; the health care agency can define a specific policy; or legislative bodies can require the screening by law as in the case of newborn hypothyroidism and PKU, or lead-screening programs in children.

PKU is a rare genetic disorder that causes the level of an amino acid, phenylalanine, to build up because of a metabolizing enzyme defect. Children who are identified as having PKU can be placed on a phenylalanine-restricted diet and medication to avoid the worst complications of PKU-related disease (neurological problems, delayed development, and intellectual disability/mental retardation). Lead screening for children is an essential

component of the well-child visit. Children younger than 6 years are at greatest risk, and once exposure has occurred, it is difficult to reverse toxic effects (Ness, 2013). A pediatrician in Flint, Michigan, who was reviewing positive lead screening test results in children alerted public health authorities and the state to the existence of high lead levels in the city water. As electronic health records become more digital, an electronic flag during well care visits ideally alerts the provider when the care recipient needs recommended screening.

**Group or mass screening** occurs when a target population is selected on the basis of an increased incidence of a condition or a recognized element of high risk within an identified group. For example, the target population may be invited to a central location on a designated day to be tested for the selected disorders (elevated levels of lipids and cholesterol, hypertension, osteoporosis, elevated blood glucose level).

A third advantage is the ability to provide one-test disease-specific screening or multiple test screenings. A **one-test disease-specific screening** is the administration of a single test that searches for a characteristic that indicates a high risk of developing a disorder. An example of this would be blood pressure screening to evaluate hypertension (Yoon et al., 2015). **Multiple test screening** is the administration of two or more tests to detect more than one disease. In some cases, one sample can be used to evaluate an individual for several conditions, saving time and money and making the process efficient and economical. For example, a blood sample can be assessed for a number of components, including glucose and cholesterol levels. The combination of the relatively low-cost screening test and flexibility makes screenings adaptable to all levels within the health care delivery system. Other multiple test screenings of importance are for substance abuse, mental health disorders and depression, and sexually transmitted infections (STIs).

A final advantage of screening is that it creates an opportunity for providing health education (see Chapter 10) to a group of individuals who may not otherwise receive it. In some situations, it is possible to establish a clinical relationship during the screening process that leads to preventive visits and includes educating people about healthy lifestyles, risk reduction, developmental needs, activities of daily living, and preventive self-care. Many of today's chronic illnesses are a result of individual health behaviors. Awareness is the first step in prevention. If better awareness is combined with health-education and health-promotion tools, individuals have a better opportunity to manage their own risks. Taking advantage of a potential health-promotion teachable moment should never be overlooked.

The commonly recommended 6-month dental screening is an example. Although the individual is at the dentist's office to be screened for cavities and to have teeth cleaned to avoid gum disease, the hygienist provides education and reminders on the correct way and the necessity to brush and floss teeth correctly, and a check is provided for oral cancer. Another example is the in the recommended counseling for tobacco cessation—ask, advise, assess, assist, arrange (Agency for Healthcare Research and Quality, 2014b). It is not enough to simply screen an individual with the question, "Do you use tobacco?" Readiness to quit should also be determined and combined with cessation treatment assistance (Centers for Disease Control and Prevention [CDC], 2014). Nurses who are familiar with community resources can then refer individuals to smoking cessation programs that fit with the person's preferences and values (Broder, 2013).

## Disadvantages

The primary disadvantages of screening stem largely from uncertainties in scientific evidence, which sets normal testing ranges and therefore also ranges of error for screening tests. When effectiveness depends on the screening program's ability to distinguish those who probably have the disease from those who do not, any margin of error can result in serious consequences. Some individuals who do not have the condition will be referred for further tests, and some who do have the disease will not get needed referrals. Those incorrectly referred (false positive) suffer needless anxiety and unnecessary medical interventions, some of which can be harmful, while awaiting more definitive diagnosis (e.g., high levels of prostate-specific antigen [PSA]). False positive osteoporosis screening results can lead to unnecessary bone building medication treatment that may have adverse effects. Some noninvasive prenatal strategies test for very rare disorders, so the predictive value may be questioned (Nickolich et al., 2016; Vora & O'Brien, 2014). Mammography screening for breast microcalcifications identifies a significant number of women (who may be false positives) who later undergo medically invasive breast biopsies. Women with false positive results bear the burden of the follow-up visits, lost time, inconvenience, and the cost for follow-up interventions to determine whether the disease is actually present.

The effects on those whose diseases have been overlooked (false negative) are even more important. For example, in maternal serum sampling for fetal DNA (cell-free DNA testing), false negative reports have occurred with twin pregnancies and cell mosaicism (possession of normal and abnormal cells) in either the baby or the placenta (Nickolich et al., 2016). These individuals have a false assurance of health that will be shattered eventually when the illness becomes obvious; they lose the opportunity to receive earlier treatment that could prevent irreversible damage. The difficulty of balancing the benefits to some against the burdens to others may be an ethical issue underlying many screening programs. The significance of this disadvantage can vary; therefore, it should be assessed for each screening program, disease, and population.

## SELECTION OF A SCREENED DISEASE

The selection of a screened disease goes beyond examination of any disease alone. The selection process must also encompass less tangible factors, such as the emotional impact (HIV infection) and the financial impact (osteoporosis) (Nayak et al., 2011) of the disease's detection on the screened population. Even after data have been gathered and the critical issues have been reviewed, the final decision of whether to screen individuals must often be reached with incomplete evidence or with answers that raise ethical issues, on an epidemiological and a personal level.

The potential uncertainties confounding the decision to screen individuals emphasize the need to conduct an analysis of available material to obtain a decision that is as objective and scientific as possible. Answers to the following questions may provide a basis for designating a disease as screenable or not screenable:

- Does the significance of the disorder warrant its consideration as a community problem?
- Can the disease be detected by screening?
- Should screening for the disease be done?
- What are the health benefits? For example, can it be treated?
- What are the tangible and intangible costs?

As simplistic as these questions may appear, the answers or lack of answers, in addition to individual preferences, may expose complex issues that determine whether a well-informed decision can be made on screening.

## Significance of the Disease for Screening

According to the CDC, epidemiology is the "method used to find the causes of health outcomes and diseases in populations. In epidemiology, the patient is the community and individuals are viewed collectively. By definition, epidemiology is the study (scientific, systematic, and data driven) of the distribution (frequency, pattern) and determinants (causes, risk factors) of health-related states and events (not just diseases) in specified populations (neighborhood, school, city, state, country, global)" (CDC, 2015).

Health information on both morbidity and mortality may be used to identify the most important diseases affecting populations. The term morbidity refers to a diseased state or disability from any cause; however, the view of morbidity can be broader, including a range or degree of the illness that affects the person. Mortality statistics (deaths) in a given population can be easier to use as end outcome indices as long as statistical collection measures are accurate.

The significance of a disease refers to the level of priority assigned to the disease as a public health concern. Although the opinions of political and public interest groups may influence this evaluation, significance is generally determined by incidence and prevalence, and by the quantity (severity) and quality of life affected by the disorder (CDC, 2012). The media may also have a role in defining a public health problem which should be screened for, or addressed, as the media provides a place for compelling storytelling about the impact of disease and potential screening (Dorfman & Krasnow, 2014). The ability of the Zika virus to infect the fetus and cause neurological problems and microcephaly is a graphic example of the media telling the story of mothers and babies infected and the spread of this virus worldwide.

Key factors in assessing the need for screening criteria are quantifying measures of disease frequency. The two measures most used in epidemiology are incidence and prevalence (CDC, 2012; Lundy & Janes, 2014). Incidence indicates the rate of a new population problem and estimates the risk of an individual developing a disease or condition during a specific period or over a lifetime. Prevalence is the proportion of a given population with the disease or condition at any one point in time. It provides the best estimate of whether a person is likely to become ill during a specific period. In short, incidence is new cases, and prevalence is all cases within a set period. Chronic conditions are usually measured by their prevalence (generally existing), whereas acute conditions are assessed by their incidence (rate of new occurrences). Both are used in assessing the need for community services and screenings, and help develop the criteria for evidence-based practice screening guidelines that include the age at which screening should be performed, the frequency and manner of screening, and the person who should perform the screening. The greater the physical and psychological harm experienced by the population, the greater is the urgency to designate the condition/disease as a priority health problem. A first step in assessing screening feasibility is evaluation of disease significance to decide if the disorder warrants the time, effort, and financial resources that must be allocated. For example, there has been a significant decline in the incidence of late-stage colorectal cancer in the United States since 1987, and this is attributed to increased rates of screening (Yang et al., 2014).

Estimating the **quality of life** affected by a disease presents problems but is also a necessary step. The perception of quality of life is subjective, and individual evaluations may differ. For example, not all people equally perceive the disability resulting from a disease; some may make adjustments and cope, whereas others do not. Those who do not may be more likely to say that the quality of their lives is significantly lower than that of other people.

Two epidemiological measures are used to estimate quality of life. A **quality-adjusted life year** (QALY) is a measurement of quality of life. It is defined as perfect health minus the disability-adjusted life year (DALY). The QALY assumes that 1 year of excellent health is 1 QALY (1 year of life times 1 utility value equals 1 QALY). It also assumes that 1 year spent in a less perfect state of health or with disease (or comorbidities) is worth less. A determination of the QALY value involves multiplication of the utility value associated with a state of health by the number of years lived in that state of health. Following this thinking, half a year lived in excellent health is 0.5 QALY (0.5 year of life times 1 utility value), which is the same as one full year of life lived in a disease state (immobile, fractured hip assuming half utility value) (1 year times 0.5 utility value).

A second measure, the **disability-adjusted life year** (DALY), refers to a year spent in less than healthy life. It is a measure of the burden of disease, and measures the gap between the current health status and excellent health status. It also accounts for life lost and life quality diminished through disability. The QALY and DALY measures may both be used depending on whether the outcome of the screening measure is intended to maximize health or minimize disability (Costello, 2014; Airoldi & Morton, 2009).

There is currently greater focus on quantifying measurements of health outcomes so as to weigh the costs of screening, treatment, and effects on populations. The QALY incorporates morbidity and mortality in a single arithmetic measure. It allows computation, estimation, and comparisons of screening decisions. However, the estimation of formulas association with utility and disability is difficult. QALYs assist in analyzing the gap between strict treatment decisions and their economic costs, informing public health decision-making (Costello, 2014).

By contrast, measures of the **quantity of life** affected by the disease are more readily obtainable. In addition to prevalence and incidence rates, disease-specific mortality rates present different aspects of the disease for analysis. Disease-specific mortality may be linked to the severity of an incident occurring or the longtime health burden cost associated with management of the disease. There is some evidence that mandatory screening of athletes reduces the incidence of sudden cardiac death in athletes who are supposedly young and fit; the cost of comprehensive cardiac screening is high and controversial (Anderson et al., 2014; Shephard, 2011); a death in a young athletically fit person is a very untoward, severe event. With other diseases, the prevalence of the disorder may not be high, but the problem requires disproportionate amounts spent on maintenance or management after the condition is fully expressed. For PKU, a case undetected at birth means a lifetime of suboptimal development and neurological disease management.

## Detection

With the relative significance of the disease established, the next step is to determine if health professionals can screen individuals for the disease. Are there well-documented diagnostic criteria for the disorder? Is there a valid and reliable screening instrument? Are sufficient community resources and treatment modalities available to support a screening program?

### Diagnostic Criteria

Detection of a disease requires knowledge of the characteristics that indicate its presence or, as in screening, its early pathogenic, asymptomatic state, and is often based on risk factors such as heredity, age, sex, and family history. For example, screening tests may be recommended for men or women (US Department of Health and Human Services, Office on Women's Health, 2012, 2013; Womenshealth.gov, 2013). Selected disease diagnostic criteria should be well documented and defined and not merely accepted as commonly used indicators. The impact of uncertainty in detecting disease is amplified when the application of the screening design is considered. Some diseases, such as sickle cell anemia or PKU, are defined by the presence or absence of a single, isolated gene or enzyme. Other conditions, such as high blood glucose levels (diabetes), are measured according to numerical values for which a normal range has been set. Although there may be some disagreements over normal parameters, diabetes is a serious disease, and early treatment has been shown to decrease the incidence of morbidity and death attributable to vascular diseases and stroke.

### Screening Measures

The next step is to determine if methods exist to detect the disease during an early stage. If screening measures are available, an analysis should determine if any of them fulfill the requirements for the screening process: available, easy to administer, safe with minimal discomfort, cost-effective, and accurate. Ultimately the decision to use a screening test will depend on how well the measure can distinguish those individuals who probably do not have and will not develop the condition from those who are likely to develop the condition. The variables that aid in a screening instrument's evaluation include reliability, validity, and reproducibility, which are a measure of the accuracy of the instrument.

**Reliability** is an assessment of the reproducibility of the test's results when different individuals with the same level of skill perform the test during different periods and under different conditions. The instrument or measure should yield consistent or stable results over time. If the same result emerges when two individuals perform the test, **interobserver reliability** is shown. If the same individual is able to reproduce the results several times, **intraobserver reliability** is demonstrated.

From this information, health professionals can determine the amount of training required for health care professionals, technicians, or personnel who administer the test. For example, if interobserver reliability is low, additional training might be required to work toward a more consistent method of screening test delivery. This is frequently necessary in blood pressure cuff hypertension screening (Ringrose et al., 2015) or in weight measurements, where the scale may not function properly. If intraobserver reliability is low, the health professional might surmise that the instrument, and not the individual, is at fault. Some screening measures are of necessity more qualitative, and intraobserver reliability may be very important in the case of substance abuse or mental health/depression screening. Finally, for a screening test to be valid, which is the next requirement, it must first be reliable, but reliability is only a necessary condition and is not entirely sufficient for validity.

**Validity** reflects the accuracy or truthfulness of the test or instrument itself. In a controlled setting, one evaluates validity by testing the instrument on a group of individuals who have positive or negative results. A valid test correctly distinguishes individuals who have preclinical disease from those without preclinical disease. The ideal result is to have the instrument identify 100% of the diseased individuals (positive reactions) and 100% of the nondiseased individuals (negative reactions).

There are also ranges of measurement for disease reliability and validity. Perfectly accurate categorization of validity rarely occurs in practice; therefore the measure of validity has been divided into two components that quantify the margin of error in screening instruments. **Sensitivity** measures the first component. This refers to the proportion of people with a condition who correctly test positive when screened. If a test has good sensitivity, the number of individuals with the disease who are missed through inaccurate categorization as false negatives will decrease. Conversely, a test with poor sensitivity will overlook individuals with the condition, and there will be a large number of false negative test results: individuals actually have the condition but were told they are disease-free or tested negative for the disease.

**Specificity** is the second component. Specificity measures the test's ability to recognize negative reactions or individuals in which disease is absent. A test with excellent specificity will rarely produce a positive result if the disease is not present. A test with poor specificity could result in false positive test results. Individuals with false positive test results are told that they have a disease or condition when in actuality they do not. Specific epidemiological formulas are used to measure both sensitivity and specificity.

In a perfect world, tests would be highly sensitive and highly specific; however, that is usually not the case, and some balance is reached between the two concepts. For some tests, there may also be an indeterminate zone in which the individual does not test strictly negative or positive. In these tests, the numerical cutoff may be subject to interpretation or a more arbitrary decision. A cutoff decision may be made so that the screening instrument is less likely to miss actual cases of disease at the cost of erroneously identifying cases of disease (false positives) that will need more diagnostic work, which may be expensive and invasive.

Consider the issues that a public health nurse faces when using a newly developed screening test with low specificity and moderate sensitivity. Low specificity means few true negative test results and more false positive test results. This is the current situation with mammography screening. The nurse and other health professionals (also health advocacy groups, such as those involved in breast cancer awareness) must then consider the cost, inconvenience, and psychological stress experienced by the people with false positive results during the period after their incorrect screening test, the unnecessary additional referrals, and the ability of the existing follow-up services to meet these needs. With only moderate sensitivity, a number of false negative results could occur, which may ignore individuals who could benefit from treatment. Medical, economic, political, and ethical issues are involved; that is, should a screening program be implemented when it is known that the tests may involve avoidable harms such as additional biopsies and excessive treatment. The use of mammography screening became a special case for inclusion under Affordable Care Act coverage as this legislation requires coverage for preventive services having a certainty of moderate or substantial benefit, and mammography science testing to date cannot meet that level of accuracy (Lin & Gostin, 2016).

A broader issue concerns large health fair screening programs; for example, where a targeted population such as older adults is sought for a mass screening. The **efficiency** and **efficacy** of such programs must be analyzed. The following are examples of questions that address efficiency and efficacy: Is the targeted population prepared in an appropriate way before engaging in the screening tests? Are the health care practitioners who are administering the test educated (and certified) according to the standard protocols of test administration? Are follow-up measures and appropriate referral access instituted in the program? There are times when an older adult lacks the cognitive ability or finances to follow-up on positive screening results. Patients and health care providers may overestimate the benefits and underestimate the harm of screening and associated treatment (Hoffmann & Del Mar, 2015). Answers to these questions challenge health care providers in the development, implementation, and follow-up processes identified so that screening efficiency and efficacy is enhanced.

Very recently, a number of for-profit genomic and biotechnology companies have marketed genetic tests (Box 9-1: Genomics) to identify genes and ancestry associated with risk factors and diseases. A number are available on the Internet. One of the most widely known, *23andme* (http://www.23andme.com), reports that its DNA analysis can provide information on about 100

⚠ **BOX 9-1** **GENOMICS**

### Detection of Maternal Malignancies via Prenatal Testing for Fetal Chromosome Abnormalities

Prenatal screening on blood samples is becoming the norm and is reducing amniocentesis testing. This less invasive blood test determines whether the fetus has a chromosomal abnormality (Down syndrome—chromosome 21, or other chromosomes—13, 18, X, and Y) by testing free DNA. If the finding is abnormal, amniocentesis is used to confirm the original result. In this study (Bianchi et al., 2015) of 125,426 blood samples, 3% were found to be abnormal.

What is interesting about this study is that this prenatal screening may identify not only problems in the fetus but also problems in the mother's cells' arrangement indicative of cancer. From the set of 3757 abnormal fetal results, 10 cases of maternal cancer were found.

The uses of genomic testing are just beginning to be realized and may lead in directions unexpected from the original purpose of the screening.

From Bianchi, D. W., Chudova, D., Sehnert, A. J., Bhatt, S., Murray, K., Prosen, T. L., et al. (2015). Noninvasive prenatal testing and incidental detection of occult maternal malignancies. *JAMA, 314*(2), 162–169.

health disorders and traits, including carrier risk, drug response, and disease risk (e.g., Parkinson disease, cholesterol levels, presence of diabetes). Noninvasive prenatal tests are currently marketed to identify neonatal chromosomal abnormalities, including Down syndrome, very early in gestation with a simple blood test (Nickolich et al., 2016); these tests are less invasive than amniocentesis, but positive test results require confirmation by amniocentesis. These tests are becoming common and dramatically less expensive.

Green and Farahany (2014) reported that the Food and Drug Administration (FDA) may be overcautious in its oversight of consumer genetic testing/genomics as the FDA is requiring stricter disclosure of information to consumers. Consumer-available tests can involve issues of standardization, cost, and privacy, and failure to make reports fully explainable or understandable. Comprehensive research on screening tests significantly influences the efficacy of the entire process. Data on the reliability and validity of individual tests and screening programs in general provides valuable information to evaluate, anticipate, and ideally control these influences, enabling the program to work effectively toward its established goal and positive health care outcomes.

### Primary Care and Community Screening Resources

Screening is often done in an outpatient primary care setting. As funding for traditional public health nursing roles is declining, the responsibility for screening often falls to nurses in other basic and advanced practice roles. Implementing a screening program depends on availability of appropriate community resources, such as funds, health care workers, and follow-up services, including access, referrals, treatment sources, and administrative personnel. Nurses can provide structure and design for screening programs as seamless organization of a program is essential to success. Knowledge of a disease's characteristics and an effective screening instrument are useless without financial and organized human support to use them. Many screening programs are of necessity complex, requiring intense efforts in the area of partner development.

A **lead agency** or group may be identified to oversee the development of the community health program. The origins of the lead agency range from a community service organization to local public health departments responding to regulations or a mandate at the state or federal level. Regardless of its origin, the agency must perform a self-evaluation to compare its level of expertise with what is required to supervise the process of the screening effort. Early identification of the lead agency, along with potential partnerships, allows the effective use of talents and the division of labor.

Some screening programs may involve intricate legal issues; for example, states have policies about HIV testing and privacy and identification of individuals. HIV screening and testing is highly recommended in high-risk individuals—those who have injected steroids or drugs, those who have unprotected sex (especially men who have sex with men), and those who have other STIs or comorbidities (e.g., hepatitis C). Consumer-controlled home screening kits may protect individual identities (CDC, 2011). In 2012, the FDA (2012) approved the first over-the-counter HIV test. This test, OraQuick (http://www.oraquick.com), requires a fluid specimen from the mouth at the upper and lower gums and gives preliminary results in 20 minutes.

For the lead agency to develop and oversee the development of any community health program, such as the delivery of a screening program, partnerships and coalitions are essential. The agency must contact and organize necessary stakeholders. **Stakeholders** are individuals or groups who have a legitimate interest in the topic. Examples of stakeholders include key community individuals; hospitals; health and social service agencies, such as primary health care centers; and community organizations, including houses of worship, community centers, schools, transportation agencies, and volunteer organizations. **Key community individuals** are those people who are considered leaders within the community. The primary rule is to never assume that what is appropriate and effective for one community will be appropriate and effective for another.

Stakeholders and partners along with nurses perform the **community assessment** together. A community assessment is a systematic method of data collection that provides a detailed account, first identifying need and subsequently determining the type, quantity, and quality of resources. Review of demographic, vital statistics, and morbidity and mortality data may identify the assessed need. Resources might come from an eclectic variety of support sources, including government entities such as public health departments, social services, and even safety and transportation in the case of car seat safety screenings. Schools, private businesses, churches, and places of social gatherings might provide resource support, either in screening support or in the actual administration of the screening.

After the assessment has been completed, the data analysis will reveal the **target community** or high-risk population, the available health care resources, and the health needs of the high-risk population. The identified partners collaborate, review, and analyze the data, leading to the development of

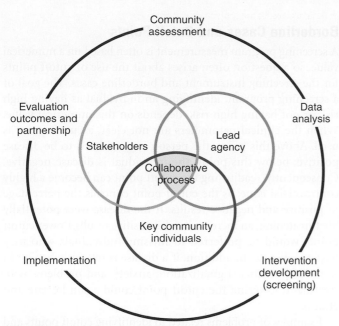

Community assessment

Evaluation outcomes and partnership

Stakeholders

Lead agency

Collaborative process

Data analysis

Key community individuals

Implementation

Intervention development (screening)

**FIGURE 9-2** Collaborative partnership: community health program development.

health-improvement strategies (in this case a screening program), with methods of implementation to move the target population smoothly through the screening process. Finally, monitoring and evaluating outcomes is essential to determine the effectiveness of the program and the achievement of stated goals. Evaluation includes monitoring of the entire process, including the successful workings of the partnership. Figure 9-2 presents a model of collaborative partnership: community health program development. Population health nursing is an important component of the partnership.

The constraints affecting the operation of a screening program include financial concerns, political issues, cultural constraints, follow-up and referral services, and accessible treatment facilities. All partners are aware that responses from the target community are affected partly by their experience with other screening programs, such as the means used to inform them, the accessibility of the location, the availability of transportation, the convenience of the program's hours, and the cultural sensitivity of the delivery and design of the program. A public health nursing approach identifies the necessary community resources and defines how these resources interact and may be mobilized to achieve maximal benefits and positive outcomes. Financial support of a screening program is a constraint that can influence all points in the system. Although some programs are delivered entirely on a voluntary basis, organizers of others must submit grant proposals to local, state, or federal departments when consideration of medical and economic ethics is involved. Planners must look beyond the screening day and investigate financial resources for follow-up care and treatment.

In addition to financial accessibility, follow-up services need to be accessible in terms of convenient locations and open hours. For example, an evening clinic may reach those who are reluctant or financially unable to miss work. Nurse practitioner clinics

facilitate access to preventive health services at convenient times for various population groups. An efficient referral system links the follow-up resources to the screening program, providing continuity of care. A method must be devised to encourage the participant to take positive action on the referral. Public health nurses will facilitate this process with a variety of communication techniques, such as e-mails, telephone or in-person counseling, mailings, and home visits.

Another example is that a college of health sciences organizes a health fair which includes screening. This also creates opportunities for **interprofessional education** and practice (Uden-Holman et al., 2015). Nursing students and medical students manage physical assessments and laboratory screenings. Pharmacists screen individuals for medical use of inappropriate or contraindicated medications. Social workers may assess individuals for mental health issues. There is a plan for continuation of care if disease issues and risks are identified; for example, individuals needing immediate referrals for hypertension control. In this instance the college may agree to assist in referrals to providers who will donate time to assist in this effort.

## Should Screening for the Disease Be Done?

After it has been determined that the disease is significant and can be screened for, establishing whether health professionals should do so is the final step. Screening for a particular disorder and ultimately treating those with the early-identified disorder improve the chances of a favorable outcome in comparison with those whose disorder is not found until signs and symptoms become evident. Therefore several questions must be considered. If a test accurately identifies a condition in the early stages, is there any benefit to the individual? Are there effective treatment modalities for the condition? The **US Preventive Services Task Force** (USPSTF) may recommend against routine screening (USPSTF, 2016a). In 2012, the USPSTF recommended against PSA screening for prostate cancer. PSA screening was rated as grade D (not recommended) because the balance of harms from early treatment (urinary incontinence, bowel control, erectile dysfunction) outweighed the benefits of early diagnosis. As noted before, recommendations for mammography screening have changed several times within the last decade because of high rates of false positive test results, overdiagnosis, too many normal/benign biopsy specimens, and overtreatment (Kidd & Colbert, 2015; Lin & Gostin, 2016; Thompson et al., 2015). A woman with microcalcifications found on mammography may have to undergo an open or core biopsy to determine if cancer cells are truly present; this may involve several days' absence from work or child care.

It is necessary for the health care provider to remain aware of changes in screening guidelines. Screening is based on the disease's asymptomatic period; therefore adequate information must exist concerning the optimal time for screening, specific intervention during this time, and knowledge regarding the effect of early detection and treatment on the prognosis. Without this knowledge, health care professionals are unable to explain how the outcomes of those with early detected disease differ from those with undetected disease, and they cannot support the health benefits derived from the screening program.

Follow-up is critical to determine if the intervention strategies prescribed are in fact happening. Should screening be done if there is no follow-up in terms of medical or social services? A prescribed follow-up regimen may be very broad and include a wide variety of intervention strategies, such as diet, exercise, and drug therapy. Follow-up services may include an evaluation and review of the literature that discusses evidence-based practice pertaining to a particular drug, as well as the identification of intervention characteristics that impair follow-up, such as cost, inconvenience, or side effects. Consideration must also be given to those factors that enhance follow-up. For example, nurses can provide ongoing counseling and education about a medication and assist individuals in lifestyle transformations that include health-promoting behaviors.

The safety of a potential intervention is a concern when the widespread application of further medical interventions or invasive diagnostic tests after a screening program is considered. Risks or harmful side effects can be costly in terms of human health and the increased medical care required to correct **iatrogenic** or interventional effects (e.g., additional surgical procedures or emotional distress). As an example, Jordana, who is aged 54 years and has a low risk of breast cancer, attends a community clinic and wants more information about the optimal interval between breast cancer screenings. She heard that there are disagreements between US government studies (USPSTF), the American Cancer Society, and other sources of reasonable medical advice. The nurse, using an evidence-based practice model, helps Jordana to find or review the most recent and best sources of information that would answer her question (Mandelblatt et al., 2016). In addition to the scientific literature, the nurse locates consumer information for Jordana. In this case the nurse would assist women to make informed health choices about screening tests.

The bottom line is that to be effective, a high-quality, cost-effective, research/evidence-based screening tool or technique is needed that identifies a real or potential "problem." Screening must provide real and workable "solutions," in which the tangible and intangible costs of the screening are less than the risk of the disease and result in measurable health benefits.

## ETHICAL CONSIDERATIONS

Improving health is considered a just and moral act integral to values endorsed throughout the care delivery system. Screening activities are separate from interventions offered for established disease (e.g., myocardial infarction). Rather than treating those who have established disease, a screening program invites seemingly well individuals to be tested to determine their disease risk and the need for follow-up. This request for voluntary participation implies an expectation of a health benefit, although at this stage nothing is said about what it will be, the cost, or what the participant must do to obtain it. Screening programs need to clarify expectations and inform participants as contingent issues occur. Screening participants need to know whether the ultimate benefit is preventive, ameliorative, or curative and what responsibility they assume to secure this outcome.

## Borderline Cases and Cutoff Points

A screening program measurement is often based on a numerical value, so a question often arises about the use of cutoff points for the screening instrument and borderline cases. The goal of a screening program, identifying an individual as having high risk or not having high risk, depends on this numerical value. When the clinical parameters are not clear, a cutoff point is used. Above this point, the person is considered to be disease positive; below this point, the individual is disease negative. Consequently, readjusting the cutoff point can become a highly controversial issue, as the cutoff point controls the percentage of positive and negative results. If the disease were potentially life threatening, an increase in false positive results (lower cutoff point) would be preferred to missing individuals who may have the disease. In addition, if a disease is relatively benign in terms of potential stigmatization, anxiety, and problems with treatment, lowering the cutoff point could again be safe and ethical.

Examples of problems related to identifying cutoff points and borderline cases are common in community nursing practice. Hypertension is a common disease in which a variance of 5 to 10 mmHg can make the difference in identifying a person as having high risk of hypertension. Lipid and cholesterol level cutoffs and ratios are always subject to further examination. Osteoporosis standards for men are debated (USPSTF, 2015). Recommendations change as new evidence emerges. Sophisticated approaches may discriminate between borderline cases that should be referred and ones that should not. Nurses can assist in identifying other risk factors associated with hypertension or lipid level evaluation, such as family history, diet, and smoking, as criteria for deciding whether to refer an individual. An updated literature review is imperative before these issues are reviewed in relation to a particular screenable disease.

## Economic Costs and Ethics

In the past, the tendency was to disregard the cost of promoting a healthy, disease-free, or disease-controlled status; this results in a philosophical stand that all care should be given to all people at all costs. There is now a fuller recognition of the enormous costs that could be involved with many screening programs. Allocating community funds to a large screening event may result in a lack of funds for other projects. Populations benefiting from a screening test will be balanced by those suffering in terms of decreases in service for other medical or social needs.

The initial operational costs must be considered, including buying or renting screening equipment, floor space, and engaging professionals or technicians to administer the tests and interpret the results. These costs are encountered a second time when individuals are referred for further evaluation. Consumer costs include follow-up visits, treatment, and time and income that are lost. Given the combined operational and consumer costs, several questions are raised. Do the costs result in improved health outcomes? Are the benefits worth the expenditures required? These answers are influenced partly by the values (other than monetary ones) attributed to the benefit. Saving lives in a young population may be judged more valuable than screening older populations with more chronic illnesses. A strictly economic approach, however, may eliminate the intangible variables and require the use of more objective data for decision-making.

When program designs are reviewed, three main approaches may be used to evaluate the economic resources affected: cost-benefit ratio, cost-effectiveness, and cost-efficiency analyses. The current relevance and use of such concepts require a basic understanding of their role in the selection of a condition for screening. They tend to be separate methods and most frequently are used independently of one another.

## Cost-Benefit Ratio

Cost-benefit ratio analysis is performed first, because it allows the comparison of various outcomes in monetary terms. This comparison is necessary in health planning when the initial consideration is dependent on whether the expected health outcome (such as reduction in the incidences of cardiovascular disease, decrease in infant mortality, or reduction of the detection of a visual problem) will be most beneficial to the community at the most reasonable cost. The cost of the screening versus the cost of long-term care management may be weighed. For example, what is the cost-benefit ratio of blood pressure screenings, compared with the medical and financial cost of a stroke caused by undiagnosed hypertension, to the individual, the community, and the health care system? The cost of screening is weighed against other factors, such as the cost and feasibility of vaccination programs, as in the case of screening individuals for human papilloma virus for cervical cancer (Maine et al., 2011). Resources available through the use of electronic data gathering tools, such as the CDC's Chronic Disease Cost Calculator version 2 (CDC, 2013), which estimates state Medicare expenditures for certain diseases, may assist in this analysis.

## Cost-Effectiveness

If the reduction of cardiovascular disease is chosen as the desired outcome, the next step is a cost-effectiveness analysis, which determines the optimal use of resources to reach a predetermined, constant end-point or the desired health outcome. The screening benefit remains the same; the best method of getting to the target outcome is the focus of the investigation. For example, for reduction of cardiovascular disease, various methods might be used. These methods include screening individuals for hypertension and cholesterol, performing electrocardiograms on all individuals aged 25 years or older who are admitted to the hospital, screening young athletes for cardiovascular disease, sponsoring an antismoking campaign, or providing nutrition counseling. Implementation of all these options would be ideal, but with limited resources some choices are made.

## Cost-Efficiency

The last approach to help bring the economic resources into perspective is cost-efficiency analysis. The purpose is to be efficient and budget a limited amount of money toward achieving as much of the desired outcome as possible. The funds are the focus, not the health benefit.

## SELECTION OF SCREENABLE POPULATIONS

The selection of a screenable population is as important as the selection of a screenable disease and is often based on incidence and prevalence data. The objective is to identify a high-risk group that, when tested, will yield a significant number of diseased individuals. With a well-planned selection approach, the efforts and cost of screening the population are minimized and the health benefit is maximized. The main criterion used to define an appropriate population is the definitive presence of risk factors related to the disorder. Within community settings, nurses can ensure a thorough examination of possible risk factors, including both person-dependent and environment-dependent factors (Box 9-2: Research for Evidence-Based Practice).

### Person-Dependent Factors

The person's age is important because of age-dependent changes in the levels of risk factors throughout the population. For example, the risk of many cancers increases as a person grows older (Weir et al., 2015). A high priority is placed on screening vulnerable populations, especially women, infants, and children, as the outcomes obtained affect long-range growth and development patterns. As the average life span increases, however, the effects of risk factors in young adults and middle-aged adults are becoming more apparent, making certain prevalent and costly chronic conditions equally important to control. The middle-aged adult population may be screened for hypertension, diabetes, breast cancer, glaucoma, and heart disease; this population is requiring earlier screening as some of these disease conditions are becoming apparent in early adulthood and even teenage years. Older adults may be screened for cognitive decline, although screening for the asymptomatic elderly is controversial because of lack of effective dementia treatment. Routine genetic screening for various biomarkers, such as amyloid amyloid $\beta_2$-microglobulin

---

### BOX 9-2  RESEARCH FOR EVIDENCE-BASED PRACTICE

#### Population-Based Research Optimizing Screening

The National Cancer Institute has developed Population-Based Research Optimizing Screening Through Personalized Regimens (PROSPR) to support research on the community-based screening processes to include experiences and outcomes for breast, colon, and cervical cancer. The overall aim is to develop coordination between the research practices conducted at multiple sites. It reviews recruitment, screening, diagnosis, referral, and treatment rates. It focuses on research translation and implementation, addressing issues such as the controversy regarding breast cancer screening and mammography by studying the comparative effectiveness and outcomes of existing and emerging research. In September 2011 the National Cancer Institute funded seven research centers and one statistical site as part of this integrated research screening program. Be on the lookout for similar new programs because the Prevention Fund supported by the Affordable Care Act supports the development of other such opportunities to discover and support evidence-based health-promotion and disease-prevention activities.

From National Cancer Institute. (2015). *PROSPR: Population-Based Research Optimizing Screening Through Personalized Regimens.* https://healthcaredelivery.cancer.gov/prospr/.

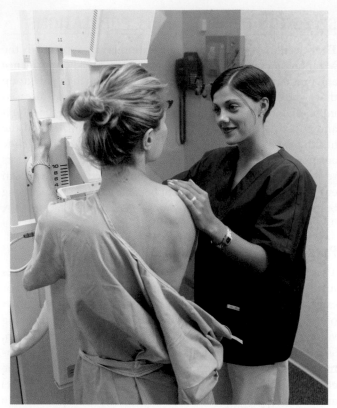

**FIGURE 9-3** Mammography screening. (Courtesy of John Foxx; from Stockbyte/Thinkstock.)

and tau proteins, amyloid plaques, and *APOE-e4* is under investigation (Alzheimer's Association, 2015; Sutphen et al., 2015).

Gender has obvious implications for screening programs. For example, women are tested frequently for two reproductive-related conditions: breast cancer and cervical cancer (Figure 9-3). Screening a population from a particular ethnic or racial group is appropriate as some disorders occur more frequently in certain racial or ethnic groups. For example, black American women are more than 35% more likely than white women to die of breast cancer, but breast cancer is diagnosed in them 10% less frequently (CDC, 2010; Kidd & Colbert, 2015). Vietnamese American women have the highest rate of cervical cancer among any racial or ethnic group in the United States, and the rate is five times higher than the rates among non-Hispanic white women (CDC, 2010). Nurses can lobby and advocate for specific groups to have more targeted screenings, particularly in communities that have large numbers of ethnic or racial minority women (Box 9-3: Diversity Awareness).

Income level has been associated repeatedly with many health disparities. According to a 2010 Gallup poll, chronic conditions are more likely to be diagnosed in low-income Americans than in high-income Americans. The physical health illness disparities were the greatest for depression, high blood pressure, and diabetes, and higher levels of obesity also place lower-income populations at greater risk (Mendez, 2010). In addition to a greater likelihood of not having adequate health insurance, low-income Americans can least afford necessary preventive care, effective treatment, and health education (Mendez, 2010).

## BOX 9-3   DIVERSITY AWARENESS

### Eliminating Health Disparities Among Ethnic Groups

The United States has been referred to frequently as a population melting pot. Diversity is acknowledged as a strength of the United States, but it is apparent that disparities exist among the various racial and ethnic groups in the attainment and maintenance of health. The minority populations of the United States include black Americans, Hispanics, Asian/Pacific Islanders, American Indians, and Alaskan Natives. These categories oversimplify the reality of the multicultural nature of assessing health status, screening, and making plans to improve health. These particular racial groupings are not absolute because there are subgroups within each.

These disparities and factors such as access to care need to be taken into consideration when screening programs are being planned. To plan, implement, and evaluate a screening program that targets a specific population, the provider must have an awareness of the target population that includes components such as lifestyle, socioeconomic characteristics, education, heredity, environmental factors, values, religious and cultural beliefs, communication style, and language. Partnering with key individuals and organizations in the community through the entire process is important for any screening program to be successful, as the following scenario illustrates.

Hospital administrators in a town located outside a city in the Northeast are concerned about the health status of a new immigrant population. Recent census data indicate that the number of immigrants from Guatemala has grown. The census data also reveal that this population is primarily young adults, male and female. The officials of the town and the hospital are aware that most of the men are day laborers, many of whom gather each morning in the town square to be transported to their jobs. The young women are mothers who work in small, privately owned businesses or are hired by local housecleaning services.

On the basis of these data, the hospital officials decide to plan a health and screening day for this population. The hospital distributes flyers in the community in the primary native language of the target population. The day of the screening arrives, and the number of participants is very low. The hospital officials are very concerned. They had good intentions. They do not know what to do next.

- What critical actions did the hospital officials perform that might be considered positive in the planning of the health and screening day?
- What critical actions did the hospital officials not perform that might have contributed to the poor turnout at the health and screening function?
- What might the hospital officials consider in their planning for the next health and screening day?
- How might they engage the community and the target population in planning the health and screening day?
- What local community agencies and groups might be invited to participate as partners when the health and screening day is being planned and implemented?
- Can you identify any creative ways to bring the health and screening day to the targeted population, making the program more accessible?

Personal behavioral characteristics related to lifestyle may suggest the need to screen a particular individual or group. When health care practitioners review lifestyle, they are looking at daily habits that affect health and wellness, such as nutrition, fitness level, tobacco use, alcohol and drug use, sexual practices (HIV), stress management, adequate rest, immunizations, periodic examinations, use of seat belts, and other safety factors. Engaging in some of these behaviors while avoiding others is essential for living a healthy life. Therefore screening for personal behavioral characteristics that are considered risky assesses the likelihood of a longer, disease-free life. Once screening recommends elimination of risky behaviors, the development of healthy behaviors via programming and transformation of lifestyles is crucial. Health care providers have a responsibility to educate and empower individuals about the next step in the evaluation of their potential condition once screening has been completed. Those being screened have a responsibility to seek treatment and follow-up services, and ultimately engage in behavioral change toward a healthy lifestyle if the screening is to serve a purpose.

Regional disparities exist and include many of the previously mentioned disparities. These disparities are of great concern, but identifying the cause is complex. Research is being done on interrelationships between the determinants of health, to include biology and genetics, individual behaviors, the social environment, the physical environment, and health services (access and quality). The Centers for Disease Control and Prevention (CDC) Racial and Ethnic Approaches to Community Health (REACH) program (http://www.cdc.gov/reach/) addresses the factors and is demonstrating success by empowering residents to "seek better health; help change local health care practices; and mobilize communities to implement evidence-based public health programs that address their unique social, historical, economic, and cultural circumstances" (CDC, 2010). Appropriate screening is integrated into the REACH program.

## Environment-Dependent Factors

The area of environmental health and protection has expanded over the years and is becoming more complex. Environmental health and protection has been defined as the science that is concerned with elements of the environment that influence people's health and well-being. These factors include conditions of the workplace, home, and communities, including chemical, physical, and psychological forces (Allender et al., 2014). Environment-related risk factors relevant to screening designs are associated with an individual's surroundings. Areas that may be considered include overpopulation; indoor and outdoor air pollution; water pollution; safe drinking water; noise pollution; radiation exposure; biological pollutants; hazardous waste management and disposal of garbage; vector and pesticide control; deforestation, wetlands destruction, and desertification; energy depletion; inadequate housing; contaminated food and foods with toxic additives; safety in the home, at the work site, and in the community; and psychological hazards (Allender et al., 2014; Roelofs et al., 2010).

In occupational health, a legitimate population for screening includes those in high-risk work areas, where harmful chemicals, airborne particles, or high-decibel machinery puts the workers at risk of cancer, respiratory conditions, or auditory problems. At the other extreme is the sedentary executive work life, where the lack of exercise is prevalent, placing the worker at risk of obesity and obesity-related conditions such as diabetes. The use of an occupational health nurse to provide individual and mass screening for such problems, in addition to routinely recommended screening, is recognized as integral in promoting better business practices.

## National Guidance and Health Care Reform

### Healthy People 2020

Many national organizations are guiding and promoting evidence-based care and screening. *Healthy People 2020* has been establishing benchmarks and monitoring progress on goals and objectives to promote health care delivery partnerships, guide individuals toward making empowered health decisions, and assess the efficacy of preventive programs (HealthyPeople.gov, 2015). This newest version of *Healthy People 2020* also includes resources for implementing community programs that support its goals and objectives, including screening. For more specific objectives related to screening, see Box 9-4: *Healthy People 2020.*

### Recommended Screenings of the US Preventive Services Task Force

More specifically, the USPSTF, part of the Agency for Healthcare Research and Quality of the Department of Health and Human

---

### ♥ BOX 9-4  HEALTHY PEOPLE 2020

#### *Objectives Related to Screening*

- (Developmental) Increase the proportion of persons with a diagnosis of hemoglobinopathies who receive early and continuous screening for complications.
- Increase the proportion of women who receive a cervical cancer screening based on the most recent guidelines.
- Increase the proportion of adults who receive a colorectal cancer screening based on the most recent guidelines.
- Increase the proportion of women who receive a breast cancer screening based on the most recent guidelines.
- Increase the proportion of adults who were counseled about cancer screening consistent with current guidelines.
- Increase the proportion of elementary, middle, and senior high schools that provide school health education to promote personal health and wellness in the following areas: handwashing or hand hygiene; oral health; growth and development; sun safety and skin cancer prevention; benefits of rest and sleep; ways to prevent vision and hearing loss; and the importance of health screenings and checkups.
- Reduce the proportion of children who experience developmental delay requiring special education services.
- Increase appropriate newborn blood-spot screening and follow-up testing.
- Increase the number of states including the District of Columbia that verify through linkage with vital records that all newborns are screened shortly after birth for conditions mandated by their state-sponsored screening program.
- (Developmental) Increase the proportion of children with a diagnosed condition identified through newborn screening who have an annual assessment of services needed and received.
- Increase depression screening by primary care providers.
- Increase tobacco screening in office-based ambulatory care settings.
- Increase tobacco screening in hospital ambulatory care settings.
- (Developmental) Increase tobacco screening in substance abuse care settings.
- Increase the proportion of preschool children aged 5 years or younger who receive vision screening.

From HealthyPeople.gov. (2015). *Healthy People 2020.* Washington, DC: US Department of Health and Human Services, Office of Disease Prevention and Health Promotion. http://www.healthypeople.gov.

Services, identifies recommendations in its *Guide to Clinical Preventive Services* (Agency for Healthcare Research and Quality, 2014a). There are recommendations for adults, children, and adolescents (USPSTF, 2016b). The recommendations evolve as new scientific evidence becomes available, so this chapter will not provide specific details on the recommended screenings. Boxes 9-5 and 9-6 list the USPSTF recommended screening services for adults (USPSTF, 2016b), children, and adolescents.

### The Affordable Care Act and Prevention Incentives

The passing of the Affordable Care Act (ACA) in 2010 catalyzed a public health movement toward prevention and health promotion,

---

with incentives and policies, including the development of the National Prevention Strategy. One result is that preventive services are required to be covered by new health insurance plans or policies, as an incentivized quality program for Medicare recipients. Medicare now also covers annual wellness visits that incorporate a personalized prevention plan according to the recommendations of the USPSTF, based on an individual's age and health status; these visits can be conducted by a variety of practitioners, including nurse practitioners, clinical nurse specialists, and certified nurse midwives (Center for Medicare Advocacy, 2015).

Among other incentives, Medicare has developed a rating guide for Medicare Advantage programs, incentivizing high-quality health plans with up to a 10% bonus. Many of the criteria that determine the highest ratings are screening and preventive services. This helps seniors identify quality insurance plans that cover preventive services and provide the necessary follow-up.

### National Prevention Strategy

In addition to increasing the funded coverage of preventive services and screenings, the ACA also created the National Prevention Council (NPC), comprising "17 heads of departments, agencies, and offices across the Federal government who are committed to promoting prevention and wellness. The Council provides the leadership necessary to engage not only the federal government but a diverse array of stakeholders, from state and local policymakers, to business leaders, to individuals, their families and communities, to champion the policies and programs needed to ensure the health of Americans prospers" (National Prevention Council, 2011, p. 3) (Box 9-7: Innovative Practice).

The resulting *National Prevention Strategy* (NPS) was released in June 2011 and "recognizes that good health comes not just from receiving quality medical care, but also from clean air and water, safe outdoor spaces for physical activity, safe work sites, healthy foods, violence-free environments and healthy homes. Prevention should be woven into all aspects of our lives, including where and how we live, learn, work and play. Everyone—businesses, educators, health care institutions, government, communities

---

### BOX 9-5   Preventive Services for Adults (Examples)

- Abdominal aortic aneurysm screening
- Alcohol misuse screening
- Aspirin for prevention of cardiovascular disease
- BRCA-related cancer in women
- Breast cancer screening
- Colorectal cancer screening
- Depression screening for adults
- Diabetes mellitus screening
- HIV infection screening
- Obesity screening and counseling
- Osteoporosis screening
- Sexually transmitted infection (STI) prevention counseling
- Syphilis infection screening for pregnant women
- Tobacco use Screening

From Agency for Healthcare Research and Quality. (2014a). *Guide to clinical preventive services. Clinical summaries, recommendations for adults, children and adolescents.* http://www.ahrq.gov/professionals/clinicians-providers/guidelines-recommendations/guide/.

---

### BOX 9-6   Preventive Services for Children and Adolescents (Examples)

- Alcohol misuse
- Blood lead levels
- Cervical cancer screening
- Child maltreatment
- Developmental dysplasia of hip
- Gonorrhea screening
- Hearing loss
- Height, weight, and body mass index screening
- Hematocrit or hemoglobin screening for children
- HIV infection screening
- High blood pressure screening in children
- Hyperbilirubinemia screening in infants
- Iron-deficiency anemia
- Major depressive disorder screening
- Obesity screening and counseling
- PKU screening
- Sexually transmitted infection (STI) prevention counseling and screening
- Speech and language delay screening
- Vision impairment screening

From Agency for Healthcare Research and Quality. (2014a). *Guide to clinical preventive services. Clinical summaries, recommendations for adults, children and adolescents.* http://www.ahrq.gov/professionals/clinicians-providers/guidelines-recommendations/guide/.

---

### ☀ BOX 9-7   INNOVATIVE PRACTICE
#### *Informatics, Technology, and Newborn Screening*

Health information technology will allow health care to better assess and manage quality health care with the streamlining of efficient and effective information. A number of US governmental sites list information about newborn screening and long-term follow-up. The results of newborn screening may include normal values and out-of-range values. Access to digital medical records allows the sharing of results and follow-up findings between clinicians, testing laboratories, and health delivery providers.

- How does access to newborn electronic screening results benefit the clinician? How does it benefit the person seeking care? How does it benefit public health?
- Where else do you think health care could benefit from similar abilities?
- What do you think is necessary for this to happen (think about differences in data collection requirements)?

From US National Library of Medicine. (2014). *Newborn screening coding and terminology guide.* http://newbornscreeningcodes.nlm.nih.gov/nb/sc/updates.

## BOX 9-8  QUALITY AND SAFETY SCENARIO

### *Pender's Health-Promotion Model*

A health care provider's responsibility is to assess, plan, implement, and evaluate a screening program. Part of this responsibility includes teaching individuals, families, and populations about the importance of participating in these programs and ultimately engaging in safe behaviors promoting health. The health-promotion model is a useful guide for practice (Pender et al., 2015). The model presents the interrelationship among behavior-specific cognitions and affective factors and individual characteristics and experiences that motivate individuals to engage in behaviors that promote health and decrease unsafe habits and practices. The health care provider may find that the application of this model in practice influences the relationship between the provider and the individual in a positive way. The model is a framework that assists the provider in assessing factors believed to influence health behavioral changes. Once the provider has an accurate assessment, obtained via questions, decisions may be made concerning factors that inhibit health-promoting behaviors and, ultimately, potential interventions to assist individuals in achieving positive health outcomes. This information will assist the provider to develop appropriate teaching methods.

**Health-Promotion Assessment Questions**

- How do you define health?
- What does health mean to you?
- How would you describe your health now?
- Do the choices you make and the actions you take affect your health?
- Can you give examples when choices and actions created a positive change in health for you?
- Can you give examples when choices and actions created a negative or unsafe change in health for you?
- What factors facilitated choices and actions that created a positive change in health?
- What factors created barriers to choices and actions that led to a negative or unsafe change in health?
- Are there any supportive personal influences in your life that would assist you in choices and actions that would create a positive change in your health (e.g., family, friends, and health care providers)?
- Are there any supportive situational influences, such as more than one plan of action, pertaining to the health change available to you?

Modified from Pender, N., Murdaugh, C., & Parsons, M. A. (2015). Health promotion in nursing practice (7th ed.). Upper Saddle River, NJ: Pearson.

and every single American—has a role in creating a healthier nation" (http://www.surgeongeneral.gov/priorities/prevention/strategy/#The Vision) (Hanna-Attisha et al., 2016) (Box 9-8: Quality and Safety Scenario).

The four strategic directions are:

- Healthy and safe community environments: Create, sustain, and recognize communities that promote health and wellness through prevention.
- Clinical and community preventive services: Ensure that prevention-focused health care and community prevention efforts are available, integrated, and mutually reinforcing.
- Empowered people: Support people in making healthy choices.
- Elimination of health disparities: Eliminate disparities, improving the quality of life for all Americans.

Under the second strategic direction, the strategy identifies six recommendations, including a focus on improving cardiovascular health, incorporating screenings, using payments and reimbursement to encourage clinical preventive services, and reducing access barriers to community preventive services (National Prevention Council, 2011) (Figure 9-4).

## THE NURSE'S ROLE

As one of the important stakeholders (Institute of Medicine, 2011), nurses play a role in every aspect of the screening program development process, including assessment, data analysis, planning, implementation, evaluation of the health outcomes, and evaluation of the process (including the workings of the partnership; see Figure 9-2). One aspect of this health process is the development and implementation of screening programs for targeted groups. As nurses use higher decision-making skills based on advancing education and expertise (Institute of Medicine, 2011), they will face questions such as "Should this condition be screened for or not?" In the role of decision maker and planner, the nurse is responsible for reviewing all issues concerned with screening individuals for an appropriate disease, including the criteria specific to the disease, the medical and economic ethics, and the community resources that are affected. If the choice is to screen individuals, the participation of nurses and other partnering groups is essential in the development of a care plan. The last step integral to the nursing role is the planning and development of an efficient referral system to enhance continuity of care and to ensure follow-up.

Because many preventive care services are provided through insurance coverage, the nurse collaborates with other health providers to ensure that preventive services (see Boxes 9-5 and 9-6), along with the required education and counseling, are available through primary care or community services such as a primary care clinic, a person-centered medical home, or a community health center or even at the work site. These services may include:

- Blood pressure, diabetes, and cholesterol tests
- Cancer screenings, including mammograms and colonoscopies
- Counseling on topics such as quitting smoking, losing weight, eating healthily, treating depression, and reducing alcohol use
- Routine vaccinations against diseases
- Flu and pneumonia immunizations
- Counseling, screening, and vaccines to ensure healthy pregnancies
- Regular well-baby and well-child visits, from birth to age 21 years

Nurses have long been responsible for screening individuals and educating people about healthy lifestyles and decreased risks as part of the ordinary primary care assessment process. Questions concerning nutrition, coping, and self-care are all assessment or screening questions, leading to moments of opportunity or "teachable moments" for health promotion. These evaluation activities are invaluable for gauging risk and potential areas for screening. Teaching individuals the meaning and limitation of screening test results is an important element of this role, as is informing them of their part in obtaining implied benefits.

Nursing staff, at all levels, are important in applying preventive services to include screening and education. The concept of the

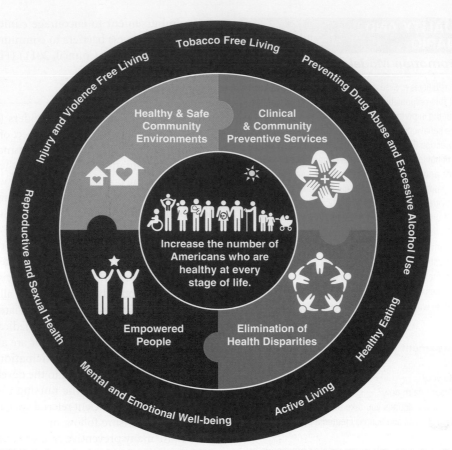

**FIGURE 9-4** America's plan for better health and wellness. (From National Prevention Council. [2011]. *National Prevention Strategy.* http://www.surgeongeneral.gov/priorities/prevention/strategy.)

person-centered medical home encourages the use of each member of the primary health care team to the highest level of their professional and licensing abilities. The combined nursing roles of health educator and screener mean that the nurse continues to educate individuals about risk factors and teach them ways to alter and reduce risks generally through lifestyle changes, such as proper diet, exercise, and stress management, and by limiting the use of alcohol, drugs, and tobacco. The role as educator is essential in the screening process because nurses provide individuals with the information necessary for choices they will make regarding healthy behavioral change. The nurse is actually practicing primary prevention interventions, but this is done in coordination with a secondary preventive role.

## RACIAL AND ETHNIC APPROACHES TO COMMUNITY HEALTH

An excellent resource is the CDC REACH website http://www.cdc.gov/nccdphp/dch/programs/reach/. This program supports effective community-level programs to reduce health disparities in minority communities across the United States. Data from the REACH Risk Factor Survey (2009), focusing on breast and cervical cancer prevention, cardiovascular health, and

diabetes management, have shown that changing health behaviors in minority communities has improved health and reduced community disparities (Box 9-9).

## SUMMARY

Screening is the administration of measures or tests to distinguish individuals who may have a condition from those who probably do not have it. It is an effective, efficient tool in preventive health care if used for conditions applicable to the screening model and specifically directed toward an at-risk population.

Implementing screening programs requires coordination and planning and provides numerous places for nursing intervention, especially within the currently evolving health care environment, which is emphasizing prevention activities. Nurses can provide individuals, communities, and populations with valuable preventive, health-promotion, and health-education support in the care of healthy individuals and populations.

## ⓔ EVOLVE CHAPTER FEATURES

http://evolve.elsevier.com/Edelman/
• Study Questions

## BOX 9-9   Racial and Ethnic Approaches to Community Health US Keys to Success

### Trust: Build a Culture of Collaboration With Communities That Is Based on Trust

- **Empowerment.** Give individuals and communities the knowledge and tools needed to create change by seeking and demanding better health and building on local resources.
- **Culture and history.** Design health initiatives that are grounded in the unique historical and cultural context of racial and ethnic minority communities in the United States.
- **Focus on causes.** Assess and focus on the underlying causes of poor community health and implement solutions that will stay embedded in the community infrastructure.
- **Community investment and expertise.** Recognize and invest in local community expertise and motivate communities to mobilize and organize existing resources.

- **Trusted organizations.** Enlist organizations within the community that are valued by community members, including groups with a primary mission unrelated to health.
- **Community leaders.** Help community leaders and key organizations forge unique partnerships and act as catalysts for change in the community.
- **Ownership.** Develop a collective outlook to promote shared interest in a healthy future through widespread community engagement and leadership.
- **Sustainability.** Make changes to organizations, community environments, and policies to help ensure that health improvements are long-lasting and community activities and programs are self-sustaining.
- **Hope.** Foster optimism, pride, and a promising vision for a healthier future.

From Centers for Disease Control and Prevention. (2016). *Racial and Ethnic Approaches to Community Health.* http://www.cdc.gov/reach.

## CASE STUDY

### Screening

Mrs. C. is an 82-year-old white widow. Six years ago, she moved from her house into a one-bedroom apartment. Her primary insurance is Medicare. She maintains her apartment and does all her errands without assistance, all of which she is very proud. She reports that occasionally she has fallen, probably because of some degree of decreasing vision, especially when moving from direct sunlight into shadows and when walking at night. The only medications she takes are an analgesic for pain management of osteoarthritis, an antihypertensive agent, and a daily vitamin and cranberry supplement. Her antihypertensive medication has recently been changed.

Today, she is going to her annual "check-up" with nurse practitioner (NP) Kelly, who is part of a new practice of "integrative medicine." The collaborative practice of registered nurses, NPs, and physicians emphasizes the role of prevention, including screenings. While Kelly is assessing Mrs. C.'s health status, she is also reflecting on how to better care for the practice's ever-enlarging older

adult population. Kelly has access to a large referral group including medical specialists.

#### Reflective Questions

- What data will nurse practitioner Kelly collect to assess Mrs. C.'s health? Why?
- What risk factors will Kelly most likely evaluate? Why?
- What screening tests will Kelly suggest? Why?
- Propose several possible nursing diagnoses for Mrs. C. What possible etiological factors from Mrs. C., her family, and her community might be involved?
- What questions will Kelly ask to evaluate Mrs. C.'s health status?
- Compare and contrast these different (individual, family, and community) approaches to health promotion, emphasizing screening and cost-effectiveness.
- Discuss the advantages and disadvantages of screening older adults.

## ◎ CARE PLAN

### Health Promotion, Emphasizing Screenings of Older Adults: Mrs. C.

Caring for older adults is challenging and rewarding. New ways of caring need to be developed especially considering the increasing number of the older "baby boomer generation" in America.

   *NURSING DIAGNOSIS: Effective community therapeutic regimen management

#### Definition

The pattern in which an individual, family, and/or community experiences (or is at risk of experiencing) difficulty integrating screening programs for the promotion of health and reduction of risk factors

#### Defining Characteristics
##### Major
- The individual, family, and/or community verbalizes the desire to manage health promotion with the assistance of the family and community including a nurse practitioner.
- The individual and family verbalize inadequate knowledge of health-promotion strategies, especially risk factors identified through screening methods.

##### Minor
- What are Mrs. C.'s screening and health-promotion needs?
- What is Mrs. C's understanding of aging and of accelerated risk factors for illness?

#### Related Factors
- Complexity, including discomfort, of some screenings (e.g., mammograms, osteoporosis testing)
- New ways of thinking about and delivering health promotion, including periodic screening recommended for older adults
- Shifts of resources and costs from individual providers to the community and family (e.g., self-screenings, transportation)

#### Interventions
- Promote attitudes of openness to new health information.
- For elevated blood pressure readings, repeat blood pressure screening on three different visits.

*Continued*

## CARE PLAN

### Health Promotion, Emphasizing Screenings of Older Adults: Mrs. C.—cont'd

- Develop a more detailed activity/experience log with special attention to physical safety (falls) and vision problems.
- Explore nutritional and activity strategies that are more appealing to each individual.
- Begin the program slowly.
- Follow up on additional risk factors.
- Offer resources to support goals and interventions.

**Expected Outcomes**
- The person may experience anxiety.
- The person may experience despair.

Mrs. C., her family, and her community will:
- Verbalize a full understanding of health promotion, especially screenings. Mrs. C. will:
- Identify and discuss her own risk factors and other data obtained from screenings.
- Establish appropriate goals to decrease the unhealthy findings of her screenings.
- Design and implement a modification program to fulfill these goals.
- Evaluate the efficacy of this care plan with nurse practitioner Kelly.

*NANDA Nursing Diagnoses—Herdman, T. H. & Kamitsuru, S. (Eds.). Nursing Diagnoses–Definitions and Classification 2015–2017. Copyright © 2014, 1994–2014 NANDA International. Used by arrangement with John Wiley & Sons Limited. In order to make safe and effective judgments using the NANDA-I nursing diagnoses it is essential that nurses refer to the definitions and defining characteristics of the diagnoses listed in this work.

## REFERENCES

Agency for Healthcare Research and Quality. (2014a). Guide to clinical preventive services. Clinical summaries, recommendations for adults, children and adolescents. http://www.ahrq.gov/professionals/clinicians-providers/guidelines-recommendations/guide/.

Agency for Healthcare Research and Quality. (2014b). Treating tobacco use and dependence—2008 Update. October 2014. Rockville, MD: Agency for Healthcare Research and Quality. http://www.ahrq.gov/professionals/clinicians-providers/guidelines-recommendations/tobacco/clinicians/update/correctadd.html.

Airoldi, M., & Morton, A. (2009). Adjusting life for quality or disability: Stylistic difference or substantial dispute? *Health Economics*, 18(11), 1237–1247.

Allender, J., Rector, C., & Warner, K. (2014). *Community health nursing: Promoting and protecting the public's health* (8th ed.). New York, NY: Lippincott, Williams & Wilkins.

Alzheimer's Association. (2015). Alzheimer's & dementia/research. http://www.alz.org.

Anderson, J. B., et al. (2014). Usefulness of combined history, physical examination, electrocardiogram, and limited echocardiogram in screening adolescent athletes for risk for sudden cardiac death. *American Journal of Cardiology*, 114(11), 1763–1767.

Botkin, J., et al. (2013). Use of residual newborn screening bloodspots. *Pediatrics*, 131(1), 120–127.

Broder, M. (2013). Communities' attitudes toward cancer screenings shed light on cultural differences. http://berkeley.edu/bh/wp-content/uploads/2013/06/cancerscreening.

Bynum, S. A., et al. (2012). Unwillingness to participate in colorectal cancer screenings: Examining fears, attitudes, and medical mistrust in an ethnically diverse sample of adults 50 years and older. *American Journal of Health Promotion*, 26(5), 295–300.

Center for Medicare Advocacy. (2015). Medicare coverage for prevention and wellness. http://www.medicareadvocacy.org.

Centers for Disease Control and Prevention (CDC). (2010). Reach U.S. finding solutions to health disparities: At a glance 2010. http://www.cdc.gov/needphp/dch/programs/reach.

Centers for Disease Control and Prevention (CDC). (2011). National HIV and STD testing resources. https://gettested.cdc.gov/.

Centers for Disease Control and Prevention (CDC). (2012). Introduction to epidemiology. http://www.cdc.gov/ophss/csels/dsepd/ss1978/lesson1/section/.html/.

Centers for Disease Control and Prevention (CDC). (2013). Chronic Disease Cost Calculator version 2. http://www.cdc.gov/chronicdisease/pdf/cdcc_user_guide.pdf.

Centers for Disease Control and Prevention (CDC). (2014). Best practices for comprehensive tobacco control programs. Atlanta, GA: US Department of Health and Human Services, Centers for Disease Control and Prevention, National Center for Chronic Disease Prevention and Health Promotion, Office on Smoking and Health.

Centers for Disease Control and Prevention (CDC). (2015). What is epidemiology. http://www.cdc.gov/excite/epidemiology.

Costello, J. (2014). Measuring benefits. https://www.givingwhatwecan.org/blog/2014-03-04/measuring-benefits.

Davis, J. L., et al. (2012). Sociodemographic differences in fears and mistrust contributing to unwillingness to participate in cancer screenings. *Journal Health Care Poor Underserved*, 23(4 Suppl.), 67–76.

Dorfman, L., & Krasnow, I. D. (2014). Public health and media advocacy. *Annual Review of Public Health*, 35, 293–306.

Food and Drug Administration. (2012). OraQuick rapid HIV-1 antibody, package insert. http://www.fda.gov/downloads/BiologicsBloodVaccines/BloodBloodProducts/ApprovedProducts/PremarketApprovalsPMAs/UCM310606.pdf.

Green, R. C., & Farahany, N. A. (2014). The FDA is over cautious on consumer genomics. *Nature*, 505, 286–287.

Hanna-Attisha, M., et al. (2016). Elevated blood lead levels in children associated with the Flint drinking water crisis: A spatial analysis of risk and public health response. *American Journal of Public Health*, 106(2), 283–290.

HealthyPeople.gov. (2015). Healthy People 2020. http://healthypeople.gov/2020/default.

Hoffmann, T. C., & Del Mar, C. (2015). Patients' expectations of the benefits and harms of treatments, screening, and tests: A systematic review. *Journal of the American Medical Association Internal Medicine*, 175(2), 274–286.

Institute of Medicine. (2011). The future of nursing: Leading change, advancing health. http://www.iom.edu/Reports/2010/The-Future-of-Nursing-Leading-Change-Advancing-Health.aspx/.

Kidd, A. D., & Colbert, A. M. (2015). Mammography: Review of the controversy, health disparities, and impact on young African American women. *Clinical Journal of Oncology Nursing*, *19*(3), E52–E58.

Lin, K. W., & Gostin, L. O. (2016). A public health framework for screening mammography: Evidence-based vs politically mandated care. *Journal of the American Medical Association*, *315*(10), 977–978.

Lundy, K., & Janes, S. (2014). *Community health nursing: Caring for the public's health* (3rd ed.). Boston, MA: Jones & Bartlett.

Maine, D., Hurlburt, S., & Greeson, D. (2011). Cervical cancer prevention in the 21st century: Cost is not the only issue. *American Journal of Public Health*, *101*(9), 1549–1555.

Mandelblatt, J., et al. (2016). Collaborative modeling of the benefits and harms associated with different US breast cancer screening strategies. *Annals of Internal Medicine*, *164*(4), 215–225.

Mendez, E. (2010). In U.S., health disparities across incomes are wide-ranging. http://www.gallup.com/poll/143696/health-disparities-across-incomes-wide-ranging.aspx?ut.

National Prevention Council. (2011). National Prevention Strategy. Washington, DC: US Department of Health and Human Services, Office of the Surgeon General. https://www.surgeongeneral.gov/priorities/prevention/strategy/report.pdf.

Nayak, S., Roberts, M., & Greenspan, S. (2011). Cost-effectiveness of different screening strategies for osteoporosis in postmenopausal women. *Annals of Internal Medicine*, *155*, 751–761.

Ness, R. (2013). Practice guidelines for childhood lead screening in primary care. *Journal of Pediatric Health Care*, *27*(5), 395–399.

Nickolich, S., et al. (2016). Aneuploidy screening: Newer noninvasive test gains traction. *Clinician Reviews*, *26*(2), 26, 29–30.

Ringrose, J., et al. (2015). Effect of overcuffing on the accuracy of oscillometric blood pressure measurements. *Journal of the American Society of Hypertension*, *9*(7), 563–568.

Roelofs, C., et al. (2010). The Boston safe shops model: An integrated approach to community environmental and occupational health. *American Journal of Public Health*, *100*(Suppl. 1), S52–S55.

Shephard, R. (2011). Mandatory ECG screening of athletes: Is this question now resolved? *Sports Medicine*, *41*(12), 989–1002.

Sutphen, C. L., et al. (2015). Longitudinal cerebrospinal fluid biomarker changes in preclinical Alzheimer's disease during middle age. *Journal of the American Medical Association Neurology*, *72*(9), 1029–1042.

Thompson, C. K., Eklund, M., & Esserman, L. J. (2015). Putting the "great mammography debate" to rest. *American Journal of Hematology/Oncology*, *11*(9), 21–22.

Uden-Holman, T. M., Curry, S. J., & Benz, L. (2015). Public health as a catalyst for interprofessional education on a health sciences campus. *American Journal of Public Health*, *105*(S1), S104–S105.

US Department of Health and Human Services, Office on Women's Health. (2012). Screening tests for men. http://www.womenshealth.gov/screening-tests-and-vaccines/screening-tests-for-men.pdf.

US Department of Health and Human Services, Office on Women's Health. (2013). Screening tests for women. http://www.womenshealth.gov/screening-tests-and-vacines/screening-tests-for-women.pdf.

US Preventive Services Task Force (USPSTF). (2015). Osteoporosis: Screening. http://www.uspreventiveservicestaskforce.org/uspstf10/osteoporosis/osteors.htm.

US Preventive Services Task Force (USPSTF). (2016a). USPSTF A and B recommendations. https://www.uspreventiveservicestaskforce.org/Page/Name/uspstf-a-and-b-recommendations/.

US Preventive Services Task Force (USPSTF). (2016b). Recommendations for primary care practice, pediatric, adolescents, adults. https://www.uspreventiveservicestaskforce.org/Search.

Vora, N. L., & O'Brien, B. M. (2014). Noninvasive prenatal testing for microdeletion syndromes and expanded trisomies: Proceed with caution. *Obstetrics and gynecology*, *123*(5), 1097–1099.

Weir, H. K., et al. (2015). The past, present, and future of cancer incidence in the US: 1975–2020. *Cancer*, *121*(11), 1827–1837.

Womenshealth.gov. (2013). Screening tests and vaccines. http://www.womenshealth.gov/screening-tests-and-vaccines/screening-tests-for-women/.

Yang, D. X., et al. (2014). Estimating the magnitude of colorectal cancers prevented during the era of screening: 1976 to 2009. *Cancer*, *120*, 2893–2901.

Yoon, S. S., Fryar, C. D., & Carroll, M. S. (2015). Hypertension prevalence and control among adults: US, 2011–2014. NCHS data brief, no 220. Hyattsville, MD: National Center for Health Statistics.

# 10

# Health Education

*Susan A. Heady*

## OBJECTIVES

*After completing this chapter, the reader will be able to:*
- Analyze the goals of health education.
- Discuss learning principles that affect health education.
- Apply teaching and learning concepts to teaching.
- Describe selected theoretical models used in health education to influence the behavior change process.
- Explain the steps in preparing a health teaching plan.
- Propose learning strategies appropriate to each learning domain.
- Discuss the importance of evaluating the educational process.

## KEY TERMS

Behavior change
Ecological model
Empowerment
Health behaviors
Health belief model
Health counseling

Health disparities
Health education
Health literacy
Health promotion
Quality and safety
Self-efficacy

Social cognitive theory
Social justice
Social marketing
Transtheoretical model (Stages of change)

 **THINK ABOUT IT**

### The Challenges of Health Education

With personal health behavior patterns linked closely to the current causes of morbidity and death, health education is fundamental to promoting lifestyle change. People may lack the knowledge needed for making lifestyle changes, such as awareness of risks. In addition, they may not be aware of effective health-promotion strategies and resources in the community. In each encounter the nurse has the opportunity to assess the learner's needs for education related to primary, secondary, and/or tertiary prevention. Whether the target audience is an individual or a community, the nurse considers these questions in addressing the health-education needs:

- What can people do to improve their health in the context of lifestyles?
- How can individuals, families, and communities make healthier choices?
- What is the nurse's role in facilitating health through education and program planning?

Reflect on the following scenario. Tonya is a 14-year-old black American who lives with her mother and older brothers in a low-income housing complex in a high-risk neighborhood. Her after-school activities focus on texting her friends and watching television. Tonya is obese for her age and height. According to the school nurse, many of her peers are also overweight or obese. Consider the following:

- What does Tonya know about healthy nutrition and exercise?
- What factors may promote or interfere with Tonya's learning or adopting a change in lifestyle?
- How can the nurse best address Tonya's health-education needs?
- What are the health-education needs of other students in the school?
- What information is relevant to teaching Tonya or planning programs for the middle school students in this neighborhood?
- Which theories can be used in planning health-education programs?
- How might families or the community be involved in supporting obesity prevention and reduction for these teens?
- What are the needs of other residents of the community?

Health education is a vital component in promoting individual and community health. Individual behaviors such as diet, physical activity level, and substance abuse play a significant role in health outcomes.

Lifestyle changes should not be viewed as only primary prevention. Chronic diseases related to health behaviors are the major causes of poor health, disability, and death, and contribute considerably to health care costs. Individual intensive lifestyle changes and strategies to address population health can be effective not only in preventing chronic diseases but also in reversing their progression and significantly reducing health care costs (Bauer et al., 2014).

Health education to promote positive behavior change, along with policies and programs that address the social determinants of health, can reduce the rates of chronic illness and disability in the United States. The *Healthy People 2020* national health objectives emphasize priorities to improve the health of individuals, groups, and communities in the United States. These priorities involve promoting positive health behaviors, increasing health literacy, and reducing health disparities (US Department of Health and Human Services [USDHHS], 2010). Achievement of these objectives provides challenges and opportunities for health promotion.

Although many health goals are affected by individual lifestyle practices, health is influenced significantly by social, economic, physical, and political factors. The *Healthy People 2020* vision for health education includes a commitment to providing early health literacy and prevention education beginning with preschool, then continuing throughout the K-12 education continuum and beyond. This involves an approach to developing healthy citizens not only by delivering basic health-promotion and disease-prevention concepts and encouraging risk-reduction behaviors but also by demonstrating the value of interrelatedness and the connection between individual and community health (Koh et al., 2011). Box 10-1: *Healthy People 2020* includes objectives related to educational programs.

Nursing, with its unique contributions to health care, is a professional resource that can help facilitate these changes through health-education strategies. Nurses, in partnership with other health care professionals, can be the link between the philosophy of *Healthy People 2020* and the people who need to hear its messages and act on those messages.

## NURSING AND HEALTH EDUCATION

Nurses as educators play a key role in improving the health of the nation. Educating people is an integral part of the nurse's role in every practice setting—schools, communities, work sites, health care delivery sites, and homes. Health education involves not only providing relevant information but also facilitating health-related behavior change. The nurse, using health-education principles, can assist people in achieving their health goals in a way that is consistent with their personal lifestyles, values, and beliefs.

*Nursing: Scope and Standards of Practice* (American Nurses Association, 2015) describes health teaching and health promotion as primary nursing responsibilities. This includes educating

 **BOX 10-1   HEALTHY PEOPLE 2020**

### Selected Health-Promotion and Disease-Prevention Objectives Related to Educational and Community-Based Programs

Goal: To increase the quality, availability, and effectiveness of educational and community-based programs designed to prevent disease and injury, improve health, and enhance quality of life

**School Setting**

- Increase the proportion of preschool programs that provide health education to prevent problems in these areas: unintentional injury; violence; tobacco use; alcohol and other drug use; unhealthy dietary patterns; and inadequate physical activity, dental health, and safety.
- Increase the proportion of elementary, middle, and senior high schools that provide comprehensive health education to prevent problems in the following areas: unintentional injury; violence and suicide; tobacco use; alcohol and other drug use; unintended pregnancy and sexually transmitted infections; unhealthy dietary patterns; and inadequate physical activity.
- Increase the proportion of elementary, middle, and senior high schools that have health-education goals or objectives that address the knowledge and skills articulated in the National Health Education Standards (high school, middle, elementary).
- Increase the proportion of elementary, middle, junior high, and senior high schools that have a nurse-to-student ratio of at least 1 : 750.
- Increase the rate of completion of high school.
- Increase the proportion of college and university students who receive information for the institution of each of the six priority health-risk behavior areas listed in the preceding fourth objective.

**Work Setting**

- Increase the proportion of work sites that offer an employee health-promotion program to their employees.
- Increase the proportion of employees who participate in employer-sponsored health-promotion activities.

**Community Setting and Select Populations**

- Increase the proportion of tribal and local health service organizations that provide population-based primary prevention services in the following areas: injury and violence prevention; mental illness; tobacco use; substance abuse; unintended pregnancy; chronic disease programs; nutrition; physical activity.
- Increase the proportion of local health departments that establish culturally appropriate and linguistically competent community health-promotion and disease-prevention programs.

From US Department of Health and Human Services. (2010). *Healthy People 2020.* http://www.healthypeople.gov.

people about healthy lifestyles, risk reduction, developmental needs, activities of daily living, and preventive self-care. *Nursing's Social Policy Statement* of the American Nurses Association (2010) also addresses health teaching and health counseling. This responsibility to teach individuals is balanced by their right to receive information about their health status, risks, and ways to reduce their risks. The nurse provides health teaching and health counseling on the basis of individual interests and decisions to enable individuals to make informed decisions about their health.

Nurses usually function as health care coordinators for individuals in their care. Depending on the interests and needs of a person, nurses establish a partnership to guide the individual in the selection and use of relevant health services. Health-education principles provide the nurse with strategies and tools for assessing an individual's readiness for health teaching, with technical information, and with help in practicing healthy behaviors in his or her daily life. These strategies also help the nurse facilitate behavior change while satisfying the person's right to relevant health information and the freedom for people to make decisions about their own health. Health education encourages self-care, self-empowerment, and, ultimately, less dependence on the health care system.

Nurses have long been involved in public health education, taking on the full-time role of coordinating the educational services provided by a health agency or institution. As a health educator, the nurse may use marketing strategies to enhance the effectiveness of health-education programs that are focused on certain target populations. The health-education specialist helps other nurses and health professionals improve their skills in developing and delivering teaching plans.

## Definition

Health education is "any combination of learning experiences designed to help individuals and communities improve their health, by increasing their knowledge or influencing their attitudes" (World Health Organization, 2016). This process involves several key components. First, health education involves the use of teaching-learning strategies. Second, learners maintain voluntary control over the decision to make changes in their actions. Third, health education focuses on behavior changes that have been found to improve health status.

Health education facilitates the development of health knowledge, skills, and attitudes through the application of theories or models. Commonly used theories of individual and community behavior change will be discussed later in this chapter. Generally, health-education strategies help ensure that individuals, as consumers of health services, are satisfied and have received the health information that is most relevant to their health risks. From a public health perspective, health-education programs are intended not only to enhance individuals' abilities to make positive lifestyle changes but also to support social and political actions that promote health and quality of life in communities.

The following scenario is an example of a therapeutic situation in which a health-education approach may be used to meet an individual's health needs.

Sada Thompson, a 21-year-old university senior, visits university health services because she wants to change her method of birth control. She has experienced side effects from the birth control pill that she has been taking for the past year and knows little about other options. She has recently started dating John after breaking up with Steven 3 months ago. Having decided to be sexually active with John, Sada is feeling uncertain about what she needs to do to take care of herself and how to discuss this uncertainty with John. She is aware of all the talk about AIDS on campus, and she knows that John is popular and has dated several other women in school, which concerns her.

Sada needs to learn new information, she may need to acquire new skills, and she needs to clarify any feelings or attitudes that affect her decision to use a new birth control method and ensure her continued safety. After recording her health assessment history and arranging for a gynecological examination and laboratory tests, the nurse develops a teaching plan. Selecting one or more strategies for helping Sada review all the birth control options, the nurse establishes an environment in which Sada can choose to try a new method or request a change in her prescription for oral contraceptives. Together they identify actions that Sada can take to use the method properly. They also anticipate and identify ways that Sada can solve problems of adjusting to the new method.

The nurse answers Sada's immediate questions about safe sex, gives her several pamphlets written for college students about this topic, and suggests that she participate in the peer counseling night on sexually transmitted diseases that will be held on campus in 2 weeks. The peer counseling hotline number and drop-in hours are given to Sada. The nurse explains that the students who provide the peer counseling are trained to help other students talk about and deal with this important issue. The nurse invites Sada to call or come back to the office for additional help, information, and problem-solving discussion.

This example illustrates that educational interventions, in addition to direct health services, are necessary to meet the individual's goal. Although health care providers and nurses prefer that people choose to take actions that will promote health and not detract from it, the individual determines the at-home application of health recommendations.

## Goals

The goal of health education is to help individuals, families, and communities achieve, through their own actions and initiative, optimal states of health. Health education facilitates voluntary actions to promote health. Another important goal of health education is improving health literacy.

Health literacy is defined as "the degree to which individuals have the capacity to obtain, process, and understand health information and services needed to make appropriate health decisions" (USDHHS, 2016). Simply stated, "health literacy is about communicating health information clearly and understanding it correctly" (Osborne, 2013). Health literacy includes the ability to read, write, speak, listen, compute, and comprehend, and to apply those skills to health situations.

According to the 2003 National Assessment of Health Literacy study, only approximately 12% of US adults had proficient health literacy. More than one-third of US adults have only basic or below basic health literacy. This means they would have difficulty with common health tasks, such as following directions on a prescription drug label or adhering to a childhood immunization schedule using a standard chart. Although half of adults without a high school education had below basic health literacy skills, even high school and college graduates can have limited health literacy. The more vulnerable members of our communities—those with lower education levels, racial/ethnic minorities, the uninsured and publicly insured, and the elderly—have the lowest levels of health literacy (USDHHS, 2016).

Nurses, through their unique responsibility for the majority of care recipient, caregiver, and community health education and communication, can also contribute to improving health literacy by assuming a lead role in reviewing and revising all types of forms and educational materials intended for care recipients, examining these materials for relevance, clarity, cultural appropriateness, and clinical accuracy (Baur, 2011). This includes materials available via the electronic health record.

Addressing health literacy and providing culturally sensitive health education are critical to reducing health disparities and achieving health equity. **Health disparities** are systematic, potentially avoidable health differences that adversely affect socially disadvantaged groups. The groups affected are those with characteristics such as race/ethnicity, skin color, religion, language, or nationality; socioeconomic resources or position; sex, sexual orientation, or gender identity; age; physical, mental, or emotional disability or illness; geography; political or other affiliation; or other characteristics that have been linked historically to discrimination or marginalization (Braverman et al., 2011). Examples of public health interventions to reduce health disparities in the United States include Vaccines for Children; Many Men, Many Voices, for black men who have sex with men; Healthy Love, to reduce the risk of HIV infection in heterosexual black women; and an initiative to reduce motor vehicle accidents in four Native American nations (Centers for Disease Control and Prevention, USDHHS, 2014).

People-centered care is an essential component of **quality and safety** whether health promotion is directed toward an individual, family, or community. In the planning and implementation of health-education programs, essential components include showing respect for values and cultural, ethic, and social diversity, empowering and actively involving the learners, promoting physical and emotional comfort, communicating in ways that are appropriate to health literacy and sociocultural background, and seeking continual self-improvement in effective education (Quality and Safety in Nursing Institute, 2014). Use of health-education strategies that are person centered can have a significant impact on the outcomes of health care recipients (Box 10-2: Quality and Safety Scenario).

Health education encourages positive, informed changes in lifestyle behaviors that prevent acute and chronic disease, decrease disability, and enhance wellness. Another goal of health education that may foster successful changes in health behavior is **empowerment**. People who believe that they can make a difference in health and who are involved in decision-making are more likely to make changes (Anderson & Fallin, 2012).

Changes in health behaviors that are related to health education help prevent disease and disability. Two main objectives of health education and health counseling are to change health behaviors and to improve health status. Information alone does not change behavior.

Health education and health counseling are mutually supportive activities. Health educators often use one-to-one and group counseling techniques as strategies for active health learning. Counselors may refer people to health-education resources or assist them in acquiring information pertinent to solving a health problem. The following example helps illustrate the goals of health education. The general principles of learning that are found in Box 10-3 are fundamental to the planning of successful health-education programs.

### BOX 10-2   QUALITY AND SAFETY SCENARIO

#### A Community-Based Person-Centered Health Promotion

The Southwest Organizing Project (SWOP) provides an example of a person-centered community-based approach designed to reduce health disparity in people of color. SWOP, a successful grassroots organization, combats childhood obesity in low-income families in Albuquerque, New Mexico, by targeting population-level causes of obesity.

SWOP tailored health promotion to the community using an innovative three lens health-promotion framework based on the Robert Wood Johnson Foundation's Communities Creating Health Environments initiative. The three lenses used to organize the community to advocate for a healthy sustainable environment included social justice, culture-place, and organizational capacity–organizing approach. **Social justice** refers to fair treatment, equal access to goods and resources, and the right to self-determination and cultural expression for all people. The social justice lens is used to identify the structural cause of the targeted health disparity. The culture-place lens, the "total way of life of a people" (values, rituals, patterns of thinking, and group identity), as well as the place characteristics (geography, history, political), determines culturally and geographically meaningful and responsive interventions to address the population cause. Organizational capacity–organizing approach, the capacity of a grassroots organization to organize resources and strategies, determines the most effective strategy to align the interventions and organization to promote health in the targeted area.

For example, in Albuquerque, application of the food justice perspective identified the structural cause of the childhood obesity as limited access to locally grown healthy foods and lack of fresh produce in school lunches. Cultural and geographical analysis indicated tailoring the project to the demographics of the children, Hispanic and blended Hispanic Native American from a historically farming culture. In addition, because of strong support from several legislators, the state legislature was targeted to support a healthy school lunch policy rather than Albuquerque city council or school board. SWOP's organizational capacity analysis revealed adult and youth leaders, alliance with key community organizations, established relationships with city and state councils, and limited relationships with school decision makers. Community interventions included involving leaders and residents in establishing an urban community garden, education in farming, gardening, and healthy eating, forming alliances with community stakeholders, and advocating a healthy school lunch policy.

SWOP used a three-lens framework to develop and implement interventions centered on the health-promotion needs of the obese children in the Albuquerque community. Community-based health-promotion interventions, such as SWOP, involving nurses and key leaders in partnering with the community, empower communities of color to take long-term action to reduce health disparities.

Data from Subica, A. M., Grills, C. T., Douglas, J. A., & Villanueva, S. (2016). Communities of color creating healthy environments to combat childhood obesity. *American Journal of Public Health, 106*(1), 78–86.

Kate Hanson, aged 22 years, visits the local family health center for fatigue and symptoms similar to influenza. During the assessment with the nurse, Kate discloses that she has missed her last two periods.

The physical examination findings, the laboratory test findings, and the health assessment pattern confirm Kate's suspicions of pregnancy. Psychosocial evaluation reveals that Kate works part-time as a secretary for a temporary agency and lives in an apartment with her recently unemployed husband, Jim. Further interviewing reveals that Kate has minimal knowledge of prenatal

---

**BOX 10-3   How to Facilitate Learning**

- Use methods that stimulate a variety of senses.
- Involve the person actively in the learning process.
- Establish a comfortable, appropriate learning environment.
- Assess the readiness of the learner, which may be affected by physical, social, emotional, and financial factors.
- Make the information relevant by connecting with the existing needs and interests of the learner.
- Use repetition. Review and reinforce concepts several times in a variety of ways.
- Make the learning encounter positive. Structure it to achieve progress recognizable by the individual and provide frequent, positive feedback.
- Start with what is known and proceed to what is unknown, moving from simple to complex.
- Apply the concepts to several settings to facilitate generalization.
- Pace the learning appropriately for the individual.

---

care; she has a diet of take-out food that is high in fat, sodium, and sugar, with infrequent consumption of fresh fruits or vegetables; and she has three or four beers on the weekends. Kate has never taken vitamin supplements, she leads a sedentary lifestyle, and she is obviously overwhelmed by the news that she is pregnant.

The nurse first takes steps to create a safe and trusting atmosphere in which Kate can feel free to share her concerns and apprehensions. When Kate expresses concerns about telling her husband about the pregnancy, the nurse discusses this with her. Kate is then taught the importance of taking a multiple vitamin with an iron supplement daily, discontinuing the consumption of alcohol, checking with her physician before taking medications, and making time for more rest during the day. Sensing that this is all that can be accomplished at this time, the nurse gives Kate two pamphlets on prenatal care and makes an appointment for her to return in 1 week with her husband. Kate acknowledges that she understands the instructions, and the nurse documents the teaching and recommendations in Kate's medical record.

During the next visit, the nurse meets Kate and Jim, explores the meaning of the pregnancy in their lives, and helps them identify actions they will need to take. The recommendations that were made during Kate's first visit are reviewed and reinforced. The nurse then details specifics of dietary changes, reinforces the need for proper rest and exercise, and helps the couple solve problems while they adjust to these new responsibilities. Most importantly, the nurse gives them information on the clinic's weekly prenatal classes and explains that because the classes are partially covered by local community funding, the charge is minimal. The classes include information about physical changes, psychosocial changes, and nutritional needs during the pregnancy, the labor and delivery period, and the newborn and postpartum periods. A nurse practitioner conducts the classes at the clinic, which are given in a group format to facilitate social support and problem-solving among expectant parents.

The nurse gives Kate and Jim several other pamphlets to read at home, makes a clinic appointment for Kate in a couple of weeks, and encourages her to call if she has questions or concerns

in the interim. A schedule of the prenatal classes is reviewed, and a date for the next session is made. The couple is encouraged to meet the social worker to explore their financial needs and options because Jim was recently laid off. Kate and Jim acknowledge that they understand what they need to do, and the nurse documents what was taught and discussed in Kate's health care record.

This example illustrates the goal of health education: to help individuals achieve optimal health and well-being through their actions and initiative. Through health education, individuals can learn to make informed decisions about personal and family health practices and to use health services in the community. The couple in this example receives educational assistance from the nurse that will promote better health and well-being for Kate and their baby.

## Learning Assumptions

Chapters 16 to 24 in this text address the factors one should consider when teaching different age groups and the learners' respective characteristics to consider when one is developing a teaching plan.

The nurse considers the developmental stage, cognitive level, and interests of the individual. The level of information to be conveyed and the skills and abilities of the individual will guide the methods and resources used.

## Family Health Teaching

The family plays an important role in health and illness. Because the family is the unit within which health values, health habits, and health risk perceptions are developed, organized, and performed, individual's health, understanding, and intervening with the family is essential to promoting health and reducing health risks in individuals and communities (Anderson & Fallin, 2012). Skills in family interviewing and assessment are valuable tools for nurses. Family health assessment and health teaching are closely related. The assessment model in Chapter 6 provides a comprehensive approach to identifying problems, strengths, and health-education needs. The goal is to help the members achieve optimal states of health while guiding them through problem-solving and decision-making. This process empowers them. Members believe they can make a difference in their own health.

In clarifying the health teaching needs of a family, the nurse might ask herself/himself the following questions: "Who is in this family? What health-related tasks are they performing? How are they functioning and how are they meeting each other's needs? How well are they communicating? What does this family need to know? What do they need to know now? What do they think they need to know? How can they learn what they need to know?"

The nurse works with the family to set a broad health-promotion goal for the family, then directs the health teaching toward a more specific area. It is essential that the family agrees with the goal and teaching needs. As the family participates in the assessment interview, perhaps members can identify their own health teaching needs. Health teaching includes all family members, with learning activities appropriate for each individual. The general teaching goal will be the same for all members, but

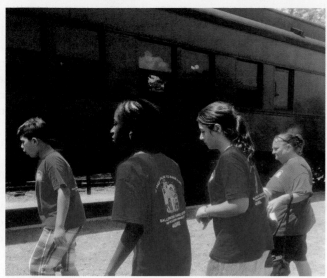

**FIGURE 10-1** School-age children will engage in safe travel.

the approaches and specific goals for each member or subsystem will be different. Children, adolescents, and elderly members pose special challenges to the nurse, who may be geared toward teaching young or middle-aged adults (Figure 10-1).

## Health Behavior Change

The process of health education directs people toward voluntary changes of their health behaviors. Viewing health behavior through an **ecological model**, the nurse recognizes the complex interaction of individuals with their environment and the multiple influences of the individual, the interpersonal group, and the community on health behavior. This section examines the use of commonly used models of individual health behavior change. Community and group models in health-education planning are addressed later in this chapter.

Individual models of health behavior help explain factors influencing and interfering with positive health behaviors. In addition, they contribute to understanding how educational intervention supports behavior change.

Beliefs, attitudes, values, and information contribute to motivation and behavior and are underlying factors in the making of any decision to change behavior (Richards, 2014). **Health behaviors** are any activities that an individual undertakes to enhance health, prevent disease, and detect and control the symptoms of a disease. Identifying and teaching people about lifestyle behaviors that need to be changed is only the first step in the process of assisting individuals in moving from knowledge to action. Nurses apply concepts from the health belief model, social learning theory, and the transtheoretical model (TTM) in subsequent steps to formulate an action plan that meets the needs and capabilities of each person in making healthy behavior changes.

## Health Belief Model

The **health belief model** is a paradigm used to predict and explain health behavior. The following components of the health belief model provide guidelines for nurses to analyze factors that contribute to a person's perceived state of health or risk of disease and to the individual's probability of making an appropriate plan of action:

- individual perceptions of susceptibility to a health condition or disease;
- perceived seriousness of the disease;
- perceived benefits of health action;
- perceived barriers to the health action;
- cues that promote action (feelings or media responses);
- perceived ability to perform the action (Rosenstock et al., 1988; Skinner et al., 2015).

Application of components of the health belief model generates data to assist nurses in choosing effective educational strategies. The nurse then determines the most appropriate interventions for a particular person through collaboration with the individual.

## Social Cognitive Theory

**Social cognitive theory** is another model that adds to the understanding of the determinants of health behavior. Bandura (1997) emphasizes the influence of self-efficacy, or efficacy beliefs, on health behavior. **Self-efficacy** refers to an individual's belief in being personally capable of performing the behavior required to influence one's own health (see the case study and the care plan at the end of this chapter). Social cognitive theory also describes the roles of reinforcement and observational learning in explaining health behavior change. Modeling, or providing opportunities for imitating the behavior of others, can be used to demonstrate the desired behavior.

## Transtheoretical Model of Change

The **transtheoretical model** (TTM) or **"stages of change model,"** is useful for determining where a person is in relation to making a behavior change (Prochaska & DiClemente, 1984). According to the TTM, health-related behavior change progresses through the following five stages regardless of whether an individual is quitting or adopting a behavior:

- Precontemplation: The person is not thinking about or considering quitting or adopting a behavior change within the next 6 months (not intending to make changes).
- Contemplation: The person is seriously considering making a specific behavior change within the next 6 months (considering a change).
- Planning or preparation: The person who has made a behavior change is seriously thinking about making a change within the next month (making small or sporadic changes).
- Action: The person has made a behavior change, and it has persisted for 6 months (actively engaged in behavior change).
- Maintenance: The period beginning 6 months after the action has started and continuing indefinitely (sustaining the change over time) (Prochaska et al., 2015).

The TTM is useful in determining the person's readiness for learning in relation to changing a behavior so that health education or behavior change interventions can be matched to the stage. Self-efficacy is a key construct in this model. This model also acknowledges the importance of continuing intervention to maintaining behavior change long term. The TTM has been used by health professionals in planning interventions with a wide variety of people at risk.

Regardless of the quality of nurses' assessment methods and educational strategies, experience in the area of health education indicates that people do not always make the choices recommended to them by health professionals or adhere to the healthy changes. Naturally, health professionals want people to choose the recommended course of action, but each individual has the right to choose not to follow advice. Enlisting the individual's partnership or cooperation achieves better results.

Attempts to influence a person's behavior through education are not always successful. Attempting to persuade people to change their behavior to something that might make them, their friends, and their family healthier can be discouraging and sometimes futile. An individual's values, beliefs, and life stresses may present obstacles to these changes. Effective health education requires an understanding of the influential factors affecting the individual's decision-making (values, beliefs, attitudes, life stresses, religion, previous experiences with the health care system, and life goals). Another key factor in the ability to comply with health education is financial constraints. The individual may not have the resources to pay for a proper diet or may not have a safe, convenient place to exercise.

Many health professionals tend to view a person's cooperation with the health care regimen as a single choice, when this cooperation often involves many choices every day. For example, following a low-fat, low-cholesterol diet involves constant, and often inconvenient, choices throughout the day. The expectation is that people will do this every day for the rest of their lives, even when the nurse cannot guarantee health as a result.

Ultimately, the nurse needs to respect a person's right to choose. However, nurses can increase an individual's motivation and capabilities to change by involving the individual in planning and goal setting, providing information that is understandable and acceptable, and assisting the person in developing new skills.

After clarifying behaviors that a person is willing to change, the nurse can use the following framework for developing interventions for behavior change:

- Assess the behavior.
- Educate the person about the need for and benefits of change.
- Motivate the person using personalized messages.
- Assess and increase the person' self-efficacy.
- Assess and offer resources to decrease barriers to change.
- Assist the person with goal setting to modify behavior.
- Practice the skills needed to change behavior.
- Plan ways to monitor and maintain the behavior change.

Theories of health behavior change are at the heart of health education. The theories presented in this section help nurses to assess an individual's stage in the behavior change process and to develop appropriate teaching plans. The goals of the teaching plans and the strategies selected will differ depending on the factors affecting the individual's readiness to learn and to change.

## Ethics

Applying principles of respect, autonomy, justice, and beneficence, nurses have an active role as advocates in empowering care recipients to make their own informed decisions about their health and care. The nurse works as a partner, facilitator, and resource for the person and family (Burkhardt & Nathaniel, 2014). Although the focus of health education may be on the behavior change process, the nurse needs to exercise caution in using tools of persuasion in communication with people because of the potential for manipulation and coercion, particularly when addressing different cultural or minority groups (Simons-Morton et al., 2012).

However, when planning health education to promote health, nurses experience several ethical dilemmas.

Choices about health care practices belong to individuals not health care providers. All competent people have the right to autonomous choice. Nurses should respect decisions made by people and their families, even when the choice is not what the nurse might do or suggest or is considered "unhealthy." The nurse and the family should work together on a mutually agreed on plan that incorporates these individual and family values and beliefs (Burkhardt & Nathaniel, 2014). When health promotion focuses on individual behavior, disregarding other social factors that may contribute significantly to the problem, this can inadvertently lead to victim blaming. Defining a problem as simply an individual problem suggests the individual is responsible for both the problem and the solution (Simons-Morton et al., 2012).

The role of the nurse is to facilitate a communicative environment in which people can exercise their right to make informed free choices. Individuals need to participate in the decision-making process when their lives may be influenced by a change.

Although each person's state of health affects family members and the community, individuals are responsible for their own health maintenance. Health professionals need to accept and welcome individual differences in meeting this responsibility. By selecting interventions that create an environment of open communication and risk-taking, individuals can better develop the problem-solving skills to direct their own growth and development.

## Genomics and Health Education

Advances in genetics and genomics present new opportunities and responsibilities for nurses in health education. Routine use of genetic and genomic technologies requires nurses to incorporate information about and implications of the technologies into educational programs for vulnerable individuals, families, and populations. Although an increasingly wide range of situations include the need for the nurse to be prepared to discuss genetics and genomics, the primary focus for nursing is health promotion, symptom management, and disease prevention. Box 10-4: Genomics describes the current role of the nurse in providing genomics education.

## Diversity and Health Teaching

The increasing racial and ethnic diversity of the US population, as well as the challenge to eliminate disparities in the health status of people of diverse backgrounds, demands that we provide culturally appropriate health education and health promotion. Individuals' cultural groups influence their beliefs about health, perceptions of disease and illness, help-seeking behaviors, and

## BOX 10-4 GENOMICS
### The Nurse's Role in Health Education

Currently the role of all nurses in providing competent genomics education involves:

- Becoming knowledgeable about basic genetic and genomics information relevant to their practice setting and population
- Identifying risks based on three-generation family history (pedigree)
- Recognizing ethical issues such as the right to determine what information to disclose to whom
- Discussing genetic or genomic factors revealed by the history that increase the risk of disease or may guide the selection of treatment options
- Explaining the difference between genetic screening and genetic testing (screening indicates a level of risk, whereas testing provides definitive diagnosis)
- Clarifying the meaning of test results and the implications for the family
- Understanding how family values and experience influence understanding of genetic/genomic facts, the difficult nature of decision-making, and the variability in personal risk interpretation
- Providing reliable sources for genetic education such as Genetics and Genomics for Patients and the Public (https://www.genome.gov/17516481)
- Cautioning the client about the use of direct-to-consumer testing because of the possible lack of information about validity, counseling, confidentiality
- Referring individuals to the appropriate level of professional help for further information

From Lea, D. H., Skirton, H., Read, C. Y., & Williams, J. K. (2011). Implications for educating the next generation of nurses on genetics and genomics in the 21st century. *Journal of Nursing Scholarship*, 43(1), 3–12.

## BOX 10-5 INNOVATIVE PRACTICE
### Empowering Rural Low-Income Mothers

Rural women often face health challenges such as limited access to care, poverty, and increased rates of obesity. A participatory project focused on empowerment by engaging mothers in designing health messages that appealed to them. The empowerment process addressed self-efficacy and personal control, positive and negative reinforcement, and barriers specific to the mothers' everyday lives.

Forty-three low-income mothers from different racial and ethnic groups from rural counties in eight states participated in focus groups. They discussed food security, physical activity, and oral health. From the discussions, the main elements of health messages preferred by the mothers emerged. They wanted the spokesperson to be a combination of a peer with facts from an authority. Most of the mothers preferred that messages focus on positive results of doing a health behavior rather than negative results of not doing it. The mothers insisted that messages be simple and fit in with and show empathy for their hectic daily lives. The voices of these rural low-income mothers illustrate how educational messages can be co-created with the target group that are culturally relevant and meaningful.

From Aldoory, L., Braun, B., Maring, E. F., Duggal, M., & Briones, R. L. (2015). Empowerment in the process of health messaging for rural low-income mothers: An exploratory message design project. *Women & Health*, 55, 297–313.

attitudes toward health providers, and play a role in their use of traditional and complementary healing practices. Prevention strategies must address each group's unique culture, experiences, language, age, sex, and sexual orientation and be culturally and linguistically appropriate for them to be effective (Perez & Luquis, 2014).

Another challenge for health professionals is to apply health-education strategies with people from diverse cultural backgrounds, people who do not speak English as their native language, and people with limited health literacy levels (Box 10-5: Innovative Practice).

Nurses also need to provide a welcoming environment for the lesbian, gay, bisexual, and transgender community. This involves, but is not limited to, using inclusive language (such as "partner" rather than "spouse" and "relationship status" instead of "marital status"), not making assumptions, and respecting each person's sexual self-identity (Perez & Luquis, 2014).

The health professional needs to take the time to assess cultural beliefs that influence social and health practices and make an effort to analyze educational interventions that are acceptable and satisfying to the individual. Social marketing processes and the diffusion of innovations model discussed in the next section help one identify characteristics, interests, and concerns of target populations.

When teaching people of different cultural, racial, and ethnic groups, the nurse endeavors to provide culturally sensitive education. Nurses recognize that the person's or group's background, beliefs, and knowledge may differ significantly from their own and seek to understand and show respect for these differences (Degazon, 2012) (Box 10-6: Diversity Awareness).

## COMMUNITY AND GROUP HEALTH EDUCATION

When nurses begin to teach groups of people, they automatically enter a program planning and administrative process. When an organization wants to offer an ongoing health-education program for a target population, social marketing provides a strategy for reaching members of the group and implementing a service that will satisfy these members as consumers. Principles of social marketing and health-education strategies are combined to promote population-based changes in behavior to improve health. Concepts from community group health behavior change models and health-education strategies are combined to promote population-based changes to improve health.

**Social marketing** is defined as "a process that uses marketing principles and techniques to influence priority audience behaviors that will benefit society as well as the individual. The process relies on creating, communicating, delivering, and exchanging offerings that have value for individuals, clients, partners, and society at large" (Joint Committee on Health Education and Promotion Terminology, 2012). The primary objective of social marketing is to change behavior. Social marketing provides a strategy for reaching members of the group and implementing a service that will satisfy these members as consumers.

Social marketing communication reaches beyond the individual level to influence social conditions, policy, legislation, and normative group behavior. Key attributes of a social marketing approach are the offering of benefits and the reduction of barriers to

---

### BOX 10-6 DIVERSITY AWARENESS
*Cultural Aspects of Health Teaching*

**When There Is a Language Barrier**
- Use courtesy and a formal approach.
- Address the person by his or her last name.
- Introduce yourself, pointing to yourself as you give your name.
- Project a friendly attitude with a smile and a handshake.
- Speak with a moderate tone and volume.
- Attempt to use words in the person's language, which indicates respect for the individual's culture.
- Use simple, everyday words rather than complex words, medical jargon, or colloquialisms.
- Use hand gestures to help the person understand.
- Instruct the person in small increments.
- Have the person demonstrate understanding of the message.
- Provide written instructions for the person to take home.
- When available, use flash cards and phrase books in other languages.
- Use qualified health care interpreters.[a]

**Areas to Consider in Cultural Assessment**
- Individual's identification with a particular cultural group
- Habits, customs, values, and beliefs
- Language and communication patterns
- Cultural sanctions and restrictions
- Healing beliefs and practices
- Cultural health practices
- Kinship and social networks
- Nutritional beliefs, food preferences, and restrictions
- Religious beliefs and practices related to health
- Attitudes, values, and beliefs about health (Andrews & Boyle, 2008)[b]

[a]For specific requirements of the Joint Commission. (2014). *Advancing effective communication, cultural competence, and patient-and family-centered care: A roadmap for hospitals.* https://www.jointcommission.org/roadmap_for_hospitals/
[b]From Andrews, M. M., & Boyle, J. S. (2008). *Transcultural concepts in nursing care* (5th ed.). Philadelphia: Wolters Kluwer/Lippincott.

---

### BOX 10-7 Steps in the Teaching-Learning Process

- Assessment
  - Learner characteristics
  - Learning needs
- Development of expected learning outcomes
- Development of a teaching plan
  - Content
  - Teaching strategies, learning activities
- Implementation of the teaching plan
- Evaluation of expected outcomes
  - Achievement of learning outcomes
  - Evaluation of the teaching process

---

influence the target group's behavior. Social marketers attempt to modify the attractiveness of specific behavioral options to favor one choice over competing alternatives. The systematic approach to understanding and responding to specific audience characteristics makes the messages more appealing (Storey et al., 2015). Social marketing strategies could be used in designing programs for health promotion (tobacco use, obesity), injury prevention (seat belt wearing, gun storage), and environmental protection (pesticides, water conservation) (Cheng et al., 2011). Any information about the target population that is generated by social marketing strategies will improve the nurse's ability to develop effective educational interventions.

Another model commonly used in community health-education planning is the diffusion of innovations model (Rogers, 2003), which explains how an idea or product is adopted and spreads through a social system. In public health, diffusion of innovations is used to address the factors that support or inhibit the adoption of effective, evidence-based interventions to improve community health. Practical application of the model involves understanding the target population and recognizing the importance of achieving a good fit among the characteristics of the innovation, the community adopting it, and the context or environment for change. (Brownson et al., 2015).

## TEACHING PLAN

Preparation for teaching a group program, such as a seminar or course, begins after the marketing and administrative plans are well under way. These activities ensure that there are enough participants for the program, and they provide the structure for developing the teaching plan—the program objectives, available time, human and material resources, and so on. When the marketing and administrative functions have been provided by others, and when educational strategies are developed for one person at a time, the nurse can concentrate efforts on developing the teaching plan.

A health teaching plan may emphasize a phase of the behavior change process that is related to the individual's or group's health-promotion needs or problems. The written teaching plan represents a package of educational services provided to a consumer or student. The plan is written from the learner's point of view (Box 10-7).

The process of generating a teaching plan helps the nurse recognize and use methods of learning that involve the individual as an active participant. The plan includes a list of specific actions or abilities that the person may perform at intervals during and at the end of the educational intervention. Teaching plans help nurses clarify these outcomes. Preparing a teaching plan involves the steps of the teaching-learning process outlined in Box 10-7.

### Assessment

Assessment, the first step in the process, involves determining the characteristics of the learner and identifying learning needs. The following characteristics of the learner are important for the nurse to identify and consider in planning:
- Age, developmental stage in the life cycle, and level of education
- Health beliefs
- Motivation and readiness to learn
- Health risks and problems
- Current knowledge and skills
- Barriers and facilitators to learning

The reader is encouraged to refer to the chapters (see Unit 4) about individual development. Assessment of the learner can be accomplished by one answering the following five questions:

- What are the characteristics and learning capabilities of the individual?
- What are the learner's needs for health promotion, risk reduction, or health problems?
- What does the person already know and what skills can the person already perform that are relevant to the health needs?
- Is the learner motivated to change any unhealthy behaviors?
- What are the barriers to and facilitators of health behavior change?

When preparing a teaching plan for one person in a primary care setting, the nurse may learn background information about the individual from that person's record and agency reports that include descriptions of the person's population group. Nurses often agree to teach health classes that others have organized. In this case the nurse asks for project reports that provide marketing and needs-assessment information about the students who are expected to attend the classes (see the care plan at the end of the chapter).

## Determining Expected Learning Outcomes

To determine the expected learning outcomes of a health-education intervention, the nurse answers the following questions:

- What broad public health and social goals guide the proposed educational program?
- What are the participant's learning goals?
- What does the learner need to know, do, and believe to progress through the behavior change process?

### Program Goals

The program goals of a health-education project reflect the desire to facilitate improvement in some health problem or social living condition. Program goals are broad statements on long-range expected accomplishments that provide direction; they do not have to be stated in measurable terms (Miller & Stoeckel, 2011).

### Learning Goals

Learning goals are best established when the student and the nurse work together. These goals reflect the health behavior or health status change that the person will have achieved by the end of an educational intervention. Learning goals relate to the program goals.

### Learning Objectives

Learning objectives indicate the steps to be taken by the individual toward meeting the learning goal, and may involve the development of knowledge, skill, or change in attitude. Objectives are most useful when stated in behavioral terms and when they contain the following components: the learner and a precise action verb that indicates what the learner will be able to do; the conditions under which the task is performed; and the level of performance expected (Bastable & Alt, 2014). Learning

objectives guide the selection of content and methods and help narrow the focus of a teaching plan to more achievable steps; they also aid in setting standards of performance and suggesting evaluation strategies.

## Selecting Content

To select appropriate content for a health-education program, the nurse considers what information, skills, and attitudes need to be taught and the level of learning to be achieved.

### Three Domains of Learning

Content is commonly divided into three domains: cognitive; psychomotor; and affective. Cognitive learning refers to the development of new facts or concepts, and building on or applying knowledge to new situations. Psychomotor learning involves developing physical skills from simple to complex actions. Affective learning alludes to the recognition of values, religious and spiritual beliefs, family interaction patterns and relationships, and personal attitudes that affect decisions and problem-solving progress.

To learn or change a health behavior, a person may need to acquire new information, practice some physical techniques, and clarify the ways in which the new behavior may affect relationships with others. The nurse's role is to select a combination of content from the three domains that is appropriate to meet the behavioral objective. To find samples of content for a teaching plan, the nurse researches resource materials, such as books, teaching guides, journal articles, pamphlets, and flyers created by nonprofit agencies and professional organizations. The nurse is careful about giving students materials with technical vocabulary that is too complex for the audience.

### Examples of Learning Objectives

In writing learning objectives, the nurse selects action verbs from the taxonomies previously mentioned that indicate observable learning. In Table 10-1 examples are given for objectives in each domain of learning. The first objective listed for each domain is incorrect because the verb does not indicate observable learning. The second example for each domain is measurable because the

| TABLE 10-1 Examples of Nonmeasurable and Measurable Objectives | |
|---|---|
| **Domain** | **Objectives** |
| Cognitive | **Not measurable:** Dan will understand the correct food choices for following a low-fat diet<br>**Measurable:** Dan will correctly **select** low-fat foods from the options provided |
| Affective | **Not measurable:** Dan will demonstrate the importance of weight loss<br>**Measurable:** Dan will **verbalize** the importance of weight loss |
| Psychomotor | **Not measurable:** Dan will know how to determine a serving<br>**Measurable:** Dan will **demonstrate** correct measurement of a one-serving portion |

verb used (indicated in boldface type) allows the learning to be observed.

When preparing a teaching plan, the nurse differentiates between information the individual needs to know and information considered helpful to know to develop appropriate learning objectives. This process provides cues to the nurse for planning effective strategies for the necessary level of learning. As the level of learning to be achieved becomes complex, the educational strategies and methods selected involve the individuals in more active application and analysis of the content.

## Designing Learning Strategies

Designing the learning strategies for an educational intervention involves selecting the methods and tools and structuring the sequence of activities. The teaching plan to this point provides the foundation on which to base the activity selection and sequence. The following questions guide the design of learning strategies:

- What are some basic considerations for selecting teaching methods for health-education programs?
- How does the nurse, as instructor, establish and maintain a learning climate?
- What actions can the nurse perform to increase the effectiveness of the learning methods?
- What are the appropriate methods for each learning domain?
- What methods tend to promote behavior change?

### Teaching Strategies

Numerous strategies for teaching are available (Table 10-2). A few of those most commonly used are listed and described here. Lecture is a well-known method in which the teacher verbally presents information and instructions to the person or audience. Lecture provides a way to present a large amount of information to a number of people in a nonthreatening way. This can be an effective method if active learning strategies such as questioning are integrated. Discussion involves interaction between the nurse educator and the individuals. The nurse prepares questions in advance to guide the discussion. This method allows an opportunity for the nurse to gain a better perception of the individuals' understanding of the topic and to clarify the information.

Demonstration and practice is used in learning psychomotor skills such as performing exercises. The nurse demonstrates the expected behavior while the person observes. Then the nurse watches and provides feedback and encouragement while the person performs the behavior. Using the actual equipment that the individual will use in his or her home facilitates successful performance. For complex tasks, teaching a few steps at a time, in sequence, aids skill development.

Simulation gaming may involve computer learning, board games, or role play. Obviously, computer learning games are dependent on the availability of hardware and software appropriate for the individual and the topic. Simple board games can be developed for cognitive learning. An example might be the development of a bingo game based on the food pyramid. Role play involves acting out a potential scenario. This allows individuals to practice appropriate responses to challenging situations. For example, a person restricted to a low-fat diet can act out a response to being offered dessert by an insistent family member or friend played by the nurse (Figure 10-2).

### Considerations for Selecting Methods

The nurse's first consideration is to promote an environment and use methods that foster self-directed learning. An active participant usually learns more.

| TABLE 10-2 Domains of Learning, Teaching Strategies, and Examples of Desired Outcomes Related to a Behavior Change | | |
|---|---|---|
| **Domain of Learning** | **Teaching Strategies** | **Examples of Desired Outcomes Related to a Behavior Change** |
| Cognitive (thinking) | Lecture<br>One-to-one instruction<br>Discussion<br>Discovery<br>Audiovisual or printed materials<br>Computer-assisted instruction | Describes and/or explains information relevant to the behavior change |
| Affective (feeling) | Role modeling<br>Discussion<br>Role playing<br>Simulation gaming | Expresses positive feeling, attitudes, values toward changing the behavior |
| Psychomotor (acting) | Demonstration<br>Practice<br>Mental imaging | Demonstrates performance of skills related to the behavior change |

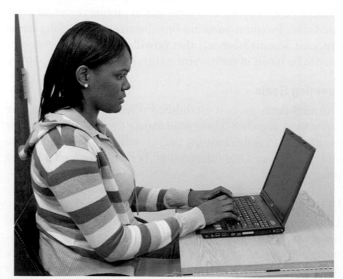

**FIGURE 10-2** Woman using the Internet as a source for health information. (From Young-Adams, A. P. [2011]. Kinn's the administrative medical assistant, an applied learning approach [7th ed.]. St. Louis: Saunders.)

There will be many learning styles in a group audience; therefore the nurse varies the teaching methods used in a given session. Taking into consideration the characteristics of the population (developmental stage, age, and knowledge of the topic), the nurse selects teaching methods that best support the goals and theme of the educational program. The order of content proceeds from simple ideas and skills to the more complex concepts, from known material toward lesser-known data. The nurse is sensitive to the energy level and anxiety of the audience when presenting content that requires strong concentration or causes anxiety.

### Learning Climate

For group presentations the nurse addresses several activities when seeking to establish an environment that is conducive to health behavior change. The first activity is creating a sense of preparedness and organization by providing physical facilities with adequate furnishings and suitable audiovisual materials and handouts. Even the instructor's appearance will lend credibility or distraction to the presentation.

The second activity involves anticipating the needs of the group and communicating information about the schedule and the facilities. This action alleviates the group's apprehension and makes the group members more comfortable.

The third activity focuses on the nurse's assessment of the individual and group learning needs, possibly through questions and dialogue. Members of the group need to believe that the program will be beneficial and relevant to their situations. The instructor watches for and reinforces signs of motivation to participate in the experience.

Fourth, having established a positive learning climate, the nurse seeks to maintain a high level of motivation, a sense of individualized attention, and a progression. As a reality check, the nurse might ask for periodic feedback from the group about the effectiveness of the program and its relevance to group needs.

Finally, the nurse works with the group to maintain the learning climate. This process involves observing group interactions, helping individuals to participate, intervening to help the group deal with controlling its members, and remaining cognizant of dynamics in the group process that will facilitate or inhibit learning.

### Teaching for Each Learning Domain

As mentioned, teaching is directed toward one or more of three learning domains: cognitive, psychomotor, and affective. Examples of appropriate teaching strategies for each domain and the expected outcomes in relation to behavior change are summarized in Table 10-2.

### Evaluating the Teaching-Learning Process

The teacher can evaluate the learning, or measure achievement of learning objectives, in all domains through the use of written or oral testing, demonstrations, observation, self-reports, and self-monitoring. Teaching methods for one domain may overlap those for another domain.

The nurse can incorporate written, verbal, and nonverbal techniques for obtaining feedback about teaching performance

into the teaching plan. End-of-program questionnaires are the usual method for obtaining written feedback. The nurse may ask for verbal feedback at various times from the group, from individual students, and from observers of the class. Nonverbal communication cues from participants may indicate their satisfaction, fatigue, or frustration with the educational intervention.

The overall process of the teaching-learning experience needs to be evaluated. The procedures used to organize and promote an educational program can affect its ultimate success. The nurse (or a program administration committee) records activities such as advertising, registration, fee collection, and availability and repair of equipment and materials. This evaluative information can then be used to improve subsequent programs. Surveys by telephone or by questionnaires help obtain the consumer's opinion about these implementation procedures. Word-of-mouth referrals to future programs and support from other community agencies and professionals may also indicate approval of the program format.

Occasionally the nurse is asked to justify a health-education program in terms of its effect on the community's public health goals or social problems. Health promotion involves a combination of health-protection activities, preventive health services, and health-education programs; therefore drawing a direct correlation between an educational intervention and the statistical improvement of the health problem can be difficult.

Nurses can often describe the theoretical influence of an educational intervention on health behaviors, health problems, and social problems. Statistics such as the number of people served each year, the percentage of the target population reached, the number of service providers used, and the number and cost of programs are important and need to be preserved. As these statistics change over time, the data will provide cues to program successes and problems.

### Referring Individuals to Other Resources

The end of a teaching plan includes resources for people to use for continuing education, counseling, peer support, and health services. Nurses encourage people to view health education as a lifelong learning process. Each person has different developmental needs and health concerns through the life cycle. Moreover, any one educational intervention may help a person move only from one phase of the behavior change process to the next. Additionally, the Internet as a health-education tool may influence a person's health practices.

## TEACHING AND ORGANIZING SKILLS

To develop teaching and organizing skills in health education, the nurse often needs to learn new behaviors. A systematic guide can be used to learn these professional skills. To perform these steps, the nurse does the following:
- Seeks self-assessment opportunities.
- Identifies, lists, and prioritizes learning needs.
- Begins to identify the resources that are available for reading, instructor training, and practice teaching.
- Drafts an initial set of learning goals.
- Selects the target population and the general topic.

- Works through the steps of the teaching-learning process, including the development of a teaching plan.
- Identifies other people or a project team to help.

After implementing the educational intervention, the nurse sets time aside to discuss what happened. Did the program go as planned? What changes were made in the teaching plan? What can be changed for the next program? The nurse reviews the self-developed learning goals and determines new ones.

In addition, health-education research evaluates teaching interventions. This contributes to the evidence base from which nurses can implement new teaching strategies or question the effectiveness of traditional approaches. For an example of a study comparing the effects of using narrative information versus traditional information to teach a high-risk group, see Box 10-8: Research for Evidence-Based Practice.

As additional programs on either an individual or a group basis are provided, the nurse will be able to clarify specific instructor teaching and organizing skills that come naturally.

These skills tend to improve a program's effectiveness and enable the logistics to run smoothly. The teacher is first a learner; this is true in health education and any other form of education.

## SUMMARY

Of all health professionals, nurses spend the most time in direct contact with individuals; they have many opportunities to recognize a need for knowledge and a readiness to learn new information and behaviors. Nurses often coordinate group programs. The more accurate the analysis of the educational aspects of a health-promotion program and the assessment of characteristics and learning needs of the target audience, the more effective an educational intervention will be in influencing health behaviors.

The principles of health education form a generic basis for implementing a variety of health topics, such as accident prevention and use of first aid, expectant parent education, hypertension education, nutrition and fitness, stress management, substance abuse, sex education, and education in areas including diabetes and arthritis. The two scenarios described in this chapter provide insights into the nurse's role in conducting educational interventions about family planning and prenatal care.

Planning to teach one person is different from planning to teach a group. One-to-one interventions tend to follow a counseling or problem-solving approach. Group interventions can range from guided discussions on concerns that evolve from the group to a more structured learning experience involving presentations, skill practice, and attitude-awareness exercises. The range of health-education strategies provides nurses and all health care professionals with techniques and methods applicable in health service settings, schools, work sites, and other community facilities.

---

## BOX 10-8    RESEARCH FOR EVIDENCE-BASED PRACTICE

### *Promoting Health Among Teens Intervention*

Because black Americans are disproportionately affected by cardiovascular disease and cancer, this health-promotion intervention targeted black American youth to address behaviors that contribute to these disparities in adults. Promoting Health Among Teens (PHAT) is a brief, culturally tailored health-education curriculum focused on dietary behaviors, physical activity, and substance use knowledge in black American teens.

A total of 1654 teens aged 14 to 17 years participated, with at least 400 from each of four mid-sized eastern cities in the United States (Macon, Georgia; Providence, Rhode Island; Syracuse, New York; and Columbia, South Carolina). The teens were randomly assigned to either the PHAT group (experimental) or a sexual-health-promotion group (control). Comparison of general health knowledge at the baseline showed no significant difference between the experimental group and the control group.

The PHAT intervention curriculum consisted of eight modules designed to increase health knowledge, develop health behavior skills, change attitudes, increase self-efficacy, explore beliefs about personal health behaviors, and address factors that interfere with healthy behavior related to diet, physical activity, and substance abuse. The program was tailed to promote cultural pride in black American teens. Workshops were held on two consecutive Saturdays for a total of 16 contact hours with 12 to 13 participants per group. Various interactive learning strategies included discussion, games, role playing, and sharing exercises implemented by trained group facilitators. At least half of the trainers were black American to promote racial concordance. The consistency of the curriculum and implementation was maintained across sites throughout the project.

Audio computer-assisted self-interview (ACASI) was used to collect demographic characteristics, and assess knowledge and behaviors. ACASI helps to reduce literacy-related challenges and social desirability in participant response. Data collection occurred at the baseline and at 3, 6, and 12 months after the intervention to measure differences between PHAT participants and the control group in health knowledge, dietary behaviors, physical activity, and substance use.

PHAT program participants had significantly greater increases in health knowledge than the control group; however, their changes in behavior were modest. Importantly participants retained the higher knowledge at least 1 year after a brief intervention, and those with higher knowledge demonstrated greater behavior change. Recommendations for the future application of PHAT are to continue the emphasis on knowledge building while increasing the number of contact hours and spreading the intervention over several more days to facilitate behavior change. A longer intervention might allow facilitators to develop increased rapport and trust, practice health behaviors, and develop increased self-efficacy to implement and maintain behavior change. Further research is suggested to explore the differences in the impact of increased knowledge on specific risk behaviors.

From Kerr, J. C., Valois, R. F., Farber, N. B., Vanable, P. A., DiClemente, R. J., Salazar, L., et al. (2013). Effects of promoting health among teens on dietary, physical activity, and substance use knowledge and behaviors for African American adolescents. *American Journal of Health Education, 44*(4), 191–202.

## CASE STUDY
### Albert

Albert Mitchell is a 36-year-old man who will be traveling to Dubai to give a business presentation in 3 months. Although he has traveled widely in the United States as a consultant, this is his first trip to the Middle East. He requests information regarding immunizations needed before his trip. Albert states that as he will be in Dubai for only a few days, he is unlikely to contract a disease in such a short time and therefore believes that it is illogical to obtain immunizations. Albert states that he has heard that the side effects of the immunizations might be worse than the diseases they prevent. He is also concerned about leaving his wife at home alone because she is 6 months pregnant.

#### Reflective Questions
- How would you address Albert's beliefs?
- What learning would be needed in each domain?
- What learning theories would you consider?
- How might his family concerns be addressed?

## ◎ CARE PLAN
### Preparing a Teaching Plan

**\*NURSING DIAGNOSIS: Deficient knowledge (specify area)**

#### Defining Characteristics
- Verbalization of inadequate information or an inadequate recall of information
- Verbalization of misunderstanding or misconception
- Request for information
- Instructions followed inaccurately
- Inadequate performance on a test
- Inadequate demonstration of a skill

#### Related Factors
- Pathophysiological states
- Sensory deficits
- Memory loss
- Intellectual limitations
- Interfering coping strategies (denial or anxiety)
- Lack of exposure to accurate information
- Lack of motivation to learn
- Inattention
- Cultural or language barriers

#### Expected Outcomes
- The individual will express an interest in learning.
- The individual will correctly state the information on the specific topic.
- The individual will correctly demonstrate skills needed to practice health-related behavior.
- The individual and the family will explain how to incorporate new information into their lifestyle.
- The individual will modify health behavior on the basis of the acquisition of new knowledge.
- The individual will list resources for more information or support.

#### Interventions
- Provide accurate and culturally relevant information related to the specific topic.
- Select teaching techniques appropriate to the individual's learning needs.
- Explore the individual's interpretation of the information and its meaning in the context of the person's life.
- Demonstrate and then have the individual practice new skills.
- Assist the person in identifying and implementing alternative strategies when initial choices are not successful.
- Include the family or significant others as appropriate.
- Provide names and telephone numbers of resource people or organizations.

\*NANDA Nursing Diagnoses—Herdman, T. H. & Kamitsuru, S. (Eds.). Nursing Diagnoses–Definitions and Classification 2015–2017. Copyright © 2014, 1994–2014 NANDA International. Used by arrangement with John Wiley & Sons Limited. In order to make safe and effective judgments using the NANDA-I nursing diagnoses it is essential that nurses refer to the definitions and defining characteristics of the diagnoses listed in this work.

## REFERENCES

American Nurses Association. (2010). *Nursing's social policy statement.* Washington, DC: American Nurses Association.

American Nurses Association. (2015). *Nursing: Scope and standards of practice* (3rd ed.). Silver Spring, MD: American Nurses Association.

Anderson, D. G., & Fallin, A. (2012). Family health risks. In M. Stanhope & J. Lancaster (Eds.), *Public health nursing: Population-centered health care in the community* (8th ed.). St. Louis: Mosby.

Bandura, A. (1997). *Self-efficacy: The exercise of control.* New York: W.H. Freeman.

Bastable, S. B., & Alt, M. F. (2014). Behavioral objectives. In S. B. Bastable (Ed.), *Nurse as educator: Principles of teaching and learning for nursing practice* (4th ed.). Burlington, MA: Jones & Bartlett.

Bauer, U. E., et al. (2014). Prevention of chronic disease in the 21st century: Elimination of the leading preventable causes of premature death and disability in the USA. *Lancet, 384,* 45–52.

Baur, C. (2011). Calling the nation to act: Implementing the national action plan to improve health literacy. *Nursing Outlook, 59*(2), 63–69.

Braverman, P. A., et al. (2011). Health disparities and health equity: The issue is justice. *American Journal of Public Health, 101*(Suppl. 1), S149–S155.

Brownson, R. C., et al. (2015). Implementation, diffusion, & dissemination of public health interventions. In K. Glanz, B. K. Rimer, & K. Viswanath (Eds.), *Health behavior and health education: Theory, research, and practice* (5th ed.). San Francisco: Jossey-Bass.

Burkhardt, M. A., & Nathaniel, A. K. (2014). *Ethics and issues in contemporary nursing* (4th ed.). Melbourne: Cengage Learning.

Centers for Disease Control and Prevention, US Department of Health and Human Services (USDHHS). (2014). Strategies for reducing health disparities—Selected CDC-sponsored interventions, US, 2014. *Morbidity and Mortality Weekly Report, 63*(1), 1–48.

Cheng, H., Kotler, P., & Lee, N. R. (2011). *Social marketing for public health: Global trends and success stories.* Sudbury, MA: Jones & Bartlett.

Degazon, C. E. (2012). Cultural diversity in the community. In M. Stanhope & J. Lancaster (Eds.), *Public health nursing: Population-centered health care in the community* (8th ed.). St. Louis: Mosby.

Joint Committee on Health Education and Promotion Terminology. (2012). Report of the 2011 Joint Committee on Health Education and Promotion Terminology. *American Journal of Health Education, 43*(2), 15.

Koh, H. K., Nowinski, J. M., & Piotrowski, J. J. (2011). A 2020 vision for educating the next generation of public health leaders. *American Journal of Preventive Medicine, 40*(2), 199–202.

Miller, M. A., & Stoeckel, P. R. (2011). *Client education: Theory and practice.* Sudbury, MA: Jones & Bartlett.

Osborne, H. (2013). *Health literacy from A to Z: Practical ways to communicate your health message* (2nd ed.). Burlington, MA: Jones & Bartlett Learning.

Perez, M. A., & Luquis, R. R. (2014). *Cultural competence in health education and health promotion* (2nd ed.). San Francisco, CA: Jossey-Bass.

Prochaska, J. O., & DiClemente, C. C. (1984). *The transtheoretical approach: Crossing traditional boundaries of change.* Homewood, NJ: Dow Jones-Irwin.

Prochaska, J. O., Redding, C. A., & Evers, K. E. (2015). The transtheoretical model and stages of change. In K. Glanz, B. K. Rimer, & K. Viswanath (Eds.), *Health behavior and health education: Theory, research, and practice* (5th ed.). San Francisco: Jossey-Bass.

Quality and Safety in Nursing Institute. (2014). *QSEN competencies.* Cleveland, OH: Quality and Safety Institute, Case Western Reserve University. http://qsen.org/competencies/pre-licensure-ksas/.

Richards, E. (2014). Compliance, motivation, and health behaviors of the learner. In S. B. Bastable (Ed.), *Nurse as educator: Principles of teaching and learning for nursing practice* (4th ed.). Burlington, MA: Jones & Bartlett.

Rogers, E. M. (2003). *Diffusion of innovations* (5th ed.). New York: Free Press.

Rosenstock, I. M., Strecher, K. J., & Becker, M. H. (1988). The social learning theory and health belief model. *Health Education Quarterly, 15,* 175–183.

Simons-Morton, B. G., McLeroy, K. R., & Wendel, M. L. (2012). *Behavior theory in health promotion practice and research.* Burlington, MA: Jones & Bartlett Learning.

Skinner, C. S., Champion, V. L., & Tiro, J. (2015). The health belief model. In K. Glanz, B. K. Rimer, & K. Viswanath (Eds.), *Health behavior and health education: Theory, research, and practice* (5th ed.). San Francisco: Jossey-Bass.

Storey, J. D., Hess, R., & Saffitz, G. B. (2015). Social marketing. In K. Glanz, B. K. Rimer, & K. Viswanath (Eds.), *Health behavior and health education: Theory, research, and practice* (5th ed.). San Francisco: Jossey-Bass.

US Department of Health and Human Services (USDHHS). (2010). Healthy People 2020. http://www.healthypeople.gov.

US Department of Health and Human Services (USDHHS). (2016). Health literacy. http://www.hrsa.gov/publichealth/healthliteracy/.

World Health Organization. (2016). Health education. http://www.who.int/topics/health_education/en/.

# 11

# Nutrition Counseling for Health Promotion

*Myrtle McCulloch and Staci McIntosh*

## OBJECTIVES

*After completing this chapter, the reader will be able to:*

- Evaluate the objectives outlined in *Healthy People 2020* nutrition and food safety issues.
- Analyze the leading diet-related causes of illness and death in the United States and the corresponding nutrients specific to each.
- Summarize and evaluate the rationale behind the recommendations contained in the *Dietary Guidelines for Americans 2015–2020*.
- Compare the number of servings and serving sizes recommended in MyPlate with serving sizes featured currently in the marketplace.
- Analyze US food aid programs for marginalized groups and older adults in the United States.
- Evaluate personal diet intakes over a 24-hour to 48-hour period using SuperTracker (https://www.supertracker.usda.gov) to learn how to plan diets for any stage in the life cycle.

## KEY TERMS

Body mass index
Botanicals
Cancer
Cardiovascular diseases
Cholesterol
Cirrhosis
Coronary heart disease
Diabetes mellitus
Dietary Approaches to Stop
    Hypertension (DASH)
Dietary Guidelines Advisory
    Committee
Dietary Guidelines for Americans
Dietary reference intakes
Dyslipidemia
Fiber
Food insecurity
Food secure

Heart disease
Hemolytic uremic syndrome
Hemorrhagic colitis
Herbals
High-density lipoprotein cholesterol
Human immunodeficiency virus
Hyperglycemia
Hyperlipidemia
Hypertension
Incidence
Lacto-ovo vegetarian
Low-density lipoprotein cholesterol
Metabolic syndrome
Micronutrients
Microbiome
MyPlate
Nutrition screening
Nutrigenomics

Nutritional genomics
Obese
Osteoporosis
Overweight
Pre-diabetes
Pre-hypertension
Prevalence
Salmonellosis
Serving sizes
Stroke
Sugar
Teratogenic
Trans fat
Triglyceride
Type 2 diabetes
Underweight
Vegan

## NUTRITION IN THE UNITED STATES: LOOKING FORWARD FROM THE PAST

### Classic Vitamin-Deficiency Diseases

Food and nutrition have always been important to health. Until as recently as the 1940s, many nutrient-deficiency diseases, such as rickets, pellagra, scurvy, beriberi, xerophthalmia (eye fails to produce tears), and goiter, were still prevalent in the United States (Carpenter, 2000). Although these conditions still persist in some developing countries, they have virtually disappeared from developed areas of the world. The availability of an abundant food supply, the fortification of some foods with critical nutrients, and the implementation of better methods of determining and increasing the nutrient contents of foods have contributed to the decline of nutrient-deficiency diseases.

The introduction of iodized salt in the 1920s, for example, contributed greatly to elimination of iodine-deficiency goiter as a public health problem. Similarly, beriberi and pellagra disappeared after the discovery that inadequate thiamine and niacin levels respectively contribute to these diseases. Today, nutrient deficiencies are mostly seen as iron and calcium deficits, with osteoporosis and anemia respectively being the most common, as well as malnutrition related to obesity and its related comorbidities. The few cases of protein-energy malnutrition that are listed annually as causes of death generally occur as secondary results of severe illness or injury, premature birth, child neglect, problems of the homebound aged, alcoholism, or some combination of these factors. Although undernutrition still occurs in some groups of people in the United States, including those who are isolated or poor, these once-prevalent diseases of nutritional deficiency have been replaced by diseases of dietary excess and imbalance (Table 11-1).

### Dietary Inadequacy

Calorie inadequacies can have devastating effects in children in developing countries leading to wasting and stunting syndromes. Although not to the same degree, many impoverished areas in the United States show some degree of these imbalances.

Although there are differences as to their causes, eating disorders are also classified as calorie imbalances. These can be seen in any sex and age group, with some starting in elementary school children. For diagnostic purposes, there are four conditions: anorexia nervosa, bulimia nervosa, binge eating disorder, and disordered eating not otherwise specified. The latter may include binge eating, compulsive overeating, or overexercising with respect to the calories consumed.

Depending on the length of time and the age of the individual, the physiological consequences, especially for anorexia nervosa, are life threatening. Long-term complications may include alterations in the heart rate and blood pressure, depletion of lean mass, anemia, bone loss, amenorrhea, hypoglycemia, and psychological symptoms. Early diagnosis and treatment are critical to the success of recovery.

### Dietary Excesses

Problems resulting from dietary imbalances (i.e., overconsumption of some foods groups and inadequate consumption of other food groups) now rank among the leading causes of illness and death in the United States. As stated in 2015 by the US Department of Health and Human Services (USDHHS) and the US Department of Agriculture (USDA) in their *Dietary Guidelines for Americans 2015–2020* (USDHHS & USDA, 2015), "the US population, across almost every age and sex group, consumes eating patterns that are low in vegetables, fruits, whole grains, dairy, seafood, and oil and high in refined grains, added sugars, saturated fats, sodium, and for some age-sex groups, high in the meats, poultry, and eggs subgroup."

Four leading causes of death directly associated with diet are coronary heart disease (CHD), some types of cancer, stroke, and diabetes mellitus (DM). Four other major causes of death—accidents, cirrhosis, suicide, and homicide—are often associated with excessive alcohol intake.

## TABLE 11-1   Health Problems Related to Poor Nutrition

| Health Problem[a] | Contributing Lifestyle and Nutrition Practices[b] |
|---|---|
| Anemia | Diet with inadequate iron, folate, or vitamin B12 intake (depending on type of anemia) |
| Cancer (breast, cervical, and colon) | Excessive calorie intake, belly fat; low fiber intake |
| Cirrhosis | Excessive alcohol intake |
| Constipation | Inadequate fiber or fluid intake; high fat intake; sedentary lifestyle |
| Dental caries | Excessive, frequent consumption of concentrated sweets or sugar-sweetened beverages; lack of fluoride; poor dental hygiene |
| Type 2 diabetes | Excessive calorie intake; excessive fat intake (in particular saturated fat, trans fat); sedentary lifestyle |
| Cardiovascular/heart disease | Excessive calorie intake; excessive fat intake (in particular saturated fat, trans fat); excessive sodium intake, inadequate fiber intake; sedentary lifestyle |
| Hypertension | Excessive sodium and insufficient potassium intake; excessive calorie intake; possible excess alcohol intake; sedentary lifestyle |
| Obesity | Excessive calorie intake; excessive fat intake; sedentary lifestyle |
| Osteoporosis | Low calcium intake; low vitamin D intake; excessive intake of protein, sodium, and caffeine; sedentary lifestyle; excessive alcohol intake |
| Underweight and growth failure | Inadequate calorie intake; poor diet |

[a]A number of health problems are caused or exacerbated by poor nutrition. Health care professionals strive to prevent or delay these health problems.
[b]Not all may apply in every case.

Current statistics show that two in three American adults and one in three children are either overweight or obese (Flegal et al., 2010). Although adult levels of overweight/obesity on their own are alarming, excess weight among the young has been linked to health problems that until now were seen only in adults: high blood pressure, type 2 diabetes, and high cholesterol levels (White House Task Force on Childhood Obesity, 2010). Although there has been a slight leveling off as compared with earlier statistics (National Center for Health Statistics, 2010), the proportion of American children who are obese is currently 17% (Ogden et al., 2014).

Reducing the incidence of obesity in any age group is vital to overall health. Although excess weight or obesity is commonly viewed as an imbalance between energy intake and energy expenditure, other factors need to be considered, such as the environment, race, and socioeconomic status. For example, genes are involved in the process of energy balance as well as in differences in fat distribution by sex and age (Bray & Champagne, 2007). The more recent interest in the human microbiome has generated studies on microbial gut alterations, obesity (Kaplanm & Walker, 2012), and diabetes (Tai et al., 2015).

The fifth guideline of the *Dietary Guidelines for Americans 2015–2020* states: "Support healthy eating patterns for all: Everyone has a role in helping to create and support healthy eating patterns in multiple settings nationwide, from home to school to work to communities." The guidelines acknowledge the importance of a coordinated, system-wide approach that engages all sectors of influence. Figure 11-1 demonstrates the complex layers of influence that shape a person's food and physical activity choices. Creating and supporting a healthy eating pattern means that such influential factors have been taken into consideration and that healthy food options should be made available and should be accessible to all individuals. In support of this guideline, the Centers for Disease Control and Prevention (CDC) has proposed

strategies for both providing healthy food and preventing obesity in the United States (see Box 11-1: Innovative Practice for examples).

Encouraging healthy choices in diet, exercise, and weight control is also one of the major themes of *Healthy People 2020* (USDHHS, 2010a) (Figure 11-2). It also includes a new framework to include additional emphasis on health disparities and health inequities, as well as focus on future measures to help healthy choices be the easy choice wherever people live, work, learn, and play.

Because dietary factors contribute substantially to the burden of preventable illness and premature death, *Healthy People 2020* aims at directing American dietary patterns toward current recommendations, especially the *Dietary Guidelines for Americans 2015–2020* (USDHHS & USDA, 2015).

## *HEALTHY PEOPLE 2020:* NUTRITION OBJECTIVES

The nutrition and weight status objectives of *Healthy People 2020* (Box 11-2: *Healthy People 2020*) reflect evidence-based science supporting the health benefits of consuming a nutritious diet and maintaining a healthy body weight. The objectives also emphasize that efforts to change diet and weight should address individual behaviors, as well as policies and environments that support these behaviors, in settings such as schools, work sites, health care organizations, and communities.

The report also contains 12 topics of leading health indicators, with "Nutrition, Physical Activity, and Obesity" being one of them. Although the importance of physical activity will be discussed in Chapter 12, combining physical activity with nutrition and obesity as one topic illustrates how interrelated they are. Details of the leading nutrition health indicators are listed in Box 11-2: *Healthy People 2020*.

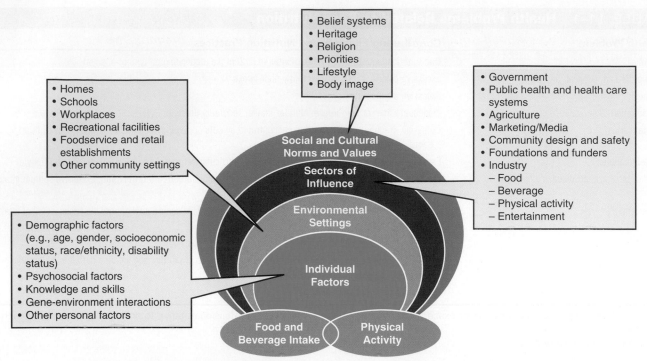

**FIGURE 11-1** Social-ecological framework for food and physical activity decisions. (From US Department of Health and Human Services & US Department of Agriculture. [2015]. *Dietary guidelines for Americans 2015–2020* [8th ed.]. http://health.gov/dietaryguidelines/2015/guidelines/.)

---

### ☀ BOX 11-1    INNOVATIVE PRACTICE

*Summary of Recommended Community Strategies and Measurements to Prevent Obesity in the United States Related to Healthy Foods*[a]

**Strategy 1**
Communities should increase availability of healthier food and beverage choices in public service venues.

*Suggested Measurement*
A policy exists to apply nutrition standards that are consistent with the *Dietary Guidelines for Americans* to all food sold (e.g., meal menus and vending machines) within local government facilities in a local jurisdiction or on public school campuses during the school day within the largest school district in a local jurisdiction.

**Strategy 2**
Communities should increase availability of affordable healthier food and beverage choices in public service venues.

*Suggested Measurement*
A policy exists to affect the cost of healthier foods and beverages as defined by the Institute of Medicine (Koplan et al., 2005) relative to the cost of less healthy foods and beverages sold within local government facilities in a local jurisdiction or on public school campuses during the school day within the largest school district in a local jurisdiction.

**Strategy 3**
Communities should increase geographical availability of supermarkets in underserved areas.

*Suggested Measurement*
The number of full-service grocery stores and supermarkets per 10,000 residents located within the three largest underserved census tracts within a local jurisdiction.

**Strategy 4**
Communities should provide incentives to food retailers to locate in and/or offer healthier food and beverage choices in underserved areas.

*Suggested Measurement*
Local government offers at least one incentive to new and/or existing food retailers to offer healthier food and beverage choices in underserved areas.

**Strategy 5**
Communities should increase availability of mechanisms for purchasing foods from farms.

*Suggested Measurement*
The total annual number of farmer-days at farmers' markets per 10,000 residents within a local jurisdiction.

**Strategy 6**
Communities should provide incentives for the production, distribution, and procurement of foods from local farms.

*Suggested Measurement*
Local government has a policy that encourages the production, distribution, or procurement of food from local farms in the local jurisdiction.

**Strategies to Support Healthy Food and Beverage Choices**

**Strategy 7**
Communities should restrict availability of less healthy foods and beverages in public service venues.

---

### ✦ BOX 11-1    INNOVATIVE PRACTICE—cont'd

*Summary of Recommended Community Strategies and Measurements to Prevent Obesity in the United States Related to Healthy Foods[a]*

**Suggested Measurement**

A policy exists that prohibits the sale of less healthy foods and beverages (as defined by the IOM; Koplan et al., 2005) within local government facilities in a local jurisdiction or on public school campuses during the school day within the largest school district in a local jurisdiction.

**Strategy 8**

Communities should institute smaller portion size options in public service venues.

**Suggested Measurement**

Local government has a policy to limit the portion size of any entree (including sandwiches and entree salads) by either reducing the standard portion size of entrees or offering smaller portion sizes in addition to standard portion sizes within local government facilities within a local jurisdiction.

**Strategy 9**

Communities should limit advertisements of less healthy foods and beverages.

**Suggested Measurement**

A policy exists that limits advertising and promotion of less healthy foods and beverages within local government facilities in a local jurisdiction or on public

school campuses during the school day within the largest school district in a local jurisdiction.

**Strategy 10**

Communities should discourage consumption of sugar-sweetened beverages.

**Suggested Measurement**

Licensed child care facilities within the local jurisdiction are required to ban sugar-sweetened beverages, including flavored/sweetened milk, and limit the portion size of 100% juice.

**Strategy to Encourage Breastfeeding**

**Strategy 11**

Communities should increase support for breastfeeding.

**Suggested Measurement**

Local government has a policy requiring local government facilities to provide breastfeeding accommodations for employees that include both time and private space for breastfeeding (or pumping of milk) during working hours.

[a]The entire report includes 24 strategies and measurements to include those related to physical activity. Because physical activity is discussed in Chapter 12, this excerpt includes nutrition advice only.
Institute of Medicine (IOM), Koplan, J.P., Liverman, C.T., & Kraak, V.I. (2005). *Preventing childhood obesity: Health in the balance*. Washington, DC: The National Academies Press; Khan, L. K., Sobush, K., Keener, D., Goodman, K., Lowry, A., Kakietek, J., et al. (2009). Recommended community strategies and measurements to prevent obesity in the United States. *MMWR. Recommendations and Reports, 58*(EE-7):1-26.

---

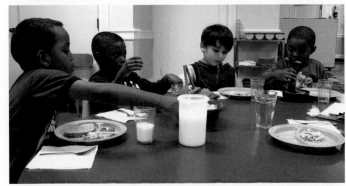

**FIGURE 11-2** Children who eat with each other in an appropriate environment often eat more nutritiously and try a wider variety of foods than when eating alone or at home. (From Mahan, L. K., & Raymond, J. L. [2017]. *Krause's food & the nutrition care process* [14th ed.]. St Louis: Elsevier.)

## Nutrition-Related Health Status

A variety of diet-related factors exact a heavy toll on the US population as the following key points illustrate (CDC, 2015; Food Research and Action Center [FRAC], 2011; National Prevention Council, 2011). The following statements give a broad-based view of the health status of Americans:

- Less than 18% of adults in each state surveyed consumed the recommended amount of fruit, and less than 14% consumed the recommended amount of vegetables (CDC, 2015).

- From 2007 to 2010, 60% of children consumed fewer cup equivalents of fruit than recommended, and 93% consumed fewer vegetables than recommended.

- Sixty-three percent of adults and 84% of adolescents consume at least one sugar-sweetened drink (e.g., soda, sport drinks, fruit drinks and punches, low-calorie drinks, sweetened tea) each day.

- Most American adults consume more than twice the recommended average daily sodium intake level (for healthy people). Nearly 80% of this sodium originates from packaged, processed, and restaurant foods.

- More than two-thirds of the adult population is overweight or obese. Approximately one in five children are overweight or obese by the time they reach age 6 years, and more than half of obese children become overweight at or before age 2 years.

- Low-income women are more likely than their higher-income counterparts to return to work earlier after childbirth and to be engaged in jobs that make it challenging for them to breastfeed. Babies who are breastfed may be less likely to become obese (USDHHS, 2011).

- Almost 50 million households (15%) experience food insecurity at least occasionally during the year, meaning that their access to adequate food is limited by a lack of money and other resources. Individuals and families who experience food insecurity may be more likely to be overweight or obese, potentially because of the relatively lower cost of calorie-dense foods (i.e., foods with a low nutrient density).

**BOX 11-2   HEALTHY PEOPLE 2020**

## Objectives Related to Nutrition and Food Safety, Healthier Food Access

- Increase the number of states with nutrition standards for foods and beverages provided to preschool children in child care.
- Increase the proportion of schools that offer nutritious foods and beverages outside school meals.
- Increase the number of states that have state-level policies that incentivize food retail outlets to provide foods that are encouraged by the *Dietary Guidelines for Americans*.
- (Developmental objective) Increase the proportion of Americans who have access to a food retail outlet that sells a variety of foods that are encouraged by the *Dietary Guidelines for Americans*.

### Health Care and Work Site Settings

- Increase the proportion of primary care physicians who regularly measure the BMI of their care recipients (both adults and children/adolescents).
- Increase the proportion of physician office visits that include counseling or education related to nutrition or weight (by diagnosis such as CVD, diabetes, hyperlipidemia, or obesity).
- (Developmental objective) Increase the proportion of work sites that offer nutrition or weight-management classes or counseling.

### Weight Status

- Increase the proportion of adults who are at a healthy weight.
- (Developmental objective) Prevent inappropriate weight gain in youth and adults.

### Food Insecurity

- Eliminate very low food security among children.
- Reduce household food insecurity and in so doing reduce hunger.

### Food and Nutrient Consumption

- Increase the contribution of fruits to the diets of the population aged 2 years and older.
- (Leading health indicator) Increase the variety of vegetables in and their contribution to the diets of the population aged 2 years or older (increase the contribution of total vegetables, including dark green vegetables, orange vegetables, and legumes).
- Increase the contribution of whole grains in the diets of the population aged 2 years or older.
- Reduce the consumption of calories from solid fats and added sugars in the population aged 2 years or older.
- Reduce the consumption of saturated fat in the population aged 2 years or older.
- Reduce the consumption of sodium in the population aged 2 years or older.
- Increase the consumption of calcium in the population aged 2 years or older.
- Reduce iron deficiency among young children and females of childbearing age (children aged 1–2 years and aged 3–4 years, females aged 12–49 years).
- Reduce iron deficiency among pregnant females.

### Objectives for Selected Diseases With Nutrition Components

#### Heart Disease and Stroke

Goal: Increase overall cardiovascular health in the US population and reduce CHD and stroke deaths.

- Reduce the proportion of adults with high total blood cholesterol levels.
- Reduce the mean total blood cholesterol levels among adults (for adults aged 20 years or older).
- Increase the proportion of adults with pre-hypertension who meet the recommended guidelines (for nutrition, BMI, saturated fat consumption, sodium intake, and moderate alcohol consumption).
- (Developmental objective) Increase the proportion of adults with hypertension who meet the recommended guidelines (for nutrition, BMI, saturated fat consumption, sodium intake, and moderate alcohol consumption).
- (Developmental objective) Increase the proportion of adults with elevated LDL cholesterol levels who have been advised by a health care provider regarding cholesterol-lowering management including lifestyle changes (such as cholesterol-lowering diet, weight control) and, if indicated, medication.
- (Developmental objective) Increase the proportion of adults with elevated LDL cholesterol levels who adhere to the prescribed LDL cholesterol–lowering management lifestyle changes (such as cholesterol-lowering diet, weight control) and, if indicated, medication.
- (Developmental objective) Increase the proportion of adults with CHD or stroke who have their LDL cholesterol level at or below recommended levels.

#### Obesity

- (Leading health indicator) Reduce the proportion of adults who are obese (to 30.6% from 34%).
- (Leading health indicator) Reduce the proportion of children and adolescents (age categories 2–5 years, 6–11 years, 12–19 years) who are considered obese (to 14.6% from almost 17%).

#### Diabetes

- Improve glycemic control among the population with diagnosed diabetes.
- Improve lipid control among people with diagnosed diabetes.
- Increase the proportion of the population with diagnosed diabetes whose blood pressure is under control.
- Increase the proportion of people with diabetes who receive formal diabetes education.
- Increase prevention behaviors in people with pre-diabetes at high risk of diabetes.

### Objectives for Food Safety

- Reduce the number of outbreak-associated infections due to Shiga toxin–producing *E. coli* O157, or *Campylobacter*, *Listeria*, or *Salmonella* species associated with food commodity groups (beef, dairy, fruits and nuts, leafy vegetables, and poultry).

#### Key Food Safety Practices

- Increase the proportion of consumers who follow key food safety practices (clean: wash hands and surfaces often; separate: do not cross-contaminate; cook: cook to proper temperatures; chill: refrigerate promptly).
- (Developmental) Improve food safety practices associated with food-borne illness in food service and retail establishments.

From US Department of Health and Human Services. (2010). *Healthy People 2020*. Washington, DC: US Government Printing Office. http://www.healhypeople.gov/2020/default.aspx.

- Each year approximately one in six Americans (48 million people) become ill. Of those who are sick, 128,000 are hospitalized and 3000 die of food-borne diseases. Reducing the number of people affected by food-borne illness by 10% would prevent illness in approximately 5 million Americans each year.

## Nutrition Objectives for the United States

As can be seen already, a considerable gap exists between public health recommendations and consumer practices. The overarching goal for nutrition in the second decade of the millennium is that food intake patterns change in the direction of the targeted goals recommended in *Healthy People 2020*, the *Dietary Guidelines for Americans 2015–2020*, and the MyPlate food guidance system.

## FOOD AND NUTRITION RECOMMENDATIONS

Food and nutrition guidelines are introduced in this chapter, with the intent of motivating the reader to achieve three principal goals. The first goal is to encourage individual interest in the health-promoting power of good nutrition and to promote self-evaluation and comparison of one's own food habits and choices with respect to the dietary recommendations presented here. The second goal is to understand the many systemic factors that have contributed to the current nutrition-related health issues. These problems are so pervasive that many health authorities believe a multisectoral approach, beyond traditional education about healthy food choices, is required. A final goal is to define the kinds and amounts of food that are generally acknowledged as essential for obtaining the necessary energy and nutrients required for health. The following reports provide the foundation for national nutrition recommendations that have been translated into law, policy, programs, and many consumer messages.

- *Dietary Reference Intakes: The Essential Guide to Nutrient Requirements* (National Research Council, 2006) and *Dietary Reference Intakes for Calcium and Vitamin D* (National Research Council, 2010)
- *Dietary Guidelines for Americans 2015–2020*, eighth edition (USDHHS & USDA, 2015)
- MyPlate food guidance system (USDA, Center for Nutrition Policy and Promotion, 2010) (Figure 11-3)

## Dietary Reference Intakes

The original dietary reference intakes (DRIs) were developed by the Institute of Medicine (IOM) of the National Academies of Sciences, Engineering, and Medicine in 1997 to reflect the latest understanding about nutrient requirements based on optimizing health in individuals and groups. They are quantitative estimates of nutrient intakes, which can be used to plan and assess the diets of healthy people in the United States, to prevent disease and deficiencies. The recommended dietary allowances (RDAs) form the basis for the DRIs. The adequate intakes are to be used whenever there is not enough evidence to include a nutrient in the RDAs. See Box 11-3: Dietary Reference Intake Components and Definitions for details on these components and suggested uses.

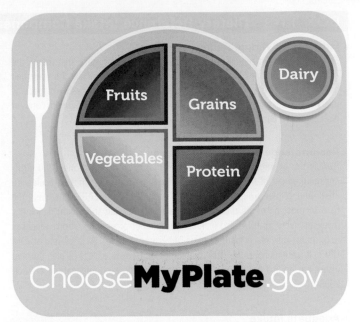

**FIGURE 11-3** Learn about healthy eating at http://www.choosemyplate.gov. (From US Department of Agriculture, Center for Nutrition Policy and Promotion. [n.d.]. *Choose MyPlate*. http://www.choosemyplate.gov.)

It is important to note that in contrast to the routine 5-year review of the *Dietary Guidelines for Americans*, the DRIs are updated only when deemed necessary. In 2008 the US and Canadian governments decided there were enough new studies as well as concern about vitamin D, in particular, to warrant the development of new DRIs for vitamin D and calcium. The latest updates were published in late 2010. The revision of the vitamin D and calcium DRIs since 1997 demonstrates that DRIs continue to be researched and revised as more information and evidence-based studies become available.

There are some controversies over DRIs because there may be limited data relating to genetic diversity in the population or specific groups such as children, pregnant women, and elderly people. However, they are a good starting point based on best available evidence and probability of harm or benefit.

As the DRIs are intended to be applied to healthy people, it is possible that a provider might override the DRI for a specific nutrient on the basis of clinical judgment and recommend more or less for a particular recipient. It is also helpful to remember that whereas DRIs may be used for individuals, ideally, they are guidelines for population groups and apply over time. So, if an individual does not meet the recommendation for a specific nutrient, such as vitamin C, on a certain day, that is not a cause for alarm. It is the trend that matters with respect to food sources as opposed to supplements.

After this discussion of DRIs, the twentieth-century anthropologist Margaret Mead's statement that "People eat food, not nutrition" seems particularly apt. Nutrition recommendations stated in terms of micrograms or milligrams of nutrients are of

## BOX 11-3 Dietary Reference Intake Components and Definitions

**Estimated Average Requirement**

Estimated average requirement (EAR) is the (median) intake that meets the estimated nutrient needs of half of the individuals in a particular life stage and gender group. It is used as a basis for developing the RDA and is especially useful for evaluating adequacy of nutrient intake of a group (or groups) and for planning how much the group(s) should consume.

**Recommended Dietary Allowance**

RDA is the average dietary intake level that is sufficient to meet the nutrient requirement of nearly all (97–98%) healthy individuals in a particular life stage and gender group. It is computed with use of the EAR. In the past, the RDA of most nutrients represented the levels needed to prevent deficiency diseases. Now an RDA also includes the goal of preventing chronic diseases (e.g., heart disease or osteoporosis, where applicable). As a variety of IOM DRI publications note, the RDA should not be used to assess or plan nutrient intake for groups but may be useful in some individual applications (Taylor, 2008).

**Adequate Intake**

An adequate intake (AI) is set to fill the gap (e.g., infants) when there is not enough scientific evidence to determine the RDA. The AI is based on estimates of observed or experimentally determined mean nutrient intake of a group (or groups) of healthy people and assumes that the amount consumed is adequate to promote health. The level is set to meet or exceed the needs of almost all people in a particular life stage and gender group. This is the most controversial component in the DRIs.

**Tolerable Upper Intake Level**

This is the highest average daily intake that can be safely eaten continuously and still be considered safe for almost all healthy individuals in a specified group. The UL is not intended to be a recommended level of intake. No established benefit exists for individuals to consume nutrients at levels above the RDA or AI. As intake increases above the UL, the potential risk of adverse health effects increases. For most nutrients the UL would include total intakes from any of the following (alone or in combination): food, fortified food, and nutrient supplements. It is important to note that ULs are set only when there is a strong pool of scientific data. In cases where the evidence is limited or inconclusive, a UL will not be established. In that case, eating levels close to the RDA or AI (as applicable) is not advised.

**Acceptable Macronutrient Distribution Range**

This is the range of intake for a particular energy source (e.g., carbohydrate, fat, and protein) that is associated with reduced risk of chronic disease while providing intakes of essential nutrients for a healthy person within an identified life stage and gender group. An intake outside the acceptable macronutrient distribution range (AMDR) carries the potential of increased risk of chronic diseases and/or insufficient intakes of essential nutrients. For example, the AMDR for carbohydrates for a 19-year-old woman (in the life stage and gender group of female, 19–30 yrs old) is 45% to 65% of calories.

**Estimated Energy Requirement**

This is the average dietary energy intake predicted to maintain energy balance in a healthy adult of a specific life stage and gender group calculated with a reference weight, height, and level of physical activity that is consistent with good health.

From the American Dietetic Association Evidence Analysis Library and based on Greer, N., Mosser, G., Logan, G., & Wagstrom Halaas, G. (2000). A practical approach to evidence grading. *The Joint Commission Journal on Quality Improvement, 26,* 700–712; Taylor, C. L. (2008). *Framework for DRI development: Components "known" and components "to be explored."* Background paper. Washington, DC: Institute of Medicine, National Academies of Science, Engineering and Medicine. http://www.nationalacademies.org/hmd/Activities/Nutrition/SummaryDRIs/~/media/Files/Activity%20Files/Nutrition/DRIs/New%20Material/11Bckgrd%20PaperFramework%20for%20DRI%20Devel; US Department of Agriculture. (2010). Appendix 16: Glossary of terms. In *Dietary guidelines for Americans* (7th ed.). Washington, DC: US Government Printing Office. http://www.cnpp.usda.gov/Publications/DietaryGuidelines/2010/PolicyDoc/PolicyDoc.pdf.

no use unless people are advised as to what types and quantities of foods should be consumed to meet the recommendations. The intent of *Dietary Guidelines for Americans 2015–2020* has been to translate science-based nutrition recommendations into optimal eating guidelines that can be adopted by the public to maximize healthy habits and minimize chronic disease.

The DRIs also form the foundation for US nutrition policy, in the design and implementation of nutrition-related programs, including federal nutrition programs for families, children, and elderly people. These guidelines also provide nutrition education initiatives for the general public of adults and children aged 2 years or older.

## Dietary Guidelines for Americans 2015–2020

Key recommendations from the 2015–2020 **Dietary Guidelines Advisory Committee** (DGAC) include recommendations to:

- Follow a healthy eating pattern across the life span. All food and beverage choices matter. Choose a healthy eating pattern at an appropriate calorie level to help achieve and maintain a healthy body weight, support nutrient adequacy, and reduce the risk of chronic disease.

- Focus on variety, nutrient density, and amount. To meet nutrient needs within calorie limits, choose a variety of nutrient-dense foods across and within all food groups in recommended amounts.

- Limit calories from added sugars and saturated fats and reduce sodium intake. Consume an eating pattern low in added sugars, saturated fats, and sodium. Cut back on foods and beverages higher in these components to amounts that fit within healthy eating patterns.

- Shift to healthier food and beverage choices. Choose nutrient-dense foods and beverages across and within all food groups in place of less healthy choices. Consider cultural and personal preferences to make these shifts easier to accomplish and maintain.

- Support healthy eating patterns for all. Everyone has a role in helping to create and support healthy eating patterns in multiple settings nationwide, from home to school to work to communities.

Other topics addressed in detail include guidance for specific population groups: children and adolescents, women of childbearing age, pregnant and breastfeeding women, and older adults, as well as adults at high risk of chronic disease. A discussion of how to build healthy eating patterns embraces USDA eating patterns with lacto-ovo vegetarian, vegan, and Dietary Approaches to Stop Hypertension (DASH) variations provided at various calorie levels. (For details, see http://health.gov/dietaryguidelines/.) For nursing professionals interested in helping themselves or others balance calories, Chapter 2 is particularly helpful. Just like *Healthy People 2020,* the report includes an emphasis on consumer aspects of food safety.

Representing the best and most current scientific evidence and advice from nutrition experts, these guidelines are intended to reduce the nation's major diet-related health problems such as CHD, certain cancers, diabetes, high blood pressure, obesity, osteoporosis, and stroke (USDA, Food and Nutrition Service [FNS], 2011c).

Nursing professionals play a key role in promoting the *Dietary Guidelines of Americans* as one component of healthful lifestyles. For more information about the articles and reports used to inform the development of the *Dietary Guidelines for Americans,* see the *Report of the Dietary Guidelines Advisory Committee* on the *Dietary Guidelines for Americans 2015–2020,* and the related USDA's Nutrition Evidence Library website (http://www.nel.gov/) (USDA, 2015).

The latest MyPlate food icon revision has retained the on-line tracker tools (now called SuperTracker for adults and BlastOff for kids) as well as Spanish language versions of educational materials.

The USDA unveiled MyPlate in June 2011 in keeping with the 2010 White House Child Obesity Task Force's call for action to provide the US public with easy to understand and useful advice. MyPlate visually reminds consumers what a healthy "plate" looks like using a familiar place setting (see Figure 11-3). It is not meant to stand alone as a teaching tool. Consumers and health professionals are directed to the website (http://www.choosemyplate.gov) for details. The new food guidance system puts four of the food groups on the plate (grains, vegetables, fruits, and protein group [which replaced the meat and bean group]) with dairy (including milk and dairy substitutes) on the side.

Although the USDA's MyPlate food guidance system reflects general eating patterns of Americans, it has enough flexibility for different cultural traditions and eating patterns, including vegetarian (see Box 11-4: Diversity Awareness).

Recognizing that in recent years almost 15 million adults and children have found it difficult to obtain enough food to meet their needs, the MyPlate website includes an emphasis on resources for eating on a budget and how to access nutrition assistance programs. The USDA also has resources available in Spanish. The website continues to be updated, so it is worth checking periodically.

## DIETARY SUPPLEMENTS AND HERBAL MEDICINES

In recent decades the popularity of supplemental vitamins, minerals, proteins, fiber, and herbs has earned a high profile in the health field. It was the explosion of the use of single-component dietary supplements in the 1980s that helped to spur the change from the old RDAs to the DRIs. New evidence indicated that perhaps ranges of nutrients could be used that were higher than the old "one size fits all" RDAs. At the same time, there appeared to be a point at which a nutrient could pose more of a risk than an advantage. As a result, tolerable upper limit (UL) guidelines were developed for specific life stages, ages, and gender (Taylor, 2008).

According to the National Institutes of Health (NIH), Office of Dietary Supplements (2012), most US adults take one or more dietary supplements either daily or occasionally. Almost 18% take other products, such as fish oil, echinacea, flaxseed oil, and ginseng (National Center for Complementary and Alternative Medicine, 2010). The 1994 Dietary Supplement Health and Education Act expanded the definition of dietary supplement to include any product intended for ingestion as a supplement to the diet. Today's dietary supplements include vitamins, minerals, herbals and botanicals, amino acids, enzymes, probiotics, and fish oils, as well as powders, energy drinks, and energy bars. People use supplements as if they were drugs. Additionally, they are marketed in the same manner as over-the-counter medications. To distinguish a dietary supplement from an over-the-counter drug, the words *dietary supplement* must appear on the product label. The labels may carry certain types of structure-function claims about certain common conditions associated with aging, pregnancy, menopause, and adolescence that do not relate to disease. These include health maintenance claims ("maintains a healthy circulatory system"), other nondisease claims ("for muscle enhancement" or "helps you relax"), and claims for common, minor symptoms associated with life stages ("for common symptoms of premenstrual syndrome" or "for hot flashes"). Such claims must be followed by the words "This statement has not been evaluated by the Food and Drug Administration. This product is not intended to diagnose, treat, cure, or prevent any disease." (Food and Drug Administration [FDA], 2008).

Because the FDA is the federal agency that oversees both dietary supplements and drugs, it might be easy to assume the federal regulations for supplements and drugs are similar. This is not the case. Dietary supplements are not regulated by the FDA in the sense that they do not require premarket review or approval by the FDA. Although a supplement manufacturer is responsible for providing evidence that its products are safe and its label claims are truthful and not misleading, it does not have to provide that evidence to the FDA before marketing the product.

Once a dietary supplement is on the market, the FDA monitors information on the product label and package insert to make sure that information about the supplement's content is accurate and that any claims made for the product are truthful and not misleading. If the FDA finds a product to be unsafe or otherwise unfit for human consumption, it may take enforcement action to remove the product from the marketplace or it may work with the manufacturer to voluntarily recall the product. Some supplements have had to be recalled because of proven or potential harmful effects. The reasons for these recalls include microbiological, pesticide, and heavy metal contamination; absence of a dietary ingredient claimed to be in the product; and the presence of more or less than the amount of the dietary ingredient claimed on the label.

## ⊕ BOX 11-4 DIVERSITY AWARENESS

### Food and Culture

The reasons why people eat the ways they do are numerous. Although it is true that without food people cannot survive, food is much more than a tool of survival. Food is also a source of pleasure ("Let's eat out tonight"), a source of comfort ("Right now, I could use some of my mother's chicken soup"), a symbol of hospitality ("Please come to my house for brunch on Sunday"), and an indicator of social status (consider an expensive T-bone steak versus a hamburger). Food also has ritual significance. Drinking champagne to celebrate an important event, the bride and groom saving the top layer of their wedding cake, and people of the Jewish faith sharing challah (braided bread) at their Sabbath (Friday evening) meal are examples.

To a large extent the environment determines what people typically eat. For example, wheat that is plentiful in the heartland of the United States is the principal grain in North America, whereas rice enjoys a similar status in Asian countries. Typical wheat-based staples in the United States and Canada include a slice of wheat bread, a bowl of wheat cereal, wheat crackers, pastries made from wheat flour, and pasta made from wheat. Rice-based foods form the backbone of the Chinese diet.

Every culture has its particular food ways, or activities related to food. Food ways include the activities that surround procuring, distributing, storing, consuming, and disposing of food, all of which define what is fit to eat, or what is edible. Factors that affect everyone's food choices and factors that affect food selections of new arrivals to a community should be examined. It is important to remember, however, that just because a person is from a specific culture does not mean the person follows his or her cultural food patterns. These general guidelines are helpful as a starting point, but do not assume—ask questions to clarify specific eating habits with individuals and families.

Among traditional Chinese people, health and disease are believed to relate to the balance between the forces of yin and yang in the body. Diseases that are caused by yang forces may be treated with yin forces to restore balance. Yin foods include low-calorie-density, low-protein foods, such as fresh fruits and vegetables. Yang foods are high in calories, cooked in oil, and irritating to the mouth, or are red, orange, or yellow. Examples include most meats, chili peppers, tomatoes, garlic, ginger, and alcoholic beverages. The hot-cold theory in Puerto Rico follows the same basic principles as do yin and yang, but the food groupings differ somewhat.

Religious beliefs affect the food choices of millions of people worldwide. Many religions, including Buddhism, Hinduism, Islam, Judaism, and Seventh Day Adventism, specify the foods that may be eaten and how they should be prepared. The following is a very basic summary of the principal dietary practices of these five major world religions (adapted from Barer-Stein, 1979, and Kittler & Sucher, 2000).

Many Buddhists practice vegetarianism. Foods of plant origin are viewed as the most appropriate for consumption, except pungent foods (garlic, leeks, scallions, chives, and onions), which are believed to generate lust when eaten cooked and to cause rage when eaten raw. For most Buddhists, however, dietary rules such as these are observed on a voluntary basis. What characterizes all Buddhists is the belief that all forms of life share a common link and are thus sacred. Therefore rather than the specific type of food eaten, more important is the attitude of the person receiving the food and the person's sincere gratitude for the lives of the plants and animals contained in the meal that have served to sustain and further enhance the life of the individual.

Many Hindus practice vegetarianism, but those who originate from the cold northern areas of India usually eat meat (except for beef, which is considered sacred and prohibited).

Many Muslims follow Islamic food laws, which include foods that are halal (permitted), haram (prohibited), and questionable (*mashbooh*). Foods believed to be unclean, or haram, are animals that are improperly slaughtered or already-dead animals such as carrion, swine/pork and its by-products (bacon, lard, shortening), carnivorous animals with fangs (dogs, cats, and lions), birds of prey, and land animals without ears (frogs and snakes). Alcohol and intoxicants are also prohibited. Halal-certified products are used.

Conservative Jews follow Judaic food laws, which prohibit the consumption of swine/pork, carrion, carrion eaters (scavengers), shellfish, animals with a cloven (split) hoof and that do not chew their cud (horses), and animals not slaughtered by the appropriate ritual method or kosher (fit). According to Jewish kosher dietary laws, meat (beef, lamb, veal, and poultry), fish, and meat products (eggs) cannot be served at the same meal or be cooked or eaten in the same vessels as dairy products. Kosher-certified products are used.

The dietary practices of Seventh Day Adventists focus on health, so many Seventh Day Adventists practice vegetarianism as the foundation of their dietary standard. They also abstain from alcohol, and many do not drink caffeine-containing beverages.

From Barer-Stein, T. (1979). Multiculturalism and nutrition counseling. *Journal of the Canadian Dietetic Association, 40*(2), 112–116; Kittler, P. G., & Sucher, K. P. (2000). *Cultural foods: Traditions and trends.* Belmont, CA: Wadsworth.

The federal government can take legal action against companies and websites that sell dietary supplements when the companies make false or deceptive statements about their products, if they promote them as treatments or cures for diseases, or if their products are unsafe. In a position paper, the Academy of Nutrition and Dietetics (formerly the American Dietetic Association) states that some people may benefit from supplements but that a diet rich in nutrients should be their major source (Marra & Bovar, 2009). It went further to say that practitioners need to keep up to date on the safety and efficacy of these supplements. Although laws exist to help protect the consumer, the reality is that it is a "buyer beware" environment because of historically low funding and resources for the FDA, along with political pressure and lack of scientific study on the overwhelming majority of supplements available in the United States (Nestle, 2002).

Although the desirable way for the general public to obtain recommended levels of nutrients is by eating a variety of foods,

if people take dietary supplements, they should avoid taking them in excess of the UL of the DRI for those nutrients for their age and gender group to preclude possible adverse effects. An example of this is a recent study of the effects of dietary as well as calcium supplementation in fracture prevention in which it was concluded that there was no such association (Bolland et al., 2015). For other types of supplements, such as herbals or botanicals, caution is also advised. Natural is not always better. For example, the National Center for Complementary and Alternative Medicine cautions against the use of products such as comfrey or kava, which can be toxic to the liver.

### Vitamin and Mineral Toxicity

Toxic levels of certain **micronutrients** can cause a host of health problems. For example, it is important to advise individuals not to overuse the fat-soluble vitamins (vitamins A, D, E, and K). Of particular concern is vitamin A, an excess of which may be

## BOX 11-5 QUALITY AND SAFETY SCENARIO

### Supplements/Vitamin A

Adele is a 32-year-old married black American woman with no children and a history of one miscarriage. She and her husband have been trying to conceive for the past 4 years and have recently started talking about going to a fertility clinic. Always one to try the "natural way" first, she read that vitamin A is important for normal fetal development and decides to take a multivitamin supplement with 25,000 IU of preformed vitamin A. Adele knows that she can get vitamin A from food, but she also makes an effort to read nutrition labels and choose fortified foods that have 20% or more vitamin A content. She comes into the physician's office for a regular routine visit. It is common knowledge that she and her husband are trying to have a baby.

#### Reflective Questions

- Why is it important to discuss the use and type of supplements (and potentially fortified food use) during preconception/pregnancy?
- What is the vitamin A DRI recommendation for a woman of her age?
- How can learning about simple changes in her eating habits/supplement use affect her risk of a spontaneous abortion or a birth defect in the event of pregnancy?
- What would your next step be in this situation?

  **Note:** One retinol activity equivalent = 1 mcg of all-*trans*-retinol = 3.33 IU from retinol = 2 mcg of supplemental all-*trans*-β-carotene = 12 mcg of dietary all-*trans*-β-carotene = 24 mcg of other dietary provitamin A carotenoids. *DRI,* Dietary reference intake.

teratogenic during pregnancy or may increase the risk of lung cancer for current or former smokers (American Dietetic Association, 2009). On the other hand, water-soluble vitamins such as vitamin C and the B-complex vitamins may pose less danger because the body is able to excrete them through the urine.

Nutrient imbalances and toxicities are rarely likely to occur when nutrients are derived from foods in a normal diet. Most nutrient toxicities occur through supplementation, and in some cases with a combination of supplementation and fortification of foods. The estimated toxic doses for daily oral consumption of vitamins and minerals by adults are as low as five times the recommended intake for selenium, and as high as 25 to 50 times or more the recommended intakes for folic acid and vitamins C and E. The toxicities of high doses of nutrients such as vitamin A, vitamin B6, vitamin D, niacin, iron, and selenium are well established. Iron supplements intended for other household members are the most common cause of pediatric poisoning deaths in the United States (National Library of Medicine, 2011).

Large doses of vitamin A may be teratogenic. Because of this risk, supplementation with preformed vitamin A should be avoided during the first trimester of pregnancy unless there is evidence of deficiency (see Box 11-5: Quality and Safety Scenario). Excess preformed vitamin A supplements (more than 10,000 international units [IU]) during the first trimester of pregnancy has been linked to birth defects of the eyes, lungs, skull, and heart (Office of Dietary Supplements, 2012). Such a risk in early pregnancy raises the need for caution about general vitamin and mineral supplement use by women of childbearing age.

Besides problems with direct toxicity of some individual nutrients, there may be problems related to nutrient imbalances or adverse interactions with prescribed medication. Often, high

doses of a single nutrient may reflect interactions that result in a relative deficiency of another nutrient (American Dietetic Association, 2009). Some examples follow:

- High doses of vitamin E can interfere with vitamin K action and enhance the effect of warfarin as one of the anticoagulant drugs. Examples such as this are one of the reasons that health care providers may ask about supplement use before surgery and recommend discontinuation of use of certain supplements for 1 week before and 1 week after surgery. Large amounts of calcium inhibit absorption of iron and possibly other trace elements.
- Folic acid can mask hematological signs of vitamin B12 deficiency, which, if untreated, can result in irreversible neurological damage. Folic acid can also interact adversely with anticonvulsant medications.
- Zinc supplementation can reduce copper levels, impair immune responses, and decrease levels of high-density lipoprotein (HDL) cholesterol ("good" cholesterol).

Nursing professionals can help people who suspect an adverse supplement effect by reporting the event to the FDA, or by encouraging the individual to file a report. This should be done as soon as possible when there is a suspected problem. Information on how to do this is available at http://www.fda.gov/food/dietarysupplements/reportadverseevent/. Another avenue is to alert the product's manufacturer or distributor to any serious side effects through the address or phone number listed on the supplement's label. By law, dietary supplement firms are required to forward reports they receive about serious adverse effects to the FDA within 15 days.

## Circumstances When Nutrient Supplementation Is Indicated

Nutrient supplements or fortified foods, or sometimes a combination of both, are sometimes necessary for specific populations to obtain desirable amounts of particular nutrients (National Research Council, 2010; USDHHS & USDA, 2015). Some examples follow:

- Folic acid (400 mcg) from fortified enriched grains or supplements in addition to folate-rich foods for women who could become pregnant to help prevent neural tube defects.
- Iron supplements during pregnancy when indicated in laboratory tests.
- Calcium and vitamin D supplements in older postmenopausal women to reduce their risk of osteoporosis (levels should not exceed the UL of 2000 mg for calcium or 100 mcg for vitamin D through either supplements or a combination of foods and supplements).
- Vitamin D for those who do not meet the recommended DRI intake (without exceeding the DRI UL of 4000 IU or 100 mcg by a combination of food, supplement, and fortified food).
- Vitamin B12 through food fortified with the crystalline form or B12 supplements for individuals older than 50 years (who may often have a reduced ability to absorb naturally occurring vitamin B12). In addition, vegans should ensure they have adequate intake of vitamin B12 through fortified foods or supplements.

People can get their nutritional requirements from foods and, when necessary, from supplements. However, the amounts needed are generalized to population studies (e.g., amounts for all women during pregnancy). These requirements do not account for individual genetic variations. In the future, it may be possible for specific nutrients to be prescribed to individuals on the basis of genomic maps. This new and exciting study of nutrigenomics explores the effects of nutrients on gene expression. However, when it comes to nutrients in foods and their effects on gene expression, the science is not ready to create diets specific to an individual's genome makeup. As this is an issue of ethics medicine as well as nutrition, it is a field that will move with caution (Pavlidis et al., 2015).

## FOOD SAFETY

Americans spend more than $1 trillion on food each year, with nearly 50% of food consumption occurring outside the home (Johnson, 2011). The combined efforts of the food industry and the regulatory agencies are often credited with making the US food supply among the safest in the world. Nonetheless, the CDC reports that each year an estimated one in six Americans—a total of 48 million people—become sick from food-borne illnesses caused by contamination by any of a number of microbial pathogens. Of these, an estimated 128,000 people require hospitalization and 3000 people die (CDC, 2011a). Food-borne illnesses are estimated to cost the United States $77.7 billion annually, not including costs to the food industry or public health agencies.

Attention to food-borne illnesses is becoming increasingly important with the globalization of the world's food supply. New disease-causing organisms have emerged, and food imports from countries without the same safety standards as the United States are on the rise. Furthermore, more consumers are demanding fresh produce and more seafood to be available throughout the year as well as accessibility to less-processed foods, such as raw milk and fresh juices that are not cooked or pasteurized to kill bacteria. Consumers may also ignore warnings about unsafe food habits because of preferences for foods such as raw oysters, rare hamburgers, fresh juices, unpasteurized cheese, and runny egg yolks, which all carry higher risks of contamination.

To protect the public from numerous sources of food contamination (physical, chemical, biological), private industry and numerous federal, state, and local agencies share responsibilities for regulating the safety of the US food supply. On the food industry side, one example of initiatives is food processors that are working on programs to better trace products through the supply chain and monitor temperatures in trucks from remote locations. In late 2010, Congress passed sweeping food safety legislation called the Food Safety Modernization Act (FSMA), which gives the FDA new powers to police food safety and focus its efforts on preventing food contamination. Subject to adequate funding, the FSMA allows the FDA to increase its inspection of imported food, set safety standards for fresh produce, force companies to recall tainted products, and require companies to keep better production records.

When the safeguards built into this system fail, however, consumers themselves must serve as the final and sometimes most important guardian against unsafe food. Therefore it is essential to be informed and educated about the potential dangers of food-borne illness and ways to avoid contaminated food products.

## Causes of Food-Borne Illness

A food-borne illness is classified according to the source of its contamination (the unintended presence of harmful substances or microorganisms). Food contaminants may be categorized as biological, chemical, or physical. Biological contaminants include bacteria, viruses, parasites, and fungi (yeasts and molds). Chemical contamination refers to the presence of pesticides, kitchen-cleaning supplies, and toxic chemicals in food that have been leached from worn metal cookware and equipment. Physical contamination includes dirt, glass chips, crockery, wood, splinters, stones, hair, jewelry, and metal shavings from dull can openers. Another unintended physical contaminant may be an unintended allergen added to a food product that typically does not include that ingredient (such as peanuts) during food processing in the same location.

## Examples of Common Food-Borne Pathogens

The safety of the US food supply is so important that there are specific objectives tied to the monitoring of common pathogens in *Healthy People 2020*. These include outbreak-associated infections attributable to Shiga toxin–producing *Escherichia coli* O157, or *Campylobacter, Listeria,* or *Salmonella* species associated with food commodity groups (e.g., beef, dairy, fruits and nuts, leafy vegetables, and poultry). Two common types are discussed next.

### Salmonellosis

The most frequently reported cause of food-borne illness is from *Salmonella* bacteria. Each year in the United States, approximately 40,000 cases of salmonellosis are reported, with 400 deaths from acute salmonellosis (CDC, 2010). The actual number of infections may be closer to 1.4 million because milder cases are often not diagnosed or reported. Although the *Salmonella* family includes more than 2300 serotypes of the bacterium, the most common in the United States are *Salmonella enteritidis* and *Salmonella typhimurium.*

The typical way humans are exposed to salmonellosis is by consuming foods contaminated with animal feces. Foods of animal origin such as beef, poultry, milk, and eggs are often the source of infection. However, *all* foods, including seafood from polluted water and vegetables, may become contaminated. Contamination may also occur from unsanitary handling of foods and utensils by infected food handlers and contact with the feces of some pets, especially those with diarrhea. Symptoms of salmonellosis (CDC, 2004) include abdominal cramping, mild to severe diarrhea, nausea, vomiting, and fever within 8 to 72 hours after infection. Symptoms may resolve within 4 to 7 days without treatment; however, infections can become life threatening for people with weakened immune systems such as infants with an immature immune system, young children, pregnant women, older adults, and people with autoimmune disorders or those being treated for cancer. Antibiotics are usually not necessary unless the infection spreads from the intestines. To prevent salmonellosis, avoid uncooked egg dishes, undercooked meat, shellfish, and unpasteurized milk and juice. Adherence to sanitary regulations, as well as proper food handling, is necessary to control salmonellosis outbreaks.

### Escherichia coli O157:H7 Infection

Theodor Escherichia, a German pediatrician, first discovered the *E. coli* bacterium in the human colon in 1885. A particularly virulent strain of *E. coli*, known as *E. coli* O157:H7, was first identified in 1982 as a food-borne pathogen during an investigation of an outbreak of severe bloody diarrhea attributable to ingestion of contaminated hamburgers. As a leading cause of food-borne illness, *E. coli* O157:H7 can produce a powerful toxin causing severe illness and damage to the intestinal lining (CDC, 2011a). The illness is characterized by severe abdominal cramping, watery to bloody diarrhea, dehydration, nausea, and vomiting with or without low-grade fever. Hemorrhagic colitis is usually self-limited and lasts for an average of 8 days. Most *E. coli* O157:H7 infections (CDC, 2004) are food-borne and associated with undercooked or raw ground beef, unpasteurized fruit juices and milk, alfalfa sprouts, lettuce, spinach, and fruits. Moreover, outbreaks can be caused by secondary person-to-person contamination in homes, day care centers, nursing homes, and hospitals. Another mode of transmission of *E. coli* O157:H7 is by hand-to-mouth contact with animals or contaminated surfaces at petting zoos and agricultural fairs. Although all people are included in *E. coli* O157:H7 target populations, children and older adults are more susceptible. In cases confirmed in children, infection may develop into hemolytic uremic syndrome, leading to permanent loss of kidney function.

### Food Safety Practices

The few examples already cited demonstrate how serious food-borne illness can be. Individuals in their own homes can reduce contaminants and keep food safe to eat by following safe food handling practices. Four basic food safety principles work together to reduce the risk of food-borne illness—clean, separate, cook, and chill. These four principles are the cornerstones of Fight BAC!, a national food safety education campaign (http://www.fightbac.org). *Healthy People 2020* included a key food safety objective designed to increase the proportion of consumers following them. As you can see from the following results of the 2006 national Food Safety Survey, there is significant room for improvement (see *Healthy People 2020*, FS-5.1–FS-5.4 for details).

- Clean: Wash hands, utensils, and cutting boards before and after contact with raw meat, poultry, seafood, and eggs (33% of the surveyed population did not do this) (USDA Center for Nutrition Policy and Promotion 2012).
  - Wash all parts of the hands thoroughly with running warm water with soap and friction for approximately 20 to 30 seconds. Teach children to sing the *Happy Birthday* song twice. If no water is available, use alcohol-based (≥60%) hand sanitizers.
  - Clean all surfaces with warm, soapy water often (including all appliances, knobs, and handles) and clean up spills immediately. A solution of one tablespoon of unscented, liquid chlorine bleach per gallon of water can be used to sanitize surfaces.

- At least once a week, discard refrigerated foods that should no longer be eaten. Cooked leftovers should be discarded after 4 days; raw poultry and ground meats should be discarded after 1 to 2 days.
- Separate: Do not cross-contaminate. Keep raw meat and poultry separated from foods that will not be cooked while shopping, preparing, or storing foods (11% of the surveyed population did not do this).
  - Rinse fresh fruits and vegetables thoroughly with running water before eating, cutting, or cooking them (unless they are prepackaged). Scrub firm surfaces (e.g., cantaloupes and cucumbers) with a produce brush. Commercial cleaners are unnecessary.
- Cook: Cook food to the proper temperatures and use a food thermometer. The appearance or smell of food does not always indicate its safety.
  - Seafood, meat, poultry, and egg dishes should be cooked to the recommended safe minimum internal temperature to destroy harmful microbes. Eggs should be cooked thoroughly, and children should not "lick" the bowls of cake mixes using fresh eggs.
  - When food is being cooked in a microwave oven, foods should be stirred, rotated, and/or flipped periodically to help them cook evenly.
- Chill: Refrigerate food promptly within 2 hours, or in 1 hour for environments that are 90°F or hotter. This includes groceries, food being prepared, and leftovers and takeout foods. Keep the refrigerator at 40°F or less and the freezer at 0°F or less and monitor temperatures with a thermometer.
  - Keep hot food hot (140°F or higher) and cold foods cold (32–40°F). Between these temperatures is the danger zone in which harmful bacteria can grow rapidly, even exponentially.
  - Thaw food properly to avoid any bad bacteria: in the refrigerator; in cold water, such as in a leak-proof bag, changing the water for cold water every 30 minutes; or in the microwave oven, never on the countertop.

These guidelines also apply to carryout meals, restaurant leftovers, and home-packed meals to go. If in doubt, discard it.

Making a food safe after it has been handled improperly may not always be possible. For example, certain bacteria found in food that has been left at room temperature too long may produce a heat-resistant toxin that cannot be destroyed by cooking. Therefore the principal point is to be careful in preparing food, including cooking foods to the right temperatures, keeping track of the time food is exposed to certain temperatures, and being vigilant when eating out. If there is any doubt about the safety of the food, it is better not to eat it.

Without exception, everyone should exercise their best judgment and care when eating out, when handling their own food, or when handling the food of others. Prevention through education is the key to promoting healthy lives that are unscathed by the potentially severe and life-threatening effects of food-borne illness. On a more positive note, normal healthy adults with healthy immune systems are able to withstand the ill effects of most contaminants from the environment and from food.

# FOOD, NUTRITION, AND POVERTY

As already noted in the discussion of *Healthy People 2020*, a current focus is on attempting to reduce health disparities and health inequities, as well as a focus on future preventive measures. This can be done by healthy food choices being made available wherever people live, work, learn, and play.

*Healthy People 2020* goal: Promote health and reduce chronic disease risk through the consumption of healthful diets and achievement and maintenance of healthy body weights.

- Eliminate very low food security among children (from 1.3% of households with children in 2008 to 0.2% in 2020).
- Reduce household food insecurity (from 14.6% in 2008 to 6% in 2020) and in doing so reduce hunger.

## Poverty and Income Distribution

For most people in the United States, income has risen over time, providing more options for personal consumption expenditures, including those on food. However, growth in income has not increased equally for all households. Moreover, in recent economic times, people who normally have never needed help have flooded food banks and other federal and community resources (USA Today Supplement, 2010).

According to the US Census Bureau, in 2010 alone, 15.1% of the US population (or 46.2 million people) lived below the poverty level set by the government to determine eligibility for various types of government programs. This was the largest number in 52 years, since the beginning of poverty surveys. Of those people, approximately one-third (35.5%) were children, followed by those with disabilities (28%) and older Americans (25%). Regionally, poverty is concentrated in the South, followed by the West, Midwest, and Northeast. It also appears higher in cities than in rural areas (Nord et al., 2010; US Census Bureau, 2011).

In 2010, the groups with particularly high poverty rates included Hispanics and black Americans, with statistically equivalent poverty rates of 20.6% and 24.3% respectively. Food assistance programs, as discussed next, are one mechanism to provide a limited safety net to keep people from falling further into poverty (Nord et al., 2010).

## Food Assistance for Low-Income Individuals

Most Americans are food secure, having enough money and resources to obtain adequate food for active, healthy lives. However, for the minority who are living at or below the national poverty line, obtaining a nutritious diet without assistance can be a challenge. Low-income families spend a significantly higher percentage of their annual income on food than other families, often with less access to healthier options such as fresh fruits and vegetables (FRAC, 2016). A variety of federal, state, and local governments and private charitable organizations work to reduce hunger in the United States. The primary responsibility at the federal level falls to the USDA, which administers 15 nutrition assistance programs through the FNS using a combination of federal funding and farm commodities. Programs target the diverse needs of different subgroups of low-income people by providing supplemental assistance through a variety of forms and settings. In 2011, federally funded outlays for nutrition assistance programs resulted in amounts as detailed in the following list (USDA, FNS, 2011a):

- Supplemental Nutrition Assistance Program (SNAP)—formerly known as Food Stamps: $71 billion (Rosenbaum, 2012)
- Child Nutrition Program (includes the National School Breakfast Program [NSBP], the National School Lunch Program [NSLP], the Special Milk Program, the Child and Adult Care Food Program, and the Summer Food Service Program): almost $19.4 billion
- Special Supplemental Nutrition Program for Women, Infants, and Children (WIC): more than $7 billion
- Commodity supplemental food programs (Food Distribution Program on Native American Reservations, Nutrition Services Incentive Program, the Emergency Food Assistance Program, and farmers' market programs): almost $153 million

One in six people in the United States receive federally funded food assistance at some point every year. The SNAP, NSLP, NSBP, WIC, and Older American Act programs are the main programs that provide food and nutrition assistance. With tightening of federal and state budgets, these programs are continually targeted for significant funding cuts. Table 11-2 provides information on the various programs, along with their website addresses. Income eligibility requirements are based on household income and will change annually. Instructions for applying to the programs may be found directly on the respective websites.

## Supplemental Nutrition Assistance Program

SNAP supplements the food-buying power of eligible low-income households and is the foundation of the nations' nutrition safety net. Benefits are provided through an electronic benefit transfer (EBT) card that participants use to purchase food at authorized stores. It is designed to help low-income families and individuals purchase nutritionally adequate foods. Households can use their EBT card to purchase any food or food product for home consumption, as well as seeds and plants for use in home gardens. Restaurants can be authorized to accept EBT cards from qualified homeless, older, or disabled people in exchange for low-cost meals. Items that recipients cannot buy with EBT cards include alcoholic beverages, tobacco, hot ready-to-eat foods, lunch-counter items, and foods to be eaten in the store, vitamins, medicines, and pet foods.

Although there is no requirement that the EBT card be used to purchase nutrient-dense food, the goal of the SNAP nutrition education program is to increase the likelihood that recipients will make healthy food choices within their limited food budget. SNAP uses multiple strategies to facilitate healthy food choices and active lifestyles. These include providing nutrition education programs; encouraging more farmers' markets, small urban markets, and bodegas to participate in the program; and offering a demonstration project to examine the impact of incentives on participant purchases of fruits and vegetables.

The program is administered nationally by the FNS and locally by state and welfare agencies in all 50 states, the District of Columbia, Guam, and the US Virgin Islands. Eligibility is based on financial factors such as income and expenses available to the household, as well as 5 years of legal immigrant status, if applicable. SNAP requires most able-bodied adults aged between

| TABLE 11-2 | Select Federal Nutrition Assistance Programs | |
|---|---|---|
| **Program** | **Mission** | **To Find Out More** |
| Child and Adult Care Food Program (CACFP) | Provide aid to child and adult care institutions and family or group day care homes for the provision of nutritious foods that contribute to the wellness, healthy growth, and development of young children, and to the health and wellness of older adults and chronically impaired disabled individuals | http://www.fns.usda.gov/cacfp/child-and-adult-care-food-program |
| Child Nutrition Program | Provide healthy food to children from low-income families through a variety of programs, including the National School Lunch Program, the National School Breakfast Program, the Child and Adult Care Food Program, the Summer Food Service Program, the Fresh Fruit and Vegetable Program, and the Special Milk Program | http://www.fns.usda.gov/school-meals/child-nutrition-programs |
| Supplemental Nutrition Assistance Program (SNAP) | Offer nutrition assistance to low-income individuals and families and provide economic benefits to communities | http://www.fns.usda.gov/snap/supplemental-nutrition-assistance-program-snap |
| Special Supplemental Nutrition Program for Women, Infants, and Children (WIC) | Provide federal grants to states for supplemental foods, health care referrals, and nutrition education for low-income pregnant, breastfeeding, and nonbreastfeeding postpartum women, and to infants and children up to age 5 years who are found to be at nutritional risk | http://www.fns.usda.gov/wic/women-infants-and-children-wic |
| Food distribution programs | To strengthen the nation's nutrition safety net by providing food and nutrition assistance to schoolchildren and families; and support American agriculture by distributing high-quality, 100% American-grown USDA foods. The programs include the following: the Commodity Supplemental Food Program, the Food Distribution Program on Indian Reservations, The Emergency Food Assistance Program, the Nutrition Services Incentive Program, the DoD Fresh Fruit & Vegetable Program, and the Child Nutrition USDA Foods Program | http://www.fns.usda.gov/fdd/food-distribution-programs |

*DoD,* Department of Defense; *USDA,* US Department of Agriculture.
Modified from US Department of Agriculture, Food and Nutrition Service. (2016). *Programs and services.* Washington, DC. http://www.fns.usda.gov/programs-and-services.

16 and 60 years (with few exceptions) to register for work, to take part in employment/training programs referred by the SNAP office, and to accept or continue in suitable employment. Households may own certain limited resources. In addition to income, the EBT allotment is also based on family size. In contrast to public perception, less than 10% of households received cash welfare in 2009, and the latest statistics from 2010 showed 40% of households had at least one wage earner. In addition, according to FNS data, most households advance from SNAP in less than 1 year (Rosenbaum, 2012). In 2011, 92% of SNAP funding went directly to 40.3 million people: 48% children, 44% adults, and 8% adult aged 60 years or older. The average monthly benefit per person was approximately $134 and almost $290 per household (USDA, FNS, 2011b).

With passage of the 2012 Farm Bill, approximately $4.5 billion will be cut from SNAP, with an estimated loss of 500,000 possible recipients and almost $90 less in benefits per household.

## Child Nutrition Program

Collectively called the "Child Nutrition Program," these programs provide cash reimbursement and commodity support for meals served to children in schools, child care facilities, and summer settings. They include the NSLP, the NSBP, the Child and Adult Care Food Program, the Summer Food Service Program, and the Special Milk Program. The general purpose of these programs is to help ensure the health and well-being of all the nation's children. The two biggest and most well-known programs are described next.

*National school lunch program.* The federally funded NSLP is administered by the FNS. On the state level, the NSLP is usually administered by the US Department of Education, which contracts with local public, nonprofit private, and residential child care centers and schools to provide balanced, low-cost or free lunches. The NSLP reaches approximately 31.6 million children each school day (FRAC, 2016), including the following:

- Children from families with incomes at or below 130% of the federal poverty level guidelines are eligible for free school meals.
- Children from families with incomes above 130% to 185% of the poverty level are eligible for reduced-price school meals.
- Children from families with incomes more than 185% of the poverty level are eligible for full-price school meals.

Schools that choose to take part in the lunch program must implement wellness policies that promote healthy eating, address obesity, and encourage physical activity. Schools are provided with cash subsidies and approved agricultural commodities from the USDA as a supplement. Up to January 2012, free, reduced-price, or full-price lunches had to meet the following federal minimum pattern requirements:

- Must provide one-third of the recommended nutrient intake of 1989 RDAs
- To the extent possible, be consistent with the *Dietary Guidelines for Americans* recommendations for reducing sugar, salt, and fat intake

Under the Healthy Hunger-Free Kids Act of 2010, the USDA gained authority to set policy and nutrition criteria for all child nutrition standards, including the NSLP. New meal standards were published in 2012 based on the 2009 IOM recommendations to move subsidized meals into line with the *Dietary Guidelines for Americans* and the DRIs (Stallings et al., 2010; USDA, FNS, 2011b). The new rules stipulate a doubling of previous amounts of fruits and vegetables served in schools, set limits on the levels of trans fats and salt, increase the amount of whole grains served, make 1% and fat-free milk the norm, and establish suitable ranges for daily calorie intake. They also require free drinkable water in food service areas and increase subsidies to schools following the new guidelines. Even with changes, the NSLP budget projections are less than the current budget by eliminating the meat/meat substitute requirement at breakfast, allowing a phase-in period for fruits and vegetables, honoring requests to take smaller portions, and discontinuing price supports for meals, including separately priced items.

*National school breakfast program.* The NSBP was designed to make it possible for all schoolchildren to receive a nutritious breakfast every day. Skipping breakfast can adversely affect children's performance potential. The NSBP provides assistance to states to initiate, maintain, or expand nonprofit breakfast programs in eligible schools and residential child care institutions. Any child attending a participating school may receive a free, reduced-price, or full-price breakfast based on the same income criteria used by the NSLP. In the 2010 to 2011 school year, 11.7 million children in almost 88,000 schools were fed every day (FRAC, 2016).

### Special Supplemental Nutrition Program for Women, Infants, and Children

WIC supplies free nutritious supplemental food, nutrition counseling, breastfeeding support, and health and social service referrals to eligible low-income pregnant or postpartum women and to children younger than 5 years old who are at nutritional risk. Congress funds WIC every year for a specific amount as a federal grant program to be administered by FNS and 90 "state" agencies (including 50 states, 34 tribes, the District of Columbia, and 5 US territories). Services are offered in a wide variety of settings: county health departments, hospitals, mobile clinics, community centers, schools, public housing sites, Indian reservations, migrant health centers and camps, and Indian Health Service facilities.

Eligibility is based on the following factors. Income must be 185% or less of the US poverty income guidelines (approximately $41,000 for a family of four in 2009), and participants must meet one of two major types of nutritional risk:
- Medically based risks, such as anemia, underweight, maternal age, history of pregnancy complications, or poor pregnancy outcome
- Diet-based risks, such as inadequate dietary pattern as determined by 24-hour recall, food frequency questionnaire, or diet history

Those who qualify usually receive monthly checks or vouchers to buy foods designed to augment their diet with specific nutrients. In addition, a growing number of state agencies issue an electronic benefit card (like a debit card), and some distribute WIC foods through warehouses or deliver WIC foods to recipients' homes.

The foods differ depending on an individual's specific food package designation but can include iron-fortified infant cereal, iron-fortified adult cereal, fruit or vegetable juice rich in vitamin C, eggs, milk, cheese, and peanut butter or dried beans. WIC recognizes and promotes breastfeeding as the optimal source of nutrition for infants. For women who do not breastfeed, WIC provides iron-fortified infant formula. Special infant formulas and medical foods may be provided when prescribed by a physician for a specified medical condition. In 2009 new foods were added and specific food packages were reformulated to improve variety, to increase flexibility for diverse cultures, and for alignment with the *Dietary Guidelines for Americans* and American Academy of Pediatrics infant feeding practice guidelines. These foods include soy-based beverages, tofu, fruits and vegetables, baby foods, whole-wheat bread, and other whole-grain options.

Each WIC participant receives vouchers with maximum monthly allowable amounts of particular components specially designed for the following categories: fully breastfeeding mother; pregnant or partially breastfeeding mother; postpartum, fully formula feeding mother; fully breastfed baby; partially breastfed baby; fully formula-fed baby; and children 1 to 5 years old (California WIC Association, 2009).

Of the 9.17 million people who received WIC benefits each month in 2011, approximately 4.86 million were children, 2.17 million were infants, and 2.14 million were women (USDA, FNS, 2011a). Financial constraints preclude WIC from serving all eligible people; therefore a system of priorities has been established for filling program openings. After a local WIC agency has reached its maximum caseload, vacancies are filled in the order of the following priority levels:
- Pregnant women, breastfeeding women, and infants determined to be at nutritional risk of serious medical problems
- Infants up to 6 months of age whose mothers participate in WIC or are eligible to participate and have serious medical problems
- Children up to age 5 years at nutritional risk of serious medical problems
- Pregnant or breastfeeding women and infants who are at nutritional risk of dietary problems
- Children up to age 5 years at nutritional risk of dietary problems
- Nonbreastfeeding postpartum women with any nutritional risk
- Individuals at nutritional risk only because they are homeless or migrants and current participants who would likely continue to have medical or dietary problems without WIC assistance

WIC funding may be inadequate in the future to fund the increased numbers of expected participants (National WIC Association, 2014). For state agencies that apply for a grant, the WIC Farmers' Market Nutrition Program (or WIC FMNP) gives additional coupons to people to use to purchase fresh fruits and vegetables at participating farmers' markets. The WIC FMNP has two goals: to provide fresh, nutritious, unprepared, locally grown fruits and vegetables from farmers' markets to WIC participants, and to expand consumers' awareness and use of farmers' markets.

The overall statistics on WIC demonstrate it is effective in improving the health of its participants. Medicaid costs for women who participate in the program during pregnancy and their infants are lower than those for women who do not participate. WIC participation is also linked to longer gestation periods, higher birth weights, and lower infant mortality rates (USDA, FNS, Office of Research and Analysis, 2012).

### Food and Nutrition Programs for Older Adults

At the other end of the life cycle, a significant number of older people face special obstacles to obtaining an optimal diet. Of particular concern are adults older than 75 years who are frail, alone, or restricted to a limited budget. Life changes such as the loss of a spouse/significant other; sensory changes in taste or smell; physical inability to obtain food; and decreasing calorie needs can make acquisition of an adequate diet challenging.

A variety of nutrition assistance programs are available to this population. They include SNAP, the Senior Farmer's Market Nutrition Program, the Child and Adult Care Food Program, The Emergency Food Assistance Program, and the Commodity Supplemental Food Program. However, the programs that most people may be familiar with are some of those provided under the Older Americans Act, collectively called the Elderly Nutrition Services Program, which are managed by the Administration on Aging (AoA) through the USDHHS. They are designed to help older adults access nutritionally sound meals, obtain nutritional services and other health-promotion services (including nutrition screening and counseling), and reduce the social isolation that may occur in old age. Priority is given to older people with the greatest social and economic need: low income, minorities, those with limited English proficiency, rural location, and frail seniors at risk of institutionalization (USDHHS, AoA, 2009).

*The older adults nutrition services program.* This program includes the Congregate Nutrition Services Program (CNSP), the Home-Delivered Nutrition Services Program (i.e., "Meals on Wheels"); and the Nutrition Services Incentive Program (NSIP), which gives states, territories, and Indian tribal organizations (ITOs) the ability to purchase food or to cover the cost of commodities from the USDA for the CNSP and the Home-Delivered Nutrition Services Program. The AoA provides funds to states, territories, and ITOs, and it awards money to Area Agencies on Aging for coordination with area food sites such as senior centers, faith-based sites, community centers, adult day care centers, and schools. For NSIP, the share of the population who received meals under CNSP or Meals on Wheels in the preceding year determines money or commodity allocation.

By law, age is the only factor used in determining eligibility. People aged 60 years or older and their spouse or caretaker, regardless of age, are eligible for benefits. ITOs may select an age younger than 60 years for the definition of an older person for their tribes because of a shorter life expectancy and higher incidence of chronic illnesses. Additionally, disabled people who live in elder care housing facilities, people who accompany older participants to congregate feeding sites, and volunteers who assist in the meal service may also receive meals. For those in the Home-Delivered Nutrition Services Program, spouses of any age and disabled persons may also participate as long as they live with the homebound elder.

Additionally, by law, there is no income requirement for meals. Each recipient may contribute as much as desired toward the cost of the meal, but meals are free to people who cannot make any contribution. As of 2011, federal money contributed only approximately 42% of the money for these programs; 15% came from state funding, with the balance coming from local, private, or participant contribution (Johnson, 2011). In recent years, many states have shifted allowable money from congregate feeding sites into Meals on Wheels or other nutrition/health-promotion programs to help keep older adults in their communities. Even so, long waiting lists for Meals on Wheels are not uncommon and volunteers to help deliver meals to stretch limited dollars are always needed. This situation is not likely to improve with continuing federal and state budget constraints.

In 2010, 92.5 million meals, or approximately 40% of total meals, were served in congregate settings to just less than 1.69 million meal participants. A 2009 report by the AoA showed 57% of those people were aged 75 years or older, 48% lived alone, 13% had annual incomes of $10,000 or less, and 57% stated the meal provided half or more of their daily food intake. Participants also said they saw friends more often because of meals (87%). For every 10 meals, 6 were delivered to homebound elderly people, for a total of 149.2 million home-delivered meals to approximately 880,000 meal participants. Of those older people, 70% were aged 75 years or older, 56% lived alone, 25% had an annual income of $10,000 or less, and 59% said the meals provided half or more of their daily food intake. Four in 10 people needed help with at least one activity of daily living, and 85% needed help with shopping, housework, and ambulating.

## NUTRITION SCREENING

**Nutrition screening** is the process of discovering characteristics or risk factors that are known to be associated with dietary or nutrition problems. Its primary purpose is to identify individuals (such as older adults and the poor) who are potentially at high risk of complex and involved problems that relate to nutrition. To serve this purpose, screening criteria must be simple, relatively straightforward, and easy to administer. Screening is also helpful in establishing priorities for the most efficient use of valuable time and money.

The single largest demographic group at disproportionate risk of malnutrition is older Americans. Nutrition screening holds a tremendous preventive health potential for older adults. The nurse should assess the need for nutrition counseling or a referral to a registered dietitian for an older person who has food-related problems that are impacting eating pleasure and quality of life (American Dietetic Association, 2010a). The pendulum has shifted to reduce unnecessary therapeutic diets for those at risk of unintentional weight loss and undernutrition. There is also controversy about the benefit of weight loss for obese older Americans except if their laboratory test results indicate risk of metabolic syndrome. A dietitian or community nutrition program might be appropriate if any of the following are identified in the individual:

- Inappropriate or inadequate food intake
- Desire by obese elderly person to lose weight—tailoring to provide adequate calories, protein, and physical activity to preserve lean body mass
- Need for nutrient/disease-specific counseling with specific food preferences, cultural taboos, or environmental constraints
- Serum cholesterol levels of more than 240 mg/dL with desire to change eating pattern
- Inability to self-feed or to prepare and purchase food, or inability to carry out food-related activities of daily living

The health care professional should refer the individual to a physician when there has been an involuntary decrease in weight of more than 10 pounds during the previous 6 months. Additional anthropometric measurements suggesting malnutrition include the following:

- Triceps skin-fold thickness less than the 10th percentile
- Mid-arm muscle circumference less than the 10th percentile
- Serum albumin level less than 3.5 g/dL
- Evidence of osteoporosis or mineral deficiency (indicated by a history of bone pain or fractures, particularly in housebound older women)
- Evidence of vitamin deficiency (indicated by long-term inadequate fruit and vegetable intake; angular stomatitis, glossitis, or bleeding gums; or pressure sores in bedridden individuals)

## NUTRITION RISK FACTORS

This section examines the role of nutrition in the cause and prevention of the leading nutrition-related chronic diseases—heart disease, stroke, some forms of cancer, osteoporosis, obesity, and type 2 diabetes—and in the early treatment of people in whom human immunodeficiency virus (HIV) infection was recently diagnosed.

### Cardiovascular Diseases

Cardiovascular diseases (CVDs), principally CHD and stroke, are among the leading killers of both men and women among all racial and ethnic groups in the United States. Approximately one-fourth of the US population has some form of CVD, including hypertension, CHD, and stroke.

CVD prevention is so important that *Healthy People 2020* has specific objectives to improve cardiovascular health and quality of life through prevention, detection, and treatment of risk factors for heart attack and stroke. Specific objectives are listed in Box 11-2: *Healthy People 2020*.

### Heart Disease
#### Diet Intervention

In an attempt to reduce the incidence of CVD, the American Heart Association (AHA) recommends that people older than 2 years adopt a well-balanced diet (Box 11-6: Research for Evidence-Based Practice), achieve and maintain a healthy body weight, and reach optimal levels for total cholesterol, high-density lipoprotein (HDL) cholesterol, low-density lipoprotein (LDL)

---

### BOX 11-6 RESEARCH FOR EVIDENCE-BASED PRACTICE
#### Dietary Risk Factors and Heart Disease[a]

Developing guidelines and recommendations for preventing heart disease is a topic that is routinely reassessed. You may ask, "Why do the recommendations change over time?" As with all things scientific, technology is ever-growing and advancing. Such scientific progress brings new findings, for which guidelines are amended. The gold standard in medicine is to base all medical intervention protocols on evidence-based practice. Evidence-based practice is the use of current evidence from available research coupled with clinical expertise to establish high-quality patient care.

CVD is the leading cause of death in the United States, and suboptimal diet quality is the single largest risk factor contributing to death and disability. The American Heart Association notes that the primary contributors to poor dietary habits are insufficient consumption of fruits, vegetables, nuts/seeds, whole grains, and seafood and an excessively high intake of sodium (Mozaffarian et al., 2016). The American Heart Association's evidence-based practice guidelines to prevent CVD encourage American's to achieve at least four of the five following key components of a healthy diet:

- Fruits and vegetables: consume more than 4.5 cups per day
- Fish: consume more than two 3.5-oz servings per week (preferably oily fish)
- Fiber-rich whole grains (>1.1 g of fiber per 10 g of carbohydrates): consume three 1-oz-equivalent servings per day
- Sodium: limit to less than 1500 mg per day
- Sugar-sweetened beverages: limit to less than 450 kcal (36 oz) total per week

Considering that only 1.5% of adults and less than 1% of children in the United States currently meet these healthy diet criteria, there is a lot of room for improvement.

[a]With contribution from Staci Nix.
From Mozaffarian, D, Benjamin, E. J., Go, A. S., Arnett, D. K., Blaha, M. J., Cushman, M., et al. (2016). Heart disease and stroke statistics—2016 update: A report from the American Heart Association. *Circulation, 133,* e38–e360.

---

cholesterol, blood pressure, and blood glucose (Lichtenstein et al., 2006). (The AHA did not set guidelines for children younger than 2 years.)

However, eating two or more servings of fish (approximately 8 ounces) every week, preferably oily varieties rich in eicosapentaenoic acid or docosahexaenoic acid, omega-3 fatty acids, such as canned light tuna, salmon, pollock, and catfish seems safe.

Smaller fish may have less mercury contaminants than larger ones.

- Limit intake of saturated fat to 10% of energy by choosing lean meats and vegetable alternatives, and fat-free (skim) or low-fat (1% fat) dairy products.
- When eating food prepared outside of the home, follow these diet and lifestyle recommendations:
  - Reduce salt intake by comparing the sodium content of similar products (e.g., different brands of tomato sauce) and choosing products with less salt or sodium; choosing versions of processed foods, including cereals and baked goods, that are reduced in salt or sodium; and limiting consumption of condiments (e.g., soy sauce, ketchup).
  - Neither antioxidant vitamin supplements nor other supplements such as selenium are recommended.

Many children, adolescents, and adults who already have unhealthy levels of lipids in their blood should receive nutrition counseling (Grundy et al., 2004). In children aged 2 to 20 years, an acceptable level of total cholesterol is less than 170 mg/dL.

Individuals with LDL cholesterol levels that are higher than 100 mg/dL should be advised to reduce their dietary intake of saturated fat and cholesterol to levels below those recommended for the general population (Expert Panel on Detection, Evaluation, and Treatment of High Blood Cholesterol in Adults, 2001). The upper limit for these individuals is less than 7% of the total energy for saturated fat and less than 200 mg of cholesterol per day. The *Dietary Guidelines for Americans 2015–2020* does not set specific quantitative limits for dietary cholesterol consumption per day. However, the healthy eating patterns that are recommended are naturally low in cholesterol, with approximately 100 to 300 mg of dietary cholesterol per day. Individuals at risk of heart disease may be advised to further limit their cholesterol intake, particularly if their LDL cholesterol levels are high. After the dietary intervention has been outlined to the individual, follow-up sessions are scheduled to monitor lipid levels and dietary adherence.

The National Cholesterol Education Program (NCEP) develops new guidelines periodically, as warranted by research advances. The most recent set of guidelines, the *Third Report of the NCEP Expert Panel on Detection, Evaluation, and Treatment of High Blood Cholesterol in Adults,* also known as the Adult Treatment Panel III (ATP III) (Table 11-3), was updated in 2004. The changes in

options for more intensive cholesterol level reduction treatment for high-risk and moderate-risk individuals were based on the review of five clinical trials of cholesterol-lowering statin treatment. The update did not change the ATP III recommendations for people at moderate or lower risk. The ATP guidelines recommend that healthy adults have a lipoprotein analysis once every 5 years. A lipoprotein profile measures levels of LDL cholesterol, total cholesterol, HDL cholesterol, and triglycerides (fat in the blood). The level at which HDL becomes a major risk factor for heart disease is less than 40 mg/dL for men and less than 50 mg/dL for women.

In addition to a low HDL level, there are other major risk factors for CHD:

- Clinical forms of atherosclerotic disease (peripheral arterial disease, abdominal aortic aneurysm, and symptomatic carotid artery disease)
- Age (≥45 years for men and ≥55 years for women)
- Cigarette smoking
- Hypertension (blood pressure ≥140/90 mmHg or taking antihypertensive medication)
- Family history of premature heart disease (heart disease in a first-degree relative at age less than 55 years for men or at age less than 65 years for women)
- Type 1 diabetes
- Obesity
- Metabolic syndrome

HDL cholesterol level greater than 60 mg/dL is considered a negative risk factor.

### Therapeutic Lifestyle Changes Treatment Plan

The therapeutic lifestyle changes (TLC) treatment plan of nutrition, physical activity, and weight control is recommended for treatment of people who present with type 2 diabetes, elevated levels of LDL, or **metabolic syndrome**.

Metabolic syndrome describes the presence of a cluster of risk factors that often occur together, which dramatically increases the risk of coronary events. The syndrome is diagnosed when an individual has three or more of the following factors:

- Excessive abdominal fat, as indicated by too large a waist measurement (>35 inches or 88 cm in women and >40 inches or 102 cm in men)
- Elevated blood pressure (higher than 130 mmHg systolic or 85 mmHg diastolic)
- Low HDL level (<40 mg/dL)
- Elevated **triglyceride** level (>150 mg/dL), which is significantly linked to the degree of heart disease risk. (The guidelines recommend even borderline high triglyceride levels be treated with therapy that includes weight control and physical activity.)

The dietary component of the TLC treatment plan includes the following daily intake:

- Less than 7% of calories from saturated fat
- Less than 200 mg of dietary cholesterol
- Up to 35% of calories from total fat, provided most of the fat is unsaturated fat, which does not raise cholesterol levels. (A higher fat intake may be needed by some individuals with high triglyceride levels or a low HDL level, or both, to prevent their triglyceride levels or HDL status from increasing.)

| TABLE 11-3 Cholesterol and Lipoprotein Profile Classification | |
|---|---|
| **Cholesterol Reading** | **Classification** |
| **Total Cholesterol (mg/dL)** | |
| <180 | Optimal |
| <200 | Near optimal |
| 200–239 | Borderline high |
| ≥240 | High |
| **Low-Density Lipoprotein Cholesterol (mg/dL)** | |
| <100 | Optimal |
| 100–129 | Near optimal |
| 130–159 | Borderline high |
| 160–189 | High |
| ≥190 | Very high |
| **High-Density Lipoprotein Cholesterol (mg/dL)** | |
| ≥60 | Optimal |
| 40–59 | Borderline/normal |
| <40 | A major risk factor for heart disease |
| **Triglycerides (mg/dL)** | |
| <150 | Optimal |
| 150–199 | Borderline high |
| 200–499 | High |
| ≥500 | Very high |

Modified from Nix, S. (2017). *Williams' basic nutrition and diet therapy* (15th ed.). St. Louis: Elsevier.

- Intake of certain foods to boost the diet's LDL-lowering power: 2 g/day of plant stanols and sterols found in cholesterol-lowering margarines and salad dressings, and 10 to 25 g/day of foods high in soluble fiber, such as cereal grains, beans, peas, legumes, and many fruits and vegetables

A primary treatment goal of the TLC treatment plan is reduction of an elevated LDL level to:

- Less than 100 mg/dL with a therapeutic option of less than 70 mg/dL in the presence of CHD or other forms of atherosclerotic disease
- Less than 130 mg/dL with a therapeutic option of less than 100 mg/dL in the presence of two or more risk factors for CHD
- Less than 160 mg/dL in the presence of fewer than two risk factors for CHD

The final goal of the TLC treatment plan includes weight control (to enhance LDL level lowering and raise HDL level) and physical activity that lasts at least 30 minutes, expending at least 200 calories per day on most days (to decrease HDL and, for some, LDL levels).

## Removing Barriers to Treatment Goals

To improve an individual's adherence to ATP III goals, treatment barriers can be eliminated by the development of protocols to encourage long-term individual adherence and follow-up, such as establishing clinic policy and developing computerized databases for those seeking care, establishing management algorithms, reinforcing and rewarding adherence, and enhancing third-party reimbursement. The nurse uses behavioral theories to identify a person's level of readiness to change and focus on counseling strategies to match that level of readiness (Snetselaar, 2004).

## Hypertension

Blood pressure, the force of blood against the walls of arteries, is recorded as the systolic pressure (as the heart beats) over the diastolic pressure (as the heart relaxes between beats). The measurement is written with one number above (or before) the other, with the systolic blood pressure (SBP) listed first and the diastolic blood pressure (DBP) listed second. For example, a blood pressure measurement of 120/80 mmHg is expressed verbally as "120 over 80." Normal blood pressure is less than 120 mmHg systolic and less than 80 mmHg diastolic. *The Seventh Report of the Joint National Committee on Prevention, Detection, Evaluation, and Treatment of High Blood Pressure* (National High Blood Pressure Education Program, 2003) added a pre-hypertension classification defined as an SBP range of 120 to 139 mmHg or a DBP range of 80 to 89 mmHg to highlight increased risk of progression to frank hypertension and CVD (National High Blood Pressure Education Program, 2003). A more recent review by the panel members appointed to the Eighth Joint National Committee (JNC 8) did not readdress the definitions of hypertension and pre-hypertension, but reexamined and redefined thresholds for drug treatment (James et al., 2014). JNC 8 also found strong evidence to address treating hypertensive 60-year-old or older individuals to a goal blood pressure of 150/90 mmHg and younger hypertensive individuals aged 30 to 59 years to a DBP of less than 90 mmHg (James et al., 2014). On the basis of this evidence, *Healthy People 2020* contains objectives related to pre-hypertension (see Box 11-2: *Healthy People 2020*).

## Epidemiology

In 2008 hypertension contributed to the deaths of approximately 348,000 Americans out of 2.4 million people. Approximately 44% were men and 56% were women (Roger et al., 2012). If a definition of hypertension as blood pressure higher than 140/90 mmHg is used, as many as 76.5 million adult Americans, or nearly one-third of all adults in the United States, have high blood pressure. NHANES data from 2005 to 2008 show that one in three people with hypertension are unaware of their condition, and over 50% of those surveyed do not have controlled high blood pressure (Egan et al., 2011). Untreated hypertension can damage arteries and increase the risk of stroke and congestive heart failure. High blood pressure is also responsible for many cases of kidney failure requiring dialysis and increases the risk of kidney failure in people with diabetes.

Non-Hispanic black and non-Hispanic white Americans are more likely to have high blood pressure than are Hispanic Americans although the rates for all ethnicities are significant. More women than men (3 in 4) have high blood pressure at age 75 years or older. It appears to affect more people with lower educational and income levels, although this may be related to other factors.

## Diet Intervention

The modifiable nutrition-related risk factors for stroke include high blood pressure, obesity, habitual high alcohol intake, and high intake of sodium (Appel et al., 2006; CDC, 2011c; Lloyd-Jones et al., 2010). However there appears to be no need to restrict salt intake to less than the suggested 2000 mg currently in the guidelines for everyone with mild hypertension. There appears to be a class of hypertensive individuals who are salt sensitive who benefit from sodium restriction (Sanada et al., 2011). No certain method exists for identifying susceptible people or ascertaining how many of them become hypertensive as a result of excessive salt intake; therefore the conservative preventive health approach recommends a daily salt intake limited to 6 g or less for adults. Sodium chloride is approximately 40% sodium by weight; therefore a diet with 6 g of salt contains approximately 2300 mg of sodium. This amount is regarded as mild sodium restriction. Ideally, the recommendations are to reduce sodium intake to approximately 1500 mg, but this is very difficult with the current prevalence of sodium in packaged and restaurant foods. More than 45 national health organizations and 20 restaurant and food packaging companies have so far joined in the National Salt Reduction Initiative, started by New York City mayor Michael Bloomberg in 2008; the initiative aims to reduce the sodium level in food by 25% over 5 years. The following are the three major sources of sodium in the US diet, in order of predominance:

- Salt added by food processing companies as an ingredient in almost all processed foods (including many foods that do not taste salty, such as baked goods); most processed foods have a high sodium content (80%)
- Salt added by consumers to food during cooking or at the table (5–6% each)

- Salt from all animal products, which are a natural source of sodium

The following recommended food tips are designed to reduce salt and sodium intake:

- Sodium occurs naturally in many foods and is also added to most processed foods; therefore add salt only sparingly in home cooking and at the table.
- Consume fewer foods that have high sodium levels, such as many cheeses; processed meats; most frozen dinners and entrees; packaged mixes; most canned soups and vegetables; salad dressings; and condiments such as soy sauce, pickles, olives, catsup, and mustard.
- Rinse canned vegetables before warming them.
- Eat salty, highly processed salty, salt-preserved, and salt-pickled foods infrequently.
- Check labels for the amount of sodium in foods and choose products lower in sodium (free, <5 mg per serving; low, <140 mg per serving; reduced or less, 25% less than standard-reference food; healthy, <480 mg per serving).

### Dietary Approaches to Stop Hypertension Eating Plan

Clinical studies show that following the DASH eating plan helps to lower blood pressure. The National Heart, Lung, and Blood Institute, with additional support by the NIH, funded the DASH research, with the final results appearing in 1997. The DASH eating plan makes consuming less salt and sodium easier because the plan includes abundant fruits and vegetables, which are lower in sodium but higher in potassium than other foods. Potassium and sodium play important roles as electrolytes in intracellular and extracellular fluid balance. People at high risk of hypertension may have a high sodium intake that may upset the sodium-to-potassium ratio, and eating more vegetables and fruits may account for the success of the DASH diet. The plan also includes more fat-free or low-fat milk and milk products, whole grains, fish, poultry, beans, seeds, and nuts, but contains less sweets, added sugars and sugar-containing beverages, fats, and red meats than the average typical American diet.

The plan is rich in magnesium, potassium, calcium, protein, and fiber. At approximately 2100 calories a day, the nutrients include 4700 mg of potassium, 500 mg of magnesium, and 1250 mg of calcium. These totals are approximately two to three times the amounts most Americans receive.

On the basis of the findings of DASH clinical studies, a combination of the eating plan and reduced sodium intake can reduce elevated blood pressure or prevent it when blood pressure is normal. The plan may even eliminate the need for medication or, in the case of severe high blood pressure, allow a reduction in medication. Other steps to control or prevent hypertension should continue to be encouraged, including exercise weight loss when necessary, not smoking, and limiting alcohol consumption. DASH may also improve health in other ways. The potassium in fruits and vegetables helps reduce hypertension (AHA, 2016) and may reduce the risk of some cancers; the calcium in dairy products may reduce fat mass and thus hypertension (Zemel, 2001). The diet may help lower the risk of osteoporosis, and a diet low in saturated fat and cholesterol can reduce CVD risk. The complete DASH eating plan entitled *Your Guide to Lowering*

*Your Blood Pressure With DASH* (USDHHS, NIH, National Heart, Lung, and Blood Institute, 2006) can be obtained from http://www.nhlbi.nih.gov/health/resources/heart/hbp-dash-index.

## Cancer
### Epidemiology

The National Cancer Institute estimates that almost one in two (41%) women and men will receive a diagnosis of some type of cancer in their lifetime. Cancer remains the second leading cause of death in the United States (American Cancer Society, 2017; Miniño, 2011).

The most common cancers in in men and women are lung, colorectal, prostate and breast; these cancers apprise approximately 46% of cancer deaths. Over 25% of cancer deaths are due to lung cancer. For men in 2017, 42% of new cases will occur at prostate, lung, and colorectal sites; in women the most common sites are breast, lung, and colorectal. Breast cancer alone accounts for 30% of newly diagnosed cases (American Cancer Society, 2017).

Approximately one-third of cancer deaths among men and women are related to diet and sedentary lifestyle factors. The introduction of a healthy diet (Figure 11-4) and exercise practices at any time from childhood to old age can promote health and likely reduce cancer risk.

### Diet Intervention for Risk Reduction

Many dietary factors can affect cancer risk: types of foods, food preparation methods, portion sizes, food variety, and overall calorie balance. An overall dietary pattern that balances calorie intake and physical activity for weight management along with inclusion of a high proportion of plant foods (fruits, vegetables, whole grains, and beans) and limited amounts of processed or red meats and whole-fat dairy products may reduce the risk of cancer. The phytochemicals in fruits and vegetables, in particular, appear to have a protective effect by themselves, but dietary supplements, in particular supplements that exceed DRIs, do not provide the same benefits.

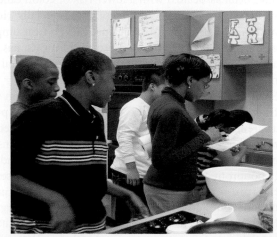

**FIGURE 11-4** Teenagers who help to prepare safe, nutritious meals become engaged in the healthy eating process. (From Mahan, L. K., & Raymond, J. L. [2017]. *Krause's food & the nutrition care process* [14th ed.]. St Louis: Elsevier.)

Based on its review of the scientific evidence, the American Cancer Society (ACS) updated its nutrition and physical activity guidelines in 2011 (Kushi et al., 2012). The ACS recommendations are very consistent with the messages of the *Dietary Guidelines for Americans 2015–2020,* the MyPlate guidelines, and the dietary recommendations of other national agencies for general health promotion and prevention of other diet-related chronic conditions. Although no diet can guarantee full protection against any disease, the ACS believes that the following recommendations offer the best nutrition information currently available to help Americans:

- For national, state, and local community action:
  - Apply policy and environmental changes that increase access to affordable, healthy foods in all places where adults and children live, work, go to school, or play and decrease access and marketing of foods and drinks of low nutritional value, particularly to youth.
- For individuals:
  - Choose most of the foods you eat from plant sources. Choose fewer and smaller portions of high-fat or calorie-dense foods and beverages. Eat at least 2.5 cups of a variety of fruits and vegetables every day. Choose whole-grain breads, cereals, pastas, brown rice, and beans. Limit consumption of processed meat (bacon, sausage, luncheon meats) and red meats such as beef, pork, or lamb. For those who do eat meat, choose leaner cuts and small portions, not more than one-quarter of the plate (similar to the MyPlate recommendation). Many scientific studies show that eating fruits and vegetables (especially green and dark yellow or orange vegetables, foods in the cabbage family, soy products, and legumes) may protect against cancers at many sites, particularly for cancers of the gastrointestinal and respiratory tracts. Consumption of at least five servings of fruits and vegetables among both smokers and nonsmokers seems to reduce the risk of lung cancer. Grains as well as fruits, vegetables, and dairy products are also an important source of many vitamins and minerals, such as folate, calcium, and selenium, which have been associated with a lower risk of colon cancer in some studies. Beans (legumes) are especially rich in nutrients that may protect against cancer. Consumption of meat, particularly red and processed meats, has been associated with an increased risk of cancer at several sites, most notably the colon, stomach, and prostate.
  - Since 1991 the 5 A Day for Better Health Program (now Fruits and Veggies—More Matters) has raised public awareness about the importance of fruits and vegetables in disease prevention. The program is jointly sponsored by the CDC and the Produce for Better Health Foundation (a nonprofit consumer education foundation representing the fruit and vegetable industry). Through its unique national public-private partnership, Fruits and Veggies—More Matters seeks to increase consumption of fruits and vegetables to five or more servings each day. The program focuses on mothers as the gatekeepers for families for the most part and provides informations, recipes, and materials for both consumers and partner organizations. It gives Americans a simple, positive message: eat more fruits and vegetables, start small, and aim for variety.

- Be physically active: achieve and maintain a healthy weight. Being overweight or obese, by itself or in combination with excess belly fat, increases the risk of cancers at several sites, such as the colon and rectum, prostate, endometrium, breast (among postmenopausal women), and kidney. Both increasing physical activity and balancing food intake to maximize nutrient density within calorie needs are essential. Keeping a healthy BMI without being underweight is ideal. If overweight, avoidance of more weight gain or even losing as little as 5% to 10% of weight can be beneficial.
- For those who drink alcohol, limit consumption. No more than one drink per day for women or two drinks per day for men should be the limit. Alcoholic beverages, along with cigarette smoking and the use of tobacco products, contribute to cancers of the oral cavity, esophagus, and larynx. Studies have also shown an association between alcohol consumption and an increased risk of breast cancer (American Cancer Society, 2009). The mechanism of this effect is not known, but the association may be related to the carcinogenic effects of alcohol or its metabolites, to changes in levels of hormones such as estrogens, or other processes. Regardless of the mechanism, studies show that the risk of breast cancer increases with an intake beginning at only a few drinks per week. Reducing alcohol consumption is a good way for women who drink regularly to reduce their risk of breast cancer.

Nurses may find it is helpful to refer to the sections in the nutrition and physical activity guidelines (Kushi et al., 2012) that refer to other aspects of food intake relating to prevention of cancer. They include more specific suggestions for particular cancers, evidence specific to nutrient supplementation, and answers to other frequently asked questions. It is available free for download (subject to copyright if used) at http://onlinelibrary.wiley.com/doi/10.3322/caac.20140/full.

## Osteoporosis
### Epidemiology

Osteoporosis, a bone disease characterized by low bone mass leading to fragile bones and an increased risk of hip, spine, and wrist fractures, is a major public health risk for an estimated 44 million individuals in the United States, or 55% of people aged 50 years or older (National Osteoporosis Foundation, 2011). Osteoporosis has already been diagnosed in 10 million people, and 34 million more people have low bone mineral density or osteopenia, placing them at increased risk of osteoporosis. Of the 10 million Americans estimated to have osteoporosis, 80% are women and 20% are men. Of those with hip fractures, 24% die within a year, men twice as often as women and black American women more often than Caucasian women. Direct financial expenditures for management of osteoporotic fracture alone were estimated at $19 billion in 2005 and will likely rise to approximately $25.3 billion by 2025. These figures underestimate significantly the true costs of osteoporosis because they fail to include the costs of treatment for individuals without a history of fractures or the indirect costs of lost wages or productivity of either the individual or the caregiver.

The National Osteoporosis Foundation recognizes the following risk factors for osteoporosis:

- Older age: as age increases, risk increases
- Female gender
- Personal history of osteoporosis or fracture as an adult
- Family history of osteoporosis or broken bones
- Low levels of sex hormones: in women, early estrogen deficiency (younger than 45 years) or low estrogen levels during menopause, missing periods (amenorrhea); in men, low levels of testosterone and estrogen
- Diet: low in calcium or vitamin D intake; high intake of protein, sodium, and caffeine
- Sedentary lifestyle
- Use of oral corticosteroid therapy for 3 months or more
- Smoking (active or passive)
- High alcohol intake (three or more drinks per day)
- Specific medications (steroids, some anticonvulsants, and other medications)
- Some diseases and conditions (anorexia nervosa, rheumatoid arthritis, gastrointestinal diseases, including celiac disease, sickle cell anemia, and lupus).

Although the prevalence of osteoporosis and the incidence of fracture differ by sex and race/ethnicity, there is a significant risk for all groups even with differences in bone mass density. The latest available facts (National Institute of Arthritis and Musculoskeletal and Skin Diseases, 2012a, 2102b) indicate that an estimated 20% of non-Hispanic Caucasian/Asian women, 10% of Hispanic women, and 5% of non-Hispanic black women 50 years or older currently have osteoporosis. Low bone density is even higher in the same groups: 52%, 49%, and 35% respectively. Currently, risk is rising most rapidly in Hispanic women although the reasons are unknown. Among men 50 years or older, an estimated 7% of non-Hispanic Caucasian/Asian men, 4% of non-Hispanic black men, and 3% of Hispanic men have osteoporosis. Low bone density is higher in the same groups: 35%, 19%, and 23% respectively (National Institute of Arthritis and Musculoskeletal and Skin Diseases, 2012a, 2012b). As there is limited information on other ethnic/racial groups, the data are not included.

## Pathophysiology

Osteoporosis develops slowly, resulting in loss of bone mass and fractures, especially in the wrist, hip, and spinal areas. It is defined as a skeletal disorder characterized by compromised bone strength predisposing to an increased risk of fracture. Bone strength reflects the integration of two main features: bone density and bone quality. Bone mineral density is expressed as grams of mineral per area or volume and, in any given individual, is determined by peak bone mass and amount of bone loss. Bone quality refers to architecture, turnover, damage accumulation (microfractures), and mineralization. Osteoporotic bone fractures more easily than healthy bone; as such, osteoporosis is a significant risk factor for fracture.

***Factors involved in building and maintaining skeletal health throughout life.*** The bone mass attained early in life, 85% to 90% of which is reached by age 18 years for girls and age 20 years for boys, is perhaps the most important determinant of lifelong skeletal health. Individuals with the highest peak bone mass after adolescence have the greatest protective advantage when there is a decline in bone density with increasing age, illness, and diminished sex steroid production.

Genetic factors exert a strong and perhaps predominant influence on peak bone mass, but physiological, environmental, and modifiable lifestyle factors can also play a significant role. Among these factors are adequate nutrition and body weight, the sex hormones of puberty, and physical activity (particularly weight-bearing activity). Therefore maximizing bone mineral density early in life presents a vital opportunity to reduce the effect of bone loss related to aging. Childhood is a critical time for development of lifestyle habits conducive to maintaining good bone health throughout life. Additionally, cigarette smoking, which may start in adolescence, may have a deleterious effect on bone mass.

## Prevention

Once thought to be a natural part of aging among women, osteoporosis is no longer considered age or sex dependent and is largely preventable, thanks to the recent progress in the understanding of its causes, diagnosis, and treatment. Optimization of bone health is a process that must occur throughout the life span in both men and women so as to prevent osteoporosis. Calcium and vitamin D are the nutrients most important for attaining peak bone mass and for preventing and treating osteoporosis. Although it is difficult to obtain an adequate amount of calcium from food sources, the alternative use of supplements is in question as there is no apparent evidence that they prevent fractures as well as dietary sources (Bolland et al., 2015).

A healthy diet, adequate in calories and appropriate nutrients, is essential for normal growth and development of all tissues, including bone. Table 11-4 suggests dietary calcium (and vitamin D) intake recommendations for various stages of life. Factors contributing to low calcium intake include restriction of consumption of dairy products because of food preferences or lactose intolerance, a generally low level of fruit and vegetable consumption, and a high intake of low-calcium beverages such as soft drinks. Lactose and vitamin D enhance calcium absorption, as does as an acidic environment, seen in superior absorption in calcium-enriched orange juice. Calcium is well absorbed from dairy foods, which are also the only source of lactose that enhances absorption.

Vitamin D is a fat-soluble vitamin encompassing two molecules—vitamin D2 (ergocalciferol) and vitamin D3 (cholecalciferol). Vitamin D3 is the form of vitamin D that best supports bone health. It is synthesized in the body when the skin is exposed to the ultraviolet rays of the sun. This process is complicated by various concerns about sunscreens, clothing, and weather changes. Vitamin D from foods, as well as that from sun exposure, then undergoes a complicated metabolic pathway through the liver and the kidneys, emerging as the hormone 1,25-dehydroxyvitamin $D_3$, the active form. Vitamin D is commonly added to milk, and other food sources of vitamin D include fatty fish (salmon and mackerel); fortified margarine; eggs; and

## TABLE 11-4 Dietary Reference Intakes for Calcium and Vitamin D

| Life Stage Group | CALCIUM | | | VITAMIN D | | |
|---|---|---|---|---|---|---|
| | EAR (mg/day) | RDA (mg/day) | UL (mg/day) | EAR (IU/day) | RDA (IU/day) | UL (IU/day) |
| Infants from birth to 6 mo | — | — | 1000 | — | — | 1000 |
| Infants from 6 to 12 mo | — | — | 1500 | — | — | 1500 |
| 1–3 yr | 500 | 700 | 2500 | 400 | 600 | 2500 |
| 4–8 yr | 800 | 1000 | 2500 | 400 | 600 | 3000 |
| 9–13 yr | 1100 | 1300 | 3000 | 400 | 600 | 4000 |
| 14–18 yr | 1100 | 1300 | 3000 | 400 | 600 | |
| 19–30 yr | 800 | 1000 | 2500 | 400 | 600 | 4000 |
| 31–50 yr | 800 | 1000 | 2500 | 400 | 600 | 4000 |
| 51–70 yr men | 800 | 1000 | 2000 | 400 | 600 | 4000 |
| 51–70 yr women | 1000 | 1200 | 2000 | 400 | 600 | 4000 |
| >70 yr | 1000 | 1200 | 2000 | 400 | 800 | 4000 |
| 14–18 yr, pregnant or lactating | 1100 | 1300 | 3000 | 400 | 600 | 4000 |
| 19–50 yr, pregnant or lactating | 800 | 1000 | 2500 | 400 | 600 | 4000 |

*EAR*, Estimated average requirement; *RDA*, recommended dietary allowance; *UL*, tolerable upper intake level.
From Food and Nutrition Board, Institute of Medicine. (2011*). Dietary reference intakes for calcium and vitamin D.* Washington, DC: National Academies Press.

some fortified, ready-to-eat cereals. Some studies are questioning whether or not most infants and young children in the United States are getting adequate calcium and vitamin D intakes. Black and colleagues (2014) concluded that the overall dietary intake of children consuming a usual diet makes it impossible to meet the vitamin D recommendations of the Institute of Medicine, Food and Nutrition Board (2011). During adolescence, when consumption of dairy products decreases, vitamin D intake is likely to be inadequate, which may affect calcium absorption adversely. Other nutrients have been evaluated relative to bone health. High dietary protein, caffeine, phosphorus, and sodium intake may adversely affect calcium balance; however, their effects appear to be offset in individuals with adequate calcium intakes.

Food should be selected to provide adequate calcium intake. Women of all ages should make sure they get adequate calcium intake by consuming more calcium-rich foods, including calcium-fortified foods such as orange juice, milk, and other dairy products as they deliver the most calcium of any food group. Low-fat (1%) and fat-free milk, low-fat yogurt, and low-fat cheeses are the dairy products of choice. Other good sources of calcium include sardines, canned salmon (if the bones are eaten), and some dark green leafy vegetables, especially collard greens. Orange juice and milk fortified with calcium are also good sources, as are soy, almond and rice milks, and other fortified food products. Supplementation with calcium tablets may be appropriate for high-risk individuals with inadequate calcium intake. However, it is particularly important for older women to be vigilant about their intakes of calcium from dietary sources, supplements, and medications such as antacids because of the

risk of exceeding the UL of any age/gender group (National Research Council, 2010). Men may also be wise to limit calcium supplementation and not exceed normal dietary levels because of an association with increased risk of prostate cancer (Kushi et al., 2012).

For those who do choose calcium supplements, calcium carbonate (40% elemental calcium), calcium citrate (24%), calcium lactate (14%), and calcium gluconate (9%) are preferred. (Dolomite and bone meal are not recommended because they may be contaminated with lead.) Calcium supplement absorption is most efficient for individuals with adequate gastric acid production at doses no greater than 500 mg at a time when taken with meals.

Anyone younger than 25 years who ingests less than the recommended DRI for calcium should be urged to develop strategies for increasing it. Children, particularly girls between the ages of 9 and 18 years, are at the highest risk of deficiency (National Research Council, 2010). By modeling appropriate behaviors, health care professionals can help prevent or delay the onset of osteoporosis in themselves, their families, and the people in their care.

## Obesity

Overweight (defined in the Body Mass Index Formulas section) can seriously affect health and longevity and is associated with the leading nutrition-related causes of death in the United States: type 2 DM, CVD, and some cancers. Obesity (defined in the Body Mass Index for Adults section) is also associated with gout and gallbladder disease and may contribute to the development of osteoarthritis in the weight-bearing joints.

## Epidemiology

Overweight and obesity are found worldwide, and the prevalence of these conditions in the United States ranks high in comparison with that of other developed nations. As already mentioned, 36.5% of American adults aged 20 years or older are obese. In children, 8.9% of those aged 2 to 5 years were classified as obese and 17.5% of those aged 6 to 11 years were classified as obese, and 20.5% of adolescents aged 12 to 19 years were classified as obese (CDC, 2016a,b). Lifestyle, genetics, hormonal factors, and social-ecological factors are among the many factors contributing to the problem.

Obesity is more common in women than in men. Among men there is a modest ethnic variation in the prevalence of being overweight, the greatest difference occurring between black men (67%) and Hispanic American men (74.6%). Among women the ethnic variation is substantial. Almost 57.6% of white women are overweight, Hispanic American and Puerto Rican women have a greater prevalence of being overweight (73%) than their white counterparts, and more than 79.6% of black women are overweight (National Center for Health Statistics, 2011). Potential contributing factors often associated with the greater propensity for adult black women becoming obese include lower levels of physical activity, higher calorie intake, and lower levels of education and socioeconomic status, as well as broader acceptance of a larger body size within the black American community (Hawkins, 2007; Sanchez-Johnson et al., 2004).

## Body Mass Index for Adults

Based on an adult's height and weight, **body mass index** (BMI) is a helpful indicator of underweight, normal weight, overweight, and obesity (USDHHS, 2010b). One can calculate a person's BMI by dividing the person's weight in kilograms by their height in meters squared (http://www.cdc.gov/healthyweight/assessing/bmi).

***Body mass index formulas.*** BMI may be used as an indicator of body fat, but it cannot be interpreted as a specific percentage of body fat. Age and sex influence the relationship between fat and BMI. For example, women are more likely to have a higher percentage of body fat than men have for the same BMI. As weight is part of the BMI calculation, it must be noted that scale weights may be inaccurate if used universally. For example, a well-trained athlete with a higher proportion of muscle to fat will weigh more because muscle weighs more than fat. By the same token, bone weight differs in people with smaller frames compared with those with larger frames and higher bone density. Additionally, older people have more body fat than do younger adults (Gallagher et al., 2000). BMI is used to screen and monitor a population to detect the risk of health or nutritional disorders. In an individual, other data must be used to determine whether a high BMI is associated with increased risk of disease and death for that person; use of BMI alone is not diagnostic. Waist circumference is a better indicator of the risk of metabolic syndrome. As mentioned previously, the latter identifies several risk factors associated with morbidity such as elevated level of triglycerides, low HDL level, high LDL level, elevated blood glucose level, and elevated blood pressure. For more details, see USDHHS (2010b).

BMI ranges are based on the effect body weight has on disease and death. A BMI from 19 to 25 kg/m$^2$ is a healthy target range for adults. BMIs higher than 25 kg/m$^2$ are associated with increased risks of developing CVD, gallbladder disease, high blood pressure, and non–insulin-dependent DM (type 2 diabetes).

BMIs for adults are expressed by one number, regardless of age or sex, using the following guidelines established by the World Health Organization (2006):
- Underweight: BMI less than 18.5 kg/m$^2$
- Healthy weight: BMI of 18.5 to 24.9 kg/m$^2$
- Overweight: BMI of 25 to 29.9 kg/m$^2$
- Class 1 obese: BMI of 30 to 34.9 kg/m$^2$
- Class 2 obese: BMI of 35 to 39.9 kg/m$^2$
- Class 3 obese (morbid obesity): BMI of 40 kg/m$^2$ or higher

## Body Mass Index Growth Charts for Children

Pediatric health care providers have used growth charts since 1977, with the newest ones released in 2000 by the CDC to more accurately reflect the nation's cultural and racial diversity. To track growth and development in children and adolescents through age 20 years, pediatricians, nurses, and nutritionists use charts widely to assist in signaling potential developmental and weight problems earlier in childhood/adolescence. They consist of a series of percentile curves that illustrate the distribution in growth of children across the United States.

The BMI is an early warning signal that is helpful as early as age 2 years to help identify children who have the potential to become overweight. Early identification of obesity risk gives parents the opportunity to modify their family eating and activity patterns before their children develop a weight problem.

The CDC's charts are based on data gathered through the NHNES, the only survey that collects data from actual physical examinations on a cross-section of Americans from all over the country. This survey shows that since the 1980s the number of overweight children and adolescents has doubled. The growth charts indicate that, in general, children are heavier today than in 1977, but height has remained virtually unchanged. The charts are available on the CDC website at http://www.cdc.gov/growthcharts.

## Diet Intervention in Weight Reduction

With the advances in **nutritional genomics** it may be possible to individualize dietary recommendations on the basis of a person's genotype, thus having a greater impact on risk reduction in diet-related diseases such as obesity (Box 11-7: Genomics). A balanced diet to support weight reduction should include appropriate **serving sizes** to meet individual nutrient needs. Additionally, exercise is particularly important from the outset, because with exercise there is less need to restrict food intake. Exercise also favors long-term maintenance of body weight (as described in Chapter 12).

Nurses make referrals to supervised or unsupervised programs as appropriate. People expect this type of advice on maintaining their health. Therefore nurses can play an important role, although not supervising individuals' weight loss efforts directly. For more information on obesity among adults, see the *Solving the Problem*

## BOX 11-7 GENOMICS

### Nutritional Genomics[a]

The relatively new field of nutritional genomics is a multidisciplinary field of research that investigates the effects a person's diet has on that person's genes (i.e., nutrigenomics) and how our genetic variations dictate our response to certain nutrients (i.e., nutrigenetics). It has long been accepted that slight variations in our genetic makeup account for the individuality of our physical appearances. Think about how you guess at what your height potential will be. We generally look to our biological parents for answers regarding our physical appearance. Likewise, the study of nutritional genomics is attempting to predict how a specific genetic identity will influence a person's response to food and the nutrients within it.

There are many examples of how such individual genetic variants alter disease treatment in health care. For example, two people with hypertension may need different medications to treat the same condition because of their biological response to certain medications. It stands to reason then that the same two people may also benefit from different dietary interventions. Obesity is one of the primary health concerns in the United States and is a significant risk factor for all other major chronic diseases. Nutritional genomics makes possible the use of personalized diet prescription based on an individual's specific genetic profile. Researchers believe that the potential for personalized dietary intervention could drastically change the prevalence of chronic disease, particularly that of obesity (Huang et al., 2015). If such diet therapies are more effective in managing or preventing disease, this will allow health care to focus more on health promotion instead of disease management. Such a shift in health care represents a significantly more sustainable and cost-effective strategy to enhance the health of the nation.

For additional information regarding nutritional genomics, refer to the website of the Center of Excellence for Nutritional Genomics at the University of California, Davis: http://nutrigenomics.ucdavis.edu.

[a]With contribution from Staci Nix.
From Huang, T., & Hu, F. B. (2015). Gene-environment interactions and obesity: Recent developments and future directions. *BMC Med Genomics, 8*(Suppl 1), S2.

of *Childhood Obesity Within a Generation: The White House Task Force on Childhood Obesity Report to the President* (White House Task Force Report on Childhood Obesity, 2010), *The Surgeon General's Vision for a Healthy and Fit Nation* (USDHHS, 2010b), and *Recommended Community Strategies and Measurements to Reduce Obesity in the United States* (Khan et al., 2009).

There are many positive effects of only relatively small amounts of weight loss (5% to 10% of body weight) for people who are obese, including the following:

- Decreased blood pressure (decreased risk of a heart attack and stroke)
- Reduced abnormally high levels of blood glucose associated with diabetes
- Reduced elevated levels of cholesterol and triglycerides associated with CVD
- Reduced sleep apnea (irregular breathing during sleep)
- Decreased risk of osteoarthritis in the weight-bearing joints
- Decreased depression
- Increased self-esteem

The acronym LEARN has been suggested as a mnemonic device for health professionals. LEARN refers to the steps nurses can take to help the person who needs to improve health-related behavior (Brownell, 2000). LEARN is particularly useful as a guideline for communicating with the clinically obese individual who has indicated dissatisfaction with his or her current weight:

L—Listen with sympathy and understanding to the person's perception of the problem.
E—Explain personal perceptions of the problem.
A—Acknowledge and discuss differences and similarities.
R—Recommend treatment.
N—Negotiate an agreement.

In 1998 an NIH-sponsored technical support conference identified the following characteristics of voluntary weight loss and weight control in the United States (USDHHS, 2010b):

- Obesity is a chronic disease.
- Obesity has many causes.
- Cure is rare; palliation is realistic.
- Weight loss is slow.
- Recidivism is common.
- Weight regain may be slow, but it is often rapid.
- Management is often more frustrating than the underlying disease.

The conference noted significant adverse effects for obese dieters who regain lost weight:

- Repeated weight gain and loss may have adverse psychological and physical effects; for example, evidence suggests that mildly to moderately overweight women who are dieting may be at risk of binge eating.
- Although data on the health effects of repeated weight gain and loss (weight cycling) are also inconclusive, weight cycling appears to affect energy metabolism and may cause faster regaining of weight.
- Depression and decreased self-esteem occur.

These findings paint a bleak outlook that one should share with caution when advising individuals.

Fad diets do not provide the best way to lose weight and should be avoided. However, recognizing that people will do almost anything to lose weight when desperate, it is helpful to be able to discuss current fads intelligently and to guide individuals as needed. The new prevention-focused model of health care, mentioned earlier, includes many facets needed to avoid and treat obesity among adults and children in the United States. On an individual basis, for people who cannot or do not choose to maintain a BMI less than 30 kg/m² as a priority, the paradigm *Health at Any Size* (Spark, 2001) is described in Box 11-8.

FDA-approved weight loss medication can play a helpful role in assisting individuals to lose weight and keep it off. As of early 2012, currently orlistat (also available as Xenical by prescription or Alli over-the-counter) is the only approved general weight loss drug. It is important to help those using it to recognize the warning signs and see a health provider if they have negative symptoms. Other non–FDA-approved weight loss supplements that are available are generally not recommended because of safety concerns.

## Diabetes

### Prevalence and Incidence

Diabetes is becoming more prevalent, especially type 2 diabetes, which is associated with obesity. The numbers of existing cases

---

BOX 11-8 **Health at Any Size**

**The Size Acceptance Nondiet Movement**

This paradigm (Spark, 2001) has replaced the question "How can fat people lose weight?" with the question "How can fat people be healthy?" The following tenets are the foundation of the movement:

- Good health is a state of physical, mental, and social well-being. People of all sizes and shapes can reduce their risk of poor health by adopting a healthy lifestyle, which includes eating a variety of healthy foods, being physically active because it is fun and feels good, and appreciating the body as it is.
- Human beings come in a variety of sizes and shapes; size diversity is a positive characteristic of the human race. Respect the bodies of others, although they might be quite different.
- There is no ideal body size, shape, BMI, or body composition that every individual should strive to achieve.
- Self-esteem and body image are strongly linked. Helping people feel good about their bodies and about who they are can help motivate them to maintain healthy behaviors.
- People are responsible for care of their own bodies.
- Appearance stereotyping is wrong. Their weight notwithstanding, all people deserve to be treated equally in the job market and on the job, to be treated equally in the media, and to receive competent and respectful treatment by health care professionals.

**How to Become a Size-Sensitive Health Professional**

- On the intake form, include a question asking whether the person is satisfied with his or her body size. If the answer is "yes," then try to avoid the issue in the future.

- When the person asks not to be weighed, the request is acknowledged without complaint and automatically taken into account on follow-up office visits. (There are a few cases in which weighing is necessary, such as when certain medications, chemotherapy, or anesthetics are administered.)
- A size-sensitive health care professional does not necessarily avoid mentioning weight but should avoid making an issue of weight, avoid lectures and humiliation, and respect the individual's wishes with regard to weight discussions.
- When weight contributes to a problem, the professional mentions this situation but also considers other diagnoses and recommends tests to determine the actual diagnosis when appropriate. If weight loss is a recommended treatment for a problem, the compassionate professional may mention this, but at minimum, and recommend and prescribe other treatments. Accept the individual's wish not to use weight loss as a treatment.
- Some health care professionals believe that overweight and obesity are not necessarily unhealthy. However, other professionals who believe that fat is unhealthy may acknowledge that weight loss is usually ineffective or that individuals have the right to direct their own treatment.
- Ideally, the waiting area, examining suite, and consultation room are equipped with armless chairs, large blood pressure cuffs, large examination gowns, and other equipment suitable for large people. If this is not the case, then the office staff acknowledges the importance of these items when told.

From Spark, A. (2001). Health at any size: The size acceptance nondiet movement. *Journal of the American Medical Women's Association,* *56*(2), 69–72.

---

(prevalence) and new cases (incidence) were increasing between 1990 and 2008, but there has been a possible decrease in diabetes incidence since 2008 (Herman & Rothberg, 2015). The CDC's diabetes maps appear to be mirroring the trends seen in state obesity maps. An estimated 25.8 million Americans (8.3% of the US population) had the disease in 2010 (CDC, 2011b). Among those, older adults and minorities were disproportionately affected. Almost 27% (or 10.9 million) of adults 65 years or older have diagnosed diabetes. After adjustment for population age differences, 2007 to 2009 national survey data of adults (aged 20 years or older) showed the risk of diagnosed diabetes. When compared with non-Hispanic white adults, the risk was 18% higher among Asian Americans, 66% higher among Hispanics, and 77% higher among non-Hispanic black Americans. It was about the same for Cubans, Central Americans, and South Americans, 87% higher for Mexican Americans, and 94% higher for Puerto Ricans. In the Native American population, just among those served by the Indian Health Service, the prevalence is almost twice the national average. Rates differ by region, ranging from 5.5% among Alaska Native adults to 33.5% among Native American adults in southern Arizona.

DM accounts for 90% to 95% of all diagnosed cases of diabetes. The risk factors include the following: having pre-diabetes (impaired glucose tolerance and/or impaired fasting glucose), being older than 45 years, being overweight or obese, not exercising regularly, having a family history of diabetes or a personal history of gestational diabetes, or giving birth to a baby of at

least 9 pounds. Other risk factors include high blood pressure, low HDL cholesterol level, high triglyceride level, and certain races or ethnic groups (Nesto, 2005).

Type 2 DM is the seventh leading cause of death among Americans and the leading cause of blindness, kidney failure, and lower extremity amputations; it also greatly increases the risk of a heart attack or stroke. In 2007, diabetes accounted for more than $174 billion in direct and indirect medical costs and lost productivity (CDC, 2011b). Much of the burden of diabetes can be prevented or delayed by early detection, improved delivery of care, and better education on disease self-management (American Diabetes Association, 2012).

### Type 2 Diabetes in Children

Although DM in children and adolescents was believed to be exclusively type 1, type 2 diabetes is now considered a sizeable and growing problem among Native Americans and an emerging public health problem among other North American ethnic groups. The epidemic of obesity among children and adolescents, the decrease in physical activity, the increase in calorie-dense foods, and the exposure to diabetes in utero are likely contributors to the increase in prevalence of type 2 DM in this population. Young children with type 1 DM or type 2 DM who are either overweight or obese should be observed for metabolic syndrome and CVD risk. The adolescent population is at higher risk because of lifestyle implications, smoking, poor diet adherence, etc., that may put them at risk of chronic disease earlier in life. Recent studies suggest that renal and CVD disease risk is approximately twice that of youth with type 1 DM (Wong et al., 2015).

Although some children and adolescents are symptomatic, others do not enter the clinical arena until they have severe ketoacidosis and may have a transient insulin requirement. Diabetic complications (**dyslipidemia** and hypertension) have been observed among Pima Indians as early as the teenage years. No evidence-based guidelines for treatment of type 2 diabetes in children and adolescents are available, and oral agents have not been tested or approved for this age group. Generally, children and adolescents with type 2 DM have poor glycemic control. Population mobility, lack of symptoms, denial of illness, absence of family support, and inadequate health care insurance coverage have all been identified as major barriers to adherence to treatment and follow-up and to successful clinical management. Because of a longer duration of disease (from earlier onset), and because glucose control and adherence are challenging during the teenage years, the lifetime complications (microvascular and macrovascular diseases and decreased quality of life) in this population will probably be considerable (Fagot-Campagna et al., 2000).

### Diet Intervention

Medical nutrition therapy (MNT) is the most critical and pivotal component of diabetes care. At the minimum, MNT involves the team efforts of a physician, a registered nurse, a registered dietitian, and, in some practice settings, a mental health professional. The purpose of MNT for people with type 2 DM is to delay or prevent the development of complications (blindness, CHD, nephropathy, and neuropathy). No single diabetic diet or American Diabetes Association diet exists. The recommended diet can be defined only as a nutrition prescription based on assessment, treatment goals, and outcomes. Nutrition advice for people with type 2 diabetes is essentially the same as that for the general population: follow the *Dietary Guidelines for Americans*. MNT for people with diabetes should be individualized, with consideration given to usual eating habits, culture, and other lifestyle factors. Nutrition recommendations are then developed and implemented to meet treatment goals and desired outcomes. Monitoring metabolic parameters, including blood glucose levels, glycosylated hemoglobin (HbA1C) levels, lipid values, blood pressure, body weight, renal function (when appropriate), and quality of life, is crucial to ensure successful outcomes. Monitoring HbA1C to less than 6.5% or 7% in most current guidelines is not always the only criterion to use. More importantly the treatment should be started early to prevent further destruction of the beta cells of the pancreas that produce insulin. Studies show that even in people with pre-diabetes or diabetes there is a loss of 50% to 80% of their beta cells (Aguilar & Zonszein, 2015). The American Diabetes Association further recommends ongoing nutrition self-management education for these individuals.

For people with **hyperglycemia**, **hyperlipidemia**, obesity, or suboptimal nutrition, start with this nonpharmacological management:

- Determine an appropriate, tailored meal plan based on energy needs for body weight goals (moderate weight loss, weight maintenance, weight gain). With that data, the determination

is made with regard to serving sizes and numbers with use of MyPlate. For children and adolescents, their growth needs must be accounted for as well.
- Encourage regular exercise.
- Evaluate the individual with use of the outcome measures listed in Table 11-5. People who have been counseled regarding diet and exercise but who have not responded satisfactorily after 4 to 6 weeks should be referred to a registered dietitian who is a diabetes educator. Those with acute complications, such as hypoglycemia, exercise-related problems, renal disease, autonomic neuropathy, hypertension, or CVD, must first see a physician.

A nutrition prescription, which is done after the physician has completed a physical and medical assessment, may be general, but it should reflect the individual's therapy goals. The following are some sample orders the nurse might write for the dietitian:

- Individualized diabetic meal plan to achieve clinical goals of diabetes MNT
- MNT to achieve blood glucose levels as near normal as possible
- Individualized meal plan to decrease diabetes control and blood lipid levels
- Diet for improved glycemic control and blood pressure measurements

The registered dietitian with a summary of the planned nutrition intervention may define the prescription further. For example, the dietitian might write:

- Weight-reduction meal plan based on general eating guidelines, 1200 to 1500 calories, three meals, and one snack
- 2300 mg sodium meal plan with weight maintenance
- Carbohydrate-counting meal plan, adjusting carbohydrate and meal timing to achieve target glucose goals

## Human Immunodeficiency Virus/Acquired Immunodeficiency Syndrome
### Epidemiology

According to the CDC in 2011, 1.2 million adults and adolescents in the United States were infected with HIV, more than ever before (CDC, 2016c). In 2015, approximately 40,000 people were diagnosed with HIV: the number of new diagnoses decreased 19% from 2005 to 2014. This represents a true decline in cases (CDC, 2016c). Whereas HIV infection can be diagnosed earlier in many more people, still as many as one-third wait until it is too late for effective prevention or treatment and advance to AIDS within 12 months of diagnosis. AIDS has been diagnosed in just more than 1 million people, since the beginning of the epidemic (CDC, 2016c).

### Diet Intervention

Attention to nutrition in early HIV intervention is essential for several reasons. People can now live for decades with HIV/AIDS as long as HIV/AIDS is diagnosed early and they are treated early. Even for those people who are HIV positive but in whom HIV infection is diagnosed late, it may still take up to 1 year before most will progress to AIDS. Nutritious diets can improve the sense of well-being, minimize disease symptoms and the side effects of medications, and reduce the risk of opportunistic

**TABLE 11-5 Goals and Recommendations of Medical Nutrition Therapy for Individuals With Type 2 Diabetes**

| Index | Goal | Recommendation |
|---|---|---|
| HbA1c | *For diagnosis must have:* ≥6.5% with a method that is NGSP certified and standardized to DCCT assay | The HbA1c test is the preferred test to diagnose diabetes in nonpregnant adults; other tests listed below may also be used |
| FPG | ≥126 mg/dL (7.0 mmol/L) Fasting is defined as no calorie intake for at least 8 h | The FPG test detects diabetes and pre-diabetes. It is most reliable when done in the morning |
| 2-h plasma glucose | ≥200 mg/dL (11.1 mmol/L) during OGTT | May also be used with a WHO-approved method and a glucose load of 75 g of anhydrous glucose dissolved in water |
| Random plasma glucose | ≥200 mg/dL (11.1 mmol/L) | In people with classic hyperglycemia or hyperglycemic crisis |
| HbA1c | A reasonable HbA1c goal for many nonpregnant adults is <7%; individualize to ≤6.5% or up to 8% depending on factors such as the level of hypoglycemia, life expectancy, duration of disease, and level of CVD | Perform HbA1c test at least twice a year in individuals who are meeting treatment goals and who have stable glycemic control. Lowering of HbA1c fraction is associated with reduction of microvascular complications of diabetes and possibly macrovascular disease |
| Weight change | For most overweight/obese people (BMI <35 kg/m$^2$) recommend modest weight loss (5–7% of body weight) | Modest weight loss has been shown to reduce insulin resistance |
| MNT | Individuals who have pre-diabetes or diabetes should receive individualized MNT as needed to achieve treatment goals, preferably provided by a registered dietitian familiar with components of diabetes MNT; meet body's daily nutritional needs and minimized risk of chronic disease | Structure the program to emphasize lifestyle changes, including education and regular physical activity. Modify macronutrient composition to individual and medical condition while meeting DRIs for micronutrients; a variety of meal patterns work (Mediterranean, a lower-fat, lower-carbohydrate pattern, or vegetarian); saturated fat intake should be <7% of total calories; intake of trans fat should be minimized |
| Physical activity | If there are no medication limitations, physical activity distributed over at least 3 days per week with no more than 2 consecutive days without physical activity; encourage the person to perform resistance training at least twice per week | Physical activity level gradually increased and sustained at target goal. To improve glycemic control, assist with weight maintenance, and reduce risk of CVD, at least 150 min of moderate-intensity aerobic physical activity per week (50–70% of maximum heart rate) |

*BMI,* Body mass index; *CVD,* cardiovascular disease; *DCCT,* Diabetes Control and Complications Trial; *DRI,* dietary reference intake; *FPG,* fasting plasma glucose; *HbA1c,* glycated hemoglobin; *MNT,* medical nutrition therapy; *NGSP,* National Glycohemoglobin Standardization Program; *OGTT,* oral glucose tolerance test.
From American Diabetes Association. (2012). Standards of medical care in diabetes. *Diabetes Care, 35*(1), S11–S63.

infections. For people who are asymptomatic, following the *Dietary Guidelines for Americans* recommendations for meal planning and food safety is suggested. Implementation of good dietary habits early in the disease may have benefits for end-stage developments such as severe weight loss. The person who receives a diagnosis of being HIV positive usually becomes depressed. Depression can lead to loss of appetite; therefore attention to nutrition is critical as soon as a diagnosis is made.

An initial nutritional assessment suggesting the extent to which nutrition counseling is needed and providing valuable baseline information for evaluation of the progression of the disease is necessary (American Dietetic Association, 2010b). Involving the person's significant others in early discussions of optimal nutrition and food safety is important. A nutrient-dense, protein-rich, well-balanced diet in line with the *Dietary Guidelines for Americans 2015–2020* should be stressed but should also include a vitamin and mineral supplement. Evidence suggests that micronutrient deficiencies are common (zinc, iron, selenium, and vitamin B12) and that those affected individuals not taking vitamin supplementation have increased morbidity and mortality (American

Dietetic Association, 2010b). Fair evidence also shows that people with HIV infection and their caregivers do not understand how to best avoid food-borne illness. Giving them practical tips, as well as reasons to avoid certain foods, is helpful (Hoffman et al., 2005). Because of a compromised immune system, illness in people with HIV/AIDS will become worse when they are exposed to food-borne organisms.

The aims of nutrition therapy and counseling specifically for asymptomatic persons who have HIV/AIDS are individualized and based on the following criteria:
- Determine how the person appeared physically before becoming HIV positive. Was the person obese or heavily muscled? Was the person inactive or athletic? Was the person eating a balanced diet high in vitamins and minerals?
- Determine the calorie intakes necessary to achieve or maintain a healthy weight.
- Determine that the protein is of high quality to help maintain or gain healthy muscle mass.
- Determine what the person knows about nutrition and its effect on the disease as well as food and water safety.

- Determine the person's knowledge of the use of food to ease some of the gastrointestinal side effects of medications.
- Determine the person's understanding of the importance of maintaining eating and medication schedules to ensure maximal absorption of medication.

Assess current knowledge when the individual has diabetes or dyslipidemia, and refer the person as appropriate for teaching about how to manage these conditions within the context of HIV/AIDS.

Breastfeeding should be avoided to prevent vertical transmission of HIV from the mother to the child. This objective is fairly easy to implement in the United States, which has a long history of safe breast milk substitutes in the form of milk-based and soy-based infant formulas. In many developing countries, however, the risks attached to feeding an infant with something other than breast milk are greater than the 20% risk of vertical transmission of the virus that causes AIDS.

## CASE STUDY

### Obesity/Overweight: Estella

Estella is a 34-year-old Hispanic single mother of three children sharing a small apartment with her 68-year-old mother in inner-city Los Angeles. She is a full-time laborer in a local manufacturing facility and attends night classes to obtain her medical assistant's license. She is receiving some government assistance but is raising her children, aged 4, 7, and 10 years, on a meager income. Most days she arrives home too tired to prepare a well-balanced meal for her family and admits to eating a lot of fast food. Her mother, despite declining vision, works part-time on evenings at a local fast food restaurant to help with financial difficulties. Her mother is responsible for most of the preparation of meals. Their diet consists mainly of inexpensive carbohydrates: flour tortillas, breads, pasta, cheese, and potatoes. The family budget does not allow for much fresh fruit or vegetables or expensive meats; therefore bologna and hot dogs are frequently served.

Estella has recently been hired at a county hospital as a nursing assistant. A required preemployment physical examination revealed several health risks.

At 5 feet, 4 inches, she weighs 185 pounds. Her resting heart rate and blood pressure are also above normal levels. She has a family history of diabetes and heart disease: her father died of a heart attack at age 55 years, and her mother has diabetes that requires daily insulin injections. She was referred to her primary care physician, who recommended immediate lifestyle changes, including walking 30 minutes per day, 4 to 5 days per week, as well as dietary counseling.

#### Reflective Questions
- What is Estella's understanding of healthy eating?
- How can learning about simple changes in her eating habits affect Estella's weight and risk of type 2 diabetes?
- What local resources promote inexpensive programs to help Estella lose weight?

## ⊚ CARE PLAN

### Obesity/Overweight: Estella

**\*NURSING DIAGNOSIS: Alteration in current weight related to diet modification and weekly monitoring**

#### Defining Characteristics
- Single mother works full-time and attends night school. Is raising three children and supporting her mother on a limited income. Income falls into poverty level for family of five.
- Is a divorced woman with limited support system and resources.
- Current weight is 185 pounds at 5 feet, 4 inches tall (84.1 kg, 162.6 cm). Her BMI is 31.8 kg/m², including her in the obesity category.
- Resting blood pressure is 164/87 mm Hg, and pulse rate is 88 beats/min.
- Father died at age 55 years of a massive heart attack.
- Mother is overweight and has type 1 diabetes and high blood pressure.
- Diet consists of processed foods and a high-fat diet with little fresh fruit or vegetables.
- Recent job change requires her to be on her feet, walking, lifting, and transporting care recipients.
- Inner-city neighborhood is unsafe to walk in alone or allow her children freedom to play outdoors.
- Single mother of three small boys; she realizes the need to improve her own health to be able to care for and enjoy her children.

#### Expected Outcomes
- Estella's overall health will improve through reduction of all of the following: weight, BMI, resting pulse rate, and blood pressure.

- Establish realistic goals with Estella to improve quality of meals on a limited income.
- Develop a realistic exercise plan that is inexpensive and not time-consuming.

#### Interventions
- Teach meal planning strategy to include *Dietary Guidelines for Americans* basic recommendations for a healthy diet and (as deemed appropriate) refer Estella to a certified diabetes educator or registered dietitian if resources permit.
- Teach Estella easy menus to prepare that use more whole grains, fruits, and vegetables and less processed or fast food. (Resources might include the USDA's Center for Nutrition Policy and Promotion's *Recipes and Tips for Healthy, Thrifty Meals;* https://www.cnpp.usda.gov/sites/default/files/usda_food_plans_cost_of_food/FoodPlansRecipeBook.pdf)
- Encourage a regular exercise program, beginning with a walking program of 30 minutes per day, four to five times per week. Gradually increase the pace and distance to intensify aerobic benefits.

Investigate safe options, such as a neighborhood YMCA or park program, for family activities; refer to SNAP or WIC as appropriate; or offer other community resources such as Share Our Strength's Cooking Matters (http://cookingmatters.org/) courses for low-income adults and children.

\*NANDA Nursing Diagnoses—Herdman, T. H. & Kamitsuru, S. (Eds.). Nursing Diagnoses–Definitions and Classification 2015–2017. Copyright © 2014, 1994–2014 NANDA International. Used by arrangement with John Wiley & Sons Limited. In order to make safe and effective judgments using the NANDA-I nursing diagnoses it is essential that nurses refer to the definitions and defining characteristics of the diagnoses listed in this work.

# SUMMARY

This chapter has introduced a wide range of subjects, including the *Healthy People 2020* and *Dietary Guidelines for Americans 2015–2020* nutrition objectives, the most current diet recommendations to reduce the risks of developing nutrition-related diseases, FDA regulations for food labeling, government nutrition assistance programs for poor and older Americans, and primary and secondary prevention strategies related to the most common nutrition-related chronic diseases. Many more primary prevention strategies are being discussed as an adjunct to secondary prevention in an effort to make all strategies more successful. Together these topics form the basis of what is known as preventive nutrition, a requisite for the promotion of the nation's public health. All the topics examined in this chapter can be studied further through use of the Internet. High-quality, up-to-date materials and continuing nutrition education literature for professionals are free and on-line.

## ⓔ EVOLVE CHAPTER FEATURES

http://evolve.elsevier.com/Edelman/
- Study Questions

## REFERENCES

Aguilar, R., & Zonszein, J. (2015). Glycemic control in type 2 diabetes—how low should you go? *Clinical Advisor.* http://www.clinicaladvisor.com/cmece-features/glycemic-control-in-type-2-diabeteshow-low-should-you-go/article/441711/.

American Cancer Society. (2009). Breast cancer facts and figures 2007–2008. http://www.cancer.org/acs/groups/content/@nho/documents/document/bcfffinalpdf.pdf.

American Cancer Society. (2017). Cancer facts and figures. http://www.cancer.org/cancer/news/news/cancer-facts-and-figures-death-rate-down-25-since-1991.

American Dietetic Association. (2010a). Position of the American Dietetic Association: Individualized nutrition approaches for older adults in health care communities. *Journal of the American Dietetic Association, 110,* 1549–1553.

American Dietetic Association. (2010b). Position of the American Dietetic Association: Nutrition intervention and human immunodeficiency virus infection. *Journal of the American Dietetic Association, 110,* 1105–1119.

American Diabetes Association. (2012). Standards of medical care in diabetes—2012. *Diabetes Care, 35*(Suppl. 1), S11–S653.

American Heart Association (AHA). (2016). Potassium power: Eating foods rich in this mineral can help reduce the effects of excess sodium. http://www.heart.org/HEARTORG/Conditions/HighBloodPressure/PreventionTreatmentofHighBloodPressure/How-Potassium-Can-Help-Control-High-Blood-Pressure_UCM_303243_Article.jsp#.WHP-ZXYo7MA.

Appel, L. J., Brands, M. W., et al. (2006). Dietary approaches to prevent and treat hypertension: A scientific statement from the American Heart Association. *Hypertension, 47,* 296–308.

Black, L. J., Walton, J., et al. (2014). Adequacy of vitamin D intakes in children and teenagers from base diet fortified foods and supplements. *Public Health Nutrition, 17*(4), 721–731.

Bolland, M. J., Leung, W., et al. (2015). Calcium intake and risk of fracture: Systematic review. *British Medical Journal, 351,* h4580.

Bray, G. A., & Champagne, C. M. (2007). The complexity of obesity: Beyond energy balance. In E. D. Schlenker & S. Long (Eds.), *Williams' essentials of nutrition & diet therapy* (9th ed.). St. Louis: Mosby.

Brownell, K. (2000). *The LEARN program for weight management 2000.* Dallas: American Health Publishing.

California WIC Association. (2009). Changes in the WIC food packages: A toolkit for partnering with neighborhood stores. Co-produced with Public Health Law & Policy (now Change Lab Solutions). http://www.hungerfreecommunities.org/resource-library/changes-in-the-wic-food-packages-a-toolkit-for-partnering-with-neighborhood-stores/.

Carpenter, K. J. (2000). *Beriberi, white rice, and vitamin B: A disease, a cause, and a cure.* Berkeley, CA: University of California Press.

Centers for Disease Control and Prevention (CDC). (2004). Diagnosis and management of foodborne illnesses: A primer for physicians and other health care professionals. *Morbidity and Mortality Weekly Report, 53*(RR04), 1–33.

Centers for Disease Control and Prevention (CDC). (2010). Salmonella. http://www.cdc.gov/salmonella/general/.

Centers for Disease Control and Prevention (CDC). (2011a). CDC estimates of foodborne illness in the United States. CDC 2011 findings. http://www.cdc.gov/foodborneburden/2011-foodborne-estimates.html.

Centers for Disease Control and Prevention (CDC) (2011b). *National diabetes fact sheet: National estimates and general information on diabetes and prediabetes in the United States, 2011.* Atlanta, GA: US Department of Health and Human Services, Centers for Disease Control and Prevention.

Centers for Disease Control and Prevention (CDC). (2011c). Usual sodium intakes compared with current dietary guidelines—United States, 2005-2008. *Morbidity and Mortality Weekly Report, 60*(41), 1413–1417.

Centers for Disease Control and Prevention (CDC), (2015). Nutrition and Dietary Guidelines. https://www.cdc.gov/nutrition/strategies-guidelines.

Centers for Disease Control and Prevention (CDC). (2016a). Adult obesity fact sheet, 2016. https://www.cdc.gov/obesity/data/adult.html.

Centers for Disease Control and Prevention (CDC). (2016b). Basics about child obesity fact sheet, 2016. http://www.cdc.gov/obesity/childhood/defining.html. https://www.cdc.gov/obesity/data/childhood.html.

Centers for Disease Control and Prevention (CDC). (2016c). HIV in the United States: At a Glance. https://www.cdc.gov/hiv/statistics/overview/ataglance.html.

Egan, B. M., Zhao, Y., et al. (2011). Uncontrolled and apparent treatment resistant hypertension in the United States, 1988 to 2008. *Circulation, 124*(9), 1046–1058.

Expert Panel on Detection, Evaluation, and Treatment of High Blood Cholesterol in Adults. (2001). Executive summary of the third report of the National Cholesterol Education Program (NCEP) Expert Panel on Detection, Evaluation, and Treatment of High Blood Cholesterol in Adults (Adult Treatment Panel III). *Journal of the American Medical Association, 285*(19), 2486–2497.

Fagot-Campagna, A., Pettitt, D. J., et al. (2000). Type 2 diabetes among North American children and adolescents: An epidemiologic review and a public health perspective. *Journal of Pediatrics, 136*(5), 664–672.

Flegal, K. M., Carroll, M. D., et al. (2010). Prevalence and trends in obesity among U.S. adults, 1999–2008. *Journal of the American Medical Association, 307*(5), 491–497.

Food and Drug Administration (FDA). (2008). FDA 101: Dietary supplements. http://www.fda.gov/forconsumers/consumerupdates/ucm050803.htm.

Food and Nutrition Service (FNS), & US Department of Agriculture (USDA). (2011). Nutrition standards in the national school lunch and school breakfast programs. Thursday, January 13, 2011/Proposed Rules. *Federal Register, 76*(9), https://www.gpo.gov/fdsys/pkg/FR-2011-01-13/pdf/2011-485.pdf.

Food Research and Action Center (FRAC). (2016). Offering free breakfast to all students. http://frac.org/wp-content/uploads/frac-facts-offering-free-breakfast-to-all-students.pdf.

Gallagher, D., Ruts, E., et al. (2000). Weight stability masks sarcopenia in elderly men and women. *American Journal of Physiology. Endocrinology and Metabolism, 279*(2), E366–E375.

Grundy, S. M., Cleeman, J. I., et al. (2004). Implications of recent clinical trials for the National Cholesterol Education Program Adult Treatment Panel III Guidelines. *Circulation, 110*(2), 227–239.

Hawkins, B. (2007). African American women and obesity: From explanations to prevention. *Journal of African American Studies, 11*, 79–93.

Herman, W., & Rothberg, A. (2015). Prevalence of diabetes in the United States, a glimmer of hope. *Journal of the American Medical Association, 314*(10), 1005–1007.

Hoffman, E. W., Bergmann, V., et al. (2005). Application of a five-step message development model for food safety education materials targeting people with HIV/AIDS. *Journal of the American Dietetic Association, 105*, 1597–1604.

Institute of Medicine, Food and Nutrition Board. (2011). *Dietary reference intakes for calcium and vitamin D*. Washington, DC: National Academies Press.

James, P. A., et al. (2014). 2014 evidence-based guideline for the management of high blood pressure in adults. Report from the panel members appointed to the Eighth Joint National Committee (JNC 8). *The Journal of the American Medical Association, 311*(5), 507–520.

Johnson, R. (2011). *The federal food safety system: A primer*. Washington, DC: Congressional Research Service. http://www.fas.org/sgp/crs/misc/RS22600.pdf.

Kaplanm, J. L., & Walker, W. A. (2012). Early gut colonization and subsequent obesity risk. *Current Opinions Clinical Nutrition Metabolic Care, 15*(3), 278–284.

Khan, L. K., Sobush, K., et al. (2009). Recommended community strategies and measurements to prevent obesity in the United States. *MMWR Recommendations and Reports, 58*(RR07), 1–26.

Kushi, L. H., Doyle, C., et al. (2012). American Cancer Society guidelines on nutrition and physical activity for cancer prevention. *CA: A Cancer Journal for Clinicians, 62*, 30–67.

Lichtenstein, A. H., Appel, L. J., et al. (2006). Diet and lifestyle recommendations revision 2006: A scientific statement from the American Heart Association Nutrition Committee. *Circulation, 114*(1), 82–96.

Lloyd-Jones, D., Adams, R. J., et al. (2010). Heart disease and stroke statistics—2010 update. A report from the American Heart Association Statistics Committee and Stroke Statistics Subcommittee. *Circulation, 121*, e1–e170.

Marra, M. V., & Bovar, A. P. (2009). Position of the American Dietetic Association: Nutrient supplementation. *Journal of the American Dietetic Association, 109*(12), 2073–2085.

Miniño, A. M. (2011). *Death in the United States, 2009. NCHS data brief, no 64*. Hyattsville, MD: National Center for Health Statistics.

National Center for Complementary and Alternative Medicine. (2010). Using dietary supplements wisely. http://www.nccam.nih.gov/health/supplements/wiseuse.htm.

National Center for Health Statistics. (2011). *Health, United States, 2011*. Hyattsville, MD: National Center for Health Statistics.

National Center for Health Statistics, & Health E-Stat. (2010). Prevalence of obesity among children and adolescents: United States, trends 1963–1965 through 2007–2008. http://www.cdc.gov/nchs/data/hestat/obesity_child_07_08/obesity_child_07_08.htm/.

National High Blood Pressure Education Program. (2003). The seventh report of the Joint National Committee on Prevention, Detection, Evaluation, and Treatment of High Blood Pressure. http://www.nhlbi.nih.gov/files/docs/guidelines/jnc7full.pdf.

National Institute of Arthritis and Musculoskeletal and Skin Diseases. (2012a). Osteoporosis and African American women. http://www.niams.nih.gov/Health_Info/Bone/Osteoporosis/Background/default.asp.

National Institute of Arthritis and Musculoskeletal and Skin Diseases. (2012b). Osteoporosis and Hispanic women. http://www.niams.nih.gov/Health_Info/Bone/Osteoporosis/Background/hispanic_women.asp.

National Institutes of Health (NIH), Office of Dietary Supplements. (2012). Reliable resources for information about dietary supplements. https://ods.od.nih.gov/factsheets/list-all/.

National Library of Medicine. (2011). Iron. http://www.nlm.nih.gov/medlineplus/druginfo/natural/912.html.

National Osteoporosis Foundation. (2011). About osteoporosis: Fast facts. https://www.nof.org/?s=facts.

National Prevention Council. (2011). *National prevention strategy*. Washington, DC: US Department of Health and Human Services, Office of the Surgeon General.

National Research Council. (2006). *Dietary reference intakes: The essential guide to nutrient requirements*. Washington, DC: The National Academies Press. http://www.nap.edu/catalog/11537/dietary-reference-intakes-the-essential-guide-to-nutrient-requirements#toc.

National Research Council. (2010). *Dietary reference intakes for calcium and vitamin D*. Washington, DC: The National Academies Press. http://www.nap.edu/catalog/13050/dietary-reference-intakes-for-calcium-and-vitamin-d.

National WIC Association. (2014). https://www.nwica.org.

Nestle, M. (2002). *In Food politics. Chapter 11: Making health claims legal: The supplement industry's war with the FDA*. Berkeley, CA: University of California Press.

Nesto, R. W. (2005). Beyond low-density lipoprotein, addressing atherogenesis lipid trial in type 2 diabetes mellitus and the metabolic syndrome. *American Journal of Cardiovascular Drugs, 5*(6), 379–387.

Nord, M., Coleman-Jensen, A., et al. (2010). Household food security in the United States, 2009. ERR-108. US Department of Agriculture, Economic Research Service, https://www.ers.usda.gov/webdocs/publications/err108/7024_err108_1_.pdf.

Office of Dietary Supplements. (2012). Health professional vitamin A fact sheet. http://ods.od.nih.gov/factsheets/VitaminA-HealthProfessional/.

Ogden, C. L., Carroll, M. D., et al. (2014). Prevalence of childhood and adult obesity in the United States, 2011–2012. *Journal of the American Medical Association, 311*(8), 806–814.

Pavlidis, C., Patrinos, G. P., & Katsila, T. (2015). Nutrigenomics: A controversy. *Applied and Translational Genomics, 4*, 50–53.

Roger, V. L., Go, A. S., et al. (2012). Heart disease and stroke statistics—2012 update: A report from the American Heart Association. *Circulation, 125*(1), e2–e220.

Rosenbaum, D. (2012). *SNAP is effective and efficient.* Washington, DC: Center on Budget and Policy Priorities. http://www.cbpp.org/sites/default/files/atoms/files/7-23-10fa.pdf.

Sanada, H., Jones, J. E., & Jose, P. A. (2011). Genetics of salt-sensitive hypertension. *Current Hypertension Reports, 13*(1), 55–66.

Sanchez-Johnson, L. A. P., Fitzgibbon, M. L., et al. (2004). Ethnic differences in correlates of obesity between Latina-American and black women. *Obesity Research, 12*, 652–660.

Snetselaar, L. (2004). Counseling for change. In L. K. Mahan & S. Escott-Stump (Eds.), *Krause's food, nutrition, and diet therapy* (11th ed., pp. 519–532). St. Louis, MO: Elsevier.

Spark, A. (2001). Health at any size: The size acceptance nondiet movement. *Journal of the American Medical Women's Association, 56*(2), 69–72.

Stallings, V. A., Suitor, C. W., & Taylor, C. L. (2010). *School meals: Building blocks for healthy children.* Washington, DC: Institute of Medicine, National Academies Press.

Tai, N., Wong, F. S., & Wen, L. (2015). The role of gut microbiota in the development of type 1 and type 2 diabetes mellitus and obesity. *Review of Endocrine Metabolic Disorders, 16*(1), 55–65.

Taylor, C. L. (2008). *Framework for DRI development: Components "known" and components "to be explored." Background paper.* Washington, DC: Institute of Medicine. http://www.nationalacademies.org/hmd/Activities/Nutrition/SummaryDRIs/~/media/Files/Activity%20Files/Nutrition/DRIs/New%20Material/11Bckgrd%20PaperFramework%20for%20DRI%20Devel.

US Census Bureau. (2011). Areas with concentrated poverty: 2006–2010. ACSBR/10-17, http://www.census.gov/prod/2011pubs/acsbr10-17.pdf.

US Department of Agriculture (USDA), Center for Nutrition Policy and Promotion. (2010). MyPlate. http://www.choosemyplate.gov/.

US Department of Agriculture (USDA). (2015). Scientific Report of the 2015 Dietary Guidelines Advisory Committee. https://health.gov/dietaryguidelines/2015-scientific-report/PDFs/Scientific-Report-of-the-2015-Dietary-Guidelines-Advisory-Committee.pdf.

US Department of Agriculture (USDA), Center for Nutrition Policy and Promotion. (2012). Nutrition Evidence Library. http://www.cnpp.usda.gov/nutritionevidencelibrary.

US Department of Agriculture (USDA), Food and Nutrition Service (FNS). (2011a). WIC nutrition program facts. http://www.fns.usda.gov/wic/wic-fact-sheet.pdf.

US Department of Agriculture (USDA), Food and Nutrition Service (FNS). (2011b). SNAP basics fact sheet. http://www.fns.usda.gov/sites/default/files/SNAP_Basics_FactSheet.pdf.

US Department of Agriculture (USDA), Food and Nutrition Service (FNS). (2011c). July 21, 2011 Audit hearing on farm bill's nutrition programs to House Subcommittee on Nutrition & Horticulture. http://agriculture.house.gov/farmbill/Questionnaire_Nutrition.pdf.

US Department of Agriculture (USDA), Food and Nutrition Service, Office of Research and Analysis. (2012). National survey of WIC participants II: Participant characteristics report, by D. M. Geller et al. Project officers: S. G. Kamara, K. Castellanos-Brown. http://www.fns.usda.gov/sites/default/files/NSWP-II.pdf.

US Department of Health and Human Services (USDHHS). (2010a). Healthy People 2020. https://www.healthypeople.gov/2020/topics-objectives.

US Department of Health and Human Services (USDHHS). (2010b). The Surgeon General's vision for a healthy and fit nation. http://www.publichealthreports.org/issueopen.cfm?articleID=2453.

US Department of Health and Human Services. (2011). The Surgeon General's call to action to support breastfeeding. http://www.surgeongeneral.gov/library/calls/breastfeeding/index.html.

US Department of Health and Human Services (USDHHS), Administration on Aging (AoA). (2009). Elderly nutrition program fact sheet. http://www.aoa.gov/AoARoot/Press_Room/Products./pdf/fs_nutrition.doc.

US Department of Health and Human Services (USDHHS), National Institutes of Health (NIH), National Heart, Lung, and Blood Institute. (2006). Your guide to lowering your blood pressure with DASH. http://www.nhlbi.nih.gov/health/resources/heart/hbp-dash-index.

US Department of Health and Human Services (USDHHS) and US Department of Agriculture (USDA). (2015). Dietary guidelines for Americans 2015-2020 (8th ed.). http://health.gov/dietaryguidelines/2015/guidelines/.

USA Today Supplement. (2010). A hunger free America. Media Planet. http://doc.mediaplanet.com/all_projects/5537.pdf.

White House Task Force on Childhood Obesity. (2010). Solving the problem of childhood obesity within a generation: The White House Task Force on Childhood Obesity Report to the President. http://www.letsmove.gov/sites/letsmove.gov/files/TaskForce_on_Childhood_Obesity_May2010_FullReport.pdf.

World Health Organization. (2006). Global database on body mass index. http://apps.who.int/bmi/index.jsp?introPage=intro_3.html.

Wong, J., Constantino, M., & Yue, D. (2015). Morbidity and mortality in young onset Type 2 diabetes in comparison to type 1 diabetes: Where are we now? *Current Diabetes Reports, 15*, 566.

Zemel, M. B. (2001). Calcium modulation on hypertension and obesity: Mechanisms and implications. *Journal of the American College of Nutrition, 5*(Suppl.), 428S–435S.

# 12

# Exercise

*Kevin K. Chui, Frank Tudini, and Sheng-Che Yen*

## OBJECTIVES

*After completing this chapter, the reader will be able to:*

- Explain the physical activity and fitness goals of *Healthy People 2020,* and the progress made toward these goals.
- Describe how physical activity positively influences physical and psychological health.
- Identify the benefits of physical activity throughout the aging process.
- Evaluate the prescriptions for and benefits of daily physical activity, aerobic exercise, and resistance training.
- Explain the interventions to promote exercise adherence and compliance.

## KEY TERMS

| | | |
|---|---|---|
| Aerobic exercise | Exercise prescription | Physical activity |
| Anaerobic exercise | Fat mass | Physical fitness |
| Arthritis | Fibromyalgia syndrome | Relaxation response |
| Borg scale | Flexibility | Resistance training |
| Cardiorespiratory fitness | Low back pain | Rheumatoid arthritis |
| Cool-down period | Muscular fitness | Tai chi |
| Cross-training | Obesity | Warm-up period |
| Exercise | Osteoporosis | Yoga |

 **THINK ABOUT IT**

### Knowing Versus Doing

*Having knowledge of the benefits of exercise does not correlate well with long-term exercise compliance. Confidence in the ability to exercise and a sense of the meaning and purpose (core desire) of exercise in life ensure better success.*

- What motivates an individual to put the effort into developing and maintaining an active lifestyle?
- Why is being active and physically fit important?

Regular physical activity and exercise enhance both physical and psychological health. Generally, people who exercise regularly, or those who naturally include physical activity in their daily routine, feel better mentally and physically, improve their health profiles, and safeguard their functional independence as they go through the aging process. A holistic approach to physical activity involves exercise for cardiorespiratory health (endurance), exercise for musculoskeletal health (strength, flexibility, and bone density), and body awareness. Body awareness and mindfulness during exercise facilitate self-inquiry and self-acceptance, helping to relieve psychological stress and preventing physical injury (Box 12-1). Not only is an active lifestyle an important component of primary prevention but regular physical activity is also an essential modality in the treatment of chronic disease, which establishes the potential for benefit in all aspects of the biopsychosocial and spiritual model of health.

## DEFINING PHYSICAL ACTIVITY IN HEALTH

To fully understand the *Healthy People 2020* objectives regarding exercise, the following definitions will be used:

Physical activity: body movement that is produced by the contraction of skeletal muscles and that substantially increases energy expenditure; includes transportation and vocational and leisure-time activity. Leisure-time activity can be further categorized into sports, recreational activities, and exercise training (Figure 12-1).

Exercise (exercise training): planned, structured, and repetitive body movement performed to improve or maintain one or more components of physical fitness.

Aerobic exercise: activity that uses large muscle groups in a repetitive, rhythmical fashion over an extended period to increase the efficiency of the oxidative energy-producing system and increase cardiorespiratory endurance; uses stored adipose tissue as a major fuel source.

## BOX 12-1  Health Impact of Physical Activity

- Improves quality of life
- Improves mood and promotes a sense of well-being
- Increases flexibility
- Builds muscle strength
- Increases endurance
- Increases the efficiency of the heart
- Increases bone density
- Helps with weight reduction
- Decreases risk of stroke
- Decreases risk of heart disease
- Decreases risk of diabetes

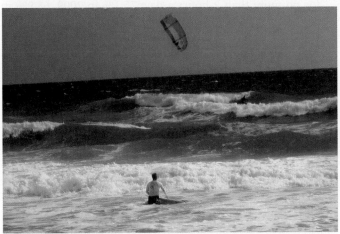

**FIGURE 12-1** Some people choose more vigorous types of exercise.

**Anaerobic exercise:** high-intensity, short-duration activity that increases the efficiency of the phosphocreatine and glycolytic energy-producing systems and increases muscle strength, power, and speed of reactivity; uses phosphagens and glucose-glycogen as major fuel sources.

**Physical fitness:** a set of attributes (**cardiorespiratory fitness,** muscular fitness, and flexibility) that people have or achieve that relates to the ability to perform physical activity without undue fatigue or risk of injury.

**Muscular fitness:** the strength and endurance of muscles that allows participation in daily activities with low risk of musculoskeletal injury.

**Flexibility:** adequate muscle length and joint mobility to allow free and painless movement through a wide range of motion (ROM).

## *HEALTHY PEOPLE 2020* OBJECTIVES

Unfortunately, only 23% of the adult population performs enough regular, sustained exercise to gain any significant health benefit, and slightly more than 10% of the population exercises at an intensity necessary to promote cardiorespiratory fitness. According to the Physical Activity and Fitness section (focus area) of *Healthy People 2020,* overall 30.3% of adults 18 years or older in 2013 reported no leisure-time physical activity (National Health Interview Survey, Centers for Disease Control and Prevention [CDC], National Center for Health Statistics) (US Department of Health and Human Services [USDHHS], 2010). Furthermore, the percentage of adults who report no leisure-time physical activity differs by race and ethnicity, sex, educational level, geographical location, disability status, age group, and the presence or absence of arthritis symptoms. The tendency to be sedentary, unfortunately, continues to increase with age and affects all the body's systems, such as the cutaneous, cardiovascular, respiratory, gastrointestinal, and urinary systems. As a result of a person being sedentary, the risk of premature morbidity, death, impairment, functional limitation, and disability increases. According to data from the 2013 Behavioral Risk Factor Surveillance System (BRFSS), the percentage of adults who engage in no leisure-time physical activity increases with age: 18.3% for 18 to 24 years, 22.5% for 25 to 34 years, 24.9% for 35 to 44 years, 27.3% for 45 to 54 years, 28.7% for 55 to 64 years, and 33.1% for 65 years or older (CDC, 2016a). The goal of the Physical Activity and Fitness focus area is to "improve health, fitness, and quality of life through daily physical activity" (USDHHS, 2010). In 2008 the USDHHS released the first-ever publication of national guidelines for physical activity, *2008 Physical Activity Guidelines for Americans* (USDHHS, 2008). These guidelines provide an evidence-based approach to assist Americans to improve their health status. They recommend that children and adolescents be active for at least 60 minutes daily and advise adults to perform at least 150 minutes of moderate-intensity activity per week or 75 minutes of vigorous activity per week. In 2012, only 20.6% of adults met the guidelines for both aerobic and muscle-strengthening activities (CDC, 2017). The importance of physical activity in the nation's health is reflected in the 15 physical activity and fitness objectives (USDHHS, 2010), a number of objectives which now emphasize traditional and nontraditional partnerships. These objectives take into account the demonstrated relationship between physical activity and an improvement in the biological markers associated with health, and they identify the reasons for the trend toward a more sedentary lifestyle. The National Physical Activity Plan has a vision that all Americans will be physically active in all aspects of their life, which includes work and play (National Physical Activity Plan, 2010). Box 12-2: *Healthy People 2020* provides a summary of the updated physical activity objectives set for 2020.

### Physical Activity Objectives: Making Progress

The review of the physical activity data from *Healthy People 2020* (http://www.healthypeople.gov) provides evidence of the progress that has been made toward achieving the original objectives and the regress that has occurred (National Center for Health Statistics, 2016; USDHHS, 2010).

Improving trends (the percentage of):

- Adults aged 18 years or older who reported no leisure-time physical activity: 36.2% in 2008, 32.3% in 2009, 32.4% in 2010, 31.6% in 2011, 29.6% in 2012, 30.3% in 2013.
- Adults who engage in aerobic physical activity of at least moderate intensity for at least 150 min/wk, or vigorous intensity for at least 75 min/wk, or an equivalent combination: 43.5% in 2008, 47.2% in 2009, 47.1% in 2010, 48.8% in 2011, 50.0% in 2012, 49.9% in 2013.

**BOX 12-2   HEALTHY PEOPLE 2020**

*Objectives for Physical Activity*

- Reduce the proportion of adults who engage in no leisure-time physical activity.
- Increase the proportion of adults who meet current federal physical activity guidelines for aerobic physical activity and for muscle-strengthening activity.
- Increase the proportion of adolescents who meet current federal physical activity guidelines for aerobic physical activity and for muscle-strengthening activity.
- Increase the proportion of the nation's public and private schools that require daily physical education for all students.
- Increase the proportion of adolescents who participate in daily school physical education.
- Increase regularly scheduled elementary school recess in the United States.
- Increase the proportion of school districts that require or recommend elementary school recess for an appropriate period.
- Increase the proportion of children and adolescents who do not exceed recommended limits for screen time.
- Increase the number of states with licensing regulations for physical activity provided in child care.
- Increase the proportion of the nation's public and private schools that provide access to their physical activity spaces and facilities for all persons outside normal school hours (i.e., before and after the school day, on weekends, and during summer and other vacations).
- Increase the proportion of physician office visits that include counseling or education related to physical activity.
- (Developmental) Increase the proportion of employed adults who have access to and participate in employer-based exercise facilities and exercise programs.
- (Developmental) Increase the proportion of trips made by walking.
- (Developmental) Increase the proportion of trips made by bicycling.
- (Developmental) Increase legislative policies for the built environment that enhance access to and availability of physical activity opportunities.

- Adults who engage in aerobic physical activity of at least moderate intensity for more than 300 min/wk, or vigorous intensity for more than 150 min/wk, or an equivalent combination: 28.4% in 2008, 31.2% in 2009, 31.7% in 2010, 33.1% in 2011, 34.3% in 2012, 34.3% in 2013.
- Adults who perform muscle-strengthening activities on 2 days or more per week: 21.9% in 2008, 22.6% in 2009, 24.2% in 2010, 24.2% in 2011, 23.9% in 2012, 24.1% in 2013.
- Adults who meet the objectives for aerobic physical activity and for muscle-strengthening activity: 18.2% in 2008, 19.0% in 2009, 20.6% in 2010, 20.8% in 2011, 20.6% in 2012, 20.8% in 2013.
- School districts that require regularly scheduled elementary school recess: 57.1% in 2006, 58.9% in 2012.
- School districts that require or recommend elementary school recess for an appropriate period: 61.5% in 2006, 63.3% in 2012.
- Children aged 2 to 5 years who view television, view videos, or play video games for no more than 2 hours a day: 75.6% in 2005 to 2008, 76.2% in 2009 to 2012.

- Physician visits made by all children and adults that include counseling about exercise: 7.9% in 2007, 8.7% in 2008, 9.6% in 2009, 9.2% in 2010.

Worsening or no change in the trend (the percentage of):

- Adolescents who meet current federal physical activity guidelines for aerobic physical activity: 28.7% in 2011, 27.1% in 2013.
- Adolescents who participate in daily school physical education: 33.3% in 2009, 31.5% in 2011, 29.4% in 2013.
- Adolescents in grades 9 through 12 who view television, view videos, or play video games for no more than 2 hours a day: 67.2% in 2009, 67.6% in 2011, 67.5% in 2013.
- Adolescents in grades 9 through 12 who use a computer or play computer games outside school (for nonschool work) for no more than 2 hours a day: 75.1% in 2009, 68.9% in 2011, 58.7% in 2013.
- Children aged 2 to 5 years who use a computer or play computer games outside school (for nonschool work) for no more than 2 hours a day: 97.4% in 2005 to 2008, 97.5% in 2009 to 2012.
- Office visits made by individuals with a diagnosis of cardiovascular disease, diabetes, or hyperlipidemia that include counseling or education related to exercise: 13.0% in 2007, 14.1% in 2008, 15.1% in 2009, 12.3% in 2010.

According to the 2014 *State Indicator Report on Physical Activity* (CDC, 2014), the US national weighted percentage of adults who reported no leisure-time activity is 25.4% (unchanged since the 2010 report), with a low of 16.5% in Colorado and a high of 36.0% in Mississippi. Furthermore, for adults nationally, 51.6% met the 150-minute aerobic activity per week guideline, 31.8% met the 300-minute aerobic activity per week guideline, 29.3% met the muscle-strengthening guideline, 20.6% met both the 150-minute aerobic activity guideline and the muscle-strengthening guideline, and 3.4% usually biked or walked to work. Nationally for youths, from the Youth Risk Behavior Surveillance System (YRBSS) data, 15.2% reported that they did not participate in at least 60 minutes of physical activity on at least 1 day (an improvement from 17.1% reported in 2010), with a low of 10.7% in Montana and Nebraska and a high of 27.7% in the District of Columbia. Furthermore, for youths nationally, 27.1% met aerobic activity guidelines and 29.4% had daily physical education (a decline from 30.3% reported in 2010). However, despite gains (indicating that the message regarding the benefits of physical activity is reaching some segments of the population), the improvements fall short, and the new goals set for *Healthy People 2020* reflect the work that remains.

The prevalence of obese children, adolescents, and adults has increased in the United States and is considered an epidemic. Children and adolescents (aged 2–19 years) are categorized as being obese if their body mass index (BMI), expressed as weight in kilograms divided by height in meters squared, is equal to or greater than the 85th percentile in age- and gender-specific BMI growth charts. According to results from the NHANES for 2011 to 2014, which is conducted by CDC's National Center for Health Statistics, 17.0% of children and adolescents are obese. By age group, 8.9%, 17.5%, and 20.5% of children and adolescents aged 2 to 5 years, 6 to 11 years, and 12 to 19 years respectively were obese, with the same pattern found in both sexes (Ogden et al., 2015). Between 1999 to 2000 and 2013 to 2014, there was a significant increase in obesity in children and adolescents; however, there was no significant increase between 2003 to 2004 and 2013 to 2014: 13.9% in 1999 to 2000, 15.4% in 2001 to 2002, 17.1% in 2003 to 2004, 15.4% in 2005 to 2006, 16.8% in 2007 to 2008, 16.9% in 2009 to 2010, 16.9% in 2011 to 2012, and 17.2% in 2013 to 2014 (Ogden et al., 2015).

Adults, those aged 20 years or older, are considered overweight if their BMI is 25.0 to 29.9 kg/m$^2$, obese if their BMI is 30.0 kg/m$^2$ or higher, and extremely obese if their BMI is 40 kg/m$^2$ or higher. According to data from the NHANES for 2011 to 2014, 36.3% of adults aged 20 years or older were obese (Ogden et al., 2015). The overall prevalence of obesity among women (38.3%) was higher than among men (34.3%). The pattern of obesity for both sexes was similar by age group and was highest (40.2%) among middle-aged adults (40–59 years) and lowest (32.3%) among younger adults (20–39 years), with older adults (60 years or older) falling in the middle (37.0%). Between 1999 to 2000 and 2013 to 2014, there was a significant increase in obesity in adults: 30.5% in 1999 to 2000, 30.5% in 2001 to 2002, 32.2% in 2003 to 2004, 34.3% in 2005 to 2006, 33.7% in 2007 to 2008, 35.7% in 2009 to 2010, 34.9% in 2011 to 2012, and 37.7% in 2013 to 2014 (Ogden et al., 2015).

The age-adjusted prevalence of overweight and extreme obesity has also been reported for adults by the NHANES (Fryar et al., 2014). The prevalence of overweight adults was 34.0% in 1999 to 2000, 35.1% in 2001 to 2002, 34.1% in 2003 to 2004, 32.6% in 2005 to 2006, 34.3% in 2007 to 2008, 33.0% in 2009 to 2010, and 33.6% in 2011 to 2012. The prevalence of extreme obesity was 4.7% in 1999 to 2000, 5.1% in 2001 to 2002, 4.8% in 2003 to 2004, 5.9% in 2005 to 2006, 5.7% in 2007 to 2008, 6.3% in 2009 to 2010, and 6.4% in 2011 to 2012.

The number of adults who combine good dietary practice with regular physical activity in an attempt to attain an appropriate body weight has decreased. This decidedly negative trend may be related to the decline in physical activity in and outside schools. According to the YRBSS data from the CDC (2014), 29.4% of adolescents participated in daily school physical education in 2014 (down from 33.3% in 2009), and the target for *Healthy People 2020* is 36.6% (USDHHS, 2010). Additional changes from the YRBSS include a significant increase in the percentage of 9th to 12th graders who report playing video or computer games or used a computer for 3 hours or more per day (31.1% in 2011 compared with 41.3% in 2013) and a decrease in the percentage who played on at least one sports team (58.4% in 2011 compared with 54.0% in 2013).

In a seminal study that tracked physical activity over time using data from the Trois-Rivières Growth and Development Study, there was a significant but weak correlation between adult and childhood physical activity (Trudeau et al., 2004). Researchers from the same institution (Larouche et al., 2012) recently examined the effects of receiving different amounts of physical education during primary school (5 hours of weekly physical education vs. 40 minutes of weekly physical education) on the amount of physical activity during four life transitions (i.e., adolescence, postsecondary studies, entry into the labor market,

and parenthood). They found a progressive nonlinear decline in the physical activity of both groups and differences between sexes during life transitions. The researchers suggest initiatives should be undertaken to maintain or increase physical activity during these transition periods. In a similar type of study based on data from the National Longitudinal Study of Adolescent Health, increased physical activity during adolescence decreased the likelihood of young adults being overweight (Menschik et al., 2008). Using data from the Canadian Physical Activity Longitudinal Study, Brien and colleagues (2007) reported that previous cardiorespiratory fitness ($\dot{V}o_{2max}$) and previous BMI measurements are significant predictors of future weight gain and obesity in adults. Finally, a meta-analysis explored the different mechanisms through which physical activity during adolescence benefits adult health, such as reducing morbidity (Hallal et al., 2006).

If a standard is to be set for the importance of physical activity throughout the life span, it needs to start with children, who have the potential to develop lifelong healthy habits.

As the health care system moves toward a preventive model, primary care providers must facilitate a wellness attitude in their care recipients, which involves not only encouraging individuals to be physically active but also leading by example. Recommending regular exercise and espousing the benefits from personal experience can have a significant influence on individual involvement. Health care practitioners are in a position to inquire about and provide counseling for the exercise habits of their care recipients. For example, for each of the preferred physical therapist practice patterns (musculoskeletal, neuromuscular, cardiovascular/pulmonary, and integumentary), the first corresponding pattern is primary prevention/risk reduction. Although some progress has been made in providing preventive care to reduce risk, data indicate a shortfall in reaching the goal set for 2020 (USDHHS, 2010). Although there has been some improvement in some areas, overall the proportion of the population reporting physical activity has remained essentially unchanged, and progress is limited. Obviously, the progress that has been made toward the physical activity objectives for the year 2020 does not reflect a significant shift in the attitude of the general population or the health care profession. There are still populations at greater risk of obesity based on race/ethnicity (National Institute of Diabetes and Digestive and Kidney Diseases, 2012; Whitson et al., 2011); school type, public versus private (Li & Hooker, 2010); and socioeconomic status (Balistreri & Hook, 2011; Scharoun-Lee et al., 2009) (Box 12-3).

## Aging

The biological changes attributed to aging closely resemble the effects of physical inactivity. The list for both aging and inactivity includes an increase in body fat and a decrease in all the following: aerobic capacity, muscle mass (sarcopenia), metabolic rate, strength and flexibility, bone mass, sexual function, mental performance, immune function, and sleep quality.

Among older adults, exercise can improve health, prevent disability and hospitalizations, improve blood lipid profiles, and reduce body fat. According to the 2010 US census, the population aged 65 years or older has grown to 40.3 million people, an increase of 15% since 2000 (US Census Bureau, 2011). In 2012

## BOX 12-3 Populations With Low Rates of Physical Activity

- Women are generally less active than men at all ages.
- People with lower incomes and less education are typically not as physically active as those with higher incomes and education.
- Black Americans and Hispanics are generally less physically active than whites.
- Adults in northeastern and southern states tend to be less active than adults in north central and western states.
- People with disabilities are less physically active than people without disabilities.
- By age 75 years, one in three men and one in two women engage in no regular physical activity.

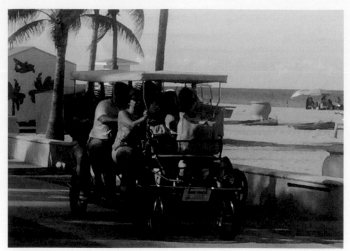

**FIGURE 12-2** Older adults can maintain functional independence while biking.

there were an estimated 43.1 million older adults aged 65 years or older, and that number is expected to almost double to 83.7 million by 2050 (Ortman et al., 2014). Projected numbers and proportions of the US population of older adults have been reported: 43.1 million or 13.7% in 2012, 56.0 million or 16.8% in 2020, 72.8 million or 20.3% in 2030, 79.7 million or 21.0% in 2040, 83.7 million or 20.9% in 2050 (Ortman et al., 2014).

Exercise is especially important for older women, who constitute the majority of the older population, because it has the potential to improve bone health (Bielemann et al., 2013; Hamilton et al., 2010; Julián-Almárcegui et al., 2015) and reduce fracture risk as part of a multidimensional approach (Kemmler et al., 2013; Perry & Downey, 2012). The percentage of female older adults aged 65 years or older has been reported and projected as 56.4% in 2012, 55.1% in 2030, and 55.1% in 2050 (Ortman et al., 2014). The percentage drastically increases for reports and projections for older adults aged 85 or older: 66.6% in 2012, 62.4% in 2030, and 61.9% in 2050 (Ortman et al., 2014).

By exercising, older people can improve levels of cardiovascular, cardiopulmonary, and metabolic functions, including muscle performance and aerobic capacity. Several researchers have reported significant increases or improvements in strength (Candow et al., 2011), physical performance such as gait speed (Chou et al., 2012), flexibility (Marquard et al., 2012), self-efficacy (Park et al., 2011), quality of life (McGrath et al., 2010), balance (Rose & Hernandez, 2010), continence (Shamliyan et al., 2008), bone density (Alghadir et al., 2015), safety (fewer falls and fall-related injuries) (Caban-Martinez et al., 2015), and the ability to live independently (Cowan et al., 2009). Additional resources are available that discuss exercise prescription considerations and guidelines for the older adult (American College of Sports Medicine [ACSM], 2013; Chodzko-Zajko et al., 2009; Elsawy & Higgins, 2010; Liu et al., 2011a; McDermott & Mernitz, 2006; O'Donovan et al., 2010).

Older adults, in particular, need to be concerned about their nutritional status because the potential for malnutrition, a common problem for older adults, is associated with a decline in muscle strength and thus poorer outcomes, such as decreased function and performance (Bauer et al., 2008; Henwood et al., 2012; Jones et al., 2009; Mithal et al., 2013; Morgan, 2012; Tarnopolsky, 2008; Walrand et al., 2011).

The health of the musculoskeletal system depends on movement and activity. Bone is a dynamic tissue, constantly changing and adapting to the stresses to which it is subjected. Bone strength depends on stresses applied by muscular and weight-bearing activity (mechanical stress during active movement). Exercise may increase or maintain bone mineral density (BMD), but recent meta-analytic data suggest that the effects of exercises on BMD may depend on the mode of exercise, body part, combination of exercises (mixed loading), and other (e.g., pharmacological, tai chi) concurrent treatments (Almstedt et al., 2011; Alperson & Berger, 2011; Guadalupe-Grau et al., 2009; Howe et al., 2011; Martyn-St James & Carroll, 2009). To stay healthy, joints must do what they are designed to do—move and bear weight. The health of the cartilage covering the joint surfaces is vital for maintaining proper joint function. The only way the cartilage can receive nourishment is through the manufacture and distribution of synovial fluid, which delivers nutrients, removes waste products, and lubricates joint surfaces. Movement is vital for the creation of this environment of blood and lymph in and out of joint structures and the adjacent soft tissues. Without the stress of weight-bearing activity, normal bone and cartilage metabolism and repair become dysfunctional, resulting in injury and disease.

### Effects of Exercise on the Aging Process

Everyone needs physical activity to be healthy. Human physiology has evolved in preparation for physical exertion. Until recently, survival through the vigor of daily living depended on a moderate degree of physical fitness. However, with mechanization and the style of living in today's society, daily life has become too sedentary. A lifestyle of inactivity places the population at risk of death and morbidity, and the literature supports exercise as an essential element of health.

Regular physical activity can help maintain functional independence and improve the quality of life throughout the aging process (Figure 12-2). Physical and psychological benefits of increased physical activity have been documented widely in healthy and in chronically ill older adults (Arne et al., 2009;

CDC, 2015; Dogra, 2011; Lin et al., 2010; Liu-Ambrose et al., 2010). Unfortunately, according to data from the BRFSS, less than 33.1% of older adults engage in physical activity (CDC, 2016a). According to the CDC (2015), older adults require at least 2.5 hours of moderate-intensity aerobic activity weekly, as well as muscle strengthening on 2 days or more per week. Considerable research has tested interventions to increase activity by younger adults and by populations of all ages. Interventions' research with older adults is being reported more frequently. The most common interventions are self-monitoring, general health education, goal setting, supervised center-based exercise, problem-solving, feedback reinforcement, and relapse prevention education. A few studies have examined multicomponent cognitive-behavioral group intervention (Zijlstra et al., 2009). Lifestyle activity in an older adult recommends the accumulation of minutes of physical activity spread over the entire day. Some evidence suggests the potential beneficial effects of lifestyle activity and the probability that some aging adults may be more receptive to lifestyle activity changes that include episodic exercise (Zijlstra et al., 2009).

## CARDIAC RISK FACTORS

The literature strongly demonstrates that the risk of coronary heart disease (CHD) decreases as physical activity increases and that a plausible relationship between the decreased risk and a number of potential physiological and metabolic mechanisms exists (Ahmed et al., 2012; Ghadieh & Saab, 2015; Li et al., 2015; Pattyn et al., 2013):

- Increasing levels of high-density lipoprotein (HDL) cholesterol
- Decreasing levels of low-density lipoprotein (LDL) cholesterol
- Decreasing total cholesterol levels
- Decreasing serum triglyceride (TRG) levels
- Decreasing high blood pressure
- Improving glucose tolerance and insulin sensitivity
- Decreasing obesity; altering the distribution of body fat
- Reducing the sensitivity of the myocardium to the effects of catecholamines, thereby decreasing the risk of ventricular arrhythmias
- Enhancing fibrinolysis and altering platelet function

### High-Density Lipoprotein and Serum Triglyceride Levels

Exercise has a major influence on lipoprotein metabolism, primarily affecting plasma levels of HDL and TRG. There is a strong negative correlation between CHD and plasma HDL levels. Increases in HDL level lower the total cholesterol to HDL ratio, thereby reducing CHD risk. Exercise, a common part of treatment of hypertriglyceridemia, may have a lowering effect on TRG levels (Cho et al., 2014; Lee & Heo, 2014; Vrablík & Češka, 2015). A meta-analysis of randomized controlled trials examined the effects of progressive resistance training on adults and found significant reductions in total cholesterol levels, the ratio of total cholesterol to HDL, and the levels of non-HDL, LDL, and TRG (Kelley & Kelley, 2009). A similar systemic review examined

exercise in obese children and found that aerobic exercise improved LDL and TRG concentrations and that combined exercise (aerobic fitness, strength, and flexibility training) improved the HDL concentration (Escalante et al., 2012). In another study of obese children, exercise significantly lowered total cholesterol, TRG, LDL, very low density lipoprotein, and insulin levels and significantly increased HDL levels when compared with no exercise (Zorba et al., 2011). A recent meta-analysis of randomized controlled trials compared the effects of diet, exercise, and both diet and exercise on total cholesterol, HDL, LDL, and TRG and found that exercise alone and when combined with diet results in positive changes in lipid and lipoprotein levels in adults (Kelley et al., 2012).

The effect of exercise on lipid metabolism may be related more to the volume (duration and frequency) than to the intensity of the exercise. In a systematic review, Tambalis and colleagues (2009) reviewed the literature for responses in the levels of blood lipids to a variety of modes and volumes of exercise. Moderate-intensity aerobic exercise training (less than 60% $\dot{V}o_{2max}$ or six metabolic equivalents) appears to have the greatest effect on HDL levels. However, stronger evidence suggested that high-intensity aerobic training promotes significant increases in HDL levels. This was observed among a wide range of 90 to 200 minutes per week. Resistance training supported a marked reduction in LDL levels, followed by a significant reduction in total cholesterol levels. The review found combining resistance and aerobic exercise can lead to remarkable reductions in LDL levels, significant increases in HDL levels, and significant decreases in total cholesterol levels (Tambalis et al., 2009).

### Hypertension

According to the CDC, the age-adjusted percentage of the US population with hypertension increased from 25.5% in 1988 to 1994 to 30.0% in 2011 to 2012. The ACSM (2009a) and the American Heart Association (Braith & Stewart, 2006) recommend **resistance training** in the prevention and treatment of hypertension (Box 12-4). Furthermore, the ACSM (Pescatello et al., 2004) summarizes evidence, of differing degrees, that supports the use of physical activity, dynamic aerobic training, dynamic exercise, and resistance training to decrease blood pressure in adults. The summary of the evidence supports regular endurance exercise to decrease blood pressure in older adults. There was no evidence to support a different blood pressure response to exercise between sexes and different ethnicities. A recent systematic review examined the effects of various forms of exercise training on resting blood pressure in healthy adults (Cornelissen & Smart, 2013). Only randomized controlled trials were included in the meta-analysis, and the results indicate that endurance, dynamic resistance, and isometric resistance training lower both systolic blood pressure and diastolic blood pressure. A similar meta-analysis reported the blood pressure–lowering effects of dynamic resistance training and isometric handgrip training (Cornelissen et al., 2011).

The ACSM recommends endurance training should include aerobic activities with use of large muscle groups on most days of the week for 30 minutes or more (ACSM, 2009a). Low- to moderate-intensity aerobic exercise also appears to be effective in

## BOX 12-4   Resistive Training Exercises

### Chest Press (Figures 1 and 2)

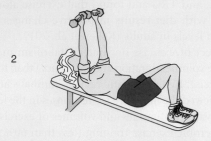

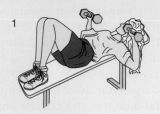

- Lie on a bench with feet flat on the bench, or lie on the floor with knees bent and feet flat, whichever is more comfortable.
- Hold weights near shoulders with elbows out and palms facing away from the body.
- Exhale while extending arms straight up, following an "A" pattern with the weights touching at the peak.
- Slowly lower the weights back to original position while inhaling.
- Repeat 8 to 12 times.

### Chest Fly (Figures 3 and 4)

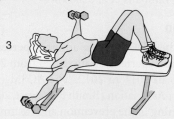

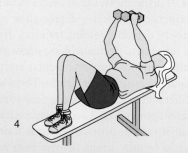

- Lie on a bench with feet flat on the bench, or lie on the floor with knees bent and feet flat, whichever is more comfortable.
- With palms facing each other, extend arms above chest, keeping elbows slightly bent at all times.
- Inhale and lower arms perpendicularly away from the body until arms are out of peripheral vision.

- Exhale while returning to starting position by visualizing arms hugging a barrel that is lying on the chest.
- Repeat 8 to 12 times.

### Bent Over Row (Figures 5 and 6)

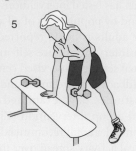

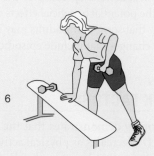

- Bend at waist while supporting the body with one hand (on table, bench, etc.) and holding a weight with the other hand in an overhand grip.
- Keep knees bent while the weight is hanging perpendicular to the torso.
- Slowly pull the weight up to the chest as if starting a lawn mower, exhaling and keeping the elbow away from the body.
- Slowly lower weight back to starting position while inhaling.
- Repeat 8 to 12 times on each side.

### Dumbbell Curl (Figures 7 and 8)

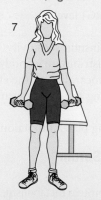
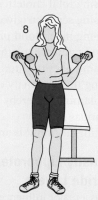

- Stand or sit with weights held at sides in an underhand grip, keeping elbows close to the body and upper arms stationary.
- Curl weights to the chin or upper chest while exhaling.
- Inhale while slowly lowering weights.
- Keep back straight throughout the duration of motion.
- Repeat 8 to 12 times.

## BOX 12-4 Resistive Training Exercises—cont'd

### Triceps Extension (Figures 9 and 10)

9  10

- While seated or standing in the neutral back position, lift the hand holding the weight straight above the head and in alignment with the ear.
- Keeping the upper arm tight, slowly bend the elbow to lower the weight between the shoulder blades.
- Use the free hand to support the elbow and to prevent movement in the upper arm.
- Raise the weight back to its original position by straightening the arm and exhaling.
- Repeat 8 to 12 times on each side.

lowering blood pressure (Cornelissen et al., 2009; Hua et al., 2009; Roussel et al., 2009). The mechanisms underlying the exercise-training effect on lowering blood pressure are not completely clear but may involve attenuation of sympathetic nervous system activity. This attenuation results in the dilation of peripheral blood vessels, which decreases systemic vascular resistance. Decreasing sympathetic nervous system activity may have a beneficial effect on the insulin resistance that is often observed in hypertensive people. The literature has also uncovered significant effects of both interval and continuous training of between 45 and 60 minutes on systolic and diastolic blood pressure (Lamina, 2010). Fagard (2011) reviewed the current literature and found inconclusive evidence for exercise intensity and its effect on blood pressure. This study observed two exercise groups, low-intensity exercise (33% of heart rate reserve) and high-intensity exercise (66% of heart rate reserve), performed three times a week for a 1 hour each time. The results revealed that systolic blood pressure decreases with both intensities but diastolic blood pressure decreases significantly after higher-intensity exercise (Fagard, 2011).

## Hyperinsulinemia and Glucose Intolerance

Hyperinsulinemia and glucose intolerance account for the various types of diabetes. Diabetes mellitus encompasses a group of metabolic disorders that have in common an increase in blood glucose levels and associated metabolic dysfunction. Type 1 involves elevated blood glucose levels that are a result of a deficiency of circulating insulin caused by destruction of the pancreatic β cells, and type 2 diabetes involves elevated blood glucose levels from insulin resistance (decreased insulin sensitivity)—largely in skeletal muscles—or impaired insulin secretion (Nathan, 2015). Approximately 90% to 95% of those with diabetes have type 2 diabetes. According to the CDC, the age-adjusted percentage of the US population with diabetes increased from 8.8% in 1988 to 1994 to 11.9% in 2011 to 2012. In addition, adiposity and poor fitness are linked with insulin resistance (Larson-Meyer et al., 2010). Complications of diabetes include heart disease and stroke, peripheral arterial disease, retinopathy, nephropathy, peripheral neuropathy, and lower-extremity amputation (Deshpande et al., 2008).

Exercise, in addition to diet, is a first-line intervention for diabetes (Gulve, 2008). In a recent meta-analysis of randomized controlled trials, both diet and lifestyle interventions including exercise and physical activity decreased 2-hour plasma glucose and fasting plasma glucose levels in individuals with impaired glucose tolerance (Gong et al., 2015). In a similar meta-analysis of randomized controlled trials, researchers examined the effects of lifestyle interventions including exercise and physical activity on risk factors in individuals with type 2 diabetes and found a significant reduction in the level of hemoglobin A1c ($HbA_{1c}$), among other risk factors (Chen et al., 2015). A randomized control trial by Belli and colleagues (2011) examined the effects of 12-week overground walking training in individuals with type 2 diabetes. The exercise group performed walking at the ventilatory threshold velocity. When compared with the control group, the exercise group had significant reductions in $HbA_{1c}$ levels (glycemic control) and body composition (body mass and BMI) and a significant increase in exercise capacity (peak oxygen uptake and exercise duration). Marcus and colleagues (2008) compared the effects of aerobic exercise with a combination of aerobic and high-force eccentric resistance exercise over the course of 16 weeks in individuals with type 2 diabetes. Both groups had a significant decrease in $HbA_{1c}$ levels, decrease in amount of intramuscular fat, and increase in 6-minute walk distance, with no between-group differences. The aerobic and high-force eccentric resistance exercise group also had a significant gain in lean tissue and greater decrease in BMI when compared with the aerobic exercise group (Box 12-5: Diversity Awareness).

In addition, several meta-analyses examined the effects of different modes of exercise on glycemic control. Strasser and colleagues (2010) examined the effect of resistance training with abnormal glucose metabolism and found significant improvements in glycemic control, with a mean $HbA_{1c}$ level reduction of 0.48%. Irvine and Taylor (2009) found the following results in individuals with type 2 diabetes: progressive resistance exercise resulted in a significant reduction in $HbA_{1c}$ level of 0.3% when compared with no exercise; there was no difference in $HbA_{1c}$ levels between resistance and aerobic exercise groups; and progressive resistance exercise resulted in significant increases in strength

### *Walk Away From Ethnic Glucose Intolerance*

The Pima Indians of the Gila River Indian Community in Arizona have the highest documented incidence rates of type 2 diabetes in the world. On the island of Mauritius in the southwest Indian Ocean, all four ethnic groups (Hindu and Muslim Asian Indians, African Creoles, and Chinese) have unusually high rates of type 2 diabetes. In the United States, type 2 diabetes is 30% more prevalent in blacks than in whites. The presence of type 2 diabetes in each of these ethnic groups provides strong support for the existence of one or more modifiable risk factors in the cause of the disease.

Excessive weight gain is a strong independent predictor of type 2 diabetes. The development of type 2 diabetes (characterized by insulin resistance, hyperinsulinemia, and glucose intolerance) is related to weight gain in adults, particularly to fat accumulation around the waist, abdomen, and upper body (android or apple shape). This type of fat distribution is also associated with a higher risk of developing CHD. Adipose tissue is a major site for insulin insensitivity, and most obese individuals have increased insulin resistance or some degree of glucose intolerance, or both.

Physical activity has an important role in the prevention and treatment of type 2 diabetes. By helping to maintain a proper lean-to-fat body mass, either by losing weight or by preventing weight gain, physical activity may indirectly protect against the development of type 2 diabetes. The modulating effect of physical activity on fat stores helps to increase insulin sensitivity and glucose tolerance. Additionally, physical activity may directly affect glucose metabolism. The shorter-term effect of exercise can lower plasma glucose levels by enhancing the effect of insulin; long-term exercise improves insulin action and increases glucose tolerance.

Epidemiological studies of ethnic groups indicate that physical inactivity is also a risk factor for type 2 diabetes. In the United States, blacks and Native Americans have a disproportionate number of poor, unemployed, and disadvantaged individuals who lack access to the health care system. The least active individuals within these populations should be given the most attention because they have the most to gain. The methods and programs that are used to relay information to the public on the importance of physical activity need to be varied, depending on the socioeconomic and cultural factors specific to ethnic populations. Promotion of physical activity by schools, communities, and government and health agencies, with these factors in mind, will significantly help achieve the goal of improving lifestyles and decreasing the incidence of type 2 diabetes.

when compared with aerobic exercise and no exercise. Chudyk and Patrella (2011) reported that aerobic exercise alone or combined with resistance training significantly reduced HbA$_{1c}$ levels, systolic blood pressure, and triglyceride levels in individuals with type 2 diabetes. Furthermore, waist circumference was significantly reduced only when aerobic exercise and resistance training were combined.

During physical activity, contracting skeletal muscles work with insulin to enhance glucose uptake into the cells (Stanford & Goodyear, 2014; Turcotte & Fisher, 2008). Insulin resistance impedes glucose mobilization into cells, increasing plasma glucose levels and setting the potential for development of type 2 diabetes. Although insulin resistance in skeletal muscles may be the primary defect, the development of disease appears to be related to elevated insulin levels, a result of the body's response to the need to mobilize glucose into the cells. Additionally, this syndrome also often involves elevated TRG levels and hypertension, which

contribute to the potential for disease. Exercise increases insulin sensitivity, improves the inherent effect of endogenous insulin, decreases obesity, and plays a role in lowering TRG levels and blood pressure; therefore it is recommended in the management of type 2 diabetes (Chen et al., 2015; Gong et al., 2015; Gulve, 2008; Nathan, 2015; Polikandrioti & Dokoutsidou, 2009; Waryasz & McDermott, 2010; Weltman et al., 2009). With diet, weight control, and exercise, preventing or decreasing the need for oral antiglycolytic agents and insulin is possible while maintaining normal blood glucose levels. Physical activity may be most beneficial in preventing the progression of type 2 diabetes during the earlier stages of the disease process, before insulin therapy is required. Overall, physical activity has a significant positive effect on a chronic disease that is associated with a high risk of developing CHD.

## OBESITY

Overweight and **obesity** are conditions of excess body fat (adipose tissue). Adults are considered overweight if their BMI is 25.0 to 29.9 kg/m$^2$ and obese if their BMI is 30.0 kg/m$^2$ or higher. Furthermore, the ACSM (Wallace & Ray, 2009) considers those with a BMI of 40 kg/m$^2$ or higher as being extremely obese.

Obesity may also be defined as body weight that is equal to or greater than 120% to 125% of the ideal body weight. **Fat mass** (body fat percentage) is also important in determining the ideal body weight. The recommended body fat levels are approximately 15% to 16% for men and 23% to 24% for women (ACSM, 2009b). The average American man and woman tend to exceed the recommended body fat level. An increase in fat mass and the development of obesity occur when energy intake exceeds total daily energy expenditure for a prolonged period. Decreased physical activity may be both a cause and a consequence of weight gain over a lifetime.

The prevalence of obesity, as well as overweight and extreme obesity, is typically reported on the basis of BMI values, as is the case with the National Health and Nutrition Examination Survey (NHANES). Unfortunately, the prevalence of obesity in the United States remains high and has been increasing. According to the NHANES data for 2009 to 2012 (CDC, 2016b), from 2009 to 2012 35.3% of the US population was obese (up from 33.9% in 2005 to 2008). A nutrition and weight status objective (NWS-9) for *Healthy People 2020* is to reduce the proportion of adults who are obese to 30.5% in 2020. In the United States, no state has met the nation's *Healthy People 2010* goal to lower obesity prevalence to 15%. In fact, no state has an obesity prevalence less than 20%. The number of states with an obesity prevalence between 30% and less than 35% actually increased from none in 2000 to 19 in 2014, including Alabama, Delaware, Georgia, Indiana, Iowa, Kansas, Kentucky, Louisiana, Michigan, Missouri, Nebraska, North Dakota, Ohio, Oklahoma, Pennsylvania, South Carolina, Tennessee, Texas, and Wisconsin (CDC, 2014). Furthermore, three states have a prevalence of obesity greater than 35%: Arkansas, Mississippi, and West Virginia.

According to the most recent NHANES data, the prevalence of obesity in women exceeds that of men in the non-Hispanic black, Hispanic, and Mexican American ethnic groups.

Furthermore, the prevalence of obesity differs by racial/ethnic group for female adults only. That is, adult females of Mexican American (49.2%), Hispanic (44.4%), and non-Hispanic black (56.6%) racial/ethnic backgrounds have a greater prevalence of obesity than do those of non-Hispanic white (32.8%) background. In contrast, the prevalence of obesity is comparable for males of Mexican American (44.0%), Hispanic (40.1%), non-Hispanic black (37.1%), and non-Hispanic white (32.4%) racial/ethnic backgrounds.

Several studies have related increased fat mass and reduced physical activity to the risk of cardiovascular disease and overall mortality (Larson-Meyer et al., 2010). Both obesity and decreased activity are related to insulin resistance, elevated blood pressure, and elevated total and LDL cholesterol concentrations, all of which reduce with weight loss and fitness (Larson-Meyer, 2010). Nevertheless, obesity should be considered an independent target for intervention in health promotion. Being overweight and being obese are major contributors to many preventable causes of death. On average, higher body weights are associated with higher death rates (USDHHS, Prevention and Wellness, 2015).

Maintaining fitness and health is closely related to controlling weight. The literature supports the positive influence that physical activity has on body weight and obesity. A meta-analysis concluded that exercise resulted in weight loss in people who were overweight or obese (Shaw et al., 2006). In fact, in comparison with no treatment, the meta-analytic data show that exercise alone produced favorable changes in body weight, BMI, diastolic blood pressure, and serum triglyceride, serum HDL, and fasting serum glucose levels. A more recent meta-analysis examined the effect of exercise on body composition in menopausal women (Yeh et al., 2011). The results showed a significant decrease in weight, BMI, and body fat in menopausal women who exercised. A recent study examined the ability of obese adolescents with diabetes to retain the benefits of a 12-week exercise intervention (Gow et al., 2016). Significant gains in aerobic fitness ($\dot{V}o_2$ peak) and time to anaerobic threshold were achieved after the intervention and were maintained for an additional 6 months.

Physical activity:
- Promotes a negative energy balance (burns calories)
- Increases metabolic rate for an extended period after the activity
- Increases metabolic efficiency for burning calories by increasing lean body mass
- Helps counteract the decrease in metabolic rate associated with low-calorie diets by preserving lean body mass
- Is a good alternative to eating when eating is a response to stress rather than to hunger

Unfortunately, most overweight people ignore exercise as a means of weight loss, or they exercise at rates below federal health guidelines (CDC, 2010).

Management of obesity involves a comprehensive program of nutrition management, behavior modification, and physical activity or exercise. The key to normalizing body fatness is long-term adherence and permanent lifestyle changes, not dieting or short-term exercise trials.

Increasingly sophisticated obesity treatments that demonstrate the best outcomes emphasize five components: behavioral techniques, cognitive strategies, social support, nutrition, and exercise. The effectiveness of physical activity is related to the frequency and duration of each activity session and the longevity of the activity program. Recommended ACSM guidelines for exercise include the following (Wallace & Ray, 2009):
- A program of low-impact aerobic exercise, increase in daily activities, and resistance training
- A frequency of 5 to 7 times a week
- A length of 40 to 60 minutes a day or 20 to 30 minutes twice daily

As long as calorie expenditure is similar, moderate lifestyle activity may be as effective as structured exercise. Moderate intensity appears to be most effective for total and fat calorie consumption during the activity.

Women tend to have a 5% to 10% lower resting metabolic rate than men and a higher percentage of body fat than men of similar weight. Consequently, women have a lower percentage of lean body mass and may not be as metabolically active as are men during exercise. Women may expend up to 40% fewer calories than do men during the same exercise protocol at the same relative intensity (Tremblay et al., 1985).

Fat in men is stored primarily in the upper body or upper abdominal region. Fat in women is primarily stored in the lower half of the abdomen, the hips, and the thighs. Adipose tissue metabolism tends to be different in various regions. The fat-metabolism response to exercise appears to be less in the femoral-gluteal region than in the upper body–abdominal region. Femoral-gluteal adipose tissue serves as an important source of energy during lactation. Women may not lose fat as easily as do men in response to exercise, because genetic differences are related to where and how fat is stored and metabolized. Consequently, women who need to lose weight may need to be more diligent about increasing the duration of their exercise training sessions and making resistance training a priority to facilitate maximal energy expenditure.

Several studies have examined parental awareness of weight status in children. A survey by the American Academy of Child and Adolescent Psychiatry (2004) of parents, 23% of whom had overweight children, reported that only 10.5% of parents with overweight children perceived their children's weight accurately compared with 59.4% of other parents. In a study by He and Evans (2007), 29.9% of the children examined were overweight or obese. However, on the basis of the parent's perception of their children's weight, only 18.3% were overweight or obese. Factors such as the child's sex, the child's ethnicity, and mother's weight contributed to the parent's inability to recognize weight status. In a study by Huang and colleagues (2007), 61% of parents correctly identified their child's weight status, and these parents were also able to correctly identify the weight status of unrelated children in 58% of reviewed photographs. The results indicate that the parent's ability to correctly identify their child's weight status depends on their child's age and weight status. Moore and colleagues (2012) examined factors that influenced parental concern about their child's weight. Their results indicate that parents were significantly more likely to be concerned about their child's weight if the child was female, they believed the child to be overweight or obese, or the child was overweight or obese on the basis of the BMI.

# OSTEOPOROSIS

Osteoporosis, or porous bone, is the most common bone disease and a major health threat. It is characterized by low bone mass and structural weakness of bone tissue, leading to bone fragility and increased risk of fractures (National Institutes of Health, Osteoporosis and Related Bone Diseases National Resource Center, 2011; Smith et al., 2009). In the United States an estimated 10 million people have osteoporosis and 44 million have low bone density and an increased risk of developing osteoporosis (National Osteoporosis Foundation, 2016). Furthermore, half of adults aged 50 years and older are at risk for breaking a bone, and one in two females and one in four males will fracture a bone due to osteoporosis. Unfortunately, the incidence of osteoporosis in women is greater than heart attack, stroke, and cancer combined (National Osteoporosis Foundation, 2016).

Some loss of bone occurs naturally after age 30 years. Twenty to thirty percent of bone mass development is regulated by environmental factors, such as nutrition and physical activity. In addition to the importance of optimizing physiological intake of calcium and vitamin D (Kalyani et al., 2010), and maintaining normal menstrual cycles for maximization of peak bone mass, physical activity plays a significant role in developing bone mass during childhood and adolescence and in maintaining skeletal mass into adulthood and old age (Bielemann et al., 2013). Two recent meta-analyses provide evidence to support the importance of the combined effects of nutrition and physical activity on bone health (Behringer et al., 2014; Julián-Almárcegui et al., 2015). Physical activities, those that involve weight-bearing in particular, increase BMD (Behringer et al., 2014; Borer, 2005) and provide support for a stronger skeletal foundation throughout aging. Additionally, systematic reviews examining the effects of different exercises in menopausal and postmenopausal women suggested that an active lifestyle and strength training may help to reduce fracture risk and preserve BMD, specifically spine and hip BMD, in osteopenic and osteoporotic women (Howe et al., 2011; Hurley & Armstrong, 2012; Martyn-St James & Carroll, 2009; Zehnacker & Bemis-Dougherty, 2007). A systematic review supports the benefits of resistance training to improve the domains of physical function and activities of daily living in those with osteoporosis or osteopenia (Wilhelm et al., 2012). Inadequate calcium intake during growth has implications for peak bone mass, which may occur as early as the late teenage years or as late as the mid-30s, and may have implications for bone health later in life (Theobald, 2005). Unfortunately, Caucasian females in North America aged 4 to 8 years, 9 to 18 years, 19 to 50 years, and older than 51 years take in 105%, 64%, 74%, and 55% of the recommended amount of calcium respectively (Borer, 2005). Although dietary sources are the preferred means of achieving adequate calcium intake, foods fortified with calcium are becoming more prevalent and are manufactured to provide approximately 300 mg of calcium in each serving (see Chapter 11).

Bone mass increases during childhood and adolescence and peaks during the third decade of life. When a person reaches age approximately 30 years, age-related bone loss occurs throughout the skeletal system, in all races and in both sexes. However, there are significant differences in bone loss patterns between the sexes, with female sex being a risk factor for osteoporosis. Women have less bone mass than men at all ages, and by their mid-thirties can expect age-related bone loss of approximately 1% annually. The rate of bone loss accelerates rapidly during the first 5 years after menopause, with annual losses of 3% to 5% being common. By the fifth decade, or during their forties, women can anticipate a 10% loss of vertebral bone mass. Cumulative bone loss can approach 40% of peak bone mass over a woman's lifetime. Unfortunately, a loss of at least 30% of bone mass is required for detection on plain film radiographs (McKinnis, 2014). Therefore it is important to detect women at risk early in the natural course of the disease and to target interventions toward lifestyle-oriented health promotion. Additional risk factors for osteoporosis include Caucasian/Asian race, family history, low body weight for height, premature menopause, lack of physical activity, long-term smoking, and excessive alcohol consumption (Mirza & Cannalis, 2015; Smith et al., 2009; Stagi et al., 2014). In addition, risk factors for osteoporotic fractures attributable to falls include sensory and coordination deficits, unsafe living situation, older age, musculoskeletal weakness, alterations in posture (e.g., increased spine kyphosis), diminished reflexes, medication use, and associated diseases (Hsu et al., 2014; Kessenich, 2007).

The ACSM recommends that osteoporotic people should engage in weight-bearing and impact exercises to promote strengthening and cardiovascular conditioning, as well as flexibility, coordination, and balance training to improve quality of life, maintain an active lifestyle, and decrease the risk of falls (Kohrt et al., 2004). Maintenance of bone mass may be related to the intensity of the physical activity and the degree to which the activity stresses the bone. Weight-bearing actions that stress the skeleton (walking, stair climbing, floor calisthenics, and aerobic dance) have a positive effect on bone density. Weight-bearing exercise, which increases mechanical stresses on the skeleton, is an important component of reducing osteoporosis risk. Such exercises should be performed for 20 to 30 minutes or more, at least three to five times per week (Smith et al., 2009). Recent intervention trials and meta-analyses suggest that low-impact to moderate-impact weight-bearing exercises combined with resistance and/or agility training facilitate the most effective gains in BMD, prevention of bone loss, and functional capacity in older men and women (Nikander et al., 2010). Aerobic exercise and resistance training have also been advocated for people with osteoporosis (Iwanto et al., 2010) and may give affected individuals more desire to participate in daily activities, promoting a more active lifestyle (Lirani-Galvao & Lazaretti-Castro, 2010). In younger women, the goal of exercise is to increase bone density; in older women who are already 30 to 40 years after menopause, a more realistic goal would be to decrease the risk of fractures through fall prevention. With respect to reducing fall risk in older postmenopausal women, Lirani-Galvao and Lazaretti-Castro (2010) found that tai chi may play a role in preventing osteoporotic fractures because of increases in muscle strength and improvements in balance and decreased risk of falling; however, research has shown that tai chi does not support increases in BMD. Furthermore, it was found that the incidence of fragility fractures was noticeably lower in middle-aged to older men and women who participated in 3 to 4 days of moderate to vigorous physical activity per week (Nikander et al., 2010). A recent review also discusses the evidence to support the use of assistive devices such as spinal and foot orthoses for fall prevention (Hsu et al., 2014). See Box 12-6: Research for Evidence-Based Practice for a recent longitudinal study that supports the benefits of exercise to reduce the incidence of falls and fractures in older women with a history of falls (Kim et al., 2014).

## ARTHRITIS

Arthritis upsets the balance of joint health. Although rheumatoid arthritis and osteoarthritis have different causes and attack different parts of the joint, impaired joint function is the result. Cartilage is destroyed, and irregularities occur in the bone ends. As proper joint alignment changes, normal ROM is decreased, normal muscle balance and activity are altered, and disfigurement and dysfunction occur; and ultimately normal movement patterns are altered. Although there is an ongoing progression in arthritis that cannot be reversed by exercise, physical activity nevertheless helps to restore health to synovium and cartilage, increase strength and flexibility, decrease joint vulnerability, and delay the onset of dysfunction. Most importantly, exercise has been shown to reduce pain and joint stiffness, reduce fatigue, and improve function and psychological well-being in individuals with arthritis (Cooney et al., 2010; Kelley et al., 2015; Kujala, 2009; Nelson et al., 2014). Further evidence is needed to determine if postponing exercise is appropriate during exacerbations of rheumatoid arthritis (Cooney et al., 2010); however, vigorous exercise is typically contraindicated in individuals with acute joint inflammation (ACSM, 2009b).

Using exercise to counteract the effects of inactivity associated with arthritis is certainly a component to effective management (ACSM, 2009b). Although researchers have concluded that regular exercise cannot relieve or cure arthritis, exercise has the following quality-of-life benefits for people with arthritis (ACSM, 2009b; Cooney et al., 2010; Kujala, 2009; Nieman, 2000):

- Improvement in joint function and increase of ROM
- Increase in muscle strength and aerobic fitness that enhance daily activities of living
- Improvement in psychological state
- Decrease in loss of bone mass, and may promote increased BMD
- Decrease in the risk of chronic disease

Consequently, exercise programs based on individual needs and interests should emphasize exercises to increase joint ROM and flexibility (performed before aerobic or strength activities) and should also include muscle-strengthening (two to three times per week) and aerobic exercises (5–10 minutes with progression to a 30-minute session 3–5 days per week) and be functionally based (ACSM, 2009a).

The collective evidence strongly and consistently suggests that exercise is beneficial for individuals with osteoarthritis. The specific aspects of exercise prescription for individuals with osteoarthritis have been studied to differing extents. In terms of the different modes of exercise, various forms of exercise have been shown to be effective for osteoarthritis. A systematic review of studies of the effect of aquatic exercise on osteoarthritis concluded that aquatic exercise produces short-term beneficial effects on function and quality of life and, to a lesser extent, pain management (Bartels et al., 2007). A more recent systematic

---

### BOX 12-6   RESEARCH FOR EVIDENCE-BASED PRACTICE

Falls and fractures in participants and excluded nonparticipants of a fall prevention exercise program for elderly women with a history of falls: 1-year follow-up study.

Objectives: To examine the effectiveness of strength and balance exercises to prevent falls in community-dwelling older adults with a history of falls.

Design: A 1-year follow-up study was conducted on 105 women older than 70 years who had experienced at least one fall in the previous year. Participants were randomly assigned to an exercise group or education group. A third group consisted of women excluded from participation. The exercise group performed strengthening and balance activities that increased in complexity in a sequential manner for 3 months. The education group received information on nutrition, cognitive function, and oral hygiene in the same period. Those excluded from the study were asked to continue their regular routines. Outcomes of interest, including falls, injuries, fractures, and function, were measured at three points in time: at the baseline, after intervention, and at 1-year follow-up. Falls, injuries, fractures, and function were measured at the baseline, after intervention, and at 1-year follow-up.

Setting: Community health promotion center.

Participants: Community-dwelling women older than 70 years with a history of falls.

Intervention: Participants were randomly assigned to one of two groups: exercise (conducted twice per week for 3 months to improve strength and balance) ($n$ = 52) and education (conducted once per month for 3 months; $n$ = 53). Both groups were also compared with a group of excluded participants ($n$ = 91).

Measurements: The primary outcome measures included fall rates, fracture rates, and odds ratios (ORs) for falls and fractures. Additional outcome measures included measures of balance, walking speed, and lower extremity strength.

Results: There was a significant difference ($\chi^2$ = 7.069, $P$ = 0.029) in fall incidences between groups: 19.6% in the exercise group, 40.4% in the education group, and 40.8% in the excluded group. There was also a significant difference (Fisher's exact test = 0.043) in fracture rate between groups: 10.0% in the exercise group, 9.5% in the education group, and 27.6% in the excluded group. When compared with the exercise group, those in the education group (OR 2.78) and the excluded group (OR 2.83) had significantly greater odds of falling, and those in the excluded group (OR 4.30) also had significantly greater odds of fractures. Additional significant differences between groups and over time included increases in one leg standing time, usual walking speed, knee extension strength, and dorsiflexion strength.

Conclusion: These findings support the use of strengthening and balance exercises to decrease the incidence of falls and fractures in those with a history of falls.

From Kim, H., Yoshida, H., & Suzuki, T. (2014). Falls and fractures in participants and excluded nonparticipants of a fall prevention exercise program for elderly women with a history of falls: 1-year follow-up study. *Geriatrics & Gerontology International, 14*(2), 285–292.

review examined the effects of aquatic exercise on symptoms and function associated with lower extremity osteoarthritis and reported significant effects for pain, self-reported function, physical functioning, stiffness, and quality of life (Waller et al., 2014). With respect to fall risk, the available evidence produces mixed results with use of aquatic exercise to reduce fall risk in individuals with hip and/or knee osteoarthritis, supporting the use of aquatic exercise in conjunction with fall risk education to effectively reduce fall risk, but not the use of aquatic exercise alone (Arnold & Faulkner, 2010; Hale et al., 2012). Lastly, an 18-week trial comparing aquatic exercise with land-based exercise found that although both modes of exercise improved function and pain management, the aquatic exercise group demonstrated a significantly greater reduction in pain level (Silva et al., 2008). Long-term effects have not been shown to date; thus, we suggest aquatic exercise either be incorporated into a broader exercise program or be modified and exercise increase regularly to promote adaptation to and avoid accommodation to the training stimulus.

With respect to non–aquatic-based exercise, an umbrella review found high-quality evidence supporting the beneficial effects of exercise on pain and function in individuals with osteoarthritis of the knee (Jamtvedt et al., 2008). Similarly, a systematic review of the effects of strength training alone, exercise therapy alone, and a combination of exercise and manual therapy in individuals with osteoarthritis of the knee concluded that these modes of treatment improved function and reduced pain to a small degree, with the addition of manual therapy to treatment producing a moderate effect on pain (Jansen et al., 2011). A systematic review incorporating adults and older adults with knee osteoarthritis supported progressive resistance exercise and aerobic exercise as having a modest beneficial effect on strength, pain, and function (Keysor & Brembs, 2011). A recent systematic review of randomized controlled trials concluded that physical therapies including strength training, tai chi, and aerobic exercises improved balance outcomes and decreased fall risk in older individuals with knee osteoarthritis (Mat et al., 2015).

Available evidence may also support a small but positive benefit from education and self-management programs as complements to exercise to improve self-efficacy (May, 2010). Furthermore, additional evidence suggests that increased belief that physical activity can be beneficial to manage arthritis leads to higher levels of participation in physical activity (Ehrlich-Jones et al., 2011) and is significantly associated with decreased pain and fatigue, increased function, and a self-perceived positive effect (Bezalel et al., 2010; Hewlett et al., 2011; Pisters et al., 2010). Exercise intensity is another important consideration for exercise prescription in individuals with osteoarthritis (OA); however, unlike the mode of exercise, intensity has received little attention. There is limited research available that compares the outcomes in individuals with OA with the intensity of training; however, some evidence supports both high-intensity and low-intensity training as being of equal benefit in individuals with knee OA with respect to pain, strength, and function, without a difference in the rate of unfavorable effects. More research is needed to determine the optimal parameters for exercise in individuals with osteoarthritis, and an impairment-based, person-centered

approach with consideration of comorbidities and accessibility is required (Bennell & Hinman, 2011).

**Rheumatoid arthritis** (RA) and **fibromyalgia syndrome** are two related arthritic conditions that have begun to be studied more. Evidence suggests that aerobic exercise in individuals with fibromyalgia can increase function and relieve some symptoms (Busch et al., 2008). However, evidence pertaining to the effectiveness of strength training to produce similar effects in individuals with fibromyalgia is of low quality (Kujala, 2009). A recent systematic review concluded that aquatic therapy can improve self-reported function capacity (Fibromyalgia Impact Questionnaire) and performance-based function (6-minute walk test) and reduce stiffness in individuals with fibromyalgia (Lima et al., 2013). In addition to evidence supporting the use of a combination of aerobic and strength exercises to improve outcomes in those with rheumatoid arthritis (Cooney et al., 2010), the use of tai chi as a form of activity in individuals with RA has also been considered. A case series study of the use of tai chi in individuals with RA supported significant reduction in swelling of joints and increase in strength and endurance as measured by the "timed sit to stand test," and suggests practicing tai chi may help individuals with RA increase their level of physical activity (Uhlig et al., 2010). Importantly, although the evidence has not shown that tai chi reduces pain or relieves other symptoms of RA, it does not appear to exacerbate these symptoms (Han et al., 2004). A meta-analysis of the effects of cardiorespiratory aerobic exercise in individuals with rheumatoid arthritis demonstrated small but meaningful effects on quality of life, function, and pain (Baillet et al., 2010). In addition, a recent systematic review examined the correlates in four categories (sociodemographic, physical, psychological, and social variables) with levels of physical activity in individuals with rheumatoid arthritis (Larkin & Kennedy, 2014). Positive correlations with physical activity were found for motivation, self-efficacy, health perception, and previous physical activity levels, whereas negative correlations were found for fatigue, a coerced regulation style (i.e., the extent to which the person believes the physical activity goal was set not by himself or herself but by others), and certain physiological variables.

Again, further evidence is needed to determine if postponing exercise is appropriate during exacerbations of RA (Cooney et al., 2010). A review of the studies of the effects of aerobic exercise, strength training, and aquatic therapy on individuals with fibromyalgia syndrome concluded there is evidence supporting benefits of exercise in this population to improve function and well-being, and decrease pain and stiffness (Busch et al., 2007; Kujala, 2009; Lima et al., 2013). Aerobic activities such as stepping and walking and strengthening exercises such as lifting weights or use of resistance exercise machines can be used in addition to stretching for flexibility. Although exercise is part of the overall management of fibromyalgia syndrome, the review by Busch and colleagues (2007) examined the effects of exercise when used separately or combined with other strategies such as education programs, biofeedback, and medications. In that review, aerobic exercises were done for at least 20 minutes once a day (or twice for 10 minutes), 2 days a week. Strength training was done two to three times a week and with at least 8 to 12 repetitions per exercise. The exercise programs lasted between 2.5 and 24 weeks. In a study by Sañudo and colleagues (2010), aerobic exercise was compared with combined exercise (aerobic, muscle strength, and flexibility exercises) and control (nonexercising) groups. Both exercise groups demonstrated significant improvements on the Fibromyalgia Impact Questionnaire and the Beck Depression Inventory. When compared with the aerobic exercise and control groups, the combined exercise group had significantly better outcomes on the SF-36 physical function, body pain, vitality, and mental health subscales and for ROM (shoulder and hip) measurements and grip strength. In a more recent study, Sañudo and colleagues (2012) examined the effect of whole-body vibration exercise on balance in women with fibromyalgia. The control group received an exercise training program, and the experimental group received the same exercise training program plus whole-body vibration exercises. The results indicated that the group with whole-body vibration demonstrated significantly better balance, as measured by the mediolateral stability index, when compared with the control group.

## LOW BACK PAIN

Low back pain is a common medical and social problem frequently associated with disability and absence from work. Low back pain is a multifactorial disorder that is unlikely to be caused by a single factor. Obesity is associated with an increased risk of low back pain, as well as an increased likelihood of seeking care for subacute and chronic low back pain (Shiri et al., 2010). The risk of low back pain increases as BMI increases: 2.9% when BMI is 20 to 25 kg/m$^2$, 5.2% when BMI is 26 to 30 kg/m$^2$, 7.7% when BMI is 31 to 35 kg/m$^2$, and 11.6% when BMI is 36 kg/m$^2$ or greater (Smuck et al., 2014). Contrary to commonly held opinion, there is a lack of evidence that a sedentary lifestyle is a risk factor for the onset of low back pain (Chen et al., 2009). However, higher levels of muscular and aerobic fitness are associated with a decreased risk of low back pain (Heneweer et al., 2012). A recent meta-analysis concluded that aerobic exercise can reduce pain and improve the physical and psychological functioning of individuals with chronic low back pain (Meng & Yeu, 2015). Roffey and colleagues (2010a) in a systematic review found strong evidence that there is no relationship between awkward occupational postures and low back pain. Specifically, it is unlikely that occupational bending and twisting (Wai et al., 2010a), occupational sitting (Roffey et al., 2010b), occupational standing or walking (Roffey et al., 2010c), occupational lifting (Wai et al., 2010b), occupational pushing or pulling (Roffey, et al., 2010d), occupational carrying (Wai et al., 2010c), and occupational manual handling and individual assistance (Roffey et al., 2010e) are independent risk factors for low back pain.

Exercise can, however, have a positive influence on low back pain. There is some evidence to support overground walking more than treadmill walking in the management of low back pain (Hendrick et al., 2010). A more recent study found a positive synergistic effect of a rehabilitation program consisting of 14 exercises and treadmill exercises on the low back extensor strength in individuals with chronic low back pain (Cho et al., 2015). A systematic review concluded that exercise can effectively reduce pain and improve function in persons with chronic low back

pain; however, there was no clear advantage for any one form of exercise (van Middelkoop et al., 2010). Staal and colleagues (2004) concluded that graded activity was more effective than usual care in reducing the number of days of absence from work because of low back pain. Olaya-Contreras and colleagues (2015) examined the effects of advising a group of people with acute severe low back pain to "stay active in spite of the pain," and they found no difference in pain intensity trajectory and a significantly higher level of physical activity when this group was compared with a group that was instructed to "adjust activity to the pain." Given the acknowledged detriments of bed rest, staying active is good advice for individuals with low back pain. A recently updated Cochrane Review found that exercise therapy for acute low back pain may be effective in reducing pain and improving function in persons with chronic low back pain and reducing absenteeism in persons with subacute low back pain (Hayden et al., 2005). Another Cochrane Review found moderate evidence that exercise following treatment for low back pain may reduce recurrent episodes of low back pain (Choi et al., 2010).

The spinal column is composed of 24 vertebrae stacked vertically, forming natural curves that allow the bony column to function with the resiliency of a spring. The intervertebral disks help with mobility and shock absorption. The health of the bony vertebrae and the cartilaginous disks depends on movement. The cartilage receives its nutrients from cyclical compression and decompression as a function of weight-bearing and non–weight-bearing movement. Similarly, repeated weight-bearing and non–weight-bearing activity stimulates vertebral bone integrity.

Muscles are intimately involved in the support and function of the spinal column. Maintaining the proper curves (anterior and posterior convexities) of lordosis in the cervical and lumbar vertebrae and kyphosis in the thoracic vertebrae is vital for sustaining the spring and shock-absorption qualities of the spine. The lumbar curve is especially influenced by three sets of muscles that are attached to the pelvis and the lumbar vertebrae. By altering the tilt of the pelvis, these muscles can increase (iliopsoas muscle) or decrease (abdominal and hamstring muscles) the lumbar curve. In addition, the deep muscles of the back (paraspinal muscles) work in controlled synergistic and antagonistic fashions to control spinal planes of motion; they are also influential in supporting the spinal curves in posture. Weakness or shortening of any of these muscles can adversely impact posture and increase stress on the back. The result can be back pain from muscle strain, altered joint function (facet joints), and abnormal force on the intervertebral disks.

In a systematic review, Hayden and colleagues (2005) concluded that in persons with various levels of low back pain, exercise was beneficial in terms of reducing pain, improving function, and decreasing absenteeism. The American Pain Society and the American College of Physicians have also jointly stated that there is good evidence for the effectiveness of exercise in reducing chronic low back pain (Chou & Huffman, 2007). Specific types of exercise that have been shown to be effective in persons with low back pain include training of the deep and superficial paraspinal muscles as well as unweighted or suspended exercise. The only systematic review of the effects of unweighted movement on persons with chronic low back pain concluded that there was consistent and strong evidence to support unweighted exercise to decrease pain and improve function (Slade & Keating, 2007). Exercise targeting specific lumbar paraspinal muscles has been shown to substantially reduce pain and restore function (Chang et al., 2015; Hwangbo et al., 2015; Koumantakis et al., 2005; Shaughnessy & Caulfield, 2004). Although walking appears to be effective in the management of chronic musculoskeletal pain, including low back pain (O'Connor et al., 2015), Rasmussen-Barr and colleagues (2009) found that graded exercises target both deep and superficial muscles that support and control the lumbar spine and pelvis and were more effective in the long term in reducing disability and the need for recurrent treatment and improving pain self-efficacy.

The goal of exercise programs for individuals with low back pain is to prevent debilitation as a result of inactivity and to increase endurance, strength, and flexibility, allowing a return to usual functional activities. Exercise recommendations and progression of activity are highly individualized on the basis of the origin, duration, and severity of pain. Strengthening exercises for trunk and extremity musculature have been demonstrated to benefit people with low back pain. Aerobic conditioning, such as walking, swimming, and stationary bicycling, is recommended to maintain endurance and prevent debilitation from inactivity (ACSM, 2013).

Advanced age, osteoporosis, arthritis, and low back pain are not reasons to exclude exercise from anyone's lifestyle. In fact, the opposite is true. These conditions are reasons to remain as physically active as possible to facilitate the ability to function throughout the aging process.

A referral to a physical therapist is warranted in most, if not all, cases of low back pain to allow there to be proper comprehensive management, which may include exercise as well as other safe and effective interventions.

## IMMUNE FUNCTION

The relationship between exercise and immune function has a fairly long history of study, and the interest that grew out of the human immunodeficiency virus (HIV) epidemic continues to stimulate investigations in this area. Several studies demonstrate that people with impaired immune function can exercise safely without risk to their health status and can enhance their physiological and psychological well-being with regular exercise (Fillipas et al., 2006; Galantino et al., 2005; Gomes-Neto et al., 2013; Sax, 2006; Terry et al., 2006). A systematic review concluded that progressive resistive exercise may increase body weight and limb girth and aerobic exercise may improve adipose levels and lipid profiles by decreasing fat in tissues and blood in individuals with HIV (Fillipas et al., 2010). Another systematic review concluded that resistance exercise may improve body composition by decreasing body fat and increasing muscle strength, aerobic exercise may also improve body composition and increase aerobic capacity, and concurrent training may improve all outcomes evaluated in individuals with HIV (Gomes-Neto et al., 2013).

Furthermore, two recently updated meta-analyses suggest that aerobic exercise, either alone or in conjunction with progressive resistance exercise, can be safely performed by adults with HIV/acquired immunodeficiency syndrome (AIDS) and may increase fitness and improve body composition and well-being (O'Brien et al., 2009, 2010). Recommended parameters include exercising at least three times per week for 20 minutes over a period of 5 weeks or more (O'Brien et al., 2010).

The effect of exercise on immune system markers (e.g., CD4 levels, CD4/CD8 ratio, or viral load) in people with HIV/AIDS is unclear. Reviews discuss the effects of exercise on immune function in individuals with HIV/AIDS and report conflicting findings (Anderson, 2006; Dudgeon et al., 2004). A meta-analysis compared aerobic exercise groups with nonexercising groups and found no significant differences in CD4 count, CD4 percentage, or viral load (Nixon et al., 2005). Similarly, meta-analytic data compared the combination of aerobic and progressive resistance exercise with no exercise and found no significant differences in CD4 count (O'Brien et al., 2004). Despite the fact that the CD4 count did not differ between exercising and nonexercising groups, there were significant beneficial changes in depressive symptoms, mean body weight, mean arm and thigh girth, and maximum heart rate for those in the exercising groups (Nixon et al., 2005; O'Brien et al., 2004). In another study, Jaggers and colleagues (2015) examined the effects of combined aerobic and resistance training on the psychological well-being of adults with HIV and found significant decreases in depression and mood states (Profile of Mood States) for the exercise group. The control group, the members of which were allowed to engage in sedentary activities, showed a significant increase in the perception of stress (Perceived Stress Scale). Evidence suggests that regular exercisers and athletes are less likely to become ill than sedentary women (Nieman, 1994) and middle-aged men and women (Matthews et al., 2002). In direct contrast, evidence also suggests that athletes are also at increased risk of infection during increased periods of training or after competition (Nieman, 1994; Nieman et al., 1990; Pedersen & Bruunsgaard, 1995; Peters-Futre, 1997). Another reported finding is that after exercise, sedentary individuals have a higher risk of infection than active individuals (Kiwata et al., 2014). A recent review concluded that immune function, both innate and acquired, of athletes under heavy training is often observed to decrease by approximately 15% to 25%, but studies on whether this change increases infection risk remain inconclusive (Walsh et al., 2015).

Classic epidemiological studies indicate that a J-curve relationship may exist between the intensity of exercise and the risk of upper respiratory tract infection (URTI) (Nieman, 1994; Pedersen et al., 1998). That is, in theory, moderate exercise may decrease the risk of URTI below that of a sedentary individual, but high-intensity exercise may raise the risk above average. In direct contrast, Lee and colleagues (1992) concluded that immune function was not linked to the risk of URTI in a group of cadets during basic training, and Pyne and colleagues (1995) reported similar rates of URTI between elite swimmers under intense training and age- and gender-matched sedentary controls. Similarly, Gleeson and colleagues (2013) reported that high-exercising (≥ 11 h/wk) and medium-exercising (7–10 h/wk) groups had more URTI episodes than the low-exercising (3–6 h/wk) group. Factors that confound studies on the relationship between exercise and URTI include failure to distinguish between new infection and the clinical manifestations of a dormant infection (Gleeson et al., 2002) and failure to distinguish between airway hyperresponsiveness and URTI (Langdeau & Boulet, 2001).

Immune system changes that are apparently related to the intensity of exercise have been identified. Moderate-endurance exercise stimulates the neuroendocrine system, which causes changes in the function and numbers of various immune system cells, such as the natural killer, CD4, and CD8 cells. Evidence also indicates that moderate exercise is associated with a prolonged improvement in the killing capacity of neutrophils (one of the most efficient phagocytes). Several immune marker changes suggest increased risk of illness in those who engage in high-intensity exercise, including a low level of salivary immunoglobulin (antibodies), low serum complement levels, low lymphocyte count, depressed natural killer cell activity, low helper and suppressor T cell ratio, and decreased neutrophil phagocytic capacity (Mackinnon, 1992; Nieman, 1994; Pedersen & Ullum, 1994). Most aspects of immunity in male and female athletes are not significantly different (Gleeson et al., 2011).

Changes in immune cell counts and activity may be related to hormonal immunoregulation. Moderate exercise increases the release of immunostimulatory hormones, such as growth hormone and endogenous opiates ($\beta$-endorphin and methionine enkephalin). The increase in the levels of $\beta$-endorphins with exercise seems to have a positive effect on natural killer cell activity. Conversely, intense exercise is associated with increases in the levels of catecholamine and corticosteroid (cortisol), which have immunosuppressive characteristics (Mackinnon, 1992). High-intensity exercise is also associated with muscle cell damage and inflammation. The immune system is involved in tissue repair. It is theorized that while immune cells are busy with the repair process, host protection may suffer. A window of opportunity for infection during recovery from high-intensity exercise appears to exist. Accordingly, rest is recommended after vigorous exercise to allow the body to recover, and moderate exercise may be the better choice for enhancement of health and well-being.

There is convincing evidence that exercise and physical activity have a significant protective effect on the gastrointestinal system, and, in particular, against colon cancer (Martin, 2011). However, there is less convincing evidence for the following conditions: gastric and pancreatic cancers, gastroesophageal reflux disease, peptic ulcer disease, nonalcoholic fatty liver disease, cholelithiasis, diverticular disease, irritable bowel syndrome, and constipation (Martin, 2011).

Evidence also suggests that physical activity is a modifiable risk factor for breast cancer (Bardi, 2007). Physical activity appears to lower the risk of developing many conditions, in particular breast cancer (Warburton et al., 2007). Unfortunately, physical activity during adolescence does not appear to play a protective role for the risk of breast cancer later in life (Gammon et al., 1998). A recent meta-analysis concluded that physical activity may reduce all-cause breast cancer–related deaths and breast cancer events in breast cancer survivors (Lahart et al., 2015). Another meta-analysis concluded that physical activity may decrease the risk of prostate cancer, and encouraged men to engage in regular physical activity (Liu et al., 2011b). A synthesis of clinical practice guidelines, systematic reviews, meta-analyses, and individual studies suggests that exercise may minimize or prevent adverse physiological effects of cancer and its treatment (Ingram & Visovsky, 2007). A recent position statement on immune function and exercise (Walsh et al., 2011) offered the following conclusion: "There is consensus that exercise training protects against some types of cancers. Training also enhances aspects of antitumor immunity and reduces inflammatory mediators. However, the data linking immunological and inflammatory mechanisms, physical activity, and cancer risk reduction remains tentative."

Preliminary findings in the area of immunosenescence, the natural decline in immune function that occurs with aging, suggest that regular exercise and increased fitness may have potential immune restorative properties and improve the "immune risk profile" in elderly people (Simpson & Guy, 2010).

## MENTAL HEALTH

People who exercise regularly generally state that they feel better, have increased self-esteem, and have a more positive outlook on life. Not only do they feel better physically, they also they feel better mentally. Epidemiological research with both men and women suggests that physical activity may be associated with improvements in positive affect and general sense of well-being (USDHHS, 2015). Much of the work has focused on depression (Cooney et al., 2013; Josefsson et al., 2014), anxiety (Bartley et al., 2013; Wegner et al., 2014), stress (Georgiades et al., 2000; Rimmele et al., 2007), and schizophrenia (Firth et al., 2015; Gorczynski & Faulkner, 2010).

Evidence from a review of the literature (prospective studies, randomized controlled trials, and meta-analyses) found that exercise protects against and is an intervention for mild to major depression (Graven et al., 2011; Nahas & Sheikh, 2011). A recent meta-analysis concluded that exercise can reduce depressive symptoms in individuals with arthritis and other rheumatic conditions (Kelley et al., 2015). Research by the National College Health Assessment examined the association between vigorous/moderate or strength-training exercises and mental health in a national sample of college women (Adams et al., 2007). Both vigorous/moderate and strength-training exercises were positively associated with perceived health. Furthermore, both vigorous/moderate and strength-training exercises were negatively associated with several indicators of mental health (e.g., depression, anxiety, and suicidal ideation). Similarly, research examined the association between exercise and mental health and concluded that mental health is modifiable through exercise (Galper et al., 2006; Windle et al., 2010).

The mental health benefits of physical activity, as an intervention, have been summarized elsewhere and include promoting mental health and well-being in healthy adults, preventing and treating mental disorders, and supporting psychosocial rehabilitation (Nyström et al., 2015; C. W. Wang et al., 2014; F. Wang et al., 2014).

Investigations have focused on populations across the life span, including children, young adults, and older adults. Based on a limited number of small trials, a recently updated Cochrane

Review concluded that, when compared with no intervention, exercise reduces anxiety and depression in children and young adults (Larun et al., 2009). Another Cochrane Review suggests that long-term exercise, of various types, is most likely to have a beneficial effect on mood in adults; however, the magnitude of the effect is indeterminate at this point (Mead et al., 2009). Researchers examining major depressive disorder recommended an exercise prescription that is supervised, individually customized, at least 30 minutes, and at least three times per week (Nyström et al., 2015). Yoga has also been shown to be effective in treating depression (Cramer et al., 2013).

In a recent systematic review of the effect of exercise on cognitive function in older adults, Tseng and colleagues (2011) suggested that there were positive benefits to adopting unimodal, simple exercises for cognitively impaired older adults and a more diversified, multimodal program for healthy older adults. They also recommended an exercise regimen of 6 weeks in duration, at least three sessions per week lasting 60 minutes each, to increase the likelihood of a positive effect on cognition.

Furthermore, the effect of exercise on individuals with various disorders or diseases, such as schizophrenia, cancer, or other chronic illnesses, has been studied. In a systematic review, Herring and colleagues (2010) concluded that although exercise in sedentary persons with a chronic illness reduces anxiety, training programs lasting as few as 12 weeks and consisting of sessions of at least 30 minutes resulted in the largest reductions in anxiety. A Cochrane Review of the psychological and physical effects of dance and movement therapy on persons with cancer was unable to arrive at a conclusion because of a dearth of high-quality studies in this area, although there may be a positive effect on quality of life in persons with breast cancer (Bradt et al., 2011). Based on a limited number of small trials, an updated Cochrane Review concluded that regular exercise may improve both physical and mental health and well-being in persons with schizophrenia (Gorczynski & Faulkner, 2010). Exercise had been shown in two meta-analyses to improve health-related quality of life in those scheduled to receive, actively undergoing, or having completed cancer treatment (Mishra et al., 2014, 2015).

Various types and modalities of exercise have been used in studies; an example of one such intervention is tai chi. Tai chi significantly improved both psychological (perceived well-being) and physical (functional capacity, knee extension strength, and flexibility) health over baseline levels (Macfarlane et al., 2005). In a systematic review and meta-analysis of the effect of tai chi on psychological well-being, Wang and colleagues (2010) demonstrated an apparent association with reductions in anxiety, depression, mood disturbance, and stress, as well as improvements in self-esteem. A more recent review examining various populations again supported the benefits of tai chi for treatment of depression, treatment of anxiety, general stress management, and exercise self-efficacy (F. Wang et al., 2014). Yoga has also been shown to decrease depression and anxiety in a variety of conditions (Cramer et al., 2013; Pascoe & Bauer, 2015). Similarly, qigong exercise has been shown to reduce stress and anxiety in healthy adults when compared with waiting list controls (C. W. Wang et al., 2014).

# EXERCISE PRESCRIPTION

The literature certainly reflects both the physiological and the psychological benefits that can be experienced with commitment to an active lifestyle. In short, regular physical activity or exercise can help people feel better, look better, and perform better. Unfortunately, as discussed, Americans have failed to embrace the concept and health value of an active lifestyle. Many have been overwhelmed by the misperception that to gain health benefits they must perform vigorous, continual exercise. The result has been discouragement in getting started and poor compliance in staying with it. "No pain, no gain" has been an unfortunate and common refrain (Box 12-7: Quality and Safety Scenario).

People need to be reminded that many of their daily physical activities are actually forms of exercise (Figure 12-3). This approach to physical activity serves as a good foundation to a healthy lifestyle. However, when possible, individuals should also be encouraged to include more formal exercise training in their overall activities to promote optimal cardiorespiratory fitness and significantly increase muscle strength and endurance. The amount of exercise required to achieve these goals is determined by the parameters of an exercise prescription:

| | |
|---|---|
| **F** (frequency) | Aerobic exercise three to five times a week |
| | Resistance training two to three times a week |
| **I** (intensity) | Moderate to vigorous, by heart rate and perceived exertion |
| | Able to complete each resistance exercise, 8 to 12 repetitions, without strain |
| **T** (time) | 20 to 60 minutes, plus warm-up and cool-down periods |
| | 15 to 30 minutes to complete a series of 8 to 10 resistance exercises |
| **T** (type) | Aerobic (walking, jogging, biking, swimming, rowing, cross-country skiing, elliptical trainer, NordicTrack, StairMaster, aerobics, dancing, skating, or rollerblading) |
| | Resistance training (weight machines, free weights, and calisthenics such as push-ups, sit-ups, or pull-ups) |
| | (ACSM, 2013) |

## Aerobic Exercise

The benefits of aerobic exercise are cumulative; therefore a frequency of three to five times a week is recommended. Every other day is a good frame of reference and allows recovery between training sessions, potentially decreasing the chance of overuse injuries. The benefits of exercising more than five times a week are outweighed by the risk of injury, especially with higher-impact activities. When more frequent exercising is a goal, cross-training is recommended. **Cross-training** means performing different types of exercise on different days of the week or performing different types of exercise within

## ☑ BOX 12-7 QUALITY AND SAFETY SCENARIO

### *Less Pain, More Gain*

In an attempt to encourage increased participation in physical activity, a panel of scientists from the CDC and the ACSM came together to review the evidence related to physical activity and to issue a public health message concerning the recommended types and amounts of physical activity. The evidence clearly indicates that the protective effects of exercise can be achieved at more moderate levels of intensity than had been recommended previously. The health and fitness benefits of exercise appear to be related more to the total amount of exercise performed (calories expended) rather than to the specific exercise intensity, frequency, and duration. The recommendations are as follows:

- Adults should perform 30 minutes or more of moderate-intensity (brisk) physical activity on most (or all) days of the week, for a weekly total of 3 to 4 hours.
- The activity need not be continuous; benefits can be realized with short bouts of activity (a minimum of 10 minutes) over the course of the day.
- This amount of activity will expend approximately 150 to 200 calories per day (the equivalent of walking 2 miles briskly) or 1000 to 1400 calories per week.

- All types of activity can be applied to the daily total (raking leaves, dancing, or gardening).
- Lower-intensity activities should be performed more often, or for longer periods, or both. More vigorous activities should be performed for shorter periods or less frequently.

Because most adults do not meet these standards, they have the most to gain by incorporating a few minutes of increased activity into their day, gradually building up to 30 minutes a day. People who are active on an irregular basis should strive to be more consistent. People who prefer more formal exercise can choose to participate in more vigorous, organized exercise regimens, sports, and recreational activities.

Sedentary individuals gain the most by increasing their activity to the recommended level. However, any person who already meets the standards can derive some additional benefit by becoming more active.

*People who do a little bit of exercise are better off than those…who do none and those who do a little more are better off still (Franklin, 1993).*

Franklin, B. (1993). How much exercise is enough? In *Encyclopedia britannica* (pp. 471–476). Los Angeles: Encyclopedia Britannica, Inc.

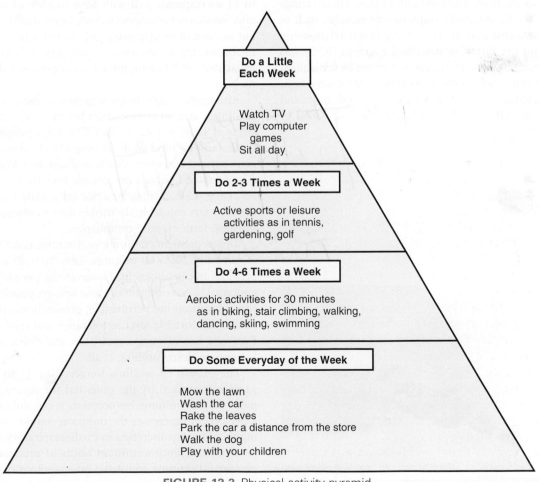

**FIGURE 12-3** Physical activity pyramid.

one session. The benefits of cross-training include a decreased risk of musculoskeletal injury, an increased potential for total body conditioning, and improved long-term compliance because variety decreases boredom and eliminates the exercise barrier of limited choices.

The intensity of exercise that results in health and fitness benefits ranges from moderate to vigorous and is comfortable, but challenging (brisk). Intensity is defined by the objective measure of heart rate (HR) and the subjective measure of perceived exertion. The increase in HR during exercise has a strong linear relationship with exercise intensity and aerobic capacity. Resting heart rate is the HR measured at rest. Maximum heart rate is the rate measured at the highest workload tolerated during exercise. Maximum heart rate also decreases with age; a generic formula for determining maximum heart rate is 220 minus age. Formulas for determining appropriate exercise HRs have been developed that take resting heart rate and maximum heart rate into consideration.

The Borg scale for rating perceived exertion is a psychophysical category scale for the subjective rating of sensations associated with the intensity of physical work (Borg, 1973, 1982) (Figure 12-4). The scale uses ratings based on the individual's overall feeling of exertion and physical fatigue. These ratings correspond well with metabolic responses to exercise, such as HR and oxygen consumption. The strong linear relationship between HR and the rating of perceived exertion (RPE) was originally suggested by Borg and has been verified by subsequent studies. Correlation coefficients from 80% to 90% have been reported consistently with use of a variety of work tasks and exercise conditions (Borg, 1973, 1982; Skinner et al., 1973). A

meta-analysis has shown the Borg scale to be a valid measure of exercise intensity with a strong link between RPE and HR (Chen et al., 2002). In addition, recent studies support use of the Borg scale for various populations, including individuals with stroke (Sage et al., 2013), obesity (Coquart et al., 2012), and fibromyalgia (Soriano-Maldonado et al., 2015), and have quantified its ability to predict $\dot{V}o_{2max}$ (or $\dot{V}o_2$ peak) (Coquart et al., 2014). However, perceptions of exertion and the relationship with HR are influenced by both physiological and psychological factors (aches, cramps, pain, fatigue, shortness of breath, anxiety, depression, and introversion or extroversion). Smutok and colleagues (1980) noted that some individuals are more accurate in regulating exercise intensity by RPE than are others and that this variability may be more the result of psychological than physiological factors. Other factors that may alter the strong relationship between HR and RPE are drug-related situations (β-blockers), age, and disease states (Hautala et al., 2013; Mampuya, 2012).

Despite this potential for variability in perception, RPE correlates well with HR clinically, and together they form a complementary means of helping individuals determine a comfortable, beneficial level of exercise intensity. An RPE of 11 to 14 corresponds well with 50% to 85% of maximum heart rate. Subjective parameters include being slightly short of breath, but not out of breath; being able to talk without difficulty, but unable to sing a song easily; being pleasantly fatigued, but not exhausted; and having mild musculoskeletal discomfort, but no pain.

Attention to RPE helps a person develop a sense of body awareness and an appreciation for the body's response to the stress of activity. Awareness of RPE helps people listen to their bodies and become aware of how it feels to move, where they carry tension, and where they have discomfort. With this increased awareness, individuals can choose how they want to respond, adjusting their exercise practice on a daily basis, making the activity more enjoyable, decreasing the risk of injury, and improving long-term exercise compliance.

The recommended duration of aerobic conditioning exercise is generally 20 to 60 minutes. Less than 20 minutes usually provides minimal benefit. However, for people who are unaccustomed to exercising or for those who are greatly deconditioned, short durations are permissible, gradually increasing to a beneficial, comfortable level as tolerance and confidence increase. Everyone has to start somewhere, and doing a little is much better than doing nothing at all.

The benefit of sessions longer than 45 to 60 minutes is again outweighed by the potential for injury. Exercising for more than 60 minutes on occasion is certainly not wrong, but a person who increases the duration should consider decreasing the intensity. Increases in cardiorespiratory fitness can also be accrued from intermittent bouts of moderate to vigorous exercise (10-minute segments) on a workout day. As discussed, longer bouts of exercise are more beneficial for weight loss. The range of acceptable duration allows greater flexibility, giving reassurance of benefit to the individual who varies exercise choices daily on the basis of capability, interests, and life demands.

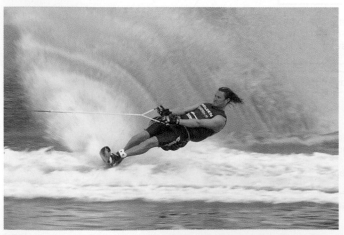

**FIGURE 12-4** Water skiing is a form of intense exercise. (From Cummings, N. H., Stanley-Green, S., & Higgs, P. [2009]. Perspectives in athletic training. St. Louis: Mosby.)

As mentioned, many different choices for the mode of aerobic exercise are available. A question that is often asked is "What is the best type of aerobic exercise?" The answer is "The one that the individual is willing to do on a regular basis." Different aerobic exercises have different benefits; they all have their advantages and disadvantages. From a cardiovascular point of view, with relative intensity, frequency, and duration being equal, the benefit is about the same for all modes. Probably the best scenario is cross-training, which results in the greatest number of optimal all-around benefits. However, the most important recommendation is that the person starts moving—choosing the person's favorite exercise will increase the likelihood of adhering to an exercise program.

Walking is probably the most accessible and popular form of aerobic exercise. Done briskly, walking provides a good cardiorespiratory challenge in 60% to 80% of the adult population. Walking is also an activity that nearly everyone can do, requires little equipment or cost, can be done almost anywhere, and can be a social or a solitary activity, depending on individual needs. Walking is often the recommended exercise of choice for people who are greatly deconditioned or for those who have physical limitations. Considered a low-impact activity, walking can be easily regulated to accommodate a wide range of fitness levels and motor abilities. Cycling, rowing, and swimming (or water walking or other water aerobics) are non–weight-bearing to low–weight-bearing activities that may be good choices for individuals with physical limitations. Aquatic exercise is a good alternative for individuals with musculoskeletal limitations who need some weight relief with exercise, such as individuals with advanced osteoarthritis. Although the buoyancy of the water provides this weight relief, the water also provides resistance to the limbs as they move, encouraging an increase in intensity and conditioning. Individuals should be encouraged to do the types of aerobic exercise that best fit their needs, interests, and lifestyles while providing reasonable benefits.

## Warm-Up and Cool-Down Periods

In addition to the endurance phase of exercise, warm-up and cool-down periods should be a regular part of the exercise session. The warm-up period usually lasts 5 to 10 minutes and may include light stretching, calisthenics, or performance of the chosen aerobic activity at a low intensity. This approach prepares both the musculoskeletal system and the cardiorespiratory system for the transition from rest to exercise by increasing blood flow, respiration, body temperature, and muscle flexibility. The warm-up period decreases the risks of injury and heart irregularities.

The cool-down period follows the endurance phase and usually lasts 5 to 10 minutes. This phase allows the body to readjust gradually from the demands of exercise back to the baseline. Stretching and slow, rhythmical movement help to increase muscle elasticity, prevent blood pooling and hypotension, and facilitate dissipation of body heat and removal of lactic acid. The result is the prevention of injury, light-headedness, fatigue, and muscle soreness.

Yoga is an excellent example of one form of exercise to use during warm-up and cool-down periods. The word yoga means union or "established in being," which implies a mind-body connection. Simply defined, yoga is mindful stretching. The mind is quiet, and awareness is focused on feeling the body as it moves. Movement into and out of yoga postures (called asanas) provides the necessary stimulation of weight-bearing activity to help keep bones strong, provides the movement to increase joint ROM, and stretches and tones muscles. The sun salute (surya namaskar), a series of 12 flexion-extension yoga postures linked together as one fluid movement by the breath rhythm, is a wonderful practice to include in the warm-up and cool-down phases of exercise, providing both physiological and mind-body benefits.

Yoga also helps develop an appreciation for the experience of the basic resting state, a mindfulness of how it feels to be relaxed physically and mentally during the activity. In this form, exercise becomes an inner experience: that is, quiet and settled on the inside, dynamic and lively on the outside. The yoga philosophy encourages an appreciation of body sensations, slow stretching, and maintenance of proper posture, all of which help to prevent injury and promote health. There is a growing body of evidence to support the use of yoga to increase ROM, reduce pain, improve posture, function, mental health, and sleep patterns, reduce disability, and improve quality of life in select populations (Alfonso et al., 2012; Bussing et al., 2012; Ebnezar et al., 2012; Holtzman & Beggs, 2013; Visceglia & Lewis, 2011).

## Flexibility

Flexibility is a basic component of physical fitness. Warm-up and cool-down periods provide the opportunity to work on stretching muscles and increasing joint ROM. A safe stretch is one that is gentle and relaxing; a little discomfort may be felt as the muscle stretches, but the discomfort should never reach the point of pain. Stretching mindfully, as in yoga, will ensure a safe stretch. Holding the position for 10 to 20 seconds and repeating the stretch three to five times will encourage optimal flexibility (ACSM, 2013).

## Resistance Training

Studies suggest that people who maintain or increase their flexibility and strength are better able to perform daily activities and avoid injury and disability (Pate et al., 1995). Resistance training increases muscle strength and endurance, increases muscle mass, increases metabolic efficiency, maintains or increases bone density, prevents limitations in performance of everyday tasks, decreases the effort required to perform these tasks, and decreases the potential for injury during physical activity.

On average, after their early 20s people lose approximately half a pound of muscle every year through lack of use. This reduction in muscle mass is largely responsible for a decrease in resting metabolic rate, which may translate into weight gain. Resistance training is recommended for the general population because it has a positive effect on many of the degenerative problems associated with the aging process.

Every individual should try to perform activities throughout the day that stimulate muscle strength and endurance. Activities that involve lifting, carrying, or performing repetitive movement against a resistance (vacuuming, raking, shoveling, or baking bread) help preserve lean body mass. If these types of activities are not performed on a regular basis, then the guidelines for resistance training provided in Box 12-4 are suggested. These guidelines are not meant to represent workouts performed by bodybuilders and competitive weight lifters; they are not meant to result in significant muscular hypertrophy. The purpose of weight training from a health perspective is to develop healthy muscles that provide the strength to do daily activities without risk of injury and to stimulate bone health.

The figures in Box 12-4 demonstrate several suggested resistance exercises for upper body strengthening. Resistance training for all major muscle groups is appropriate, but individuals often choose to concentrate on the upper body because these muscles tend to be neglected in daily activity and other exercise regimens. The ACSM (2013) recommends the incorporation of bilateral and unilateral, and single-joint and multijoint exercises, including total body exercises. Although many people believe that they need to do three sets of each exercise, excellent results can be attained by doing one set (Hass et al., 2000). A recent meta-analysis of the effect of single versus multiple sets on muscle hypertrophy showed multiple sets yielded a 40% greater increase in muscle hypertrophy (Krieger, 2010). The ACSM recommends three to five sets of 8 to 12 repetitions (ACSM, 2013). The weight that is lifted should result in near muscle fatigue at the end of each set (this differs substantially depending on the muscle being trained, the amount of resistance, and the fitness level of the athlete) and should be performed without strain and while maintaining proper form. Once 12 to 15 repetitions can be completed without fatigue, the resistance can be increased (by 5% or less), or the same weight can be used to do an additional set to fatigue. The movements should be performed slowly, preferably coordinated with the breath. Rest intervals differ substantially in the literature; however, a review suggested that 3 to 5 minutes allows hypertrophy and power development and 1 to 3 minutes allows endurance gains (de Salles et al., 2009). The ACSM suggests 1 to 3 minutes of rest between sets to develop endurance and 3 to 5 minutes to develop strength and power. Slow, controlled movements result in greater benefits, lower risk of injury, and more appreciation of how the body feels as its muscles are challenged. The recommended frequency depends on the individual and should be two to three times per week for novice levels, three to four times per week for intermediate levels, and four to five times per week for advanced levels (ACSM, 2013). The exercise variables that constitute the exercise prescription must always be chosen to meet the specific needs and limitations of each individual.

## EXERCISE THE SPIRIT: RELAXATION RESPONSE

Exercise should not be considered merely a physical regimen with objective outcomes (calories burned and repetitions completed). Exercise is also a process of challenging the body and the mind to gain a sense of well-being and a feeling of accomplishment, an opportunity to learn about who we really are.

Most people understand the physical benefits of exercise, and some people enjoy the challenge of being physically active, but few realize the learning potential inherent in physical activity. Success in embracing a physically active lifestyle may involve a change in focus from the mechanics of exercise to an appreciation for how it feels and what it means to move. Physical activity can be time spent in meditation that fuels both the body and the spirit.

The **relaxation response** (RR) is an inborn set of physiological changes that offset those of the fight-or-flight (stress) response. When elicited, the RR results in a "letting go" of physical, emotional, and mental tension. It is a physiological response inborn in everyone and, although it can sometimes occur without the individual being aware of it, people generally need to develop techniques that help them let go on a more regular basis. Some techniques that are used commonly to elicit the RR include diaphragmatic breathing, meditation, imagery, mindfulness, yoga stretching, and repetitive exercise.

The RR can be combined with exercise to facilitate the release of tension and improve self-awareness and the feeling of well-being. However, a shift in attitude about exercise is also involved, with the focus becoming the process and awareness of movement. Successful elicitation of the RR involves two basic components: a repetitive focus (the breath, a mantra, and the cadence or rhythm of physical activity) and a nonjudgmental attitude (about everyday thoughts and the quality of performance) (Benson & Stuart, 1992). Berger and Owen (1988) have developed exercise characteristics that facilitate stress reduction and support an exercise environment that allows the successful elicitation of the RR. Activities must:

- Be pleasant and enjoyable.
- Be noncompetitive (competition implies judgment about the self and others).
- Be predictable (elicitation of the RR involves a shift in awareness from the external to the internal environment that will happen only with a sense of safety and reliability).
- Be repetitive and rhythmical (the cadence of activity provides a focus for awareness).
- Facilitate abdominal breathing (watching the breath serves to anchor thoughts in the moment; in combination with cadence, it provides a focused awareness).
- Continue for 20 to 30 minutes at a comfortable intensity on most days of the week (continuity restores a sense of serenity).

All forms of exercise can be used to gain this experience. As discussed, yoga involves mindful stretching with a breathing focus, providing an environment for successful elicitation of the RR. **Tai chi** is another exercise practice with roots in Eastern philosophy. Known as moving meditation, tai chi combines movement with focused awareness, involving a physical and cognitive focus for moving in choreographed forms that become a meditation.

The quality of body awareness can also be brought into a more traditional exercise practice. Aerobic exercise lends itself well to the elicitation of the RR, because it has rhythmical and repetitive form and because it facilitates abdominal breathing. The practitioner can focus on the breath rhythm, the step cadence of walking or jogging, the pedaling cadence of bicycling, or the stroke cadence of swimming. Mantras can be used to create a positive mindset and to focus the mind in the present moment as the experience unfolds. Resistance training takes on new meaning when coordinated with the breath. Focusing on the muscles and how it feels to move through the ROM enhances the knowledge of what feels good and what does not, providing feedback on accepting physical challenge.

Exercise focus can and should vary on a daily basis depending on need, mood, and intent. Some days it feels right to focus on the more physical aspects of the activity, appreciating the challenge of working harder or longer. Other exercise sessions may be more contemplative, letting creativity run, working through the tension of a lingering stressor, quieting the mind for relaxation, listening to music, or appreciating nature. Focusing on the process rather than the outcomes brings meaning and purpose to the activity and helps achieve something more valuable than mere physical outcomes.

When exercise integrates mind and body, it stops being something that has to be done and instead becomes something desired. Being mindful during physical activity and exercising in the moment increase awareness. With awareness comes choices in the possibilities of self-care. Exercise for fitness of the spirit, walk for the soul, and just let the body do the work. There is a growing body of evidence to support the use of tai chi to improve balance in confidence, decrease pain, improve cognitive function, mental health, and functional mobility, decrease disability, increase self-efficacy and quality of life, and reduce fall risk in select populations (Hall et al., 2011; Huang et al., 2011; Leung et al., 2011; Rand et al., 2011; Wayne et al., 2014).

## MONITORING THE INNER AND THE OUTER ENVIRONMENT

The primary purpose of exercise is to enhance health. However, because exercise involves stress to the body, the potential to cause or exacerbate health problems is inherent. When a person is not feeling well, the exercise effort should be decreased or stopped until the individual is feeling better. With an infection, a cold, or influenza, the body is under stress, and overexertion will only increase that stress and possibly lengthen the healing time. The level of activity should be adjusted to accommodate how the individual feels, slowly progressing to normal workout levels until strength and energy return. This philosophy also holds true for chronic diseases such as arthritis and HIV infection. During an acute exacerbation, activity should be limited to necessary activities of daily living, but on a regular basis staying active is important, adjusting activity levels as tolerated. Exercise can be a useful tool in coping with chronic illness.

Missing an occasional workout will not affect the fitness level; choosing to stop or reduce the amount of exercise when not feeling well is the right choice. However, after missing workouts for 2 weeks, a decline in fitness is inevitable. When one starts again, resumption of the activity should be slow, gradually working back to the usual level of activity. Inactivity for 3 to 5 months results in the loss of all conditioning benefits gained, and resumption of exercise involves starting over (ACSM, 2013). Being aware of the external exercise environment is also important. Extremes of heat and cold affect performance as the body adjusts to different temperatures and wind conditions. Changing the time of day for exercise (early morning and later evening are better choices

for humid days), adjusting fluid intake, and varying the length of warm-up and cool-down periods will increase tolerance for environmental conditions and enhance exercise safety.

### Fluid News

Proper hydration before, during, and after exercise is an important component of a good fitness program. Extra fluid is needed to support physiological homeostasis during exercise, especially during hot weather. The following hydration recommendations are from the ACSM (2011). Before exercising, recommendations include drinking 16 to 20 ounces of water or sports beverage at least 4 hours before exercise and then drinking 8 to 12 ounces of water 10 to 15 minutes before exercise. According to the ACSM, a sports beverage should generally contain 4% to 8% carbohydrate, 20 to 30 meq of sodium per liter, and 2 to 5 meq of potassium per liter. During exercise, hydration recommendations include drinking 3 to 8 ounces of water every 15 to 20 minutes when exercising for less than 1 hour or drinking 3 to 8 ounces of a sports beverage every 15 to 20 minutes when exercising for more than 1 hour. The ACSM also recommends not drinking more than 1 quart per hour during exercise. After exercise, the ACSM recommends drinking 20 to 24 ounces of water or sports beverage for every 1 pound lost. As noted earlier, under certain circumstances the ACSM recommends consuming beverages containing electrolytes and carbohydrates during exercise over water alone. For exercise routines lasting longer than 1 hour, a sports beverage with carbohydrates and electrolytes enhances performance and is recommended (Sawka et al., 2007). This type of liquid provides muscles with energy and helps delay fatigue while meeting fluid needs. Sports beverages containing a 4% to 8% carbohydrate concentration are designed to replace carbohydrates at the proper rate during exercise. They also contain sodium, which promotes fluid retention, enhances flavor, and protects against hyponatremia, which can occur with lengthy exercise sessions. Most sports drinks provide 14 to 20 g of carbohydrate per 8-ounce serving. The recommended intake is 5 to 12 ounces every 15 to 20 minutes. Which sports drink is the best? Several brands should be tried to determine personal preference in taste, but one should be chosen that contains approximately 50 to 80 calories per 8-ounce serving; any more and the carbohydrate concentration will inhibit fluid absorption. Table 12-1 provides choices for sports drinks that both hydrate and energize individuals.

## SPECIAL CONSIDERATIONS

Most adults do not need to consult a physician before starting a moderate-intensity physical activity program. However, men older than 40 years and women older than 50 years who plan a vigorous program (intensity more than 60% of maximum heart rate or $\dot{V}O_{2max}$) or who have either chronic disease or risk factors for chronic disease should consult an appropriate health care provider before starting exercise (Table 12-2 and Box 12-8).

People with CHD or diabetes have special exercise needs. Earlier in this chapter the ways in which exercise and physical activity positively affect primary and secondary prevention in both disease processes were discussed. Limitations in the ability to exercise are related to the severity of the disease and the signs

## TABLE 12-1　Sports Drinks That Hydrate and Energize Individuals

| Brand | Calories | Carbohydrate (g) |
|---|---|---|
| All Sport (20-oz size) | 150 | 40 |
| Cytomax | 95–100 | 20 |
| Endura | 120 | 29 |
| Gatorade | 104 | 27 |
| Hydra Fuel | 100 | 17 |
| Isostar | 148 | 35 |
| MET-Rx ORS | 148 | 38 |
| Perform | 100 | 25 |
| Powerade | 109 | 27 |
| Power Surge | 200 | 48 |
| Race Day | 100 | 28 |
| Vitamin Water | 100 | 26 |
| SoBe | 80 | 20 |
| Propel | 20 | 6 |

All values are for 16 oz unless noted otherwise.

## BOX 12-8　Symptoms and Signs Suggestive of Cardiopulmonary Disease

- Pain, discomfort (or other anginal equivalent) in the chest, neck, jaw, arm, or other areas that may be ischemic in nature
- Shortness of breath at rest or with mild exertion
- Dizziness or syncope
- Orthopnea or paroxysmal nocturnal dyspnea
- Ankle edema
- Palpitations or tachycardia
- Intermittent claudication
- Known heart murmur
- Unusual fatigue or shortness of breath with usual activities

These symptoms must be interpreted in the clinical context in which they appear because they are not all specific to cardiopulmonary or metabolic disease.

## TABLE 12-2　American College of Sports Medicine Recommendation for Medical Examination and Exercise Testing Before Beginning an Exercise Program

| | APPARENTLY HEALTHY | | | INCREASED RISK | |
| | Younger[a] | Older | No Symptoms | Symptoms | Known Disease[b] |
|---|---|---|---|---|---|
| Moderate exercise[c] | No | No | No | Yes | Yes |
| Vigorous exercise[d] | No | Yes | Yes | Yes | Yes |

[a]Younger implies age 40 years or younger for men, and 50 years or younger for women.
[b]Individuals with known cardiac, pulmonary, or metabolic disease.
[c]Moderate exercise is defined by an intensity of 40% to 60% of $\dot{V}O_{2max}$, or if the intensity is uncertain, an effort well within the individual's current capacity and that can be comfortably sustained for a prolonged period (60 minutes), slow progression, and generally noncompetitive.
[d]Vigorous exercise is defined by an intensity of more than 60% of $\dot{V}O_{2max}$, or if the intensity is uncertain, exercise intense enough to represent a substantial cardiorespiratory challenge or result in fatigue within 20 minutes.
From American College of Sports Medicine. (2014). *Guidelines for exercise testing and prescription* (9th ed.). Philadelphia: Lippincott Williams & Wilkins.

and symptoms of intolerance. For people with CHD and diabetes mellitus, safety with starting a new exercise program requires supervision and guidance from knowledgeable health care providers. Before starting the program, these individuals should have a medical evaluation, including an exercise tolerance test, to determine functional capacity and the severity of disease.

### Coronary Heart Disease

Exercise plays a strong role in rehabilitation after a cardiac event such as myocardial infarction (MI), coronary artery bypass surgery, percutaneous transluminal coronary angioplasty or stent placement, and angina. Increased physical activity appears to benefit individuals from all these groups. The benefits include the following (Cornelissen et al., 2011; Heran et al., 2011; Lavie & Milani, 2011; Menezes et al., 2012; Milani et al., 2011; Oerkild et al., 2011):

- Reduction in blood pressure (systolic and diastolic)
- Reduction in total and cardiovascular mortality
- Reduction in hospital admissions
- Reduction of symptoms
- Reduction in obesity
- Increase in exercise tolerance and functional capacity
- Increase in the confidence and ability to carry out usual activities of daily living
- Improvement in psychological well-being and quality of life

Despite the numerous benefits noted previously, cardiac rehabilitation and exercise training is underused by older adults (Menezes et al., 2012).

Generally, people with CHD demonstrate a reduction in $\dot{V}O_{2max}$ and the ability to do submaximal levels of work. With exercise training, the increase in $\dot{V}O_{2max}$ in persons with CHD averages approximately 20% after 3 months. This improvement in conditioning is the result of both central (cardiac) and peripheral (muscular) changes (ACSM, 2009b). Some of the most significant increases in exercise tolerance have been noted in individuals with angina. With a decrease in submaximal HR or a decrease in systolic blood pressure resulting from conditioning, myocardial oxygen demand is decreased and individuals are able to do a greater amount of work before reaching the anginal threshold. This boost is reflected in an observed increase in the heart rate–pressure product (RPP: HR × SBP) at the anginal threshold (ACSM/AHA, 2007). An increase in functional capacity allows progression of exercise tolerance and progression with daily activities and leisure or vocational activities.

Appropriately prescribed and conducted exercise training programs increase exercise tolerance and physical fitness in individuals with CHD. Moderate and vigorous regimens are of value, but care must be taken to determine safe exercise parameters for each individual. The parameters of the exercise prescriptions are the same as those for the general population, including frequency, intensity, duration, and mode of exercise.

Aerobic exercise increases cardiorespiratory fitness and functional capacity. Any of the aforementioned aerobic exercises are acceptable for this population, depending on the level of fitness and musculoskeletal limitations. Traditionally, resistance training was not commonly recommended for individuals with CHD. The belief was that lifting weights resulted in a disproportionate rise in blood pressure, increased the myocardial oxygen demand, and increased the risk of angina and MI. However, data from several studies indicate that moderate, supervised weight training is feasible, tolerable, and beneficial for individuals with hypertension and CHD. Strength training can keep the heart healthy by helping to control body weight, reduce cholesterol levels, and regulate blood glucose levels. Guidelines for determination of appropriate individual training include an aerobic capacity of at least four to five metabolic equivalents, an ejection fraction of greater than 30%, and the absence of severe, symptomatic aortic stenosis. However, clinical experience demonstrates that people with severer disease can use small hand weights to increase muscle tone without risk of cardiovascular compromise.

The exercise intensity for persons who have had a cardiac event but who have not had a symptom-limited exercise tolerance test should be kept at a low level based on an elevated heart rate of 20 to 30 beats per minute above the resting heart rate and an RPE of less than 12. After an exercise tolerance test has been performed, intensity should then be prescribed on the basis of 50% to 85% of maximum heart rate and an RPE of 11 to 14, or below the ischemic, anginal, or arrhythmic threshold. The duration and frequency recommendations are similar to those for the general population. People who are the most deconditioned may need to exercise at lower intensities, for short durations, and more frequently throughout the day. Generally, a reasonable goal is three to five times per week for 20 to 40 minutes, plus 5 to 10 minutes for each warm-up and cool-down period (ACSM/AHA, 2007).

## Diabetes

Exercise has long been regarded as part of the triad in the management of diabetes in conjunction with diet and medication (insulin or oral medication). In the early 1900s it was determined that exercise lowers the blood glucose concentration of people with diabetes. After the introduction of insulin, studies revealed that exercise can potentiate the hypoglycemic effect of injected insulin. More recently, findings suggest that in individuals who have poor control (i.e., excessive blood glucose levels), exercise may induce a further increase in blood glucose levels, resulting in ketosis. On average, people with diabetes have a lower maximum heart rate, achieve a lower cardiac output at maximal exercise, and have a higher blood pressure during exercise, resulting in lower maximal oxygen consumption. However, these individuals can increase their exercise capacity with training and can experience the benefits related to overall fitness and cardiorespiratory training similar to the benefits gained by people without diabetes.

Apparently, both benefits and risks from exercise exist for people with diabetes. The overall goals regarding physical activity should be to teach individuals to incorporate activity into their daily life, pursue an exercise program if they wish, and develop strategies to avoid the complications of exercise.

As discussed, in addition to diet and weight loss, regular physical activity is an important modality in the prevention and treatment of type 2 diabetes. Regular physical activity can prevent or delay type 2 diabetes, with up to a 58% risk reduction in high-risk individuals when combined with modest weight loss, as well as positively affecting lipid levels, blood pressure, cardiovascular events, mortality, and quality of life (Colberg et al., 2010). Furthermore, a recent meta-analysis found that lifestyle modifications, such as diet, exercise, and education significantly reduced risk factors (i.e., lower cholesterol, high blood pressure, and diabetes) associated with the development of CHD in individuals with type 2 diabetes (Chen et al., 2015).

People with type 2 diabetes should monitor their blood glucose levels and determine their responses to exercise. However, individuals with type 2 diabetes can usually follow the same exercise prescription parameters as those of the general population. Although the same exercise benefits can be achieved by people with type 1 diabetes, the inherent behavior and function of endogenous insulin makes exercising a more difficult proposition for these individuals. The major functions of insulin are to promote glucose uptake into the cells and to control metabolic homeostasis during exercise, working in synergy with the counterregulatory hormones. With exercise, insulin secretion decreases slightly and the concentrations of counterregulatory hormones increase. This increase stimulates hepatic glucose production, which balances the increased use of glucose by the working muscles, maintaining normoglycemia. However, with injected insulin the plasma insulin concentration does not decrease with exercise, hepatic glucose is not produced as quickly as it is used, and a decrease in blood glucose concentration results. In contrast, people who have poorly controlled diabetes with decreased plasma insulin concentrations already have elevated blood glucose levels because there is insufficient insulin to assist glucose transport into cells. During exercise the liver is stimulated to produce more glucose, which causes a further elevation in blood glucose levels, worsening the hyperglycemic condition. Ketosis may also result from increased mobilization and incomplete combustion of free fatty acids in muscle cells and accelerated ketone body formation in the liver (Federici & Benedetti, 2006).

Although each person with diabetes should be evaluated and given individual exercise recommendations, the goals of an exercise program are universal:

- Maintain or increase cardiovascular fitness to prevent or minimize long-term cardiovascular complications.

- Increase flexibility that is impaired as muscle collagen becomes glycosylated.
- Increase muscle strength, which may deteriorate as a result of neuropathy.
- Allow people with type 1 diabetes to safely participate in and enjoy physical activities or sports.
- Assist with weight control for people with type 2 diabetes.
- Allow people with diabetes to experience and gain the same benefits and enjoyment from regular exercise as do people without diabetes.

Box 12-9: Innovative Practice presents a list of recommendations and precautions for people with diabetes who are interested in regular physical activity and exercise. Table 12-3 presents recommended food adjustments when exercising. Table 12-4 presents the peak effects of different medications for diabetes. Box 12-10: Genomics presents findings from a meta-analysis that examines the association between genetics and the odds/risk of type 2 diabetes.

## BUILDING A RHYTHM OF PHYSICAL ACTIVITY

Participation in regular physical activity increased gradually from the 1960s to the 1980s but seems to have plateaued in recent years. The progress made toward the *Healthy People 2020* physical

---

### BOX 12-9  INNOVATIVE PRACTICE

**Recommendations and Precautions for People With Diabetes Who Are Interested in Regular Physical Activity and Exercise**

- Notify primary care physician, ophthalmologist, and podiatrist of intent to exercise.
- Monitor blood glucose level before and 20 to 30 minutes after exercise to determine the response to exercise.
- Be sure blood glucose level is less than 300 mg/dL in those with type 1 diabetes or less than 400 mg/dL in those with type 2 diabetes, and urine test results are negative for ketones (if blood glucose level is greater than 240 mg/dL). If blood glucose level is consistently equal to or greater than 250 mg/dL, improved control must be established before continuing exercise.
- If possible, exercise approximately 1 hour after meals, when blood glucose level is highest. This plan helps with weight loss, because extra food will not have to be eaten to ward off hypoglycemia. When exercising before meals, a snack may be necessary. (See Table 12-3 for suggestions on food adjustments to maintain blood glucose balance with exercise.)
- Know the action and peak times of insulin dosage and avoid exercising at the peak. (Table 12-4 shows the peak action of insulin preparations.)
- Consider adjusting oral medication or insulin dosage to prevent low blood glucose level during exercise. The adjustment will depend on the intensity of the exercise, the duration of the exercise session, and the type of insulin that is used during exercise.
- Be alert to the hypoglycemic lag effect that may occur 12 to 24 hours after vigorous exercise; an extra snack after exercise will help.

- Avoid injecting insulin into a muscle area that will be active during exercise; the pumping action of the muscle may accelerate absorption of the insulin and cause a rapid decrease of blood glucose level.
- Use proper footwear and frequently inspect the feet.
- Avoid high-impact activity when prone to neuropathy in the legs or feet or when there is a history of neuropathy.
- Keep systolic blood pressure below 180 to 200 mmHg in the presence of eye or kidney disease.
- Exercising every day is best, but should be done at least three to four times per week. Start with 10 to 20 minutes and gradually increase to 30 to 40 minutes at 50% to 75% of maximum heart rate. Continuous aerobic activity helps maintain good blood glucose level control better than intermittent activities. Do not forget the 5-minute to 10-minute warm-up and cool-down periods.
- Avoid high-intensity anaerobic exercise, but low- to moderate-intensity resistance training is acceptable.
- Carry a concentrated form of carbohydrate (sugar packets, glucose tablets, or hard candy) when exercising.
- Wear some form of diabetes identification.
- People with type 2 diabetes need to test blood glucose levels with exercise and potentially adjust oral medications. Consider decreasing medication if blood glucose level is less than 80 mg/dL after exercise. For weight loss, plan the best time to exercise so that snacks can be avoided.

---

### TABLE 12-3  Food Adjustments

| Duration and Intensity | Blood Glucose (mg/dL) | Suggested Food Adjustment |
|---|---|---|
| <30 min of moderate activity. Examples: walking 1 mile or bicycling for <30 min | <100 | 1 fruit + 1 bread + 1 meat |
| | 100–180 | 1 bread or 1 fruit |
| | >180 | May not need snack |
| 30–60 min of moderate activity. Examples: tennis, swimming, jogging, bicycling, yard work, or housework | <100 | 1 fruit + 1 bread + 1 meat |
| | 100–180 | 1 bread or 1 meat |
| | >180–240 | 1 bread or 1 fruit |
| | >240 | May not need snack |
| 60 min of moderate- to high-intensity activity. Examples: competitive sports, strenuous bicycling, long-distance running, heavy shoveling | — | |

If you are doing strenuous activity or playing sports, consult a physician or exercise physiologist for advice on blood glucose level management. Insulin adjustment may be required in addition to food adjustments (see Table 12-4). Blood glucose level should be tested hourly: 1 bread or 1 fruit per hour unless blood glucose level is 180 mg/dL or higher (snack may not be needed for that hour).
Modified from Beaser, R. S., & Campbell, A. (2005). *The Joslin guide to diabetes* (2nd ed.). New York: Simon & Schuster.

## TABLE 12-4  Peak Action of Insulin Preparations

| Rapid Acting | Intermediate Acting | Long Acting |
|---|---|---|
| Regular insulin peak action 2–4 h | Isophane insulin peak action 6–12 h | Glargine peak action 5–24 h |
| Aspart peak action 0.6–0.8 h | Insulin zinc peak action 8–12 h | Extended insulin zinc action 18–24 h |
| Lispro peak action 0.5–1.5 h | | |
| Glulisine peak action 0.5–1.5 h | | |

From Ciccone, C. D. (2014). *Pharmacology in rehabilitation* (4th ed.). Philadelphia: F.A. Davis.

### BOX 12-10  GENOMICS

Type 2 diabetes accounts for most diabetes cases, and it is affected by both genetic and environmental factors. A recent meta-analysis examined the effect of the hemochromatosis gene (HFE) on the odds/risk of type 2 diabetes. Findings from 23 studies were included, of which 23 examined the C282Y variant and 18 examined the H63D variant. The meta-analytic data included 5528 individuals with type 2 diabetes and 6920 controls from a variety of countries, races, and ethnicities. The results from the meta-analysis showed that the H63D variant significantly increased the odds of having type 2 diabetes (OR 1.20, 95% confidence interval [CI] 1.03–1.41) in a comparison of individuals carrying the D allele with those carrying the H allele. In contrast, the C282Y variant was not significantly associated with diabetes risk (OR 0.96, 95% CI 0.82–1.12). In conclusion the authors found that the H63D variant was associated with a moderate increase in the odds/risk of type 2 diabetes.

From Chen, L., Pei, J. H., Kuang, J., Chen, H. M., Chen, Z., Li, Z. W., et al. (2015). Effect of lifestyle intervention in patients with type 2 diabetes: A meta-analysis. *Metabolism: Clinical and Experimental,* 64(2), 338–347.

activity goals indicates that most of the population has not embraced a physically active lifestyle (USDHHS, 2010). Although the benefits of physical activity are common to all people, patterns of physical activity differ among population subgroups defined by sex, age, racial background, income, and body fat. The following generalities are true:

- Men are more active than women.
- Physical activity declines with age.
- Ethnic minorities are less active than white Americans.
- Higher education and income are associated with more leisure-time activity.
- People who are obese are usually less active than their leaner counterparts.

## Adherence and Compliance

Physiological, behavioral, and psychological variables all influence the decision to adhere to diabetes treatment, including physical activity and medications. Each person is unique, and success with exercise over the long term comes from recognition of personal motivation or core desire and support from the social environment. Core desire defines the purpose behind putting the effort into developing and maintaining an active lifestyle; it

is what motivates the individual to exercise. People should be encouraged to spend some quiet time meditating on why being adherent is important to them.

Finding meaning and purpose in an active lifestyle can enhance behavior. Biopsychosocial and spiritual variables need to be considered in promoting physical activity. An individual's biopsychosocial factors and spiritual beliefs affect the behavioral and attitudinal factors that influence the motivation and ability to adhere to an active lifestyle. Generally, however, physical activity is more likely to be initiated and maintained if the individual (Pentecost & Taket, 2011):

- Perceives a net benefit
- Chooses an enjoyable activity
- Feels competent doing the activity
- Feels confident in overcoming barriers that may interfere with the activity
- Feels safe doing the activity
- Can access the activity easily on a regular basis
- Perceives no significant negative financial or social cost
- Experiences minimal musculoskeletal discomfort
- Is able to address competing time demands
- Is readily able to fit the activity into the daily schedule
- Balances the use of labor-saving devices with activities that involve physical exertion

In addition, measures to increase satisfaction and increase adherence to medication use have been explored and include (García-Pérez et al., 2013):

- Complexity of dosing regimens: reducing the complexity of therapy by fixed-dose combination pills and less frequent dosing regimens
- Safety and tolerability: using medications that are associated with fewer adverse events (e.g., hypoglycemia or weight gain)
- Perceptions of medication: educational initiatives
- Care recipient-provider interaction: improved care recipient–health care provider communication
- Economic considerations: social support to help reduce costs

Educating the public about physical activity helps to provide guidelines for safe and effective exercise, to reinforce potential benefits, and to alleviate misperceptions that may interfere with the decision to change behavior. However, knowledge of exercise and the intent to exercise do not correlate well with long-term compliance. Confidence in the ability to be physically active—and the confidence that overcoming barriers produces positive benefits that are related to personal goals (self-efficacy)—is strongly related to participation and compliance (Figure 12-5). Exercise self-efficacy is increased when people perform exercise successfully, receive positive feedback about success, view exercise role models, and learn more about the relationships among exercise, health, and body awareness (see the case study and care plan at the end of this chapter).

### Creating a Climate That Supports Exercise

Clearly exercise and fitness need to be social norms. A climate that supports and encourages physical activity should be fostered. Other people and organizations in the individual's social environment can influence the adoption and maintenance of physical activity.

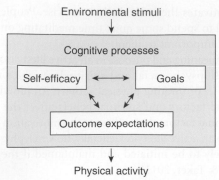

**FIGURE 12-5** Three interacting cognitive processes of Bandura's social-cognitive theory. (Modified from Dzewaltowski, D. A. [1995]. Physical activity determinants: A social-cognitive approach. *Medicine and Science in Sports and Exercise, 26,* 1395–1399.)

## Health Care Professionals

People are more likely to increase their physical activity if counseled to do so by clinicians. Clinicians inquire about exercise habits, communicate the benefits of increased activity, assist the person in initiating activity, and provide adequate follow-up. Challenging perceived individual barriers to exercise and offering alternative viewpoints can help create new exercise paradigms (Lascar et al., 2014; Leone & Ward, 2013; Veldhuijzen van Zanten et al., 2015). Teixeira and colleagues (2012) published an informative systematic review that summarizes the evidence for self-determination theory, which can be used to improve our understanding of exercise motivation and the importance of autonomous regulations in promoting physical activity. Clinicians also serve as role models by demonstrating enthusiasm for and the health benefits of being physically active.

Recognizing the stages of behavioral change helps in meeting people at their stage of readiness to change behavior. Providing information on physical activity designed for specific stages of readiness enables people to move from stages of contemplation and preparation into action. An individual in precontemplation is not ready to actively change behavior. This person may respond better to support and information about the benefits of changing behavior rather than being placed in an action environment. The decision to change may come gradually. After an individual has made the commitment to change, the action phase lasts approximately 6 months. Continued follow-up throughout the action phase into maintenance is valuable in helping the individual stay committed until the termination phase is reached and the behavior is secure.

## Family and Friends

Social support can be a valuable resource for behavioral change. Significant others or friends can serve as buddies, providing a source of companionship and motivation. These people can offer to share daily responsibilities to make time for exercise (e.g., provide child care). Parents can support their children's activity by having family outings and providing transportation, praise, and encouragement. Joining a fitness club or an exercise group at work provides various forms of stimulation and socialization, which increases the potential for new friendships grounded in an appreciation of the rewards of exercise.

## Schools

Schools are one of the most important resources for increasing physical activity. Strategies must be developed to facilitate increased activity in children because it is clear that children are becoming less active and more obese. Schools are providing less opportunity and poorer quality time for physical activity during school hours. All schools should provide opportunities for physical activity that:

- Are appropriate and enjoyable for children of all skill levels and are not limited to competitive sports or physical education classes
- Appeal to girls and boys and to children from diverse backgrounds
- Are offered daily
- Can serve as a foundation for activities throughout life

Schools can also serve as a resource for the community. Expanding operating hours at either end of the school day creates a safe, indoor environment for hall walking.

## Communities

Participation in regular physical activity at the community level depends in large part on the availability and proximity of facilities and safe environments. Community government agencies, local health agencies, schools, and places of worship have the potential to provide activity resources to the population at large. Churches seem to be particularly successful in reaching ethnic minorities and older adults. Making neighborhoods safe for outdoor activities can have a major effect on improving activity habits, especially among low socioeconomic and disadvantaged populations, who report lower levels of daily physical activity.

Recognizing that many of the previous recommendations require a financial commitment, government agencies must respond to reports by health agencies and establish public policies that support the importance of physical activity for the general population. Individuals should make a personal commitment to be physically active, but that commitment needs to be supported by a social and political environment that values this type of lifestyle choice.

## SUMMARY

It is important that people incorporate increased activity into their lifestyles on a long-term basis; exercise in the short term is of little overall benefit. Helping individuals gain the knowledge (benefits of exercise and recommended parameters for exercise), skills (self-monitoring), and attitude (core desire) increases compliance. People need to be motivated enough to start the activity, enjoy the activity enough to want to continue, and appreciate the value enough to start again if they lapse. Lapses should be anticipated to avoid the unrealistic sense of total success or total failure. Behavioral change is cyclical rather than linear; success often comes with repeated movement through stages of change, and it helps to explore the reasons for the lapse and to view the lapse as a learning experience rather than a failure. The

## CASE STUDY

### Exercise Self-Efficacy: Sharon G.

Sharon G. is a 53-year-old account executive who is 2 years after menopause, has insomnia, and has chronic low back pain and knee pain.

*History:* Motor vehicle accident (2012), resulting in bone graft to left leg (her left leg is shorter than her right leg). As part of rehabilitation, Sharon started jogging, which was more comfortable than walking with chronic right-sided sacroiliac joint pain. She started running marathons in 2014 and continued until 2015. In 2015 she began to add more variety to exercise and decreased her running, but she still identified herself as being an athlete.

In 2016 Sharon had a fall that resulted in chronic low back pain, and she was unable to continue aerobic exercise. She began to experience depression and insomnia; exercise had been a significant coping mechanism in the past, and now her whole sense of well-being was being affected. As Sharon attempted to rebuild her exercise practice, she would alternate between overexercising, exacerbating symptoms, and then having to stop and recuperate, reinforcing her negative self-image. Magnetic resonance imaging studies showed mild arthritis in her knees.

#### Reflective Questions

- What are some of her barriers to exercise?
- How will a regular practice of mindfulness and the relaxation response benefit Sharon's exercise practice?
- How would she benefit from cross-training?
- What exercise is she doing that is beneficial for helping to prevent osteoporosis?

## CARE PLAN

### Exercise Self-Efficacy: Sharon G.

*NURSING DIAGNOSIS: Altered sleep pattern related to low back pain, depression, and recent weight gain

#### Medications

- Serax (oxazepam) 30 mg, four to six times a week
- Ginkgo biloba

#### Defining Characteristics

- Insomnia
- Chronic low back and knee pain
- Depression
- Upset about recent weight gain of 10 lb (61.5 inches, 118 lb); sees her ideal body weight as 108 lb

#### Expected Outcomes

- Walking, treadmill, bicycling, and low-impact aerobics (30 minutes, three to four times per week)
- Weights three to four times per week
- Stretching three to four times per week
- Daily relaxation response
- Build mindfulness into exercise practice

#### Interventions

- Treadmill and walking daily for 30 minutes
- Weights two to three times per week
- Yoga and stretching daily

*NANDA Nursing Diagnoses—Herdman, T. H. & Kamitsuru, S. (Eds.). Nursing Diagnoses–Definitions and Classification 2015–2017. Copyright © 2014, 1994–2014 NANDA International. Used by arrangement with John Wiley & Sons Limited. In order to make safe and effective judgments using the NANDA-I nursing diagnoses it is essential that nurses refer to the definitions and defining characteristics of the diagnoses listed in this work.

goal is to prevent a relapse that results in a more permanent noncompliance.

The benefits and enjoyment derived from a physically active lifestyle have a significant effect on the quality of life. However, this lifestyle is successful only when it is supported by a degree of self-awareness and self-care. People must realize that they are worth the effort of doing something good for themselves, that they have the right to be happy and healthy, and that exercise can help them achieve that end. By adding a mind-body component to physical activity and not regarding it solely as a physical regimen, people can experience true health rather than mere fitness. A great deal of body exercise is not required; 30 minutes a day can make a significant difference. Success comes with building a rhythm of physical activity into everyday life. The following are some suggestions for a lifestyle approach to exercise:

- Something is better than nothing.
- Attempt small changes over time (gradualism).
- Emphasize moderate intensity.
- Make activity an integral part of life.
- Focus on the process rather than the outcome.

- Clinicians can provide a knowledgeable, supportive, and enthusiastic environment to encourage the change to a healthier, more active way of life.

## EVOLVE CHAPTER FEATURES

http://evolve.elsevier.com/Edelman/
- Study Questions

## REFERENCES

Adams, T. B., Moore, M. T., & Dye, J. (2007). The relationship between physical activity and mental health in a national sample of college females. *Women and Health*, *45*(1), 69–85.

Ahmed, H. M., et al. (2012). Effects of physical activity on cardiovascular disease. *American Journal of Cardiology*, *109*, 288–295.

Alfonso, R. F., et al. (2012). Yoga decreases insomnia in postmenopausal women: A randomized clinical trial. *Menopause*, *19*(2), 186–193.

Alghadir, A. H., Gabr, S. A., & Al-Eisa, E. (2015). Physical activity and lifestyle effects on bone mineral density among young adults:

Sociodemographic and biochemical analysis. *Journal of Physical Therapy Science, 27*(7), 2261–2270.

Almstedt, H. C., et al. (2011). Changes in bone mineral density in response to 24 weeks of resistance training in college-age men and women. *Journal of Strength and Conditioning Research, 25*(4), 1098–1103.

Alperson, S. Y., & Berger, V. W. (2011). Opposing systematic reviews: The effects of two quality rating instruments on evidence regarding t'ai chi and bone mineral density in postmenopausal women. *Journal of Alternative and Complementary Medicine, 17,* 389–395.

American Academy of Child and Adolescent Psychiatry. (2004). Obesity in children and teens, no. 79. http://www.aacap.org/aacap/Publications/Home.aspx.

American College of Sports Medicine (ACSM). (2009a). American College of Sports Medicine position stand. Progression models in resistance training for healthy adults. *Medicine & Science in Sports & Exercise, 41,* 687–708.

American College of Sports Medicine (ACSM). (2009b). *ACSM's exercise management for persons with chronic diseases and disabilities* (3rd ed.). Champaign, IL: Human Kinetics.

American College of Sports Medicine (ACSM). (2011). Selecting and effectively using hydration for fitness. ACSM's Consumer Information Committee.

American College of Sports Medicine (ACSM). (2013). *ACSM's guidelines for exercise testing and prescription* (9th ed.). Philadelphia: Lippincott Williams & Wilkins.

American College of Sports Medicine, & American Heart Association (ACSM/AHA). (2007). Exercise and acute cardiovascular events: Placing the risks into perspective. *Medicine & Science in Sports & Exercise, 39*(5), 886–897.

Anderson, S. L. (2006). Physical therapy for patients with HIV/AIDS. *Cardiopulmonary Physical Therapy Journal, 17*(3), 103–109.

Arne, M., et al. (2009). Physical activity and quality of life in subjects with chronic disease: Chronic obstructive pulmonary disease compared with rheumatoid arthritis and diabetes mellitus. *Scandinavian Journal of Primary Health Care, 27*(3), 141–147.

Arnold, C. M., & Faulkner, R. A. (2010). The effect of aquatic exercise and education on lowering fall risk in older adults with hip osteoarthritis. *Journal of Aging and Physical Activity, 18,* 245–260.

Baillet, A., et al. (2010). Efficacy of cardiorespiratory aerobic exercise in rheumatoid arthritis: Meta-analysis of randomized controlled trials. *Arthritis Care & Research, 62*(7), 984–992.

Balistreri, K. S., & Hook, J. V. (2011). Trajectories of overweight among US school children: A focus on social and economic characteristics. *Maternal and Child Health Journal, 15,* 610–619.

Bardi, A. (2007). Can physical activity reduce the risk of breast cancer? *Clinical Nutrition Insight, 33,* 1–3.

Bartels, E. M., et al. (2007). Aquatic exercise for the treatment of knee and hip osteoarthritis. *The Cochrane Database of Systematic Reviews,* (4), CD005523.

Bartley, C. A., Hay, M., & Bloch, M. H. (2013). Meta-analysis: Aerobic exercise for the treatment of anxiety disorders. *Progress in Neuro-Psychopharmacology and Biological Psychiatry, 45,* 34–39.

Bauer, J. M., Kaiser, M. J., & Sieber, C. C. (2008). Sarcopenia in nursing home residents. *Journal of the American Medical Directors Association, 9*(8), 545–551.

Behringer, M., et al. (2014). Effects of weight-bearing activities on bone mineral content and density in children and adolescents: A meta-analysis. *Journal of Bone and Mineral Research: The Official*

*Journal of the American Society for Bone and Mineral Research, 29*(2), 467–478.

Belli, T., et al. (2011). Effects of 12-week overground training at ventilatory threshold velocity in type 2 diabetic women. *Diabetes Research and Clinical Practice, 93*(3), 337–343.

Bennell, K. L., & Hinman, R. S. (2011). A review of the clinical evidence for exercise in osteoarthritis of the hip and knee. *Journal of Science and Medicine in Sport, 14,* 4–9.

Benson, H., & Stuart, E. (1992). *The wellness book: The comprehensive guide to maintaining health and treating stress-related illness.* New York: Simon & Schuster.

Berger, B., & Owen, D. (1988). Stress reduction and mood enhancement in four exercise modes: Swimming, body conditioning, hatha yoga, and fencing. *Research Quarterly for Exercise and Sport, 59*(2), 148–159.

Bezalel, T., Carmeli, E., & Katz-Leurer, M. (2010). The effect of a group education programme on pain and function through knowledge acquisition and home-based exercise among patients with knee osteoarthritis: A parallel randomised single-blind clinical trial. *Physiotherapy, 96,* 137–143.

Bielemann, R. M., Martinez-Mesa, J., & Gigante, D. P. (2013). Physical activity during life course and bone mass: A systematic review of methods and findings from cohort studies with young adults. *BMC Musculoskeletal Disorders, 14,* 77.

Borer, K. T. (2005). Physical activity in the prevention and amelioration of osteoporosis in women: Interaction of mechanical, hormonal, and dietary factors. *Sports Medicine, 35*(9), 779–830.

Borg, G. A. (1973). Perceived exertion: A note on "history" and methods. *Medicine & Science in Sports & Exercise, 5*(2), 90–93.

Borg, G. A. (1982). Psychophysical bases of perceived exertion. *Medicine & Science in Sports & Exercise, 14*(5), 377–381.

Bradt, J., Goodill, S. W., & Dileo, C. (2011). Dance/movement therapy for improving psychological and physical outcomes in cancer patients. *The Cochrane Database of Systematic Reviews,* (10), CD007103.

Braith, R. W., & Stewart, K. J. (2006). Resistance exercise training: Its role in the prevention of cardiovascular disease. *Circulation, 113*(22), 2642–2650.

Brien, S. E., et al. (2007). Physical activity, cardiorespiratory fitness and body mass index as predictors of substantial weight gain and obesity. *Canadian Journal of Public Health, 98*(2), 121–124.

Busch, A. J., et al. (2007). Exercise for treating fibromyalgia syndrome. *The Cochrane Database of Systematic Reviews,* (4), CD003786.

Busch, A. J., et al. (2008). Exercise for fibromyalgia: A systematic review. *Journal of Rheumatology, 35*(6), 1130–1140.

Bussing, A., et al. (2012). Effects of yoga intervention on pain and pain-associated disability: A meta-analysis. *Journal of Pain, 13*(1), 1–9.

Caban-Martinez, A. J., et al. (2015). Leisure-time physical activity, falls, and fall injuries in middle-aged adults. *American Journal of Preventive Medicine, 49*(6), 888–901.

Candow, D. G., et al. (2011). Short-term heavy resistance training eliminates age-related deficits in muscle mass and strength in healthy older males. *Journal of Strength and Conditioning Research, 25*(2), 326–333.

Centers for Disease Control and Prevention (CDC). (2010). State indicator report on physical activity, 2010. Atlanta, GA: US Department of Health and Human Services.

Centers for Disease Control and Prevention (CDC). (2014). State indicator report on physical activity. Atlanta, GA: US Department of Health and Human Services.

Centers for Disease Control and Prevention (CDC). (2015). Physical activity for everyone: Older adults. Atlanta, GA: US Department of Health and Human Services.

Centers for Disease Control and Prevention (CDC). (2016a). Behavioral Risk Factor Surveillance System. Atlanta, GA: US Department of Health and Human Services.

Centers for Disease Control and Prevention (CDC). (2016b). National Health and Nutrition Examination Survey. Atlanta, GA: US Department of Health and Human Services.

Centers for Disease Control and Prevention (CDC). (2017). National Center for Health Statistics. Atlanta, GA: US Department of Health and Human Services.

Chang, W. D., Lin, H. Y., & Lai, P. T. (2015). Core strength training for patients with chronic low back pain. *Journal of Physical Therapy Science*, 27(3), 619–622.

Chen, L., et al. (2015). Effect of lifestyle intervention in patients with type 2 diabetes: A meta-analysis. *Metabolism: Clinical and Experimental*, 64(2), 338–347.

Chen, M. J., Fan, X., & Moe, S. T. (2002). Criterion-related validity of the Borg ratings of perceived exertion scale in healthy individuals: A meta-analysis. *Journal of Sports Sciences*, 20(11), 873–899.

Chen, S. M., et al. (2009). Sedentary lifestyle as a risk factor for low back pain: A systematic review. *International Archives of Occupational and Environmental Health*, 82, 797–806.

Cho, H. C., et al. (2014). Effects of combined exercise on cardiovascular risk factors and serum BDNF level in mid-aged women. *The Journal of Exercise Nutrition and Biochemistry*, 6(1), 61–67.

Cho, Y. K., et al. (2015). Synergistic effect of a rehabilitation program and treadmill exercise on pain and dysfunction in patients with chronic low back pain. *Journal of Physical Therapy Science*, 27(4), 1187–1190.

Chodzko-Zajko, W. J., et al. (2009). American College of Sports Medicine: Position stand. Exercise and physical activity for older adults. *Medicine & Science in Sports & Exercise*, 41(7), 1510–1530.

Choi, B. K. L., et al. (2010). Exercises for prevention of recurrences of low-back pain. *The Cochrane Database of Systematic Reviews*, (1), CD006555.

Chou, C. H., Hwang, C. L., & Wu, Y. T. (2012). Effect of exercise on physical function, daily living activities, and quality of life in frail older adults: A meta-analysis. *Archives of Physical Medicine and Rehabilitation*, 93(2), 237–244.

Chou, R., & Huffman, L. H. (2007). Nonpharmacologic therapies for acute and chronic low back pain: A review of the evidence for an American Pain Society/American College of Physicians clinical practice guideline. *Annals of Internal Medicine*, 147(1), 492–504.

Chudyk, A., & Patrella, R. J. (2011). Effects of exercise on cardiovascular risk factors in type 2 diabetes. A meta-analysis. *Diabetes Care*, 34(5), 1228–1237.

Colberg, S. R., et al. (2010). Exercise and type 2 diabetes: The American College of Sports Medicine and the American Diabetes Association: Joint position statement executive summary. *Diabetes Care*, 33(12), 2692–2696.

Cooney, G. M., et al. (2013). Exercise for depression. *The Cochrane Database of Systematic Reviews*, (9), CD004366.

Cooney, J. K., et al. (2010). Benefits of exercise in rheumatoid arthritis. *Journal of Aging Research*, 13, 1–14.

Coquart, J. B., et al. (2012). Relevance of the measure of perceived exertion for the rehabilitation of obese patients. *Annals of Physical and Rehabilitation Medicine*, 55(9-10), 623–640.

Coquart, J. B., et al. (2014). Prediction of maximal or peak oxygen uptake from ratings of perceived exertion. *Sports Medicine*, 44(5), 563–578.

Cornelissen, V. A., et al. (2009). Influence of exercise at lower and higher intensity on blood pressure and cardiovascular risk factors at older age. *Journal of Hypertension*, 27(4), 753–762.

Cornelissen, V. A., et al. (2011). Impact of resistance training on blood pressure and other cardiovascular risk factors: A meta-analysis of randomized, controlled trials. *Hypertension*, 58(5), 950–958.

Cornelissen, V. A., & Smart, N. A. (2013). Exercise training for blood pressure: A systematic review and meta-analysis. *Journal of the American Heart Association*, 2(1), e004473.

Cowan, D., et al. (2009). A community-based physical maintenance program for frail older adults: The Stay Well program. *Topics in Geriatric Rehabilitation*, 25(4), 355–364.

Cramer, H., et al. (2013). Yoga for depression: A systematic review and meta-analysis. *Journal of Depression and Anxiety*, 30(1), 1068–1083.

de Salles, B. F., et al. (2009). Rest interval between sets in strength training. *Sports Medicine*, 39, 765–777.

Deshpande, A. D., Harris-Hayes, M., & Schootman, M. (2008). Epidemiology of diabetes and diabetes-related complications. *Physical Therapy*, 88(11), 1254–1264.

Dogra, S. (2011). Better self-perceived health is associated with lower odds of physical inactivity in older adults with chronic disease. *Journal of Aging and Physical Activity*, 19(4), 322–335.

Dudgeon, W. D., et al. (2004). Physiological and psychological effects of exercise interventions in HIV disease. *AIDS Patient Care and Stds*, 18(2), 81–98.

Ebnezar, J., et al. (2012). Effects of integrated approach of Hatha yoga therapy on functional disability, pain, and flexibility in osteoarthritis of the knee joint: A randomized controlled study. *Journal of Alternative and Complementary Medicine*, 18(5), 463–472.

Ehrlich-Jones, L., et al. (2011). Relationship between beliefs, motivation, and worries about physical activity and physical activity participation in persons with rheumatoid arthritis. *Arthritis Care & Research*, 63(12), 1700–1705.

Elsawy, B., & Higgins, K. E. (2010). Physical activity guidelines for older adults. *American Family Physician*, 81(1), 55–59.

Escalante, Y., et al. (2012). Improvement of the lipid profile with exercise in obese children: A systematic review. *Preventive Medicine*, 54(5), 293–301.

Fagard, R. H. (2011). Exercise intensity and blood pressure response to endurance training. *Hypertension*, 28(1), 20–23.

Federici, M. O., & Benedetti, M. M. (2006). Ketone bodies monitoring. *Diabetes Research & Clinical Practice*, 74, S77–S81.

Fillipas, S., et al. (2006). A six-month, supervised, aerobic and resistance exercise program improves self-efficacy in people with human immunodeficiency virus: A randomized controlled trial. *Australian Journal of Physiotherapy*, 52(3), 185–190.

Fillipas, S., et al. (2010). The effects of exercise training on metabolic and morphological outcomes for people living with HIV: A systematic review of randomised controlled trials. *HIV Clinical Trials*, 11, 270–282.

Firth, J., et al. (2015). A systematic review and meta-analysis of exercise interventions in schizophrenia patients. *Psychological Medicine*, 45, 1343–1361.

Fryar, C. D., Carroll, M. D., & Ogden, C. L. (2014). Prevalence of overweight, obesity, and extreme obesity among adults: United States, 1960–1962 through 2011–2012. *Health E-Stats*. http://

www.cdc.gov/nchs/data/hestat/obesity_adult_11_12/obesity_adult_11_12.htm.

Galantino, M. L., et al. (2005). The effect of group aerobic exercise and t'ai chi on functional outcomes and quality of life for persons living with acquired immunodeficiency syndrome. *Journal of Alternative and Complementary Medicine*, *11*(6), 1085–1092.

Galper, D. I., et al. (2006). Inverse association between physical inactivity and mental health in men and women. *Medicine & Science in Sports & Exercise*, *38*(1), 173–178.

Gammon, M. D., et al. (1998). Recreational physical activity and breast cancer risk among women under age 45 years. *American Journal of Epidemiology*, *147*(3), 273–280.

García-Pérez, L. E., et al. (2013). Adherence to therapies in patients with type 2 diabetes. *Diabetes Ther*, *4*, 175–194.

Georgiades, A., et al. (2000). Effects of exercise and weight loss on mental stress-induced cardiovascular responses in individuals with high blood pressure. *Hypertension*, *36*, 171–176.

Ghadieh, A. S., & Saab, B. (2015). Evidence for exercise training in the management of hypertension in adults. *Canadian Family Physician Médecin De Famille Canadien*, *61*(3), 233–239.

Gleeson, M., et al. (2002). Epstein-Barr virus reactivation and upper-respiratory illness in elite swimmers. *Medicine & Science in Sports & Exercise*, *34*(3), 411–417.

Gleeson, M., et al. (2011). Sex differences in immune variables and respiratory infection incidence in an athletic population. *Exercise Immunology Review*, *17*, 122–135.

Gleeson, M., et al. (2013). Influence of training load on upper respiratory tract infection incidence and antigen-stimulated cytokine production. *Scan J Med Sci Sports*, *23*(4), 451–457.

Gomes-Neto, M., et al. (2013). A systematic review of the effects of different types of therapeutic exercise on physiologic and functional measurements in patients with HIV/AIDS. *Clinics (São Paulo, Brazil)*, *68*(8), 1157–1167.

Gong, Q.-H., et al. (2015). Lifestyle interventions for adults with impaired glucose tolerance: A systematic review and meta-analysis of the effects on glycemic control. *Internal Medicine (Tokyo, Japan)*, *54*(3), 303–310.

Gorczynski, P., & Faulkner, G. (2010). Exercise therapy for schizophrenia. *The Cochrane Database of Systematic Reviews*, (5), CD004412.

Gow, M. L., et al. (2016). Sustained improvements in fitness and exercise tolerance in obese adolescents after a 12-week exercise intervention. *Obesity Research & Clinical Practice*, *10*(2), 178–188.

Graven, C., et al. (2011). Are rehabilitation and/or care co-coordination interventions delivered in the community effective in reducing depression, facilitating participation and improving quality of life after stroke? *Disability and Rehabilitation*, *33*(17/18), 1501–1520.

Guadalupe-Grau, A., et al. (2009). Exercise and bone mass in adults. *Sports Medicine*, *39*(6), 439–468.

Gulve, E. A. (2008). Exercise and glycemic control in diabetes: Benefits, challenges, and adjustments to pharmacotherapy. *Physical Therapy*, *88*(11), 1297–1321.

Hale, L. A., Waters, D., & Herbison, P. (2012). A randomized controlled trial to investigate the effects of water-based exercise to improve falls risk and physical function in older adults with lower-extremity osteoarthritis. *Archives of Physical Medicine and Rehabilitation*, *93*, 27–34.

Hall, A. M., et al. (2011). Tai chi exercise for treatment of pain and disability in people with persistent low back pain: A randomized controlled trial. *Arthritis Care & Research*, *63*(11), 1576–1583.

Hallal, P. C., et al. (2006). Adolescent physical activity and health: A systematic review. *Sports Medicine*, *36*(12), 1019–1030.

Hamilton, C. J., Swan, V. J., & Jamal, S. A. (2010). The effects of exercise and physical activity participation on bone mass and geometry in postmenopausal women: A systematic review of pQCT studies. *Osteoporosis International*, *21*, 11–23.

Han, A., et al. (2004). Tai chi for treating rheumatoid arthritis. *The Cochrane Database of Systematic Reviews*, (3), CD004849.

Hass, C. J., et al. (2000). Single versus multiple sets in long-term recreational weightlifters. *Medicine & Science in Sports & Exercise*, *32*(1), 235–242.

Hautala, A. J., et al. (2013). Peak exercise capacity prediction from a submaximal exercise test in coronary artery disease patients. *Frontiers in Physiology*, *4*, 1–6.

Hayden, J. A., et al. (2005). Exercise therapy for treatment of non-specific low back pain. *The Cochrane Database of Systematic Reviews*, (3), CD000335.

He, M., & Evans, A. (2007). Are parents aware that their children are overweight or obese? *Canadian Family Physician*, *53*, 1494–1499.

Hendrick, P., et al. (2010). The effectiveness of walking as an intervention for low back pain: A systematic review. *European Spine Journal*, *19*, 1613–1620.

Heneweer, H., et al. (2012). Physical fitness, rather than self-reported physical activities, is more strongly associated with low back pain: Evidence from a working population. *European Spine Journal*, *21*(7), 1265–1272.

Henwood, T., Keogh, J., & Climstein, M. (2012). Sarcopenia in older adults. *Australian Nursing Journal*, *19*(9), 39–40.

Heran, B. S., et al. (2011). Exercise-based cardiac rehabilitation for coronary heart disease. *The Cochrane Database of Systematic Reviews*, (7), CD001800.

Herring, M. P., O'Connor, P. J., & Dishman, R. K. (2010). The effect of exercise training on anxiety symptoms among patients: A systematic review. *Archives of Internal Medicine*, *170*, 321–331.

Hewlett, S., et al. (2011). Self-management of fatigue in rheumatoid arthritis: A randomised controlled trial of group cognitive-behavioural therapy. *Annals of the Rheumatic Diseases*, *70*, 1060–1067.

Holtzman, S., & Beggs, R. T. (2013). Yoga for chronic low back pain: A meta-analysis of randomized controlled trials. *Pain Research & Management*, *18*(5), 267–272.

Howe, T. E., et al. (2011). Exercise for preventing and treating osteoporosis in postmenopausal women. *The Cochrane Database of Systematic Reviews*, (7), CD000333.

Hsu, W. L., et al. (2014). Balance control in elderly people with osteoporosis. *Journal of the Formosan Medical Association Taiwan Yi Zhi*, *113*(6), 334–339.

Hua, L. P. T., et al. (2009). Effects of low-intensity exercise conditioning on blood pressure, and autonomic modulation of heart rate in men and women with hypertension. *Biological Research for Nursing*, *11*(2), 129–143.

Huang, J. S., et al. (2007). Parental ability to discriminate the weight status of children: Results of a survey. *Pediatrics*, *120*(1), e112–e119.

Huang, T. T., Yang, L. H., & Liu, C. Y. (2011). Reducing the fear of falling among community-dwelling elderly adults through cognitive-behavioural strategies and intense tai chi exercise: A randomized controlled trial. *Journal of Advanced Nursing*, *67*(5), 961–971.

Hurley, B., & Armstrong, T. J. (2012). Bisphosphonates vs exercise for the prevention and treatment of osteoporosis. *Journal for Nurse Practitioners*, *8*(3), 217–224.

Hwangbo, G., et al. (2015). The effects of trunk stability exercise and a combined exercise program on pain, flexibility, and static balance in chronic low back pain patients. *Journal of Physical Therapy Science*, 27(4), 1153–1155.

Ingram, C., & Visovsky, C. (2007). Exercise intervention to modify physiologic risk factors in cancer survivors. *Seminars in Oncology Nursing*, 23(4), 275–284.

Irvine, C., & Taylor, N. F. (2009). Progressive resistance exercise improves glycaemic control in people with type 2 diabetes mellitus: A systematic review. *Australian Journal of Physiotherapy*, 55(4), 237–246.

Iwanto, J., et al. (2010). Effectiveness of exercise in the treatment of lumbar spinal stenosis, knee arthritis, and osteoporosis. *Aging Clinical and Experimental Research*, 22(2), 116–122.

Jaggers, J., et al. (2015). Aerobic and resistance training improves mood state among adults living with HIV. *International Journal of Sports Medicine*, 36(02), 175–181.

Jamtvedt, G., et al. (2008). Physical therapy interventions for patients with osteoarthritis of the knee: An overview of systematic reviews. *Physical Therapy*, 88(1), 123–136.

Jansen, M. J., et al. (2011). Strength training alone, exercise therapy alone, and exercise therapy with passive manual mobilisation each reduce pain and disability in people with knee osteoarthritis: A systematic review. *Journal of Physiotherapy*, 57, 11–20.

Jones, T. E., et al. (2009). Sarcopenia—mechanism and treatments. *Journal of Geriatric Physical Therapy*, 32(2), 39–45.

Josefsson, T., Lindwall, M., & Archer, T. (2014). Physical exercise intervention in depressive disorders: Meta-analysis and systematic review. *Scandinavian Journal of Medicine and Science in Sports*, 24, 259–272.

Julián-Almárcegui, C., et al. (2015). Combined effects of interaction between physical activity and nutrition on bone health in children and adolescents: A systematic review. *Nutrition Reviews*, 73(3), 127–139.

Kalyani, R. R., et al. (2010). Vitamin D treatment for the preventions of falls in older adults: Systematic review and meta-analysis. *Journal of the American Geriatrics Society*, 58, 1299–1310.

Kelley, G. A., & Kelley, K. S. (2009). Impact of progressive resistance training on lipids and lipoproteins in adults: A meta-analysis of randomized controlled trials. *Preventive Medicine*, 48(1), 9–19.

Kelley, G. A., et al. (2012). Comparison of aerobic exercise, diet or both on lipids and lipoproteins in adults: A meta-analysis of randomized controlled trials. *Clinical Nutrition: Official Journal of the European Society of Parenteral and Enteral Nutrition*, 31(2), 156–167.

Kelley, G. A., Kelley, K. S., & Hootman, J. M. (2015). Effects of exercise on depression in adults with arthritis: A systematic review with meta-analysis of randomized controlled trials. *Arthritis Research & Therapy*, 17(21).

Kemmler, W., Häberle, L., & von Stengel, S. (2013). Effects of exercise on fracture reduction in older adults: A systematic review and meta-analysis. *Osteoporosis International: A Journal Established as Result of Cooperation between the European Foundation for Osteoporosis and the National Osteoporosis Foundation of the USA*, 24(7), 1937–1950.

Kessenich, C. R. (2007). Nonpharmacological prevention of osteoporotic fractures. *Journal of Clinical Interventions in Aging*, 2(2), 263–266.

Keysor, J. J., & Brembs, A. (2011). Exercise: Necessary but not sufficient for improving function and preventing disability? *Current Opinion in Rheumatology*, 23, 211–218.

Kim, H., Yoshida, H., & Suzuki, T. (2014). Falls and fractures in participants and excluded nonparticipants of a fall prevention exercise program for elderly women with a history of falls: 1-year follow-up study. *Geriatr Gerentol Int*, 14(2), 285–292.

Kiwata, J., et al. (2014). Effects of aerobic exercise on lipid-effector molecules of the innate immune response. *Medicine and Science in Sports and Exercise*, 46(3), 506–512.

Kohrt, W. M., et al. (2004). American College of Sports Medicine Position stand: Physical activity and bone health. *Medicine & Science in Sports & Exercise*, 36(11), 1985–1996.

Koumantakis, G. A., Watson, P. J., & Oldham, J. A. (2005). Trunk muscle stabilization training plus general exercise versus general exercise only: Randomized controlled trial of patients with recurrent low back pain. *Physical Therapy*, 85(3), 209–225.

Krieger, J. W. (2010). Single vs. multiple sets of resistance exercise for muscle hypertrophy: A meta-analysis. *Journal of Strength & Conditioning Research*, 24, 1150–1159.

Kujala, U. M. (2009). Evidence on the effects of exercise therapy in the treatment of chronic disease. *British Journal of Sports Medicine*, 43, 550–555.

Lahart, I. M., et al. (2015). Physical activity, risk of death and recurrence in breast cancer survivors: A systematic review and meta-analysis of epidemiological studies. *Acta Oncologica*, 54(5), 635–654.

Lamina, S. (2010). Effects of continuous and interval training programs in the management of hypertension: A randomized controlled trial. *Journal of Clinical Hypertension*, 12(11), 841–849.

Langdeau, J. B., & Boulet, L. P. (2001). Prevalence and mechanisms of development of asthma and airway hyperresponsiveness in athletes. *Journal of Sports Medicine*, 31(8), 601–616.

Larkin, L., & Kennedy, N. (2014). Correlates of physical activity in adults with rheumatoid arthritis: A systematic review. *Journal of Physical Activity and Health*, 11(6), 1248–1261.

Larouche, R., et al. (2012). Life transitions in the waning of physical activity from childhood to adult life in the Trois-Rivières study. *Journal of Physical Activity & Health*, 9(4), 516–524.

Larson-Meyer, D. E., et al. (2010). Caloric restriction with or without exercise: The fitness versus fatness debate. *Medicine & Science in Sports & Exercise*, 42(1), 152–159.

Larun, L., et al. (2009). Exercise in prevention and treatment of anxiety and depression among children and young people. *The Cochrane Database of Systematic Reviews*, (3), CD004691.

Lascar, N., et al. (2014). Attitudes and barriers to exercise in adults with type 1 diabetes (T1DM) and how best to address them: A qualitative study. *PLoS ONE*, 9(9), e108019.

Lavie, C. J., & Milani, R. V. (2011). Cardiac rehabilitation and exercise training in secondary coronary heart disease prevention. *Progress in Cardiovascular Diseases*, 53(6), 397–403.

Lee, D. J., et al. (1992). Immune responsiveness and risk of illness in US Air Force Academy cadets during basic cadet training. *Aviation, Space, and Environmental Medicine*, 63(6), 517–523.

Lee, H. C., & Heo, T. (2014). Effects of exercise therapy on blood lipids of obese women. *Journal of Physical Therapy Science*, 26(11), 1675–1677.

Leone, L. A., & Ward, D. S. (2013). A mixed methods comparison of perceived benefits and barriers to exercise between obese and non-obese women. *J Phys Act Health*, 10(4), 461–469.

Leung, D. P., et al. (2011). Tai chi as an intervention to improve balance and reduce falls in older adults: A systematic and meta-analytical review. *Alternative Therapies in Health and Medicine*, 17(1), 40–48.

Li, C. S., et al. (2015). Motivating patients to exercise: Translating high blood pressure into equivalent risk of inactivity. *Journal of Hypertension, 33*(2), 287–293.

Li, J., & Hooker, N. H. (2010). Childhood obesity and schools: Evidence from the National Survey of Children's Health. *Journal of School Health, 80*(2), 96–103.

Lima, T. B., et al. (2013). The effectiveness of aquatic physical therapy in the treatment of fibromyalgia: A systematic review with meta-analysis. *Clinical Rehabilitation, 27*(10), 892–908.

Lin, Y., Yeh, M., & Huang, L. (2010). Physical activity status and gender differences in community-dwelling older adults with chronic diseases. *Journal of Nursing Research, 18*(2), 88–96.

Lirani-Galvao, A. P. R., & Lazaretti-Castro, M. (2010). Physical approach for prevention and treatment of osteoporosis. *Arquivos Brasileiros de Endocrinologia and Metabologia, 54*(2), 171–178.

Liu, C. K., & Fielding, R. A. (2011a). Exercise as an intervention for frailty. *Clinics in Geriatric Medicine, 27*(1), 101–110.

Liu, Y., et al. (2011b). Does physical activity reduce the risk of prostate cancer? A systematic review and meta-analysis. *European Urology, 60*, 1029–1044.

Liu-Ambrose, T. Y., Ashe, M. C., & Marra, C. (2010). Independent and inverse association of healthcare utilisation with physical activity in older adults with multiple chronic conditions. *British Journal of Sports Medicine, 44*(14), 1024–1028.

Macfarlane, D. J., Chou, K., & Cheng, W. (2005). The effect of tai chi on the physical and psychological well-being of Chinese older women. *Journal of Exercise Science & Fitness, 3*(2), 87–94.

Mackinnon, L. T. (1992). *Exercise and immunology.* Champaign, IL: Human Kinetics.

Mampuya, W. M. (2012). Cardiac rehabilitation past, present and future: An overview. *Cardiovasc Diagn Ther, 2*(1), 38–49.

Marcus, R. L., et al. (2008). Comparison of combined aerobic and high-force eccentric resistance exercise with aerobic exercise only for people with type 2 diabetes mellitus. *Physical Therapy, 88*(11), 1345–1354.

Marquard, J. L., et al. (2012). Evaluation of a volunteer-led in-home program for home-bound older adults. *Work (Reading, Mass.), 41*(3), 339–354.

Martin, D. (2011). Physical activity benefits and risks on the gastrointestinal system. *Southern Medical Journal, 104*, 831–837.

Martyn-St James, M., & Carroll, S. (2009). A meta-analysis of impact exercise on postmenopausal bone loss: The case for mixed loading exercise programmes. *British Journal of Sports Medicine, 43*(12), 898–908.

Mat, S., et al. (2015). Physical therapies for improving balance and reducing falls risk in osteoarthritis of the knee: A systematic review. *Age and Ageing, 44*(1), 16–24.

Matthews, C. E., et al. (2002). Moderate to vigorous physical activity and risk of upper-respiratory tract infection. *Medicine & Science in Sports & Exercise, 34*(8), 1242–1248.

May, S. (2010). Self-management of chronic low back pain and osteoarthritis. *Nature Reviews. Rheumatology, 6*, 199–209.

McDermott, A. Y., & Mernitz, H. (2006). Exercise and older patients: Prescribing guidelines. *American Family Physician, 74*(3), 437–444.

McGrath, J. A., O'Malley, M., & Hendrix, T. J. (2010). Group exercise mode and health-related quality of life among healthy adults. *Journal of Advanced Nursing, 67*(3), 491–500.

McKinnis, L. N. (2014). *Fundamentals of orthopedic radiology* (4th ed.). Philadelphia, PA: F.A. Davis.

Mead, G. E., et al. (2009). Exercise for depression. *The Cochrane Database of Systematic Reviews, (3),* CD004366

Menezes, A. R., et al. (2012). Cardiac rehabilitation and exercise therapy in the elderly: Should we invest in the aged? *Journal of Geriatric Cardiology, 9*, 68–75.

Meng, X. G., & Yue, S. W. (2015). Efficacy of aerobic exercise for treatment of chronic low back pain: A meta-analysis. *American Journal of Physical Medicine & Rehabilitation/Association of Academic Physiatrists, 94*(5), 358–365.

Menschik, D., et al. (2008). Adolescent physical activities as predictors of young adult weight. *Archives of Pediatric & Adolescent Medicine, 162*(1), 29–33.

Milani, R. V., et al. (2011). Impact of exercise training and depression on survival in heart failure due to coronary heart disease. *American Journal of Cardiology, 107*, 64–68.

Mirza, F., & Canalis, E. (2015). Management of endocrine disease: Secondary osteoporosis: Pathophysiology and management. *European Journal of Endocrinology/European Federation of Endocrine Societies, 173*(3), R131–R151.

Mishra, S. I., et al. (2014). Are exercise programs effective for improving health-related quality of life among cancer survivors? A systematic review and meta-analysis. *Oncology Nursing Forum, 41*(6), 326–342.

Mishra, S. I., et al. (2015). The effectiveness of exercise interventions for improving health-related quality of life from diagnosis through active cancer treatment. *Oncology Nursing Forum, 42*(1), E33–E53.

Mithal, A., et al. (2013). Impact of nutrition on muscle mass, strength, and performance in older adults. *Osteoporosis International, 24*(5), 1555–1566.

Moore, L., Harris, C., & Bradlyn, A. (2012). Exploring the relationship between parental concern and the management of childhood obesity. *Maternal and Child Health Journal, 16*(4), 902–908.

Morgan, K. T. (2012). Nutrition, resistance training, and sarcopenia: Their role in successful aging. *Topics in Clinical Nutrition, 27*(2), 114–123.

Nahas, R., & Sheikh, O. (2011). Complementary and alternative medicine for the treatment of major depressive disorder. *Canadian Family Physician, 57*(6), 659–663.

Nathan, D. M. (2015). Diabetes: Advances in diagnosis and treatment. *JAMA: The Journal of the American Medical Association, 314*(10), 1052–1062.

National Center for Health Statistics. (2016). Vital statistics rapid release, quarterly provisional estimates of infant mortality. https://www.cdc.gov/nchs/index.htm.

National Institute of Diabetes and Digestive and Kidney Diseases. (2012). Overweight and obesity statistics. Bethesda, MD: US Department of Health and Human Services.

National Institutes of Health, Osteoporosis and Related Bone Diseases National Resource Center. (2011). Osteoporosis. http://www.niams.nih.gov/Health_Info/Bone/Osteoporosis.

National Osteoporosis Foundation. (2016). Fast facts about osteoporosis. https://cdn.nof.org/wp-content/uploads/2016/04/Fast-Facts-About-Osteoporosis.pdf.

National Physical Activity Plan. (2010). National Physical Activity Plan. http://www.physicalactivityplan.org/.

Nelson, A. E., et al. (2014). A systematic review of recommendations and guidelines for the management of osteoarthritis: The Chronic Osteoarthritis Management Initiative of the U.S. Bone and Joint Initiative. *Seminars in Arthritis and Rheumatism, 43*(6), 701–712.

Nieman, D. (1994). Exercise, upper respiratory tract infection, and the immune system. *Medicine & Science in Sports & Exercise, 26*(2), 128–139

Nieman, D. (2000). Exercise soothes arthritis: Joint effects. *ACSM's Health & Fitness Journal*, 4(3), 20–28.

Nieman, D. C., et al. (1990). Infectious episodes in runners before and after the Los Angeles Marathon. *Journal of Sports Medicine and Physical Fitness*, 30(3), 316–328.

Nikander, R., et al. (2010). Targeted exercise against osteoporosis: A systematic review and meta-analysis for optimising bone strength throughout life. *BMC Medicine*, 8(47), 1–16.

Nixon, S., et al. (2005). Aerobic exercise interventions for adults living with HIV/AIDS. *The Cochrane Database of Systematic Reviews*, (2), CD001796.

Nyström, M. B. T., et al. (2015). Treating major depression with physical activity: A systematic overview with recommendations. *Cognitive Behaviour Therapy*, 44(4), 341–352.

O'Brien, K., et al. (2004). Progressive resistive exercise interventions for adults living with HIV/AIDS. *The Cochrane Database of Systematic Reviews*, (4), CD004248.

O'Brien, K., et al. (2009). Progressive resistive exercise interventions for adults living with HIV/AIDS. *The Cochrane Database of Systematic Reviews*, (4), CD004248, pub2.

O'Brien, K., et al. (2010). Aerobic exercise interventions for adults living with HIV/AIDS. *The Cochrane Database of Systematic Reviews*, (8), CD001796.

O'Connor, S. R., et al. (2015). Walking exercise for chronic musculoskeletal pain: Systematic review and meta-analysis. *Archives of Physical Medicine and Rehabilitation*, 96(4), 724–734.

O'Donovan, G., et al. (2010). The ABC of physical activity for health: A consensus statement from the British Association for Sport and Exercise Sciences. *Journal of Sports Sciences*, 28(6), 573–591.

Oerkild, B., et al. (2011). Home-based cardiac rehabilitation is as effective as centre-based cardiac rehabilitation among elderly with coronary heart disease: Results from a randomised clinical trial. *Age and Ageing*, 40, 78–85.

Ogden, C. L., et al. (2015). Prevalence of obesity among adults and youth: United States, 2011–2014. NCHS data brief, no 219. Hyattsville, MD: National Center for Health Statistics.

Olaya-Contreras, P., et al. (2015). The effect of the stay active advice on physical activity and on the course of acute severe low back pain. *BMC Sports Science, Medicine and Rehabilitation*, 7, 19.

Ortman, J. M., Velkoff, V. A., & Hogan, H. (2014). An aging nation: The older population in the United States. US Department of Commerce.

Park, Y. H., et al. (2011). The effects of an integrated health education and exercise program in community-dwelling older adults with hypertension: A randomized controlled trial. *Patient Education and Counseling*, 82(1), 133–137.

Pascoe, M. C., & Bauer, I. E. (2015). A systemic review of randomized control trials on the effects of yoga on stress measures and mood. *Journal of Psychiatric Research*, 68, 270–282.

Pate, R. R., et al. (1995). Physical activity and public health. A recommendation for the Centers for Disease Control and Prevention and the American College of Sports Medicine. *Journal of the American Medical Association*, 273(5), 402–407.

Pattyn, N., et al. (2013). The effect of exercise on the cardiovascular risk factors constituting the metabolic syndrome: A meta-analysis of controlled trials. *Sports Medicine*, 43(2), 121–133.

Pedersen, B., Rohde, T., & Ostrowski, K. (1998). Recovery of the immune system after exercise. *Acta Physiologica Scandinavica*, 162(3), 325–332.

Pedersen, B., & Ullum, H. (1994). NK cell response to physical activity: Possible mechanisms of action. *Medicine & Science in Sports & Exercise*, 26(2), 140–146.

Pedersen, B. K., & Bruunsgaard, H. (1995). How physical exercise influences the establishment of infections. *Sports Medicine*, 19(6), 393–400.

Pentecost, C., & Taket, A. (2011). Understanding exercise uptake and adherence for people with chronic conditions: A new model demonstrating the importance of exercise identity, benefits of attending and support. *Health Education Research*, 26, 908–922.

Perry, S. B., & Downey, P. A. (2012). Fracture risk and prevention: A multidimensional approach. *Physical Therapy*, 92(1), 164–178.

Pescatello, L. S., et al. (2004). American College of Sports Medicine position standard. Exercise and hypertension. *Medicine & Science in Sports & Exercise*, 36(3), 533–553.

Peters-Futre, E. M. (1997). Vitamin C, neutrophil function, and upper respiratory tract infection risk in distance runners: The missing link. *Exercise Immunology Review*, 3, 32–52.

Pisters, M. F., et al. (2010). Exercise adherence improving long-term patient outcome in patients with osteoarthritis of the hip and/or knee. *Arthritis Care & Research*, 62(8), 1087–1094.

Polikandrioti, M., & Dokoutsidou, H. (2009). The role of exercise and nutrition in type II diabetes mellitus management. *Health Science Journal*, 3(4), 216–221.

Pyne, D. B., et al. (1995). Effects of an intensive 12-wk training program by elite swimmers on neutrophil oxidative activity. *Medicine & Science in Sports & Exercise*, 27(4), 536–542.

Rand, D., et al. (2011). Interventions for addressing low balance confidence in older adults: A systematic review and meta-analysis. *Age & Aging*, 40(3), 297–306.

Rasmussen-Barr, E., et al. (2009). Graded exercise for recurrent low-back pain: A randomized, controlled trial with 6-, 12-, and 36-month follow-ups. *Spine*, 34, 221–228.

Rimmele, U., et al. (2007). Trained men show lower cortisol, heart rate and psychological responses to psychosocial stress compared with untrained men. *Psychoneuroendocrinology*, 32, 627–635.

Roffey, D. M., et al. (2010a). Causal assessment of awkward occupational postures and low back pain: Results of a systematic review. *Spine Journal*, 10(1), 89–99.

Roffey, D. M., et al. (2010b). Causal assessment of occupational sitting and low back pain: Results of a systematic review. *Spine Journal*, 10(3), 252–261.

Roffey, D. M., et al. (2010c). Causal assessment of occupational standing or walking and low back pain: Results of a systematic review. *Spine Journal*, 10(3), 262–272.

Roffey, D. M., et al. (2010d). Causal assessment of occupational pushing or pulling and low back pain: Results of a systematic review. *Spine Journal*, 10(6), 544–553.

Roffey, D. M., et al. (2010e). Causal assessment of workplace manual handling or assisting patients and low back pain: Results of a systematic review. *Spine Journal*, 10(7), 639–651.

Rose, D. J., & Hernandez, D. (2010). The role of exercise in fall prevention for older adults. *Clinics in Geriatric Medicine*, 26(4), 607–631.

Roussel, M., et al. (2009). Influence of a walking program on the metabolic risk profile of obese postmenopausal women. *Menopause (New York, N.Y.)*, 16(3), 566–575.

Sage, M., et al. (2013). Validity of rating of perceived exertion ranges in individuals in the subacute stage of stroke recovery. *Topics in Stroke Rehabilitation*, 20(6), 519–527.

Sañudo, B., et al. (2012). Effect of whole-body vibration exercise on balance in women with fibromyalgia syndrome: A randomized controlled trial. *Journal of Alternative and Complementary Medicine*, 18(2), 158–164.

Sañudo, B., et al. (2010). Aerobic exercise versus combined exercise therapy in women with fibromyalgia syndrome: A randomized controlled trial. *Archives of Physical Medicine & Rehabilitation*, 91(12), 1838–1843.

Sawka, M. R., et al. (2007). American College of Sports Medicine position stand: Exercise and fluid replacement. *Medicine & Science in Sports & Exercise*, 39(2), 377–390.

Sax, P. E. (2006). Strategies for management and treatment of dyslipidemia in HIV/AIDS. *AIDS Care*, 18(2), 149–157.

Scharoun-Lee, M., et al. (2009). Obesity, race/ethnicity and life course socioeconomic status across the transition from adolescence to adulthood. *Journal of Epidemiology & Community Health*, 63(2), 133–139.

Shamliyan, T. A., et al. (2008). Systematic review: Randomized, controlled trials of nonsurgical treatments for urinary incontinence in women. *Annals of Internal Medicine*, 148(6), 459–473.

Shaughnessy, M., & Caulfield, B. (2004). A pilot study to investigate the effect of lumbar stabilisation exercise training on functional ability and quality of life in patients with chronic low back pain. *International Journal of Rehabilitation Research*, 27(4), 297–301.

Shaw, K., et al. (2006). Exercise for overweight or obesity. *The Cochrane Database of Systematic Reviews*, (4), CD003817.

Shiri, R., et al. (2010). The association between obesity and low back pain: A meta-analysis. *American Journal of Epidemiology*, 171, 135–154.

Silva, L. E., et al. (2008). Hydrotherapy versus conventional land-based exercise for the management of patients with osteoarthritis of the knee: A randomized clinical trial. *Physical Therapy*, 88(1), 12–21.

Simpson, R. J., & Guy, K. (2010). Coupling aging immunity with a sedentary lifestyle: Has the damage already been done? A mini-review. *Gerontology*, 56, 449–458.

Skinner, J. S., et al. (1973). The validity and reliability of a rating scale of perceived exertion. *Medicine & Science in Sports & Exercise*, 5(2), 94–96.

Slade, S. C., & Keating, J. L. (2007). Unloaded movement facilitation exercise compared to no exercise or alternative therapy on outcomes for people with nonspecific chronic low back pain: A systematic review. *Journal of Manipulative and Physiological Therapeutics*, 30(4), 301–311.

Smith, S. S., Wang, C. H., & Bloomfield, S. A. (2009). *Osteoporosis. ACSM's exercise management for persons with chronic diseases and disabilities* (3rd ed., pp. 270–279). Champaign, IL: Human Kinetics.

Smuck, M., et al. (2014). Does physical activity influence the relationship between low back pain and obesity? *The Spine Journal: Official Journal of the North American Spine Society*, 14(2), 209–216.

Smutok, M., Skrinar, G., & Pandolf, K. (1980). Exercise intensity: Subjective regulation by perceived exertion. *Archives of Physical Medicine & Rehabilitation*, 61(12), 569–574.

Soriano-Maldonado, A., et al. (2015). Validity and reliability of rating perceived exertion in women with fibromyalgia: Exertion-pain discrimination. *Journal of Sports Sciences*, 33(14), 1515–1522.

Staal, J. B., et al. (2004). Graded activity for low back pain in occupational health care: A randomized, controlled trial. *Annals of Internal Medicine*, 140(2), 77–84.

Stagi, S., et al. (2014). The ever-expanding conundrum of primary osteoporosis: Aetiopathogenesis, diagnosis, and treatment. *Italian Journal of Pediatrics*, 40(55), 1–18.

Stanford, K. I., & Goodyear, L. J. (2014). Exercise and type 2 diabetes: Molecular mechanisms regulating glucose uptake in skeletal muscle. *Advances in Physiology Education*, 38(4), 308–314.

Strasser, B., Siebert, U., & Schobersberger, W. (2010). Resistance training in the treatment of the metabolic syndrome. *Sports Medicine*, 40(5), 397–415.

Tambalis, K., et al. (2009). Responses of blood lipids to aerobic, resistance, and combined aerobic with resistance exercise training: A systematic review of current evidence. *Angiology*, 60(5), 614–832.

Tarnopolsky, M. A. (2008). Nutritional consideration in the aging athlete. *Clinical Journal of Sport Medicine*, 18(6), 531–538.

Terry, L., et al. (2006). Exercise training in HIV-1-infected individuals with dyslipidemia and lipodystrophy. *Medicine & Science in Sports & Exercise*, 38(3), 411–417.

Teixeira, P. J., et al. (2012). Exercise, physical activity, and self-determination theory: A systematic review. *International Journal of Behavioral Nutrition and Physical Activity*, 9(78), 1–30.

Theobald, H. E. (2005). Dietary calcium and health. *Nutrition Bulletin*, 30(3), 237–277.

Tremblay, A., Despres, J. P., & Bouchard, C. (1985). The effects of exercise-training on energy balance and adipose tissue morphology and metabolism. *Sports Medicine*, 2(3), 223–233.

Trudeau, F., Laurencelle, L., & Shephard, R. J. (2004). Tracking of physical activity from childhood to adulthood. *Medicine and Science in Sports and Exercise*, 36(11), 1937–1943.

Tseng, C. N., Gau, B. S., & Lou, M. F. (2011). The effectiveness of exercise on improving cognitive function in older people: A systematic review. *Journal of Nursing Research*, 19, 119–131.

Turcotte, L. P., & Fisher, J. S. (2008). Skeletal muscle insulin resistance: Roles of fatty acid metabolism and exercise. *Physical Therapy*, 88(11), 1279–1296.

Uhlig, T., et al. (2010). Exploring tai chi in rheumatoid arthritis: A quantitative and qualitative study. *BMC Musculoskeletal Disorders*, 11(43), 1–7.

US Census Bureau. (2011). 2010 Census shows nation's population is aging. Washington, DC: US Census Bureau.

US Department of Health and Human Services (USDHHS). (2008). 2008 physical activity guidelines for Americans. Washington, DC: US Department of Health and Human Services.

US Department of Health and Human Services (USDHHS). (2010). Healthy People 2020. http://www.healthypeople.gov.

US Department of Health and Human Services (USDHHS). (2015). Prevention and Wellness. https://www.hhs.gov/programs/prevention-and-wellness/index.html.

van Middelkoop, M., et al. (2010). Exercise therapy for chronic nonspecific low-back pain. *Best Practice & Research in Clinical Rheumatology*, 24, 193–204.

Veldhuijzen van Zanten, J. J., et al. (2015). Perceived barriers, facilitators and benefits for regular physical activity and exercise in patients with rheumatoid arthritis: A review of the literature. *Sports Medicine (Auckland, N.Z.)*, 45, 1401–1412.

Visceglia, E., & Lewis, S. (2011). Yoga as an adjunctive treatment for schizophrenia: A randomized, controlled pilot study. *Journal of Alternative & Complementary Medicine*, 17(7), 601–607.

Vrablík, M., & Česka, R. (2015). Treatment of hypertriglyceridemia: A review of current options. *Physiological Research / Academia Scientiarum Bohemoslovaca*, 64(Suppl. 3), S331–S340.

Wai, E. K., et al. (2010a). Causal assessment of occupational bending or twisting and low back pain: Results of a systematic review. *Spine Journal*, 10(1), 76–88.

Wai, E. K., et al. (2010b). Causal assessment of occupational lifting and low back pain: Results of a systematic review. *Spine Journal*, *10*(6), 554–566.

Wai, E. K., et al. (2010c). Causal assessment of occupational carrying and low back pain: Results of a systematic review. *Spine Journal*, *10*(7), 628–638.

Wallace, J. P., & Ray, S. (2009). Obesity. In *ACSM's exercise management for persons with chronic diseases and disabilities* (pp. 192–200). Champaign, IL: Human Kinetics.

Waller, B., et al. (2014). Effect of therapeutic aquatic exercise on symptoms and function associated with lower limb osteoarthritis: Systematic review with meta-analysis. *Physical Therapy*, *94*(10), 1383–1395.

Walrand, S., et al. (2011). Physiopathological mechanism of sarcopenia. *Clinics in Geriatric Medicine*, *27*(3), 365–385.

Walsh, J. N., et al. (2015). Impact of short- and long-term tai chi mind-body exercise training on cognitive function in healthy adults: Results from a hybrid observational study and randomized trial. *Global Advances in Health and Medicine*, *4*(4), 38–48.

Walsh, N. P., et al. (2011). Position statement. Part one: Immune function and exercise. *Exercise Immunology Review*, *17*, 6–63.

Wang, C., et al. (2010). Tai chi on psychological well-being: Systematic review and meta-analysis. *BMC Complementary and Alternative Medicine*, *10*, 23.

Wang, C. W., et al. (2014). Managing stress and anxiety through qigong exercise in healthy adults: A systematic review and meta-analysis of randomized controlled trials. *BMC Complementary and Alternative Medicine*, *14*(8).

Wang, F., et al. (2014). The effects of tai chi on depression, anxiety, and psychological well-being: A systematic review and meta-analysis. *International Journal of Behavioral Medicine*, *21*(4), 605–617.

Warburton, D. E., et al. (2007). Evidence-informed physical activity guidelines for Canadian adults. *Canadian Journal of Public Health*, *98*(Suppl. 2), S16–S68.

Waryasz, G. R., & McDermott, A. Y. (2010). Exercise prescription and the patient with type 2 diabetes: A clinical approach to optimizing patient outcomes. *Journal of American Academy of Nurse Practitioners*, *22*, 217–227.

Wayne, P. M., et al. (2014). The impact of tai chi on cognitive performance in older adults: A systematic review and meta-analysis. *Journal of the American Geriatrics Society*, *62*(1), 25–39.

Wegner, M., et al. (2014). Effects of exercise on anxiety and depression disorders: Review of meta analyses and neurobiological mechanisms. *CNS and Neurological Disorders Drug Targets*, *13*, 1002–1014.

Weltman, N. Y., et al. (2009). The use of exercise in the management of type 1 and type 2 diabetes. *Clinics in Sports Medicine*, *28*(3), 423–439.

Whitson, H. E., et al. (2011). Back-white disparity in disability: The role of medical conditions. *Journal of the American Geriatrics Society*, *59*(5), 844–850.

Wilhelm, M., et al. (2012). Effect of resistance exercises on function in older adults with osteoporosis or osteopenia: A systematic review. *Physiotherapy Canada*, *64*(4), 386–394.

Windle, G., et al. (2010). Is exercise effective in promoting mental well-being in older age? A systematic review. *Aging & Mental Health*, *14*(6), 652–669.

Yeh, M. L., et al. (2011). The effect of exercise on body composition in menopausal women: A systematic review and meta-analysis. *Journal of Nursing and Health Care Research*, *7*(1), 44.

Zehnacker, C. H., & Bemis-Dougherty, A. (2007). Effect of weighted exercises on bone mineral density in post menopausal women without hormone replacement therapy. *Journal of Geriatric Physical Therapy*, *30*(2), 79–88.

Zijlstra, G. A. R., et al. (2009). Effects of a multicomponent cognitive behavioral group intervention on fear of falling and activity avoidance in community-dwelling older adults: Results of a randomized controlled trial. *Journal of the American Geriatrics Society*, *57*(11), 2020–2028.

Zorba, E., Cengiz, T., & Karacabey, K. (2011). Exercise training improves body composition, blood lipid profile and serum insulin levels in obese children. *Journal of Sports Medicine and Physical Fitness*, *51*(4), 664–669.

# 13

# Stress Management

*June Andrews Horowitz*

## OBJECTIVES

*After completing this chapter, the reader will be able to:*
- Analyze concepts of stress, stressor, eustress, and distress.
- Evaluate physical, psychological, social, spiritual, and behavioral stressors that are potential contributors to physical and mental health disorders.
- Analyze the pathophysiology of the stress response and effects on health and illness.
- Examine primary and secondary cognitive appraisals of stress.
- Develop evidence-based stress-management interventions that can be used in clinical practice.
- Explain the nurse's role in stress management and crisis intervention.

## KEY TERMS

Active listening
Acupuncture
Affirmation
Anxiety sensitivity
Aromatherapy
Assertive communication
Burnout
Caregiver stress/burden
Cognitive restructuring
Coping
Diabetes
Distress
Empathy
Eustress
Exercise
Expressive writing
Fight-or-flight response

Goal setting
Healthy diet
Healthy pleasures
Homeostasis
Homeodynamics
Humor
Hypnosis
Interplay
Journal writing
Meridian
Mindfulness
Mini relaxations
Presence
Primary appraisal
Reflexology
Reiki
Relaxation response

Sandwich generation
Secondary appraisal
Self-awareness
Sleep hygiene
Social support
Sociophysiology
Spillover stress
Spiritual practice
Stress
Stress management
Stress response
Stress warning signs
Stressor
Values clarification
Yoga

## 💡 THINK ABOUT IT

### *Do We Live to Work or Work to Live?*

*When asked about yourself, what is your first response? Do you say what you do for work, or do you describe your characteristics? For most of us, our work roles, including being students, define us to a great extent. For most adults who live in industrialized countries and many other societies, employment is a primary source of income and social connection; working also contributes to a personal sense of accomplishment. However, how much work is too much? Americans take fewer yearly vacation days than their counterparts in other industrialized countries, and workplace pressures can increase the risk of a variety of disorders. Work-related stress can be a significant problem.*

- What aspects of work typically create stress?
- How do people manage work-related stress? Which strategies are effective and which strategies increase health risks?
- How do people manage the work–home life balance (**spillover stress**)?
- What health-promotion strategies could you implement to reduce your own work-related stress?
- What could you do to promote workplace health in your own practice?

Stress is an excellent paradigm for understanding the relationships among the determinants of health, the leading health indicators, and health outcomes. Stress has been shown to cause or exacerbate many of the leading health problems in the United States today, such as those related to obesity, alcohol and drug abuse, poverty, and sexually transmitted diseases (US Department of Health and Human Services [USDHHS], 2011). Consequently, helping individuals, families, and communities to find more effective ways to respond to stress is an important health-promotion goal. The Centers for Disease Control and Prevention (CDC) healthy communities program works to support people in making healthy choices where they live and work (CDC, 2012a).

Stress management has been an effective intervention framework for health promotion, disease prevention, and symptom management. Stress-management strategies such as relaxation and imagery, self-monitoring, goal setting, cognitive restructuring, mindfulness, and problem-solving have long been staples of community health-promotion programs, including Alcoholics Anonymous, Smokenders, YMCA (Y-USA), and Weight Watchers. These strategies help people to modify health risk behaviors and thereby improve quality of life. However, national health data (CDC, 2012b) indicate the need for continued and expanded use of these modalities across the life span. Although the United States health care system provides excellent, expensive, heroic care, it provides poor-quality low-cost health-promotion/preventive care, including stress management. Moreover, to ameliorate many harmful effects of stress, community-level health promotion is essential. Although shifting focus from providing acute care for individuals to enhancing the health of communities requires a revolution in our health care delivery systems and outlook, successful community health-promotion initiatives hold promise for the future (Fawcett & Ellenbecker, 2015).

The goal of stress management is to improve quality of life by increasing healthy, effective coping, thereby reducing unhealthy consequences of distress. This process produces a dynamic interaction of mind, body, and spirit, which influences physical health and well-being. Stress management is thus an essential tool for expert nursing practice, which recognizes the interface of knowledge on behavior change. The use of critical reasoning to examine multiple factors contributing to symptom development provides a valuable contribution to meeting the goals of *Healthy People 2020*. Stress management can have a significant impact on the following leading health indicators in *Healthy People 2020*: physical activity, obesity, tobacco use, substance abuse, responsible sexual behavior, mental health, injury and violence, environmental quality, immunization, workplace wellness, and access to health care (USDHHS, 2011). (See Chapter 1 for additional discussion of *Healthy People 2020*.) This chapter outlines the multifaceted psychophysiological aspects of stress, examines strategies shown to mediate its harmful effects, reviews examples of clinical situations in which stress management has been effective, and explores the unique perspective nurses bring that helps individuals identify healthy stress-management strategies.

## SOURCES OF STRESS

A stressor is any psychological, social, environmental, physiological, or spiritual stimulus that disrupts the tendency of a system, especially the physiological system of higher animals, to maintain internal stability, owing to the coordinated response of its parts to any situation or stimulus that would tend to disturb its normal condition or function. Although in use for more than 100 years, the term has suggested balance and stability but has also denoted interchange and continuous regulated or balanced change (Bortz, 2015). In other words, homeostasis has connoted a state of balance thereby requiring change or adaptation—not a static state (Figure 13-1). To reflect advances in science that underscore the continuously changing nature of and interaction among life processes in all of its manifestations, the term homeodynamics has emerged in the past decade (Bortz, 2015) as a better descriptor:

*Homeodynamics extends homeostasis into a more inclusive term. It is evident that there is no stasis in life. All of life is dynamic. 98% of a body's atoms are replaced each year. The Krebs cycle turns over 2.66×10^21 times per minute. The half-life of an intestinal cell is measured in days. Stasis is nowhere to be found. Life is a verb rather than a noun.*

Then stress is understood as a state of threatened homeostasis/homeodynamics that triggers an array of adaptive physiological, behavioral, and even social responses in an effort to reestablish homeostasis or relative balance to avoid chaos. These descriptions of stress underscore important ideas: even welcome events, such as a child's wedding, are stressors because they precipitate change. Nonetheless, stress is not intrinsically bad or unhealthy, and stress is experienced psychophysiologically and socially (i.e., as an *interplay* across all domains of individual and communal living). Stress is an essential component of being alive. Stress can be situational or maturational. One's coping strategies and resources will determine the outcomes of each stressful experience. Moreover, family and communal/social response will also affect many responses to shared

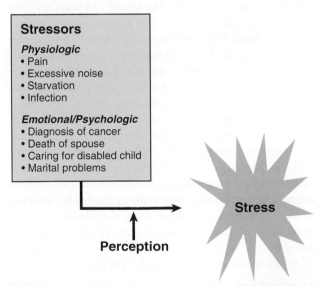

**FIGURE 13-1** Stressors can be physiological or emotional/psychological. Perception of the stressors will determine whether they cause stress. (From Lewis, S. L., Dirksen, S. R., Heitkemper, M. M., & Bucher, L. [2014]. *Medical-surgical nursing: assessment and management of clinical problems* [9th ed.]. St Louis: Mosby.)

stress. In this age of instant messaging and 24/7 news cycles, the communal shared nature of stress is intensified.

Individuals encounter a variety of physical, psychological, social, spiritual, and environmental stressors. These stressors are not simply an additive but rather have an interactive effect within a homeodynamic human-ecological system. Stressors range from health and illness experiences, such as childbirth, physical illness, trauma, or blood loss, to activities of daily living, such as caring for children, meeting work deadlines, and cleaning or repairing the house, to less common events, such as taking a critical examination, experiencing the death of a relative, losing possessions in a fire, losing a job, getting a divorce, or getting married, and environmental contexts. As a useful rubric, stressors can be organized into three categories: stressors over which people have no control (extrinsic factors), such as the weather, a traffic jam, or the death of a spouse; stressors that individuals can modify by changing their environment, social interactions, or behaviors; and stressors created or exacerbated (intrinsic factors) by poor time management, procrastination, poor communication, catastrophic negative thinking (expecting the worst), or struggling with self-defeating behaviors. However, stressors can never be neatly boxed into simple categories: Stress is a person-environment process. The person-environment fit model indicates that the person appraises a situation as taxing or as exceeding his or her resources and endangering well-being. Moreover, links between biological pathways and social adversity to subsequent adverse health outcomes underscore the importance of stress as a health determinant (Berger et al., 2015; Lazarus & Folkman, 1984; Weber, 2011).

Stress appraisal is an important concept that helps to explain why two people react in different ways to the same situation. In addition, models of stress have evolved from an individualistic perspective to consideration of family-level and community-level stress and coping (Weber, 2011).

*The shared situation of Ms. Hernandez (86 years old) and Ms. Goldman (86 years old), both in good health, provides a case in point. Both individuals are about to become new residents at an assisted living retirement community in their hometown. Ms. Hernandez perceives this move as an opportunity to increase the ease of her socializations and activities of daily living, and is looking forward to making new friends and participating in new recreational activities. In contrast, Ms. Goldman views this move as abandonment by her family and fears that the available resources will be inadequate. Although the event is virtually the same for both Ms. Hernandez and Ms. Goldman, the homeodynamic consequences are personalized because each woman perceives her situation differently. Even though the move to the new environment is the same, each woman has different coping styles and each has different support systems, so the experience will differ in its perception and thereby its level of stress.*

Stress is the physical, psychological, social, or spiritual effect of life's pressures and events. Stress is an interactive hemodynamic process that involves appraisal and response to loss or the threat of loss of well-being at individual, family, and community levels (Weber, 2011). Canadian physiologist Hans Selye (1950, 1974,

1982) first introduced the general adaptation syndrome, which led the way to continual interest in stress and the effect on the body. Selye reported that, to a certain extent, stress can be challenging and useful, which he identified as eustress. Selye also observed that when stress becomes chronic or excessive, the body is unable to adapt and maintain homeostasis, and thus the process becomes distress. Stress can be both useful and harmful. As stress increases, efficiency and performance also increase, but not endlessly. At a certain point performance and efficiency start to decrease significantly if stress continues unabated. It is important to understand the many causes of stress and the negative physical, psychosocial, and spiritual consequences of distress. Understanding the many-sided sources of stress provides the rationale for a multifaceted approach to its management. It is noteworthy that even in its early understanding, scientists and clinicians recognized the dynamic changing nature of stress and its many human system responses (Box 13-1).

In nursing we have operated within multiple frameworks to understand stress and its outcomes. Historically nursing has been grounded in the biological and medical sciences because of our long-standing roles in health promotion and caring for people experiencing illness. Yet over many decades nursing frameworks have also embraced concepts of continuous change and interaction in human-environmental fields. Most notably Martha Rogers's science of unitary human beings (Phillips, 2015; Willis et al., 2015), Neuman's systems model, and Roy's adaptation model (Willis et al., 2015) have stressed the dynamic, interactive nature of human life. As a result, nurses have learned to balance and integrate the worldviews of traditional medical and bench science with the evolving and sometimes rather heretical nursing frameworks that focused more on continual change and interaction within and among human-environmental systems. Thus in this chapter, examining stress, its manifestations, and approaches to ameliorate distress and associated health problems involves weaving knowledge and understanding generated from diverse and sometimes conflicting perspectives.

The models for understanding human stress are multifaceted and complex. In the past, scientists and clinicians tended to examine and understand stress from their own disciplinary or scientific silos. In other words, understanding stress was typically split into neurobiological and psychosocial camps. However, in recent decades "sociophysiology" has emerged as a multidisciplinary perspective to integrate the "social" and "biological" worlds and answer the following question (Barchas & Barchas, 2011): "How do social processes impact the physiology of the organism and how does that altered physiology affect future social behavior?"

Nursing science has long held an interest in the dynamic interaction among human systems. Outstanding among nurses' voices calling for innovative perspectives to topple the traditional and accepted mechanistic, medical worldview was Martha Rogers's theory of unitary human beings (Phillips, 2015). Phillips, a valued colleague of Rogers, described her as a heretic and heroine because of her then revolutionary view about nursing and health and illness. Today her ideas resonate well with contemporary understandings of the rapidly evolving interplay across all spheres of human life.

## BOX 13-1 Relationship Between Stress and Development of Breast Cancer and Survivorship

Nurses appreciate the multiple factors in the development of breast cancer and other diseases. Researchers exploring the relationship between stress and breast cancer have demonstrated a relationship among stress (personality traits, stressful life events, and responses to stress), the immune system, genetics, and environmental factors. The physiological influences of stress on breast cancer may be mediated by the immune system. Although women may be unable to prevent stress in their lives, they can learn stress-management strategies. Dealing positively with stress may improve the quality of life for individuals and their families with or at risk of breast cancer.

Growing research evidence supports this understanding of the complex interactions between life stress and breast cancer risk. For example, Kruk (2012) examined the relationship between severe life events and breast cancer risk. Kruk used case-control examination of 858 Polish invasive breast cancer patients and 1095 controls matched for age and place of residence. Data on life events, sociodemographic characteristics, reproductive factors, family history of breast cancer, current weight and height, and lifestyle habits were collected via a self-administered questionnaire. Unconditional logistic regression analyses with odds ratios with 95% confidence intervals were estimated. After adjustment for potential breast cancer risk factors, women with four to six individual major life events had 5.33 times higher risk of breast cancer compared with those in the lowest quartile. Similarly, women with a high lifetime life change score had approximately five times higher risk compared with women with corresponding scores in the lowest range. Several life events (death of a close family member, personal injury or illness, imprisonment/trouble with the law, retirement) were significantly associated with breast cancer risk. Those findings suggest that major life events may have an important etiological role in the development of breast cancer. Surviving breast cancer also poses ongoing challenges to women who experienced breast cancer and their partners (Gregorio et al., 2012).

From Gregorio, S. W., Carpenter, K. M., Dorfman, C. S., Yang, I. L. C., Simonelli, L. F., & Carson III, W. E. (2012). Impact of breast cancer recurrence and cancer-specific stress on spouse health and immune function. *Brain, Behavior, & Immunity, 26*(2), 228–233; Kruk, J. (2012). Self-reported psychological stress and the risk of breast cancer: A case-control study. *Stress, 15*(2), 162–171; National Cancer Institute. (n.d.). *Psychological stress and cancer: Questions and answers.* http://www.cancer.gov/cancertopics/factsheet/Risk/stress.

Thus understanding stress and its management involves attention to the *interactions* of social and biological life at individual and family/communal levels. It follows that stress-management strategies/interventions need to be multifaceted and could be aimed at neurophysiological and interpersonal/social stressors and/or interactions and responses. Establishing empathy by the nurse in understanding stress is beneficial in designing interventions aimed at primary, secondary, and tertiary levels of prevention.

## PHYSICAL, PSYCHOLOGICAL, SOCIOBEHAVIORAL, AND SPIRITUAL/HOMEODYNAMIC CONSEQUENCES OF STRESS

To begin, it is necessary to set the groundwork for understanding stress and its multifaceted/interactive consequences. In the discussion that follows, facets of human responses are artificially categorized and discussed to assist the learner to discern the many aspects of stress responses. In no way should this content be interpreted as meaning that stress responses are isolated to specific human systems or simply additive. Growing understanding of the homeodynamic interplay, including epigenetics, within individuals and across human and ecological systems forces us to examine the ever-changing nature of our knowledge of our world. As a startling example, in 2016 the Zika virus emerged on the global stage to pose multiple human health risks, with a specific threat to pregnant women and their fetuses for microcephaly, a devastating birth anomaly: the effects reverberated across continents with lightning speed and had global effects on health, travel, and prevention efforts (Sifferlin, 2016). Thus we all must remain cognizant of the ongoing interplay within and among human, social, and ecological systems, even as we examine knowledge focused predominantly at specific response areas (i.e., human systems). Nevertheless, understanding stress effects at a variety of micro to macro levels is needed to comprehend a holistic picture. The future challenges to do so are indeed exciting!

## Physiological Effects of Stress

An individual's homeodynamic response to stress provides a model to examine changes across biopsychosocial-spiritual domains. In response to a perceived threat (i.e., stressor), the body prepares to meet the challenge. Perception of threat stimulates a physiological pattern of neuroendocrine activation and behavioral changes mediated by the central nervous system. Moreover, chronic stressful life circumstances likely exacerbate conditions favorable to adverse heath outcomes (Figure 13-2) (Berger et al., 2015). Nonetheless, in most cases this reaction is an adaptive, short-term, acute response to a stressor. First termed the **fight-or-flight response** (Cannon, 1914) and later called the **stress response** (Selye, 1950, 1974, 1982), the individual's reaction to a real or imagined threat prepares the body for emergency reaction and fosters survival in circumstances of immediate, time-limited threat. The hypothalamus signals the sympathetic nervous system to release epinephrine and norepinephrine, along with other related hormones. A resultant state of arousal is characterized by increased metabolism, pulse rate, blood pressure, respiration rate, and muscle tension. This physiological arousal proceeds along three main pathways: the musculoskeletal system, the autonomic nervous system, and the psychoneuroendocrine system.

The musculoskeletal system responds by increasing tension and tone. At the same time, the autonomic nervous system, via the sympathetic branch, orchestrates a generalized arousal that includes increases in heart rate, blood pressure, and respiration rate. Additionally, a heightened awareness of the environment is triggered, and blood shifts from the visceral organs to the large muscle groups. Concurrently the psychoneuroendocrine system stimulates the hypothalamic-pituitary-adrenal axis and the secretion of corticosteroids (primarily cortisol) and other neuroendocrine substances into the systemic circulation, increasing blood glucose levels, influencing sodium retention, and, in the acute phase, increasing the antiinflammatory response.

Study findings (CDC, 2012b) have shown that maladaptive stress can cause or exacerbate disease or symptoms of diseases.

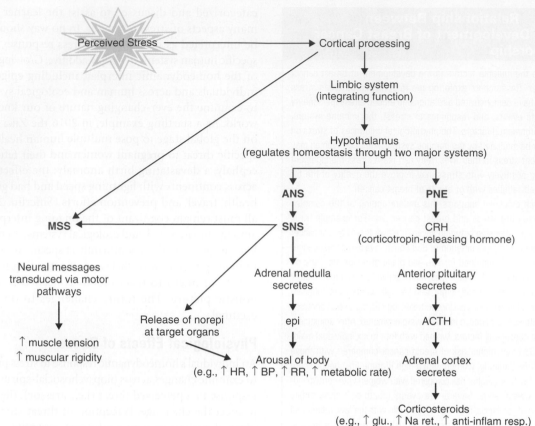

FIGURE 13-2 The stress response. *ACTH,* Adrenocorticotropic hormone; *ANS,* autonomic nervous system; *anti-inflam resp.,* antiinflammatory response; *BP,* blood pressure; *CRH,* corticotropin-releasing hormone; *epi,* epinephrine; *glu.,* blood glucose level; *HR,* heart rate; *MSS,* musculoskeletal system; *Na ret.,* sodium retention; *norepi,* norepinephrine; *PNE,* pituitary-neuroendocrine system; *RR,* respiration rate; *SNS,* sympathetic nervous system. (From Wells-Federman, C., Stuart-Shor, E., Deckro, J., Mandle, C. L., Baim, M., & Medich, C. [1995]. The mind/body connection: The psychophysiology of many traditional nursing interventions. *Clinical Nurse Specialist, 9,* 60.)

Proinflammation associated with stress is emerging as a common pathway in a variety of diseases, such as asthma, angina, cardiac arrhythmias, pain, tension headaches, insomnia, depression, and gastrointestinal disorders. Additionally, stress can produce hyperreactivity or hyporeactivity of hormones regulated by the psychoneuroendocrine system (Bonfiglio et al., 2011).

As mentioned previously, in most cases the stress response is a beneficial adaptive pattern that increases the efficiency and quality of performance, but it can prove maladaptive when a stressor continues indefinitely. Maladaptive stress (distress) is an enduring and sometimes self-sustaining cascade of responses that degenerate physical, psychosocial, and spiritual well-being. Not surprisingly, stress and specifically depression have been associated with increased susceptibility to cardiovascular disease, as well as poor response to its treatment. Inflammation has been suggested as one of the processes underlying the association between cardiovascular disease and depression, two debilitating conditions (Nikkheslat et al., 2015). Nonetheless, indirect influences of stress and depression on self-care health behaviors also help to explain associations between these diseases. Needless to say, further investigation is needed to demonstrate direct causal links, as well as effectiveness of psychological interventions, for people with cardiovascular disease (Whalley et al., 2011).

## Psychological Effects of Stress

The psychological effects of stress are best illustrated by its contributory role in negative mood states, including anxiety, depression, hostility, and anger. Exposure to stressful stimuli is associated with elevated cortisol levels and resultant effects on the immune system. The duration, intensity, and timing of a stressor have been shown to affect immune responses in animals. Although systematic studies to explain different patterns of immune response with humans are not yet adequate, the interactive nature of the mind and immune system is an exciting area of investigation that may contribute to future evidence-based practice (Hou & Baldwin, 2012).

A growing body of clinical research outcomes illustrates the interplay of stress and various health outcomes. For example, research evidence is convincing that individuals with eating disorders experience a high rate of stress, and that appraisal is more important than the nature of any stressful event itself (Courbasson & Jeyarajan, 2011). The relationship between stress and cardiac symptoms also is well documented. Closa and colleagues (2010) demonstrated that for individuals awaiting angiography, stress and lack of social support predicted self-reported cardiac symptoms, regardless of actual disease severity. Clinical implications include reducing perceived stress and ruminative, angry coping styles by encouraging reappraisal and support seeking. In conclusion, the evidence to date demonstrates a strong association between chronic stress and negative health effects for individuals and their family members.

## Sociobehavioral Effects of Stress

In response to stress, individuals often revert to or increase their reliance on less healthy behaviors, such as overeating, excessive use of alcohol or drugs, and smoking. Recognizing that such behaviors are inconsistent with the healthy behaviors needed to cope with stress is easy; however, stopping these behaviors and using health-promoting strategies instead is not. Risky behaviors and traits such as a sedentary lifestyle, obesity, overeating high-fat foods, smoking, substance abuse, and social isolation have been linked to morbidity and mortality (USDHHS, 2011). Conversely, exercise, healthy diet, smoking cessation, healthy weight maintenance, and social interaction have been identified as leading indicators of health in the United States (USDHHS, 2011). Encouraging these health behaviors supports the goals of *Healthy People 2020*. However, unless we understand how psychosocial factors affect health behaviors, promotion of effective self-care is an unrealistic goal (Box 13-2: *Healthy People 2020*).

## Spiritual Effects of Stress

Interest in the connection between spirituality and health is significant. Spirituality is defined in many ways, but key components are typically that spirituality comprises feelings, thoughts, experiences, and behaviors that arise from a search for meaning and may include interconnectedness with self, others, nature, and a higher force called God, a life-force/higher power, nature, or the transcendent. Spirituality and religion intersect for many, yet they are not synonymous. Many individuals feel spiritual without a formal religious affiliation or practice. In response to stress, people often feel disconnected from life's meaning and purpose; harmful effects on their health and well-being can result.

Stressful events can shatter individuals' spiritual center or conversely can move individuals to seek comfort in spirituality or religious practice, beliefs, or community. Encouraging involvement with one's religious/spiritual practices is recommended as a helpful intervention for stress-related problems (Weber, 2011).

Examination of spiritual healing in the aftermath of men's childhood mistreatment through nursing research unearthed the following themes (Willis et al., 2015):

- Exploring spiritual faith traditions as a foundation for spiritual healing
- Being in spiritual community serves as a foundation for spiritual healing
- Being in spiritual community facilities healing connections with other human beings and the transcendent
- Cultivating spiritual consciousness through prayer, music, yoga, nature, and reading spiritual material expands awareness of one's spiritual being
- Loving and letting go reflects one's spirituality and humanity
- Believing in a cosmic energy, divine purpose, or higher power can bring a sense of healing

These themes provide foundations for nursing interventions to be tested (Willis et al., 2015). Engaging a pastoral counselor of the individual's choice in the treatment team can be an effective strategy to promote spiritual healing. However, the source of mistreatment must be carefully explored sensitively with the individual in advance to determine the acceptability of engaging a member of the clergy.

The previous section discussed how stress can adversely affect biological, cognitive, emotional, behavioral, and spiritual well-being. This understanding of the psychophysiology of the mind-body-spirit connection is fundamental to the application of stress management in nursing and provides an obvious rationale for a multifaceted approach. Further support is provided from research endorsing the health-promoting effects of managing stress (Gregorio et al., 2012) (Box 13-3: Research for Evidence-Based Practice).

## HEALTH BENEFITS OF MANAGING STRESS

A growing body of evidence underscores the importance of controlling stress to promote health and quality of life for people with a variety of health problems. "The association between stressors and biomarkers specific to physiological systems (i.e., cardiovascular, neuroendocrine, immune, etc.) is an emerging area of interest in biomedical research…with evidence that specific stressors may differentially affect various physiological systems" (Paradies, 2011). Thus interventions that reduce the stress response are an important component of comprehensive disease prevention and management. Psychotherapeutic approaches, such as interpersonal and cognitive-behavioral psychotherapies that focus on perception and management of life stressors, are effective treatments for depression and related mental health disorders (Sadock & Sadock, 2015). These psychotherapies have been incorporated into a range of treatment and secondary prevention programs, such as cardiac rehabilitation, with great potential for wider adapted use (Menezes et al., 2011). Targeting primary

 ## BOX 13-2 HEALTHY PEOPLE 2020

### *Health-Related Quality of Life and Well-Being*

Health-related quality of life (HRQoL) is a "multi-dimensional concept that includes domains related to physical, mental, emotional and social functioning." HRQoL is a new topic in *Healthy People 2020* and goes beyond "direct measures of population health, life expectancy and causes of death, and focuses on the impact health status has on quality of life. A related concept of HRQoL is well-being, which assesses the positive aspects of a person's life, such as positive emotions and life satisfaction." As explained in this chapter, stress is a challenge to HRQoL. Stress management is a key strategy to improving HRQoL.

From US Department of Health and Human Services. (2014). *Health-related quality of life & well-being.* http://healthypeople.gov/2020/topicsobjectives2020/overview.aspx?topicid=19.

## BOX 13-3 RESEARCH FOR EVIDENCE-BASED PRACTICE

### Impact of Breast Cancer Recurrence and Cancer-Specific Stress on Spouse Health and Immune Function

Spouses of people with cancer are often primary informal caregivers for their partners. As a group, they experience a variety of poor health outcomes. This study examined the relative contributions of cancer recurrence—a cancer-specific stressful event—and the subjective experience of cancer-specific stress in a sample of male spouses of breast cancer survivors. The investigators hypothesized that stress would contribute to poorer physical health and compromised immune function. Given the difficulty of random assignment for this type of study, the researchers used a matched-control design, comparing spouses of women with recurrence to a cohort of spouses whose wives were disease-free but had a history of breast cancer. Spouses of women experiencing a first recurrence were matched to spouses of women with no evidence of disease. The results showed that cancer recurrence status was not a significant predictor of spouses' physical health or immune function; however, among all spouses, cancer-specific stress symptoms were associated with increased physical symptoms and altered T-cell blastogenesis. These findings suggest that health effects for these caregiving spouses were more strongly connected to their subjective experience of cancer as stressful, rather than their partners' current disease status. A practice implication is that exploring spouses' appraisals of the experience should be an essential component of family care when one partner has breast cancer.

From Gregorio, S. W., Carpenter, K. M., Dorfman, C. S., Yang, H. C., Simonelli, L. E., & Carson III, W. E. (2012). Impact of breast cancer recurrence and cancer-specific stress on spouse health and immune function. *Brain, Behavior, & Immunity, 26,* 228–233.

prevention programs is the aim of nurses in assisting individuals with stress reduction before becoming symptomatic.

Promoting a positive attitude and development of skills to cope with stress is foundational to many stress-management interventions. As early as 1982, Kobasa and colleagues (1982) made a groundbreaking contribution to our understanding of the stress-illness relationship when they identified characteristics of hardiness. They described individuals with stress-hardy characteristics who, when exercising and accessing social support, were less vulnerable to stress-related symptoms and diseases. The characteristics of stress hardiness are control, challenge, and commitment. For stress-hardy individuals, stress is viewed as a challenge rather than a threat; they feel in control of situations in their lives, and they are committed to rather than alienated from work, home, and family. Hardiness continues to be assessed (recognized) by nurses in assisting individuals and families dealing with a crisis and promoting the strengths of survivorship in dealing with new stressors. Another term that is used is resiliency.

Stress management is especially important in situations such as caregiving that extend over long periods. Caregiver stress/burden can be described as the appraisal of the experience of caregiving including the taxing nature of behaviors of the recipient of care, role conflict or strain, and physical and mental health effects on the caregiver (McLennon et al., 2011). As the setting for care increasingly is the home and family members take on mounting responsibility for care of loved ones (i.e., children, spouses, or aging parents with chronic conditions), the importance of caring for the caregiver to prevent significant burnout grows. As a result of current trends of delayed parenting and increased life span, the "sandwich generation" of middle-aged adults who have concurrent responsibility for their children and aging parents is at particular risk of severe caregiver burden. Research evidence supports the usefulness of interventions aimed at helping caregivers to find meaning in their activities and role in buffering caregiver stress (McLennon et al., 2011; Quinn et al., 2011; Wood et al., 2015). Moreover, the quality of the caregiver–care recipient relationship can affect the caregiver's well-being (Quinn et al., 2011).

In summary, the evidence is conclusive that thoughts, feelings, behaviors, beliefs, and biological activity are interrelated. Perceptions, or the way individuals view situations, can lead to stress and, in turn, adversely affect biological activity, emotions, behavior, and the connection with life meaning and purpose. This interaction among perceptions, stress, and multifaceted effects, in turn, can increase stress and foster a negative stress cycle. The remainder of this chapter presents assessment of stress relating to the homeodynamic framework, including the facets of physical, psychosocial, and spiritual health and well-being of individuals, and describes the application of a variety of strategies shown to help break the negative stress cycle and mitigate its harmful effects across the biological, psychosocial, and spiritual domains.

## ASSESSMENT OF STRESS

Assessment of the stress-coping abilities of an individual, family, or community is part of a comprehensive health assessment that includes past and present subjective and objective data. Collection of these data enables the individual and the nurse to determine the status of the person's stress-coping pattern, and actual and potential strengths and weaknesses.

The nurse thoroughly collects data during the history, physical examination, and health patterns assessment (see Chapters 7–9). Identifying the stress-coping pattern is especially important. Asking for specific examples of events with probes to elicit the person's thoughts, feelings, and actions leads to discussion of appraisal and ideas for alternative actions in the future (see Chapter 4, Box 4-12 and Figure 4-4). Each individual is the primary data source; no other person can explain accurately the individual's perceptions of the stressors, stress responses, and resources to prevent or alleviate the stress.

Stress is experienced across biological, psychosocial, and spiritual domains; therefore all perceptions are important for the assessment. Throughout the assessment process, individuals may become aware of information of which they were previously unaware, or they may identify information related to their perceived problems. For example, a man may be aware of the stress of his job but may be unaware that his high blood pressure was caused at least in part by this stress.

Lazarus and Folkman (1984) proposed a theory comprising primary and secondary appraisals of stressful events, situations, or demands and the effectiveness of an individual's coping skills. Primary appraisal of coping includes descriptions of perceived actual and potential positive and negative outcomes. Negative outcomes refer to harm, whereas positive outcomes refer to the challenges resulting from stressors that an individual perceives can be overcome. Examples of negative outcomes include physical injury; disease; loss of a cherished relationship, position, or possession; and death. Positive outcomes include graduation, promotion, and development of important relationships (see the case study and care plan at the end of this chapter).

Secondary appraisal follows primary appraisal. Secondary appraisal consists of the individual's identification of choices to cope with the actual or potential harm, threat, or challenge. The choices may be internal or external resources and responses. For example, a social resource in coping with the needs of a toddler might be learning strategies in a parent-effectiveness training course. A coping response to the challenges of parenting a toddler might be restructuring the toddler's and parent's schedules to allow for more frequent cycles of activities and rest.

The individual's primary and secondary appraisals of stress provide opportunities to consider the stress experiences in different ways. Resources that had been forgotten may be remembered, or a threat may be newly viewed as a challenge and an opportunity for enhanced development and status. The appraisal process mediates stress responses. This understanding supports use of cognitive-behavioral therapy (CBT) as an effective intervention approach for stress-related problems (Wood et al., 2015). Nurses appropriately may refer individuals for CBT and are also encouraged to obtain advanced training in CBT to integrate this evidence-based intervention into their practice. Use of good-quality health texts aimed at the general population is also an effective psychoeducational approach. For example, Marchant's (2016) highly readable book *Cure: A Journey Into the Science of Mind Over Body* and Kaku's (2014) interesting text *The Future of the Mind* are examples of materials that can serve as springboards for discussion of ways to adjust the meaning of life stressors, responses, and ways to cope.

Measuring stress and related symptoms/responses is important in assessment and evaluation of treatment outcomes. By using measurement instruments with established reliability and validity, nurses can improve assessment of an individual's stress and coping. Tools can help nurses distinguish between diagnoses that have many signs and symptoms in common. For example, disturbances in thinking and feeling processes can be difficult to distinguish and may have confounding clinical pictures. These disturbances can occur separately or simultaneously in the same person. An example of this complexity is the overlapping symptoms of depression and dementia. The nurse determines whether one health problem is actually the cause of the other so as to develop an effective plan of care (see the case study and care plan at the end of this chapter).

A wide variety of instruments are available to help nurses assess orientation, attention, cognitive skills and patterns, traits and states of emotions, symptoms of mental health distress and disorders, and overall quality of life. For example, the Schedule of Recent Experiences (Holmes, 1981) and the Impact of Event Scale (Horowitz et al., 1979) are two well-established instruments used widely in clinical assessment and research to measure stress associated with life changes and events. Burnout, be it work

related or personal, is understood as emotional exhaustion, depersonalization, and a sense of reduced personal accomplishment. The Maslach Burnout Inventory (Maslach & Jackson, 1986) is a psychometrically robust instrument to assess perceptions about work-life balance. Before using any instrument, clinicians and researchers need to check information about its reliability and validity, updates/revisions, training requirements, and copyright restrictions (e.g., purchase requirements) that can affect access to its use. Older instruments typically have a long-established record of demonstrated reliability and validity; however, phenomena may evolve with time, and revised versions may have been developed and tested for specific populations. Therefore exploration of the literature to seek updated information to inform use is always wise. Additionally, the seeking of consultation from clinical experts/researchers regarding instrument selection is recommended.

Use of standardized instruments promotes accuracy in developing diagnoses and care plans and assists in evaluating the effectiveness of care. For example, a nurse may compare an individual's self-evaluation and/or symptom preintervention scores with postintervention scores and revise the care plan accordingly. Additionally, nurses may analyze population baseline scores for relevant characteristics and develop programs of research and quality improvements aimed at improving outcomes.

Assessment at the family and community levels is also recommended. Family assessment consists of three major categories: structural, developmental, and functional components of the family (Wright & Leahey, 2013). Environmental factors also contribute to the determinants of health and thus to stress, so a thorough nursing assessment requires consideration of the community. For example, examination of community-level data for unemployment, population density, housing, school quality, crime, suicide incidence, and disease occurrence patterns (i.e., health profiles of the community), as well as availability of various amenities such as green space and access to transportation and healthy foods, provides a more complete stress assessment than does individual assessment alone (DeMarco & Segraves, 2011). Moreover, family and community assessment can point to possible stress-reduction interventions, such as marshaling available social support or engaging in outdoor activities and exercise.

## STRESS-MANAGEMENT INTERVENTIONS

Stress-management strategies are beneficial to people across a broad spectrum of chronological, gender, cultural, and ethnic characteristics. Men and women, young and old, from divergent socioeconomic, cultural, and ethnic backgrounds can benefit from stress-management interventions. Sensitivity to the needs and values of individuals and communities, particularly for high-risk groups (i.e., vulnerable populations), guides assessment and intervention techniques. The language, belief system, and cultural distinctions of individuals and families in the community guide the choice and adoption of stress-management strategies. Understanding stress and its management involves attention to the *interactions* of social and biological life at individual and family/communal levels (Barchas & Barchas, 2011); therefore interventions may need to encompass a variety and combination of psychosocial and biological approaches at the primary, secondary, and tertiary levels of prevention. Population-based interventions may be expanded from the individual to the community and to a system- or population-focused practice (Harkness & DeMarco, 2012).

## Developing Self-Awareness

Self-awareness is one of the most effective stress-management tools. Self-awareness helps people learn about interactions among mind, body, and spirit; increases a sense of control; and counters self-defeating perceptions. Interventions that promote self-awareness help people make sense of life events and circumstances that may be bewildering or discomforting. Many experiences in life lead to feelings of emptiness and disharmony because people are unable to connect the experience with thoughts, feelings, actions, and physiological responses. Self-awareness helps individuals recognize stress that they create through negative, exaggerated, unrealistic thinking. This recognition affords an opportunity to change these negative thought patterns, thereby decreasing stress and increasing control. Strategies that increase self-awareness can empower individuals to make new connections and to reframe and reinterpret their experiences in light of their own inner strengths and wisdom.

A closely related concept is mindfulness, nonjudgmental self-awareness characterized by intentional acceptance of the unfolding of experience in the moment. Mindfulness can be understood as having two components: "the intentional self-regulation of attention so that it remains focused on present-moment experiences (i.e., thoughts and feelings) as they arise" (Baer, 2014) and "an attitude of openness, acceptance, and curiosity toward whatever arises" (Baer, 2014). Mindfulness requires dedicated practice both to achieve and to use to reduce negative stress effects. A variety of mindfulness approaches have been proposed and tested. Those with the best empirical support are mindfulness-based stress reduction, dialectical behavior therapy, and acceptance and commitment therapy (Baer, 2014). Mindfulness interventions can be combined with other efficacious treatments or can serve as primary interventions for stress management. Mindfulness as both a state and an intervention is not simple although it may appear so at first. Therefore nurses are urged to obtain specialized training in mindfulness approaches so they can use them in their practice. Mindfulness interventions have shown promise to improve quality of life in coping with various health conditions. For example, Lengacher and colleagues (2015) demonstrated the cost-effectiveness and efficacy of a mindfulness stress-reduction program in improving quality of life for breast cancer survivors.

The neuroscience basis of mindfulness remains a fruitful field of investigation. As is common to new areas of research, the studies to date generally lack robust methods and offer only speculative conclusions (Tang et al., 2015). Nonetheless, there is developing evidence that mindfulness meditation may precipitate neuroplastic changes "in the structure, and function of brain regions involved in regulation of attention, emotion and self-awareness" (Tang et al., 2015). The horizons are vast and exciting for future nurse scientists to engage in team science to explore the underpinnings of interventions such as mindfulness.

## Techniques for Developing Self-Awareness

*Monitoring stress warning signs.* The negative stress cycle can be difficult to interrupt. Recognizing warning signs of stress is a necessary first step. Often individuals have long ignored physical, emotional, or behavioral cues or reactions to a stressor that are stress warning signs. A man who has chronic, intermittent backaches and ignores the daily muscle tension caused by poor posture that precedes the backaches provides an example. If he had attended to his early stress warning signs of poor posture and muscle tension, he might have avoided the backache that kept him from exercising and socializing. Becoming aware of these stress warning signs is the first step. Attending to these cues is the next step. After this connection has been made, the development of skills to reduce negative mood states, unhealthy behaviors, and physical symptoms becomes much easier. Furthermore, some people misinterpret physiological signs of anxiety (e.g., shortness of breath, racing heartbeat) as indicative of serious physical danger (e.g., suffocation, myocardial infarction). This tendency to misinterpret physical anxiety cues is referred to as anxiety sensitivity, a belief that body sensations associated with anxiety indicate imminent and dangerous outcomes, and is associated with various anxiety disorders and health anxiety. In a study of gender differences in anxiety sensitivity, Thompson and colleagues (2011) found that distraction worked better than sensation focusing in reducing stress for males. By assisting individuals who are prone to anxiety sensitivity to interpret body sensations accurately or to distract from the sensation, nurses can help reduce individuals' misinterpretations, as well as the likelihood of escalation of anxiety symptoms and possibly even development of anxiety disorders.

Nurses teach people to identify their warning signals of stress and to stop, take a few breaths, and break the cycle. Figure 13-3 shows a sample form for identifying and recording this information. These signals or cues differ among individuals and can be physical, emotional, behavioral, cognitive, relational, or spiritual. When asked to monitor their responses to a particular event, individuals become more consciously aware of these cues. Although this heightened awareness initially may increase an individual's consciousness of physical pain or emotional discomfort, awareness is a necessary first step in recognizing the negative effects of stress and the relationship of thoughts, feelings, behavior, and biological processes. In addition, nurses and other clinicians have a responsibility to screen individuals for emotional distress to help them recognize and monitor their own physical and mood states. For individuals with health conditions such as coronary artery disease, which is known to have high comorbidity with emotional distress and specifically depression, routine screening should be the standard of care (Menezes et al., 2011).

Try this: Ask an individual to identify a stressful experience and the physical or emotional reactions (stress warning signals) to that particular experience. For example, after being instructed to stop, take a breath, and notice the physical and emotional response to a stressful situation, one woman related the following:

*On my way to work yesterday, I sat in a huge traffic jam. I noticed that my heart was racing, my breathing had changed,*

**Physical Symptoms**

____ Headaches
____ Indigestion
____ Stomachaches
____ Sweaty palms
____ Sleep difficulties
____ Dizziness

____ Back pain
____ Tight neck and shoulders
____ Racing heart
____ Restlessness
____ Tiredness
____ Ringing in ears

**Behavioral Symptoms**

____ Excess smoking
____ Bossiness
____ Compulsive gum chewing
____ Attitude critical of others

____ Grinding of teeth at night
____ Overuse of alcohol
____ Compulsive eating
____ Inability to get things done

**Emotional Symptoms**

____ Crying
____ Nervousness and anxiety
____ Boredom (no meaning to things)
____ Edginess (ready to explode)
____ Feeling powerless to change things

____ Overwhelming sense of pressure
____ Anger
____ Loneliness
____ Unhappiness for no reason
____ Easily upset

**Cognitive Symptoms**

____ Trouble thinking clearly
____ Lack of creativity
____ Memory loss
____ Forgetfulness

____ Inability to make decisions
____ Thoughts of running away
____ Constant worry
____ Loss of sense of humor

**Spiritual Symptoms**

____ Emptiness
____ Loss of meaning
____ Doubt
____ Unforgiving
____ Martyrdom
____ Looking for magic
____ Loss of direction
____ Cynicism
____ Apathy
____ Needing to "prove" self

**Relational Symptoms**

____ Isolation
____ Intolerance
____ Resentment
____ Loneliness
____ Lashing out
____ Hiding
____ Clamming up
____ Lowered sex drive
____ Nagging
____ Distrust
____ Lack of intimacy
____ Using people

**FIGURE 13-3** Stress warning signals. (From Medical symptom reduction clinic patient notebook. [n.d.]. Boston: The Benson-Henry Institute for Mind Body Medicine of Massachusetts General Hospital, Harvard Medical School.)

*and my hands were gripping the steering wheel. I felt angry and frustrated because I was going to be late for work.*

Although these responses seem quite obvious, most people are unaware of the effects of stress on their minds and bodies. In the preceding example, the building of the woman's stress may continue to escalate at work, influencing her interactions with coworkers. Once individuals become aware of these effects, they may be able to release tension more easily, countering the negative effects of stress and increasing a sense of control. Techniques that help to reduce negative effects of stress include use of distraction by purposefully shifting focus to pleasant thoughts or engaging in a diversion activity, and use of a **relaxation response** technique, as described in the following section.

***Learning and practicing a relaxation response technique.***
Eliciting the relaxation response is another technique to help people develop awareness and counter the negative effects of stress. Relaxation response techniques oppose the stress response by reducing sympathetic arousal (Benson, 1975). The immediate physiological effects of relaxation are decreases in heart rate, blood pressure, respiration rate, and muscle tension. The long-term physiological effect is a decrease in central nervous system arousal with a concomitant decrease in musculoskeletal system, autonomic nervous system, and psychoneuroendocrine system arousal. To the extent that stress causes or exacerbates a symptom, elicitation of the relaxation response can break this stress-symptom cycle. In addition to these physiological changes, psychological changes such as improved mood and behavioral changes, including a reduction in risky behaviors, can occur. The relaxation response can counteract stress-related disease processes, particularly processes associated with immunological, cardiovascular, and neurodegenerative disorders (Walsh, 2011).

The relaxation response is an innate physiological response (Benson, 1975); therefore a number of techniques that involve mental focusing can be used. Details on these techniques and guidelines for clinical applications can be found in Chapter 14. All of these techniques have two basic components:
- The repetition of a word, sound, phrase, prayer, image, or physical activity
- The passive disregard of everyday thoughts when they occur Electronic recordings (e.g., DVDs, CDs, MP3/MP4 files, and mobile apps/downloads) can be used to help guide this process of focusing, especially during the initial learning phase.

Nurses can often introduce individuals to the immediate calming effects of the relaxation response in less than 5 minutes. One effective way is to have the person make a fist and notice what happens to the breathing pattern. Most people have a tendency to hold their breath while tensing a body part. Now ask the person to take a few deep diaphragmatic breaths while making a fist. Most people will notice that the tension is much harder to maintain while taking a deep breath. This awareness helps to recognize the relationship between breath and tension. Lamaze techniques for helping women manage pain during labor and delivery are based on this connection between breathing and relaxation. Most people hold their breath when they perceive a threat (stress), feel anxious, or become angry. By stopping and taking a few deep breaths when they become aware of physical changes (holding the breath or clenching the jaw) or emotional changes (feeling anxious or angry), individuals can elicit the relaxation response, reduce sympathetic arousal, calm negative mood states, and gain a sense of control. Yoga and deep breathing can assist with mindfulness (i.e., awareness of perception) and promote relaxation.

***Using mini relaxations.*** Mini relaxations can be taught quickly and used throughout the day to help develop awareness and to counter the negative effects of stress on the mind, body, and spirit. Individuals can be taught to monitor minor stress warning signs (jaw and shoulder tension) and to use a mini-relaxation exercise to keep these initial symptoms of stress from developing into an incapacitating tension headache. A mini-relaxation exercise can be anything from a few conscious, deep diaphragmatic breaths

---

### BOX 13-4  QUALITY AND SAFETY SCENARIO

#### A Stress-Management Strategy for Nurses

Develop the skill of personal presence. Presence is the gift of self through availability and attention to needs. Presence means "being there" for another person. To be available to others in this way, first practice the skill of being present with yourself. One effective way of developing this skill is through mindfulness, which is the ability to focus attention on what you are experiencing from moment to moment. Mindfulness encompasses the abilities of slowing down and bringing your full attention (thoughts, feelings, and body sensations) to the action in which you are engaged at the moment. The practice can be particularly useful in allowing yourself to extend the benefits of eliciting the relaxation response in more areas of your daily life.

The following are some ideas for practicing personal presence (mindfulness):
- When you awaken each morning, bring your full attention to your breathing. Allow your awareness to expand gradually into the room and then slowly begin to listen to the sounds of the outdoors.
- On your way to work, focus on how you walk, drive, or ride the transit. Take some deep diaphragmatic breaths and relax your body as you travel.
- Take a moment to attend to your breath, relax your body, and focus your mind before entering a care recipient's room.
- As you eat a meal, carefully examine it through all of your senses—the sight, smell, touch, taste, and the sound of each bite. Mindfully enjoy this new experience.
- Recurring events of the day can become cues for a mini relaxation (the ringing telephone; auscultating a heartbeat; answering a call light, before, during, and after rounds or report).
- Make the transition home from work mindful. Leave thoughts and worries of work at work and be conscious of your home environment each day.

Once again, focus on your breathing and become completely aware of your surroundings as you go to sleep. Practice mindfully letting go of today and tomorrow as you allow your mind and body to get some much-needed rest.

Modified from Benson-Henry Institute for Mind Body Medicine of Massachusetts General Hospital. (n.d.). *Stress*. https://www.bensonhenryinstitute.org/

---

to several minutes of sitting quietly (Box 13-4: Quality and Safety Scenario). Practice is needed to elicit the response quickly when stress, pain, or tension is recognized. The power of using relaxation, including visualization, and breathing techniques is illustrated by the personal experience of a nurse who had coached pregnant women and partners in Lamaze preparation for childbirth for 10 years before having her third baby. During pitocin induction due to a postdate determination, the woman was experiencing significant contractions. Her very experienced labor nurse commented that she was an advertisement for childbirth preparation. The woman managed a smile in response. The woman reflected:

*The contractions were tough. I think that the pitocin escalated the process so that contractions increased quickly from mild to intense. Did my Lamaze relaxation techniques help? Oh yes. Was it still painful—Oh yes. However, I was able to make it through this and two previous labors and deliveries without an epidural by using relaxation techniques that I had taught and practiced. I cannot emphasize enough that relaxation techniques including breathing, visualization, distraction, and partner/nurse coaching support are powerful tools. These techniques require practice to be called upon in an instant of pain or stress. Medication and/or anesthesia remain as helpful tools in situations of acute pain such as labor, surgery, injury, or ongoing stress, but the power of our capacities to harness our own abilities are powerful and should not be overlooked. Let's empower ourselves so that pharmacotherapeutics is not the immediate go-to solution for stress and pain!*

***Alternative and complementary therapies.*** A variety of alternative and complementary therapies can prevent and reduce harmful effects of stress (Snyder & Lindquist, 2010). These therapies include acupuncture, hypnosis, aromatherapy, reflexology, reiki, and chiropractic and herbal therapies. These approaches have developed outside the mainstream of traditional Western medicine; however, developing evidence of efficacy has promoted growing acceptance of some of these approaches. People are increasingly using alternative and complementary practices as self-help measures, and research to study their effects has exploded in recent years. Nurses can help individuals evaluate the safety and efficacy of various alternative and complementary therapies. In particular, herbal remedies require cautious use because they can have harmful, as well as beneficial, effects, and they sometimes interfere with other treatments and medications. Among the alternative therapies available, there is strong evidence of effectiveness of acupuncture and hypnosis, and they are becoming widely accepted within mainstream health care.

Acupuncture is an ancient Chinese technique used to reduce pain and to prevent and manage various disorders by placement of fine needles at specific meridian points on the body. Acupuncture is not a self-help approach, so seeking treatment from an experienced acupuncturist is required. The Western scientific community cannot explain why acupuncture works but acknowledges its effectiveness. Even the World Health Organization has listed illnesses that can be managed with acupuncture (Stuart, 2013), and some health insurance plans provide reimbursement for acupuncture treatments.

*Hypnosis* comes from a Greek word meaning sleep. Hypnosis narrows consciousness and elicits relaxation, inertia, and passivity, like sleep, yet awareness is never lost completely and the hypnotized person can respond (Brann et al., 2011). The exact mechanisms through which hypnosis works are not known, although perhaps its ability to induce deep relaxation and its possible action in shifting brain activity from the "analytical" left side to the "nonanalytical" right side might be explanatory. Nevertheless, its effectiveness in managing a variety of conditions, notably smoking and anxiety-related problems, and managing pain is well recognized. Trained therapists provide hypnotherapy to manage stress and various mental health problems, including phobias, addictions, and posttraumatic stress disorder. Self-hypnosis, a form of deep relaxation similar to the relaxation techniques described in this chapter, can be a useful stress-reduction tool. Self-help guides provide safe and easy-to-follow guidelines. One note of caution is warranted: hypnosis is not recommended for people with organic brain disorders, psychotic disorders, or other severe mental disorders. For individuals with trauma histories, practice with an expert clinician is recommended.

Reiki (pronounced ray-kee) is made up of two Japanese words: *rei*, or universal spirit (sometimes thought of as a supreme being), and *ki*. Thus the word reiki means universal life energy. Reiki is a therapy that uses energy fields with the intent to affect health. To transmit ki, believed to be a life-force energy, the reiki practitioner places hands on or near the person receiving treatment. In the United States, reiki is designated as a form of complementary and alternative medicine (National Center for Complementary and Alternative Medicine, n.d.; Snyder & Lindquist, 2010).

***Expressive writing.*** Transforming thoughts and emotions related to stressful experiences into written language has demonstrated positive effects on health (North et al., 2011). In its therapeutic meaning, expressive writing involves telling a "story" about traumatic, emotionally charged, or stressful events and personal reactions. Journal writing—more specifically, self-confessional writing—is a form of expressive writing that is typically done via entries in a journal over time that describe unfolding personal responses to life events. Expressive writing is useful in disclosing and processing emotions, and in measurably improving physical and mental health.

Expressive writing, including journaling, can help people reflect on stressful events and their reactions to these events. Such reflection is an opportunity to reform perceptions and to consider alternative ways to manage stress. Individuals may find resolutions to conflicts that work uniquely for them. These resolutions may then increase a sense of control and mediate negative consequences of stress. This self-reflective process shares elements of CBT—an intervention effective in reducing harmful effects of stress. (See Chapter 4, Figure 4-4.)

Nurses can advise people to get a special notebook or a journal (or use an electronic tablet or computer) and write about a stressful event for 15 minutes a day in a setting in which they will not be interrupted. From a health perspective, people will be more effective when they make themselves the only audience. The nurse should warn the individual that he or she may feel sad or depressed immediately after the writing session, but these feelings usually dissipate within an hour. Nonetheless, exploring deep thoughts and feelings on paper is not a panacea. When an individual is coping with death, divorce, or some other major stressor, feeling better instantly after writing cannot be expected. A person can, however, develop a clearer understanding of feelings and of the situation through journal writing. In other words, journal writing helps people objectify experiences, identify the influence of stress on symptoms, and develop insights into more effective problem-solving. Some individuals may recognize the need for psychotherapeutic support through journal writing, and an appropriate referral can then be made. Nurses can use the same approaches to examine their own stressful work-related situations to reflect, analyze their responses/reactions, and generate effective responses to similar experiences in the future.

## Nutrition: Healthy Diet

Countering negative effects of stress requires caring for physical health and well-being. The mind and body are connected;

therefore paying attention to one while ignoring the other does not promote overall health. The body requires rest, a healthy diet of balanced food choices, and exercise. In the last few decades, nutrition has moved to the forefront as a major component of health promotion, disease prevention, and symptom management. Food is now viewed as a positive influence on health, physical performance, and state of mind rather than simply a fuel needed to prevent disease and sustain life. Adaptive eating is characterized by balanced eating patterns and calorie intake as well as appropriate body weight for height. Nutrition is an important component of early intervention strategies to improve physical, cognitive, emotional, social, and spiritual functioning.

However, the American lifestyle has made practicing healthy eating habits increasingly difficult. Americans frequently replace nutritionally balanced meals with readily available high-fat, high-calorie food (US Department of Agriculture, 2012). One of the frustrations that nurses experience is trying to help children and adults develop healthy eating habits. This effort requires planning and correctly choosing a variety of foods and eating a diet low in fat, saturated fat, and cholesterol, with plenty of vegetables, fruits, and grain products. The current US dietary guidelines (US Department of Agriculture, 2012) are based on the following two overarching concepts: focus on calorie balance over time to achieve and maintain a healthy weight; focus on consuming nutrient-dense foods and beverages. Daily food choices should be made from the five food groups. Key recommendations also highlight the importance of calorie control and physical activity. Guidelines continue to undergo evaluation and revision; for example, guidelines about "healthy foods" are under ongoing review, so nurses are urged to check for updated guidelines. A detailed discussion of the health benefits of balanced nutrition and guidelines throughout the life span can be found in Chapter 11.

Encouraging healthier dietary choices helps people to recognize that control over their health and well-being is possible. This knowledge, in turn, helps counter the negative effects of stress and lower the stress-disinhibition effect that can influence poor dietary choices. Nurses encourage people to monitor their daily dietary patterns to gain awareness of how they use food in times of stress. Tools such as food diaries (24-hour recall) help people to monitor the amount and quality of what they eat and drink and to set realistic goals. An example of an on-line free program is MyFitnessPal (2015), which combines nutrition tips and a way to monitor exercise in a journal format.

## Physical Activity

Combining a healthy diet with a regular exercise routine has many health benefits and can positively affect quality of life. For example, one of the most effective ways to lose weight and improve self-esteem is to combine exercise with nutritious eating. Exercise (physical activity that increases strength and flexibility and improves conditioning) and balanced nutrition serve as protective factors against several major chronic diseases. Regular physical activity decreases the risk of death from heart disease, lowers the risk of developing diabetes, and is associated with a decreased risk of colon cancer (USDHHS, 2011). Exercise helps prevent high blood pressure and helps lower blood pressure in people with elevated levels. Regular physical activity, even at moderate levels, is associated with lower death rates for adults of any age. Psychological well-being is enhanced, and the risk of developing depression can be reduced; regular physical activity appears to reduce symptoms of depression and anxiety and to improve mood.

Additionally, children and adolescents need weight-bearing exercise for normal skeletal development, and young adults need this type of exercise to achieve and maintain peak bone mass (USDHHS, 2011). Regular physical activity also increases the ability of older people, and those with certain chronic, disabling conditions, to perform activities of daily living. Nevertheless, high stress could increase injury risk for athletes, and injured athletes may experience greater stress than noninjured peers when they are sidelined from competition. Chapter 12 provides a comprehensive discussion of the benefits of exercise and its clinical application throughout the life span.

Regular physical activity helps people adopt a more active lifestyle as they begin to feel better physically and emotionally, thereby breaking the negative stress cycle (Figure 13-4). Positive effects can be obtained with exercise of only moderate intensity. For example, a brisk walk of 30 to 60 minutes, 3 to 5 times a week, promotes fitness and decreases the risk of disease. Being physically active on a daily basis is extremely important; therefore nurses can help individuals increase their physical activity by suggesting a variety of activities in which they might engage each day (Box 13-5). An exercise diary can generate a baseline for usual activity to set realistic goals and monitor progress. By simply changing a few daily routines, individuals can gain enormous physical, psychosocial, and spiritual rewards that promote health and break the negative stress cycle.

## Sleep Hygiene

Health and the ability to meet life's many demands and manage stress effectively require proper rest. Many people experience sleep deprivation and sleep disorders (e.g., sleep apnea) that can cause or exacerbate conditions such as depression and fatigue and contribute to poor concentration and ineffective problem-solving. Insomnia can be induced by stress or other cognitive-behavioral factors, such as unrealistic expectations, inappropriate scheduling of sleep, trying too hard to sleep, consuming caffeine,

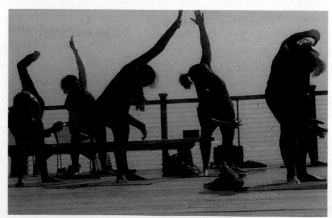

**FIGURE 13-4** Regular physical activity helps individuals adopt a more active lifestyle.

## BOX 13-5  Helping Individuals Increase Physical Activity

Nurses can suggest ways for individuals to increase physical activity throughout the day, including:

- Have fun and play active games with children.
- Engage in a sport.
- Find a friend with whom to walk or jog.
- Take a class in yoga or tai chi.
- Get and walk a dog.
- Garden on the weekends.
- Walk or bicycle to school or work.
- Take the stairs, never the elevator.
- Park the car at the farthest point in the parking lot at work, at school, or when shopping.

  By simply changing a few daily routines, a person can gain enormous physical, psychosocial, and spiritual rewards that promote health and break the negative stress cycle.

## BOX 13-6  Sleep Hygiene Strategies

Nurses find the following suggestions to be helpful for individuals with sleep disturbance resulting from behavioral or stress-related issues:

- Keep a sleep diary, which helps determine sleep patterns more accurately, assess progress, and reinforce behavior change.
- Challenge irrational beliefs.
- Reduce consumption of alcohol and caffeine. (Chapter 11 gives some tips.)
- Avoid use of sleeping pills.
- Have a regular sleep-wake schedule, even on the weekends.
- If you are unable to fall asleep within 20 to 30 minutes, or if you wake up and are unable to fall back to sleep within that time, get out of bed and do something until you are groggy and sleepy again.
- Focus on relaxation, not sleep. Use a relaxation tape, and practice diaphragmatic breathing. Limit naps during the day to less than 45 minutes. Longer naps reset the biological clock and disturb nighttime sleep.
- Exercise within 3 to 6 hours of bedtime. Exercise improves sleep by producing a significant rise in body temperature, followed by a compensatory drop a few hours later, making it easier to fall asleep and stay asleep. Furthermore, because exercise is a physical stressor, the brain compensates for this by increasing the amount of deep sleep.
- Take a hot bath 2 hours before bedtime. The temperature drop after the bath helps to induce sleep.
- Sleep in a cool room. Individuals become sleepier and less active when body temperature falls.

From Stuart, G. W. (2013). *Principles and practice of psychiatric nursing* (10th ed.). St. Louis: Mosby.

getting inadequate exercise, and a number of other factors, including illness, alcohol use, or drug use (Stuart, 2013). Determining the extent to which sleep disturbance is the result of behavior or stress-related issues is a necessary assessment. Overcoming sleep disturbances cannot be done quickly. Changing these behaviors requires patience and persistence. Once the factors associated with sleep disturbance have been identified, nurses can help individuals improve their sleep patterns by counseling them to follow several sleep hygiene or behavior guidelines (keeping a sleep diary, having a regular sleep-wake cycle, and making prudent dietary changes). Referral for appropriate evaluation of possible disorders such as sleep apnea is also a necessary nursing intervention. Assisting people to make healthy behavior changes in their sleep habits provides another opportunity for people to increase self-regulation, confidence, and control, thereby reducing stress and improving quality of life. Box 13-6 presents several sleep hygiene strategies.

## Cognitive-Behavioral Restructuring

Many stressful situations can be created or exacerbated by negative, exaggerated, catastrophic thinking. CBT is a conceptually based short-term intervention to modify this thinking and related behaviors, and thereby reduce stress. In the context of therapy, cognitive-behavioral restructuring is a technique or a series of strategies that help people evaluate their thoughts, challenge them, and replace them with more rational cognitive and behavioral responses (Beck, 1976, 1979; Clark & Beck, 2012; Dowd et al., 2015). Although advanced training is needed to provide CBT and nurses are encouraged to do so, nurses can safely and effectively use basic strategies. A helpful resource for nurses is the Beck Institute for Cognitive Behavior Therapy (2012).

Appraisal, or the way in which a situation is viewed, can be a major cause of stress, making CBT especially suited for stress management. When situations are viewed in a negative, distorted, or illogical manner, such perceptions can adversely affect emotions, behaviors, beliefs, and physiological parameters. Cognitive-behavioral restructuring teaches people to recognize that negative thinking often causes emotional distress and associated behaviors. This recognition, in turn, alters problematic thinking and behavior, reduces the negative consequences of stress, and enhances health (Stuart, 2013).

Cognitive-behavioral restructuring does not gloss over or deny misfortune, suffering, or negative feelings. Many circumstances exist in peoples' lives for which it is appropriate to feel sad, anxious, angry, or depressed. More accurately, cognitive-behavioral restructuring is a technique that helps some people become unstuck from these moods so that they can experience a broader range of feelings and try out new behaviors (Stuart, 2013). In this structured method, individuals are asked to consider their cognitive appraisal of a situation and how this assessment affects feelings, behaviors, and physiological processes. Reframing, or cognitive reappraisal, educates individuals in monitoring thoughts and replacing those that are negative and irrational with those that are more realistic and helpful. Adding behaviors that are consistent with reframed thinking follows.

For example, a woman may have had plans to meet a friend for lunch on a day she woke up with a migraine headache. She might begin to think such thoughts as "This always happens to me when I have plans," "This headache will never go away," "I shouldn't have to deal with this," or "My day is ruined." The result of this negative, irrational self-talk is disappointment, frustration, and anger. This emotional arousal will, in turn, increase muscle tension and a variety of other stress-related symptoms, which may exacerbate the headache. To help individuals develop the skill of cognitive-behavioral restructuring, nurses can teach them to examine a stressful situation using the four-step innovative practice CBT approach highlighted in Box 13-7: Innovative Practice.

## ☀ BOX 13-7 INNOVATIVE PRACTICE

### The Four Step Approach to Cognitive Restructuring Enhanced With Technology

To help individuals develop the skill of cognitive restructuring, nurses can teach them to examine a stressful situation using the following four-step approach:

- *Stop* (break the cycle of escalating, negative thoughts).
- *Breathe deeply* (elicit the relaxation response and release tension).
- *Reflect* (ask "What is going on here? What am I thinking? Is the thought true? Is the thought helpful? Am I jumping to conclusions or magnifying the situation?").
- *Choose* a more realistic, rational response. Try out the alternative response in a future situation.

#### Alternative Approach

Teaching/coaching can be done face-to-face or can be provided via technology (e.g., a website and/or smartphone application that shows the previous steps with a feedback interface). Via technology, feedback can be given via text or e-mail messages to correct negative thoughts and to provide suggestions and positive reinforcement for steps 2 to 4 when success is reported. Phone and/or face-to-face interaction can augment contact via technology when possible. Tracking successful cognitive restructuring via on-line entry can provide useful outcome data. As Internet and smartphone penetration increase and costs decrease, use of such technological interventions will increasingly be cost-effective ways to reach more individuals and can be applied across a range of technological platforms (e.g., computers, smartphones, and tablets). Reminder generic affirmations also can be added via text messaging at very low cost to encourage practice of the steps.

Modified from Clark, D. A., & Beck, A. T. (2012). *The anxiety and worry workbook: The cognitive behavioral solution.* New York: Guilford Press; Stuart, G. W. (2009). Psychophysiological responses and somatoform and sleep disorders. In G. W. Stuart & M. T. Laraia (Eds.), *Principles and practice of psychiatric nursing* (9th ed., p. 241). St Louis: Mosby; Stuart, G. W. (Ed.) (2013). *Principles and practice of psychiatric nursing* (10th ed.). St. Louis: Mosby.

In the previous example, the woman may reflect that "I am having a migraine headache, and I hate that it is on a day that I had made plans, but I will take my medication, listen to my relaxation tapes, and rest. I'll call my friend and see if we can change our plans. Perhaps she can come over to visit me for tea this afternoon if I feel better." Although it is understandable that anyone would be disappointed and upset over this situation, application of the four-step cognitive restructuring technique can help individuals identify healthy choices and gain a sense of control.

Based on the work of pioneers such as Aaron Beck (1976, 1979) and Albert Ellis (Ellis, 1962; Ellis & Dryden, 1987), cognitive therapy has emerged during the past several decades as a treatment designed to alter dysfunctional beliefs and thoughts associated with depression, anxiety disorders, and other emotional problems (Clark & Beck, 2012). Over time, theorists, clinical researchers, and clinicians recognized the effectiveness of this approach for many people, as well as the value of linking helpful alterations in thinking to complementary behavioral changes. As a result, CBT emerged. CBT is an efficacious treatment approach for many stress-related and mental health disorders. For example, researchers have shown that CBT is effective, alone or with other

## 🌐 BOX 13-8 DIVERSITY AWARENESS

### Social Stressors Can Lead to Discrimination for Vulnerable Populations

Health is perceived through one's spiritual beliefs, holistic practice, and biomedical perspectives. Nurses understand cultural sensitivity when providing care and the importance of clear communication in multicultural care. Greater concern for health literacy and improved coordination with support organizations are needed. Barriers such as discrimination and geopolitical tension may affect the ability to cope through frustration and may influence health care outcomes. *Healthy People 2020* identifies the need to close the gap and supports health equity by addressing chronic disease and infant mortality rates. For example, social stressors have been linked to increased depressive symptoms among antepartum black American women (Dailey et al., 2011). Thus in addition to the need for universal symptom screening, it is essential that nurses develop and test interventions to ameliorate effects of social stressors such as discrimination for vulnerable populations.

From Dailey, D. E., Dawn, E., & Humphreys, J. C. (2011). Social stressors associated with antepartum depressive symptoms in low-income African American women. *Public Health Nursing, 28,* 203–212.

therapies or medication, in alleviating postpartum depression (Bobo & Yawn, 2014). Evidence provides strong support for use of cognitive-behavioral restructuring as a stress-management approach. A comparison of an on-line mindfulness-based cognitive therapy intervention (Mindfulness in Action) with on-line pain management psychoeducation showed positive outcomes in self well-being from both approaches, yet Mindfulness in Action was associated with more pronounced positive outcomes (Dowd et al., 2015). Although the results were promising, more research is needed to demonstrate efficacy. Sensitivity to stress appraisals is also situated within a person's culture and experience. Cultural sensitivity to such influences is critical to providing quality care. Box 13-8: Diversity Awareness presents relevant information related to the effects of racial/ethnic discrimination on cognitive appraisals of interactions as threatening and harmful, resulting in increased overall stress burden.

### Affirmations

**Affirmations** can be an effective stress-management and cognitive-behavioral restructuring skill because they are a method of countering self-defeating negative thoughts and attitudes in addition to being helpful in addressing spiritual needs. An affirmation is a positive thought, in the form of a short phrase or saying, which has meaning for the individual. By reinforcing new ways of thinking or behaving in the present moment, affirmations are statements that people can use to reaffirm new intentions and to clarify goals.

Nurses coach individuals to create an affirmation as a way of developing a more helpful, realistic belief system. For example, thoughts such as "I can't handle this" and "My day is ruined" can be countered with "I can handle this" and "I know ways to increase my comfort." Repeating an affirmation often throughout the day, perhaps after elicitation of the relaxation response or as part of a breathing exercise, can become second nature and can help to enhance self-esteem and reduce stress.

## Social Support

Having supportive family, friends, and coworkers is for many individuals an important contributor to effective coping and stress hardiness (Kobasa et al., 1982). Many people believe that confiding in others and talking out problems can be a helpful way to get good advice or uncritical support. Social support comprises a network of close family, friends, coworkers, and professionals. The social support literature notes that both the number of supports and the quality of the relationships are important (van Woerden et al., 2011).

Research outcomes demonstrate the protective health effects of social support. However, influences may differ by type or source of support. For example, van Woerden and colleagues (2011) examined the effects of social support from personal, professional, and community networks and other factors in relation to self-rated health using a cross-sectional postal and Web-based survey with a random sample of 10,000 households in Wandsworth, London. The results demonstrated that social support from family or friends, at work, and by civic participation was associated with a lower likelihood of poor self-rated health, but that social support from neighbors was associated with a higher likelihood of reporting poor health. The outcomes suggest that most of the health effects of social support are complementary. Nonetheless, the finding that the health effects of family social support were insignificant after the other social support variables had been controlled for suggests that it can be compensated by support from other sources. Sociodemographic variables (e.g., sex, age, being married, being employed, and owning a home) were also associated with better self-rated health. The principal message is that a variety of sources of social support may promote health and that nurses should ask individuals about all types of social support so as to help them cultivate and use support from many sources. In addition, substituting support from a different source when it is lacking from one usual source such as the family can be a helpful strategy.

Nursing interventions are aimed at facilitating social support to promote effective coping and reduce stress. Using information available in their local communities or through national organizations, nurses suggest support groups (see Chapter 8), website chat rooms, social networking sites, educational classes, and exercise facilities. Individuals and their families are often referred to volunteer organizations such as the American Lung Association, the American Heart Association, the American Cancer Society, and the Arthritis Foundation for resources related to specific health-promotion/maintenance needs that also may provide social support opportunities.

## Assertive Communication

Effective communication is an important stress-management skill. An important coping and problem-solving skill, communication can be adversely affected by exaggerated negative thoughts and deeply held negative beliefs and assumptions (Stuart, 2013). (See Chapter 4 for additional discussion of communication.) People who have difficulty with communication usually have one or all of the following problems:

- Disparity between what they say (statement) and what they want (intent)
- Confusion about or resistance to stating clearly how they feel, what they want, or what they need (lack of assertiveness), with either a tendency to deny their own feelings (passiveness) or indifference toward the feelings of others (aggressiveness)
- Difficulty listening to others

The importance of matching the statement with intention is illustrated by the following example:

*As Timothy is leaving for his basketball game on a Saturday afternoon, his mother tells him, "Remember to be home early tonight." When Timothy arrives home at 9:00 pm, his mother, who is waiting at the front door, yells, "Where were you? Is this your idea of early? You know your father and I had plans tonight. We were counting on you. You think only of yourself. This always happens. You'll never change. You'll always be irresponsible and selfish."*

The first guideline for effective communication is that people need to be clear about what they want and what they need (intent) in statements to others. Although it would be wonderful if a son or daughter, spouse, friend, or others were great mind readers, assuming that people automatically know what is meant does little to help with communication. Nurses help individuals match statements with intentions. This process requires that individuals recognize distorted, exaggerated thoughts and emotions and take responsibility for their part of the conversation. Communicating effectively is a learned art and skill.

In our reviewing the previous example, it is helpful to note that if the mother's intention was to have her son home before 8:00 p.m., then her statement needed to indicate this. She could have said "I hope you enjoy the game, but remember your father and I are going out tonight. We need to have you home before 8:00 p.m. to take care of your sister." It is important that the person understands that the other person in the conversation is not obligated to respond as one would wish. However, a request can be much clearer when the statement reflects the intent.

The next guideline for effective communication is to be assertive. Assertive communication, in most cases, is the most effective way to communicate. An assertive statement is nonjudgmental, expresses feelings and opinions, and reaffirms perceived rights. The general format of an assertive statement is: *I feel* [emotion], *when you* [the behavior], *because* [explanation].

The formula requires that all three elements be included. Cognitive restructuring, as described earlier, facilitates assertive communication because it requires individuals to identify their thoughts and feelings. In the previous example, Timothy's mother could:

- *Stop* (breaking the cycle of escalating, negative thoughts)
- *Breathe deeply* (releasing physical tension; promoting relaxation)
- *Reflect:*
  - How do I feel emotionally? (e.g., frustrated)
  - What are my automatic thoughts? ("If he cared about us, then he would have been home on time. He's always selfish and irresponsible. He's never going to change.")
- *Choose:*
  - A more realistic, helpful way of thinking ("He's not always selfish and irresponsible. Even though it feels like he doesn't care about us when he does this, I know he cares.")

Becoming aware of her automatic thoughts and feelings would help Timothy's mother plan an assertive statement when Timothy comes home. She could then say "I feel frustrated [emotion] when you are late [behavior] because I expected you would be home in time to care for your sister while your father and I went out, or that you would have called if you were going to be late [explanation]." This statement both makes her feelings clear and explains why she feels this way, which in turn provides a better opportunity to work on problem-solving. When people cannot verbalize both their feelings and their needs, others are forced to figure out what they are. When others fail to do so correctly, individuals may feel victimized and blame the others for not understanding. Nurses help people recognize that they have a right and a responsibility to speak up and to do so in an assertive manner. The nurse helps individuals in matching their emotions with the explanation (frustration equals unmet expectation). It is important to remind them that this way of communicating may feel awkward and uncomfortable at first. Practicing this technique many times will be required before communication improves. Role play can be a useful technique to practice. Other people need time to become accustomed to the changes. Effective communication takes both practice and patience with everyone involved.

## Empathy

**Empathy** is an effective stress-management intervention because it assists with communication. Empathy is the ability to consider another person's perspective and to communicate this understanding back to that person. Empathy guides individuals to become better listeners.

Empathy can be facilitated through the technique of active listening. **Active listening** requires conscious, empathic, non-judgmental awareness. Listening also helps clarify the issues involved and can deescalate many emotional exchanges. The use of focus groups can assist the nurse in understanding concerns, such as a parent group concerned about nutrition choices in the lunch room. For example, during a situation in which a parent announces "I'm fed up with the food selection in the cafeteria," the response may be important to resolving the issues without promoting further miscommunications and increasing problems. Rather than being caught by a defensive, emotional reaction, individuals can learn to communicate empathetically using the four-step approach:

- *Stop* (breaking the cycle of escalating, negative thoughts)
- *Breathe deeply* (releasing physical tension; promoting relaxation)
- *Reflect*:
  - How do I feel emotionally? (hurt, angry)
  - What are my automatic thoughts? ("How could [person] say that? It's not my fault. I have things to do. [Person] always accuses me. This is never going to change.")
  - What are the thoughts and emotions being expressed by the other person?
- *Choose*:
  - "My feelings are hurt, but I don't have to react defensively."
  - "I'm going to try to understand [person's] perspective using this phrase: 'You sound ____ about ____' and listen to [person's] response."

By using this phrase ('You sound ____ about ____'), an individual can gain awareness from another person's perspective (Rogers, 1951). If we continue with the scenario, the response might be "You sound upset about the choice of food available…." Possible responses to this empathetic statement might include "It's not just about that. Everything went wrong today, and this was just one more thing when my child complains about lunch" and "You're right. I hate having to pay for food that my child will not eat."

When one uses active listening, the other person often feels heard. An opportunity to clarify any misunderstanding becomes available. This exercise may help reduce emotional arousal, defensive behavior, and conflict. Active listening allows the individual to buy time and to get a better perspective on what the other person is thinking and feeling. Individuals can then make a choice as to how they want to respond. They may choose to use assertive communication or to step away from the interaction. Active listening promotes empathic, objective, and nonjudgmental communication. Nurses recommend use of stress-management skills that include active listening techniques to facilitate effective communication, which, in turn, reduces conflict and stress.

## Healthy Pleasures

Engaging in **healthy pleasures** (activities that bring feelings of peace, joy, and happiness) is, for most individuals, an important part of life. However, for individuals who are feeling overwhelmed with daily hassles of work-life balance, illness, or loss, this practice may have been lost. Individuals may feel that they do not deserve to have pleasure or that they are waiting for happiness until they feel better, until the stressors are resolved, or until they go away. This belief makes breaking the stress cycle even more challenging; however, rewards motivate behavior (Stuart, 2013). By nurses asking people to pursue a healthy and pleasurable activity every week, motivating them to become more involved in their lives and break this cycle is often easier. The activity can be simple, and it need not cost money. For example, people often find pleasure in enjoying nature, spending time with a friend, reading a book, or watching a movie. Hobbies are purposeful leisure-time activities that can balance hectic, stressful lives. A hobby should be chosen from interest and/or talent. Many hobbies have added benefits of increasing activity (e.g., gardening) or promoting social engagement (e.g., a book club or chorus). Nurses advise individuals to make leisure-time activities a regular part of the week as a purposeful and conscious plan to break the stress cycle.

## Spiritual Practice

In response to stress, people can feel disconnected from life's meaning and purpose, which in turn affects spiritual health and well-being. Meeting spiritual needs may be facilitated by **spiritual practice** or activities that help people find meaning, purpose, and connection. For example, individuals may choose to elicit the relaxation response through prayer. This focused, relaxed state of mind might help them develop a spiritual perspective that can engender a shift in values and beliefs to help them cope with a stressor they cannot change, such as chronic illness or loss of a loved one. Expression of anger or confusion in the face of difficulties, trauma, or tragedy also can provide a therapeutic outlet, but conversely may engender spiritual or religious doubt, or a sense of alienation from one's beliefs. Nurses suggest a referral to a chaplain or clergy member, provide spiritual music or art work, recommend spiritual reading material, and provide personal presence (see Box 13-4: Quality and Safety Scenario). Willis and colleagues (2015) explicated how spiritual healing manifested itself in the aftermath of childhood maltreatment and point out the potential helpfulness of "constructing caring-healing interventions aimed at both cultivating spiritual consciousness and facilitating loving-kindness and acts of letting go in the healing process."

Nurses propose activities that provide a sense of meaning and purpose. Keeping a journal can be an important strategy to help individuals focus on aspects of life that are more positive and that become clouded from view when a person is feeling overwhelmed by stress. Finding ways of helping others (e.g., tutoring children, reading to the blind, or visiting an older adult) can have a positive influence on spiritual health and well-being. Altruism, generosity, kindness, and service to others are more than moral virtues. These attributes not only help to make the world a better place but also help people find meaning and purpose in life. Religious and existential well-being has provided some defense against depression for people with chronic and life-threatening conditions. Older, chronically ill, and homebound people can be encouraged to produce written or oral histories that can be a legacy or, when able, to contact others needing care or to make telephone calls to raise funds for a favorite charity. In addition, nurses and other health care professionals can assist individuals and families to describe and clarify their personal religious and spiritual perspectives, especially in light of evolving practices/meaning structures and high rates of interfaith marriages/partnerships (Walsh, 2011). Spirituality and religious affiliation cannot be equated. Additionally, being part of a "faith community" may provide an important source of social support for many people. Within faith communities, nurses (also known as "parish" nurses) act as facilitators, educators, and referrers to individuals and families in promoting holistic care. Nurses can encourage individuals to search for a community that is comfortable, accepting, and supportive.

## Clarifying Values and Beliefs

To manage stress and develop a balanced lifestyle, people must recognize the things and values that are important to them, reflect on where they are in life, evaluate what needs to be changed, and generate an action plan for that change (see Chapter 4). This process is known as values clarification. The first step is to identify what is important, meaningful, and valuable so as to assess whether actions are consistent with beliefs. What people believe and value guides their actions by endorsing certain behaviors and changing others. When people assess their values and beliefs, they use the ability to make their own choices rather than relying on beliefs and values dictated to them by others.

One method nurses use to help people identify what they value and, ultimately, to help them clarify the relationship between their beliefs and actions is to ask them to identify what is important or meaningful to them. The form in Figure 13-5 is an example of questions used in the Medical Symptom Reduction Program at the Benson-Henry Institute for Mind Body Medicine

of Massachusetts General Hospital (n.d.) in Boston. Individuals are asked to identify what is important and meaningful to them in eight domains. Nurses change the domains to reflect more accurately the values and beliefs of the individuals they are counseling. After reviewing the results, individuals may find that they have not been doing certain things that are important to them (becoming more physically active, eating a healthier diet, volunteering, or spending time with their children). When people detect inconsistencies between their values and their actual living habits, they can begin to develop a working plan for correcting these inconsistencies. This process enables them to make conscious choices and to have more control (see Figure 13-5).

## Setting Realistic Goals

Developing an action plan for change to work toward a more balanced health-promoting lifestyle that is consistent with a person's values and beliefs is an important stress-management strategy. Setting realistic, attainable goals facilitates this exercise. Goal setting is a dynamic process that involves both the individual and the nurse. Goals should be specific, concrete, measurable, and achievable. Nurses facilitate this process by respecting the individual's input and using a values clarification exercise (such as the one mentioned) to facilitate a more complete database to guide individuals to identify and prioritize problems to be addressed, and set mutually agreed on long-term and short-term goals. Nurses encourage individuals to challenge themselves when their behaviors are not consistent with what they identified as important and meaningful to them. For example, when an overweight man with hypertension and high cholesterol levels continues to smoke and eat high-fat foods, nurses help him to look at these behaviors relative to what is meaningful to him, such as his family. The cost and benefit are usually clear, and the responsibility for the change is with the individual, not the nurse. Nurses ask the following questions to help individuals clarify long-term goals:

- What is important to you?
- What would you like to change about your life?
- What can you do to start that change?
- When will you take that action?
- How will you measure success?
- How will you maintain the desired change?
- How can I help you to reach your goal?

Setting realistic, attainable goals helps to create a sense of confidence and achievement and to build enthusiasm to set future goals. This process, in turn, increases a sense of control and mitigates the negative effects of stress.

## Humor

Humor is an enjoyable and effective antidote to stress for many people. Humor can have health-promoting properties (Konradt et al., 2013; Stuart, 2013). When acting as a stress reducer, humor produces laughter. Laughter creates predictable physiological changes in the body. Similarly to how it behaves with other forms of exercise, the body responds in two stages: an arousal phase with an increase in physiological parameters, and a resolution phase, during which these parameters return to resting values or lower values (Wooten, 2009).

## "What Is Important and Meaningful to You in Life?"

In each of the following areas, what do you want for yourself, today, next week, a year from now?

Under each of the following categories, please ask yourself these important questions.

*Professional, educational, and intellectual*
Today _____
Next week _____
A year from now _____

*Relationships*
Today _____
Next week _____
A year from now _____

*Creative things*
Today _____
Next week _____
A year from now _____

*Spiritual*
Today _____
Next week _____
A year from now _____

*Volunteer and altruistic*
Today _____
Next week _____
A year from now _____

*Health*
Today _____
Next week _____
A year from now _____

*Fun and play*
Today _____
Next week _____
A year from now _____

*Material objects*
Today _____
Next week _____
A year from now _____

**FIGURE 13-5** What is important and meaningful to you in life? (From Medical symptom reduction program patient notebook. [n.d.]. Boston: The Benson-Henry Institute for Mind Body Medicine of Massachusetts General Hospital, Harvard Medical School.)

Humor can open different perspectives on problems and facilitate objectivity, which increases a sense of self-protection and control. Finding humor in a stressful situation can help people to reframe perceptions of the event. Some hospital staffs are using laughter libraries, humor rooms, comedy carts that can be wheeled into an individual's hospital room, and clowns to bring laughter and joy to the bedside. Humor has potential as an accessible, enjoyable, and inexpensive stress-reduction strategy that can offer people new perspectives on their world and themselves. Nevertheless, recognizing that humor can mask conflict or be hurtful is critically important in judging when and how to use it in clinical and work setting encounters (Box 13-9).

## Engaging in Pleasurable Activities

A variety of activities can promote the relaxation response. Finding activities that are enjoyable to the person can be a key strategy to reduce stress and promote healthy behaviors. For example, Wong in her engaging book *Scales to Scalpels* (Wong & Viagas,

## BOX 13-9 Humor Strategies for Stress Reduction

Nurses help individuals use humor for health promotion and stress reduction in a variety of ways, including:

- Keeping a humor journal: looking for the unintentional amusing remark, watching for funny things young children say or do, and looking in the newspaper for humorous grammatical errors or an inappropriate choice of words and writing them in a journal
- Looking on the Internet for humorous resources
- Creating a scrapbook of humorous cartoons, pictures, stickers, poems, and songs
- Reading a cartoon or joke in the newspaper every day and sharing it with a friend
- Watching funny movies or reruns of old television programs
- Finding and spending time with funny, light-hearted people

For more information about using humor to reduce stress, see Box 6-4.

## BOX 13-10 GENOMICS

Epigenetic regulators modify gene expression without changes in DNA sequence. Nutrition is such a regulator that affects the brain throughout life, with profound implications for cognitive decline and dementia. Effects are mediated by changes in expression of multiple genes, and responses to nutrition are in turn affected by individual genetic variability. Epigenetic mechanisms are central to brain development, structure, and function. Epigenetics promote cell-specific and age-related gene expression that can be highly stable but also reversible in response to factors such as nutrition. Health and brain function, in particular, result from highly complex interactions between numerous genetic and environmental factors, including nutrition, physical activity, age, and stress. The interplay of genetic and environmental factors, including nutrition and stress, is critical to our understanding the causes of many health disorders and developing effective interventions.

Modified from Dauncey, M. J. (2014). Nutrition, the brain and cognitive decline: Insights from epigenetics. *European Journal of Clinical Nutrition, 68*(11), 1179–1185.

2012) described how the Longwood Symphony Orchestra in Boston, a talented group of medical professionals who practice at an elite center of health care and research, helps them to thrive as artists. Carving out the time to create music within this ensemble in the midst of demanding clinical and academic lives allows these musician/clinicians to practice the healing art of music for themselves and in turn to be better healers. Wong's engaging narrative underscores the value of integrating various art therapies into our care plans as a valuable strategy for health promotion and stress reduction. Additionally, it points to the importance of self-care for clinicians.

## EFFECTIVE COPING

When people believe that they can cope effectively, the harmful effects of stress can be minimized. The stressful situation is perceived as a challenge rather than a threat. This often elusive difference has vital mind, body, and spirit effects. When people believe that their lives are more balanced and under control, they are productive, but not driven; are aroused, but not anxious; and may even be physically or mentally tired, but not exhausted.

Effective coping helps people face great adversity (such as illness) and recognize the opportunity that the situation often presents. First and foremost, individuals must recognize that coping is the ability to find a balance between acceptance and action, between letting go and taking control. Many stress-management strategies help individuals distinguish these differences by providing a format for observing or objectifying their experiences. Other strategies such as exercise and balanced nutrition help individuals promote physical health and well-being to counter the harmful effects of stress. In addition, epigenetics (i.e., how environmental factors such as nutrition and stress trigger or mute the expression of genetic traits) is a vast canvas for the exploration of causes and intervention across a variety of physical and mental health disorders for individuals and populations (Dauncey, 2014) (Box 13-10: Genomics).

Nurses help individuals improve effective coping by guiding them in the art of choosing the right strategy at the right time. In doing so, people gain a sense of control that minimizes or

buffers harmful effects of stress. Nurses use the interventions described in this chapter to assist individuals to manage extrinsic and intrinsic stressors.

When individuals cannot control or influence the situation (extrinsic stressors), nurses advise them to do the following:

- Take care of physical health and well-being: exercise; eat healthy, balanced meals; and practice sleep hygiene.
- Accept: learn to accept that some situations or people cannot be changed or avoided. Forgiveness and letting go of resentment are often a part of acceptance.
- Use distraction: distraction involves putting a worry aside, when necessary, until the situation can be dealt with directly. This prioritizing is quite different from procrastinating or denial, because it is a necessary delay rather than avoidance.
- Reduce emotional arousal: practice mini relaxations, listen to a relaxation recording, use the four-step cognitive-behavioral restructuring technique, exercise, seek social support, pray, meditate, use humor and affirmations, write in a journal, or engage in a healthy pleasure.

When individuals can alter or influence the situation, or when they are contributing to or creating the stress (intrinsic stressors), nurses advise them to do the following:

- Take care of physical health and well-being: exercise; eat healthy, balanced meals; and practice sleep hygiene.
- Reduce emotional arousal: practice mini relaxations, listen to music or a relaxation DVD or CD, engage in exercise, seek social support, pray, meditate, use humor and affirmations, write in a journal, engage in a healthy pleasure, and/or use the four-step cognitive-behavioral restructuring strategy:
  - *Stop* (breaking the cycle of escalating, negative thoughts)
  - *Breathe deeply* (eliciting the relaxation response and releasing tension)
  - *Reflect* (asking "What is going on here? What am I thinking? Is the thought true? Is the thought helpful? Am I jumping to conclusions or magnifying the situation?")
  - *Choose* a more realistic, rational response and related behavioral reaction.

- *Problem-solve:*
  - Clarify values, beliefs, and expectations.
  - Gather information.
  - Seek advice, support, assistance, or information.
  - Use assertive communication and empathy.

- Set realistic goals, design action strategies, and determine the best steps to handle the problem.
- Take action.

See the care plan for John DeMarco for an example of a plan for effective coping.

## CASE STUDY

### Health Assessment: John DeMarco

John DeMarco, a 29-year-old man separated from his wife, walked into the health maintenance organization stating he had a severe sore throat, could not eat, had not worked for a day, and was feeling "awful." He wanted to see the physician and get a prescription for an antibiotic. The medical record revealed two episodes within the last 9 months of reports of a sore throat, culture of organism, and antibiotic treatment. The separation from his wife occurred 1 year ago. He had not had a physical examination in 2 years. During the assessment interview, the nurse gathered the following information: John DeMarco appeared tired; he presented his problem in short, terse statements; he was irritable about the clinic's slow service; and he expressed a need to get back to work. Within the last 3 weeks he had been required to work overtime because he faced deadline penalties, and his boss said that Mr. DeMarco's promotion, due in 2 months, depended on his performance now. The company is struggling, and layoffs may be pending. Mr. DeMarco said that, in general, things were fine.

His wife was apparently happy without him, and he was too busy to care or to think about that relationship. He made one remark about his boss: "What do you do with a nervous boss?" He described his diet as fast food "taken on the run." He said he gets about 6 hours of sleep per night and awakens one to two times near morning. He has infrequent contact with family members, who live in the area. In accordance with the clinical protocol for the health center, the nurse collects a throat culture.

#### Reflective Questions

- As Mr. DeMarco's nurse, how would you comprehensively assess his health?
- What are several different diagnoses and possible individual, family, and etiological factors to consider?
- What work-related health issues may be a concern?
- What other issues may impact the community where Mr. DeMarco is employed?

## CARE PLAN

### Plan for Effective Coping: John DeMarco

**\*NURSING DIAGNOSIS: Ineffective coping related to increased stress at work and limited coping strategies**

#### Defining Characteristics to Assess

- Physiological disturbances
- Abuse of alcohol or drugs
- Participation in potentially dangerous activities
- Engaging in lifestyle with risk to health
- Impairment of social role functioning:
  - Nonproductive lifestyle
  - Failure to function in usual social roles
  - Nonperformance of activities of daily living
  - Inappropriate behaviors in social situations
  - Self-absorption
  - Lack of concern for or detachment from usual social supports
- Poor morale:
  - Unhappiness
  - Lack of future orientation
  - Hopelessness
  - Unacceptable quality of life
  - Pessimism
- Defensive patterns:
  - Inflexibility
  - Hypervigilance
  - Avoidance
  - Inertia
  - Refusal or rejection of help

#### Expected Outcomes

Mr. DeMarco will:

- Report increased information on and consequences to himself of stressors experienced.
- Practice the relaxation response for 20 to 30 minutes every day through prayer or contemplation; use multiple mini relaxations throughout each day.
- Report increasing weekly exercise or activity and healthy changes in nutrition and sleep or rest patterns.
- Develop effective coping and problem-solving abilities to manage stress, beginning with the stress at work.
- Evaluate the result of throat culture and consult with his primary care provider if the result is positive and an antibiotic is indicated.

#### Interventions

- Promote an attitude of openness to new information.
- Enroll him in a cognitive-behavioral group program to learn stress-management strategies and health promotion.
- Monitor his daily practice of relaxation response.
- Monitor his changes in exercise or activity, nutrition, sleep or rest patterns, and mood.
- Guide him to develop two coping strategies through cognitive-behavioral restructuring.
- Schedule a follow-up appointment or telephone check-in to monitor his well-being.

*NANDA Nursing Diagnoses—Herdman T. H. & Kamitsuru, S. (Eds.). Nursing Diagnoses–Definitions and Classification 2015–2017. Copyright © 2014, 1994–2014 NANDA International. Used by arrangement with John Wiley & Sons Limited. In order to make safe and effective judgments using the NANDA-I nursing diagnoses it is essential that nurses refer to the definitions and defining characteristics of the diagnoses listed in this work.

## SUMMARY

Health and the ability to cope effectively with the many demands of work-life balance require management of stress. Combining careful assessment and choice of strategies, thoughtful and honest feedback, and continued support, nurses assist people to cope more effectively with the innumerable actual and potential stressors they may encounter. Research to discern the interplay of homeodynamic physiological, psychological, social, and spiritual responses to stress has yielded important knowledge for practice. However, uncovering the intricate workings of the brain within the context of human stress and coping experiences is a daunting and critical challenge for today's health researchers.

Stress-management strategies provide an opportunity for individuals to acquire the necessary skills to cope more successfully and become confident in self-management. Such awareness enables the individual to challenge and change perceptions, decrease stress reactivity, improve self-management skills, and minimize the harmful consequences of stress. This process positively influences health promotion, disease prevention, and symptom management. Challenges remain to expand intervention testing to families and communities. Understanding the influences of stress on health and illness is essential to all nursing practice.

## ⓔ EVOLVE CHAPTER FEATURES

http://evolve.elsevier.com/Edelman/
- Study Questions

## REFERENCES

Baer, R. A. (2014). *Mindfulness-based treatment approaches: Clinician's Guide to evidence base and applications.* Cambridge, MA: Academic Press.

Barchas, P. R., & Barchas, J. D. (2011). Sociophysiology 25 years ago: Early perspectives of an emerging discipline now as part of neuroscience. *Annals of the New York Academy of Sciences, 1231,* 1–16.

Beck, A. T. (1976). *Cognitive therapy and the emotional disorders.* New York: International Universities Press.

Beck, A. T. (1979). *Cognitive therapy of depression.* New York: Guilford Press.

Beck Institute for Cognitive Behaviour Therapy. (2012). Beck Institute for Cognitive Behaviour Therapy. http://www .beckinstitute.org/.

Benson, H. (1975). *The relaxation response.* New York: William Morrow & Co.

Benson-Henry Institute for Mind Body Medicine of Massachusetts General Hospital. (n.d.). Stress. https://www.bensonhenryinstitute.org/.

Berger, M., Juster, R. P., & Samyi, Z. (2015). A mental health consequences of stress and trauma: Allostatic load markers for practice and policy with a focus on Indigenous health. *Australasian Psychiatry, 23*(6), 644–649.

Bobo, W. V., & Yawn, B. (2014). Concise review for physicians and other clinicians: Postpartum depression. *Mayo Clinic Proceedings, 89*(6), 835–844.

Bonfiglio, J., Inda, C., et al. (2011). The corticotropin-releasing hormone network and the hypothalamic-pituitary-adrenal axis: Molecular and cellular mechanisms involved. *Neuroendocrinology, 94*(1), 12–20.

Bortz, W. M. (2015). Updating homeostasis. *Biological Systems: Open Access, 4,* 138.

Brann, L., Owens, J., & Williamson, A. (2011). *The handbook of contemporary clinical hypnosis: Theory and practice.* Chichester, England: John Wiley & Sons.

Cannon, W. (1914). The emergency function of the adrenal medulla in pain and the major emotions. *American Journal of Physiology, 33,* 356–372.

Centers for Disease Control and Prevention (CDC). (2012a). The guide to community preventive services: The community guide; what works to promote health. http://www.thecommunityguide .org/index.html.

Centers for Disease Control and Prevention (CDC). (2012b). National prevention strategy: America's plan for better health and wellness. http://www.cdc.gov/Features/PreventionStrategy/.

Clark, D. A., & Beck, A. T. (2012). *The anxiety and worry workbook: The cognitive behavioral solution.* New York: Guilford Press.

Closa, L. T., Nouwen, A., et al. (2010). Anger rumination, social support, and cardiac symptoms in patients undergoing angiography. *British Journal of Health Psychology, 15,* 841–857.

Courbasson, C., & Jeyarajan, J. (2011). Individuals with eating disorders and stress. In A. P. Barnes & J. E. Montefuscio (Eds.), *Role of stress in psychological disorders* (pp. 99–111). New York: Nova Science Publishers.

Dauncey, M. J. (2014). Nutrition, the brain and cognitive decline: Insights from epigenetics. *European Journal of Clinical Nutrition, 68*(11), 1179–1185.

DeMarco, R., & Segraves, M. M. (2011). Community assessment. In G. Harkness & R. DeMarco (Eds.), *Community and public health nursing: Evidence for practice* (pp. 175–191). Philadelphia: Lippincott Williams & Wilkins.

Dowd, H., Hogan, M. J., et al. (2015). Comparison of an online mindfulness-based cognitive therapy intervention with online pain management psychoeducation: A randomized controlled study. *The Clinical Journal of Pain, 31,* 517–527.

Ellis, A. (1962). *Reason and emotion in psychotherapy.* New York: L. Stuart.

Ellis, A., & Dryden, W. (1987). *The practice of rational emotive therapy (RET).* New York: Springer.

Fawcett, J., & Ellenbecker, C. H. (2015). A proposed conceptual model of nursing and population health. *Nursing Outlook, 63,* 288–298.

Gregorio, S. W., Carpenter, K. M., et al. (2012). Impact of breast cancer recurrence and cancer-specific stress on spouse health and immune function. *Brain, Behavior, & Immunity, 26,* 228–233.

Harkness, G., & DeMarco, R. (Eds.), (2012). *Community and public health nursing: Evidence for practice.* Philadelphia: Lippincott Williams & Wilkins.

Holmes, T. H. (1981). *The schedule of recent experiences.* Seattle: University of Washington Press.

Horowitz, M., Wilner, N., & Alvarez, W. (1979). Impact of event scale: A measure of subjective stress. *Psychosomatic Medicine, 41*(3), 209–218.

Hou, R., & Baldwin, D. (2012). A neuroimmunological perspective on anxiety disorders. *Human Psychopharmacology, 27*(1), 6–14.

Kaku, M. (2014). *The future of the mind.* New York: Doubleday.

Kobasa, S. C., Maddi, S. R., & Kahn, S. (1982). Hardiness and health: A prospective study. *Journal of Personality and Social Psychology, 42,* 391–404.

Konradt, B., Hirsch, R. D., et al. (2013). Evaluation of a standardized humor group in a clinical setting: A feasibility study for older patients with depression. *International Journal of Geriatric Psychiatry, 28*(8), 850–857.

Lazarus, R., & Folkman, S. (1984). *Stress, appraisal, and coping.* New York: Springer.

Lengacher, C. A., Kip, K. E., et al. (2015). A cost-effective mindfulness stress reduction program: A randomized control trial for breast cancer survivors. *Nursing Economics, 33*(4), 210–232.

Marchant, J. (2016). *Cure: A journey into the science of mind over body.* New York: Crown Publishers.

Maslach, C., & Jackson, S. E. (1986). *Burnout inventory* (manual research ed., 2nd ed). Palo Alto, CA: Consulting Psychologists Press.

McLennon, S. M., Habermann, B., & Rice, M. (2011). Finding meaning as a mediator of burden on the health of caregivers of spouses with dementia. *Aging & Mental Health, 15*, 522–530.

Menezes, A. R., Lavie, C. J., et al. (2011). Psychological risk factors and cardiovascular disease: Is it all in your head? *Postgraduate Medicine, 123*, 165–176.

MyFitnessPal. (2015). Free calorie counter. http://www.myfitnesspal.com/.

National Center for Complementary and Integrative Health. (n.d.). https://nccih.nih.gov.

Nikkheslat, N., Zunszain, P. A., et al. (2015). Insufficient glucocorticoid signaling and elevated inflammation in coronary heart disease patients with comorbid depression. *Brain, Behavior, and Immunity, 48*, 8–18.

North, R. J., Pai, A. V., et al. (2011). Finding happiness in negative emotions: An experimental test of a novel expressive writing paradigm. *Journal of Positive Psychology, 6*, 192–203.

Paradies, Y. (2011). A theoretical review of psychosocial stress and health. In A. B. Barnes & J. E. Montefuscio (Eds.), *Role of stress in psychological disorders* (pp. 1–19). New York, NY: Nova Science Publishers.

Phillips, J. R. (2015). Martha E. Rogers: Heretic and heroine. *Nursing Science Quarterly, 28*, 42–48.

Quinn, C., Clare, V., & Woods, R. T. (2011). The impact of motivation and meanings on the wellbeing of caregivers of people with dementia. *International Psychogeriatrics, 22*, 43–55.

Rogers, C. (1951). *Client-centered therapy.* Boston, MA: Houghton Mifflin.

Sadock, B. S., & Sadock, V. A. (2015). *Kaplan & Sadock's synopsis of clinical psychiatry* (11th ed.). Philadelphia: Wolters Kluwer.

Selye, H. (1950). *Stress.* Montreal: Acta Inc.

Selye, H. (1974). *Stress without distress.* Philadelphia: J. B. Lippincott & Co.

Selye, H. (1982). History and present status of the stress concept. In L. Goldberger & S. Breznitz (Eds.), *Handbook of stress: Theoretical and clinical aspects* (pp. 7–17). New York: Free Press.

Sifferlin, A. (2016). What you need to know about Zika: How to beat the virus and the mosquitoes that carry it. *Time, 187*(18), 32–41.

Snyder, M., & Lindquist, R. (Eds.), (2010). *Complementary/alternative therapies in nursing* (6th ed.). New York: Springer.

Stuart, G. W. (Ed.)., (2013). *Principles and practice of psychiatric nursing* (10th ed.). St. Louis: Mosby.

Tang, Y. Y., Holzel, B. K., & Posner, M. I. (2015). The neuroscience of mindfulness meditation. *Nature Reviews. Neuroscience, 16*, 213–225.

Thompson, T., Keogh, E., & French, C. C. (2011). Sensory focusing versus distraction and pain: Moderating effects of anxiety sensitivity in males and females. *Journal of Pain, 12*, 849–858.

US Department of Agriculture. (2012). Dietary guidelines for Americans. http://www.cnpp.usda.gov/dietaryguidelines.htm.

US Department of Health and Human Services (USDHHS). (2011). Healthy People 2020. http://https://www.healthypeople.gov/2020/topics-objectives.

van Woerden, H. C., Poortinga, W., et al. (2011). The relationship of different sources of social support and civic participation with self-rated health. *Journal of Public Mental Health, 10*, 126–139.

Walsh, A. (2011). The relaxation response: A strategy to address stress. *International Journal of Athletic Therapy & Training, 16*(2), 20–23.

Weber, J. G. (2011). *Individual and family stress and crises.* Thousand Oaks, CA: Sage Publications.

Whalley, B., Rees, K., et al. (2011). Psychological interventions for coronary heart disease. *The Cochrane Database of Systematic Reviews,* (8), CD002902.

Willis, D. G., DeSanto-Madeya, S., et al. (2015). Spiritual healing in the aftermath of childhood maltreatment: Translating men's lived experiences utilizing conceptual models and theory. *Advances in Nursing Science, 38*, 162–174.

Wong, L., & Viagas, R. (2012). *Scales to scalpels.* New York: Pegasus Books.

Wood, A. W., Gonzales, J., & Barden, S. M. (2015). Mindful caring: Using mindfulness-based cognitive therapy with caregivers of cancer survivors. *Journal of Psychosocial Oncology, 33*, 66–84.

Wooten, P. (2009). Humor, laughter, and play: Maintaining balance in a serious world. In B. Dossey, L. Keegan, & C. Guzzetta (Eds.), *Holistic nursing: A handbook for practice* (5th ed., pp. 239–249). Sudbury, MA: Jones & Bartlett.

Wright, L. M., & Leahey, M. (2013). *Nurses and families: A guide to family assessment and intervention* (6th ed.). Philadelphia: F.A. Davis.

# 14

# Complementary and Alternative Strategies

*Donna Dellolacona*

## OBJECTIVES

*After completing this chapter, the reader will be able to:*

- Compare holistic, allopathic, and complementary and alternative health modalities.
- Describe the nursing role in complementary health therapies.
- Explain the origin and practice of selected holistic health strategies.
- Identify complementary and alternative medicine resources and guidelines.
- Discuss complementary and alternative medicine safety and effectiveness.

## KEY TERMS

| | | |
|---|---|---|
| Acupressure | Genetics | Pet therapy |
| Acupuncture | Healing touch | Physical therapy |
| Affordable Care Act | Health | Polarity therapy |
| Allopathic medicine | Herbal therapy | Prayer |
| Allopathy | Holism | Presence |
| Alternative therapy | Holistic health | Probiotics |
| American Holistic Nurses Association | Homeopathy | Qi |
| Aromatherapy | Hydrotherapy | Qigong |
| Attunement | Hypnotherapy | Reflexology |
| Ayurvedic medicine | Imagery | Reiki |
| Biofeedback | Integrative therapy | Shiatsu |
| Centering | Jin Shin Jyutsu | Spinal or bone manipulation |
| Chi | Massage | Tai chi |
| Chiropractic medicine | Meditation | Therapeutic presence |
| Complementary and alternative medicine | Meridians | Therapeutic touch |
| | Moxibustion | Touch therapies |
| Complementary therapy | Music therapy | Traditional Chinese medicine |
| Cranial and craniosacral therapies | National Center for Complementary and Integrative Health | Visual or guided imagery |
| Dance therapy | | Wellness |
| Distant healing | National Prevention Strategy | Whole medical systems |
| Energy healing or therapy | Naturopathy | Yoga |
| Energy therapy | Nursing presence | |
| Energy work | Nutritional counseling | |

**THINK ABOUT IT**

*Ms. Gonzalez is 45 years old in her usual state of good health working as a teacher, until she receives a diagnosis of with lung cancer. She has never smoked, has no family history of smoking, but worked as a waitress in a diner for 10 years as a young woman. Smoking in restaurants was not restricted at that time. Her presenting symptoms were hemoptysis, low-grade fever, fatigue, and persistent cough. Her family and friends are very concerned and have provided her with various complementary and alternative medicine (CAM) modalities to help to treat her. She goes to the preoperative clinic for surgery, and in addition to 650 mg aspirin she has been taking coenzyme $Q_{10}$, amygdalin/laetrile, milk thistle, and green tea as treatment for her cancer and kava kava to help her relax and rest since her diagnosis. She has begun yoga classes at a local spa. She is frightened, and she believes that she feels less fatigued since starting these therapies. She has never taken prescription medications and is afraid of addiction if she takes prescribed pain medication. The local hospital offers a center for wellness classes involving alternative and complementary therapies, including reiki, yoga, acupuncture, massage, and dietary supplements, to assist with treatment effects. She understands that these complementary therapies may help relieve her symptoms, but she believes they will also treat her cancer. After looking at sites on the Internet, including http://cam.cancer.gov and http://www.nccih.gov, she feels overwhelmed and confused as to what is best for her.*

- What is the difference between reiki and massage?
- What occurs in a usual visit for acupuncture or a reiki session?
- How do these therapies work?
- Are these therapies evidence-based?
- What is the best understanding of the biological and physiological mechanisms for these therapies?
- What is the best understanding of the safety of these therapies?
- Which therapies are covered by her insurance?
- Would Ms. Gonzalez's therapies be considered complementary, alternative, or integrative?

## BACKGROUND

Although many complementary and alternative therapies date back more than 5000 years to the Han Dynasty, Hippocrates, and Indian cultures with Ayurveda, only a few have been evaluated with well-conducted research (National Center for Complementary and Integrative Health [NCCIH], 2015b). In the United States the CAM movement is far more modern, with herbal agents used by Native Americans, chiropractic, meditative, and a variety of therapies beginning in the 19th century. The first center for alternative medicine, the Office of Alternative Medicine, was commissioned by Congress only in 1991(NCCIH, 2015b). The working definition of CAM at that time was "a group of medical, health care, and healing systems other than those included in mainstream health care in the United States" (NCCIH, 2015b). CAM now includes an ever-increasing array of theories, modalities, products, and practices that are used to treat illnesses and/or promote health and well-being.

The field is broad and constantly changing, but an authoritative and governmental source, the National Institutes of Health's **National Center for Complementary and Integrative Health** (NCCIH), currently defines CAM as "a group of diverse medical and health care systems, practices, and products that are not generally considered part of conventional medicine or Western allopathic medicine and the traditional medical providers in the United States health care system" (NCCIH, 2015b). NCCIH has separate definitions of complementary, alternative, and integrative therapy. It defines **complementary therapy** as the use of CAM in conjunction with and as a complement to allopathic traditional medicine. One example is the use of acupuncture to help lessen some side effects of cancer treatment. **Alternative therapy** uses CAM instead of standard medicine. One example is the use of a special diet or herbs to treat cancer instead of anticancer drugs prescribed by an oncologist. **Integrative therapy** is a total approach to medical care that combines standard medical and surgical interventions with the CAM practices that have been shown to be safe and effective. They treat the client's mind, body, and spirit. There is an emphasis on safety and effectiveness (NCCIH, 2015c). Complementary and alternative therapies are more holistic than traditional medicine practices have been in

the past. The most common of these from a national survey can be seen in Figure 14-1.

Although heterogeneous, the major CAM systems have many common characteristics, including a focus on individualizing treatments, treating the whole person, promoting self-care and self-healing, and recognizing the spiritual nature of individuals. A large gap exists between our current level of scientific evidence and what we need to provide to clients in terms of evidence-based advice. More rigorous scientific research is being conducted by many countries to enrich our knowledge base.

### Some Known Facts

- The World Health Organization estimates that more than 80% of the world's population uses some form of herbal medicine.
- Seventy-five percent of Americans use some herbal supplement; most do not report them to providers.
- Approximately 26% of people scheduled for surgery use herbal products that have an adverse impact on their surgical outcome; 19 agents are associated with abnormal bleeding (Wong et al., 2012).
- Accurate risk assessments are unknown as there is:
  - No regulation of these agents.
  - No standard manufacturing process.
  - No method to determine ingredients.
  - No quality controls.
  - No protection against contamination.
  - No Food and Drug Administration (FDA, 2015) required reporting of adverse reactions from alternative therapies.
  - No evidence base for most of the claims.
- A large national survey found that:
  - Seventy-seven percent of Americans believed that the government reviewed the safety of supplements and approved them before they were marketed.
  - Sixty-eight percent of Americans believed that supplements had to list potential side effects on their labels.
  - Fifty-five percent of Americans believed that supplement labels could not make claims of safety without scientific evidence.

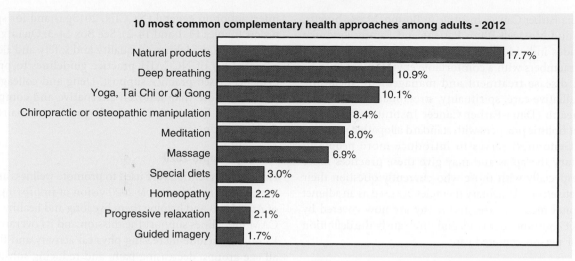

**10 most common complementary health approaches among adults - 2012**

| Approach | Percentage |
|---|---|
| Natural products | 17.7% |
| Deep breathing | 10.9% |
| Yoga, Tai Chi or Qi Gong | 10.1% |
| Chiropractic or osteopathic manipulation | 8.4% |
| Meditation | 8.0% |
| Massage | 6.9% |
| Special diets | 3.0% |
| Homeopathy | 2.2% |
| Progressive relaxation | 2.1% |
| Guided imagery | 1.7% |

**FIGURE 14-1** Ten most common complementary health approaches among adults. (From Clarke, T. C., Black, L. I., Stussman, B. J., Barnes, P. M., & Nahin, R. L. [2015]. *Trends in the use of complementary health approaches among adults: United States, 2002–2012. National health statistics reports no. 79.* Hyattsville, MD: National Center for Health Statistics. http://www.cdc.gov/nchs/data/nhsr/nhsr079.pdf.)

- Americans were unaware that herbal-pharmaceutical interactions occur (Clarke et al., 2015).

## WHAT IS THE DIFFERENCE BETWEEN HOLISM AND ALLOPATHY?

Health care and delivery in the United States is most often **allopathic medicine,** a system in which physicians and other health care professionals, such as nurses, pharmacists, and therapists, treat symptoms and diseases using medications, radiation, lasers, or surgical interventions. **Allopathy** is also called biomedicine, conventional medicine, mainstream medicine, orthodox medicine, and Western medicine (NCCIH, 2015c).

Holistic health considers the whole person and how he or she interacts with his or her environment. It emphasizes the connection of mind, body, and spirit. **Holistic health** is a system of preventive care that takes into account the whole individual, one's own responsibility for one's well-being, and the total influences—social, psychological, environmental—that affect health, including nutrition, exercise, and mental relaxation. **Holism** entails a focus on proactive, healthy living and considers not only prevention of illness but also the root cause of the illness. When disease occurs, holistic practitioners seek to support the person's natural healing systems, to consider the whole person, and to consider the environment, both physical and mental, surrounding the person. This movement in the healing arts reflects the theory of holism and recognizes that all aspects of the person must be considered when care is being planned and delivered (NCCIH, 2015c).

### Person-Centered Care

There are a variety of reasons why people seeking care seek a more holistic approach to care, and use CAM. Those receiving traditional medicine therapies are often disappointed in the lack of effective treatments or cures for many disorders, have fear of

the safety and long-term effects of "drugs" or treatments, believe herbal products are safe because they are derived from "nature," and have a desire to have control of their own health, so they choose alternative and/or complementary methods. There is a great deal of advertising, media, and peer influence that impacts their holistic choices.

Many people are seeking alternative styles of health care that focus on seeing care recipients as whole people, increasing well-being, and giving them greater control over self-care. The 2012 National Health Interview Survey (NHIS) (Clarke et al., 2015) identified that people in the United States use CAM modalities and they spent $33.9 billion out-of-pocket on CAM. CAM costs are 11.2% of total out-of-pocket expenditures on health care. The $14.8 billion spent on nonvitamin, nonmineral, natural products is equivalent to approximately one-third of the total out-of-pocket spending on prescription drugs ($47.6 billion), and the $11.9 billion spent on CAM practitioner visits is equivalent to approximately one-fourth of the total out-of-pocket spending on physician visits ($49.6 billion) (NCCIH, 2015d).

CAM practices are moving into mainstream medical practice. Many traditional medical centers now include a holistic viewpoint and integrative therapies, including Harvard, Stanford, Duke, and the Mayo Clinic. Most of them offer acupuncture, massage, healing gardens, and nutrition counseling. The Van Elslander Cancer Center at St. John Hospital and Medical Center in Detroit, Michigan, has a clinic that also offers qigong, tai chi, yoga classes, hypnotherapy, and guided imagery (St. John Providence, 2015). With a vision "to promote health and healing of body, mind, and spirit," the Woodwinds Health Campus located in Woodbury, Minnesota, offers complementary therapies, including the use of essential oils, energy-based therapies, imagery, music, acupuncture, acupressure, and massage (Woodwinds Health Campus, 2015). The Birchtree Center in western Massachusetts offers professional holistic development classes for nurses that can help them prepare for holistic nursing certification (Birchtree Center, 2015).

At the Dana Farber Cancer Institute in Boston, Massachusetts, the Eleanor and Maxwell Blum Patient and Family Resource Center provides individuals undergoing cancer therapies and their family members with a comfortable environment to learn more about disease treatment and management, including nutrition, palliative care, spirituality, stress management, and emotional health (Dana-Farber Cancer Institute, 2016). This integration of holistic practices with standard allopathic medicine (Box 14-1: Genomics) serves to introduce more people to complementary therapies and may give these practices more credibility, especially with those who currently question their value. Alternative/complementary therapies are used as an adjunct to conventional medical care, and many are now covered by insurers, meet consumer demand, and thus satisfy the definition of patient- or person-centered care.

## Health and Wellness

The World Health Organization's timeless definition of **health** is "a state of complete physical, mental and social well-being and not merely the absence of disease or infirmity" (World Health Organization, 1948). The Wellness Initiative (Substance Abuse and Mental Health Services Administration, 2015) defines **wellness** as "overall well-being. It includes the mental, emotional, physical, occupational, intellectual, and spiritual aspects of a person's life." Working toward health and wellness is an ongoing process that includes self-knowledge and self-care (Definition of Wellness, 2015). The wellness-related reasons that people use a variety of nontraditional therapies analyzed for this report include:

- Treatment of a specific health condition
- General wellness or disease prevention
- Improve immune function
- Improve energy
- Focus on the whole person—mind, body, and spirit
- Improve memory or concentration

Use of holistic modalities can also help meet the goals of *Healthy People 2020* (United States Department of Health and Human Services, 2015). This includes increasing quality and number of years of life, improving nutrition, increasing physical activity, and decreasing illegal substance abuse and harassment throughout the life span (Box 14-2: *Healthy People 2020*). The Affordable Care Act includes provisions that allow CAM providers to participate in health care delivery teams.

## Health Policy

### Clinical Practice Guidelines

Clinical practice guidelines for CAM modalities exist to identify and describe evidence-based recommended courses of

intervention in general (NCCIH, 2015g,i) and for specific disorders (Tables 14-1 and 14-2). See Box 14-3: Quality and Safety Scenario for guidelines on quality and safety and Box 14-4 for a partial list of NCCAIH practice guidelines to provide best evidence-based practice support. Deng and colleagues (2013) provided more than a dozen alternative and complementary therapies to be included in the diagnosis and management of the disease process.

### Healthy People 2020

Holistic interventions are used to promote wellness and are used to meet the *Healthy People 2020* vision of improving the health of Americans and helping them live long and healthy lives. Many CAM modalities support the mission and its overarching goals. Examples include increasing physical activity and flexibility in all age groups, decreasing pain, and reducing substance abuse (http://www.healthypeople.gov).

### Affordable Care Act and National Prevention Strategy

The **Affordable Care Act** (https://www.healthcare.gov) mandates that insurers not discriminate against licensed health care providers, including those who practice alternative medicine, such as naturopaths, massage therapists, and acupuncturists. CAM practitioners and integrative practices are mentioned in several areas of the law, including workforce planning; patient-centered medical homes; wellness, prevention, and health-promotion services; comparative effectiveness research; and birthing services. The **National Prevention Strategy,** released in June 2011 as a result of the Affordable Care Act, has the following four strategic directions:

- Healthy and safe community environments: Create, sustain, and recognize communities that promote health and wellness through prevention.
- Clinical and community preventive services: Ensure that prevention-focused health care and community prevention efforts are available, integrated, and mutually reinforcing.
- Empowered people: Support people in making healthy choices.
- Elimination of health disparities: Eliminate disparities, improving the quality of life for all Americans.

The second direction has a holistic objective: "enhance coordination and integration of clinical, behavioral, and complementary health strategies." Inclusion of CAM into future research and evaluation and integration into care are mentioned several times throughout the document (National Prevention Council, 2011).

### Nursing and Nursing Education

A variety of holistic, complementary, and alternative practices are now very prevalent and part of mainstream health care practice; therefore nurses must understand the nature of these interventions to provide safe, effective care and to discuss these practices with individuals who are using them so as to facilitate integrative care. Nurses who understand holistic practices will be able to make appropriate referrals to alternative/complementary practitioners. Nurses also find that holistic interventions such as **energy work**, bodywork, aromatherapy, prayer, meditation, massage, imagery, music therapy, and the movement arts of yoga, tai chi, and qigong provide a useful adjunct to current nursing theory (Dossey & Keegan, 2013) and practice.

---

**BOX 14-1   GENOMICS**

**Genetics** contributes to people's risk of developing many common diseases. Diet, lifestyle, and environmental exposures are factors in many conditions, and risk factors for many types of cancer. A better understanding of the interface of CAM practices with genetics may identify measures to mitigate health risks. Mapping the genetic components of cells, explaining how all the various elements work together to affect the human body in both health and disease, and developing targeted therapies will help providers better educate and advise those in their care.

**BOX 14-2 HEALTHY PEOPLE 2020**

### Selected National Health and Wellness Objectives

- (Developmental) Increase the proportion of insured persons with coverage for clinical preventive services.
- (Developmental) Increase the proportion of persons who receive appropriate evidence-based clinical preventive services.
- Increase the proportion of adolescents who have had a wellness checkup in the past 12 months.
- Increase the proportion of schools with a school breakfast program.
- Reduce the proportion of adolescents who have been offered, sold, or given an illegal drug on school property.
- Increase the proportion of adolescents whose parents consider them to be safe at school.
- (Developmental) Increase the proportion of middle and high schools that prohibit harassment on the basis of a student's sexual orientation or gender identity.
- Increase the proportion of elementary, middle, and senior high schools that provide comprehensive school health education to prevent health problems in the following areas: unintentional injury; violence; suicide; tobacco use and addiction; alcohol or other drug use; unintended pregnancy, HIV/AIDS, and infection with sexually transmitted diseases; unhealthy dietary patterns; and inadequate physical activity.
- Increase the proportion of elementary, middle, and senior high schools that provide school health education to promote personal health and wellness in the following areas: hand washing or hand hygiene; oral health; growth and development; sun safety and skin cancer prevention; benefits of rest and sleep; ways to prevent vision and hearing loss; and the importance of health screenings and checkups.
- Increase the proportion of college and university students who receive information from their institution on each of the priority health risk behavior areas

- (all priority areas; unintentional injury; violence; suicide; tobacco use and addiction; alcohol and other drug use; unintended pregnancy, HIV/AIDS, and infection with sexually transmitted diseases; unhealthy dietary patterns; and inadequate physical activity).
- (Developmental) Increase the proportion of work sites that offer an employee health-promotion program to their employees.
- Increase the proportion of persons who report that their health care providers always involved them in decisions about their health care as much as they wanted.
- (Developmental) Increase the proportion of individuals whose physician recommends personalized health information resources to help them manage their health.
- Increase the proportion of adults who meet current federal physical activity guidelines for aerobic physical activity and for muscle-strengthening activity.
- Increase the proportion of adolescents who meet current federal physical activity guidelines for aerobic physical activity and for muscle-strengthening activity.
- Increase the proportion of physician office visits that include counseling or education related to physical activity.
- Health-related quality of life and well-being is a new topic area for *Healthy People 2020*. Health-related quality of life is a multidimensional concept that includes domains related to physical, mental, emotional, and social functioning. It goes beyond direct measures of population health, life expectancy, and causes of death, and focuses on the impact health status has on quality of life. A concept related to health-related quality of life is well-being, which assesses the positive aspects of a person's life, such as positive emotions and life satisfaction.

From US Department of Health and Human Services. (2011). *Healthy People 2020.* http://www.healthypeople.gov/2020/about/default.aspx.

| TABLE 14-1 | Herbs as Medicine |
|---|---|
| **Drug Name** | **Plant/Tree** |
| Digitalis (heart drug) | Foxglove plant |
| Paclitaxel (cancer drug) | Pacific yew tree |
| Aspirin | Willow tree |
| Quinine (malaria drug) | Cinchona tree |
| Morphine | Opium poppy |
| Galantamine (Alzheimer disease drug) | Daffodil bulb |
| Vincristine (cancer drug) | Rosy periwinkle |
| Reserpine (blood pressure drug) | Indian snakeroot plant |

What are herbs? An herb (also called a botanical) is a plant or plant part used for its scent, flavor, and/or therapeutic properties. An herbal supplement is a type of dietary supplement that contains herbs, either alone or in mixtures.
From National Center for Complementary and Integrative Health. *Herbs at a glance.* http://nccam.nih.gov/sites/nccam.nih.gov/files/herbs/NIH_Herbs_at_a_Glance.pdf.

The **American Holistic Nurses Association** (AHNA) defines holistic nursing as nursing practice that heals the whole person. It is a "specialty practice that draws on nursing knowledge, theories, expertise and intuition to guide nurses in becoming therapeutic partners with people in their care. This practice recognizes the totality of the human being—the interconnectedness of body, mind, emotion, spirit, social/cultural, relationship, context, and environment" by integrating CAM modalities into clinical practice to broaden and enrich nursing treatment of physiological, psychological, and spiritual needs. Florence Nightingale is thought to be one of the first holistic nurses because she believed in care of the person, focusing on unity, wellness, and the interrelationship of human beings with their environment. Holistic therapy is considered an "attitude, a philosophy, a way of being" although some holistic nurses specialize in one or more modalities (AHNA, 2015a,b; Dossey & Keegan, 2013).

The AHNA "advances the profession of holistic nursing by providing continuing education in holistic nursing, helping to improve the health care workplace through the incorporation of the concepts of holistic nursing, educating professionals and the public about holistic nursing and integrative health care, and promoting research and scholarship in the field of holistic nursing" (AHNA, 2015a). The AHNA website offers a variety of resources, including a directory of holistic practitioners based on modality and location, descriptions of healing modalities (AHNA, 2015a,d), and guidance on starting a holistic private practice.

## INTERVENTIONS

NCCIH divides CAM modalities into several loose domains and an additional "whole medical system category" that incorporates

## TABLE 14-2 Commonly Used Herbs: Safety Profile

| Herb | Uses | Side Effects | Interactions | Evidence |
|------|------|--------------|--------------|----------|
| St. John's wort | Depression | Dizziness, restlessness, sensitivity to sunlight, sleep disturbances, constipation | Seizure medications, alcohol, warfarin, calcium channel blockers, digoxin, oral contraceptives, statins | No statistically significant effect other than placebo effect on depression scores |
| Ginseng | Depression, anxiety, energy, concentration, immunity | Chest pain, headache, hypertension, impotence, palpitations, | Diabetic agents, including insulin | Some evidence for concentration, no benefit for energy, mood, or immune modulation |
| Milk thistle | Liver ailments | Laxative effects | Flagyl | Cirrhosis; patients may have longer survival; may be protective against hepatotoxic agents |
| Black cohosh | Menopausal symptoms | Low blood pressure; dizziness | Iron, antihypertensive drugs, warfarin, aspirin | No better than placebo |
| Echinacea | Immune system booster | Well tolerated | Immunosuppressants | Decreases time to resolution of symptoms; no preventative effect |
| Saw palmetto | Benign prostate hyperplasia | Abdominal issues headache, urinary retention | Hormones: leuprolide, birth control agents | As effective as many prescribed medications for benign prostate hyperplasia |
| Gingko biloba | Memory, asthma, vision | Gastrointestinal upset, seizures, bleeding or bruising | Anticoagulants, warfarin, aspirin, acetaminophen, seizure medications, antidepressants | No measurable long-term benefit |
| Garlic | Asthma, diabetes, high cholesterol level, cancer | Dizziness, rash, diaphoresis, bleeding | Antiplatelet drugs, warfarin, aspirin, HIV medications | No long-term benefits |
| Cranberry | Urinary tract infection, cancer | Diarrhea | None | Reduces risk of infection; no effect on treatment |
| Soy | Menopause, cancer, heart disease | | Antibiotics, estrogens, warfarin, tamoxifen, losartan, carvedilol, levothyroxine | No effect on blood pressure Inconclusive results for hot flashes to date |
| Fish oil | Cholesterol; blood pressure, and heart disease | Prolonged bleeding, negative impact on immunity | Anticoagulants, birth control agents | May worsen depression |
| Glucosamine | Joint health | Gastrointestinal upset | Blood thinners, insulin, heart medications | Those with a shellfish allergy should avoid it |
| Coenzyme Q$_{10}$ | Heart, fatigue, immunity | Rash, gastrointestinal upset | Chemotherapy, blood pressure medications, coumadin | |
| Ephedra | Weight loss | Heart attack; respiratory depression, death | Theophylline, digoxin, caffeine, but available on the Internet | Banned by the US Food and Drug Administration in 2003 |

From National Center for Complementary and Integrative Health. (2015). *Herbs at a glance.* http://nccam.nih.gov/health/herbsataglance.htm.

all domains. The domains are not formally defined but include biologically based practices, mind and body techniques, manipulative body-based practices, energy therapies, and ancient medical systems. See Table 14-3 for examples of these categories. These domains are neither mutually exclusive nor mutually inclusive because many could belong to several categories.

Because each modality has its own identified guidance for purpose, efficacy, and safety, this section will not be specific but will briefly define many of the modalities and highlight a few of the more common ones with current known evidence.

## Whole Medical Systems

Whole medical systems are complete systems of theories and practices that have evolved culturally over time, and because

they are different from Western allopathic medicine, they are considered CAM. Examples include traditional healers and traditional or folk healers. The 2012 NHIS (Clarke et al., 2015) found that although there was less use of traditional healers than in 2007, there was an increase in the use of most other CAM modalities.

## Ayurvedic Medicine

Ayurvedic medicine has evolved over thousands of years in India. This treatment utilizes herbs in their natural state, as prepared herbal drugs, massage, and special individualized diets, based on the seasons of one's life and one's constitutional type; there are ten. Ayurvedic supplements can be made either of herbs only or a combination of herbs, metals, and minerals. Some of these

## ☑ BOX 14-3  QUALITY AND SAFETY SCENARIO

### *How Should Complementary and Alternative Medicine Be Evaluated?*

- What standards of proof should the nurse require before adopting an alternative/complementary therapy in clinical practice?
- Have all (or even some) of the alternative/complementary therapies commonly used by nurses today been subjected to these standards?
- Have all (or even most) of the standard therapies commonly used by nurses and medicine today been subjected to these standards?
- Government and consumer advocates are beginning to require the same oversight, regulation, and monitoring of some CAM practices.

From Coakley, A. B., & Barron, A. (2012). Energy therapies in oncology nursing. *Seminars in Oncology Nursing, 28*(1), 55–63; Faculty of Harvard Medical School & Natural Standard. (2008). *Complementary and alternative medicine: Therapeutic touch.* http://www.intelihealth.com/IH/ihtIH/WSIHW000/8513/34968/358873.html?d=dmtContent; Herman, P. M., D'Huyvetter, K. D., & Mohler, M. J. (2006). Are health services research methods a match for CAM? *Alternative Therapies in Health and Medicine, 12*(3), 78–83.

## BOX 14-4  Complementary and Alternative Medicine Clinical Practice Guidelines: Featured Guidelines

### Allergy and Immunology
- Diagnosis and Management of Food Allergy (*Journal of Allergy and Clinical Immunology*)
- Guidelines for the Diagnosis and Management of Asthma (National Heart, Lung, and Blood Institute)
- 2011–2012 Influenza Antiviral Medications: Summary for Clinicians (Centers for Disease Control and Prevention)

### Cardiology
- Soy and Cardiovascular Health (*Circulation*)

### Family Medicine
- Clinical Use of Dietary Supplements and Nutraceuticals (*Endocrine Practice*)
- Dietary Reference Intakes for Calcium and Vitamin D (Institute of Medicine of the National Academies)
- Herbs and Supplements in Managed Care (*The Permanente Journal*)
- Evaluation and Management of Chronic Insomnia in Adults (*Sleep*)
- Psychological and Behavioral Treatment of Insomnia (*Sleep*)
- Adjunctive Therapies for Dermatitis (American Academy of Dermatology)
- Vitamin Supplementation to Prevent Cancer and Cardiovascular Disease (Unites States Preventative Services Task Force)
- Dietary Reference Intakes for Calcium and Vitamin D (Institute of Medicine of the National Academies)

### Gastroenterology
- Probiotics and Children (*Journal of Pediatric Gastroenterology and Nutrition*)

### Neurology
- Alternative Therapies for Parkinson's Disease (*Neurology*)
- Migraine Headaches in Children and Adolescents (*Journal of Pediatric Health Care*)
- Complementary and Alternative Medicine in Multiple Sclerosis (American Academy of Neurology)
- NSAIDs and Other Complementary Treatments for Episodic Migraine Prevention in Adults (*Neurology*)

### Oncology
- Complementary Therapies for Patients With Lung Cancer (American College of Chest Physicians)
- American Cancer Society Guidelines on Nutrition and Physical Activity for Cancer Prevention (*Cancer*)
- Exercise Guidelines for Cancer Survivors (*Medicine & Science in Sports & Exercise*)

- Integrative Oncology: Complementary Therapies and Botanicals (Society for Integrative Oncology)
- Integrative Oncology in Lung Cancer (*Chest*)
- Use of Integrative Therapies as Supportive Care in Breast Cancer Patients (*Journal of the National Cancer Institute*)

### Pain Management
- Chiropractic Management of Fibromyalgia (Council on Chiropractic Guidelines and Practice Parameters)
- Chronic Pain Management (*Anesthesiology*)
- Diagnosis and Treatment of Low-Back Pain (*Annals of Internal Medicine*)
- Management of Fibromyalgia Syndrome in Adults (University of Texas, School of Nursing)
- Osteopathic Manipulative Treatment for Low-Back Pain (*Journal of the American Osteopathic Association*)
- Pain Management Task Force Final Report (Office of The Army Surgeon General)

### Pediatrics
- Migraine Headaches in Children and Adolescents (*Journal of Pediatric Health Care*)
- Probiotics and Children (*Journal of Pediatric Gastroenterology and Nutrition*)
- The Use of Complementary and Alternative Therapies in the Treatment of Fragile X Syndrome (The Fragile X Clinical and Research Consortium)

### Psychiatry and Mental Health
- Management of Post-Traumatic Stress Disorder and Acute Stress Reaction (Department of Veterans Affairs/Department of Defense)
- Posttraumatic Stress Disorder—Associated Nightmares (*Journal of Clinical Sleep Medicine*)

### Rheumatology/Orthopedics
- Osteoarthritis of the Hip and Knee (*Osteoarthritis Cartilage*)
- Osteoarthritis of the Knee (*The Journal of the American Academy of Orthopaedic Surgeons*)
- Manual Manipulation for Musculoskeletal Injuries (Academy for Chiropractic Education)
- Vitamin D and Calcium Supplementation to Prevent Fractures in Adults (US Preventive Services Task Force)
- Nonpharmacologic and Pharmacologic Therapies for Osteoarthritis of the Hand, Hip, and Knee (American College of Rheumatology)

### Women's Health
- Botanicals for Menopausal Symptoms (*Obstetrics and Gynecology*)

From National Center for Complementary and Integrative Health. (2015). *Clinical practice guidelines.* http://nccam.nih.gov/health/providers/clinicalpractice.htm.

## TABLE 14-3 Categories and Examples of Complementary and Alternative Therapies

| Whole medical systems | Chinese, ayurvedic, traditional/folk healers, naturopathy, homeopathy |
|---|---|
| Biologically based practices | Herbal remedies, vitamins, dietary supplements, diets, probiotics, chelation therapy, hydrotherapy, aromatherapy |
| Manipulative and body-based practices | Massage, reflexology, chiropractic, craniosacral therapies, physical therapy |
| Mind-body techniques | Meditation, guided imagery, hypnosis, music, biofeedback, yoga, tai chi, qigong, acupuncture, dance |
| Energy therapies | Magnetic field therapy, reiki, therapeutic touch, prayer |

products may be harmful if used improperly or without the direction of a trained practitioner (NCCIH, 2015a).

The goals are treatment of disease, prevention of disease, and improving a person's quality of life, by balancing the body, mind, and spirit. Basic premises include the beliefs that all living and nonliving things in the universe are joined together and good health is achieved when one's mind and body are in harmony (NCCIH, 2015a). Two ancient books, more than 2000 years old and written in Sanskrit, are considered the heart of the practice and identify eight branches of ayurvedic medicine: internal medicine; surgery; treatment of head and neck disease; gynecology/obstetrics; pediatrics; toxicology; care of the elderly and rejuvenation; and sexual vitality. Treatment practices include eliminating impurities, decreasing symptoms, increasing resistance to disease, and reducing worry and increasing harmony. Nearly 80% of the Indian population continues to use ayurvedic medicine. No states in the United States currently license ayurvedic practitioners.

### Traditional Chinese Medicine

Traditional Chinese medicine (TCM) has evolved over thousands of years in China and includes herbs, acupuncture, and other CAM treatments. The theoretical framework includes the complementary yet opposing yin and yang life forces, and the balance and harmony of the vital energy, or life force (qi), circulating through the body's pathways. TCM describes the organs and tissues in the body through corresponding elements of fire, earth, metal, water, and wood. It also uses eight principles to analyze symptoms and categorize conditions, including cold/heat, interior/exterior, excess/deficiency, and yin/yang (NCCIH, 2015e).

### Naturopathy

Naturopathy, also called naturopathic medicine, evolved from a combination of traditional and other modalities in 19th-century Europe guided by the healing power of nature (NCCIH, 2015f). The underlying principles are first do no harm; illness is seen as a purposeful process of the organism; symptoms are viewed as life forces attempting to heal the organism. Practitioners do not use prescription drugs, injections, X-rays, or surgery, but instead implement a variety of CAM modalities, emphasizing the adoption of a healthy lifestyle, strengthening and cleansing

the body, special diets, therapies, and use of manipulation and exercise (NCCIH, 2015f).

### Homeopathy

Homeopathy principles have been documented since at least the time of Hippocrates, but not until early in the 19th century were they brought into modern usage. Samuel Hahnemann, a German physician and chemist, is credited with founding homeopathy (National Center for Homeopathy, 2015). When Hahnemann first named the discipline in 1807, mainstream medicine involved ineffective practices such as bloodletting and purging. Homeopathy treats the whole person and believes that symptoms are a body's effort to rid itself of disease. It is based on four principles: the law of similars, or like cures like; the minimum dose, determining the least amount of medicine needed to treat a disease; totality of symptoms, matching the complete symptom profile of the person to the symptom profile of the remedy; and single remedy, administration of one remedy at a time (National Center for Homeopathy, 2015).

Homeopathy is based on the whole person rather than on the symptoms. Treatment stimulates the body's healing ability through the administration of small amounts of dilute substances that are believed to cause illness or symptoms. There is wider acceptance of homeopathy in other countries, including France, Germany, Mexico, Argentina, India, and Great Britain. The World Health Organization estimates that homeopathy is currently practiced by more than 500 million people worldwide. In April 2015 (National Center for Complementary and Integrative Health, 2015) the FDA held a hearing on homeopathic product regulation, safety, and efficacy. Most of the testimony cited the lack of scientific evidence, the lack of consumer understanding, the lack of regulation, and the harm that has come from some of these practices. Further analysis and decisions may be forthcoming.

### Biologically Based Practices/Natural Products

Biological or natural products are the oldest form of CAM. Medicinal herbs were found in the personal effects of a mummified prehistoric man in the Italian Alps (NCCIH, 2015b). Botanical remedies were inventoried in great detail in the Middle Ages. The 2012 NHIS found that nearly 40% of American adults use natural products as CAM. This area of CAM includes nutritional counseling, herbs, vitamins, minerals, probiotics, and aromatherapy. According to NCCIH, daily multivitamin and calcium supplements are not thought of as CAMs.

According to the US *National Nutritional Research Roadmap* (Interagency Committee on Human Nutrition Research, 2015), nutritional counseling uses education and diet and supplementation therapeutically as the primary or adjunctive measure to prevent or treat illness. Multiple studies have demonstrated the efficacy of nutritional interventions, vitamins, therapeutic diets, and individual instruction. Diet teaching for those receiving hemodialysis showed efficacy in stabilization of laboratory values (Garagarza et al., 2015), and nutritional interventions for those undergoing chemotherapy not only helped people maintain weight and muscle mass but also improved survival over the control group (De Waele et al., 2015).

Herbal therapy is the use of herbs or their chemical properties to treat specific conditions or to enhance the function of various body systems, such as boosting the immune system, treating allergies, or preventing a cold. Herbal medicines may act on the body like prescription drugs and may interact with prescription medications; thus it is important to elicit a full profile of what care recipients are taking and in what doses as part of medication reconciliation. A table of common agents, their common uses, side effects, and interactions, and the current evidence has been compiled from NCCIH data (NCCIH, 2015h); see Table 14-2.

Probiotics are live microorganisms found in the human digestive tract, such as "friendly bacteria." They are taken to enhance the digestive system either as a supplement or in natural forms, such as yogurt or other fermented foods.

Hydrotherapy, or water therapy, is the use of water at various temperatures or as ice or steam to relieve discomfort and promote physical well-being. Treatments include full-body immersion, hydrotherapy, steam baths, saunas, spas, and the application of hot and/or cold compresses.

Aromatherapy, also referred to as essential oil therapy, is defined by the National Association for Holistic Aromatherapy (2015) as the art and science of using naturally extracted oils from plants to balance, harmonize, and promote the health of body, mind, and spirit. The therapeutic use of the oils may be via inhalation, external application, or ingestion. The use of aromatherapy, like that of many CAMs, without professional clinical training is strongly discouraged. Individuals must be trained to know the specific warnings and contraindications for each oil, as well as to understand how to handle the oils.

## Manipulative and Body-Based Practices

Manipulative and body-based practices focus on the manipulation of bones and joints, soft tissues, and the circulatory and lymphatic systems. According to the 2012 NHIS (Clarke et al., 2015) these ranked in the top 10 CAM therapies.

### Spinal or Bone Manipulation

Spinal or bone manipulation is the application of controlled force on a bone or joint and is performed by chiropractors, physical therapists, osteopathic physicians, and some conventional physicians. Spinal manipulation was recorded in ancient Greece and became foundational to chiropractic and osteopathic medicine in the late 19th century.

Chiropractic medicine focuses on manipulation of the spine and joints, focusing on spinal alignment for optimal functioning. Chiropractors often integrate other CAMs such as massage, nutrition, and specialized kinesiology into their practice.

Cranial and craniosacral therapies also focus on a natural configuration of the skeletal system, focusing on the skull and flow of cerebrospinal fluid for the treatment of body imbalances. Craniosacral therapy originated in osteopathy and focuses on the bones of the cranium, spine, and sacrum, using gentle pressure to restore free movement of cerebrospinal fluid, allowing normal functioning.

Physical therapy integrates a variety of modalities, including massage, manipulation, heat and cold, movement, and electrical impulses, to treat the body after damage or injury, reduce swelling, relieve pain, and restore function and range of motion to the body.

### Massage

Massage incorporates different techniques in the manipulation of muscles and soft tissues of the body, such as rubbing or kneading, to increase circulation, facilitate healing, and reduce stress and increase relaxation. It is one of the oldest therapies and is referred to in writing in ancient China, Japan, India, Egypt, Greece, and Rome. Even Hippocrates mentions it in his writings. Different types of therapies have different techniques and purposes, such as lymphatic therapy, neuromuscular therapy, and trigger point therapy.

Reflexology is mixed method of CAM as it involves a type of manipulation and the concept of energy fields. A reflexologist applies pressure with the thumbs to mapped points on the feet or hands, or both, by pressing deeply into the point to release tension and stimulate circulation of blood, lymph, and energy. Reflexology is more than massage because practitioners believe that the points correspond to the organs of the body and that stimulating the points will stimulate the organs to heal (Reflexology Association of America, 2015).

## Mind-Body Medicine

Mind and body practices focus on the interactions between the brain, the body, and behavior, using the mind to affect the body and the body to affect the mind. Categories include meditation, imagery, and various methods of body movement. This concept dates back 2000 years to TCM and ayurvedic medicine practices (NCCIH, 2015a). Hippocrates noted that treatment relied on attitude, environmental influences, and natural remedies. Deep breathing, meditation, yoga, guided imagery, and progressive relaxation were in the top CAM therapies according to the 2012 NHIS (Clark et al., 2015). Visual or guided imagery encourages individuals to relax by focusing on calming thoughts or experiences. Imagery is "a gentle but powerful technique that focuses and directs the imagination" so as to, among other things, promote a sense of well-being and to help people relax (http://www.healthjourneys.com/what_is_guided_imagery.asp). In a randomized control study (Bozas et al., 2015), men with prostate cancer and women with breast cancer undergoing chemotherapy had a better quality of life and less depression and there was some positive impact on laboratory values if they used relaxation training and guided imagery as compared with the control group.

### Meditation

Meditation is a method of focused attention to increase relaxation, quiet the mind, and reduce stress. Although it is often a part of many religious cultures, it is not necessarily a religious activity and can be practiced while one is still or while one is active, such as during walking. Like massage, different types have a variety of purposes and techniques. Breath meditation is the simplest because it can be done anywhere and can evoke the relaxation response (Box 14-5). It can be taught and is useful for anyone. Centering focuses on a chosen word. Mindfulness meditation is a way of paying attention to or being mindful of a variety of topics, such as thoughts, actions, or the environment. Walking meditation is a form of mindfulness because the individual is mindful of the interaction of the inner body, the external body, and the environment with each step.

## BOX 14-5 Teaching the Technique of Breath Meditation

- You may stand, sit, or lie quietly as you begin to focus on your breath.
- Inhale and feel the air come into your nostrils, move down your throat, and into your lungs. Do not try to control the breath. Just observe it.
- Exhale and feel the air move up from your lungs and into your throat. Feel the warmth of the exhaled air in your nostrils.
- Breathe. Feel the air move in and out. Concentrate on the breath. Do not try to control the breath. Just observe it.
- Continue watching the breath for 5 to 10 minutes. As other thoughts come into focus, notice them and let them go. Focus again on the breath.
- As you become comfortable with breath meditation, you may easily add simple imagery to this technique.
- As you inhale, imagine breathing in peace or love or wellness.
- As you exhale, imagine breathing out pain or sorrow or grief.
- As you inhale, breathe in whatever it is that you need.
- As you exhale, breathe out whatever you wish to be free of in your life.

## BOX 14-6 Feel Your Own Energy

This exercise will help you feel your own energy, or chi.
- Sit quietly, back straight, feet touching the floor.
- Place your hands in your lap.
- Take a few deep breaths. Become quiet and still.
- Breathe slowly in and out for a few minutes.
- Slowly raise your hands in front of you, palms facing you, hands approximately 15 inches apart. Cup your fingers as though you are holding a basketball between your hands.
- Concentrate on the space between your hands. What is there? Can you feel anything?
- Slowly bring your palms closer together, focusing on the space between your hands.
- Can you feel warmth? Does it feel spongy? Can you move your hands around a shape?
- What you are feeling is the energy coming from the energy centers in your hands. Focus on the energy. Try to increase the sensation of fullness in the space between your hands.
- If you do not feel anything immediately, bring your hands back out to 15 inches apart and slowly move your hands together again. Try this no more than three times each time you attempt the exercise.

**Hypnotherapy** is a form of guided relaxation and focused attention of the unconscious mind. It is used with differing success for memory recall of suppressed events and for behavior changes such as discontinuation of the use of tobacco products. **Biofeedback** is a relaxation technique concentrating on vital functions such heart rate, breathing rate, and blood pressure. This visualization identifies which actions can change the rates and is used for stress and an irregular heart rate. Neurolinguistic programming changes behavior by changing patterns of thinking and speaking (NCCIH, 2015a).

### Movement Therapy

Movement therapies use movement and bodywork to promote physical, mental, emotional, and spiritual well-being. The movement arts such as qigong, tai chi, and yoga are helpful for body, mind, and spirit, and, although technically not energy work, do manipulate life energies. **Qigong** (pronounced chee gung) is part of TCM, combining relaxed movements with a meditative aspect and controlled breathing to move qi energy through the energy channels and increase vital energy. **Tai chi** (pronounced tie chee) began as a Chinese martial art and combines physical movement, breath control, and meditation in a dance-like sequence of poses based on the movements of animals. One pose flows into the next in a slow, relaxed, gentle, unbroken rhythm, bringing an awareness of the moment-to-moment state of the body and producing a meditative state.

**Yoga** is a meditative movement practice that originated in India as a form of spiritual practice and aids in flexibility, agility, balance, and relaxation. The postures have names such as proud warrior, waterfall, runner's pose, downward-facing dog, mountain pose, and eagle pose. There are many types and branches of yoga. Several studies of individuals with a variety of diagnoses have documented several health-related benefits from the practice of yoga, including reducing stress and anxiety, improving pain management, increasing flexibility, and increasing strength (Clarke et al., 2015; McCall et al., 2015). The 2012 NHIS (Clarke et al., 2015) reported yoga use up from 6% in 2007 to almost 10% in 2015. Given the increase in this practice in traditional medicine centers, the prevalence of yoga will likely rise.

**Dance therapy** is another movement-based mind-body modality, using dance to allow the body and mind to move freely in response to music.

### Energy Therapies

**Energy healing or therapy** is practiced in many cultures and involves the use of assumed energy fields to heal and maintain wellness (Box 14-6). Believers in energy therapy describe disruptions in the energy field as a cause for illness and teach that balancing energy can aid in healing when this is done by an energy practitioner. Certain types of body energy are well known. Electrical energy in the body is reflected in diagnostic studies, including electrocardiographic, electromyographic, and electroencephalographic tracings. Nerves and cells have an electromagnetic action potential. Magnetic resonance imaging uses powerful magnets to measure the array of charged particles in the human body and produce diagnostic images. People can be affected by the energy of their environments, including the energy of other people. For example, anxiety is contagious and moves readily and quickly from person to person.

There are medical uses for energy that come from the environment. The energy of radiation is used to shrink tumors; sound energy, in the form of ultrasound waves, is used to break kidney stones. Lasers, focused light energy, are used in many types of surgery and to treat disorders such as psoriasis (Neumayer & Vargo, 2012). Light energy is useful in treating seasonal affective disorder. Color, another form of light energy, has been shown to have an effect on emotions and behaviors.

Energy fields may be characterized as measurable or as yet unmeasured. Practices based on measurable forms of energy include those involving electromagnetic fields such as magnet therapy and light therapy. Practices based on other energy fields, also called biofields, generally reflect the concept that human beings are infused with subtle forms of energy, and various CAM therapies aim to treat these biofields (NCCIH, 2015b).

## BOX 14-7 DIVERSITY AWARENESS

### Hot and Cold Diseases

- Hispanic culture considers disease causation as an imbalance between hot and cold. Specific diseases are classified by their causation, and the treatments (food, home remedies, and medications) used to ameliorate disease are generally temperature opposites; for example, a cold treatment is used for a hot disease. Some examples of hot diseases are constipation, diarrhea, fever, pregnancy, ulcers, and rashes. Examples of cold diseases include arthritis, a cold, indigestion, menstrual cramps, stomachaches, and muscle spasms.

- Hispanic use of complementary and alternative therapies is substantial; these therapies are often used to support chronic conditions. Diabetes is a hot disease. Hypertension, which is considered to be caused by anger, fear, nervousness, and thick blood, is a hot disease. It is treated by the cold treatments of lemon juice and various teas. Asthma is a cold disease, treated by traditional herbal mixtures and by massage. Home treatments traditionally complement traditional therapies and include cactus, aloe vera, and bitter gourd. If home treatments, which are generally initiated by an influential female in the home, are not successful, family and friends are consulted for advice. A spiritual leader (curanderismo) may also be consulted to perform a healing ritual for an especially recalcitrant problem. If this treatment fails to resolve the problem, an allopathic physician may be consulted.

- Because there is potential for drug interactions between allopathic medicines and the traditional medicines of the Hispanic population, it is especially important that allopathic providers understand the home treatments that this population is using. One way to ease the assessment of the use of home treatments is with an open mind and with acceptance of folk practices.

From Dayer-Berenson, L. (2010). *Cultural competencies for nursing.* Sudbury, MA: Jones & Bartlett Learning; Tabur, M. M., Crowe, T. K., & Torres, E. (2009). A review of curanderismo and healing practices among Mexicans and Mexican Americans. *Occupational Therapy International, 16*(1), 82–88; Ortiz, B. I., Shields, K. M., Clauson, K. A., & Clay, P. G. (2007). Complementary and alternative medicine use among Hispanics in the United States. *Annals of Pharmacotherapy, 41*, 994–1004.

## BOX 14-8 RESEARCH FOR EVIDENCED-BASED PRACTICE

A meta-analysis of acupuncture's effectiveness as well as advances in the understanding of acupuncture's physiological action have led to the acceptance and broader use for this modality and new research directions (MacPherson et al., 2016). Acupuncture efficacy has been demonstrated in pain control and nausea suppression. In a melding of new technologies with this ancient tradition, acupuncture neuroimaging research has not only identified a novel brain-based marker for clinical pain perception but has also demonstrated brain image changes due to acupuncture therapy (MacPherson et al., 2016). Patients with fibromyalgia treated with acupuncture showed elevation of the level of a brain marker that correlates with pain intensity that normalized after treatment; positron emission tomography detected an increase of mu-opioid receptor–binding potential in multiple brain regions that correlated with reported relief of fibromyalgia pain.

Another study used functional magnetic resonance imaging to demonstrate a return to normal mapping after acupuncture treatment of carpal tunnel syndrome that correlated with subjective and objective symptom relief. This and other research has led to the development of clinical guidelines, health policy, and reimbursement practices for acupuncture therapies (MacPherson et al., 2016).

From MacPherson, H., Hammerschlag, R., Coeytaux, R. R., Davis, R. T., Harris, R. E., Kong, J. T., Wayne, P. M. (2016). Unanticipated insights into biomedicine from the study of acupuncture. *Journal of Alternative and Complementary Medicine, 22*(2), 101–107.

Any illness, stress, emotional upset, or spiritual distress can affect the flow of life energy. These disruptions in the flow of life energy can cause or exacerbate illness in the physical body and can increase emotional and spiritual distress (Box 14-7: Diversity Awareness). The basic goal behind the various modalities of energy therapy is to release blockages of energy flow, stimulate deficient life energy, and rebalance life energy.

## Acupuncture

Acupuncture manipulates life energy, referred to as chi or qi in some cultures, by stimulating precisely mapped points on the skin surface (Box 14-8: Research for Evidence-Based Practice). The points overlie the channels, called meridians, through which chi travels. The channels are named for the organs they affect, such as the lung meridian, heart meridian, and kidney meridian. Acupuncture may be used to diagnose disharmony; the points become tender to palpation in the presence of a disturbance in energy flow. The acupuncture points act as valves in the meridian system. When the points are stimulated, acupuncture acts as a treatment modality to correct disturbances in flow. When stimulated, the valve may open to release blocked or excess chi or close to allow chi to collect if chi is deficient. Stimulation of the points may be accomplished in several ways: by inserting fine needles into the points, by electrostimulation, by laser, by light stimulation, and by burning herbs on or over the points to increase point stimulation, a technique called moxibustion. Acupuncture is one of the oldest healing practices in the world. Good evidence exists for the efficacy of acupuncture in a variety of realms, and the cost of treatment is often covered by insurance providers.

Acupressure is a form of acupuncture, where the meridian points are stimulated with pressing, rubbing, squeezing, and stretching movements. The technique is taught in some massage schools because it is often used along with massage to move and balance the body's energies. Shiatsu uses a sequence of rhythmic pressure on acupressure meridians. A systematic review revealed that auricular point acupressure is a promising treatment for chronic pain management (Lin et al., 2015; Zhao et al., 2015).

## Touch Therapies

In touch therapies, such as therapeutic touch, healing touch, and reiki, practitioners use their hands to direct life energies drawn from the environment to the individual in an effort to restore balance and harmony within the human energy system (Figure 14-2). Reiki comes from Japanese tradition and requires training by a reiki master. In addition to teaching the hand placements and symbolic gestures used in reiki, the master attunes the student (Box 14-9: Innovative Practice). Attunement opens the energy channel, enabling the student to bring universal energy through the body and to the recipient. Reiki is a form of energy therapy and has been evaluated in several clinical trials for

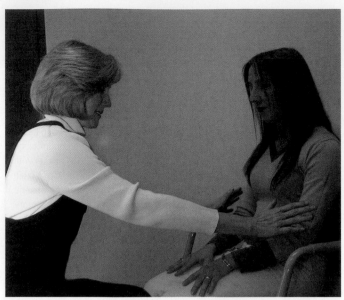

FIGURE 14-2 The assessment phase of therapeutic touch. The practitioner is attempting to sense disturbances or imbalances in the person's energy field.

treatment of anxiety and improvement of well-being in people undergoing cancer treatments (Fleisher et al., 2014). During these therapies the hands can be placed directly on the person's body or at a distance from the body.

**Therapeutic touch** was conceptualized by nursing theorist Martha Rogers. She felt humans are composed of energy fields that interact with the energy fields of their environments (Phillips, 2015). Therapeutic touch practice comprises three essential elements. The first element is centering by the practitioner. **Centering** is a process of becoming calm, present in the moment, and connected with the individual being treated, allowing the practitioner to give the person undivided attention

(Hover-Kramer, 2011). The centered practitioner is able to let go of personal feelings and emotions and is more open to inner perceptions. During assessment, the second element, the practitioner's hands move over the individual's body at a height of approximately 3 inches above the skin in an attempt to sense disturbances or imbalances in the person's energy field. The final element is a series of techniques to change the patterns in the human energy field, unruffling, to direct energy to the person to replenish depleted energy, modulation, and to balance or redistribute the individual's energies. **Healing touch** is similar to therapeutic touch but adds full-body techniques for moving energy and disorder-specific energetic interventions to the modulation phase of therapeutic touch (Hover-Kramer, 2011).

**Jin Shin Jyutsu** uses fingertips pressed on specific healing point combinations to balance energy along specific pathways. **Polarity therapy** is a combination of energy work, caring intention, movement exercises, and dietary regimens and is aimed at clearing energy blockages and building health (American Polarity Therapy Association, 2015). Many practitioners use magnets or magnet therapy to control magnetic fields around many body systems to aid in healing and in the functioning of the systems.

### Other Energy Modalities

Although the basis for many religious faiths, **prayer** focuses on the subtle energy life force known by different names. Prayer has different meanings to different people. A prayer may be a request for divine intervention, a type of meditation, or a form of intentionality that is useful in healing. Praying for others may be a form of **distant healing.** Although a recent meta-analysis (Radin et al., 2015) of high-quality experiments failed to show reliable effects, many who practice energy work believe that their efforts are effective over long distances. One method of participating in distance healing is the healing circle. The members of the healing circle join hands. Each member sends healing energy to his or her neighbor on the right until the energy is flowing around the circle. When the energy is flowing readily, each member of the group focuses the energy on one group member, who acts to send the energy to someone that person knows who is in need of healing. Each member of the circle may, in turn, receive energy from the group and send it to an individual in need of healing.

**Music therapy** uses a variety of methods in a therapeutic relationship to address physical, emotional, cognitive, and social needs of individuals. Music influences the limbic system, the area of the brain involved with emotions and feelings. Music is a form of sound energy, and this energy can be relaxing or stimulating, and has been used to decrease pain, depression, and disability. Dependent on the person and the mood desired, all forms of music can be used. In a randomized controlled trial in an ICU setting, harp music significantly decreased pain perception by 27% but did not significantly affect vital signs (Chiasson et al., 2013). Music has been successfully used to reduce distress in people with dementia (Mitchell & Agnelli, 2015).

Two-thirds of US households have at least one pet; nearly half of older Americans own a pet, but research on the therapeutic benefit of pets has been limited or not well designed. Cherniak and Cherniak (2014) provided an overview of international research findings that indicate reported benefits to older participants in the management of agitation, some benefit with regard to the level of depression, the degree of loneliness, and a variety of physical activity benefits. Only one study demonstrated that older people with a pet may be more likely to fall or have an economic burden in caring for them. Cherniak and Cherniak (2014) conclude there is a need for more well-conducted research.

## NURSING PRESENCE

Nurses have the potential to alleviate suffering and improve health care outcomes through their therapeutic presence (Carlson & Lowe, 2013; Ross, 2015). By connecting deeply with individuals and their families, nurses are in a unique position to facilitate their journey toward recovery or a peaceful death. When using nursing presence as a holistic intervention and establishing a therapeutic relationship, nurses are fulfilling the definition of nursing as an art and a science. Aiken and colleagues (Shang et al., 2013) at the University of Pennsylvania have provided a plethora of evidence about positive outcomes, lower mortality and morbidity, decreased readmission rates, and improved patient and nurse satisfaction scores when nurses are able to be present in meaningful ways.

Holistic health involves knowing the physical self, the emotional self, the mental self, and the spiritual self, seeking a comfortable balance among these aspects of being (Table 14-4), and knowing what changes need to be made to achieve this balance (AHNA, 2012c). This knowledge is vital to both the nurse attempting holistic practice and the individual interested in pursuing holistic health.

The *Wellness Quiz* can assist both nurses and individuals in the exploration of self that begins the process of self-care (Box 14-10).

When self-knowledge is gained, one or more of the holistic health strategies mentioned in this chapter, as well as emerging therapies, can be useful in helping people achieve optimal wellness. Every person is a whole, unique being; therefore each person needs to explore the possible strategies and individually decide which modalities are the best methods to achieve an improved state of wellness. People beginning this self-exploration and the practice of holistic health strategies may find that the practice changes their lives. Using presence and giving the gift of self enhances personal growth in the caregiver.

### Safety and Effectiveness

Most CAM therapies lack a strong scientific evidence base, as many have not been studied with rigorous, well-designed clinical trials. The National Institutes of Health is sponsoring research to fill the knowledge gap and build this foundation for safety, efficacy, and suitability for specific conditions.

The US FDA regulates dietary supplements, but the regulations are less strict than those for prescription or over-the-counter medications. For example, safety and efficacy do not have to be proven before a product is marketed, although once the product is on the market, the FDA does monitor label claims and inserts.

Most CAM providers are not credentialed in a standardized national system, so credentialing regulations and standards differ nationally (NCCIH, 2015i). Some require training, testing, and continuing education, but most do not. Many practitioners belong to professional organizations that establish the requirements for their profession (Box 14-11).

It is imperative that nurses and other health care professionals have knowledge of CAM practices, safety, and guidelines for use to inform and protect users. Many medical and nursing schools now include alternative/complementary therapies in their curricula. To help ensure client safety, practitioners and users should review the following principles:

- Carefully select CAM practitioners with appropriate training and experience. The US National Library of Medicine (2016), a division of the National Institutes of Health, provides a directory of providers, services, and facilities (https://www.nlm.nih.gov/medlineplus/directories.html).
- Take time to research and understand the treatment and its effectiveness.
- Be aware of scams and fraudulent claims.
- Know the costs and if the treatment is covered by insurance.
- Quality is not always regulated for dietary supplements, and they may have side effects or react dangerously with other medications and supplements. In addition, they may not have been tested on children or pregnant women, so check labels with care.
- Some energy treatments may have side effects and cause inflammation that can affect other conditions and may not have been tested on children or pregnant women.

### TABLE 14-4 Being There Versus Being With

| The Nurse Who Is There | The Nurse Who |
| --- | --- |
| Is attentive | Is available with whole self |
| Is task oriented | Enters the person's world |
| Does the right thing | Becomes vulnerable |
| Fulfills a role | Is present as a whole person |
| Assists with coping | Alleviates suffering |
| Provides security | Enables growth |

### BOX 14-10 Wellness Quiz

- Do you wake up with enthusiasm for the day ahead?
- Do you have the high energy you need to do what you want?
- Do you laugh easily and often, especially at yourself?
- Do you confidently find solutions for the challenges in your life?
- Do you feel valued and appreciated?
- Do you appreciate others and let them know it?
- Do you have a circle of warm, caring friends?
- Do the choices you make every day get you what you want?

  If you answered "no" to any of these questions, congratulations! You have identified areas in your life that you may want to change. This can be valuable information.

From Caton, S. (Ed.). (2003). *Wellness from within: The first step.* Anaheim, CA: American Holistic Health Association.

---

**BOX 14-11** **More Website Information**

- The NCCIH webpages at http://nccih.nih.gov/health/provide further guidance on how to be an informed consumer, how to obtain information for the health care professional, and how to find and select a CAM practitioner.
- The NCCIH Clearinghouse (http://nccih.nih.gov) provides information on CAM and NCCIH, including publications and searches of federal databases of scientific and medical literature. The NCCIH Clearinghouse does not provide medical advice, treatment recommendations, or referrals to practitioners. The Office of Dietary Supplements (https://ods.od.nih.gov) seeks to strengthen knowledge and understanding of dietary supplements by evaluating scientific information, supporting research, sharing research results, and educating the public. Its resources include publications (such as *Dietary Supplements: What You Need to Know*), fact sheets on a variety of specific supplement ingredients (such as vitamin D and black cohosh), and the *PubMed Dietary Supplement Subset.*
- PubMed (http://www.ncbi.nlm.nih.gov/sites/entrez) is a service of the US National Library of Medicine (2016) and contains publication information and (in most cases) brief summaries of articles from scientific and medical journals.
- The National Library of Medicine's MedlinePlus provides resources that help answer health questions. MedlinePlus brings together authoritative information from the National Institutes of Health as well as other government agencies and health-related organizations (see http://www.medlineplus.gov).
- The National Guideline Clearinghouse (http://www.guideline.gov) provides evidence-based clinical practice guidelines and includes the use of CAM practices.
- Institute of Medicine *Clinical Practice Guidelines We Can Trust* (http://iom.nationalacademies.org/Reports/2011/Clinical-Practice-Guidelines-We-Can-Trust.aspx).

---

- Always inform the care providers and both traditional and holistic practitioners about the use of CAM therapies.

The American Nurses Association recognizes holistic nursing as an official nursing specialty with its own defined scope and standards of practice. The AHNA (2015a) defines holistic nursing as "all nursing that has healing the whole person as its goal and integrates **complementary and alternative medicine** (CAM) approaches into clinical practice." According to the AHNA, a holistic nurse:

- Is a legally licensed nurse who takes a mind-body-spirit-emotion approach to the practice of nursing
- Serves as a bridge between conventional healing and complementary and alternative healing practices, and is trained in both health care models
- Works in a variety of settings—from hospitals to universities to private practice
- May specialize in one or more modalities (or methods of healing), such as acupuncture, chiropractic, or energetic healing (AHNA, 2015a)

Let us return to Ms. Gonzalez and review what is known about her CAM options and their safety and efficacy for her. To review, lung cancer has recently been diagnosed in Ms. Gonzalez. She has never smoked and has never taken prescription medications. Her family and friends have counseled her about various CAM modalities. She is also scheduled to receive traditional allopathic lung cancer treatment.

**Teaching Points for Ms. Gonzalez:**

- Aspirin prolongs bleeding, so she should stop taking aspirin 5 days before surgery.
- Coenzyme $Q_{10}$ is claimed to have three main possible benefits: possible anticancer effect; protect the heart from toxic damage caused by chemotherapy drugs; and counteract chronic fatigue. Evidence to support coenzyme $Q_{10}$ working as an anticancer agent is lacking (Rottorf et al., 2014).
- Amygdalin/laetrile has been banned in the United States (Stapf et al., 2015).
- Milk thistle may have protective effects for her liver if she needs chemotherapy.
- Green tea has antioxidant properties and may counteract her chemotherapy, and uses oxidation to work on cancer cells.
- Kava kava may have an effect or it may have a placebo effect, but it may interact with anesthetic agents, and thus its use must be stopped 1 week before her surgery.
- Yoga, reiki, and acupuncture have demonstrated positive outcomes, and she should be referred to licensed practitioners.
- A careful assessment of her dietary supplements is necessary, as many inhibit therapies, including radiation therapy. Antioxidants are useful for prevention of cancer, but with some cancer treatments, they are counterproductive (Shang et al., 2013).

Now see if you can answer these questions.

- What is the difference between reiki and massage?
- What occurs in a usual visit for acupuncture or a reiki session?
- How do these therapies work?
- Are these therapies evidence-based?
- What is the best understanding of the biological and physiological mechanisms for these therapies?
- What is the best understanding of the safety of these therapies?
- Which therapies are covered by her insurance?
- Would Ms. Gonzalez's therapies be considered complementary, alternative, or integrative?

Therapeutic touch was offered to David P. Although he was skeptical that this treatment would be effective, he agreed to treatment to please his daughter. Increased heat was noted in the neck and shoulder areas. A 30-minute therapeutic touch treatment was performed, with special attention given to the neck and shoulder area. Immediately following the therapeutic touch, David P. rated his pain as 0 on a scale of 1 to 10 and reported that he "couldn't remember when he'd been so relaxed"; and the excess heat had dissipated. David P. was also given some simple yoga exercises for the neck and advised to perform the exercises twice a day, five gentle repetitions each time. David P. was seen in the clinic a total of eight times for therapeutic touch and was given increasingly difficult yoga stretches for the neck and shoulders. His pain rating at the end of treatment remained at 0 on the 1 to 10 scale. He had stopped taking ibuprofen, saying, "I don't need it anymore." His neck range of motion had increased, and he was driving and working in his garden again. He continues his yoga stretches and has started performing daily qigong exercises.

## SUMMARY

Holistic health strategies are designed to view the individual as a biopsychosocial-spiritual whole being. Many holistic health strategies have been practiced in other cultures for thousands of years; some began as religious practices. Many of these strategies can be used to help nurses and those they serve reach the *Healthy People 2020* goals. However, high-quality evidence-based research is lacking, although there is an increased awareness of the practices and more studies are being done. Holistic health practitioner and many consumers are convinced that these practices help promote and maintain health or cure a variety of health conditions. Believing is sometimes therapy in itself. The placebo effect is not well understood but has a strong influence on the results of any research study, whether in conventional or complementary medicine.

Every person is a unique, individual being; therefore some exploration of self, the various strategies, and the practitioner will be necessary before it is determined which strategy is the right fit for each individual. Nurses must understand holistic health strategies because individuals are using them in increasing numbers, and they are evolving and expanding into new methods, such as hot yoga, where the therapy is conducted in a heated room at a temperature above 90° F. Nurses who begin to practice holistic interventions may find them a useful and exciting adjunct to their nursing practice and their personal lives.

## CASE STUDY

### Use of Therapeutic Touch: David P.

David P., an 82-year-old white man, came to the clinic reporting neck pain and stiffness of approximately 4 months' duration. He was previously treated with ibuprofen (Motrin), acetaminophen, and oxycodone (Percocet) as well as with physical therapy. At the time of the initial clinic visit, David P. was still taking ibuprofen but had stopped taking oxycodone because the pain "isn't bad enough to take drugs [narcotics]." He rated his neck pain as 5 on a scale of 1 to 10. Neck range of motion had increased, but he had problems when driving. David P. lives next to a very busy street and did not feel that he could turn his neck well enough to see the traffic coming. He was afraid to pull out into the street. His daughter had driven him to the clinic. She said, "Pop is still in pain. He has little interest in doing anything. He walks like an old man, and he can't work in his garden because of the pain." The goal of treatment for David P. is pain relief and increased range of motion.

#### Reflective Questions

- What holistic health strategies might be used to relieve David's pain and to help him increase his range of motion?
- After the treatment goals have been reached, what holistic health strategies would you recommend to assist David P. in maintaining and improving his health?

## ◎ CARE PLAN

### Use of Therapeutic Touch: David P.

**\*NURSING DIAGNOSIS: Disturbed energy field disturbance related to slowing or blocking of energy flow secondary to repetitive motion injury**

#### Defining Characteristics
- Perceptions of changes in patterns of energy flow, such as:
- Temperature change: warmth, coolness
- Visual changes: image, color
- Disruption of the field: vacant, hole, spike, bulge
- Movement: wave, spike, tingling, dense, flowing
- Sounds: tone, words

#### Related Factors
- Pathophysiological: illness, injury
- Treatment-related: immobility, perioperative experience, labor and delivery
- Situational: pain, fear, anxiety, grieving
- Maturational: age-related developmental difficulties or crises

#### Expected Outcomes
- The person will report increased sense of relaxation.
- The person will report decreased anxiety and tension.
- The person will demonstrate evidence of physical relaxation (e.g., decreased blood pressure, pulse, respiratory rate, and muscle tension).
- The person will report an increased sense of well-being.

#### Interventions
- Provide privacy if possible.
- Explain energy therapy (therapeutic touch, reiki, healing touch) and obtain permission to treat the person.
- Position the person comfortably.
- Become quiet and still (centered) and bring the focus to the person.
- Assess (scan) the energy field for openness and flow.
- Clear the exterior energy field by combing through the field from head to toe (unruffling).
- Move the palms of the hands toward the person, 2 to 4 inches over the person's body, from head to feet in a smooth, light movement.
- Sense the cues to energy imbalance (i.e., warmth, coolness, tightness, heaviness, tingling, emptiness).
- Focus on perceived areas of imbalance to repattern the energy flow.
- Reassess and smooth the exterior energy field, ensuring that the energy flow is open in the feet.
- Gently stop the treatment and allow the person time to rest.
- Encourage the person to discuss the experience.

*NANDA Nursing Diagnoses—Herdman, T. H. & Kamitsuru, S. (Eds.). Nursing Diagnoses–Definitions and Classification 2015–2017. Copyright © 2014, 1994–2014 NANDA International. Used by arrangement with John Wiley & Sons Limited. In order to make safe and effective judgments using the NANDA-I nursing diagnoses it is essential that nurses refer to the definitions and defining characteristics of the diagnoses listed in this work.

## ⓔ EVOLVE CHAPTER FEATURES

http://evolve.elsevier.com/Edelman/
• Study Questions

## REFERENCES

American Holistic Nurses Association (AHNA). (2015a). About us. http://www.ahna.org.

American Holistic Nurses Association (AHNA). (2015b). What is holistic nursing? http://www.ahna.org.

American Holistic Nurses Association (AHNA). (2015c). Fact sheet: What is holistic nursing? http://www.ahna.org .

American Holistic Nurses Association (AHNA). (2015d). Description of healing modalities. http://www.ahna.org.

American Polarity Therapy Association. (2015). About polarity therapy. http://www.polaritytherapy.org/.

Birchtree Center. (2015). Professional development for nurses: Preparation for certification in holistic nursing (HNC). http://www.birchtreecenter.com/prof_dev.html.

Bozas, E., et al. (2015). A randomized controlled trial for the effectiveness of progressive muscle relaxation and guided imagery as anxiety reducing interventions in breast and prostate cancer patients undergoing chemotherapy. *Evidence-based Complementary and Alternative Medicine, 2015,* 270876.

Carlson, N., & Lowe, N. (2013). A concept analysis of watchful waiting among providers caring for women in labour. *Journal of Advanced Nursing, 7*(3), 511–522.

Cherniack, E. P., & Cherniack, A. R. (2014). The benefit of pets and animal-assisted therapy to the health of older individuals. *Current Gerontology and Geriatrics Research, 2014,* 623203.

Chiasson, A. M., et al. (2013). The effect of live spontaneous harp music on patients in the intensive care unit. *Evidence-based Complementary and Alternative Medicine, 2013,* 428731.

Clarke, T. C., et al. (2015). *Trends in the use of complementary health approaches among adults: United States, 2002–2012. National health statistics reports no. 79.* Hyattsville, MD: National Center for Health Statistics. http://www.cdc.gov/nchs/data/nhsr/nhsr079.pdf.

Dana-Farber Cancer Institute. (2016). Patient and family resource centers. http://www.dana-farber.org/Adult-Care/Treatment-and-Support/Patient-and-Family-Support/Patient-and-Family-Resource-Centers.aspx.

Definition of Wellness. (2015). Definition of wellness. http://www.definitionofwellness.com/.

Deng, G. E., et al. (2013). Complementary therapies and integrative medicine in lung cancer: Diagnosis and management of lung cancer, 3rd ed: American College of Chest Physicians evidence-based clinical practice guidelines. *Chest, 143*(5 Suppl.), e420S–e436S.

De Waele, E., et al. (2015). Nutrition therapy in cachectic cancer patients. The Tight Caloric Control (TiCaCo) pilot trial. *Appetite, 91,* 298–301.

Dossey, B. M., & Keegan, L. (2013). *Holistic nursing: A handbook for practice* (6th ed.). Sudbury, MA: Jones & Bartlett Learning.

Fleisher, K. A., et al. (2014). Integrative Reiki for cancer patients: A program evaluation. *Integrative Cancer Therapies, 13*(1), 62–67.

Garagarza, C., et al. (2015). Effect of personalized nutritional counseling in maintenance hemodialysis patients. *Hemodialysis International, 19*(3), 353–481.

Hover-Kramer, D. (2011). *Creating healing relationships: Professional standards for energy therapy practitioners.* Santa Rosa, CA: Energy Psychology Press.

Interagency Committee on Human Nutrition Research. (2015). National Nutritional Research Roadmap. https://prevention.nih.gov/docs/nnrr/ICHNR-NNRR-Draft-Report.pdf.

Lin, W. C., et al. (2015). The anti-inflammatory actions of auricular point acupressure for chronic low back pain. *Evidence-based Complementary and Alternative Medicine, 2015,* 103570.

McCall, M., et al. (2015). Yoga in adult cancer: An exploratory, qualitative analysis of the patient experience. *BMC Complementary and Alternative Medicine, 15,* 245.

Mitchell, G., & Agnelli, J. (2015). Non-pharmacological approaches to alleviate distress in dementia care. *Nursing Standards, 30*(13), 38–44.

National Association for Holistic Aromatherapy. (2015). National Association for Holistic Aromatherapy. https://www.naha.org.

National Center for Complementary and Integrative Health (NCCIH). (2015a). Ayurvedic medicine: An introduction. http://nccih.nih.gov.

National Center for Complementary and Integrative Health (NCCIH). (2015b). What is complementary and alternative medicine? http://nccih.nih.gov.

National Center for Complementary and Integrative Health (NCCIH). (2015c). What's in a Name? ttps://nccih.nih.gov.

National Center for Complementary and Integrative Health (NCCIH). (2015d). The use of complementary and alternative medicine in the United States: Cost data. http://nccih.nih.gov.

National Center for Complementary and Integrative Health (NCCIH). (2015e). Traditional Chinese medicine: An introduction. http:/nccih.nih.gov/.

National Center for Complementary and Integrative Health (NCCIH). (2015f). Naturopathy: An introduction. http://nccih.nih.gov.

National Center for Complementary and Integrative Health (NCCIH). (2015g). Clinical practice guidelines. http://nccih.nih.gov/health/providers/clinicalpractice.htm.

National Center for Complementary and Integrative Health (NCCIH). (2015h). Herbs at a glance. http://nccih.nih.gov/health/herbsataglance.htm.

National Center for Complementary and Integrative Health (NCCIH). (2015i). How to find a CAM practitioner. http://nccih.nih.gov/health/howtofind.htm.

National Center for Homeopathy. (2015). National Center for Homeopathy. http://www.nationalcenterforhomeopathy.org.

National Prevention Council. (2011). National Prevention Strategy. http://www.healthcare.gov/prevention/nphpphc/strategy/report.pdf.

Neumayer, L., & Vargo, D. (2012). Principles of preoperative and operative surgery: Surgical devices and energy sources. In C. M. Townsend, R. D. Beauchamp, et al. (Eds.), *Sabiston textbook of surgery* (19th ed.). Philadelphia, PA: Saunders. chap 11.

Phillips, J. R. (2015). Martha E. Rogers: Heretic and heroine. *Nursing Science Quarterly, 28*(1), 42–48.

Radin, D., Schlitz, M., & Baur, C. (2015). Distant healing intention therapies: An overview of the scientific evidence. *Global Advances in Health and Medicine, 4*(Suppl.), 67–71.

Reflexology Association of America. (2015).Definition of Reflexology. http://reflexology-usa.org/information/raas-definition-of-reflexology/.

Ross, J. (2015). Assessing the whole person to improve outcomes. *Journal of Perianesthesia Nursing, 30*(2), 157–159.

Rottorf, M., Cooke, H., & CAM-Cancer Consortium. (2014). Coenzyme Q10. http://www.cam-cancer.org/CAM-Summaries/Dietary-approaches/Co-enzyme-Q10.

Shang, J., et al. (2013). Nursing practice environment and outcomes for oncology nursing. *Cancer Nursing, 36*(3), 206–212.

Stapf, A., et al. (2015). Amygdalin/laetrile. http://www.cam-cancer.org/CAM-Summaries/Dietary-approaches/Amygdalin-Laetrile.

St. John Providence. (2015). Van Elslander Cancer Center. http://www.stjohnprovidence.org/vanelslander/.

Substance Abuse and Mental Health Services Administration. (2015). Wellness Initiative. http://www.samhsa.gov/wellness-initiative.

US Department of Health and Human Services. (2015). Healthy People 2020. http://www.healthypeople.gov/2020/about/default.aspx.

US Food and Drug Administration. (2015). Homeopathic product regulation: Evaluating FDA's regulatory framework after a quarter-century. http://www.fda.gov/Drugs/NewsEvents/ucm430539.htm.

US National Library of Medicine. (2016). Directories: MedlinePlus. http://www.nlm.nih.gov/medlineplus/directories.html.

Wong, W. W., et al. (2012). Bleeding risks of herbal, homeopathic, and dietary supplements: A hidden nightmare for plastic surgeons? *Aesthetic Surgery Journal, 32*(3), 332–346.

Woodwinds Health Campus. (2015). Healing arts therapy. http://www.healtheast.org/bethesda/about-bethesda/healing-arts.html.

World Health Organization. (1948). Preamble to the Constitution of the World Health Organization as adopted by the International Health Conference, New York, 19 June–22 July 1946; signed on 22 July 1946 by the representatives of 61 States (Official Records of the World Health Organization, no. 2, p. 100) and entered into force on 7 April 1948. http://www.who.int/about/definition/en/print.html.

Zhao, H. J., et al. (2015). Auricular therapy for chronic pain management in adults: A synthesis of evidence. *Complementary Therapies in Clinical Practice, 21*(2), 68–78.

# 15

# Overview of Growth and Development Framework

*Elizabeth Connelly Kudzma*

## OBJECTIVES

*After completing this chapter, the reader will be able to:*
- Define the terms growth, development, and maturation.
- List factors that influence growth in an individual.
- Explain the importance of growth and development theory as a framework for assessing and promoting health.
- Outline Erikson's theory of psychosocial development.
- Differentiate Piaget's and Vygotsky's theories of cognitive development.
- Compare Kohlberg's and Gilligan's theories of cognitive moral development.
- Analyze individual growth and development, distinguishing normal and abnormal processes.

## KEY TERMS

Cephalocaudal
Denver Developmental Screening Test
Development
Developmental patterns
Differentiation
Erikson's theory of psychosocial development

Gilligan's theory of moral development
Growth
Growth charts
Growth patterns
Kohlberg's theory of moral development
Learning

Maturation
Piaget's theory of cognitive development
Proximodistal
Scaffolding
Vygotsky's theory of cognitive development
Zone of proximal development

## ? THINK ABOUT IT

### Vaccine Issues and Controversies

*A 4½-year-old child begins to scream as the nurse approaches with her "kindergarten shots." The mother tries to comfort her child, as she turns anxiously to the nurse and states, "I've heard vaccinations can be dangerous. No wonder she's frightened. Are they really necessary?"*
- What influence might the mother's anxiety have on the child's behavior?
- What approaches and information can the nurse have for the mother?
- What resources might the mother use to review recommendations for childhood vaccinations?
- What approaches can the nurse take to gain the child's cooperation?

Unit 4 introduces growth and development as a framework for health assessment and promotion throughout the life span. Understanding human growth and development facilitates nursing assessment of health knowledge and behavior. Furthermore, health education is more effective when the nurse acknowledges and incorporates growth and developmental needs, as well as the individual's prior understanding of and beliefs about health and health-related concepts.

Growth and development theory is incorporated in many places in *Healthy People 2020*. Throughout Unit 4, specific topics and objectives from *Healthy People 2020* will be examined in chapters appropriate to the age and individual developmental

## TABLE 15-1   GROWTH AND DEVELOPMENT

### Developmental Periods at a Glance

| Period | Age | Characteristics |
|---|---|---|
| Infant | Birth to 12 months | Fully dependent on others for basic needs<br>Ends as infant begins to explore environment, walks alone, and develops basic communication skills |
| Toddler | 12 months to 3 yr | Motor development progresses significantly<br>Child achieves a degree of physical and emotional autonomy while maintaining a close identity with the primary family unit |
| Preschool child | 3–5 yr | Child has increased interest in and involvement with peers and may have social interactions with many people |
| School-age child | 5–12 yr | Marked by entry to elementary school; interests turn away from family toward peers |
| Adolescent | 12–18 yr | Period of transition, adjustment, and personal exploration; ends when adolescent demonstrates readiness to assume full adult responsibilities of financial, emotional, and social independence |
| Young adult | 18–35 yr | Establishing an occupation or career, finding and learning how to live with a partner, and starting and rearing a family |
| Middle-aged adult | 35–65 yr | Being established in a marriage, an occupation or career, and a community; may continue to be a time of transition; adjusts to physiological changes of middle age |
| Older adult | >65 yr | May be a time of continued involvement in work and active socializing; adjusts to decreased physical strength and health; retirement; reduced income; decreasing independence; and deaths of spouses, friends, and self |

level in the life span under discussion. Although these objectives will serve as guides for the promotion of health care at each level, the topic "access to health services" crosses all levels and the entire life span. The first four objectives that increase access to health services for all people and families include increasing the proportion of individuals with health insurance; increasing the proportion of insured individuals with coverage for clinical preventive services; increasing the proportion of individuals with a usual primary care provider; and increasing the number of practicing primary care providers, including nurse practitioners (US Department of Health and Human Services, 2016). Without access to health services, health promotion cannot occur and a person has difficulty achieving and maintaining health. This chapter focuses on the study of health promotion at individual developmental levels by exploring basic concepts foundational to growth and development, as well as providing an overview of representative theories of development. Each of the following nine chapters provides health-assessment and health-promotion strategies appropriate for selected age groups across the life span. The age groups described are the childbearing period, infant, toddler, preschool child, school-age child, adolescent, young adult, middle-aged adult, and older adult (Table 15-1).

## OVERVIEW OF GROWTH AND DEVELOPMENT

Fuller understanding of growth and development has continued to expand with advances in science. Currently, the genomic era is intersecting with the digital age, and nursing educators are racing to integrate genomic content (Read & Ward, 2016). The contribution of genomic knowledge to growth and development is huge, and there is an explosion of findings on genetic and long-term impacts of early development on later health and health-related behaviors.

Individuals continue to evolve throughout the life span, and developmental transitions occur beyond childhood and

adolescence, extending into the early, middle, and later adult years. Aging adults are receiving increased attention as the average life expectancy increases, and the adult population older than 85 years has become the fastest growing age group, providing new challenges for health protection and promotion.

### Growth

Growth refers to a quantifiable change in structure size. In the body this change increases the number and/or size of the cells, resulting in an increase in the size and weight of the whole, or any of its parts. During childhood, physical changes in height, weight, and head circumference, or growth parameters, are measured and recorded regularly. Growth refers to both the obvious changes in the whole individual and to the increases (and as we age, decreases) in the size of specific organs and systems. The health history and physical assessment of an individual should include all body systems and should emphasize systems undergoing the most change. Table 15-2 outlines growth as it occurs throughout the body systems and life span. The growth of some systems, such as the skeletal and muscular systems, is more influenced by sex, whereas the growth of other systems, such as the nervous and respiratory systems, is less dependent on sex. Growth changes that occur in young, middle-aged, and older adults should be noted. Thinking of growth only as it applies to infants, children, and adolescents misses important changes that occur from conception and throughout all the stages of adulthood.

Influences on an individual's potential for growth include genetic factors, prenatal and postnatal exposures, nutrition, and environmental factors (see the case study and care plan at the end of this chapter). Other influences include emotional health and traditional cultural practices that influence childrearing, lifestyle, and health care practices (Box 15-1: Diversity Awareness). Although much of the potential for growth is primarily

*Text continued on p. 357*

## TABLE 15-2 GROWTH AND DEVELOPMENT

### Growth Changes Throughout the Life Cycle

| Overview of Developmental Changes | Prenatal Period → | Infancy → | Childhood → | Puberty and Adolescence → | Adulthood → | Middle Age → | Old Age |
|---|---|---|---|---|---|---|---|
| **Heart and Circulatory System** | | | | | | | |
| Action of heart and circulatory system is under the control of autonomic nervous system. Throughout life cardiac rate is responsive to organ needs and emotional states (fear, anxiety, tension, depression) | Heart formed and begins to beat about third week | Heart grows somewhat more slowly than rest of body (weight doubled by 1 yr, body weight triples). Grows steadily during childhood. With birth, considerable change in paths and relative volumes of blood flow, reflected in loss of certain fetal structures and changes in heart and major vessels | At puberty, heart takes part in rapid growth, reaching mature size with rest of body | | Heart weight remains relatively constant after age 25 yr (only organ other than prostate that does not decrease in weight with age). Capacity to increase rate and strength of beat during physical work is diminished with aging. Cardiac strength lessens with age, whereas expenditure of energy is more than in youth | | |
| | Heart rate high, ≈150 beats/min | Heart rate falls steadily throughout childhood | | | At maturity, women have slightly higher pulse rate than men, 65 beats/min (girls' temperature remains stationary, higher than boys'); men maintain same pulse rate in maturity (slightly lower body temperature than women) | | |
| | | 130 beats/min | 70–80 beats/min | 60 beats/min in adolescence, rate differs with sex | | | |
| | | | Heart rate more variable during childhood—regular | | | | |
| | | | Not until middle childhood does peripheral blood picture become same as adult | | | | |
| **Urinary System** | | | | | | | |
| Parallels growth as a whole. Proportion of body water and solids follows pattern related to growth—tendency for human organism to dry out as life progresses. Function of kidneys, with other organ systems, is to help in regulation of internal environment of body | Young fetus is approximately 90% water. Urinary system begins in first month | Newborn is approximately 70% water. Urinary system does not complete full development until end of first year. All renal units immature at birth; thus fluid and electrolyte imbalance occurs readily. Kidney function adequate at birth if not subjected to undue stress | Composition of urine in healthy child (after age 2 yr) changes very little as child matures; thus renal function and urinalysis can be used as monitor of well-being | | Adult is approximately 58% water. Glomerular filtration rate decreases by approximately 47% from age 20 yr to age 90 yr | | |

**Digestive System**

As a whole, grows as total body grows, although evidence suggests that various parts of gastrointestinal system undergo separate periods of growth, maturity, and senescence

| | | |
|---|---|---|
| Before birth nutrients are supplied through placental circulation; digestion and absorption do not occur in gastrointestinal tract | Stomach size increases rapidly in first few months, then grows steadily throughout childhood | All actions of gastrointestinal tract (food intake, digestion, absorption, elimination) not only respond to physiological needs but from birth to old age are also sensitive to tensions and anxiety |
| | Spurt of growth at puberty | |
| | Digestive apparatus immature at birth (food passes through rapidly, reverse peristalsis common). Acidity of gastric juices varies over life span; low during infancy, rises during childhood, plateaus approximately age 10 yr, rises during puberty. Free gastric acid (HCl) more marked in boys | Data suggest generalized atrophy of entire gastrointestinal tract with advancing age. Nutritional needs differ according to individual variation—decreasing metabolism—tone of large intestine may become impaired until decrease with senescence (also diminished taste) |
| Salivary glands small at birth | Increase rapidly during first 3 months; reach relative adult proportions by age 2 yr | |

**Special Senses**

Most are well developed at birth, although their association with higher centers comes about gradually during early life and diminishes with advancing age

| | |
|---|---|
| Begin very early in embryonic development—3-6 wk | Sense of touch is developed first, then hearing and vision. Vision: infant can perceive simple differences in shape but not complex patterns (greater proportion of total growth before birth); various dimensions of vision develop at various ages, eye muscles function at mature level in first year, fusion begins at 9 months until 6 yr; refractive power changes over life cycle—hyperopia increases until eyeball reaches adult size (≈8 yr), then reverses trend toward myopia until 30 yr, when myopia decreases and hyperopia increases |

*Continued*

## TABLE 15-2   GROWTH AND DEVELOPMENT—cont'd

### Growth Changes Throughout the Life Cycle—cont'd

| Overview of Developmental Changes | Prenatal Period → | Infancy → | Childhood → | Puberty and Adolescence → | Adulthood → | Middle Age → | Old Age |
|---|---|---|---|---|---|---|---|
| **Adipose Tissue** <br> Although adipose tissue differs greatly among individuals, an overall lifetime pattern exists. Fat accumulation differs greatly with body build and constitution. Relationship between caloric intake, amount of exercise, and utilization or accumulation of fat is not yet fully understood but is the basis of much interrelated research | Accumulates rapidly before birth; peaks at seventh gestational month. Premature infant may look wrinkled and scrawny because of lack of adipose tissue | Increases rapidly during first 6 months | Decreases from first to seventh year in both sexes | Begins to increase slowly to puberty. Fat begins to accumulate slowly and continues to accumulate uninterrupted in girls, producing feminine curves, and accounts for much of weight gain | Some girls become slim after full maturation; many maintain approximately the same amount of adipose tissue as at puberty | Typically, both sexes tend to gain weight in their 50s and 60s but do not maintain the same body contours of earlier years at same weight (increased deposit on abdomen and hips) | Usually fat stores are lost after the seventh decade in both sexes. Sharpness in contours, increasingly prominent bony landmarks |
| | | Sex differences are not noted in body shape of prepubescent children | | Deposition of fat differs in body—amount decreases sharply at time of maximal growth spurt (increased weight caused by increase in muscle mass and bones) | After full maturation, fat accumulation begins | | |
| **Lymphoid Tissue** <br> Lymphoid tissue is scattered widely throughout the body and includes lymph nodes, tonsils, adenoids, thymus, spleen, and lymphocytes of blood; follows unique pattern of growth, rapid in infancy and begins to atrophy at puberty | Begins during last month of uterine life—crosses placenta at levels equal to mother's and remains for several months after delivery | Grows most rapidly during infancy and childhood, reaching maximal size a few years before puberty; parallels development of immunity | | Atrophies and is smaller in volume at full maturity than during childhood | | | Thymus is small and difficult to locate in older people |
| | | Increased incidence of disease with increasing age of child | | | | | |

## Respiratory System

| General | Prenatal | Infancy/Childhood | Adolescence/Adulthood | Older Adulthood |
|---|---|---|---|---|
| Growth parallels that of total body. Respiratory apparatus is a highly-organized system of organs under nervous system and hormonal regulation, which functions in coordination with rest of body. Sex difference in gas exchange becomes apparent during puberty | Before birth, air sacs do not contain air; oxygen is supplied through maternal circulation | When umbilical cord is cut, infant must use own breathing apparatus—breathing irregular at first, both in rate and in depth—fast in infancy and gradually slowing through childhood until maturity is reached | Respiratory exchange gradually becomes more efficient as life advances. Actual volume of air inhaled with each breath increases as lung size expands with general body growth. Vital capacity and maximal breathing capacity rise gradually in both sexes, increasing more in boys during puberty; adult men have more efficient respiratory exchange, are capable of greater feats of muscular exertion without exhaustion than women. No sex difference in respiratory rate at any time of life | Basal metabolic rate declines (rate higher in men than in women) |

## Skeletal System

| General | Prenatal | Infancy | Childhood | Adolescence/Puberty | Adulthood | Older Adulthood |
|---|---|---|---|---|---|---|
| Bone growth passes through successive stages of development from connective tissue to cartilage to osseous tissue; completion of calcification indicates end of growing period and is thus a useful measure of growth rate and physiological maturity. Most growth ceases during adolescence | Follows cephalocaudal law of development; 70% of head growth before birth; bones of hands and wrist laid down in cartilage | At birth, shafts of metacarpals are ossified (and visible by radiography); carpal bones begin to ossify. After first year, legs grow fastest; 66% of total increase in height; the longer puberty is delayed, the greater the leg length | Trunk fastest growing, 60% of total increase | Length of trunk and depth of chest reach peak growth. Growth of both sexes is nearly even until onset of puberty in girls first (≈10 yr). Boys begin ≈2 yr later, but growth is markedly greater. Peak in height comes before peak in weight. Reserved during growth spurt | Maximal height in early 20s to 30s. Gradual decline until onset of senescence | Thinning of vertebral disks beginning in middle years; most rapid in last decade. Spinal column shortens (osteoporosis) with thinning vertebrae—shortening of trunk with long extremities—reversal of growth proportions in infancy |

*Continued*

## TABLE 15-2 GROWTH AND DEVELOPMENT—cont'd

### Growth Changes Throughout the Life Cycle—cont'd

| Overview of Developmental Changes | Prenatal Period → | Infancy → | Childhood → | Puberty and Adolescence → | Adulthood → | Middle Age → | Old Age |
|---|---|---|---|---|---|---|---|
| **Muscle System** Number of striated muscle fibers is roughly the same in all humans. Tremendous difference in size, not only from fetus to adult but also among adults, is caused by ability of individual muscle fibers to increase in size | Muscle formation begins early, assuming final shape by end of second month | Increases rapidly during infancy but slowly during childhood | Growth in both sexes is same in childhood | With onset of puberty, muscle strength is greater in boys (when muscle growth is stimulated by testosterone)<br><br>Greatest increase begins in puberty; muscle size precedes muscle strength in boys<br><br>Increase in muscle size means increasing strength in children; increase in skill is more intimately related to maturation of nervous system | Muscle mass continues to increase gradually—maximal strength attained in early adulthood—then declines slightly—according to use and genetic constitution. Will increase in bulk and strength as used until onset of senescence | | Atrophy and loss of muscle tone |
| **Nervous System** Growth and maturation of central and peripheral nervous systems (brain, spinal cord, peripheral nerves, many sense organs) reflected by changing size of head | Growth very rapid during intrauterine development; head grows at greater rate than rest of body | In first year has all the brain cells, which will continue to increase in size; number and complexity of axons, dendrites, and synapses will continue to increase<br><br>All neural tissues grow rapidly during infancy and early childhood<br><br>Brain grows rapidly after birth, reaching 90% of total size by age 2 yr | By middle childhood almost reaches adult size | (No neural growth spurt at puberty)<br><br>Slow increase to full maturity | Function continues with use<br><br>Brain weight decreases with age | | Depletion of fully functioning brain cells, whether they are lost, shrink, or lose connections<br><br>Decrease in myelin sheath, impulses decrease; slowed down speed of action and reaction |

Segmented spinal nerves are mature, fully myelinated, and functioning at term (e.g., knee jerk), but acquisition of myelin in cortex, brainstem, and spinal cord is closely correlated with observed behavior (myelination of this tract follows cephalocaudal, proximodistal rules)

Equipment for sense of taste and smell present at birth and perhaps most acute at that time

Taste less acute, less discriminatory with advancing age

Structural changes in central nervous system result in impaired perception

**Reproductive System**

Organs of reproductive system show little increase during early life but rapid development just before and coincident with puberty. Maturation and fulfillment of reproductive functions of maturity (in female) are followed by involution in later years

| | | | | |
|---|---|---|---|---|
| Genital organs form during uterine life; uterus undergoes growth spurt before birth (hormonal stimulation from mother) | Female sex organs well formed but not functioning at birth (but have full quota of sensory nerves) | Quiescent during childhood → | Maturation at puberty (menstruation) → | Involution after menopause |
| | Uterus undergoes involution to half its birth weight | Regained size by age 10–11 yr → | Adult size at puberty → | Maximum increase with pregnancy → |
| | In males, testes, as with ovaries, remain dormant and small, not even growing in proportion to rest of body (with sensory nerves) | Until puberty, interstitial cells of Leydig reappear and secrete testosterone, so testes and penis continue to increase in size; pubic hair appears | | Begins to atrophy with advancing age |
| Mammary glands develop in both sexes during fetal life | Enlargement of breasts at birth (both sexes) → | Nonsecretory during childhood until puberty → | Development rapid → | Enlarge during pregnancy, developing alveoli → Atrophy with advanced age |

Sex hormones: until puberty girls and boys produce male hormones (androgens) and female hormones (chiefly estrogens) in small and roughly equal amounts

*Continued*

## TABLE 15-2   GROWTH AND DEVELOPMENT—cont'd

*Growth Changes Throughout the Life Cycle—cont'd*

| Overview of Developmental Changes | Prenatal Period → | Infancy → | Childhood → | Puberty and Adolescence → | Adulthood → | Middle Age → | Old Age |
|---|---|---|---|---|---|---|---|
| **Integumentary System** Includes skin and its appendages and adnexa (nails, hair, sebaceous glands, eccrine and apocrine sweat glands). Although all skin is similar, this organ shows considerable variability in different parts of body (and from individual to individual) and varies greatly during life span | Hair, skin, and sebaceous glands fully formed in utero | Skin contains all its adult structures at birth but immature in function | Matures slowly until puberty (children prone to rashes) | Rapid spurt in maturation of skin and all its structures | | | Changes in skin most obvious sign of aging (exposure and environmental conditions) |
| | Lanugo begins to decrease before birth and continues regression for a few weeks postnatally → | | Replaced by body hair, less extensive distribution; marked difference in type and distribution of hair at puberty → | | | | |
| | Activity of sebaceous glands decreases after birth → | | | Increases rapidly at puberty (more prone to acne) | | | Regenerative and growth power decrease and skin loses elasticity |
| **Endocrine System** Consists of a number of glandular structures scattered throughout body. Although small in size, their hormones influence all growth and development of whole organism | Immaturity of entire endocrine system puts infant at a disadvantage if required to adjust to wide fluctuations in concentration of water, electrolytes, glucose, and amino acids. All are interrelated, but each organ develops at its own rate:<br>• Thyroid—increases in size from midfetal life to maturity; slightly larger in boys than girls; growth spurt at adolescence<br>• Adrenals—after birth decrease in size and this continues throughout first year, increase again during childhood (but smaller than at birth); spurt at puberty, reaching maturity with rest of body; greater increase in male gonads and testes and female ovaries (endocrine glands as well as reproductive organs), follow genital type of growth pattern<br>• Hypophysis, or pituitary gland—produces or stimulates hormones that influence growth<br>• Parathyroid—produces hormones that maintain homeostasis of calcium and phosphorus<br>• Islets of Langerhans—dispersed throughout pancreas; produce insulin and glucagon | | | | With age, decline occurs in all endocrine gland functions | | |

NOTE: This table indicates only general trends in growth and development; it is not all-inclusive. No distinct ages, absolute values, or ranges of normal variations are intended in this table. Modified from a format originally developed in Sutterly, D. C., & Donneley, G. F. (1973). *Perspectives in human development: Nursing throughout the life cycle.* Philadelphia: J. B. Lippincott. Further modified from Papalia, D. E. & Feldman, R. D. (2011). *Experience human development* (12th ed.). New York: McGraw Hill. Physiological adaptations updated from McCance, K. L., Huether, S. E., Brashers, V. L., & Rote, N. S. (2014). *Pathophysiology: Biological basis for disease in adults and children.* St. Louis: Mosby.

## 🌐 BOX 15-1   DIVERSITY AWARENESS

### Childhood Lead Poisoning and Latino Families

Whereas the United States has made tremendous progress in eliminating some of the more significant sources of lead (lead paint was banned in 1978; leaded gasoline was phased out in the early 1990s), lead poisoning remains a significant threat to today's children. Lead exposure results in behavior and learning problems, decreased intelligence, attention problems, lower academic achievement, impaired growth, poor eye-hand coordination, and hearing loss. The CDC (2014) now uses a reference level of 5 mcg/dL to identify children with lead exposure, and this reference value is lower than in past years. As a consequence, more children will likely be identified as having lead exposure. The National Safety Council emphasizes that lead poisoning is a totally preventable disease. During the past 2 decades, public health and provider efforts have resulted in a 90% decline in the overall number of children affected in the United States. The Flint, Michigan, water contamination crisis that started in April 2014 illustrates the importance of lead testing during childhood and prompt treatment of children who demonstrate high lead levels (Bosman & Smith, 2016).

However, there are more specific risks for Latino families. One-third of the Latino population resides in Western states and is exposed to pesticides, fertilizers, and chemical residues contaminating the water. Food and culturally defined health practices pose additional risks of lead exposure to this population (CDC, 2011). Foods packaged or canned outside the United States (especially in Mexico or South America), foods cooked in, stored in, eaten from, or drunk from ceramic containers or pottery made outside the United States (especially in Mexico or South America), Mexican or South American raisins, and wrapped Mexican candies may all contain lead.

*Empacho,* a common Hispanic term for stomach or intestinal upset or obstruction, is often treated with a folk remedy that contains 70% to 90% lead. It is known by many names, including *alarcon, azarcon, coral, greta, liga, Maria Luisa,* and *rueda.* Another common Hispanic folk remedy containing lead is *pay looah.*

An often-overlooked risk is the use of warm, hot, or boiled tap water from contaminated pipes. Many Hispanics feel that heating the water removes contaminants, although any heat mobilizes the lead and makes it easier to absorb. This is also true of pottery that is heated by cooking in it, placing heated fluids in it, or heating it in a microwave oven. Although typical instruction pamphlets teach that tap water should be run for a full minute before it is consumed, they fail to state that the water consumed should come from the cold tap if it is to be consumed.

When screening for lead poisoning in Hispanic children, the nurse remembers to ask about the use of folk remedies, pottery, imported foods, and candies, as well as the use of boiled or hot tap water. In addition, the nurse encourages a diet with less fat, because lead is retained in fat, and a greater vitamin C, calcium, and iron intake, which reduces the amount of lead in the body.

For more information about the health effects of lead on children, or how to identify children with elevated lead levels visit the following webpages:

- National Safety Council: Lead Poisoning Is Not Yesterday's News (http://www.nsc.org/learn/safety-knowledge/Pages/Lead-Poisoning-Prevention.aspx)
- CDC: What Do Parent's Need to Know to Protect Their Children (http://www.cdc.gov/nceh/lead/faq/acclpp/blood_lead_levels.htm)
- Environmental Protection Agency: Protect Your Family From Exposure to Lead (http://www.epa.gov/lead/protect-your-family)
- Environmental Protection Agency: Learn About Lead (http://www.epa.gov/lead/learn-about-lead)
- Natural Resources Defense Council. Environmental Threats in the Latino Community (http://www.nrdc.org)

From Bosman, J. & Smith, M. (2016). Gov. Rick Synder of Michigan apologizes in Flint water crisis. *New York Times*, January 19, 2016. http://www.nytimes.com/2016/01/20/us/obama-set-to-meet-with-mayor-of-flint-about-water-crisis.html?r=00.; Centers for Disease Control and Prevention (CDC). (2011). Lead poisoning of a child associated with use of a Cambodian amulet—New York City, 2009. *Morbidity and Mortality Weekly Report (MMWR)*, 60(3), 69–71; Centers for Disease Control and Prevention (CDC). (2014). *Lead: Prevention tips*. http://www.cdc.gov/nceh/lead/tips.htm.

---

determined by individual genetics, health and environmental exposures influence the attainment of that potential (CDC, 2011a,b). The timing of contact with environmental hazards and stressors may determine to a great extent the amount and kind of effects of these influences. If a pregnant mother is exposed to a virus in utero (e.g., the Zika virus), the developing fetus is more vulnerable than either the mother or an older child, especially during the first trimester, when all organs systems are in a stage of rapid growth and development. Teens who fracture a limb at the bone's growth plate also have more difficulty healing than older teens and young adults who have completed their growth spurt.

### Growth Patterns

Expected **growth patterns** exist for all people. Growth is not steady or uniform throughout life. The periods of extremely rapid growth—childbearing period, infancy, and adolescence—are contrasted with slower rates of growth during the toddler, preschool, and school-age periods. Infants typically double their birth weight by 6 months of age and triple their birth weight by 1 year of age. The well-known early adult "growth spurt" in height typically occurs early in adolescence for girls and later in adolescence for boys.

Different parts of the body increase in size at different rates. For example, during early life the head is the fastest growing section, followed by the trunk, and then the arms and legs. Newborns' heads account for one-quarter of their overall length, as opposed to adults' heads, which account for one-ninth of their overall height. The growth changes in proportions of body parts from infancy to adulthood are demonstrated in Figure 15-1.

### Growth Charts

Growth is one of the most important indications of a child's overall health and well-being. Accurate growth assessment depends on precise measurement of growth parameters with proper equipment, correct and consistent techniques, careful plotting of measurements, and thoughtful interpretation of the data.

On the basis of input from an expert panel, the Centers for Disease Control and Prevention (CDC) recommended that health practitioners in the United States use the 2006 World Health Organization (WHO) international **growth charts** for

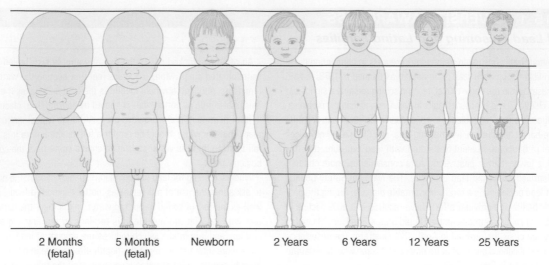

2 Months (fetal)   5 Months (fetal)   Newborn   2 Years   6 Years   12 Years   25 Years

**FIGURE 15-1** Changes in body proportions from birth to adulthood. (From McKinney, E. S., Smith Murray, S., James, S. R., & Ashwill, J. [2009]. *Maternal child nursing* [3rd ed.]. St Louis Saunders.)

children from birth to 24 months, and continue to use the revised 2000 CDC growth charts (including the body mass index [BMI] and the 3rd and 97th percentiles) for children aged 2 to 20 years. This recommendation was based on the fact that WHO growth charts were compiled from healthy breastfed infants living in optimal conditions and achieving the greatest potential of growth possible, which was recognized as the desired standard against which to compare the growth of all other infants (CDC, 2010). In creating the WHO growth charts, researchers gathered data from six countries (Brazil, Ghana, India, Norway, Oman, and the United States) using longitudinal and cross-sectional methods (Mei & Grummer-Strawn, 2011). The exceptional strength of the WHO growth charts is that they are globally representative (Ziegler & Nelson, 2012). The CDC and the WHO growth charts both describe weight for age, length (or stature) for age, weight for length, and BMI for age, and include the 5th and 95th and the 3rd and 97th percentiles (CDC, 2010). The WHO and the CDC growth charts for each sex with percentile curves can be viewed at the CDC website: http://www.cdc.gov/growthcharts/. These charts have been used by pediatricians, nurses, and parents to compare infant, child, and adolescent growth since 1977.

When one is assessing growth data for use in the growth charts, it is important to remember that a single measurement taken at one point in time, although helpful in providing a baseline, does not allow the best assessment of a child's growth. Serial measurements plotted over time on a growth chart best reflect a child's pattern of growth. Slowed growth, plateaus, or decreases in height, weight, and head circumference, as well as rapid increases, raise questions for health care providers about the adequacy of a child's nutritional intake, disease states, neglect, or emotional problems. See Box 15-2: Research for Evidence-Based Practice on the use of the new growth charts and young children.

## Concept of Development

**Development** refers to change and expansion of ability and advancement in skill from a lower to a more advanced capability. In contrast to growth, which is a quantitative or precisely measurable change, development is a qualitative change. Qualitative changes are more challenging to describe because they cannot be easily measured in precise units. Development has best been conceptualized as a process that can be assessed because it follows certain sequencing or patterns, although the timing of this advancement is individual.

### Developmental Patterns

All individuals follow similar **developmental patterns**, with one stage of development building on and leading to the next. Early development proceeds as follows:

- **Cephalocaudal**, from head to toe
- **Proximodistal**, from midline to periphery
- **Differentiation** follows a pattern: simple to complex, and general to specific

The following are examples of patterns of development:

- Cephalocaudal: Infants advance in neck and head control before controlling the movements of the extremities.
- Proximodistal: Infants' central nervous systems develop before peripheral nervous systems.
- Differentiation: Infants use a whole-hand grasp before learning the finer control of the pincer grasp, and they coo or babble before they speak.

Although the sequence of development is predictable, the exact timing of the sequencing depends on the individual. Individuals develop at their own rate, on their own schedule. For example, infants creep and crawl before they walk and their primary teeth erupt in a predictable sequence, but each will walk and develop primary teeth on an individual schedule. However, there are

## BOX 15-2 RESEARCH FOR EVIDENCE-BASED PRACTICE

### Comparing the New Growth Charts: Prediction of Future Obesity From Childhood Weight Status

The CDC and WHO growth charts use the same indicators for growth, and comparative studies have been done to indicate differences when each chart is used. These studies are critical to provide better support for public health prevention efforts addressing the increasing prevalence of childhood obesity (Mei & Grummer-Strawn, 2011).

From the beginning, it was recommended that when the WHO growth charts are used to screen individuals for abnormal or unhealthy growth that the narrower ranges of the 3rd and 97th percentiles should be used instead of the 5th and 95th percentiles respectively. This would identify fewer children as underweight as slower growth among breastfed infants is normal within the first 6 months.

Rapid weight gain during the first year of life is predictive of obesity in 2-year-olds to 3-year-olds, and there is need to promote parental awareness regarding the actual weight of their children (Vallejo et al., 2015). Maalouf-Manasseh and colleagues (2011) also reported that gaining weight more rapidly in the first year than directed by the WHO growth charts may be an early sign of later obesity.

Ziegler and Nelson (2012) observed in their comparative studies that the weight percentiles of the WHO growth charts were higher in the first 6 months and lower between 6 and 24 months when compared with the same age range CDC percentiles. Their conclusion was explained not only by their appreciating that

breastfed infants grow somewhat slower than formula-fed infants but also by their realizing the attrition rate of low-weight-gaining breastfed infants that occurred when data were being compiled for the WHO growth charts.

Whereas the WHO growth charts may be used for national and international observations of malnutrition, it is imperative that additional data be obtained before the WHO standards can be applied for local public health interventions. The low weight of the WHO growth charts should not be used to misclassify a child as overweight or obese with the use of corrective interventions (Ziegler & Nelson, 2012).

Although the new WHO growth charts furnish health care providers and researchers with an improved tool to assess and track the growth of children from birth to 24 months of age, care must be taken not to misinterpret the results for each individual child. As indicated by the evidence presented, it is too early to use the WHO growth chart as the magic bullet of early identification of and intervention for future obesity in children during the first year of life. Mothers' underestimation of the weight of their own children was common in both overweight and children of normal weight (Vallejo et al., 2015). Continued investigation in this area is promising for planning of health care education to counter factors contributing to the child and later adult obesity epidemic.

From Maalouf-Manasseh, Z., Metallinos-Katsaras, E., & Dewey, K. G. (2011). Obesity in preschool children is more prevalent and identified at a younger age when WHO growth charts are used compared with CDC charts. *Journal of Nutrition, 141,* 1154–1158; Mei, Z., & Grummer-Strawn, L. M. (2011). Comparison of changes in growth percentiles of U.S. children on CDC 2000 growth charts with corresponding changes on WHO 2006 growth charts. *Clinical Pediatrics, 50*(5), 402–407; Vallejo, M., Cortes-Rodrigues, B. A., & Colin-Ramirez, E. (2015). Maternal underestimation of child's weight status and health behaviors as risk factors for overweight in children. *Journal of Pediatric Nursing, 30*(6), e29–e33; Ziegler, E. E., & Nelson, S. E. (2012). The WHO growth standards: Strengths and limitations. *Current Opinion Clinical Nutrition Metabolic Care, 15*(3), 298–302.

guidelines or parameters that assist parents and health care providers in assessing whether children are progressing in an acceptable developmental sequence within a reasonable time frame. Areas of assessment usually focus on personal and social, gross and fine motor, and language development. The **Denver Developmental Screening Test**, which was revised in 1992 (now known as Denver II), is a screening tool that assists health care providers in monitoring children's development in each of these areas from birth to 6 years of age.

Social expectations can influence developmental tasks with expectations that an individual achieve certain landmarks during each period of development. However, the age at which a child is expected to master certain developmental tasks is determined partly by cultural expectations. Some cultures are comfortable with breastfeeding their children well into childhood, whereas others expect the transition to self-feeding with a cup much earlier. When assessing a child's abilities, nurses are aware that a child who has never been given the opportunity to learn or master a skill may be developmentally capable but fails when tested. For example, a child who is capable of learning colors or numbers can do so only if taught, just as the child who was breastfed well into childhood, never having been offered a cup, may well be developmentally capable of drinking from a cup but probably will fail in early attempts.

Development is closely interrelated with the concepts of both learning and maturation. **Learning** is the process of gaining specific knowledge or skills that result from exposure, experience,

education, and evaluation. **Maturation** is an increase in competence and adaptability that reflects understandings in the complexity of a structure that makes it possible for that structure to begin to function or to function at a higher level. Maturation of a structure, system, or individual refers to the emergence of the genetic potential of that structure, system, or individual. Learning cannot occur unless the individual is mature enough to understand and control behavior. Children can be toilet trained only when their bodies have matured to the point of developing internal and external sphincter control. Earlier attempts will be frustrating for both the child and the parent.

Growth and development are complex, interrelated processes that are influenced by and, in turn, influence the health of an individual. The nurse who understands this relationship is aware of the need for age-specific health-assessment, health-protection, and health-promotion strategies (Box 15-3: Quality and Safety Scenario).

## THEORIES OF LIFE SPAN DEVELOPMENT

Specific aspects of development of the person have been studied for centuries. Many theories of development are used in the study of individuals throughout the life span; the nurse may wish to refer to a text on developmental psychology to become familiar with some of these theories. In this unit, five theories are discussed to gain a holistic view of the progression of individual development throughout the life span. These theories

## BOX 15-3 QUALITY AND SAFETY SCENARIO

### Anticipatory Guidance

The nurse is often in a position to provide anticipatory guidance to parents, which involves teaching parents ways to handle a situation before it becomes an issue or problem. Knowledge of normal growth and development provides a foundation for this teaching. For example, the toddler period is one of intense exploration of the environment, when locomotion is the major gross motor skill acquired. The nurse, knowing the number one cause of death in toddlers is accidents, provides the following teaching to the parents of a child who is entering the toddler period:

- Use a federally approved car restraint/car seat and check for proper installation and placement.
- Supervise a child closely near any source of water, including buckets, bathtubs, toilets, and especially swimming pools.
- Move pot handles toward the back of the stove and use the back burners whenever possible.
- Place toxic substances in a locked cabinet and have the poison control contact number easily accessible. Avoid the use of syrup of ipecac unless advised by a poison control representative to use it.
- Move a toddler from the crib to a bed.
- Provide barriers on open windows.
- Decrease water temperature to avoid scald burns from tap water.
- Avoid foods that pose a choking hazard such as nuts, hard candies, raisins, fresh carrots, whole grapes, chewing gum, hot dogs, and fish with bones.
- Guard against the toddler running into the street when walking and playing outside.

## TABLE 15-3 GROWTH AND DEVELOPMENT

### Erikson's Eight Stages of Human Development

| Age Group | Psychosocial Stage | Lasting Outcomes |
|---|---|---|
| 1. Infancy | Basic trust versus basic mistrust | Faith and hope |
| 2. Toddler stage | Autonomy versus shame and doubt | Self-control and willpower |
| 3. Preschool stage | Initiative versus guilt | Direction and purpose |
| 4. School age | Industry versus inferiority | Method and competence |
| 5. Adolescence | Identity versus role confusion | Devotion and fidelity |
| 6. Young adulthood | Intimacy versus isolation | Affiliation and love |
| 7. Middle adulthood | Generativity versus stagnation | Production and care |
| 8. Older adulthood | Ego integrity versus despair | Renunciation and wisdom |

Modified from Erikson, E. H. (1995). *Childhood and society* (35th anniversary ed.). New York: Norton; Erikson, E. H., & Erikson, J. M. (1998). *The life cycle completed.* New York: Norton.

reflecting on the crises of early development and coping with the physical and mental changes of aging (Perry et al., 2015). These stages are summarized in Table 15-3 and are discussed more fully in the chapters on each developmental age group. See the case study at the end of this chapter about a potentially disabled infant girl and how hospitalization could affect her stage of psychosocial development.

## Cognitive Development

Another aspect of development is cognitive development. Jean Piaget, a Swiss psychologist, also trained in biology and philosophy, is well known for his theory of cognitive development. He viewed children as biological organisms interacting with their environment, and his theory contends that cognitive development reflects children's attempts to make sense of their worlds. Piaget developed his cognitive theory by observing his own children (Piaget, 1950). Hence the major criticism of his work is that he underestimated children's capabilities and gave little or no consideration to cultural differences. Lev Vygotsky, a Russian contemporary, was also trained in both the physical sciences and psychology. His theory of cognitive development maintains that a child's development cannot be separated from the social and cultural context in which it occurs. He also credited children with more innate ability to learn and emphasized the importance of language (Vygotsky, 1986). The theories of Piaget and Vygotsky are presented in more detail in the following sections.

## Cognitive Development: Piaget's Theory

Jean **Piaget's theory of cognitive development** is concerned primarily with structure rather than content, with how the individual mind works rather than with what it does. Piaget uses the word scheme to describe a pattern of action or thought. A scheme is used to take in or assimilate new experiences or may

were originally advanced by Erikson, Piaget, Vygotsky, Kohlberg, and Gilligan. Whereas these theories can assist in understanding developmental tasks, they are not definitive, and individuals may exhibit variations and stage activities may overlap.

## Psychosocial Development: Erikson's Theory

Erik Erikson described the development of identity of the self through successive stages that unfold throughout the life span (Erikson, 1968, 1995; Erikson & Erikson, 1998). Although he studied with Freud and supported the psychosexual theory of development, **Erikson's theory of psychosocial development** is based on the need of each person to develop a sense of trust in self and others and a sense of personal worth. Erikson described a healthy personality in positive terms, not merely through the absence of disease.

According to Erikson, psychosocial development is composed of critical stages, each requiring resolution of a conflict between two opposing forces (e.g., intimacy versus isolation). Each stage depends on the preceding stage, which must be accomplished successfully for the person to proceed. Erikson's use of a psychosocial framework acknowledges the influence of socialization and the environment but maintains that it is ultimately the individual who must master each of the conflicts. Although each of the conflicts is predominant at a certain stage in life, it is important to recognize that all the conflicts exist in each person, to some extent, at all times and that a conflict, once resolved, may emerge again in appropriate situations. For example, the renunciation and wisdom of old age is accomplished by a person

## TABLE 15-4 GROWTH AND DEVELOPMENT

### Piaget's Stages of Cognitive Development

| Stage | Age | Characteristics |
|---|---|---|
| Sensorimotor | Birth to 2 yr | Begins with a predominance and reliance on reflexes that permit the body to learn<br>Reflexes decrease and voluntary acts develop<br>Imitation predominates<br>Thought is dominated by physical manipulation of objects and events<br>Develops the concept of object permanence and the ability to form mental representations |
| Preoperational | 2–7 yr | Advancing use of language and movement<br>Development of egocentric, animistic, and magical thinking<br>Uses representational thought to interpret and learn, not in terms of general properties but in terms of the relationship or use to themselves<br>No cause-and-effect reasoning<br>Thought is dominated by the senses—what is seen, heard, or experienced |
| Concrete operations | 7–11 yr | Mental reasoning processes assume logical approaches to solving concrete problems, including cause and effect<br>Collecting; mastering facts<br>Can consider other points of view<br>Thought influenced by social contacts<br>Language is perfected |
| Formal operations | 11–15 yr | True logical thought and manipulation of abstract concepts emerge<br>Morality established |

Modified from Piaget, J. (1959). *Language and thought of the child.* New York: Routledge; Piaget, J., & Inhelder, B. (2000). *The psychology of the child.* New York: Basic Books; Schuster, C. S., & Ashburn, S. S. (1992). *The process of human development: A holistic life span* approach (2nd ed.). Boston: Lippincott.

be modified or accommodated by new experiences. Each person is striving to maintain a balance, or equilibrium, between assimilation and accommodation (Phillips, 1975; Piaget, 1950).

Piaget described the stages of cognitive development throughout the developmental years. Through a natural unfolding of ability, the child acquires sequentially predictable cognitive abilities. Given adequate environmental stimuli and an intact neurological system, the child gradually matures toward full conceptualized reasoning. Piaget's theory of cognitive development encompasses the time from birth to approximately 15 years of age. Each of the four distinct stages is summarized in Table 15-4 and is discussed more fully in the specific chapters on each developmental age. Piaget suggests that quantitative, but no further qualitative, changes in cognitive function occur after approximately age 15 years. Although more recent developmental theorists may dispute some of Piaget's findings, this scheme of cognitive development assists the nurse in assessing growth and development in children and adolescents (Carey et al., 2015).

## Cognitive Development: Vygotsky's Theory

One of the significant differences between the cognitive theories of Piaget and Vygotsky is that Piaget believed that development precedes learning. Piaget proposed that a level of cognitive development must be reached *before* learning can occur. Vygotsky thought that by viewing development and learning in this way, adults would teach to the lowest ability, aiming instruction at those mental functions or intellectual operations that had already matured in the child (Wink & Putney, 2002). In contrast, Vygotsky proposed that learning precedes development. He states that

learning pulls development, which is in stark contrast to Piaget, who felt children are not capable of learning something until they are developmentally ready.

Vygotsky argued that, while learning may be similar among children at certain times or phases of development, it is not identical in all children because of their differing social and cultural experiences (Vygotsky, 1978). He felt Piaget overemphasized the intellectual and biological universality of developmental stages. Vygotsky was more interested in the cultural and social influences on learning and development, as well as how individual children actively internalize what they learn from others. For Vygotsky, development begins as an interpersonal process of "meaning making," which then becomes an individualized process of "making sense." There are no predetermined levels of development; rather, experience is in the front—leading and expanding development in unlimited ways.

Although **Vygotsky's theory of cognitive development** is less known to health care professionals, educators have embraced his theory, especially what he refers to as the zone of proximal development. The **zone of proximal development** is the distance between the actual developmental level and the potential developmental level (Wink & Putney, 2002). In this zone, children are pulled toward new learning through their interaction with others and the environment. The guidance given by others in this zone is referred to as **scaffolding**. According to Vygotsky, all people need to understand not only the way in which an individual learns and develops but also the social, cultural, and political context in which that learning and development occur. This difference can profoundly impact how the nurse approaches teaching and learning (Box 15-4: Innovative Practice).

---

### ✴ BOX 15-4   **INNOVATIVE PRACTICE**
#### *How to Raise a Genius*

The American Academy of Pediatrics (AAP, 2013) recommends *no screen time (television/video/computer/tablet/phone) for children younger than 2 years* and recommends limits on screen time for children older than 2 years. The AAP reports that active, not passive, adult-child communication is important to expand learning experiences for children (Boyce et al. 2015). Recent studies have associated television watching with decreased language development. A study of 329 children ranging in age from 2 to 48 months found that even audible television that decreased the child's exposure to discernible adult speech led to decreased child vocalizations and delayed speech development (Christakis et al., 2009). In a similar study, television viewing by itself was significantly negative for the child younger than 2 years, but this negative result disappeared with the inclusion of two-sided adult-child conversations (Zimmerman et al., 2009). Previous studies reported that infants and toddlers learn faster and better when they are able to interact with adults, rather than just watch and listen (Boyce et al., 2015).

A later study of 3- to 5-year-olds refined these findings and indicated that the amount of television viewing negatively affected vocabulary and executive functioning, but this affect disappeared when the home learning environment was removed as a background variable (Blankson et al., 2015). A systematic review (Carson et al., 2015) of 37 studies of cognitive development in healthy children from birth to 5 years reported that the type of sedentary behavior, particularly television screen time as opposed to reading, may have differential effects on cognitive development. This study reported that further studies need to investigate the whole range of cognitive domains (language, spatial skill, executive function, and memory) to fully investigate the relationship between cognitive development and television viewing. Since the AAP guidelines were introduced in 2013, there has been an explosion in the use of digital devices including iPads, tablets and smartphones, and apps created for young children. Professional policy advice in this area may lag behind digital innovation (Brown et al., 2015). The nurse needs to convey to parents that the evidence supporting the recommendation for less television viewing for children from birth to age 5 years is evolving as this is studied further and access to digital devices increases.

- How can nurses talk to parents about the recommendation for television viewing for children younger than 2 years?
- How can nurses use the results of this study when teaching parents that face-to-face interaction and two-way conversations with their children promote cognitive development more than watching television, videos, or other virtual media?
- Nurses should emphasize that role modeling is important and young children should observe the parent's on-line politeness and use of media
- How can nurses reinforce a focus that content matters and content quality is more influential than the media platform?

From American Academy of Pediatrics (AAP). (2013). Limiting screen time. *Pediatrics, 132*, 958–961; Blankson, A. N., O'Brien, M., Leerkes, E. M., Calkins, S. D., & Marcovitch, S. (2015). Do hours spent viewing television at ages 3 and 4 predict vocabulary and executive functioning at age 5? *Merrill-Palmer Quarterly, 61*(2), 264–289; Boyce, J. S., Riley, J. G., & Patterson, L. G. (2015). Adult-child communication: A goldmine of learning experience. *Childhood Education, 91*(3), 169–173; Brown, A., Shifrin, D. L., & Hill, D. L. (2015). Beyond 'turn it off': How to advise families on media use. *AAPNews, 36*(10). http://www.aappublications.org/content/36/10/54; Carson, V., Kuzik, N., Hunter, S., Wiebe, S. A., Spence, J. C., Friedman, A., Tremblay, M. S., Slater, L. G., & Hinkley, T. (2015). Systematic review of sedentary behavior and cognitive development in early childhood. *Preventive Medicine, 78*, 115–122; Christakis, D. A., Gilkerson, J., Richards, J. A., Zimmerman, F. J., Garrison, M. M., Xu, D., et al. (2009). Audible television and decreased adult words, infant vocalizations, and conversational turns. *Archives of Pediatric and Adolescent Medicine, 163*(6), 554–558; Zimmerman, F. J., Gilkerson, J., Richards, J. A., Christakis, D. A., Xu, D., Gray, S., et al. (2009). Teaching by listening: The importance of adult-child conversations to language development. *Pediatrics, 124*(1), 342–349.

---

## Moral Development: Kohlberg's Theory

Another aspect of cognitive development is the development of moral thinking and judgment. Lawrence **Kohlberg's theory of moral development** is based on interviews that focused on hypothetical moral dilemmas such as: Should a man steal an expensive drug that would save his dying wife? This question forms the basis of Kolhberg's classic Heinz dilemma. From interviews with boys, Kohlberg developed his theory, which is outlined in Table 15-5 (Kohlberg, 1969, 1981). The three stages of moral development—preconventional, conventional, and postconventional—were based on Piaget's theory of cognitive development and emphasize the ethics of rights and justice. Progression through the successive stages of moral development generally occurs during the school-age, adolescent, and young-adult years. Beyond the young-adult years, stabilization or increased consistency of thought and perhaps an increased correlation between moral judgment and moral action occur (Kohlberg, 1981).

## Moral Development: Gilligan's Theory

Carol **Gilligan's theory of moral development** (Gilligan, 1982, 2013; Gilligan et al., 1988) suggests that the process of moral development differs in women. While a doctoral student, Gilligan conducted research with Lawrence Kohlberg at Harvard University.

### TABLE 15-5   **GROWTH AND DEVELOPMENT**
#### *Kohlberg's Stages of Moral Development*

| Stage | Goal |
|---|---|
| Preconventional | Avoiding punishment<br>Gaining reward |
| Conventional | Gaining approval<br>Avoiding disapproval |
| Postconventional | Agreeing upon rights<br>Establishing personal moral standards<br>Achieving justice |

From Kohlberg, L. (1981). *The philosophy of moral development* (Vol. 1). San Francisco: Harper & Row.

She discovered that Kohlberg's original research was conducted with only men and that women often scored lower in Kohlberg's scaling of moral levels. She asserted that women were not inferior in their moral development, just different. In developing her own research with women, she proposed an alternative theory of moral development, which, like Kohlberg's, has three stages (Table 15-6). Gilligan concluded that the transitions between stages are based on changes in one's sense of self rather than on changes in cognitive development, as Kohlberg proposed. Gilligan

## TABLE 15-6 GROWTH AND DEVELOPMENT
### Gilligan's Stages of Moral Development (for Women)

| Stage | Characteristics | Goal |
|---|---|---|
| Preconventional | What is practical to others and best for self, realizing connection to others | Individual survival |
| Conventional | Sacrifices wants and needs to fulfill others' wants and needs | Self-sacrifice is goodness |
| Postconventional | Moral equal of self and others | Principle of nonviolence, do not hurt self or others |

From Gilligan, C. (1982). *In a different voice: Psychological theory and women's development.* Cambridge, MA: Harvard University Press; Gilligan, C. (2013). *Joining the resistance.* Malden, MA: Polity Press; Gilligan, C., Ward, J. V., & Taylor, J. M. (Eds.). (1988). *Mapping the moral domain: A contribution of women's thinking to psychology and education.* Cambridge, MA: Harvard University Press.

more clearly differentiated the "voice of care" from the "voice of justice." She also reported that women think and act more from a base of caring and relationships than do men, who are more inclined to think in terms of justice, rights, and rules. The voice of justice promotes legislative policies (e.g., immigration) and development of codes of ethics (McThomas, 2015); the voice of caring speaks to the importance of social relationships, which directs health practitioners to pay more attention to individual moral situations (Campbell, 2015).

## BEHAVIORAL BIOLOGICAL DEVELOPMENT

All the preceding theories discuss the importance of experience and environmental exposure on behavior and learning. One of the fundamental questions in the nature versus nurture debate is understanding how environmental stress (physical and behavioral) alters biological development (epigenetics). Evidence in animals and from human epidemiological studies indicates that experiences and the environment change the functioning of genes, and thus provide a basis for a model of gene-environment interaction. Early life experiences and social exposures may alter the way in which genes direct cell activities (Box 15-5: Genomics); early life adversity, including living in poverty, appears to result in DNA changes in the brain and other body tissues (Szyf et al., 2016). Recent studies suggest that even parental experiences can affect the behavior of children; brain plasticity theory describes brain cell development that can potentially modify ways individuals learn and experience their outside environment. This has implications for physical disease as well as attention and behavioral and mental disorders, and even the transmission of behavioral traits to the next generation (Szyf, 2015) (see Box 15-5: Genomics).

## SUMMARY

Individuals make many choices that affect their health each day, and a number of factors influence how these choices are made.

## BOX 15-5 GENOMICS
### Epigenetics

- What Is Epigenetics?
- What are the associations between environmental stressors and physical and behavioral disorders?
- How can stressors, including poverty, affect more than one generation?

Epigenetics is the scientific investigation of the capacity of cells to react differently to variations in environmental stimuli that are not related to the DNA code itself. The term epigenetics means "above genetics." Variations in cell response were historically attributed to changes in DNA gene sequences and the manufacture of cellular proteins with RNA transcription. However, this description does not fully explain why cells sharing identical DNA sequences can have differing appearances and effects. Some of this was attributed to cell mutations or alternative forms of genes (alleles). Again, this did not fully explain the full variety of appearances seen. Further scientific investigations showed that in two cells having identical DNA, the genes may be expressed differently. Cells are capable of regulating gene expression via the presence of regulatory proteins that wrap around DNA and RNA and can change cell function negatively or positively. Some of these regulatory proteins may turn off (repress) or silence cell function (methylation). Methylation and cell regulatory proteins are stable and heritable and separate from DNA genomic patterns. Epigenetic investigations have shown that these regulatory changes can be long-lasting and passed from one generation to the next. Stressors and/or maltreatment affecting one generation may have lasting behavior effects on subsequent generations. It is estimated that many of these epigenetic regulatory changes occur early in childhood and brain development (before the age of 3 years), and that poor early development influences risks of adult diseases (diabetes, obesity, heart disease, mental health and addiction problems) (Szyf et al., 2016; van Dijk, et al., 2015). There are also associations with attention deficit disorders, learning problems, and acquisition of language and numeral skills. Studies have linked poverty to brain impairment in early child development (Boivin et al., 2015). Whereas this science is in its infancy, and it is difficult to study human generational effects, there is no question that various stressors and physical and learning disorders affecting parents and children may be a problem for the next generation (Szyf, 2015), even when the original precipitating stressors are removed.

From Boivin, M. J., Kakooza, A. M, Warf, B. C., Davidson, L. L., & Grigorenko, E. L. (2015). Reducing neurodevelopmental disorders and disability through research and interventions. *Nature, 527*(7578), S155–S160; Szyf, M. (2015). Nongenetic inheritance and transgenerational epigenetics. *Trends in Molecular Medicine, 21*(2), 134–144; Szyf, M., Tang, Y., Hill, K. G., & Musci, R. (2016). The dynamic epigenome and its implications for behavioral interventions: A role for epigenetics to inform disorder prevention and health promotion. *Translational Behavioral Medicine, 6*(1), 55–62; van Dijk, S. J., Molloy, P. L., Varinli, H., Morrison, J. L., Muhlhausler, B. S., & Members of EpiSCOPE. (2015). Epigenetics and human obesity. *International Journal of Obesity, 39*, 85–97.

The stage of growth and development, as well as the context in which learning occurs, influences how individuals experience different situations and realize the choices available. Understanding the most widely used theories of human growth and development assists nurses to have a clear understanding of the challenges an individual is likely to encounter, as well as the skills the individual is likely to need, for successful growth, development, and maturation throughout the life span. Theories provide nurses with frameworks, resources, and comparisons for health assessment, promotion, and intervention.

## CASE STUDY

### Birth of a Disabled/Chronically Ill Child: Avery

Avery is a 33-year-old woman pregnant with her third child; her other two children are aged 5 and 10 years. At 26 weeks' gestation, Avery is hospitalized for contractions. Despite pharmacological attempts to stop labor, Avery's labor continues to the active phase. Avery and her partner just learned that a baby born this prematurely may have many problems, including cerebral palsy. As the perinatologist leaves the room, Avery turns to the nurse and starts to cry.

#### Reflective Questions

- What is the nurse's role when the parents learn a child has a chronic disease and/or disability?
- What can the nurse anticipate for these new parents during the labor? At the birth of the baby?
- What can the nurse anticipate in the first 2 weeks after birth? Over the baby's first year of life? Over the first 5 years?
- How will this child's growth, development, and goals for health promotion be affected? What about those of the parents? What about those of the siblings?
- What factors might contribute to Avery's development of chronic sorrow?
- If Avery becomes depressed, how might this affect the growth and development of the new baby? What effect might this have on her relationship with her partner? What effect might her depression have on her other children?
- What will be the impact of this child's disabilities on the siblings?
- How might the nurse intervene to lessen the effects of chronic sorrow?

## ◎ CARE PLAN

### Birth of a Disabled/Chronically Ill Child: Avery

**\*NURSING DIAGNOSIS: Chronic sorrow (parental) related to missed opportunities and unending caregiving for a new child**

#### Definition
Cyclical, recurring, and potentially progressive pattern of pervasive sadness experienced (by a parent, caregiver, individual with chronic illness or disability) in response to continual loss, throughout the trajectory of an illness or disability

#### Defining Characteristics
- Parental expression of disparity between preconceived notions of parenting and reality
- Parental expression of an ongoing or recurrent sense of sadness or loss
- Parental expressions of negative feelings (e.g., anger, depression, disappointment, emptiness, frustration, self-blame, helplessness, hopelessness, loneliness, overwhelmed) that are often triggered by health care crises or conflict with expected social norms for child or family

#### Related Factors
- Change in family structure
- Change in parental role expectation
- Parental coping styles

#### Goal
- Assist family unit to attain, maintain, or regain optimal health

#### Expected Outcomes
- Grief resolution: *Adjustment to actual or impending loss.* For example, parents verbalize reality of loss, progress through stages of grief, decreasing preoccupation with loss, verbalize acceptance of loss, resolve feelings about loss.

- Hope: *Optimism that is personally satisfying and life-supporting.* For example, parents express inner peace, expectation of a positive future.
- Psychosocial adjustment: *Adaptive psychosocial response of an individual to a significant life change.* For example, parents set realistic goals, maintain productivity, verbalize optimism about present, use effective coping strategies, report feeling socially engaged.

#### Nursing Interventions
- Grief work facilitation: *Helping another cope with painful feelings of actual or perceived responsibility.* For example, listen to expression of grief, encourage identification of fears, assist in identifying needed modifications in lifestyle.
- Hope inspiration: *Enhancing the belief in one's capacity to initiate and sustain actions.* For example, help identify areas of hope in their lives, demonstrate hope by recognizing the disability or illness as only one facet of the child, provide parents with opportunities to be involved with support groups, especially with other parents of children who are disabled/chronically ill who have transcended.
- Coping enhancement: *Assisting a person to adapt to perceived stressors, changes, or threats that interfere with meeting life demands and roles.* For example, provide an atmosphere of acceptance, seek to understand each parent's perspective of the situation, appraise and discuss alternative responses to the situation, foster constructive outlets for negative feelings, assist the parents to identify positive strategies to deal with limitations and manage necessary lifestyle changes.
- Resiliency promotion: *Assisting individual, families, and communities in development, use, and strengthening of protective factors to be used in coping with environmental and societal stressors.* For example, encourage positive health-seeking behavior, facilitate development and use of neighborhood resources.

\*NANDA Nursing Diagnoses—Herdman T. H. & Kamitsuru, S. (Eds.). Nursing Diagnoses–Definitions and Classification 2015–2017. Copyright © 2014, 1994–2014 NANDA International. Used by arrangement with John Wiley & Sons Limited. In order to make safe and effective judgments using the NANDA-I nursing diagnoses it is essential that nurses refer to the definitions and defining characteristics of the diagnoses listed in this work.
Sources Bulechek, G. M., Butcher, H. K., Dochterman, J. M., & Wagner, C. (Eds.). (2013). *Nursing interventions classification (NIC)* (6th ed.). St Louis: Mosby; Johnson, M., Moorhead, S., Bulechek, G., & Butcher, H. (2011). *NANDA, NOC, and NIC linkages* (3rd ed.). St Louis: Mosby; Kao, B., Plante, W., & Lobato, D. (2009). The use of the impact on sibling scale with families of children with chronic illness and developmental disability. *Child: Care, Health and Development, 35*(4), 505–509; Masterson, M. K. (2010). *Chronic sorrow in mothers of adult children with cerebral palsy: An exploratory study.* Doctoral dissertation (UMI AA13408137). Kansas State University; Marcella-Brienza, S., & Mennillo, T. (2015). Back to work: Manager support of nurses with chronic sorrow. *Creative Nursing, 21*(4), 206–210; Moorhead, S., Johnson, M., Maas, M., & Swanson, E. (Eds.). (2013). *Nursing outcomes classification (NOC)* (5th ed.). St. Louis: Mosby; Patrick-Ott, A., & Ladd, L. D. (2010). The blending of Boss's concept of ambiguous loss and Olshansky's concept of chronic sorrow: A case study of a family with a child who has significant disabilities. *Journal of Creativity in Mental Health, 5,* 74–86.

## ⓔ EVOLVE CHAPTER FEATURES

http://evolve.elsevier.com/Edelman/
• Study Questions

## REFERENCES

Campbell, T. (2015). Voicing unease: Care ethics in the professionalization of social care. *The New Bioethics*, *21*(1), 33–45.

Carey, S., Zaitchik, D., & Bascandziez, I. (2015). Theories of development: In dialog with Jean Piaget. *Developmental Review*, *38*, 36–54.

Centers for Disease Control and Prevention (CDC). (2010). Use of World Health Organization and CDC growth charts for children aged 0–59 months in the United States. *MMWR. Recommendations and Reports*, *59*(rr09), 1–15.

Centers for Disease Control and Prevention (CDC). (2011a). CDC health disparities and inequalities report—United States, 2011. *MMWR. Recommendations and Reports*, *60*(Suppl.), 1–116.

Centers for Disease Control and Prevention (CDC). (2011b). Ten great public health achievements—United States, 2001—2010. *MMWR. Recommendations and Reports*, *60*(19), 619–623.

Erikson, E. H. (1968). *Identity, youth, and crisis.* New York: Norton.

Erikson, E. H. (1995). *Childhood and society* (35th anniversary ed.). New York: Norton.

Erikson, E. H., & Erikson, J. M. (1998). *The life cycle completed.* New York: Norton.

Gilligan, C. (1982). *In a different voice: Psychological theory and women's development.* Cambridge, MA: Harvard University Press.

Gilligan, C. (2013). *Joining the resistance.* Malden, MA: Polity Press.

Gilligan, C., Ward, J. V., & Taylor, J. M. (Eds.), (1988). *Mapping the moral domain: A contribution of women's thinking to psychology theory and education.* Cambridge, MA: Harvard University Press.

Kohlberg, L. (1969). Continuities and discontinuities in childhood and adult moral development. *Human Development*, *12*, 93–120.

Kohlberg, L. (1981). *The philosophy of moral development* (Vol. 1). San Francisco: Harper & Row.

McThomas, M. (2015). Engendering attitudes toward immigration policy: The impact of justice and care. *Public Integrity*, *17*(2), 177–188.

Mei, Z., & Grummer-Strawn, L. M. (2011). Comparison of changes in growth percentiles of USchildren on CDC 2000 growth charts with corresponding changes on WHO 2006 growth charts. *Clinical Pediatrics*, *50*(5), 402–407.

Perry, T. E., et al. (2015). Applying Erikson's wisdom to self-management practices of older adults. *Research on Aging*, *37*(3), 253–274.

Phillips, J. L. (1975). *The origins of intellect: Piaget's theory* (2nd ed.). San Francisco: W. H. Freeman.

Piaget, J. (1950). *The psychology of intelligence.* London: Routledge and Kegan Paul.

Read, C. Y., & Ward, L. D. (2016). Faculty performance on the genomic nursing concept inventory. *Journal of Nursing Scholarship*, *48*(1), 5–13.

Szyf, M. (2015). Nongenetic inheritance and transgenerational epigenetics. *Trends in Molecular Medicine*, *21*(2), 134–144.

Szyf, M., et al. (2016). The dynamic epigenome and its implications for behavioral interventions: A role for epigenetics to inform disorder prevention and health promotion. *Translational Behavioral Medicine*, *6*(1), 55–62.

US Department of Health and Human Services. (2016). Healthy People 2020 Topics and Objectives—Objectives A–Z. http://www.healthypeople.gov.

Vygotsky, L. S. (1978). *Mind in society: The development of higher psychological processes.* Cambridge, MA: Harvard University Press.

Vygotsky, L. S. (1986). *Thought and language.* Cambridge, MA: MIT Press.

Wink, J., & Putney, L. (2002). *A vision of Vygotsky.* Boston, MA: Allyn & Bacon.

Ziegler, E. E., & Nelson, S. E. (2012). The WHO growth standards: Strengths and limitations. *Current Opinion in Clinical Nutrition and Metabolic Care*, *15*(3), 298–302.

# 16

# The Childbearing Period

*Susan Scott Ricci*

## OBJECTIVES

*After completing this chapter, the reader will be able to:*

- Differentiate fetal development and the newborn transition to extrauterine life.
- Analyze changes in the maternal system during pregnancy on the basis of their influences on pregnancy adaptation.
- Interpret the role of the nurse in promoting the physical, mental, and spiritual health of the childbearing family.
- Compare and contrast fetal problems caused by maternal drinking, smoking, drug use, and viral exposure during pregnancy.
- Outline the nursing role during labor and birth with a focus on the physical, emotional, spiritual, and educational needs of the woman giving birth and her family.
- Evaluate the influence of factors such as ethnicity, legislative priorities, and the sociopolitical context of the health care delivery system on prenatal and childbirth care and the needs of families.

## KEY TERMS

Acquired immunodeficiency syndrome
Amniocentesis
Amniotic membranes
Anemia of pregnancy
Apgar scoring system
Bacterial vaginosis
Bradycardia
*Candida albicans*
Cervical effacement
Chlamydia
Chloasma
Chorionic membranes
Chorionic villi
Colostrum
Conception
Congenital defect
Cytomegalovirus
Dilation
Diversity
Down syndrome
Embryo
Endometrium
Estrogen
Fertilization
Fetal alcohol spectrum disorder
Fetal alcohol syndrome
Fetal heart monitor

Fetus
First stage of labor
Fourth stage of labor
Fundus
Gestation
Gestational hypertension
Gonococcus
Group B streptococcus
Health outcomes
Hepatitis B
Hepatitis B virus
Herpes simplex
Human chorionic gonadotropin
Human immunodeficiency virus
Infant mortality rate
Infertility
Labor
Lamaze
Linea nigra
Meconium
Miscarriage
Neonatal abstinence syndrome
Obesity
Pica
Placenta
Polyhydramnios
Positive signs of pregnancy

Prejudices
Premature delivery
Presumptive signs of pregnancy
Preterm birth
Probable signs of pregnancy
Progesterone
Quickening
Rh blood group incompatibility
Risk factors
Rubella
Second stage of labor
Sexually transmitted infections
Spontaneous abortion
Stages of labor
Station
Stillbirth
Striae gravidarum
Syphilis
Tachycardia
Teratogen
Third stage of labor
Toxoplasmosis
Trimesters
Ultrasound
Zika virus
Zygotic cells

The process of conception, pregnancy, and birth involves a complex interaction of many factors, including the physiological and psychological changes in the woman and family and the development of a fetus into a viable newborn. The nurse's role during the pregnancy cycle should encompass evidence-based practice recommendations for effective health-promotion interventions prenatally, intranatally, and postnatally to improve maternal and newborn health outcomes. The focus of this chapter is on the pregnant woman, her family, and the developing fetus; discussing one without the others is impossible. The nurse must consider all three entities when seeking to promote a healthy pregnancy and healthy family system after birth.

## BIOLOGY AND GENETICS

Cells are the basic units of life. Pregnancy begins with fertilization, the fusion of a sperm from a male and an egg from a female. Each one contains half of the genetic material to form a new individual. Fertilization is the first embryonic event in a series that culminates in the birth of an infant. The physical changes during pregnancy include natural processes involving fertilization of the egg by the sperm, implantation of the fertilized egg into the uterus, embryonic or fetal growth and development, placental development and function, and maternal changes related to the pregnancy process.

### Duration of Pregnancy

Pregnancy begins with the union of a sperm and an egg, a process called fertilization. Under normal healthy circumstances, a full-term pregnancy lasts approximately 9 solar months, 10 lunar months, or 40 weeks. An accurate estimated date of delivery is determined by use of Nägele's rule. One does this by adding 7 days to the date of the first day of the last normal menstrual period and subtracting 3 months. A usual pregnancy consists of 9 months, divided into three equal periods called trimesters. Often these trimesters form the basis for discussion of expected fetal and maternal changes during pregnancy.

### Fertilization

The union of a sperm and an egg requires several crucial factors, many of which are not fully understood. When a sperm cell penetrates an egg in the ampulla of the fallopian tube, the beginning of a human being (called a *zygote*) results. Early cell divisions occur while the zygote is slowly being transported through the fallopian tube toward the uterus. Additional division of zygotic cells results in more differentiated structures that eventually produce an embryo and subsequently a fetus.

An absence of one or more critical factors may cause infertility (failure of the couple to become pregnant despite usual sexual activity in a period of 1 year). For example, both a sperm cell and an egg cell must be mature and in the fallopian tube for approximately 5 hours for union of the sperm and egg to occur (the process of conception). The sperm must be of uniform size, be normally formed, possess high motility, and have an ability to secrete enzymes that dissolve the membrane surrounding the egg. Cellular changes within the egg prevent other sperm from entering the ovum after the sperm penetrates it (Mattson & Smith, 2015). The woman attempting pregnancy must have a certain basal body temperature and fallopian tubes free of adhesions or obstructions. A woman will likely conceive within 24 hours after ovulation.

### Implantation

The process of attachment and placental formation is called implantation. A pregnancy has not occurred until successful implantation has happened. The placenta is an organ that serves to prevent the direct exchange between the blood of the fetus and the blood of the mother. It also functions as an endocrine gland, manufacturing and secreting hormones that play a vital role in maintaining the pregnancy. Transplantation of the fertilized egg in the uterine cavity after its trip through the fallopian tube requires approximately 6 days (Mader & Windelspecht, 2015). Once the zygote reaches the uterus, it stays there for up to 5 days, receiving nutrition from the endometrium, the inner lining of the uterus (El-Mazny, 2014). The process of fertilization and implantation triggers the production of large amounts of the hormone progesterone, which stimulates the formation of endometrial cells known as the decidua, meaning "to shed." The decidua provides nutrition for the embryo, a term that defines the growing conceptus up to 8 weeks of age.

### Fetal Growth and Development

Much is known about the stages of physical development in each structural system of the embryo. However, metabolic functions, particularly those relevant to the endocrine and neurological systems, are less well defined. Appropriate fetal development depends on these events occurring in a specified period and order during each trimester of pregnancy. If this does not occur, an abnormality in structure or function (a congenital defect) may result. This defect may be noted at birth, did not occur at conception (called a genetic defect), but most likely resulted from some disruption that occurred after conception and during fetal development.

## Placental Development and Function

After implantation of the zygote, the placenta develops through an integration of embryonic and decidual cells. The chorionic membranes and amniotic membranes, which surround the fetus throughout gestation, also begin to form. The amniotic fluid, manufactured by the amniotic membrane, supports the developing fetus and protects it from injury.

The basic structure of the placenta allows maternal-fetal blood exchange to nourish the fetus and allow excretion of fetal waste products. Throughout most of gestation, increasing placental development allows maternal blood to flow through the intervillous spaces and fetal blood to flow through the chorionic villi (Cunningham et al., 2014). The unique structure of the placenta permits the exchange of certain molecules but prevents fetal and maternal blood supplies from mixing for most of the pregnancy. Substances with larger and heavier molecules (such as heparin or insulin) normally do not pass through the placenta to the fetus, but lighter molecules (such as anesthetic gases, oxygen, carbon dioxide, and electrolytes) readily cross the placenta. Because of the difficulty involved in predicting exactly which substances will cross the placenta, the nurse needs to encourage pregnant women and those contemplating pregnancy to avoid any substance that might cause harm to the fetus.

The placenta manufactures and secretes four hormones throughout pregnancy. The primary hormones produced by the placenta include estrogen, progesterone, human chorionic gonadotropin (hCG), and human placental lactogen (hPL). Estrogen's role is to increase uterine blood flow and increase uterine and breast growth. Progesterone maintains the uterus in a quiet state throughout the pregnancy to prevent labor contractions occurring too early. hCG's main role is to sustain estrogen and progesterone production in early pregnancy, and it is also the hormone detected in pregnancy tests. hPL ensures adequate fetal nutrition, increases insulin resistance, and stimulates production of growth hormones (King et al., 2015).

The fetus, which continues to gain strength and maturity during the later weeks of gestation, generally rests its head in the lower maternal pelvis by the end of pregnancy (Figure 16-1).

The membranes protect the fetus from infection and act as a container for the amniotic fluid. As birth begins, the membranes may rupture, causing the loss of amniotic fluid and stronger uterine contractions, reflective of the labor process. If the membranes rupture more than 24 hours before birth, uterine infection and potential fetal harm may result.

As gestation nears completion, placental function gradually decreases, which may serve as a stimulus for the onset of labor. When pregnancy continues beyond 42 weeks, or 2 weeks beyond the calculated due date, placental function decreases even more, posing concerns about the well-being of the fetus (Blackburn, 2014).

The discussion of fetal development provides only a brief glimpse of the prenatal period. It is also important to address maternal changes and culmination of the prenatal period, labor, and birth.

## Maternal Changes

A woman experiences various physiological effects based on a combination of hormonal and mechanical changes during pregnancy. Hormonal influences tend to increase as the pregnancy progresses. The mechanical (hemodynamic) changes reach a peak in the seventh or eighth month and then gradually decline as the pregnancy nears completion (Cunningham et al., 2014). Clinical symptoms will manifest themselves during this peak stress time.

### Signs of Pregnancy

A woman may assume that she is pregnant because she has skipped her menstrual period or experiences nausea and vomiting, changes in breast sensations and size, or increased urinary frequency (presumptive signs of pregnancy). Presumptive signs of pregnancy are the least reliable indicators of pregnancy because any one of them can be caused by conditions other than pregnancy. If she suspects she is pregnant, the woman should undergo a pregnancy test. If it is performed too early, a home pregnancy test may produce a false negative result attributable to a low level of human chorionic gonadotropin (hCG). This hormone, produced by the placenta and found in a pregnant woman's urine and blood, triggers a positive pregnancy result. These home pregnancy tests have a high degree of accuracy (97%) if the instructions are followed exactly. If the pregnancy test is positive, a prenatal visit should be scheduled to estimate gestational age and for the woman to receive appropriate pregnancy counseling, which should include taking folic acid supplementation to prevent neural tube defects (NTDs), if she has not already started taking it preconceptually. All women of reproductive age should supplement their diet before conception with 0.4 to 1.0 mg of folic acid daily as part of their multivitamins. The incidence of NTDs (~1 in 1000 live births in the United States) has fallen since the inclusion of folic acid supplementation, but recent research suggests folic acid supplementation is underused because of low adherence (Chitayat et al., 2016). As the pregnancy progresses, the woman may experience presumptive signs of pregnancy, which are subjectively experienced; probable signs of pregnancy, which are objectively observed by the health care provider; and positive signs of pregnancy, which are positive signs that verify

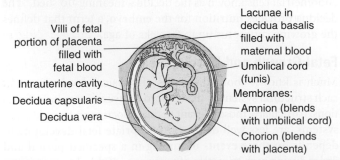

**FIGURE 16-1** Relationship of fetus, placenta, membranes, and uterus during gestation. (From Lowdermilk, D., Perry, S., Cashion, K., & Alden, K. R. [2016]. *Maternity and women's health care* [11th ed.]. St. Louis: Mosby.)

Labels in figure:
Villi of fetal portion of placenta filled with fetal blood
Intrauterine cavity
Decidua capsularis
Decidua vera
Lacunae in decidua basalis filled with maternal blood
Umbilical cord (funis)
Membranes:
Amnion (blends with umbilical cord)
Chorion (blends with placenta)

## BOX 16-1 Signs of Pregnancy and Time of Occurrence

**Presumptive**

- Breast changes (e.g., tenderness) (3–4 weeks)
- Fatigue (12 weeks)
- Urinary frequency (6–12 weeks)
- Nausea and vomiting (4–14 weeks)
- Amenorrhea (4th week)
- Quickening (16–20 weeks)

**Probable**

- Enlargement of the uterus (12–14 weeks)
- Softening of the uterine isthmus (Hegar sign) (6th –12th week)
- Bluish or cyanotic color of cervix and upper vagina (Chadwick sign) (6th–8th week)
- Softening of the cervix (Goodell sign) (5th week)
- Ballottement of the fetus (16th –28th week)
- Positive test result for hCG in the maternal urine or blood serum (4th –12th week)
- Changes in skin pigmentation (chloasma and linea nigra) (2nd half of pregnancy)

**Positive**

- Detection of fetal heart tones by auscultation, ultrasonography, or a Doppler scan (8–17 weeks)
- Palpation of fetal body parts with Leopold maneuvers (19–22 weeks)
- Fetal movements visible and detected by examiner (late pregnancy)
- Radiological or ultrasonographic demonstration of fetal parts (6–16 weeks)

*hCG,* Human chorionic gonadotropin.

that a pregnancy exists (Box 16-1). During the first trimester of pregnancy, using sophisticated testing with **ultrasound**, health care providers can determine fetal presence and placental adequacy early in pregnancy. This technology, which uses high-frequency sound waves that bounce off the fetus and are interpreted by a computer, allows visualization of the fetus and gestational structures throughout pregnancy (Norwitz & Schorge, 2015).

Nausea and vomiting in pregnancy occurs in up to 80% of women, and there is a tendency for many health care providers to minimize it. The Food and Drug Administration has approved Diclegis to treat nausea and vomiting in women whose symptoms have not abated with a change in diet or other nonmedical treatments. It is a delayed-release medication containing a combination of doxylamine (antihistamine) and pyridoxine (vitamin $B_6$). The major side effect is drowsiness (Brucker & King, 2017).

### Adaptive Changes of Other Systems

In addition to pregnancy-related changes in the reproductive system, adaptive changes in other body systems occur. The urinary system undergoes dramatic changes during gestation as follows:

- A 50% increase in glomerular filtration rate occurs related to the influences of **estrogen** and progesterone.
- Ureters increase in diameter by 25% secondary to progesterone influence.
- Urinary output increases by approximately 80% related to the total body water increase.

- Bladder capacity increases to approximately 1500 mL to accommodate extra fluids.

The cardiovascular system changes also begin early in pregnancy as follows:

- Cardiac output increases by up to 50% to meet the demands of pregnancy.
- Total blood volume increases by up to 45% during pregnancy. Physiological anemia of pregnancy may result because of a greater increase in the volume of plasma compared with the volume of red blood cells.
- Heart rate increases by 10 beats per minute to compensate for the increase in blood volume.

Respiratory system changes include the following:

- Tidal volume (volume of air inspired) increases by 30% to 40% to increase the effectiveness of air exchange. Total oxygen consumption increases by approximately 20%.
- The diaphragm is displaced upward secondary to the enlarging uterus and causes shortness of breath during the last trimester.

Increased elasticity and softening of connective tissue of the musculoskeletal system cause the following changes during pregnancy:

- The joints relax, especially the pelvic joints that support the pregnancy and create pliability at the time of birth.
- Lumbar and dorsal curves of the spine increase late in pregnancy and contribute to low back pain and the waddle of pregnancy.
- Separation of the symphysis pubis occurs secondary to the influence of the hormone relaxin.

Changes in the integumentary system occur, which may include the following:

- Hormonal changes and stretching of the connective tissue of the abdomen attributable to an enlarging uterus lead to stretch marks (**striae gravidarum**).
- A narrow, brownish line (**linea nigra**) divides the abdomen, running from the umbilicus to the symphysis pubis. The linea nigra fades after the pregnancy ends.
- An increase in pigmentation caused by melanocyte-stimulating hormone causes darkened areas on the face termed the mask of pregnancy (**chloasma**).

The gastrointestinal system undergoes dramatic changes during pregnancy, such as the following:

- The enlarging and space-occupying uterus cramps the intestinal region, causing a slowing of peristalsis and an increase in the emptying time of the stomach.
- Relaxin causes a decrease in gastric motility leading to constipation.
- Frequent "heartburn" results from reflux of stomach contents into the esophagus secondary to upward displacement of the stomach and a relaxed gastroesophageal sphincter (King et al., 2015; Tharpe et al., 2016).

### Reproductive System

The effects on the reproductive system include changes in the uterus, breasts, vagina, vulva, and ovaries. The prepregnant uterus is approximately the size of a closed fist. The uterus at term has the capacity to contain a 3.2 to 4.5 kg (7–10 lb) infant and the

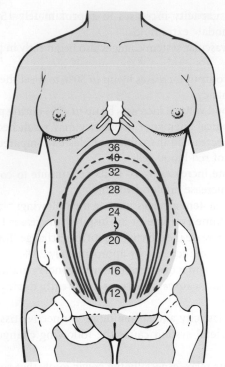

**FIGURE 16-2** Upper level of enlarging uterus by weeks of normal gestation with a single fetus. (From Seidel, H. M., Ball, J. W., Dains, J. E., Flynn, J. A., Solomon, B. S., & Stewart, R. W. [2015]. *Mosby's guide to physical assessment* [8th ed.]. St. Louis: Mosby.)

placenta. As the uterus enlarges, the **fundus** (the upper uterine segment) moves higher in the abdomen (Figure 16-2). The breasts begin enlarging early in the pregnancy, and in late pregnancy they may secrete small amounts of **colostrum**, a precursor of mature breast milk. The vagina and vulva receive a greater blood supply and appear darker (cyanotic) as a result. Some women will notice an increase in vaginal secretions and experience a whitish discharge (Mattson & Smith, 2015).

Hormones such as hCG and estrogen, secreted by the placenta and the fetus, create an optimal intrauterine environment for the fetus and stimulate many changes in the pregnant woman's body. The developing fetus contributes to the provision of an adequate environment for its own growth and nourishment, despite the possibility of creating discomforts for the pregnant woman.

## Preconception Care of Women

Preconception health promotion is a primary intervention that benefits reproductive-age women and their potential children. Prenatal care has been used as secondary prevention to improve the health of the woman during her pregnancy, but by the time prenatal care has generally started at weeks 8 to 12, a considerable amount of fetal development has already occurred. The fetus is most sensitive to maternal health and environmental exposures from weeks 4 to 10 of pregnancy, and many women may not know they are even pregnant then. The rates of adverse birth outcomes (preterm and low birth weight, infant deaths, and

birth defects) and maternal pregnancy complications in the United States are all higher than the goals in *Healthy People 2020*. Given the adverse trends seen in preterm birth rates and related infant death rates, a comprehensive public health research agenda that investigates the social, genetic, and biomedical factors contributing to these adverse outcomes was convened by the Centers for Disease Control and Prevention (CDC). The Action Plan for the National Initiative on Preconception Health and Health Care (Johnson et al., 2014) put forth the following objectives:

- Improve the knowledge, attitudes, and behaviors of men and women related to preconception health.
- Create health equity and eliminate disparities in adverse maternal, fetal, and infant outcomes.
- Ensure that all women of childbearing age receive preconception care services and enter their pregnancy in optimal health.
- Reduce risks among women who have prior adverse maternal, fetal, or infant outcomes through interventions during the postpartum and interconception periods.

The key points introduced included that preconception health is a gateway for broader conversations about women's wellness, that health practices and policies with an individual focus have finite success, and that researchers have been advocating broadening the spectrum of improving health using life course for more than a decade (CDC, 2015a).

Not all couples who seek preconception care are able to conceive on their own. Conception requires ovulation of a mature ovum, normal fallopian tubes, the presence of progressively motile sperm in the female reproductive tract, and an endometrium favorable for implantation. For many couples the experience of fertility problems and aspects of the care with uncertain outcomes can be stressful and distressing. Infertility is defined as a failure to conceive after 1 year of regular and unprotected sexual intercourse. Infertility affects more than 7 million American couples (Frankford et al., 2015). Frequently couples will seek treatment for their infertility issues and undergo testing that may include a semen analysis, assessment of ovulation, evaluation of tubal patency, and tests for ovarian reserve (Galliano & Pellicer, 2015). The nurse's role is that of support and education of the couple. The nurse can assist in educating the couple about the various methods to treat infertility and allow them to make their own decision as to which method is best for them. Infants conceived through in vitro fertilization (IVF) technologies have a higher risk of genetic abnormalities, being part of a multiple pregnancy, and being born prematurely (Green et al., 2015). The nurse must be knowledgeable to be able to respond to questions that will come up throughout the treatment experience. One of the greatest risks of assisted reproduction is the risk of obtaining a multiple pregnancy after intrauterine insemination with more than one embryo. Compared with a single pregnancy, the risks of a multiple pregnancy include iron- and folate-deficiency anemia, gestational hypertension, preeclampsia, polyhydramnios, gestational diabetes, and a high surgical birth rate (De Sutter, 2015). Most couples need a great deal of emotional support, and it is important for the nurse to be able to act as an advocate for them, particularly those using gestational surrogacy as a means of achieving parenthood.

Surrogacy is an arrangement in which a woman carries and gives birth to a child for another couple. The fundamental nature of families has changed over the years, whereby gestational surrogacy as an option for infertile couples is widely accepted. Gestational surrogacy, where the surrogate is not genetically related to the embryo, has become the norm. Surrogate motherhood is treated as a form of adoption in many countries: the birth mother and her partner are presumed to be the parents of the child, whereas the intended parents have to adopt the infant once it is born. Other than compensation for expenses related to the pregnancy, payments to surrogates are not allowed. The legal aspects of surrogacy are very complex and differ among countries (Jalili, 2015).

Preconception care before a pregnancy implies health-promotion activities that are conducted before a pregnancy occurs to address risk factors across the life span—including during adolescence. Although most pregnancies during adolescence are unintended, health behaviors initiated during this period can have a great impact, not only on future reproductive outcomes but also on present and future health.

Preconception care offers an effective and efficient means to reduce complications of pregnancy for both the mother and her newborn. Women should be made aware that certain preconception interventions may improve not only the outcomes of pregnancy but also the overall health of the woman as well. The following interventions may be included:

- Folic acid supplementation to reduce the risk of NTDs
- Rubella vaccination to reduce the risk of severe congenital defects
- Diabetes management to reduce the risk of birth defects threefold
- Hypothyroidism management to promote healthy fetal neurological development
- Hepatitis B vaccination for at-risk women to prevent chronic liver disease
- Human immunodeficiency virus (HIV)/acquired immuno-deficiency syndrome (AIDS) screening and treatment to prevent transmission to the fetus
- Healthy diet instruction throughout pregnancy
- Physical activity needs throughout pregnancy
- Substance use and medication safety
- Intimate partner violence screening
- Counseling women about immunizations for themselves and their infants
- Assessment of chronic health conditions such as diabetes, hypertension, and thyroid disease
- Screening and treatment for sexually transmitted infections (STIs) to reduce the risk of ectopic pregnancy and/or fetal anomalies
- Oral antiepileptic medication management to minimize birth defect potential
- Cessation of acne treatment with isotretinoin (Accutane) to prevent defects
- Smoking cessation counseling to reduce negative perinatal outcomes
- Screening and treating of depression to reduce the risk of postpartum depression
- Elimination of alcohol use to prevent fetal alcohol spectrum disorders
- Obesity control to reduce the risk of cerebrovascular disease, diabetes, or surgical births (CDC, 2015a)

As a group, nurses are challenged to effectively translate the concept of preconception care to all women in their practice setting. By informing women that existing health conditions and medications can affect pregnancy outcomes, nurses can provide a positive environment for the woman's future pregnancy and improve overall health practices.

## Normal Discomforts of Pregnancy

Changes in the woman's body during pregnancy support a nursing diagnosis of *alteration in comfort with relevant interventions* for most women. Women may feel a sense of relief that other pregnant women have these concerns and that interventions exist to increase their comfort at various points during gestation. Particularly for those experiencing a first pregnancy, the nurse serves as a valuable support person to help expectant couples adjust to the challenges and discomforts of pregnancy, a goal for the earlier-stated diagnosis.

## Teaching the Woman About Changes to Expect in the Body During Pregnancy

In addition to serving as a caregiver, advocate, and support person, the nurse serves as a teacher throughout the pregnancy care process. Active teaching responsive to an individual's concerns about pregnancy may occur in the clinic, physician's office, or other care environments. Nursing interventions should address recommended professional practice guidelines for education during the prenatal period to prevent complications for the family. For example, the nurse may offer textbooks, pamphlets, DVDs, and referrals to websites and other media to increase a couple's knowledge of fetal, maternal, and family changes during gestation and then encourage and answer any questions based on the material. Going beyond one-to-one teaching, the nurse may also refer couples to early pregnancy and Lamaze childbirth preparation classes to enlarge their social support network and increase knowledge of labor and birth. Throughout the care process the nurse is sensitive to the cultural and ethnic beliefs and behaviors of the individual or family. By incorporating knowledge of these beliefs and behaviors, the nurse protects the pregnant woman and her baby by providing individualized care addressing the childbearing rituals practiced by various cultural groups (Table 16-1). A summary of perinatal care guidelines is provided in Table 16-2.

Prenatally, pregnant women experience a wide variety of physiological adaptations. Nurses must possess a broad and deep understanding of these changes combined with accurate and early risk assessment to identify deviations. This knowledge base is vital for nurses caring for women during the childbearing cycle.

## Total Weight Gain

Total weight gain during pregnancy reflects not only the growth of the baby and placenta but also the growth of the uterus and breasts, the storage of maternal fat, and the increased amounts

| TABLE 16-1 | **Cultural Values Related to Pregnancy and Birth** |
|---|---|
| Filipino | Structured prenatal care for those who can afford it. Pregnancy normal event with family focused on pregnant woman's needs. Pregnant woman encouraged to eat well, sleep often, and not to work out of home. Sexual intercourse taboo during last 2 wk of pregnancy. Pregnant woman encouraged to eat fresh eggs close to delivery to help baby "slide out" with birth. Woman very modest about body needs and care during pregnancy. Father passive with birth process; pregnant woman active participant with birth. Breastfeeding encouraged until child is a toddler |
| American Indian | In many tribes, women are expected to seek prenatal care with pregnancy; some tribes accept late care. Dialogue with women in tribal community important to maximize pregnancy and birth process. Meditation, self-control practice, and indigenous plants (herbal teas) used for discomforts of pregnancy and birth. Pregnant woman stoic about birth process; father present but not active participant. Female kin present to support woman in labor; breastfeeding and bottle feeding encouraged after birth. Father may avoid hunting immediately after birth or until infant's umbilical cord detaches |
| Arab American | Pregnancy normal event; may not access prenatal care because of that belief. Much family support given to pregnant woman to allow maximal rest and minimal work. Present orientation: little preparation for birth, fears labor pains but responds once they come. Expressive with labor but not active with control of pain; relies on family members for support; father not active, may feel powerless with birth process. Very modest about care, especially with opposite-sex health care provider. Prefers bottle feeding; colostrum believed to harm baby |
| Black | Most access prenatal care after first trimester or seek care earlier with problems. Female kin provide most of support with pregnancy and birth; male support less visible. Open expression of pregnancy and birth discomfort; active participant in birth process. May self-medicate with cultural remedies for pregnancy complaints. May avoid being in photographs because of fear of stillbirth. May crave certain foods: chicken, greens, clay, starch, or dirt (pica). If of Muslim faith, may wish to have head covered during labor and birth process. Breastfeeds if given information on the benefits of this method |
| Mexican American | Often face barriers to prenatal care because of lack of insurance, fear of health care system, lack of transportation to clinic. May consider prenatal care not necessary because childbirth is normal life event. Education and acculturation influence prenatal care access. Pregnancy considered to follow marriage; family supports respect of and assistance to pregnant woman. Pregnant woman does not smoke, work, drink alcohol, or use drugs; pregnancy a time to rest, walk, eat well, sleep, drink chamomile tea, and avoid cold air. Grandmother may move into the home close to delivery time to help and provide folk remedies after birth. Modest about care and needs; same-sex health care provider encouraged. Generally, walks during labor to enhance birth; wants family for support; woman active and father delegates support to female members of family. Generally, breastfeeds for up to 1 yr |
| Vietnamese | Generally early prenatal care unless immigrant status, then depends on family for care. Encouraged to eat healthy foods, get rest, avoid strenuous activity during last trimester. Focus on keeping pregnant woman warm, encouraging salt water for oral care, and maintaining good hygiene. Sexual intercourse taboo with pregnancy. Father present but not active with pregnancy. Birth a time of hot and cold imbalance; mother "suffers in silence," may moan or grunt; mother depends on female relatives for support and guidance. Mother breastfeeds for up to 1 yr; avoids cold foods for this period |

NOTE: General ideas about beliefs and behaviors of each of these cultural groups have been given with no intent to stereotype all individuals who represent these groups' beliefs or behaviors. It is hoped that this information will provide direction to the nurse, who will continue to assess each individual to render care that meets each person's traditional values in a biomedical model of health care in the United States today.

From Ceballos, K. & Dunwoody, M. E. (2015). Cultural perspectives in childbearing. *Nursing Spectrum.* http://ce.nurse.com/ce263-60/cultural-perspectives-in-childbearing/; Callister, L. (2011). Global and cultural perinatal nursing research: Improving clinical practice. *Journal of Perinatal & Neonatal Nursing, 25*(2), 139–143; Haas, A. (2011). Cultural diversity in childbirth education. *Midwifery Today with International Midwife, 97,* 39; Lewallen, L. (2011). The importance of culture in childbearing. *Journal of Obstetric, Gynecologic, and Neonatal Nursing, 40*(1), 4–8; Purnell, L. D. (2014). *Guide to culturally competent health care* (3rd ed.). Philadelphia: F.A. Davis; Spector, R. E. (2012). *Cultural diversity in health & illness* (8th ed., pp. 101–137). Upper Saddle River, NJ: Prentice Hall.

of blood and other body fluids. It has been nearly 2 decades since guidelines for how much weight a woman should gain during pregnancy were issued by the Institute of Medicine (IOM). More research has been conducted on the effects of weight gain in pregnancy on the health of both the mother and her baby. Excessive weight gain is one of the most important potentially modifiable factors associated with adverse pregnancy outcomes. The IOM released new weight gain guidelines in 2009 that are based on revised body mass index (BMI) categories and now have a recommendation for obese women. However, the IOM did not differentiate women by age, race/ethnicity, or subclasses of obesity. As a result, the weight-gain guidelines span a wide range, and nurses are challenged to individualize their dietary counseling for the obese individual. To meet the recommendations of the report, women need to gain weight within the weight-gain ranges for their BMI category. Achieving the recommended weight gain will require individualized attention and support from a woman's care providers, as well as her family and community. Nurses are uniquely positioned to educate pregnant women about the IOM guidelines for weight gain in pregnancy and the importance of a healthy diet and adequate physical exercise. In addition, the Internet, social media, and eHealth technologies provide unprecedented opportunities to efficiently reach and educate influential family members, friends, and the media. Utilization of these modalities can quickly transform unhealthy cultural norms and prevent significant morbidity among generations of at-risk women and children (Chang & Moniz, 2015).

| TABLE 16-2 | Perinatal Care Guidelines | | | |
|---|---|---|---|---|
| **First Trimester** | **Second Trimester** | **Third Trimester** | **Labor Stages** | **Postpartum** |
| Complete assessment to identify risk factors | Assess adaptation to pregnancy and fetal well-being | Review physiological changes | Admission to birthing facility | Complete a head-to-toe physical assessment: breasts, uterus, bladder, bowels, lochia<br>Emotional status<br>Circulatory status<br>Episiotomy |
| Awareness of subtle or overt physical, sexual, or emotional abuse | Update heath history | Monitor changes related to pregnancy | *First stage:*<br>Complete maternal/fetal assessments<br>Determine labor progress<br>Assist with comfort measures<br>Monitor fetal heart rate<br>Support family in their efforts<br>Praise efforts | Assess mother for postpartum blues/depression |
| Assess physical and psychosocial progress in adaptation to pregnancy | Continue to recognize cultural influences | Assess expectant family's readiness for labor, birth, and parenting role | *Second stage:*<br>Offer encouragement<br>Assist with pushing efforts<br>Document activities | Encourage bonding and attachment |
| Inquire about physical changes and discomforts; explain causes and identify appropriate relief measures | Encourage informed decision-making and positive health care practices | Review finalized birth plan | *Third stage:*<br>Provide care as needed<br>Document time of placental delivery<br>Administer medications as ordered | Demonstrate breastfeeding techniques |
| Provide anticipatory guidance appropriate for the woman's individual needs<br>• Educational needs: hazards during pregnancy<br>• Use of drugs, alcohol, and smoking<br><br>Seat belts, high-risk behaviors<br>Warning/danger signs to report<br>Nutrition and weight management<br>Sexuality | Review potential risk factors and when to report them<br>Ensure community referrals/ resources as needed.<br>Educational needs: Oral hygiene Nutritional needs<br>Safety issues in workplace<br>Discomforts of pregnancy. Relief of common discomforts of pregnancy<br>Prepared childbirth classes | Identify community resources available to the family<br>Explain any diagnostic tests ordered. Meet educational needs: needs for newborn care<br><br>Monitoring fetal movements<br>Strategies to cope with discomforts<br>Promote family safety<br>Including partner in process<br>Childbirth preparation | *Fourth stage:*<br>Monitor vital signs; fundus, assess bladder status<br>Encourage parental-infant interaction<br>Monitor newborn's well-being<br>Provide perineal care, food, fluids<br>Provide family support | Provide anticipatory guidance needed for the family<br><br>Educational needs: Nutrition Fatigue Child care<br><br>Immunizations<br>Sexuality<br>Family planning<br>Breast engorgement<br>Family adaptation<br>Follow-up care needed<br>Danger signs to report<br>Sibling readiness for new member<br>Self-care activities |

From King, T. L., Brucker, M. C., Kriebs, J. M., Fahey, J. O., Gegor, C. L., & Varney, H. (2015). *Varney's midwifery* (5th ed.). Burlington, MA: Jones & Bartlett Learning; Macones, G. (2015). *Management of labor and delivery* (2nd ed.). Somerset, NJ: Wiley-Blackwell; Norwitz, E. R., & Schorge, J. O. (2015). *Obstetrics and gynecology at a glance* (4th ed.). Malden, MA: Blackwell Publishing.

The new IOM guidelines reflect changing US demographics, particularly the surge in the number of women who are overweight or obese. The new guidelines advise that healthy women at a normal weight for their height (BMI of 18.5–24.9 kg/m$^2$) should gain 25 to 35 pounds during pregnancy. Underweight women (BMI less than 18.5 kg/m$^2$) should gain more, 28 to 40 pounds, and overweight women (BMI of 25–29.9 kg/m$^2$) should gain less, 15 to 25 pounds. Obese women (BMI greater than 30 kg/m$^2$) should limit their gain to 11 to 20 pounds (IOM, 2015).

**Obesity** is a public health concern worldwide and has reached alarming proportions. It is arising from multifaceted and complex causes that relate to individual choice and lifestyle, and the influences of wider society. In addition to a long-standing focus on both childhood and adult obesity, there has been more recent concern relating to maternal obesity. Infants of obese mothers are more likely to be born prematurely, to be stillborn, or to die in the first 28 days of life. Obesity increases the risk of obstetrical complications during the prenatal, intrapartum, and postnatal periods, as well as contributing to technical difficulties with fetal assessment. In addition, infants of obese mothers are more likely to be born with a congenital abnormality (Lim & Mahmood, 2015). Overweight and obese women are at increased risk of several pregnancy complications that include abortion, gestational diabetes, hypertension, preeclampsia, thromboembolism, surgical birth, and postpartum weight retention. Despite the serious health implications of obesity in pregnancy, the current level of awareness of such risks among childbearing women is limited (Liat et al., 2015).

Ideally, all women with a BMI greater than 30 kg/m² should be provided with accurate and accessible information about the risks associated with obesity in pregnancy at a preconception visit. Weight-loss interventions would be most appropriately used before pregnancy, but if that is not possible, nurses need to recognize the need for opportunistic health promotion aimed at disseminating information about the risks of obesity in pregnancy to overweight and obese women of childbearing age. Most women are highly motivated to have healthy infants, and this could be a key factor in health-promotion discussions that inform women of the risks of obesity in pregnancy and promote healthy lifestyle choices and weight-loss strategies preconceptually and between pregnancies.

## Labor and Birth

Pregnancy culminates with labor and giving birth. Giving birth is a life-changing event, and the care that a woman receives during labor has the potential to affect her both physically and emotionally for a long period. The process of giving birth elicits a significant emotional response from the delivering family. A description of the events of a usual labor and birthing process must occur to establish a background for considering the physiological changes in the mother and the infant.

Several theories offer explanations for the cause of labor. Many factors likely interact, including uterine distention, mechanical irritation, progesterone deprivation, placental aging and hormones, and posterior pituitary activity. Labor usually begins at approximately 40 weeks of gestation, suggesting that hormonal control similar to that regulating the menstrual cycle also contributes to its onset (Cunningham et al., 2014).

Labor may be divided conveniently into the following four distinct stages:

- Dilation stage—lasts from the onset of true labor contractions to complete dilation of the cervix. It is divided into three phases: latent (0–3 cm dilation); active (4–7 cm dilation); and transition (8–10 cm dilation)
- Pushing stage—lasts from complete dilation (10 cm) of the cervix to birth
- Placental stage—lasts from the time of birth of the newborn to delivery of the placenta and membranes, which can range from 2 to 15 minutes
- Recovery stage—defined as the first 4 hours after childbirth, where physiological and psychological adjustments begin to occur

---

| BOX 16-2 | Signs of Beginning Labor |
|---|---|

- Bloody show or loss of the mucous plug that seals cervical canal during pregnancy
- Regular uterine contractions
- Contractions increasing in intensity, duration, and frequency
- Palpable hardening of the uterus during contractions
- Pain in the lower back radiating to the front of the abdomen

---

The first stage of labor starts with regular timing of uterine contractions and ends with complete **dilation** (opening) and **cervical effacement** (thinning of the cervix). The signs of beginning labor include those listed in Box 16-2. The cervix, the lower portion of the uterus, must dilate from a closed position (0 cm) to a totally open position (10 cm or 4 in, in diameter). During the first stage the cervix must also completely efface or shorten from a length of 1 to 2 inches to a barely palpable (paper-thin) thickness. For most women, painless Braxton Hicks contractions throughout pregnancy cause some cervical dilation and thinning, or at least cervical softening, before the onset of active labor.

During the **first stage of labor** the presenting part of the fetus begins to press on the cervix, lower uterine segment, and nerve endings around the cervix and vagina. Women's responses to this process differ; pain thresholds and cultural perceptions of and responses to pain differ among laboring women (see Table 16-1). The fundus, the active contractile part of the uterus, becomes thicker as labor progresses, retracts the lower uterine segment and cervix, and helps push the fetus toward the cervix and eventually through the vagina for birth (Macones, 2015). The first stage lasts an average of 8 to 12 hours for women experiencing a first birth and somewhat less for women having a second or additional child. On the basis of a laboring woman's needs, various pain medications, nonpharmacological measures, Lamaze breathing, and other distractive techniques may alleviate the discomfort associated with first-stage labor. Periodic vaginal examinations by the nurse or other health care provider indicate a laboring woman's cervical dilation and effacement and descent of the fetus into the birth canal (a concept called **station**). In a full-term pregnancy, loss of the amniotic membrane usually increases pressure of the fetal head against the cervix, making dilation and effacement more efficient, and tends to augment the labor process.

During the **second stage of labor** the fetus descends through the lower birth canal toward the woman's perineum. It is the time elapsing from the full cervical dilation to the birth of the newborn. The upper uterine segment greatly thickens, and the abdominal muscles assist in the descent and expulsion of the fetus. Women who have attended childbirth classes are often better prepared to actively push the baby through the pelvis and perineum during contractions. Cultural practices may support pushing from a squatting or upright position and not in a supine one. Nurses must acknowledge that the maternity health care system has a unique culture that may clash with the cultures of many of our care recipients. For many women an overwhelming urge to bear down during uterine contractions occurs at this time. The fetal head accommodates to the mother's pelvis and vaginal structure and, finally, the head becomes flush with the vaginal opening on the woman's perineum. The woman at this point actively pushes to expel the newborn.

The **third stage of labor** begins after the birth of the newborn and lasts until placental expulsion. Placental separation usually occurs within 2 to 30 minutes after completion of the second stage. After delivery of the placenta the health care provider examines the placenta to determine that all placental tissue is intact and to detect any abnormalities that could affect the infant's condition and adaptation to extrauterine life.

The **fourth stage of labor** generally consists of the first 2 hours after childbirth, during which the mother faces the greatest risk of postpartum hemorrhage. An expected blood loss of 250 to 500 mL may cause the mother to experience a moderate decline in blood pressure, but nurses should not wait or rely on this change to intervene (Pavord & Maybury, 2015). The mother may also experience an increase in pulse rate (tachycardia) to compensate for blood loss during the early postpartum period. The care plan at the end of this chapter addresses the nurse's role in managing the stages of labor.

## Overview of Care

Professional members of the health care team (nurses, midwives, physicians) play an important role in labor and birth, but a woman's family, partner, or significant other (i.e., husband, friend, family) also inherently contributes to her care during labor and birth, particularly in certain cultures (see Table 16-1). Many practitioners suggest that the expectations and beliefs of a birthing couple have a great effect on how the woman fulfills the mothering role. Therefore the nurse needs to collaborate with the people who care for the pregnant woman to meet that family's needs during pregnancy, labor, and childbearing.

With increasing numbers of lesbian/gay/transgender couples getting married, and the availability of alternative methods of conception, these couples are coming in contact more with nurses and health care providers throughout the birthing process (preconception, pregnancy, and postpartum period). Nurses need to have a better understanding of their needs and ways to improve the overall experience for this population. Many challenges that lesbian, gay, bisexual, and transgender couples face include making complex childbearing decisions, navigating a health care system designed for heterosexual couples, and confronting barriers such as health insurance issues and uncertain legal rights. Changes in health care settings to address the needs of this population might include the need to display equality signs, use of gender-neutral language on medical records, in-service education for all health care personnel to confront any heterosexist bias, and discussion of privacy issues throughout the perinatal period (Ellis et al., 2015; Holley & Pasch, 2015).

The importance of the nurse's knowledge, caregiving, and support cannot be underestimated during the first stage of labor. Active emotional and physical nursing support decreases the length of many women's labors, use of analgesics and anesthetics, and number of operative deliveries and may help women reach their birthing goals (Sawant, 2015). Provided that they are accepted by a woman's culture, independent nursing interventions to increase comfort (e.g., giving backrubs or massages, offering ice or warm fluids by mouth, assisting with ambulation and position changes, and providing a clean and dry environment) may help the laboring woman cope with the challenges of labor. Many women will request medication to diminish the pain of labor and birth, and the nurse may need to review the options for medication with each woman or couple. During the first stage the mother must not bear down, because this may cause cervical swelling; often, active nursing support and distractive techniques, such as breathing and visual refocus, can prevent pushing before the second stage of labor. A woman may depend on the nurse to model breathing techniques to relieve labor discomfort. The nurse may need to explain usual interventions during this stage of labor, including the use of a **fetal heart monitor** (a machine that detects and records fetal heart rate and activity during labor), intravenous fluids, a digital blood pressure machine, and a urinary catheter. Open and clear communication among the health care providers and laboring woman and her significant others, particularly during frequent and difficult uterine contractions, will improve coping before the pushing stage begins.

Contemporary childbearing has benefited from many medical and technical advances, but the current high rate of maternity care interventions may bring about many disadvantages for the healthy majority. Current understanding suggests that safely avoiding unneeded interventions would be wise. Promoting and supporting physiological births, which are low-technology health and wellness approaches to childbearing, would yield better outcomes. Today, physiological childbearing refers to childbearing conforming to healthy biological processes. Evidence-based research reveals that physiological childbearing facilitates better outcomes by promoting fetal readiness for birth and safety during labor, enhances labor effectiveness, provides physiological help with labor stress and pain, promotes maternal and newborn transitions, and optimizes breastfeeding and maternal-infant attachment (Buckley, 2015). Selected physiological principles include limiting use of maternity care interventions, providing prenatal care that reduces stress and anxiety in women, fostering the physiological onset of labor, not artificial intervention, encouraging hospital admission in active labor, providing privacy and reducing anxiety in labor by continuous support, making nonpharmacological pain measures available, using pharmacological measures sparingly, fostering spontaneously vaginal births, and supporting continuous skin-to-skin contact between the mother and the newborn and early breastfeeding after birth (Lewitt, 2015).

During the second stage of labor the woman needs reassurance and support for her pushing efforts. Constant reinforcement and education by the nurse about labor progress, fetal heart monitor tracings, and other interventions will give the mother and her support system the guidance needed to give birth to the infant. Throughout labor the nurse considers the specific cultural and ethnic needs to support nursing assessment and positive responses to labor by the childbearing family.

Active nursing support during the third and fourth stages of labor includes observing the woman for excessive vaginal bleeding after the placenta has been expelled, assisting the woman in breastfeeding her new baby, monitoring vital signs, and implementing uterine massage if the uterus becomes boggy or fails to contract over the placental site. Emotional support during assessments and delivery of information to explain the rationale for assessments are also important nursing roles supported by professional practice standards.

Current hospital guidelines call for mother-baby dyad care on postpartum units. Nurses must therefore be competent in caring for both populations and be able to share a large amount of information in a short time (typically 1–3 days) to prepare mothers for discharge. Although teaching and support related to breastfeeding take priority, other topics nurses must address before discharge include bathing, car seat safety, jaundice, safe sleep, postpartum mood disorders, and nutrition for both the mother and the baby. Having a standard discharge checklist and pamphlets to give the mother to read will help nurses ensure a successful transition from the hospital to the home.

Throughout the entire labor and birth process, the nurse carefully observes the laboring woman and fetus so that she can detect early any difficulties with the progress of labor or with maternal or fetal health. Problems may include unusual fetal or uterine activity, the presence of meconium (fetal stool) in the amniotic fluid, fetal tachycardia (heart rate greater than 160 beats per minute) or fetal bradycardia (heart rate less than 110 beats per minute) in a full-term infant, and fetal heart rate decreases with uterine activity during labor (Mattson & Smith, 2015). These events must be reported immediately to the health care provider, with a complete oral and electronic description of the event. The nurse must be aware that abnormal fetal and maternal signs and patterns may be related to factors such as maternal diabetes or hypertension; the type, timing, or dosage of labor medications; uterine contraction pattern; maternal or fetal infections; maternal anemia; preeclampsia; the presence and character of amniotic fluid; bleeding in the pregnant woman or fetus; or early gestational age of the infant (Spong, 2015).

Our major role as nurses is to provide safe and evidence-based care to promote optimal birth outcomes for all women. Nurses need to remember there is more than one way to provide this care. Nurses are educated to assess every woman as an individual and to plan care with mutual goal setting for the best outcomes. By assisting all people seeking care from diverse cultures and by adopting our practices as much as possible to embrace the cultural traditions of others, we will enhance the childbearing experience and promote the health of women, newborns, and families.

## CHANGES DURING TRANSITION FROM FETUS TO NEWBORN

Most newborns experience a smooth transition from intrauterine to extrauterine life. The fetus to newborn transition is complex and depends on several factors, including maternal health and chronic medical conditions, the status of the placenta, gestational duration, the presence of fetal anomalies, and birthing room care. When difficulty occurs, however, the newborn's viability depends on the nurse's understanding of the fine balance of chemical, physiological, and anatomical changes that occurs as it makes the transition to postnatal life (Swanson & Sinkin, 2015).

### TABLE 16-3  Apgar Scoring

| SIGN | SCORE | | |
|---|---|---|---|
| | 0 | 1 | 2 |
| **Heart rate** | **Absent** | **Slow (<100)** | **>100** |
| Respiratory effort | Absent | Weak cry, hypoventilation | Good strong cry |
| Muscle tone | Flaccid, limp | Some flexion of extremities | Active motion, extremities well flexed |
| Reflex irritability | No response | Grimace | Cry |
| Color | Blue, pale | Body pink, extremities blue | Completely pink |

From Bier, D., Mann, J., Alpers, D. H., Vorster, E., & Gibney, M. J. (Eds). (2015). *Nutrition for the primary care provider.* Basel, Switzerland: Karger Medical and Scientific Publishers; Whitney, E. N., & Rolfes, S. R. (2015). *Understanding nutrition* (14th ed.). Boston, MA: Cengage Learning.

### Nursing Interventions

Nursing activities during this adaptation process include assessment and interventions aimed at specific protection of the infant and prevention of complications. Cold stress should be avoided by the newborn being kept dry and warmly wrapped and by avoidance of environments that cause heat loss. Overall, the nurse should minimally disturb, but maximally observe and document, the newborn's behavior during reactive periods.

### Apgar Score

Assessment of the newborn after the first few hours of life is essentially the same as assessment of the young infant (see Chapter 17). One technique, specific to timing after birth, is the Apgar scoring system. This scoring system has historically been used to provide a simple clinical measure to evaluate the newborn's general condition at birth. The Apgar score, obtained at 1 and 5 minutes of age, may be obtained again at 10 minutes of age until the infant's condition has stabilized. A total score is calculated by addition of the values allotted to the categories noted in Table 16-3. The highest possible score is 10. A score of 8 to 10 indicates that the baby is adapting well. The Apgar score does not predict the neurological development of an infant but may relate to the infant's risk of illness or death during the first year of life, which is important information for parents of an infant with a low Apgar score (Apgar, 2015).

### Sex

Sex differences occur in fetal growth. Generally, boys grow faster than girls in the third trimester, and at birth boys are slightly heavier, are longer, and have a larger head circumference than girls (Lissauer et al., 2015). Although more boys are conceived, they tend to be aborted spontaneously more often than girl embryos; the two X chromosomes possessed by female embryos may protect them from the early hazards of pregnancy. After birth, boys continue to have a lower survival rate than do girls (Stevenson et al., 2015).

## Race and Culture

Race may affect the health of the fetus in several ways. For example, in the United States, nonwhites (mainly blacks) have more fraternal twin pregnancies than whites (Cunningham et al., 2014). Because their organs are less mature, twin fetuses face an increased risk of **premature delivery** as a result of gestational factors in the mother. Currently the United States is 49th in the world ranking for **infant mortality rate (IMR)**, with a rate of 5.87 per 1000 live births (Central Intelligence Agency, 2015). This rate reflects the number of infants who die before the end of their first year of life and is the leading indicator of a nation's health. It reveals the higher IMRs and low-birth-weight outcomes of blacks, American Indians, and other ethnic minority populations in the United States. This rate illustrates the complex sociopolitical issues that produce birth outcomes in the United States and those needing attention to reduce the IMR (US Department of Health and Human Services [USDHHS], Office of Minority Health, 2015; CDC, 2015b).

Race is also a factor in the frequency of certain genetic and congenital malformations (Box 16-3: Genomics). For example, more babies of Native American, Latino, or Asian descent have cleft palates (an opening in the oral palate) than do black babies (Tewfik et al., 2015). Black babies have higher rates of sickle cell anemia (abnormally shaped red blood cells) than white babies. The total proportion of malformations tends to be approximately the same in all races that have been studied (whites, blacks, Hispanics, and Asians) (March of Dimes, 2015).

A woman's ethnic background may also influence the health of her fetus on the basis of a link to socioeconomic status. For increasing numbers of homeless pregnant women, income may support family survival needs but not prenatal care. Minority group pregnant women may have fewer economic resources to obtain a nutritious diet or early and consistent high-quality prenatal care. These outcomes may relate to access to health care factors or cultural beliefs that do not support recommended foods or prenatal care (Box 16-4: *Healthy People 2020*).

## Genetics

The science of genetics has expanded recently to genomics (the science that studies genes that make up the human genome). The completion of the mapping and sequencing of the human genome led to the expansion of research technologies that are now used to identify genetic and genomic factors that have an influence on people's health. Genetic influences affect the survival and later well-being of the child through several known mechanisms. **Down syndrome** (trisomy 21) remains the most recognized and most commonly occurring example of an extra chromosome. Extra chromosomes, deleted chromosomes, or translocations usually cause multiple malformations incompatible with life, causing early loss of the fetus via **spontaneous abortion**. Single malformations in an otherwise normal fetus (e.g., clubfoot, cleft palate, or NTD) probably result from a combined effect of many genes (March of Dimes, 2015). These defects, found at birth, may be surgically corrected or managed during the child's life. Invasive techniques of **amniocentesis**, chorionic villus sampling, and chromosome analysis have expanded genetic counseling

---

### BOX 16-3 GENOMICS
#### *Genetic Testing May Lead to Ethical Dilemmas*

Prenatal genetic testing provides important opportunities for assessment of genetic risk and diagnosis. However, some genetic tests do not identify all the possible gene mutations that can cause a particular condition, or they have limited predictive value. Because some genetic tests may not provide all the information that families may want, the test may subsequently require difficult decisions without providing full information. As an example, a cystic fibrosis carrier test can identify couples who are both carriers. When the cystic fibrosis mutations are identified in the parents, prenatal diagnosis can be performed to determine whether a fetus has inherited a cystic fibrosis gene mutation from each parent. Knowing that a fetus has inherited two cystic fibrosis mutations, however, does not, at this time, predict the severity of the disease in the infant. For couples in this situation, the ethical dilemma involves the decision to continue or to end a pregnancy without having knowledge of the severity of the disorder.

#### Should the Information Be Obtained if No Treatment or Intervention Exists?

Genetic testing can lead to specific treatments or interventions for some conditions but not for others. This is the case with some disorders that can be detected in expanded newborn screening. When phenylketonuria is identified, dietary intervention allows individuals with this condition to lead healthy and productive lives. Currently, however, not all conditions can be adequately treated. Genetic testing for some conditions for which there are no treatments might have the potential to cause psychological harm, stigmatization, and discrimination. Genetic testing for Huntington disease, a progressive motor and cognitive disorder with onset in midlife, is one example. There are no effective treatments or preventive measures currently available. Thus choosing to have genetic testing for Huntington disease is highly personal, and it is recommended that individuals consider extensive pretest counseling. These tests may lead to decisions that cannot be reversed and are based on a woman's best guess as to what would be the best course of action for her and her family. The dilemma that occurs then is whether a newborn should be tested for disorders that we cannot treat.

Ethical decision-making models/frameworks are valuable tools that can assist nurses in addressing ethical dilemmas. Principles of autonomy, informed consent, privacy/confidentiality, beneficence, nonmaleficence, and justice are applicable to use in the ethics involved in genetic testing. These principles should be sensitive to human needs, should be responsive to contextual considerations, and should emphasize the uniqueness of each situation.

- What might be the nurse's role in assisting the family in the decision-making process?
- What assurances can be made regarding privacy and confidentiality of the genetic information to prevent future employment or health insurance discrimination?
- What resources are available to nurses to keep current on prenatal genetic testing?

---

options and interventions for women facing possible fetal genetic defects. Nurses now will have to deal with the challenges of the explosion of genomic information to provide personalized health care based on genomics. The nurse, as a vital member of the health care team, needs to assist in informing these women and couples of genetic and high-risk screening resources when family history or other factors indicate that a fetal genetic defect may be likely.

**BOX 16-4** **HEALTHY PEOPLE 2020**

### Selected National Health-Promotion and Disease-Prevention Objectives for the Prenatal Period

- MICH-1.1: Reduce the rate of fetal deaths at 20 or more weeks of gestation to no more than 5.6 per 1000 live births. (Baseline: 6.2 per 1000 live births in 2005; target, 5.6 deaths per 1000 live births and fetal deaths in 2020—10% reduction.)
- MICH-1.2: Reduce the rate of fetal and infant deaths during the perinatal period (28 weeks of gestation to 7 days after birth) to no more than 5.9 per 1000 live births. (Baseline: 6.6 per 1000 live births in 2005—10% reduction.)
- MICH-1.4: Reduce the rate of neonatal deaths (within the first 28 days of life) to 4.1 per 1000 live births. (Baseline: 4.5 per 1000 live births in 2006—10% reduction.)
- MICH-5: Reduce the rate of maternal deaths to 11.4 maternal deaths per 100,000 live births. (Baseline: 12.7 per 100,000 live births in 2007—10% reduction.)
- MICH-6: Reduce the rate of maternal illness and complications due to pregnancy (complications during hospitalized labor and birth) to 28%. (Baseline: 31.1% of pregnant women experienced complications during hospitalized labor and delivery in 2007—10% reduction.)
- MICH-7.1: Reduce the rate of cesarean births among low-risk (full-term, singleton, vertex presentation) women to 23.9%. (Baseline: 26.5% of low-risk women giving birth for the first time had a cesarean birth in 2007—10% reduction.)
- MICH-8.1: Reduce the rate of low-birth-weight newborns to 7.8%. (Baseline: 8.2% of live births were low-birth-weight births in 2007.)
- MICH-8.2: Reduce the rate of very low-birth-weight newborns to 1.4%. (Baseline: 1.5% of live births were very low-birth-weight births in 2007.)
- MICH-9.1: Reduce the rate of total preterm births to 11.4%. (Baseline: 12.7% of live births were preterm births in 2007—10% reduction.)
- MICH-9.2: Reduce the rate of late preterm births or live births at 34 to 36 weeks of gestation to 8.1%. (Baseline: 9.0% of live births were late preterm births or occurred at 34 to 36 weeks of gestation in 2007—10% reduction.)
- MICH-10.2: Increase the proportion of pregnant women who receive early and adequate prenatal care to 77.6%. (Baseline: 70.5% of pregnant women received early and adequate prenatal care in 2007—10% increase.)
- MICH-11: Increase abstinence from alcohol, cigarettes, and illicit drugs among pregnant women to 98.3% for alcohol, 98.6% for cigarette smoking, and 100% for illicit drugs. (Baselines: 89.4% of pregnant females aged 15 to 44 years reported abstaining from alcohol in the previous 30 days in 2007–08; 89.6% of females delivering a live birth reported abstaining from smoking cigarettes during pregnancy in 2007; and 94.8% of pregnant females aged 15 to 44 years reported abstaining from illicit drugs in the previous 30 days in 2007–08—10% increase.)
- MICH-14: Increase the proportion of women of childbirth potential with intake of at least 400 mcg of folic acid from fortified foods or dietary supplements to 26.2%. (Baseline: 23.8% of nonpregnant females aged 15 to 44 years reported a usual daily total intake of at least 400 mcg of folic acid from fortified foods or dietary supplements in 2003–06—10% increase.)
- MICH-16: Increase the proportion of women delivering a live birth who received preconception care services and practiced key recommended preconception health behaviors to following values: 33.1% for taking vitamins prenatally; 85.4% for not smoking cigarettes before pregnancy; 56.4% for not drinking alcohol before pregnancy; and 53.4% for maintaining a healthy weight before pregnancy. (Baselines: 30.1% of women delivering a recent live birth took multivitamins/folic acid every day in the month before pregnancy as reported in 2007; 77.6% of women delivering a recent live birth did not smoke in the 3 months before pregnancy as reported in 2007; 51.3% of women delivering a recent live birth did not drink alcohol in the 3 months before pregnancy as reported in 2007; and 48.5% of women delivering a recent live birth had a normal weight [i.e., a BMI of 18.5–24.9 $g/m^2$] before pregnancy as reported in 2007—10% increase.)

## GORDON'S FUNCTIONAL HEALTH PATTERNS

Box 16-5 provides an example of a pregnancy assessment using Gordon's (2016) functional health patterns.

### Health Perception–Health Management Pattern

On the basis of her culture and life experience, a woman may view pregnancy as an illness, as a completely natural and healthy state, or as a combination of the two. This perception will influence her view of her changing body, her attitude toward the usual discomforts of pregnancy such as fatigue or backache, her choice of health-oriented or illness-oriented care, and her decision to seek prenatal care. The woman who sees herself as healthy and pregnancy as a normal part of her life most likely will seek a health care provider with a similar outlook. Another woman with the same perception may seek help from a socially approved group, as defined by her culture, and avoid standard Western medicine during pregnancy (e.g., Roma [gypsies]). Generally, women with a positive view of pregnancy will continue with active participation in their respective social circles and careers. However, the woman who sees her pregnancy as a time of illness may use this as a reason to withdraw from her work and social obligations.

A woman's acceptance of her pregnancy influences her health-management practices and choices. The woman who denies or has strong negative feelings about her pregnancy may fail to eat properly, get enough rest and exercise, breastfeed, or seek prenatal care. A woman may deny a pregnancy because she never intended to become pregnant despite having sexual intercourse without birth control. Approximately 50% of American pregnancies are unintended, particularly among vulnerable aggregates such as adolescents, women older than 40 years, women with low income, and women who lack health care access, cultural acceptance, and education, experience sexual violence, and lack financial resources to purchase or use contraceptives. A decrease in the unintended pregnancy rate by 30% was promoted as one of the first *Healthy People* goals in 2000, but has been changed to a more modest 7% reduction rate in *Healthy People 2020* (Hewitt & Cappiello, 2015; USDHHS, 2010). These women, faced with an unplanned or a closely spaced pregnancy, may expose a fetus to alcohol, tobacco, and **sexually transmitted infections** (STIs), abuse a child who was never wanted, or fail to obtain follow-up care

## BOX 16-5  Assessment for Pregnancy According to Gordon's Functional Health Patterns

*Health perception–health management pattern:* Aware of or participates in management of pregnancy, or both; expects an uncomplicated pregnancy on the basis of the woman's or significant other's active involvement in her own care; able to state complications of pregnancy that mandate physician notification; engages in health-promotion behaviors specific to pregnancy.

*Nutritional-metabolic pattern:* Follows diet changes of pregnancy as recommended by nurse; has appropriate weight for height and has gained adequate weight for gestational age of pregnancy; eats three meals a day and two snacks (afternoon and evening), focusing on increased amounts of vegetables and fruits; drinks healthy fluids, including at least eight glasses of water per day; has elastic skin turgor.

*Elimination pattern:* Experiences occasional constipation from progesterone influence of gastrointestinal peristalsis relaxation, usually corrected by increased fluids, nightly walking, and more diet roughage; voids 7 to 10 times a day, depending on amount of fluids consumed; no known hemorrhoids or difficulty in elimination; voiding without excess frequency, urgency, or burning; understands signs of UTI.

*Activity-exercise pattern:* Walks three times a week for 20 minutes without reports of unusual fatigue or soreness; active at home with housework and at work teaching in a primary school; swam two times a week before pregnancy and moved to current residence.

*Sleep-rest pattern:* Generally, sleeps 7 to 8 hours a night; has increased total daily sleep somewhat with fatigue of pregnancy—naps for 1 hour on weekends and 30 minutes after work; sleeps on side and with two pillows for comfort; uses no sleep aids; generally able to relax and initiate sleep without difficulty; occasionally has headache at end of workday and takes acetaminophen (Tylenol) for relief or listens to soft music after work to enhance relaxation.

*Cognitive-perceptual pattern:* Realizes the need to decrease work activity and increase rest periods as she nears end of pregnancy; answers questions in appropriate tone and words during pregnancy visits; has intact memory (alert and remote); reads about pregnancy and early parenthood to prepare for the birth.

*Self-perception–self-concept pattern:* States she is excited about pregnancy after 1 year of trying to conceive; well groomed, wears maternity clothes because "I want to"; believes she looks "nice" because of pregnancy.

*Roles-relationships pattern:* Lives with husband of 3 years; visits extended family, 60 miles away, every month; shares family roles with husband, accepts this balance; has many friends who support her pregnancy; perceives extensive employee and employer support with pregnancy and time off after delivery.

*Sexuality-reproductive pattern:* States, "I have a satisfying love life and enjoy my husband"; before pregnancy, engaged in sexual intercourse four to five times a week with desire to become pregnant; with pregnancy and fatigue, has intercourse generally two to three times a week, with pattern acceptable to both partners; no known STIs in past or present.

*Coping–stress tolerance pattern:* Concerned about fatigue affecting performance as primary school teacher; walks three times a week for 20 minutes to "center myself and feel good"; smiles often, good sense of humor; supportive family excited about her pregnancy.

*Values-beliefs pattern:* Protestant religion; prays daily and gains strength from religion.

*Other data:*
- Medication history:
  Prenatal vitamin, one tablet each morning
  Ferrous sulfate, one tablet each morning
  Acetaminophen (Tylenol) 650 mg for occasional headaches
- Physical examination:
  5 feet, 4 inches tall
  Weight 140 lb (at 14 weeks of pregnancy; weight gain of 5 lb with pregnancy)
  29 years of age
  Pupils equally round and reactive to light and accommodation
  Temperature 98.2°F; pulse 76 beats per minute; respiration 16 breaths per minute
  Blood pressure 114/78 mmHg right arm (sitting, left arm)
  Peripheral pulses equal, strong bilaterally
  Skin warm, dry, elastic turgor; mucous membranes intact, moist; alert, oriented

Modified from Gordon, M. (2010). *Manual of nursing diagnosis* (12th ed.). Sudbury, MA: Jones & Bartlett Learning; Peterson, R. (2012). *Clinical companion for fundamentals of nursing* (8th ed.). St. Louis: Mosby.

for a high-risk child (i.e., experienced complications from childbirth) (USDHHS, 2010; US Preventive Services Task Force, 2015a).

Nurses encounter women with reproductive health needs and concerns in all practice settings and play an important role in caring for them as an integral member of the health care team. The nurse who works with a pregnant population must be sensitive to a wide range of views expressed by these women and work with each to effectively manage their pregnancies. For example, Hispanic women are less likely to receive early prenatal care because of a belief that pregnancy is not an illness. The nurse targets interventions that focus on this group's needs and beliefs while adhering to professional practice standards that will improve their outcomes.

## Nutritional-Metabolic Pattern

A woman's nutritional status should be assessed preconceptually with the goal of optimizing maternal and fetal health.

Pregnancy-related dietary changes should begin before conception, with needed modifications during pregnancy and lactation. Most nutritional requirements of pregnant and lactating women can be met by their consuming a variety of foods according to government-endorsed guidelines. Massive amounts of literature support the importance of optimal nutrition during pregnancy for maternal and fetal well-being. The key components of nutritional management during pregnancy include consumption of a variety of foods, appropriate weight gain, appropriate micronutrient supplementation, physical activity, and avoidance of alcohol, tobacco, and other harmful substances. Maternal malnutrition before and during pregnancy may exert a teratogenic effect on the fetus. A **teratogen** is an agent that causes either a functional or a structural disability in the organism as a result of exposure to that agent (Merriam-Webster, 2015). Teratogens principally affect the central nervous system of the fetus, leading to impaired intelligence and performance later in life. They are discussed more in the Environmental Processes section later in the chapter.

Various factors influence the quality of nutrition needed for positive fetal development and birth outcome. Fetal development suffers in cases of adolescent pregnancy or in pregnancies of older women who experience poor nutrition between and during several pregnancies. Maternal nutritional deficiencies during a woman's own fetal, infant, and childhood periods also contribute to the development of structural and physiological disadvantages to supporting a growing fetus. For example, women who are severely underweight before pregnancy often experience higher rates of low-birth-weight infants and preterm labor than do women of appropriate prepregnant weight (Cunningham et al., 2014). Inherited maternal stature and pelvic development may influence pregnancy and efficiency of labor and delivery. A lack of income to buy healthy food may also exist, and sometimes cultural values related to food intake influence the quality of nutrition during pregnancy.

To meet increased metabolic, energy, and structural needs for pregnancy, most nutritionists recommend that a pregnant woman increase her intake by approximately 300 calories each day (USDHHS, 2010). This results in a total weight gain of approximately 25 to 35 pounds (Figure 16-3). If at the end of 20 weeks of gestation the woman has not gained at least 10 pounds, she risks delivering an ill infant with fetal growth restriction. This risk also exists when a woman continues to gain insufficient weight throughout the pregnancy or in a woman who was underweight or overweight before pregnancy. Although the rate of gain and the total gain during pregnancy differ among women, a correlation exists between an erratic pattern of weight gain or a too-rapid weight gain and a lack of fetal well-being (Bier et al., 2015). The nurse advises the pregnant woman to eat a well-balanced diet.

A well-balanced diet for a pregnant woman parallels that needed by all human beings, with increases in the amounts of certain components as recommended by the Food and Nutrition Board of the National Academy of Science (IOM, 2015; USDHHS, 2010). The nurse recommends that the entire family eat a healthy diet. The nurse encourages the pregnant woman to drink 8 to 10 glasses of water per day to develop amniotic fluid and prevent urinary tract infections (UTIs) often seen with pregnancy. The nurse may also need to encourage the woman to modify her diet to include more fiber and roughage to avoid constipation during pregnancy (Table 16-4).

Protein requirements during pregnancy increase to approximately 70 g per day, or a daily increase of 25 g above normal (Whitney & Rolfes, 2015). This ensures an adequate supply of amino acids for fetal growth and development, blood volume expansion, and maternal tissue growth. Other protein sources, such as cheese, cream soups, puddings, tofu, and yogurt, may

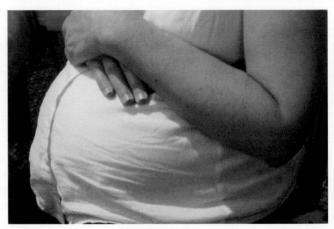

**FIGURE 16-3** Many practitioners recommend a weight gain of 25 to 35 pounds for women at normal weight for their height.

## TABLE 16-4 Nutritional Needs for Pregnant and Lactating Women

| Nutrient | Pregnancy | Lactation | Sources | Comments |
|---|---|---|---|---|
| Calories | +300 | +500 | Eat a variety from all food groups | Begin to increase calories in second and third trimesters |
| Protein | 70 g | 70 g | Lean meat, fish, eggs, poultry, milk, and dairy products | Supports fetal growth and development; formation of placenta and amniotic fluid; and expanded blood volume |
| Calcium | 1000 mg/day | 1000 mg/day | Milk, cheese, dark green leafy vegetables, nuts, and dried fruit | Women with low calcium intake require calcium supplements with vitamin D |
| Iron | 27 mg/day | 9 mg/day | Lean meats, dark green leafy vegetables, eggs, whole grain, dried fruit, and shellfish | Provides iron for fetal liver storage, which sustains infant for first 4–6 months of life |
| Folic acid | 600 mcg | 500 mcg | Fresh green leafy vegetables, liver, peanuts, whole-grain breads, and cereals | All women of childbearing age should take 400 mcg of folic acid daily to prevent neural tube defects in first trimester |
| Fats | 30% of daily calories | 30% of daily calories | Low-fat dairy products and lean cuts of meat | Provide a valuable source of energy for the body during pregnancy |
| Carbohydrates | 7–11 servings daily | 7–11 servings daily | Dairy products, fruits, vegetables, whole-grain cereals, and breads | Provide fiber necessary for proper bowel functioning. Carbohydrate intake needs to be sufficient to prevent ketoacidosis from protein use for energy |

From Thompson, J., & Manore, M. (2012). *Nutrition: An applied approach* (3rd ed.). San Francisco: Benjamin Cummings.

be better tolerated by some women and by those from cultures (Hispanic) that do not drink milk. Animal protein and less expensive legume sources provide protein and, if combined with other healthy food sources, provide high-quality meals (e.g., tuna and rice, peanut butter, and whole-wheat bread). Protein foods cost more than other foods; therefore the nurse may need to teach pregnant couples about economical ways to meet protein needs for fetal development.

Mineral intake must also increase during pregnancy. Increased protein intake usually provides the extra needed essential minerals, particularly phosphorus and calcium. The rapid deposit of calcium in fetal bones and teeth during the third trimester of pregnancy requires adequate maternal calcium stores from early pregnancy and continued calcium intake to prevent maternal bone demineralization. Other calcium sources include green, leafy vegetables and calcium-fortified foods, sources more acceptable to cultures with a history of lactose intolerance (African, Mexican, and some European groups).

Sufficient iodine intake by pregnant and lactating women is crucial for thyroid hormone production, which contributes to the offspring's neurocognitive development. Approximately one-third of pregnant women are marginally deficient in iodine. The American Academy of Pediatrics calls for pregnant and lactating women to use iodized salt and take a supplement of 150 mcg of iodine daily, which typically is not contained in prenatal vitamins. As processed and convenient foods make up a large portion of American diets today, women need to be informed that the salt used in them is not iodized (American Academy of Pediatrics, 2014).

A woman who eats a well-balanced diet should gain sufficient vitamins and minerals for maternal and fetal needs during pregnancy. However, most health care providers recommend that the pregnant woman include 30 mg of elemental iron daily to benefit both herself and the fetus, particularly during the last trimester. **Anemia of pregnancy** is a global health problem affecting nearly half of all pregnant women worldwide. High fetal demands for iron, increased erythrocyte mass, and in the third trimester, expanded maternal blood volume render iron deficiency the most common cause of anemia of pregnancy. In certain geographical populations, human pathogens such as hookworm, malarial parasite, and HIV are important factors contributing to anemia of pregnancy. The hemoglobinopathies—sickle cell disease and thalassemia—represent diverse causes of anemia of pregnancy, requiring specialized care. Iron-deficiency anemia is common among pregnant women, and anemia contributes to hemorrhage, postpartum infection, and **preterm birth**. Anemia occurs more often among pregnant adolescent, black, and older white women (Cantor et al., 2015).

There are almost universal recommendations for periconceptual folic acid supplementation to prevent NTDs. NTDs are congenital malformations that include anencephaly, encephalocele, and spina bifida caused by the failure of fusion of the neural tube, which normally closes between the 22nd and 28th days after conception (at an average of 40–42 days after the first day of the last menstrual period). The occurrence of NTDs differs among the population, ranging between 0.8 per 1000 births and 3 per 1000 births, and it is estimated that more than 300,000 pregnancies are affected every year worldwide. According to the World Health Organization (WHO), increased consumption of folic acid can decrease the risk of NTD to 0.6 per 1000 births (Cordero et al., 2015). To decrease the risk of NTD, it is recommended that all women capable of becoming pregnant should consume more folic acid. The goal is that every woman could start her pregnancy with an optimal folate status. Evidence-based research thus supports that women planning pregnancy and those in their first trimester take 0.4 mg of folic acid in a daily multivitamin supplement to prevent NTDs and anemia. This is particularly important for women with multiple gestations, who experience a greater risk of anemia. However, research has shown that only 25% of women of childbearing age consume the recommended amount of folic acid, which is critical for early fetal development (USDHHS, 2010).

Fats and carbohydrates must supply the caloric requirements during pregnancy. Although increased protein intake provides more calories, the body-building requirements of pregnancy and fetal growth demand most of the added protein. Fats and carbohydrates remain the most important sources of energy and essential vitamins and minerals. Supplemental vitamins and minerals, although not known to cause maternal or fetal harm if taken in reasonable doses, probably cost the pregnant woman more to meet the nutritional needs of pregnancy than does a well-balanced diet.

The practice of **pica**, a psychobehavioral disorder characterized by the ingestion of nonfood substances such as dirt, clay, laundry starch, ashes, plaster, raw rice, paint chips, coffee grounds, and ice, may negatively influence the quality of a pregnant woman's nutrition during pregnancy. No one knows what causes these cravings, but a combination of biochemical, psychological, and cultural factors may be at work. Pica in humans can be classified by the type of ingested substance. The three main substances consumed by pregnant women are soil or clay (geophagia), ice (pagophagia), and laundry or corn starch (amylophagia). Other pica cravings include burned matches, stones, charcoal, mothballs, soap, sand, plaster, coffee grounds, baking soda, paint chips, and glue (Jyothi, 2015). Common in rural pregnant black women, this practice may contribute to iron-deficiency anemia and interfere with nutrient absorption, particularly among women of lower economic status. Other potential complications may include lead poisoning, fecal impaction, gastrointestinal reflux, parasitic infections, prematurity, perinatal death, low-birth-weight infants, and anemia in the infant (Miao et al., 2015). Pica is often practiced by black American women, usually in the rural southern United States. It is thought to occur as a result of an iron deficiency that leads to the craving and/or a carryover from behaviors practiced in Africa (Mattson & Smith, 2015). The nurse completes a nutritional assessment on any pregnant woman. The nurse identifies instances of pica and suggests a culturally sensitive diet that will better meet the needs of the woman and her developing fetus. It is essential that the nurse remain nonjudgmental but stress the importance of an adequate diet, folic acid, iodine, and iron supplements, and the dangers of pica.

The best time to teach a woman about prenatal nutrition is before she becomes pregnant. Most women do not seek prenatal care until they suspect pregnancy. Therefore the nurse often delivers information about optimal nutrition to the pregnant woman after critical fetal development has already begun. If all schoolchildren received nutrition information as part of their kindergarten through 12th grade curriculum (a primary prevention approach), women might have better overall personal nutrition established through lifestyle practices of individuals and families that would support high-quality prenatal nutrition later in their lives. Without such a primary prevention approach, secondary prevention intervention during pregnancy occurs through laboratory monitoring of iron levels, assessment of the woman's feelings of well-being, determination of the woman's actual intake of essential nutrients, and assessment of her pattern and total weight gain during the pregnancy. Many pregnant women work outside the home and may be among the increasing numbers of American families who spend 40% of their food budgets on food eaten outside the home (USDHHS, 2010). The nurse alerts the pregnant woman and her family to the documented high amounts of cholesterol, calories, sodium, and fat and low amounts of iron and calcium that these foods contain so as to improve nutritional intake during pregnancy.

In June 2011, the US Department of Agriculture (USDA) unveiled a new food icon, MyPlate, which replaces MyPyramid as the government's primary food group symbol. MyPlate is meant to serve as a simple guide to help consumers choose healthful foods. To build a "healthy plate," MyPlate suggests that consumers choose fruits, vegetables, whole grains, low-fat dairy products, and lean protein foods to get essential nutrients without excess calories. The strategies for creating such a plate include filling half your plate with fruits and vegetables, using whole grains for at least half of your daily grains consumed (e.g., 100% whole-grain cereals, breads, and pasta), switching from whole milk to skim or 1% milk, and choosing a variety of protein sources (e.g., seafood, small portions of lean meat and poultry, and beans). It also recommends that women should avoid shark, swordfish, king mackerel, or tilefish when they are pregnant or breastfeeding. These fish contain high levels of mercury and should be avoided. In summary, the pregnant woman needs to follow the USDA Daily Food Plans for Moms as follows:

- Fruits and vegetables—seven or more servings daily (three servings of fruit and four of vegetables)
- Whole-grain or enriched breads/cereals—six to nine servings daily
- Dairy products—three to four servings of low-fat or nonfat milk, yogurt, or cheese daily
- Meat and beans—three servings daily (one serving is equivalent to 2 ounces) (USDA, 2015).

See Chapter 11 for more information on nutrition, including MyPlate.

## Elimination Pattern

### Fetus

The fetus accomplishes all essential elimination functions through the placenta. Carbon dioxide, water, urea, and other waste products pass through the placenta, to be eliminated by the mother's body. By the end of the first trimester, the fetus swallows, makes respiratory movements, and urinates. However, these abilities become truly functional only after birth.

### Pregnant Woman

The pregnant woman experiences changes in her elimination pattern because of the enlarging uterus and hormonal influences. These changes (urinary frequency during the first and third trimesters, constipation, and hemorrhoids) cause normal, minor discomforts. Anticipatory guidance by the nurse helps the pregnant woman cope with these changes and prevent complications of pregnancy. For example, teaching the pregnant woman commonsense measures (Box 16-6: Innovative Practice) may prevent UTIs, typically a problem that is more common during pregnancy. With a known correlation between UTIs and premature labor, a focus on preventing and managing these infections must occur during pregnancy.

---

### ☀ BOX 16-6 INNOVATIVE PRACTICE

**Evidence-Based Practice for Preventing Urinary Tract Infections and Promoting Genitourinary Health**

- Increase fluid intake to approximately 8 to 10 glasses per day; plain water is best to flush the body's systems of potential toxins; drink a glass of water before sexual intercourse to allow urinary output afterward to prevent UTIs.
- Avoid bladder irritants such as caffeine products, alcohol, artificial sweeteners, spicy foods, and carbonated beverages.
- Make urination a regular habit; avoid waiting to urinate until bladder is full.
- Urinate before and after sexual intercourse to cleanse the urethra and empty the bladder.
- Be aware that vigorous or frequent intercourse may contribute to increased risk of UTIs.
- Maintain consistently good perineal hygiene, including wiping from front to back after urination and defecation.
- Take all prescription medications given for UTIs, even when the symptoms of the infection have been alleviated.
- Drink cranberry juice to acidify the urine or take cranberry pills; these products may relieve some of the symptoms of a UTI. Cranberry *(Vaccinium macrocarpon)* has demonstrated antiinflammatory, antiadhesive, and antioxidant properties.
- Seek health care advice for a vaginal infection, which may contribute to development of a UTI.
- Nurses need to be aware that most UTIs are caused by *Escherichia coli*, and most women may be asymptomatic. Obtaining a urine specimen and culture is needed with any degree of suspicion of a UTI.
- Approximately half of UTIs in pregnancy occur in women with preexisting asymptomatic bacteriuria, and these UTIs have poor outcomes, including preterm rupture of membranes, preterm birth, neonatal infection, preeclampsia, maternal anemia, amnionitis, and maternal septic shock.
- The nurse should assess the woman for increased risk of developing a UTI: congenital or structural abnormalities of the genitourinary system, previous surgery to the genitourinary system; pregnancy; previous UTIs; high intake of carbonated beverages; and poor intake of water.

From Matuszkiewicz-Rowińska, J., Małyszko, J., & Wieliczko, M. (2015). Urinary tract infections in pregnancy: Old and new unresolved diagnostic and therapeutic problems. *Archives of Medical Science, 11*(1), 67–77; Sheerin, N. S. (2015). Urinary tract infection. *Medicine, 43*(8), 435–439.

## Activity-Exercise Pattern

### Fetus

Early spontaneous movements of the fetus may be reflexive, stimulated by passive uterine movement. Ultrasonographic observation of fetal movement shows repetitive movements early in pregnancy; at approximately 16 weeks, the pregnant woman feels these movements, termed **quickening**. By the end of the second trimester, fetal movement occurs less frequently because of lack of space in the uterus. The woman and her partner look forward to the regular daily cycle of movements, indicators of fetal well-being. An absence of or a dramatic increase in fetal movements for more than 8 hours may indicate fetal distress. The nurse routinely teaches a pregnant woman to count the number of fetal movements each day typically starting at 28 weeks' gestation and report any decrease in fetal activity to the health care provider.

### Pregnant Woman

The physical changes during pregnancy and the rigors of labor and delivery require that a pregnant woman be in the best physical condition of her life. Fortunately, many pregnant women view pregnancy as a normal, natural state, and they often participate actively in physical activities or sports enjoyed before pregnancy. Generally, a woman should avoid high-risk sports, such as sky diving and high-altitude climbing, because these could cause trauma to the fetus from low oxygen pressure or a maternal fall. Nurses encourage each woman to choose activities on the basis of her interests, comfort, and good judgment. When a sport or activity causes exhaustion or pain, it should be modified or discontinued. Later in pregnancy the woman should be encouraged to choose safe physical activities because of changes in her center of gravity attributable to the enlarging uterus and in the musculoskeletal system.

The woman with a sedentary lifestyle before pregnancy should slowly increase her activity level during pregnancy. A daily swim or 30-minute walk provides a good introduction to a regular exercise program. Regular exercise contributes to joint flexibility, increased cardiovascular and gastrointestinal fitness, decreased uterine tone for an efficient labor, fewer pregnancy discomforts, weight control and a lower risk of diabetes by maintaining glycemic control, and overall feelings of well-being in the pregnant woman (USDHHS, 2010). For the self-directed woman, prenatal classes or a consumer-oriented book of prenatal exercises will facilitate an adequate exercise program. For most women, group exercise with other pregnant women is more enjoyable than exercising alone. The benefits of physical activity in the general population are established, and research suggests regular physical activity following childbirth is linked to improved health outcomes. However, many women do not resume pre-pregnancy exercise levels. The nurse encourages women to enter a structured diet and exercise program sponsored by the birthing hospital to help women lose weight after childbirth (Spencer et al., 2015).

In an uncomplicated pregnancy, a couple may continue their usual sexual activity. However, threatened abortion or a history of abortion in the first trimester, early rupture of membranes, and other complications may call for restrictions on sexual intercourse or orgasm.

## Sleep-Rest Pattern

### Fetus

Electroencephalographic studies have shown four cyclical states of activity in the fetus: complete wakefulness, drowsy wakefulness, rapid eye movement sleep, and quiet sleep. Evidence suggests that a diurnal (day-night) pattern exists during the fetal period. Sleep is required for somatic and brain growth and development. Sleep-wake patterns change with central nervous system maturation. In one research study the median relative percentage of time spent in a quiet state was 26%. The median duration of time spent in a quiet state was 15.7 minutes within a 1-hour recording. Both quiet states and active states were established in 84% of the fetuses studied (Piontelli et al., 2015). Infant development entails increasing amounts of quiet sleep as well as increasing periods of quiet alertness. Both states require remarkable neural organization; thus sleep-wake patterns are an excellent window to the infant's neurological status.

### Pregnant Woman

Fatigue reflects the significant physical and emotional changes occurring in the pregnant woman. The nurse counsels a woman that fatigue usually subsides by the fourth month but may return later in pregnancy. Rest breaks during the day and 8 hours of sleep each night help prevent fatigue and increase the pregnant woman's comfort. The nurse encourages each pregnant woman to rest when her body signals it is tired because of the rapidly growing fetus and the woman's needs for physical renewal. This encouragement must be directed particularly toward working women, who may need a physician's note for their employer that validates the need for rest during the workday.

Women experience significant sleep disruption and inadequate sleep throughout pregnancy. Many pregnant women do not sleep well because they need to urinate several times a night during the first and third trimesters. In addition, some women experience positional discomfort in late pregnancy that prevents effective sleep and, therefore, increases their fatigue. Fatigue may influence a woman's evaluation of her role as a pregnant woman, her body changes, and her cultural beliefs related to her ability to succeed in pregnancy. The nurse helps the woman express her thoughts and feelings and find ways to support better sleep and rest patterns (e.g., sleeping upright in a chair at night for easier breathing).

## Cognitive-Perceptual Pattern

### Fetus

During the prenatal period, although motor functions lag behind, all fetal sensory systems function or nearly function. These systems include vision, hearing, taste, smell, touch, and proprioceptive and vestibular senses (Blackburn, 2014). The fetus with all senses intact experiences the discomfort of pregnancy and the pain of labor contractions. The visual system matures relatively late in gestation, especially compared with the tactile, olfactory, and auditory systems. Although capable of seeing by 30 weeks of age, the fetus has little opportunity to use this ability in utero because of the absence of light (Blackburn, 2014). After approximately 25 weeks, pregnant women note that their babies respond to a loud, sudden noise. Some pregnant women and their partners offer sensory stimulation to the fetus by singing or rubbing the woman's abdomen. This parental behavior may assist in the bonding process between the parent and the baby. Thus the nurse may wish to include this kind of information in prenatal teaching sessions.

## Pregnant Woman

Physical and psychological processes remain closely intertwined as pregnancy progresses. Psychological stresses and normal emotional growth affect the physical status of the pregnancy, interactions of the family members, and the eventual relationship between the mother and the infant. When considering the emotional aspects of pregnancy, the nurse recognizes that the woman's personality, environment, physical state, family, and sociocultural and spiritual background affect the ways in which she handles the psychological changes (Figure 16-4).

Two major categories of psychological influences are normal psychological growth required of parents to emotionally and physically prepare them for parenthood, and internal or external stressors on the pregnant woman that decrease her ability to provide the best environment for the developing fetus. The pregnant woman undergoes many cognitive changes that ultimately result in her psychological readiness for motherhood.

*Emotional changes.* Hormonal and other physical changes assist the woman in the psychological work of pregnancy. Progesterone level increases affect the woman's general mood, causing her to be more introverted and passive. These mood changes help her to focus her energy on the growing child and her own growth and development. In addition to hormonal changes, the presence, growth, and movements of the fetus become more a part of the woman's experiential self. According to Rubin (1984), the classic researcher on maternal-infant bonding, the pregnant woman receives immediate sensations of touch, motion, and weight from the fetus that she can share only partially with others. These support a maternal feeling of separateness and

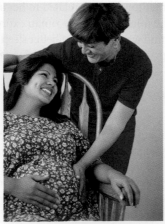

**FIGURE 16-4** The pregnant woman enjoys time with her family while pregnant.

uniqueness that causes the woman to turn inward. She frequently worries that the shift in energy away from the world toward herself and her child may cause her to lose contact, drift away from valued relationships, and lose feelings of competence in her areas of achievement. She spends time analyzing her experiences and their possible influence on her effectiveness as a future parent. She constantly studies the qualities of human relationships and shows increased sensitivity and perceptiveness to many people. To others, the woman may seem overly sensitive and analytical during pregnancy (Stockwell, 2015).

Although a woman's mood varies on the basis of a variety of factors and at different times during the pregnancy, many women experience wide mood swings, emotional lability, irritability, and changes in sexual desire. Physical discomforts, hormonal changes, feelings about altered body image, cultural considerations, work and relationship adjustments, and demanding cognitive maturational processes may also cause these emotional changes.

Rubin's classic work stimulated nurses to look beyond the physiological and pathological aspects of childbearing to the intricate process of becoming a mother, and to identify areas for providing help. Current research identifies two simultaneous processes in the transition to motherhood: engagement and growth and transformation. Engagement is making a commitment and being engrossed in mothering through active involvement in the child's care. At the same time, the woman's engagement leads to the woman's growth and transition as she becomes a mother. The bond between a mother and her newborn is one of strength, power, and potential (Hughes, 2015).

Current descriptions for the stages in the process of establishing a maternal identity in becoming a mother include the following:

- Commitment, attachment, and preparation for the pregnancy
- Acquaintance, learning, and physical restoration during the first 6 weeks after birth
- Moving toward a new normal from 2 weeks to 4 months

Nurses can promote the maternal-newborn bond through encouraging skin-to-skin contact, breastfeeding, eye contact, and newborn massage during the first hour after childbirth.

*Stressors influencing development.* The mother's age, fears related to a previous fetal loss, feelings about the pregnancy, life situation and culture, degree of stress, loss of control at times, and unintended pregnancy, the presence of other children, and the influence of loved ones may serve as stressors that influence the ways in which the mother completes the developmental tasks of motherhood. Women with unwanted pregnancies have multiple risk factors and would benefit from targeted interventions (Hall et al., 2015; Mori, 2015). A young pregnant woman facing the additional developmental task of adolescence may have difficulty incorporating the pregnant body or the role of mother into her still undefined self-image. Cognitively, she may still be unable to make plans for the baby or even accept the pregnancy until she feels the baby move. Anticipatory guidance is critical when an adolescent faces overlapping developmental challenges of age and pregnancy.

On the other hand, a pregnant woman older than 35 years may feel more isolated by her situation than does the pregnant woman in her 20s. Frequently established in career and family, the older pregnant woman needs to learn to balance her growth and development in these valued areas with her new sense of self. Fears related to being considered at high risk because of age may increase her anxiety and ambivalence about the pregnancy, even if she was previously infertile. As a first-time mother, she may worry about managing the physical demands of labor and delivery, sleeplessness of motherhood, the chances of having an abnormal child, and the need to juggle conflicting life responsibilities and relationships.

A woman with other children moves through the developmental tasks differently from a woman who is pregnant for the first time. Even with a desired pregnancy, the woman may worry about incorporating the new infant into her relationships and managing the time needed for a new baby. She may have fears and anxieties about labor and delivery because of a previous negative experience. She may be much more aware of the problems involved with caring for a new infant and may not be excited about another pregnancy experience that demands a redefinition of motherhood or additional childrearing expenses.

## Developmental Tasks

Rubin (1967, 1977, 1984) describes four major developmental tasks that a woman seeks to accomplish as she learns to become a mother. These include ensuring safe passage through pregnancy and childbirth, ensuring acceptance of the child by significant people in her family, binding to her unknown child, and learning to give of self. According to Rubin, all four tasks must be confronted simultaneously, but each task assumes greater priority at certain times than do other tasks. Each woman works through these tasks on the basis of her unique style, cultural values, and life priorities. At the end of pregnancy, however, all tasks must be integrated to create a presentation, similar to a tapestry (Rubin, 1984).

### Ensuring safe passage

- The woman engages in a variety of prenatal care options appropriate to her culture and life experience. For example, pregnant Cambodian women rely on older same-culture women to give prenatal care and advice and rely little on prenatal classes or visits. Some Hispanic American women, on the basis of their view that pregnancy is a healthy, natural experience, may not seek prenatal care but seek a strong matriarchal support system for a positive outcome.
- The woman becomes more protective of herself and the fetus by avoiding crowds, revolving doors, small spaces, and people believed to place the mother at risk. She tires of being pregnant but fears the effect of delivery on her safety and that of her child (Rubin, 1972, 1984). Although sharing fears and desires with her partner, family, or health care provider helps, only the safe delivery of a normal child can fully free a pregnant woman from her fears to meet this developmental task (Rubin, 1972, 1977).

### Ensuring acceptance of the child

- The woman must believe that her child will be accepted into her family based on her definition of family. According to Rubin (1984), the partner's receptivity to the child is

particularly important, and many women fantasize about the sex of their child on the basis of a partner's preference.

- The woman frequently judges her partner's degree of receptivity to the infant by the amount of love and attention that she, herself, receives from him during her pregnancy.
- She may desire support from other women, rather than her partner, on the basis of her life experience, values, and cultural background.

### Binding into her unknown child

- This task is the most complex cognitive process for the pregnant woman (Rubin, 1984). To accomplish this task, the woman must integrate the fetus as an integral part of herself but also as a separate being. Completion of this task occurs with birth of the baby.
- Initially, the woman fantasizes about the baby through associative images: when she eats an egg, she thinks of the baby. Fantasies in the second and third trimesters relate more specifically to what the child will be like; the woman may imagine the baby in little girl or little boy clothes.
- During the eighth month the woman begins nesting activity by preparing the nursery and thinking increasingly of the baby as an external reality in her home.

### Learning to give of herself

- Although the actual mothering activity occurs after birth, the learning process to become a mother begins during pregnancy.
- The woman begins the task by examining what she will gain and lose by becoming a mother.
- She then explores the meaning of giving by examining how others give to her and to others and how she has given to others in the past (Rubin, 1984).
- Gifts for herself and the baby represent meaningful manifestations of her own and others' acceptance of her motherhood and her ability to give to her child and develop her identity as a mother (Rubin, 1967, 1972).

## Self-Perception–Self-Concept Pattern

To develop a maternal identity, the woman must first accept the pregnant body image. Initially she may show ambivalence based on her need to "fit" the pregnancy with her perception of self. She may dislike the physical changes of pregnancy or gladly "show off" her pregnant body to others. During the second trimester, however, the woman frequently begins to feel more positive about her changing womanly image as she feels the baby move, and increased amounts of estrogen and progesterone enhance her sense of vitality, inner peace, and acceptance. Her body begins to look pregnant, and generally others respond positively to this change (Rubin, 1972).

By the third trimester, however, the woman frequently tires of the pregnancy. Her sense of awkward moments supersedes feelings of well-being. She may experience uncomfortable, sleepless nights, the constant need to urinate, Braxton Hicks contractions, and other discomforts. Some women experience infant movement or mild contractions as pleasurable, sensual sensations, whereas others find them extremely uncomfortable. By pregnancy's end, these women yearn to have their former body boundaries back, to hold the baby in their arms, or to have someone else carry the baby.

After birth the woman gradually sees the infant more and more as a separate individual, dependent on her care. The mother starts to bond with her baby on the basis of her self-perception. If she feels good about herself, she will show love toward the infant; when she feels ugly or unlovable, she may make uncomplimentary remarks about the infant's appearance (Rubin, 1984).

## Maternal Role

The pregnant woman's personality, maturity level, and psychological development influence her readiness to assume the role of a mother. The way in which society in general and her culture in particular perceive motherhood and the role of women, as well as the way in which her own views mesh with these perceptions, will affect the ease of the transition. The family situation, the availability of peer role models, and the relationship with her mother are also significant. Internalization of the mother role occurs only after the birth, when the woman interacts with the infant in a reciprocal relationship (Rubin, 1977).

## Nursing Interventions

The woman may feel overwhelmed by her feelings and thoughts during pregnancy. Although others acknowledge her physical changes, only she experiences the psychological changes of excitement, ambivalence, or confusion associated with being pregnant.

During prenatal assessment, the nurse should address expected cognitive changes and self-image issues with each pregnant woman and respond nonjudgmentally to concerns expressed in this area. In one-to-one sessions or group prenatal classes, women and their partners should be encouraged to discuss their ideas and feelings related to the emotional and relationship changes expected during pregnancy, because these changes influence the future intimate relationship.

Education on and practice of the maternal role and being a mother is an effective intervention in increasing self-confidence in caring and maternal identity. During their transition to motherhood, pregnant women want attentive, proactive, professional psychosocial support from nurses. They expect nurses to oversee the transition period and to be capable of supporting them in dealing with changes in pregnancy and in preparing them for birth and motherhood.

## Roles-Relationships Pattern

The pregnant family changes throughout the pregnancy and postpartum period as each family member explores and responds to new roles and relationships. A pregnant woman without a partner may feel isolated during pregnancy and depend on family or friends as she adjusts to her situation. Cultural beliefs and traditions may produce stresses during pregnancy, change roles and relationships, or provide emotional and physical support to the pregnant family as it prepares for the baby.

The partner of the pregnant woman faces many new situations that influence that person's parental development. The pregnant woman may seem to be a different person to others because of her emotional response to the pregnancy, introspection, fantasies,

need for more rest, and changes in sexual drive. The partner may feel a rivalry with the fetus and baby because the mother is devoting increasing amounts of time to the baby. He may resent the attention that she receives during the pregnancy and the additional demands that she may make on his time. He may experience more financial pressure because of baby expenses and his partner's need to stop working on a short-term or long-term basis. These perceptions may lead him to batter or otherwise abuse his partner, possibly causing poor pregnancy and newborn outcomes (Box 16-7: Quality and Safety Scenario). The nurse assesses each pregnant woman for abuse and intervenes appropriately to protect the safety and health of the family during gestation.

The male partner may be concerned about his ability to fulfill the father role and support his wife or significant other. His fathering role models may be limited because of a lack of contact with his own father or because he spends time with men who are not actively parenting. He may never have held a baby before and may worry that he might drop or harm his own child. If his partner experiences pregnancy complications, he may feel guilty about causing the pregnancy. Table 16-5 gives a more complete list of both the father's and the mother's emotional responses to a first pregnancy. The nurse must work with the pregnant family to help the family adapt to a first pregnancy, because this one affects how the family will cope with subsequent pregnancies.

Children in the family also experience role changes during and after the pregnancy. The very young child, unaware of the concept of a new baby before the infant arrives, may experience a changed relationship with his pregnant mother. She may have less time to play, be more irritable from fatigue, or limit or stop active play late in pregnancy because of increased awkwardness and concern about her safety. After the baby has arrived, the child may be kept away from both the baby and the mother by well-meaning friends and relatives, have to share parents with others, or may want to breastfeed from the mother as the baby does. When permitted to see the newborn, the child may be admonished to "be careful" or "don't touch the baby." Thus a young child may not accept the baby with open arms.

The older child understands the newborn's significance more clearly but still experiences apprehensions about the effects of the baby on the family. Older children may have been told that they will become a big brother or sister, but does this mean they will lose toys and time with their parents and have to give up a private bedroom? Older children may worry about their mother, who seems more tired, less available, and perhaps even sick at times. Her enlarging abdomen may appear frightening. With help from the nurse, parents can make pregnancy an exciting time of learning and growing for the family (Box 16-8). Chapter 18 discusses the sibling relationship in greater detail.

In extended families, expectant grandparents also experience changes during the pregnancy of their daughter or daughter-in-law. The maternal grandmother, seeing her daughter assume the mother role, may now view her daughter as a rival because they are both mothers. The grandparents may be reminded of their own aging, resenting when their advice about pregnancy and parenting goes unheeded. A positive outcome of a pregnancy may be a new closeness between the woman and her mother if

## BOX 16-7 QUALITY AND SAFETY SCENARIO

### Birth Outcomes in Abused Pregnant Women

Nurses and other providers who deliver health care to women must address the issue of abuse of the pregnant woman by an intimate partner. Intimate partner violence is a significant public health problem with negative physical and psychological outcomes. It has been associated with increased levels of STIs, preterm labor, low-birth-weight infants, anxiety, substance abuse behaviors, and postpartum depression (Alhusen et al., 2015). Consider the following research study and the questions that follow to understand the issue further.

Several studies have attempted to identify risk factors associated with experiencing violence during pregnancy. However, all these studies compared women who were abused during pregnancy with nonabused pregnant women. To further the understanding of risk factors for experiencing violence during pregnancy, it may be useful to investigate factors that differentiate female victims of intimate partner violence who were and were not victimized during pregnancy. This will allow us to shed light on unique aspects of pregnancy violence. In addition, the current study examines risk factors using a nationally representative sample. The **risk factors** identified included young age, less than a high school education, unemployment of mother and/or father, dissatisfaction with relationships alcohol problems, and violence in the family of origin; unmarried status increased the risk of violence during pregnancy, but the relative risk was even greater if the women separated or divorced while pregnant; paternal uncertainty and accusations of infidelity have been associated with an increased risk of violence among pregnant women (Slep et al., 2015). Male partners may develop paternal assurance tactics, such as the use of violence to establish control, to combat paternal uncertainty, and to increase the probability that the children they raise are their own and there is no infidelity on the part of the woman. Patriarchal domination has also been linked to an increased risk of violence against women. Pregnancy may symbolize a time when the woman assumes more control over her own body and may represent a degree of independence from her male partner; violence against the pregnant partner may represent a male partner's attempt to reassert control. Many women who are abused during pregnancy have reported that their partners attempt to socially isolate them from family, friends, and other social support systems. Most women reporting physical violence during pregnancy are also victims of verbal abuse and psychological aggression. Psychological abuse may be the predominant form of abuse during pregnancy in some cultures. Women who had a partner with a drinking problem were more than three times as likely to be abused during pregnancy compared with women whose partner did not have a drinking problem.

The **health outcomes** of violence against pregnant women include being kicked, punched, thrown down stairs, threatened with knives, choked, scalded, pushed out of moving cars, and having objects thrown at them. A number of violence-related injuries also include cuts, bruises, fractures, concussions, dental injuries, stab wounds, vaginal bleeding, and persistent headaches. Mental health issues include depression, stress, distress, fearfulness, anxiousness, and feelings of isolation.

### Nursing Implications

Overall, this study indicates a need for nurses to screen women for high-risk factors prenatally, to be aware of the health risks secondary to violence, and to tailor nursing interventions supportive of pregnant women facing abuse. Nurses need to be aware of the issues surrounding pregnancy violence and have the ability to provide pregnant women with the resources and information necessary to ensure their safety.

### Questions

- How do the current health care system and the sociopolitical context of care in the United States contribute to the high numbers of pregnant women facing abuse from their intimate partners?
- What kind of interventions do you believe would be effective for these abused women?
- How should US health care policy ethically and legislatively address the problem of intimate partner abuse during pregnancy?

From Alhusen, J. L., Ray, E., Sharps, P., & Bullock, L. (2015). Intimate partner violence during pregnancy: Maternal and neonatal outcomes. *Journal of Women's Health, 24*(1), 100–106; Brownridge, D. A., Taillieu, T. L., Tyler, K. A., Tiwari, A., Ko Ling, C., & Santos, S. C. (2011). Pregnancy and intimate partner violence: Risk factors, severity, and health effects. *Violence Against Women, 17*(7), 858–881; Slep, A. M. S., Foran, H. M., Heyman, R. E., Snarr, J. D., & USAF Family Advocacy Research Program. (2015). Identifying unique and shared risk factors for physical intimate partner violence and clinically-significant physical intimate partner violence. *Aggressive Behavior, 41,* 227–241.

the woman turns to her mother to seek advice and share feelings. The nurse may encourage expectant parents to use pregnancy as a transition time for their own parents, which can enhance extended family cohesion in the future.

During pregnancy and after birth, each family member begins to establish an emotional attachment to the imagined or real new baby. Research shows that when the mother has a strong support system to develop deep feelings of attachment to the fetus, she will most likely attach to the baby after birth. Therefore the nurse assesses the support system of each pregnant woman and implements primary and secondary interventions to increase family bonding with a new baby.

## Sexuality-Reproductive Pattern

The pregnant woman's body image and merging of this body image with her definition of femininity greatly influence her feelings about her sexuality. For a previously infertile couple, achieving pregnancy may be a blessed event, despite the need for technology that affects a woman's concept of self and femininity and a man's concept of self and masculinity. The reflections of others, particularly those of a pregnant woman's husband, partner, or friend, help a woman to accept changes in her body, leading to better adjustment in their sexual relations.

On the other hand, women may experience different sexual feelings during pregnancy. Some women experience an increase in desire, but many worry about intercourse during pregnancy, fearing that it will cause **miscarriage**, infection, or an early birth. Other women may experience nausea during pregnancy or simply lack sexual interest. Physical discomfort, fatigue, and awkwardness as well as fear of membrane rupture, infection, or harm to the fetus may also diminish the woman's interest in sexual relations. Sexual dissatisfaction of the couple may result from restrictions in sexual positions, pain on penetration, increased vaginal discharge, breast tenderness, or the other physical discomforts of pregnancy such as fatigue and heartburn. In some cases, the enlarging uterus will require the couple to modify the positions for intercourse, particularly during the latter part of pregnancy. The couple's feelings about the woman's changing body may

### TABLE 16-5   Possible Responses to First Pregnancy

| Phase of Pregnancy | Father's Response | Mother's Response |
|---|---|---|
| First trimester | Fear of losing wife or child<br>Self-doubt as a future father<br>May develop new hobby outside of partner as way of distancing self | Loss of interest in coitus<br>Possible less sexual effectiveness<br>Sleepiness and chronic fatigue<br>Nausea<br>Increased dependence<br>Feels ambivalent toward reality of pregnancy<br>Anxious about process of labor and prospect of caring for a child<br>Worries about miscarriage<br>Becomes aware of physical changes in her body<br>May develop a closer relationship with her mother with a common experience of motherhood |
| Second trimester | Increased respect<br>Awe as quickening comes<br>Names for fetus coined<br>May give partner extra attention she desires<br>Feeling of change, accepting the reality of the pregnancy | Solemnity, hilarity, and playfulness about fetal movements<br>Talks about and with fetus<br>Increased eroticism<br>Expects partner to demonstrate interest in caring for her and baby<br>Feels movement and thinks of child as an individual |
| Third trimester | Fear of coitus hurting fetus<br>Abstinence difficult<br>Envy or pride, or both, at wife's creativity<br>Concern about identity as a "father"<br>Worry about birth<br>Keen awareness of male-female differences<br>May show a greater level of tenderness and protectiveness | Abstinence (often recommended by physician)<br>Sleepiness<br>Backache<br>Abdominal discomfort<br>Sexual isolation<br>Heightened sense of femininity<br>Assembles items needed for care of infant and selects possible names |
| Postpartum period | Eagerness to resume marital relations<br>Concern over endangering wife's recovery<br>Sense of triumph in becoming a father<br>Tenderness toward wife and baby | Pain and fear of harm from too early coitus<br>Low eroticism<br>Concern about effect on husband of continued abstinence<br>Sense of completion as a mother |
| Pregnancy as a whole | Increased romanticism<br>Increased nurturance<br>Increased family life participation<br>Financial stress<br>Concern about lack of skills in baby care | Increased romanticism<br>Increased optimism<br>Family roles replacing marital emphases<br>Fear of miscarriage or problems with baby<br>Pride of accomplishment<br>Emotional stress, feeling overloaded |

From Golian Tehrani, S., Bazzazian, S., & Dehghan Nayeri, N. (2015). Pregnancy experiences of first-time fathers: A qualitative study. *Iranian Red Crescent Medical Journal, 17*(2), 12271–12273; Nierenberg, C. (2015). Mood swings & mommy brain: The emotional challenges of pregnancy. *Live Science.* http://www.livescience.com/51043-pregnancy-emotions.html; Rigby, F. B. (2015). Common pregnancy complaints and questions. *Medscape.* http://emedicine.medscape.com/article/259724-overview.

### BOX 16-8   Nursing Strategies to Help Parents Prepare Siblings for the Neonate

- Explain the pregnancy and birth appropriate to the child's age.
- Answer all the child's questions.
- Use relevant literature to educate the child about the coming baby.
- Encourage discussion and questions by talking about the new baby during relaxed family times rather than during busy, rushed times.
- Have the child participate in decisions, such as choosing a name, clothes, and toys for baby.
- When sibling classes are available as part of the childbirth education process, encourage parents and the child to attend.
- Suggest that the child go with the mother during clinic or office visits.
- Allow and discuss negative comments about the pregnancy or baby.
- Encourage the child to make drawings or give small gifts to the baby when it is born.

alter their sexual relationship. The nurse's first step in primary prevention intervention in this area is to support the couple's needs and to relate, in a sensitive fashion, accurate information that facilitates couple intimacy during pregnancy.

Some women experience a decreased desire for sexual intercourse but an increased desire for holding, touching, and other signs of physical affection from their husbands or partners. The nurse encourages the couple to explore other activities for mutual sexual satisfaction.

In summary, the nurse can use the following guidelines concerning sexual activity:

- Sex is generally considered safe in pregnancy.
- Abstinence should be recommended only for women who are at risk of preterm labor, multiple gestation, premature rupture of membranes, unexplained vaginal

bleeding, or antepartum hemorrhage because of placenta previa.

- There is little evidence to show that sex at term may help induce labor, but this practice is considered safe in women with low-risk pregnancies (Zakšek, 2015).
- The resumption of intercourse postpartum should be dictated by a woman's level of comfort.

## Coping–Stress Tolerance Pattern

Physical and psychological adaptations of the woman to pregnancy affect her perception of stressors and her ability to cope with all aspects of her life. Even normal discomforts of pregnancy may be stressful for a woman, mandating her to modify her usual routine to cope more effectively. Anxiety tends to be high during the first trimester as the woman adapts to pregnancy and anticipated life changes. During the second trimester the woman feels less anxious, but anxiety returns during the third trimester with impending labor and delivery. Throughout pregnancy women may demonstrate their anxieties through psychosomatic complaints and behaviors, such as nausea and vomiting after the first trimester, excessive eating, food cravings, sleeplessness, and fainting. Realistically, every pregnant woman probably experiences some degree of stress. However, many women have considerable stress or ongoing stress, such as poverty, marital difficulties, or unsatisfactory living or working conditions, that influences their coping abilities.

A pregnant woman's anxieties may be reflected in her dreams and fantasies. Many pregnant women report dreams about their babies being deformed or dead, themselves dying, or a family member being injured. Many women at the end of their pregnancies express fears about body mutilation with delivery. Other women may manifest their anxiety by smoking, drinking, or using drugs (legal or illegal), all of which can harm the fetus. Prenatal depression and/or anxiety has been associated with excessive activity and growth delays in the fetus, as well as prematurity, low birth weight, disorganized sleep, and less responsiveness to stimulation in the neonate. Infants of depressed/anxious mothers have difficult temperaments, and later in development attentional, emotional, and behavioral problems have been noted during childhood and adolescence, as well as chronic illnesses in adulthood. Caring for a newborn requires energy, patience, and emotional presence, which are all lacking in a depressed mother (Rode & Kiel, 2016). The nurse must direct a pregnant woman who is not coping well to relevant resources for assistance. The nurse must also assess each woman's progress in taking on the mothering role as the pregnancy nears term. This information can be shared with the postpartum nursing staff to encourage discussion in this important area.

The nurse encourages the pregnant woman to use tension-relieving strategies such as listening to soft music, using humor, crying, sleeping, talking to a friend, meditating, exercising, and fantasizing during times of stress. These strategies are safe for the fetus and provide relief from many normal tensions and anxieties during pregnancy and afterward. Overall, the nurse plays a key role by responding nonjudgmentally and promoting the coping of women during pregnancy.

## Values-Beliefs Pattern

Although pregnancy has been described as the fulfillment of the deepest and most powerful wish of a woman, this fulfillment often coincides with a woman's fear of losing part of herself. She gives up some relationships and pleasures to assume other anticipated satisfactions. She may find that she values friendships with other mothers now, whereas before pregnancy her friendships focused on work or school colleagues. She may discover much to her husband's confusion that she values different qualities in him than she did before anticipating birth. Her husband may also experience a shift in his values.

Pregnant women and their partners may experience changes in their spiritual values. For women with strong spiritual needs related to their cultural backgrounds, spiritual interventions will help them integrate various dimensions of their lives, develop the ability to parent successfully, and find meaning in the changes and goals of pregnancy. Seen as a mystical event or miracle, conception may lead to an increased faith in God or a favorite saint. Nonreligious couples may start to attend church after the baby's birth because they want religion to be part of their child's life. Religious beliefs may influence a woman's decision to undergo certain tests or procedures, such as amniocentesis or abortion. Some women may feel forced to reproduce because their religious or cultural mores forbid contraception or encourage large families. In these groups, each pregnancy may be seen as another unwanted, but unavoidable, burden or may be valued because having more children signifies a stronger family.

# ENVIRONMENTAL PROCESSES

## Physical Agents

A healthy infant is the outcome of most pregnancies. However, genetic abnormalities and environmental hazards may cause fetal harm, spontaneous abortion (natural loss of conceptive products), or minor or serious congenital defects. Diagnostic methods that identify an early pregnancy or a fetal loss may assist couples in practicing healthy decisions to prevent loss or congenital abnormalities. The WHO (2015) estimates that congenital defects affect 3% to 4% of all live births and contribute to infant mortality rates by causing structural or functional disability incompatible with life. Every year an estimated 276,000 infants worldwide die of congenital anomalies within 1 month after their birth. Real-time ultrasonography identifies approximately 85% of fetal anomalies by 36 weeks of gestation. The best time for a fetal scan is at 18 to 20 weeks of gestation (Rayburn et al., 2015). This knowledge, gained before giving birth, permits expectant couples and the health care delivery team to access resources for improving the baby's life or to support a grieving family if the baby is not expected to live. With progress made in diagnostic tools and the Human Genome Project, some couples may be able to prevent fetal defects or manage them during pregnancy to improve the quality of their baby's life after birth (see the case study at the end of this chapter). Unfortunately, even when no genetic or congenital defects exist, the fetus may still be injured during process of labor and delivery and face a lesser quality

## TABLE 16-6    TORCH Perinatal Infections

| Infection | Agent | Source | Fetal-Neonatal Risks | Comments |
|---|---|---|---|---|
| **T**oxoplasmosis | Protozoan *Toxoplasma gondii* | Raw or undercooked meat; unpasteurized goat's milk; feces of infected cats | Fetal growth restriction, hydrocephaly, seizures, neurological and cognitive effects, chorioretinitis, intracranial calcifications | Instruct mother to not eat undercooked or raw meat; avoid exposure to cat litter |
| **O**ther/hepatitis B | Hepadnavirus | Blood or blood products; sexually transmitted via body fluids | Generally asymptomatic, but majority become chronically infected | Newborn should receive HBIG within 12 h after birth and hepatitis B vaccine postpartum |
| **R**ubella | Rubella virus | Direct or indirect contact with droplets of infected person | CNS defects, developmental delay, deafness, cataracts, IUGR, microcephaly, cardiac defects, glaucoma | Screen all pregnant women with rubella antibody titers |
| **C**ytomegalovirus | Herpes virus | Transmitted by droplet infection from person to person | Microcephaly, fetal growth restriction, CNS abnormalities, deafness, blindness, jaundice, gastrointestinal defects, seizures | Prevention of maternal primary infection in early pregnancy; stress good personal hygiene |
| **H**erpes simplex | HSV-1 and HSV-2 | Sexually transmitted infection to mother; fetus contacts it during birth from genital lesions | Intense herpetic lesions on eyes, mouth, and skin; keratitis; conjunctivitis | Practice safer sex; careful handwashing; surgical birth if active lesions |

*CNS,* Central nervous system; *HBIG,* hepatitis B immune globulin; *HSV-1,* herpes simplex virus type 1; *HSV-2,* herpes simplex virus type 2; *IUGR,* intrauterine growth restriction.
From Neu, N., Duchon, J., & Zachariah, P. (2015). TORCH infections. *Clinics in Perinatology, 42*(1), 77–103; Smith, B. (2015). Neonatal-perinatal infections: An update. *Clinics in Perinatology, 42*(1), 77–104; Suliman, S., & Seopela, L. (2015). Congenital and neonatal infections: Review. *Obstetrics and Gynecology Forum, 25*(2), 27–32.

Teratogens are environmental agents that cause spontaneous abortions or congenital defects. Unlike genetic abnormalities, which occur only at conception, environmental agents may affect the developing infant at any point during gestation. Fetal organs have critical periods of development, and if affected at that time by a teratogen, the infant may have a defect in that organ system. Teratogens normally do not cause a congenital defect during the first 14 days after conception. However, the embryo may be lost later during early gestation (a spontaneous abortion). Therefore as a primary prevention strategy, any woman contemplating or attempting pregnancy should be counseled to avoid teratogens that might cause fetal loss or damage.

### Physical Factors and Diagnostic Tools

Modern diagnostic tools, such as ultrasonography, amniocentesis, chorionic villus sampling, and alpha-fetoprotein screening have been used to identify a number of fetal problems. Certain risk factors, some of which may be found in the family history, or maternal and paternal age, maternal illness, or previous fetal abnormalities, may indicate the need for these diagnostic tools during a woman's pregnancy. These tools commonly identify problems related to abnormal size or rate of fetal growth, chromosomal abnormalities, NTDs, and fetal lung immaturity. The nurse, in consultation with the health care team, must participate in providing informed consent to women before these diagnostic tools are used.

### Biological Agents

Biological processes in the fetal environment, which include infections and other health problems of the mother, may affect fetal growth and development. A pregnant woman who acquires an asymptomatic viral infection may not seek health care because she believes that the fetus will not be harmed. However, viral agents may cause fetal damage early in pregnancy. The woman with a health problem, such as diabetes, may also cause fetal damage if she fails to adhere to her health care provider's directives.

When the nurse discusses with pregnant couples the effects of biological processes on the fetus, she must emphasize that the timing of the maternal infection or illness is critical to predicting fetal defects. Maternal infections during the first trimester of pregnancy may cause severe fetal defects or death, depending on the organism. Infections later in pregnancy may also seriously affect the fetus, but less often. Unfortunately, pregnancy renders many women more susceptible to viral illness, supporting an argument for all women of childbearing age to be fully immunized. Many vaccines (measles, mumps, rubella, and polio) cannot be given during pregnancy because of potential risk to the fetus, but others present no risk (tetanus and diphtheria). A TORCH (*t*oxoplasmosis, *o*ther agents, *r*ubella, *c*ytomegalovirus, *h*erpes simplex; other infections include *Treponema pallidum*, hepatitis viruses, HIV, varicella, parvovirus B19, and enteroviruses) screen may be done to detect the presence of teratogenic perinatal infections: toxoplasmosis, hepatitis B, rubella, cytomegalovirus infection, and herpes simplex (Table 16-6). TORCH infections are major contributors to prenatal, perinatal, and postnatal morbidity and death. Evidence of infection may be seen at birth, in infancy, or years later. For many of these pathogens, treatment or prevention strategies are available, but early recognition, including prenatal screening, is essential.

## Toxoplasmosis

Toxoplasmosis is caused by a protozoan that infects people through consumption of undercooked meat, handling of feces of cats that become infected by eating infected rodents and birds, and exposure to contaminated soil, in countries outside the United States (CDC, 2015c). An infected pregnant woman is usually asymptomatic but may have flulike symptoms or mild to severe upper respiratory tract symptoms believed to be unrelated to an infection. Vertical transmission from an infected pregnant woman to the fetus predominantly occurs when infection is acquired for the first time during pregnancy. Overall, approximately one-third of infected pregnant women give birth to an infant with toxoplasmosis, and the risk of vertical transmission rises sharply with gestational age at maternal infection. However, fetuses infected during an early pregnancy period are much more likely to show clinical signs of infection, such as chorioretinitis, hydrocephalus, or intracranial calcification (King et al., 2015). Approximately 60% of maternal infections acquired during the third trimester will result in fetal infection, which might manifest itself as rashes, enlarged lymph nodes and liver, inflammation of the heart, pneumonia, jaundice, or severe central nervous system damage after birth or years later (CDC, 2015c). Nurses can offer some simple hygiene suggestions that reduce the risk of infection. For example, humans can acquire toxoplasmosis from eating undercooked or raw meat (especially lamb and pork), from being exposed to contaminated soil or water, or from consuming uncooked vegetables. Clearly, nurses should advise pregnant women to cook meat thoroughly and wash and scrub vegetables well, especially those eaten raw. Pregnant women should use good handwashing hygiene, avoid eating raw meat, wear gloves when gardening, and avoid handling cats or cleaning cat litter boxes to avoid exposure to *Toxoplasma*.

## Syphilis

Syphilis is an STI that can be transmitted through oral, anal, or vaginal contact. An infected mother transfers syphilis, caused by a bacterium, to her fetus. The causative organism, *Treponema pallidum*, can be transferred across the placenta and can infect the developing fetus as early as at 9 weeks of gestation. The risk of vertical transmission and infection in the newborn is directly related to the stage of maternal syphilis during pregnancy; transmission occurs more frequently during primary or secondary syphilis in the mother than during latent stages of the disease. Although syphilis is preventable and treatable, the number of congenital and neonatal syphilis cases has increased in the last several years (CDC, 2015d). Maternal risk factors for acquiring syphilis include homelessness, human immunodeficiency virus (HIV) positive status, single marital status, and a history of STIs. Maternal syphilis has been associated with complications such as polyhydramnios, spontaneous abortion, and preterm births. Fetal complications such as fetal syphilis, fetal hydrops, prematurity, fetal distress, and stillbirth also occur. Neonatal complications can include congenital syphilis, seizures, neonatal death, and late sequelae (Singh & McCloskey, 2015). The infant may be born with localized mucocutaneous lesions, nasal congestion, anemia, and generalized septicemia, but may appear healthy at birth only to have symptoms appear later. Routine testing of high-risk women for syphilis at the first prenatal visit and during the third trimester and antibiotic treatment (benzathine penicillin G) for affected women and their partners have reduced the number of infants with congenital syphilis (King & Brucker, 2016).

## Rubella

Despite the broad use of the measles, mumps, and rubella vaccine, or MMR, and the resulting immunity to rubella, approximately 20% of women reach their childbearing period without immunity to this disease (USDHHS, 2010). The risk of vertical transmission from a nonimmune mother with primary rubella infection in the first trimester of pregnancy is considerably high at 80% to 90%. Beyond the first 12 weeks of gestation, fetal organogenesis is nearly complete, and deafness may be the only consequence in the infected infant. Deafness, cataracts, and cardiac defects are the classic congenital anomalies associated with a rubella infection (Silasi et al., 2015). The symptoms of rubella may cause the mother to think she has a minor viral infection, but rubella during the first trimester may cause improper fetal development of the ears, eyes, and heart and deafness. No treatment exists for an infected fetus; however, a pregnant woman may receive the vaccine to protect future pregnancies if she has no history of rubella infection. After giving birth, new mothers often receive the vaccine before being discharged with a recommendation to avoid pregnancy for at least 3 months to prevent fetal harm from the vaccine.

## Cytomegalovirus

Cytomegalovirus (CMV) is a virus in the herpes virus family and is a leading cause of congenital infections and long-term neurodevelopmental disabilities among children. Contacts with young children have been identified as the main source of virus transmission to mothers. It is the most common infection that can cause serious fetal complications. CMV infects an estimated 1% to 2% of all infants born in the United States. Most mothers infected with CMV have mild, often nonspecific symptoms, but their infants may experience hearing loss, blindness, enlarged liver and spleen, seizures, intracranial calcifications, and neurodevelopmental disabilities (Kovacs & Briggs, 2015). Unfortunately, no means exist to prevent or manage this viral infection. Perhaps an immunization similar to that for rubella will be developed in the future. Until vaccines and nontoxic antiviral agents are available, hygienic measures are important as prophylaxis and should be emphasized by all nurses to their prenatal clients.

## Herpes Simplex Virus

Herpes simplex virus infections remain extremely common today, with many people unaware that they have the disease. It is estimated that 16% of adults in the United Sates are infected with herpes simplex virus. Herpes is lifelong infection that has the potential for transmission throughout the life span (King et al., 2015). Herpes simplex may cause spontaneous abortion or fetal neurological damage. Infants infected at birth may show localized or generalized disease with symptoms of vesicular skin lesions, microcephaly, hydrocephalus, chorioretinitis, conjunctivitis, seizures, respiratory distress, or gastrointestinal bleeding. These symptoms may cause newborn death. An infant delivered vaginally by a woman with active genital herpes has a 40% to 60% chance of being infected (CDC, 2015e), supporting a decision for a cesarean delivery for any women with active vaginal or perineal herpes lesions. Risk factors for the transmission of herpes from the mother to the newborn have been detailed. The pregnant woman who acquires genital herpes as a primary infection in the latter half of pregnancy, rather than before pregnancy, is at greatest risk of transmitting this virus to her newborn. This is true for both herpes simplex virus type 1 and herpes simplex virus type 2 (Kovacs & Briggs, 2015). Generally, an antiviral agent is recommended during pregnancy for treatment of viral lesions. The nurse educates the infected woman about comfort measures at this time, including ways to keep the lesions dry and application of comfort measures to reduce the pain of the lesions (Queenan et al., 2015).

### Zika Virus Disease

Zika virus is transmitted to humans primarily through the bite of an infected *Aedes* species mosquito during the daytime. The most common symptoms of Zika virus disease are fever, rash, headaches, bone pains, joint tenderness, and conjunctivitis. The illness is typically mild, with symptoms lasting for several days to a week after the person has being bitten. Up to 80% of people infected with the virus have no symptoms (CDC, 2016). The virus is in the Caribbean, as well as parts of Central America and South America. The virus has been reported to be spread through blood transfusions and sexual contact and can also be passed from a pregnant woman to her fetus, and has been linked to a serious birth defect of the brain termed microcephaly. The CDC, WHO, and other scientific organizations are working to understand this possible link.

In 2016 the World Health Organization (2016) declared Zika virus a public health emergency of international concern. The CDC recommends abstaining from oral, anal, or vaginal sexual contact with anyone who has traveled to areas with active infections. Pregnant women are also discouraged from traveling to regions with active infections (CDC, 2016). At this time there is no vaccine given to prevent Zika virus disease or antiviral medication to treat the infection. Prevention measures would include better housing construction, use of insect repellents, wearing long-sleeved shirts and pants, regular use of air conditioning, use of window screens, avoidance of traveling to mosquito-infested areas, and state and local mosquito control efforts.

### Chlamydia, Gonococcus, Group B Streptococcus, Bacterial Vaginosis, and *Candida albicans*

Infections caused by chlamydia, gonococcus, group B streptococcus, and yeast *(Candida albicans)* may occur in the woman's vagina or cervix, infecting the infant during a vaginal birth. Chlamydia, the most common bacterial STI, appears most often among poor women with little access to care. Although few symptoms are seen, infection may cause preterm labor, premature rupture of membranes, low-birth-weight infants, or newborn conjunctivitis or pneumonia. Routine treatment of the newborn's eyes after birth with erythromycin or other effective antibiotic ointment destroys the organisms. Maternal gonococcus (GC) infection can be transmitted to the newborn from the mother's genital tract at the time of birth and can cause ophthalmia neonatorum, a systemic neonatal infection, maternal endometritis, or pelvic infection. The risk of transmission from an infected mother to her infant is nearly 50% (Hotchin, 2015). Newborn infants often receive an antibiotic ointment in the eyes to prevent GC infection. Screening at 36 to 37 weeks of pregnancy for group B streptococcus infection has been recommended because this infection causes preterm rupture of the amniotic membranes, preterm labor, fetal respiratory distress syndrome, fetal septicemia, and meningitis (Michihata et al., 2015). Bacterial vaginosis may also cause preterm labor (Sangkomkamhang et al., 2015). *Candida albicans*, the cause of a common vaginal fungal infection, may also cause an oral infection called thrush in the newborn. Routine assessment of pregnant women, and occasionally their sexual partners (GC), for these bacterial and yeast infections must occur during pregnancy so that treatment can occur and prevent fetal infection at the time of birth.

### Human Immunodeficiency Virus

*Acquired immunodeficiency syndrome.* The US Public Health Service and the US Preventive Services Task Force recommend that all pregnant women in the United States be tested for HIV infection, ideally at the first prenatal visit (Ross et al., 2015). Any woman in a high-risk group (e.g., intravenous drug users, women who have bisexual partners or multiple sexual contacts, women with a history of STIs, women who engage in sex for money or drugs, or black or Hispanic women living in poverty) should be tested for antibodies to HIV. For the HIV-positive woman or one who engages in high-risk sexual practices, counseling must occur before conception. Counseling should include both the direct effect of the virus on pregnancy and the effect of pregnancy on HIV disease progression. Although unclear, it appears that HIV infection becomes worse during pregnancy because of a woman's altered immune status. Some early pregnancy discomforts, such as fatigue, anorexia, and weight loss, may mask the early symptoms of HIV infection and thus postpone a definitive diagnosis.

Infants born to HIV-positive women who have taken antiretroviral medications during their pregnancy, in whom the virus is undetectable, and who have avoided breastfeeding have a less than 1% perinatal transmission rate (CDC, 2015f). Affected infants may not be seropositive for HIV for many months after birth and then later develop the disease. The use of antiretroviral medications throughout pregnancy has improved the prognosis of an HIV-positive woman and has decreased viral transmission to the fetus, although the drug remains expensive and may be inaccessible for women who do not receive prenatal care.

The pregnant woman who has acquired immunodeficiency syndrome (AIDS) or who is HIV positive should be carefully monitored by a health care team for opportunistic infections that occur frequently. The nurse can be instrumental in helping this woman coordinate her contacts with care providers, answering her questions, and working as a member of the team to provide optimal care for the woman and her child. Frequently the pregnant woman with AIDS does not seek care because of fears of being reported for her disease. Involving the woman in continuous prenatal care decreases her risk of preterm rupture of membranes, problems with fetal growth, postpartum infection, drug and alcohol abuse, and difficulty in addressing sociocultural barriers to a better life (Adam, 2015).

Although important in decreasing the transmission of any disease, astute preventive measures are mandatory for nurses who are exposed to HIV-infected body fluids, such as blood, amniotic fluid, and vaginal secretions (standard precautions should be followed). All health care providers must follow hospital and birth center policies regarding the use of gloves and gowns and the disposal of needles and other potentially contaminated equipment to prevent the transmission of this disease in particular.

## Hepatitis B

Hepatitis B virus (HBV) is a serious global public health problem with more than 2 billion people infected and more than 1 million deaths occurring annually because of cirrhosis and liver carcinoma (Reddy et al., 2015). HBV infection remains a significant concern during pregnancy because it affects the maternal liver and has a high fetal transmission rate (40%) if present during the third trimester. High-risk groups for HBV infection include women from Asia, Pacific Islands, and sub-Saharan Africa, as well as health care workers, intravenous drug users, and women with multiple sexual partners (CDC, 2015g). On the basis of the large number of infected women who fail to show symptoms until liver damage has occurred, all pregnant women early in pregnancy and those at risk should be screened routinely for HBV (Queenan et al., 2015). HBV immunization (three injections over a period of 6 months) may be given before or during pregnancy to a mother who is seronegative (CDC, 2015g). According to Jhaveri (2015), most women harboring HBV transmit it vertically through the placenta to the fetus or through contaminated urine, feces, saliva, or vaginal fluids during birth. Many women carrying HBV deliver prematurely, and some infants may have acute hepatitis or later develop liver cancer.

## Other Health Concerns

Pregnant women may also develop any of the infections of nonpregnant women. For example, pregnant women frequently experience upper respiratory tract and gastrointestinal tract infections, adding to the discomforts of pregnancy. However, there is no evidence the viruses causing these infections have a teratogenic effect on the fetus.

Fever frequently occurs with illness. A high temperature for a prolonged time (hyperthermia) in a pregnant woman may harm the fetus, especially during the first trimester. Some literature indicates that fever is associated with miscarriages, low birth weight, stillbirths, and preterm births (Silasi et al., 2015). Whether the fever or an underlying illness causing the fever has created the problem must be determined. Some reports have also correlated prolonged use of a sauna or hot tub, causing hyperthermia, with birth defects such as microcephaly, anencephaly, and hypotonia (Biswas et al., 2015). Until health care providers understand this issue better, the nurse should advise pregnant women to avoid prolonged sauna or hot tub use and spending time with people who are ill or carrying disease. When a pregnant woman develops a fever, she should be advised to contact her health care provider immediately.

Pregnant woman may have other health problems that influence their physiological processes and thus harm the developing fetus. Black women experience twice the rate of hypertension and diabetes mellitus of white women. These higher rates may account for the three to four times higher maternal mortality rate seen among pregnant black women as compared with white women (CDC, 2015h). Overall, US women are more likely to die during childbirth than women in any other developed country, leading the United States to be ranked 33rd among 179 countries on the health and well-being of women and children (Robeznieks, 2016).

***Diabetes.*** Diabetes mellitus is approaching epidemic proportions worldwide, and the effects and treatment of it are still not well understood by the medical community. Diabetes may exist before pregnancy (preexisting diabetes) or start during pregnancy (gestational diabetes), affecting both the mother and the fetus. Pregnancy increases the need for maternal insulin to balance the woman's blood glucose level. Currently the American College of Obstetricians and Gynecologists recommends that all pregnant women complete a glucose tolerance test at 28 weeks of gestation to identify abnormal blood glucose utilization and the need for additional monitoring. Complications from diabetes during pregnancy include polyhydramnios (excessive amniotic fluid volume), acidosis, increased rate of infection, vascular complications, and increased risk of pregnancy-induced hypertension. Because of an increased incidence of intrauterine death after 36 weeks of gestation attributable to an aging placenta, close monitoring in the last month is essential. Neonatal complications from diabetes include hypoglycemia, respiratory distress syndrome, hyperbilirubinemia, and hypocalcemia. Infants of mothers with diabetes also have a higher incidence of congenital anomalies, such as a heart lesion or meningocele (Langer, 2015). The diabetic pregnant woman needs close health care team supervision and ongoing health teaching, including diet and exercise management, to control her disease effectively for an optimal pregnancy outcome.

***Heart disease and hypertension.*** The physiological changes that occur in pregnancy can place extra demands on cardiac function. Cardiac disease complicates approximately 4% of all pregnancies in the United States (Gandhi & Martin, 2015). Heart disease and hypertension are two serious maternal cardiovascular problems during pregnancy. Rheumatic heart disease, a common problem that affects more than 34 million people annually, contributes to congestive heart failure, threatening the lives of both the mother and the fetus. The greatest tragedy of all is that it is eminently preventable (Carapetis, 2015). The fetus may require preterm birth to prevent complications. Chronic hypertension, seen more frequently in first-time mothers older than 35 years, increases the chances of stillbirths, preterm births, preeclampsia, chronic hypertension, and development of gestational hypertension, which increase both maternal and infant mortality rates. Mothers with these problems must be monitored closely throughout pregnancy to prevent complications (Raio et al., 2015).

***Rh blood group incompatibility.*** Rh blood group incompatibility, which is a rare occurrence today because of implementation of anti-D immune globulin prophylaxis given to the mother prenatally and postnatally, sometimes affects fetal development. This problem usually occurs when the mother has Rh-negative red blood cells and the fetus has Rh-positive red blood cells, inherited from a father who has Rh-positive blood. In this disorder, maternal antibodies develop, cross the placental membranes, and destroy the Rh-positive red blood cells of the fetus. Depending on the severity of the response, the infant may develop various levels of hyperbilirubinemia after birth or may die in utero from the anemia of erythroblastosis fetalis (hemolytic disease of the newborn).

All women should be assessed for blood type, Rh factor, and development of antibody to Rh-positive cells at their first prenatal care visit and again at 24 to 28 weeks of pregnancy unless the father of the baby is Rh negative (Moise, 2015). Rh incompatibility between a mother and a future fetus may be prevented by administration of Rho(D) immune globulin (RhoGAM) to a Rh-negative mother at 28 weeks of gestation and within 72 hours after birth. The immunization prevents the mother's sensitization to fetal Rh-negative cells by inactivating fetal red blood cells in the mother before she can develop an antibody response. The ideal injection time is after the mother's first birth of an Rh-positive infant, miscarriage, or therapeutic abortion. The incompatibility generally does not occur during the first pregnancy, and the immunization prevents problems with later pregnancies.

## Chemical Agents

Substance abuse in pregnancy remains a major public health problem. The use and abuse of alcohol and other mind-altering drugs has political, legal, socioeconomic, health, mental health, and familial impact felt widely around the world. Drugs ingested by the mother may be teratogenic to the fetus. The tragic experience with the tranquilizer drug thalidomide, which caused limb deformities during the early 1960s, led to a recommendation that medications should be avoided during pregnancy unless absolutely necessary (Box 16-9: Research for Evidence-Based Practice). The fact remains, however, that during the most critical early weeks of fetal development and growth, when many women do not know they are pregnant, ingested drugs may seriously affect the fetus. Depending on fetal gestational age and drug metabolism, drugs may alter the placenta itself or directly affect

---

## BOX 16-9 RESEARCH FOR EVIDENCE-BASED PRACTICE

### Substance Use in Pregnancy

**Objective:** To improve awareness and knowledge of problematic substances (alcohol, tobacco, illicit substances of opioids, amphetamine-type stimulants, cocaine, marijuana, and unprescribed prescription drugs) used in pregnancy and to provide evidence-based recommendations for the management of this challenging clinical issue for all health care providers.

**Options:** This guideline reviews the use of screening tools, general approach to care, and recommendations for clinical management of problematic substance use in pregnancy.

**Outcomes:** Evidence-based recommendations for screening and management of problematic substance use during pregnancy and lactation.

**Evidence:** Medline, PubMed, CINAHL, and the Cochrane Library were searched for articles published from 1950 with use of the following keywords: substance-related disorders, mass screening, pregnancy complications, pregnancy, prenatal care, cocaine, cannabis, methadone, opioid, tobacco, nicotine, solvents, hallucinogens, and amphetamines. The results were initially restricted to systematic reviews and randomized controlled trials/controlled clinical trials. A subsequent search for observational studies was also conducted because there are few randomized controlled trials in this field of study. Articles were restricted to human studies published in English.

**Recommendations**
- All pregnant women and women of childbearing age should be screened periodically for alcohol, tobacco, and prescription and illicit drug use.
- When testing for substance use is clinically indicated, urine drug screening is the preferred method. Informed consent should be obtained from the woman before maternal drug toxicology testing is ordered.
- The 5As of intervention (ask, advise, assess, assist, and arrange) can be a useful framework for encouraging women to quit substance use.
- Pregnant women may require a medically supported inpatient setting to assist them in their recovery from substance abuse.

- Policies and legal requirements with respect to drug testing of newborns may differ by jurisdiction, and caregivers should be familiar with the regulations in their region.
- Health care providers should use a flexible approach to the care of women who have substance use problems, and they should encourage the use of all available community resources.
- Women should be counseled about the risks of periconception, antepartum, and postpartum drug use.
- Women seeking help should be provided with counseling and substance abuse treatment option referrals.
- Smoking cessation counseling should be considered as a first-line intervention for pregnant smokers. Nicotine replacement therapy and/or pharmacotherapy can be considered if counseling is not successful.
- Methadone maintenance treatment should be a standard of care for opioid-dependent women during pregnancy. Other slow-release opioid preparations may be considered if methadone is not available.
- Opioid detoxification should be reserved for selected women because of the high risk of relapse to opioids.
- Opiate-dependent women should be informed that neonates exposed to heroin, prescription opioids, methadone, or buprenorphine during pregnancy are monitored closely for symptoms and signs of neonatal withdrawal (neonatal abstinence syndrome).
- The risks and benefits of breastfeeding should be weighed on an individual basis because methadone maintenance therapy is not a contraindication to breastfeeding.

**Nursing implications:** Using these guidelines, nurses can assist in helping pregnant women improve access to health care, and assistance with appropriate addiction care leads to reduced health care costs and decreased maternal and neonatal morbidity and mortality.

From Mental Health and Drug & Alcohol Office. (2014). Substance use during pregnancy clinical guidelines. http://www.health.nsw.gov.au/mhdao/programs/da/Pages/substance-use-during-pregnancy-guidelines.aspx; Wong, S., Ordean, A., & Kahan, M. (2011). Substance use in pregnancy. Journal of Obstetrics & Gynaecology Canada, 33(4), 367–384.

development and growth of the fetus. The drugs that most commonly cause congenital defects are prescription medications, over-the-counter (OTC) drugs, street drugs, nicotine (cigarettes), caffeine, and alcohol.

## Prescription Medications

Women frequently become pregnant while taking medications for illnesses diagnosed before pregnancy, such as hypertension, or they may receive medication to treat an illness acquired during pregnancy, such as a UTI. Some of the more common drugs that have been studied for fetal effects include antibiotics and anticonvulsants.

Most short-term and usual-dose antibiotics do not cause fetal harm. The tetracyclines are harmful to baby teeth formation because they combine with calcium ions and are deposited in deciduous teeth (causing discoloration) and bones (inhibiting bone growth and causing deformities) (King & Brucker, 2016). Primary teeth seem most affected, but when the antibiotic is given near the time of delivery, the permanent teeth may also be damaged.

On the basis of our current state of knowledge, the vast majority of antibiotics do not cause serious harm to the unborn child if used properly and at the appropriate doses during pregnancy. The treatment with an antibiotic that is contraindicated does not justify termination of pregnancy. However, ultimately no medicine, including antibiotics, can be described as absolutely safe (Doulatram et al., 2015).

The prevalence of antiepileptic drug use in pregnant women is very low. Although their main indication is for management of epilepsy, antiepileptic drugs are increasingly being used in the treatment of bipolar mood disorders, migraine, and neuropathic pain syndrome, which means their prevalence will increase (Tomson & Klein, 2015). The effects of anticonvulsants on the fetus have been documented thoroughly. Women with seizure disorders have carried infants to term while being treated with hydantoin, barbiturates, and other antiseizure medications. Infants born to mothers taking hydantoin (Dilantin) may have fetal hydantoin syndrome, reflected in microcephaly, retardation, cleft lip and palate, and congenital heart disease. Barbiturates, such as phenobarbital, may cause newborn addiction. Women with seizure disorders should discuss their medication requirements with their physicians before becoming pregnant and have close health care team monitoring throughout pregnancy.

## Over-the-Counter Drugs

Pregnant women frequently choose to treat minor illnesses with OTC drugs. Research on acetylsalicylic acid (aspirin) and acetaminophen (Tylenol) indicates that both medications are safe in the recommended dosages. However, aspirin alters platelet function and may cause maternal and newborn bleeding if taken close to delivery. Acetaminophen can be toxic to the liver. Certain ingredients in common cold remedies have been associated with fetal irritability (King & Brucker, 2016). Ibuprofen has been known to prolong labor on the basis of its antiprostaglandin effect. Any drug may harm a fetus, so all drugs should be avoided during pregnancy unless prescribed by the health care provider.

The nurse includes information on the known and probable effects of medications on the fetus in prenatal teaching of couples. Discussion of herbal treatments is included, because little research exists on their effects and interactions with OTC and prescribed medications. The nurse recognizes that many cultural groups use these nontraditional agents because they believe that they will effectively manage pregnancy-related concerns. The nurse may need to encourage an individual to reconsider the use of herbs when evidence exists that these may harm the fetus or mother.

## Drug Abuse

Given the prevalence of drug use and abuse in our society, it is imperative that nurses be able to recognize, manage, and refer as appropriate substance abuse problems for their care recipients. Substance abuse during pregnancy poses a significant risk because all substances consumed by the mother pass freely through the placenta, and thus the fetus as well as the mother experiences substance use, abuse, and addiction. All pregnant women and women of childbearing age should be screened periodically for alcohol, tobacco, and prescription and illicit drug use.

Maternal use of narcotics, tranquilizers, cocaine, amphetamines, marijuana, and other drugs may cause serious health problems to both the mother and the unborn child. These drugs represent an enormous cost to society by causing increased risks of low-birth-weight infants and preterm infants, as well as deficits in child development, if the mother ingests them during pregnancy (National Institute on Drug Abuse [NIDA], 2015).

*Narcotics.* Long-term narcotic use during pregnancy is increasing in prevalence. Signs of narcotic withdrawal in the newborn include tremors, irritability, hyperactivity, vomiting, diarrhea, sweating, poor feeding, and possibly convulsions. No evidence suggests withdrawal in infants whose mothers used cocaine or amphetamines, although there is an increased risk of preterm births, neonatal irritability, placental abruption, premature rupture of membranes, and fetal distress (Kremer & Arora, 2015). Frequent maternal marijuana use during pregnancy may cause fetal immunological problems, but evidence conflicts with an unclear impact. Current research has shown that some infants born to women who used marijuana during their pregnancies display altered responses to visual stimuli, increased tremulousness, and a high-pitched cry, which could indicate problems with neurological development (NIDA, 2015). To avoid these problems, nurses must recognize women who abuse drugs and assist them in seeking appropriate help. This task may be difficult because drug abusers often try to hide their habit, fear being reported to the police, and may be unable to change their lifestyle without extensive intervention.

Drug and substance misuse is a serious public health issue in the United States, especially among women of childbearing age. The problem of drug abuse during pregnancy has affected women in all communities, races, and cultures and of all ages and socioeconomic levels. As a result, many infants are born exposed to illicit substances in utero, are addicted, and develop the complex disorder known as **neonatal abstinence syndrome**. This is a drug withdrawal syndrome that most commonly occurs after an in utero exposure to addictive prescriptive or illicit drugs, such as opioids, which has been increasing in prevalence during the last decade (Tolia et al., 2015). Infants with neonatal abstinence syndrome have prolonged hospital stays, they experience serious medical complications, and their treatment is very costly. Any prenatal substance abuse can have lifelong consequences for the newborn.

For early identification of newborns needing interventions, the nurse should observe newborns with a history of maternal drug abuse for the following: hyperactivity, shrill cry, muscle tension, tremors, seizures, sneezing, yawning, restless sleep, disorganized suck, vomiting, diarrhea, poor feeding, tachypnea, scratches on face, flushing, and sweating. Supporting care for these infants with neonatal abstinence syndrome includes placing them in a quiet area with dim lights, using a tight swaddling position on the side or back, using calming techniques and rocking, clustering infant-care activities with gentle handling, encouraging nonnutritive sucking, providing small, frequent feedings, and administering pharmacological agents as ordered to control withdrawal symptoms.

Nurses need to possess knowledge in the area of chemical dependency, as many women continue to consume nonprescribed drugs during pregnancy. Additionally, knowledge of how to recognize symptoms of withdrawal in infants during the immediate newborn period can lead to improved outcomes if they are treated appropriately during their withdrawal period. Nurses can also help children learn about the negative effects of consuming alcohol and other illicit drugs, especially during pregnancy. By understanding child development and appropriate strategies for teaching children, nurses can play an important role in the prevention of alcohol and illicit drug use among women during pregnancy.

*Alcohol.* Alcohol is the most widely used recreational substance worldwide. Many women in today's society drink alcohol regularly. Research has demonstrated that alcohol is a teratogen, a substance that can cause abnormal development in a growing fetus, as it crosses the placenta readily. Recognition of the effects that even low levels of prenatal alcohol exposure can have on the physical and cognitive development of a child led to the coining of the umbrella term **fetal alcohol spectrum disorder** (FASD). Fetal exposure to alcohol throughout pregnancy may cause **fetal alcohol syndrome** (FAS) or fetal alcohol spectrum disorder (FASD), a collection of symptoms including intrauterine growth restriction, increased risk of facial anomalies, structural brain abnormalities, mental health problems, attention-deficit/hyperactivity disorder, and retardation. It is clinically proven that alcohol consumption during all stages of pregnancy puts the fetus at risk of being born with lifelong alcohol-related brain damage (Viteri et al., 2015). Recent studies have reported symptoms of fetal alcohol disorder in children whose mothers may have consumed just a couple of drinks a day at certain stages of pregnancy. Another study confirmed that fetal alcohol syndrome is not the only problem connected with drinking during pregnancy: it is also a risk factor for early alcohol abuse and dependence in the child (Straussner & Fewell, 2015). Numerous studies have shown that no safe level of alcohol use exists during pregnancy; therefore alcohol consumption should be avoided during this time and when conception is being

attempted. The consequences of prenatal alcohol exposure are often grave, inhibiting both physical and intellectual development, societal acceptance, and adult success. The evidence is clear—alcohol can be more damaging to the developing fetus than heroin, cocaine, or any other drug, producing by far the most serious neurobehavioral effects in the fetus. Prenatal alcohol exposure is the leading preventable cause of intellectual disability in the United States. As many as 1 in 20 infants born today are affected by prenatal exposure to alcohol (Bingham, 2015). Nurses need to stress this finding to make all women aware of avoiding alcohol consumption during their pregnancy. Nurses can help deliver the message that alcohol poses grave risks during pregnancy. Eliminating alcohol consumption during pregnancy is an important measure to take to provide future generations with a healthy start in life and reach their full potential in life.

*Nicotine.* In the United States it is estimated that approximately 16% of pregnant women smoke during their pregnancies. Carbon monoxide and nicotine from tobacco smoke may interfere with the oxygen supply to the fetus. Nicotine also readily crosses the placenta, and concentrations in the fetus can be as much as 15% higher than maternal levels. Nicotine concentrates in fetal blood, amniotic fluid, and breast milk. Combined, these factors can have severe consequences for the fetuses and infants of mothers who smoke (NIDA, 2015). The US Preventive Services Task Force (2015b) recommends that clinicians ask all pregnant women about tobacco use and provide an augmented, pregnancy-tailored counseling framework for engaging women in smoking cessation discussions:

- Ask the woman about tobacco use.
- Advise the woman to quit through clear, personalized messages.
- Assess the woman's willingness to quit.
- Assist the woman to quit.
- Arrange follow-up and support.

Evidence indicates that maternal smoking causes increased rates of spontaneous abortion and ectopic pregnancy, decreased fertility, fetal growth restriction, increased numbers of low-birth-weight or preterm infants, placental abnormalities, vaginal bleeding, congenital anomalies, perinatal death, and premature rupture of the membranes. The best advice for pregnant mothers or women considering pregnancy is to cease all use of tobacco products, decreasing smoking if the woman is a heavy smoker, and avoiding places where smoking occurs. The nurse needs to understand the context of smoking in a woman's life and the complexity of her choice to quit smoking so as to propose solutions to decrease fetal exposure to nicotine (Box 16-10: Research for Evidence-Based Practice).

*Caffeine.* Caffeine is a widely consumed psychoactive substance. It is a stimulant found in tea, coffee, cola, chocolate, and some OTC medications. Caffeine is an addictive substance. Gene mutations have been found in laboratory animals exposed to moderate amounts of caffeine; however, these defects have not been found in human beings. One study found an association between excess caffeine intake (> 300 mg daily) and a higher risk of low-birth-weight infants (James, 2015). Until additional research clarifies the relationship between caffeine intake and

---

**BOX 16-10  RESEARCH FOR EVIDENCE-BASED PRACTICE**

*Nicotine Replacement Therapy in Pregnancy*

Maternal tobacco smoking during pregnancy is the most significant preventable cause of poor health outcomes for women and their babies, with morbidity resulting from placental abruption, miscarriage, stillbirth, prematurity, low birth weight, neonatal or sudden infant death, and asthma. Frequently, clinicians use nicotine replacement therapy (NRT) in attempts to help pregnant smokers stop smoking. However, although NRT is an effective smoking cessation treatment for nonpregnant smokers, its efficacy and safety in pregnancy have not been demonstrated adequately.

The purpose of this study was to determine the efficacy and safety of nicotine replacement therapy with or without behavioral support when used to support smoking cessation in pregnancy.

**Design, setting, and participants:** In a systematic review of randomized controlled trials in which NRT was used with or without behavioral support to promote smoking cessation, trials providing unequal behavioral support to different trial groups were excluded. Included were randomized controlled trials with designs that permitted independent effects of any type of NRT (e.g., patch, gum) for smoking cessation to be isolated. Five trials were identified that met the criteria, giving a total of 525 enrolled pregnant smokers.

**Findings:** There is currently some evidence to demonstrate that NRT, used by pregnant women for smoking cessation is either effective or safe for long-term use. Although birth outcomes were generally better among those infants born to women who had used NRT, none of the observed differences reached statistical significance. By ensuring that the only difference between the arms of the included trials was the provision of NRT to all participants, the independent effects of NRT that are of most importance to clinicians were isolated. Clinical guidelines assume that when pregnant women are heavily dependent on nicotine, use of NRT will be less harmful to them and their babies than continued smoking; however, these findings have not produced evidence for this assumption. Additional studies are needed to determine the safety and efficiency of NRT.

**Nursing implications:** In the absence of sufficient evidence for either the effectiveness or the safety or long-term use of NRT in pregnancy, nurses should perhaps emphasize the importance of the use of proven, behavioral strategies to promote smoking cessation in pregnancy to ensure optimal outcomes.

From Dhalwani, N. N., Szatkowski, L., Coleman, T., Fiaschi, L., & Tata, L. J. (2015). Nicotine replacement therapy in pregnancy and major congenital anomalies in offspring. *Pediatrics, 135*(5), 859–867; Prochaska, J. J. (2015). Nicotine replacement therapy as a maintenance treatment. *JAMA, 314*(7), 718–719.

fetal effects, nurses should teach pregnant women to avoid excess caffeine intake.

## Chemical Substances

The influence of chemicals on human development remains unclear. Some natural substances found to be teratogenic in animals, but not necessarily in human beings, include insect and bacterial toxins, insecticides, herbicides, and fungicides, including dichlorodiphenyltrichloroethane (DDT). Fish is a source of several nutrients that are important during pregnancy for healthy fetal development, including iodine, omega-3 polyunsaturated fatty acids, and vitamins A, D, and $B_{12}$. Recent studies involving pregnant women who eat large amounts of fish with high mercury levels (shark, swordfish, king mackerel, canned tuna, or tilefish) support evidence that mercury negatively affects fetal development, particularly brain development, and may be associated with preterm labor (Starling et al., 2015). Women can safely eat up to 12 ounces of cooked fish weekly. Some studies report stillbirths, abortions, preterm births, and mental retardation in fetuses exposed to lead. This area needs more study, particularly with more women working in traditional male workplaces where there are environmental contaminants. Nurses assess and provide women in their first trimester with information on environmental agents that are potentially damaging throughout gestation and counsel them on ways to avoid exposure.

## Medications Given During Childbirth

The final time that the fetus encounters drugs through the mother is during the birthing process. Many women desire medications for labor discomforts, and usually only medications deemed safe and monitored closely during labor and birth have been used (e.g., epidural anesthetics, opiate agonists in small doses). Some analgesic drugs administered during labor can cause neonatal sedation and respiratory depression and can influence the rate and quality of the infant's adaptation to extrauterine life. Studies of visual attentiveness and sucking behavior, as well as neurological tests and electroencephalography, suggest that fetal depressant effects may last as long as days after birth (Halpern & Garg, 2015).

## Mechanical Forces

The amniotic fluid reservoir protects the fetus during pregnancy and during mild to moderate trauma to the mother's abdomen. However, major trauma to the mother's abdomen, such as that sustained in a severe car accident, may cause maternal bleeding, preterm labor, and other concerns. The nurse instructs the pregnant woman in the proper way to wear both a lap belt and a shoulder harness to protect her and her fetus while driving. All women in the second and third trimesters should be encouraged to seek medical care following an accident believed to influence the health of mother or fetus.

The uterus, another mechanical force, also influences the fetus. Near the end of pregnancy, the fetus outgrows the uterus and becomes molded by it, particularly in cases of multiple pregnancy. Some children have congenitally dislocated hips from uterine pressure and fetal position in utero. Most deformities resolve either naturally or with repositioning after birth. Fetal malposition cannot be prevented; therefore the neonate is assessed for problems and support is provided to the parents about the newborn's appearance.

The actual labor and birth process represents the final mechanical force. Few newborns experience injury during this process, and those who do usually recover with limited effect. It is difficult to predict and prevent birth traumas, such as when delivery of an infant who is larger than expected requires vacuum extraction, which may injure the child. In these cases, on the basis of health care team assessment, the mother may undergo cesarean section to protect herself and the baby.

## Radiation

Radiation exposure during pregnancy has been debated for years, but various experiences are continuing to show that there are increasingly negative effects on the growing fetus, as well as effects later in life. Scientific evidence indicates that exposure to X-rays, especially early in pregnancy during organogenesis, may cause chromosomal changes, spontaneous abortion, growth restriction, microcephaly, fetal loss, or malignancy later in life (Abdalla & Elshikh, 2015). The fetus is most sensitive to radiation effects between 8 and 15 weeks of pregnancy, and thus should be spared any radiation exposure during that period (Gök et al., 2015). The literature supports a greater incidence of leukemia in children of women exposed to X-rays during pregnancy compared with children whose mothers were not exposed. Unless the benefits of radiographic information clearly outweigh the risks of exposing the fetus to X-rays, these examinations should not be performed during gestation. If radiography is deemed necessary, the wearing of a lead apron, use of as low a radiation dose as possible, and application of other recommendations made by the National Council on Radiation Protection and Measurements should be used to protect the developing fetus.

# DETERMINANTS OF HEALTH

## Social Factors and Environment

### Community and Work

Women now constitute a significant portion of the workforce. Many more women now work outside the home, either in careers or in jobs needed for family economic survival. As each woman considers or experiences pregnancy, she will need to ask herself questions that will optimize her pregnancy outcome. These questions include the following: Is my work strenuous or possibly dangerous to my baby because of exposure to toxic substances? Do I need to work for long periods, influencing my need for rest? Will workplace stressors influence my coping with pregnancy and my family needs?

A safe workplace environment (one that does not involve exposure to hazardous substances or organisms and provides adequate breaks for worker rest and body movement) will allow a pregnant woman to work until her baby is due, unless her health becomes impaired. The nurse helps each woman assess the safety of her workplace and suggests ways to decrease hazards in that setting. These hazards include exposure to viruses, fungi, industrial products (hydrocarbons or pesticides), second-hand smoke, radiation emitted by medical diagnostic equipment, air pollutants, and asbestos and the possibility of workplace violence, mental and physical stress, and even noise pollution. The nurse encourages the pregnant worker to consider workplace ergonomics, addressing how the current work space will meet her changing physical needs.

Some employers in the United States have been designated creators of "family friendly" work environments, because they have willingly made accommodations to support breastfeeding and pregnant workers and their families. These accommodations allow women to prioritize their pregnancy and family needs. Evidence indicates that such approaches reduce pregnancy complications and increase work productivity. Although few in number, family friendly employers offer health-promotion programs focusing on healthy nutrition, stress management, and exercise for employees, who experience better health outcomes.

As a rule, however, too few employers support flexible work schedules for prenatal care visits, rest periods for pregnant workers, or removal of vending machines to support optimal nutrition for pregnant working class women. Some working women, regardless of status, believe that once they announce their pregnancy, they will face workplace pressure to stop working or change positions in the company to suit their gestational needs. On the basis of experience, some employers fear that their pregnant employees will overuse sick time or seek a reduced workload.

In a recent study of pregnancy within the workplace, two factors were identified that may be challenging. In many workplaces, pressures on women to "ignore" pregnancy and to "push on" through sickness and exhaustion may relate to certain workplace cultures referred to as "male norms." The partiality for male norms could be seen as creating problems for these pregnant women, who feel obliged to downplay their "inherent femaleness" by minimizing their pregnancy so as to fit in with workplace notions of reliability and presence.

Secondly, health advice on pregnancy might also be difficult to implement within women's workplaces because of underlying assumptions, reflected in health advice, that women's care is most appropriately performed in the home. It is significant that health guidance on pregnancy care work makes little reference to place and offers slender guidance on how pregnancy care work might be implemented at work. Common sense suggests that instructions about napping during the day and using ice packs to relieve hemorrhoids would be entirely inappropriate within most workplaces, whatever the occupation of the pregnant woman (Fox & Quinn, 2015).

Research suggests that pregnant women are discriminated against in the workplace and that a significant number of new mothers leave the workforce. The pregnant woman must deal with these situations by being factual and assertive about her ability to continue working. National law dictates that it is illegal to discriminate against a woman because she is pregnant. If a woman believes that she has been treated unfairly because of her pregnancy, she may pursue the issue legally or become active in local women's rights organizations to gain support. However, when a woman leaves a job that did not support her pregnancy, she often gives up accrued leave time or takes a lower salary in another job. These outcomes influence her choices during pregnancy and early parenting.

Workplaces differ greatly in allowing leave time during and after pregnancy. Federal legislation, the Family and Medical Leave Act, obligates employers of at least 50 people to provide up to 12 weeks of paid leave for new parents or women who have medical problems during pregnancy. Ideally a woman who desires children should explore the issue of leave during a job interview, but many women fail to do this until they are already pregnant. A woman often requires written verification from her physician if she needs a leave of absence from her job attributable to pregnancy complications. Although she may wish to return to work shortly after giving birth, the woman is counseled to allow sufficient time to regain her strength and adapt to parenting. The nurse may help the couple make reasonable decisions related to locating resources for child care, exploring "shared time" with other new mothers or part-time employees (e.g., middle-age adults caring for their older parents), or finding ways of balancing work and family needs.

## Culture and Ethnicity

With the increasing diversity in the United States populations, nurses are challenged to develop culturally competent skills that meet the social, cultural, and linguistic needs of those for whom they care. Cultural competence is not static and requires frequent relearning and unlearning about diversity. Nurses must acknowledge the implications of their own "cultural lens" and continuously reflect on their own assumptions, biases, and stereotypes. Nurses must adopt an attitude of open-mindedness and respect for all cultures. Cultural groups have unique ideas and beliefs related to pregnancy, childbirth, and childbearing that must be understood by the nurse so as to render individualized care to each pregnant woman. As part of the assessment, the nurse determines the cultural attachment of a woman by asking the following question: Do you think that some or most of the childbearing ideas of your culture are old-fashioned, and do you feel obligated to follow these ideas, at least superficially, because of family pressure? In this situation, the nurse may need to be a confidant for the woman who needs to vent her frustrations about cultural restrictions.

Nonconscious stereotyping and prejudice contribute to racial and ethnic disparities in health care. Contemporary training in cultural competence is insufficient to reduce these problems because even educated, culturally sensitive nurses can activate and use their biases without being aware they are doing so. Research in social psychology shows that over time stereotypes and prejudices become invisible to those who rely on them. Automatic categorization of an individual as a member of a social group can unconsciously trigger the thoughts (stereotypes) and feelings (prejudices) associated with that group. This implies that, when activated, implicit negative attitudes and stereotypes shape how nurses evaluate and interact with minority groups. This makes minority group care recipients uncomfortable and discourages them from seeking or adhering to treatment (Tucker et al., 2015).

Nurses need to be very cognizant of their stereotyping and prejudices and "park them at the door-stop" before interacting with minority women. Have nurses ever thought about why pregnant women do not seek prenatal care or do not return for follow-up care once they have encountered a negative reception? If nurses would reverse roles with minority women and just imagine how it feels to encounter negative attitudes when needing health care, perhaps biased attitudes would change dramatically (Villarreal, 2015).

Nurses need an awareness of how culture, tradition, and acculturation may affect the women for whom they provide care, as this is the first step toward understanding diverse cultural behavior. The next step is for nurses to be aware of the three "levels" of culture when offering health advice and planning health care for various diverse groups:

- The *primary* level of culture refers to rules that are known by all and obeyed by all and may be almost unconsciously performed by women (e.g., health, healing and health-belief systems, or how illness, diseases, and their causes are perceived by that specific culture).
- The *secondary* level is the underlying rules and guidelines known by the group but not generally relayed to outsiders. This may include taboos and rituals relating to behavior, which may be followed depending on the individual.
- A *tertiary* level is visible to the outsider, such as traditional dress, foods, and religious ceremonies (Darnell & Hickson, 2015).

Intercultural caring by nurses is complex. However, nurses need to have a positive attitude and demonstrate acceptance of different cultures. This can be achieved by nurses taking the stance of respecting and understanding diversity, as well as acknowledging any barriers such as culture. Nursing support may assist the individual in adjusting both her needs and those of the culture she represents to experience a satisfactory pregnancy.

The nurse has an obligation to read about and seek information on cultures encountered in practice and to become active in community organizations that represent cultures whose members get prenatal care from the nurse. Above all, the nurse must be open to a variety of viewpoints, judging them not against personal beliefs but rather in relation to the general concept of health promotion and today's goal to provide culturally competent care to a variety of cultural groups. All nurses want to deliver care that is inclusive, that is sensitive to the care seeker's and the family's needs, and that respects the values of their health beliefs and practices. To do this, nurses need to learn about the most common minority cultures with which they interact (Box 16-11: Diversity Awareness).

## Levels of Policy Making and Health

Both legislative actions and social movements influence childbearing. In some countries, such as China, the government decrees the number of children a couple may have and imposes economic or social sanctions to enforce these restrictions. Although Americans may have as many children as they desire, various coalitions lobby strongly for families. The Family and Medical Leave Act validates the federal government's commitment to prioritizing family issues by giving new parents time off from work during the early months of parenthood, while supporting these individuals' professional work goals and needs.

The US government remains concerned about the health of pregnant women and ways to decrease fetal and infant morbidity and mortality. Historically, states have used federal monies from Medicaid and Title V maternal and child health block programs to provide services for pregnant women and children. Many countries provide universal access to prenatal care, but in the

---

🌐 **BOX 16-11** **DIVERSITY AWARENESS**

### Nursing Roles in Providing Culturally Competent Care

In recent years, greater emphasis has been placed on nurses recognizing and appreciating **diversity** so as to acquire cultural competency. Cultural knowledge is the most important construct of cultural competence for nurses, being crucial for the accurate appreciation of a care recipient's worldview. Delivery of culturally competent care implies that a nurse acknowledges and acts on the unique history that a pregnant woman and her family bring to a health care interaction. The essence of both the client centeredness and competence for the nurse is the importance of seeing the woman as a unique individual. The nurse supports culturally competent care by:

- Recognizing that cultural diversity exists and affects the process and outcome of health care
- Respecting people as unique individuals who, by their differences from the majority, bring a broadened definition of appropriate health care
- Using data gained from a cultural assessment for completion of a care plan
- Encouraging cultural behavior that protects the biopsychosocial, spiritual, and safety needs of the individual
- Gaining insight into the nurse's own beliefs and values about people who may be different from or have needs different from those of the majority or those of the nurse's own culture; understanding how these beliefs and values influence the outcomes of health care delivery with childbearing families
- Recognizing the values of the health care system reflected in the customs and practices of birthing facilities
- Providing interpreters to improve communication between the individual and health care providers
- Becoming literate in languages, customs, and cultural practices of people commonly seen in the health care environment
- Developing cultural humility by maintaining an interpersonal stance as it relates to the other person from a different culture
- Recognizing and valuing the diversity of those seeking care and entering all therapeutic relationships acknowledging that nurses are always in the process of learning and growing

From Foronda, C. L., Baptiste, D., Reinholdt, M. M., & Ousman, K. (2016). Cultural humility: A concept analysis. *Journal of Transcultural Nursing, 27*(3), 210–217; Garneau, A. B. (2016). Critical reflection in cultural competence development: A framework for undergraduate nursing education. *Journal of Nursing Education, 55*(3), 125–132.

United States low-income women rely on Medicaid, a joint federal-state program, to cover most of the cost of prenatal care. With constraints on state and federal budgets, many of which fund community prenatal clinics, concerns have been expressed about whether there will be sufficient money to fund women and children's care programs. Local health departments may offer free or low-cost prenatal care for women who are pregnant, but again the extent of services depends on state government or local allocation of funds. Despite this free or low-cost care and Affordable Care Act health insurance with subsidies, more than 36 million Americans lack health insurance and therefore face barriers that affect their easy access to prenatal care (Levy, 2015; USDHHS, 2010). Many ethnically diverse populations, and in particular Hispanic groups, lack insurance and a level of education that increases their understanding of health-related information (low health literacy) for family health promotion. Educating women during the childbearing cycle is particularly important to increase the chances of families obtaining and understanding health-promotion information for healthier behaviors (USDHHS, 2010).

With the nurse's help in data collection, consumers should be encouraged to express their views and opinions on pregnancy and parenting topics to their elected governmental representatives. This expression indeed works; many states recently legislated hospital stays of at least 48 hours for women with vaginal deliveries and even longer stays for women with cesarean deliveries. These laws evolved from public concern over premature discharges of new mothers as part of managed care insurance directives. Longer stays help health care providers identify potential problems in the mother or the baby before discharge, such as difficulty breastfeeding. Continued legislative work on insurance reform may improve family planning services so that couples can plan pregnancies to better meet their sociocultural and financial goals and needs (USDHHS, 2010). The Patient Protection and Affordable Care Act of 2010 was the most sweeping health care legislation in a generation and impacted women's health tremendously. Insurance reform, driven by legislative change, may also improve health care coverage for underinsured individuals who lack a consistent source of prenatal care or report difficulties in receiving care because of communication, structural, or personal barriers within their insurance system (Armstrong, 2015).

### Economics

When the pregnant woman begins prenatal care, personal financial resources influence the kind of care she receives, the need to remain employed during or after a pregnancy, the acceptance of her pregnancy, her nutritional status, and other choices. The expenses of planning and experiencing a pregnancy may determine whether the woman or her family faces a financial crisis. The nurse needs to understand the financial history and priorities of the couple because this information will affect access to and use of prenatal care.

The nurse inquires in a sensitive fashion about a woman's or a couple's finances to make appropriate referral to resources for care (e.g., Title V or Medicaid programs). Until recently, Medicaid provided no adolescent family planning services, a situation that may have influenced high rates of pregnancy in some sectors of this country (USDHHS, 2010). Many low-income women qualify for the USDA's Special Supplemental Nutrition Program for Women, Infants, and Children. This program provides essential foods such as milk, cheese, and eggs to pregnant and lactating women. During prenatal visits, the nurse may help a woman or family plan a budget for food and other essential requirements based on individual family needs, cultural values, the need for a healthy diet during pregnancy, and income level. Local food banks and second-hand clothing and baby supply stores may provide needed items for these families. Occasionally women may access free transportation and child care at the prenatal clinic if the nurse provides information about this program.

### Health Services/Delivery System

Options for care during pregnancy range from medical-based care by a health care professional to more health-promotion–focused care by a nurse practitioner or midwife. Globally, 80%

of people alive today have been born with the assistance of midwives (Midwives Alliance of North America, 2015). Midwives have a long tradition that includes watchful waiting, sharing empirical knowledge, protecting the normal, nonmedicalized birth process, and engaging in research to incorporate the findings into evidence-based practice. Midwifery is distinguished by characteristics that define a partnership with women by listening, being sensitive to cultural, sexual, and generational needs, encouraging shared decision-making, and practicing patience to be "with women" during their most vulnerable periods (King et al., 2015). Several national organizations provide oversight for practicing midwives. The American College of Nurse-Midwives [ACNM] is the professional association that represents certified nurse-midwives and certified midwives in the United States to set the standards in midwifery education and practice (ACNM, 2015). The National Association of Certified Professional Midwives [NACPM] is the membership organization specifically representing certified professional midwives to be a powerful voice to influence maternity health policies (NACPM, 2015). Geographical availability of options, finances, previous experience, partner's preference, cultural or social acceptability of certain options, and preexisting or newly recognized risk factors will influence a woman's choice of care. Because of her culture and the belief that pregnancy is not an illness, a woman may not seek Western medical prenatal care, but rather may rely on individuals from her culture to provide care until the actual labor, when she will go to a hospital.

Unless complications arise a woman generally chooses where she will labor and give birth and the extent of labor and birthing process intervention. The movement toward home birth that began during the early 1970s continues to meet some women's needs for a more family-oriented, natural, health-focused experience. However, most couples choose a hospital birth setting because of the availability of emergency equipment and personnel in the case of complications. Some insurance companies will reimburse only births that occur in hospitals and in birth centers or birthing rooms attached to a hospital. The nurse helps expectant couples become aware of the care and birthing alternatives to make an informed choice for a positive labor and birth experience. Women who lack resources to access the health care delivery system and teaching by the nurse during regular prenatal visits are generally less able to make informed decisions that affect their childbearing experiences.

Many expectant couples also make an informed choice about the actual process of labor and birth by developing a birth plan—those components of care and intervention that the couple desires for the birth experience. A pregnant woman and her partner may choose natural childbirth or a method of analgesia or anesthesia. The nurse helps the pregnant woman and her partner choose the most appropriate method by providing information about options and encouraging questions about each option. Collaboration between the nurse and the woman or couple in meeting their birth plan goals is important because research shows that women remember their labor and birthing experiences for a long time. A positively viewed birth experience may support a couple's involvement as active health care consumers, thus facilitating the future health of their family.

The nurse may encourage the pregnant couple or woman to attend prenatal classes. These provide valuable information and preparation for birth for many couples. The International Childbirth Education Association, the American Society for Psychoprophylaxis in Obstetrics (ASPO), and many local groups offer a variety of classes for the expectant couple. These classes may include information on early pregnancy, Lamaze-ASPO or Bradley methods, cesarean birth, breastfeeding, infant cardiopulmonary resuscitation, and parenting. Sibling classes for the newborn and involvement of children in the birth experience may also increase sibling bonding.

## NURSING APPLICATION

Teaching the pregnant woman and her partner during the prenatal period is the most important role of the nurse. Even the woman who has previously given birth or who has a high degree of education may need or want information from the health care team that will assist her family to adapt effectively to changes of pregnancy to support a healthy birth outcome.

To provide appropriate teaching, the nurse performs a comprehensive assessment that involves the entire family. Assessment, the first step in the nursing process, allows the nurse to determine maternal and fetal physical and psychological risks, the woman's informational base for pregnancy and birth, and cultural and family needs. Assessment should also include physical, spiritual, emotional, and sociocultural inspection and recognition of abuse. Battering increases during pregnancy and may be detected by physical, emotional, behavioral, and history assessment of the woman. Pregnant women at high risk of abuse include adolescents, those with low incomes, and those with a history of alcohol or drug abuse, as well as those with a partner with a similar history (Bohra et al., 2015; Copelon, 2015). In cases of suspected abuse, the nurse, in consultation with other members of the health care team, provides support and resources for the woman to make an informed decision about protecting herself and her fetus during pregnancy. The nurse may also want to refer the woman to a professional counselor for a brief counseling outreach intervention or abuse shelter for personal safety (Jewkes & Penn-Kekana, 2015).

As discussed in this chapter, assessment may also be made by use of Gordon's (2016) functional health patterns, a common conceptual framework for clinical assessment (see Box 16-5). Data used in the assessment process will likely be collected during the prenatal visit and may change depending on life occurrences of the pregnant woman. A woman may be defined as high risk during her pregnancy if she experiences heavy bleeding, premature labor, elevated blood pressure, or extreme anxiety; if there is fetal distress; or if the woman shows unexpected behavior or symptoms. After noting these high-risk conditions, the nurse should refer the pregnant woman to an obstetrical specialist or other resources for pregnant women and their families (see the case study at the end of this chapter).

After a complete assessment during each prenatal visit, the nurse develops a teaching plan for the individual. Throughout the prenatal course, the nurse collaborates with the woman and her partner to assess their learning and support needs. For example, literature on bottle feeding or breastfeeding may be provided to help a woman decide on a method, and books, videos, and websites may help couples understand more about birth and therefore feel that they have more control during labor and in meeting their birthing goals. If the woman plans to attend group prenatal classes, the nurse should coordinate her teaching content and process with those expected in the classes, thereby preventing undue repetition. The nurse teaching prenatal classes should provide a list of topics to participants in the class to share with their health care providers. A woman may be knowledgeable in some areas, and the nurse can use this knowledge as a foundation for further individualized teaching. Box 16-12 covers relevant topics to be covered by the nurse during prenatal care interactions with pregnant women. These topical areas relate to nursing interventions discussed earlier in this chapter. Basic handouts detailing danger signs of pregnancy can be posted in the home to consult if the woman experiences unexpected complications of pregnancy.

---

### BOX 16-12   Topics for Prenatal Care Teaching

- Rationale for and interpretation of physical findings and laboratory results
- Value of keeping appointments
- Danger signs that should be reported
- Breast care to prepare for lactation
- Breastfeeding versus bottle feeding
- Exercise and rest
- Fetal growth and development
- Physical and psychological changes during pregnancy and relief measures
- Effects of smoking, drinking, and drugs on the fetus
- Nutrition
- Work and play
- Body mechanics
- Personal hygiene
- Sex during pregnancy
- Preparation for labor and birth
- Superstitions and old wives' tales
- Signs of impending labor
- Supplies and preparations for the baby
- Partner's and siblings' responses

---

## CASE STUDY

### *Active Labor: Susan Wong*

Mrs. Wong, a first-time mother, is admitted to the birthing suite in early labor after spontaneous rupture of membranes at home. She is at 38 weeks of gestation with a history of abnormal alpha-fetoprotein levels at 16 weeks of pregnancy. She was scheduled for ultrasonography to visualize the fetus to rule out an open spinal defect or Down syndrome, but never followed through. Mrs. Wong and her husband disagreed about what to do (keep or terminate the pregnancy) if the ultrasonography indicated a spinal problem, so they felt they did not want this information.

#### Reflective Questions

- As the nurse, what priority data would you collect from this couple to help define relevant interventions to meet their needs?
- How can you help this couple if they experience a negative outcome in the birthing suite? What are your personal views on terminating or continuing a pregnancy with a risk of a potential anomaly? What factors may influence your views?
- With the influence of the recent Human Genome Project and the possibility of predicting open spinal defects earlier in pregnancy, how will maternity care change in the future?

#### Prediction of Human Disease

An organism's complete set of DNA is called its genome. Virtually every single cell in the body contains a complete copy of the approximately 3 billion DNA base pairs, or letters, that make up the human genome. The Human Genome Project (completed in 2003), conducted by the National Human Genome Research Institute, produced a very high-quality version of the human genome sequence that is freely available in public databases. Researchers have been able to use DNA sequencing to search for genetic variations and/or mutations that may play a role in the development or progression of a range of diseases. Clearly, there are implications and ethical considerations for the health sciences here. Along with the important information uncovered by the Human Genome Project, a great controversy arose. Even though blood tests are now available for the detection of various fatal diseases such as Huntington disease, cystic fibrosis, and colon cancer, many people would rather live with uncertainty than know they have an incurable life-threatening disease. Sadly, the tests, which have been developed, are to detect the disease and not cure it.

Another consideration is the use of genetic information by existing and prospective employers. Imagine a situation where employment preference is given to those who can demonstrate they are "genetically free" of future diseases that might limit their capacity to work. Still, three major unsolved problems in perinatal and neonatal health are preterm birth; the neonatal consequences of vaginal versus cesarean birth; and neonatal gastrointestinal disease, specifically necrotizing enterocolitis. Hopefully soon, the Human Genome Project's research will be able to address all three to improve pregnancy outcomes.

In just 1 decade, the Human Genome Project has sparked an explosion of information that has proved useful to basic and clinical scientists. We must remain cautious as to how and when this new information and technology are used in the future to ensure they are used for the betterment of humankind.

## ⊚ CARE PLAN

### *Nursing Management for Stages of Labor: Susan Wong*

**\*NURSING DIAGNOSIS: Ineffective coping related to active labor status**

#### Defining Characteristics

- Initiation of labor at 2:00 a. m. with spontaneous rupture of membranes
- First-time mother who did not attend childbirth classes
- Supportive spouse
- Current gestational age of 38 weeks
- Contraction pattern defined as moderate intensity, frequency every 2 minutes, 60 seconds in duration
- After 6 hours of labor, 4 cm dilated, 100% effaced, and stage active phase
- Moaning, moving around in bed, and stating, "I can't take this much longer; it hurts too much!"

#### Related Factors

- Prenatal history of abnormal alpha-fetoprotein levels at 16 weeks
- Prenatal care since 12 weeks pregnant
- History of depression in college
- Works as an engineer with large manufacturing firm
- Gravida 1, parity 0
- Recent resident of city, moved from East Coast approximately 4 months ago
- 25 years of age, Asian family history, married for 1 year

#### Expected Outcomes

- Mother will state level of pain to be less than 4 on a scale of 1 to 10 during labor.
- Mother will successfully use visual imagery techniques, massage, and slow deep breathing for relaxation during labor.
- Mother will state early in labor at least three ways to cope effectively with pain and will implement these strategies as relevant.
- Fetus will demonstrate an expected heart rate pattern and will experience no compromise during labor.
- Mother and family will verbalize their needs during labor and delivery to the health care team.

#### Interventions

- Assess level of labor discomfort every 20 to 30 minutes and as needed according to pain scale rating of 1 to 10.
- Implement and document nursing interventions (backrubs, heat and cold applications, position changes, back pressure and massage, and birth pool therapy, among others) to relieve labor discomforts.
- Assess cultural beliefs with labor and delivery management and implement interventions as needed to meet practice standards.
- Provide teaching about labor and delivery progress and breathing, visual imagery, and massage techniques that may decrease labor discomfort.
- Provide verbal and nonverbal reassurance during labor.
- Teach about fetal response during labor and rationale for nursing interventions to support fetal health, such as use of left side position to increase placental blood flow.
- Throughout labor, answer any questions from the mother and family members about needs and responses to labor process.
- Involve family members as much as possible during labor and as requested by the mother to improve her ability to cope.

*NANDA Nursing Diagnoses—Herdman T. H. & Kamitsuru, S. (Eds.). Nursing Diagnoses–Definitions and Classification 2015–2017. Copyright © 2014, 1994–2014 NANDA International. Used by arrangement with John Wiley & Sons Limited. In order to make safe and effective judgments using the NANDA-I nursing diagnoses it is essential that nurses refer to the definitions and defining characteristics of the diagnoses listed in this work.

## SUMMARY

Dramatic changes occur during pregnancy: a new life forms and develops and the expectant family members (mother, father, siblings, and other close members) experience major changes in their roles and relationships with each other. Although all fetal development processes, changes in pregnant women's bodies, and role transitions among family members share common elements, each family uniquely experiences pregnancy because of life experience and personal values. The focus is the entire family, although the nurse most often deals directly with the pregnant woman. The nurse provides valuable resources and information that the family may use to meet its specific needs. The overall nursing goal involves assisting each family to have a healthy pregnancy and birth outcome, to lay the foundation for satisfactory parenting and family life.

## ⓔ EVOLVE CHAPTER FEATURES

http://evolve.elsevier.com/Edelman/

- Study Questions

## REFERENCES

Abdalla, I., & Elshikh, M. (2015). Effect of radiation on pregnancy. *International Journal of Medicine and Medical Sciences, 7*(5), 98–101.

Adam, S. (2015). HIV and pregnancy: Review. *Obstetrics and Gynecology Forum, 25*(2), 19–22.

American Academy of Pediatrics. (2014). AAP recommendations on iodine nutrition during pregnancy and lactation. *Pediatrics, 134*(4), 1282–1283.

American College of Nurse-Midwives. (2015). About American College of Nurse-Midwives. http://www.midwife.org/About-ACNM.

Apgar, V. (2015). A proposal for a new method of evaluation of the newborn infant. *Anesthesia and Analgesia, 120*(5), 1056–1059.

Armstrong, J. (2015). Women's health in the age of Patient Protection and the Affordable Care Act. *Clinical Obstetrics and Gynecology, 58*(2), 323–335.

Bier, D., et al. (2015). *Nutrition for the primary care provider.* Basel: Karger Medical and Scientific Publishers.

Bingham, R. J. (2015). Latest evidence on alcohol and pregnancy. *Nursing for Women's Health, 19*(4), 338–344.

Biswas, J., et al. (2015). Fetomaternal outcome of pyrexia in pregnancy: A prospective study. *International Journal of Women's Health and Reproductive Sciences, 3*(3), 132–135.

Blackburn, S. T. (2014). *Maternal, fetal, and neonatal physiology: A clinical perspective* (4th ed.). Philadelphia: Elsevier Health Sciences.

Bohra, N., et al. (2015). Violence against women. *Indian Journal of Psychiatry, 57*(6), 333–338.

Brucker, M. C., & King, T. L. (2017). *Pharmacology for women's health* (2nd ed.). Burlington, MA: Jones & Bartlett Learning.

Buckley, S. (2015). *Hormonal physiology of childbearing: Evidence and implications for women, babies and maternity care.* Washington, DC: Childbirth Connection.

Cantor, A. G., et al. (2015). Routine iron supplementation and screening for iron deficiency anemia in pregnancy: A systematic review for the US Preventive Services Task Force. *Annals of Internal Medicine, 162*(8), 566–576.

Carapetis, J. R. (2015). The stark reality of rheumatic heart disease. *European Heart Journal, 36*(18), 1070–1073.

Centers for Disease Control and Prevention (CDC). (2015a). Preconception health and health care. http://www.cdc.gov/preconception/hcp/.

Centers for Disease Control and Prevention (CDC). (2015b). Minority health. https://www.cdc.gov/MinorityHealth/index.html.

Centers for Disease Control and Prevention (CDC). (2015c). Toxoplasmosis and pregnant women. http://www.cdc.gov/parasites/toxoplasmosis/gen_info/pregnant.html.

Centers for Disease Control and Prevention (CDC). (2015d). Syphilis during pregnancy. http://www.cdc.gov/std/tg2015/syphilis-pregnancy.htm.

Centers for Disease Control and Prevention (CDC). (2015e). Genital herpes. http://www.cdc.gov/std/herpes/stdfact-herpes.htm.

Centers for Disease Control and Prevention (CDC). (2015f). HIV among pregnant women, infants, and children. http://www.cdc.gov/hiv/group/gender/pregnantwomen/index.html.

Centers for Disease Control and Prevention (CDC). (2015g). Hepatitis B – perinatal transmission. http://www.cdc.gov/hepatitis/hbv/perinatalxmtn.htm.

Centers for Disease Control and Prevention (CDC). (2015h). Pregnancy-related deaths. http://www.cdc.gov/reproductivehealth/MaternalInfantHealth/Pregnancy-relatedMortality.htm.

Centers for Disease Control and Prevention (CDC). (2016). Zika virus. http://www.cdc.gov/zika/pregnancy/protect-yourself.html.

Central Intelligence Agency. (2015). Country comparison: Infant mortality rate. The world factbook. https://www.cia.gov/library/publications/resources/the-world-factbook/geos/us.html.

Chang, T., & Moniz, M. H. (2015). Pregnancy and weight gain: We have observed enough. *Obstetrics and Gynecology, 126*(1), 215.

Chitayat, D., et al. (2016). Folic acid supplementation for pregnant women and those planning pregnancy–2015 update. *Journal of Clinical Pharmacology, 56*(2), 170–175.

Copelon, R. (2015). Violence against women: The potential and challenge of a human rights perspective. *Women's Health Journal, 2–3*, 62–67.

Cordero, A. M., et al. (2015). Optimal serum and red blood cell folate concentrations in women of reproductive age for prevention of neural tube defects: World Health Organization guidelines. *MMWR. Morbidity and Mortality Weekly Report, 64*(15), 421–423.

Cunningham, F. G., et al. (2014). *William's obstetrics* (24th ed.). New York: McGraw-Hill Medical Education.

Darnell, L. K., & Hickson, S. V. (2015). Cultural competent patient-centered nursing care. *The Nursing Clinics of North America, 50*(1), 99–108.

De Sutter, P. (2015). The challenge of multiple pregnancies. In R. Mathur (Ed.), *Reducing risk in fertility treatment* (pp. 1–17). London: Springer.

Doulatram, G., Raj, T. D., & Govindaraj, R. (2015). Pregnancy and substance abuse. In A. D. Kaye, N. Vadivelu, & R. D. Urmaneds (Eds.), *Substance abuse* (pp. 453–494). New York: Springer.

Ellis, S. A., Wojnar, D. M., & Pettinato, M. (2015). Conception, pregnancy, and birth experiences of male and gender variant gestational parents: It's how we could have a family. *Journal of Midwifery & Women's Health, 60*(1), 62–69.

El-Mazny, A. (2014). *Human reproduction: Basic anatomy and physiology.* Charleston, SC: Amazon CreateSpace.

Fox, A. B., & Quinn, D. M. (2015). Pregnant women at work: The role of stigma in predicting women's intended exit from the workforce. *Psychology of Women Quarterly, 39*(2), 226–242.

Frankford, D. M., et al. (2015). Womb outsourcing: Commercial surrogacy in India. *MCN. The American Journal of Maternal Child Nursing, 40*(5), 284–290.

Galliano, D., & Pellicer, A. (2015). Potential etiologies of unexplained infertility in females. In *Unexplained infertility* (pp. 141–147). New York: Springer.

Gandhi, M., & Martin, S. R. (2015). Cardiac disease in pregnancy. *Obstetrics and Gynecology Clinics of North America, 42*(2), 315–333.

Gök, M., et al. (2015). Prenatal radiation exposure. *Proceedings in Obstetrics and Gynecology, 5*(1), 1–10.

Gordon, M. (2016). *Manual of nursing diagnosis* (13th ed.). Burlington, MA: Jones & Bartlett Learning.

Green, J., et al. (2015). Desperately seeking parenthood: Neonatal nurses reflect on parental anguish. *Journal of Clinical Nursing, 24*, 1885–1894.

Hall, K. S., et al. (2015). Social discrimination, stress, and risk of unintended pregnancy among young women. *The Journal of Adolescent Health, 56*(3), 330–337.

Halpern, S. H., & Garg, R. (2015). Evidence-based medicine and labor analgesia. In *Epidural labor analgesia* (pp. 285–295). Cham, Switzerland: Springer International Publishing.

Hewitt, C., & Cappiello, J. (2015). Essential competencies in nursing education for prevention and care related to unintended pregnancy. *Journal of Obstetric, Gynecologic, and Neonatal Nursing, 44*(1), 69–76.

Holley, S. R., & Pasch, L. A. (2015). Counseling lesbian, gay, bisexual, and transgender patients. In *Fertility counseling* (pp. 180–196). Cambridge, United Kingdom: Cambridge University Press.

Hotchin, R. (2015). The forgotten link between sexual health and pregnancy. *The Practicing Midwife, 18*(5), 32–34.

Hughes, V. (2015). The baby-friendly hospital initiative in US hospitals. *Infant, Child & Adolescent Nutrition, 7*(4), 182–187.

Institute of Medicine (IOM). (2015). Healthy weight gain during pregnancy. http://iom.nationalacademies.org/Reports/2009/Weight-Gain-During-Pregnancy-Reexamining-the-Guidelines.aspx.

Jalili, M. (2015). The analysis of financial and non-financial rights of children who were born by the method of surrogacy. *The Iranian Journal of Medical Law, 8*(30), 37–63.

James, J. E. (2015). Review: Higher caffeine intake during pregnancy increases risk of low birth weight. *Evidence-Based Nursing, 18*(4), 111.

Jewkes, R., & Penn-Kekana, L. (2015). Mistreatment of women in childbirth: Time for action on this important dimension of violence against women. *PLoS Medicine, 12*(6), e1001849.

Jhaveri, R. (2015). Prevention of hepatitis B virus vertical transmission: Time for the next step. *Pediatrics, 135*(5), e1286–e1287.

Johnson, K. A., et al. (2014). Action Plan for the National Initiative on Preconception Health and Health Care (PCHHC). A report of the PCHHC Steering Committee 2012–2014. http://www.cdc.gov/preconception/documents/ActionPlanNationalInitiativePCHHC2012-2014.pdf.

Jyothi, N. (2015). Case study on post pregnancy related complication of pica. *International Journal of Nursing Care, 3*(1), 42–45.

King, T. L., & Brucker, M. C. (2016). *Pharmacology for women* (2nd ed.). Burlington, MA: Jones & Bartlett Learning.

King, T. L., et al. (2015). *Varney's midwifery* (5th ed.). Burlington, MA: Jones & Bartlett Learning.

Kovacs, G., & Briggs, P. (2015). Infections during pregnancy–Varicella, herpes, cytomegalovirus, toxoplasma, Listeria, group B streptococcus. In *Lectures in obstetrics, gynecology and women's health* (pp. 133–137). Cham, Switzerland: Springer International Publishing.

Kremer, M. E., & Arora, K. S. (2015). Clinical, ethical, and legal considerations in pregnant women with opioid abuse. *Obstetrics and Gynecology, 126*(3), 474–478.

Langer, O. (2015). *The diabetes in pregnancy dilemma: Leading the change with proven solutions* (2nd ed.). Shelton, CT: People's Medical Publishing House.

Levy, J. (2015). In U.S., uninsured rate drops to 12% in first quarter. Gallup. http://www.gallup.com/poll/182348/uninsured-rate-dips-first-quarter.aspx.

Lewitt, M. (2015). Promoting normal physiologic birth through partnership with consumers, providers, and hospitals. *Journal of Obstetric, Gynecologic, and Neonatal Nursing, 44*, S21.

Liat, S., et al. (2015). Obesity in obstetrics. *Best Practice & Research. Clinical Obstetrics & Gynaecology, 29*(1), 79–90.

Lim, C. C., & Mahmood, T. (2015). Obesity in pregnancy. *Best Practice & Research. Clinical Obstetrics & Gynaecology, 29*(3), 309–319.

Lissauer, T., et al. (2015). *Neonatology at a glance* (3rd ed.). Somerset, NJ: Wiley-Blackwell.

Macones, G. (2015). *Management of labor and delivery* (2nd ed.). Somerset, NJ: Wiley-Blackwell.

Mader, S., & Windelspecht, M. (2015). *Human biology* (14th ed.). New York: McGraw-Hill Higher Education.

March of Dimes. (2015). Birth defects. http://www.marchofdimes.org/baby/birth-defects.aspx.

Mattson, S., & Smith, J. E. (2015). *Core curriculum for maternal-newborn nursing* (5th ed.). St. Louis, MO: Saunders.

Merriam-Webster. (2015). Merriam-Webster's medical dictionary online. http://www.merriam-webster.com/browse/medical/a.htm.

Miao, D., Young, S. L., & Golden, C. D. (2015). A meta-analysis of pica and micronutrient status. *American Journal of Human Biology, 27*(1), 84–93.

Michihata, N., et al. (2015). Group B streptococcus immunization during pregnancy for improving outcomes. *The Cochrane Database of Systematic Reviews*, (1), CD011496.

Midwives Alliance of North America. (2015). Midwives in the United States. http://mana.org/about-midwives/what-is-a-midwife.

Moise, K. J. (2015). Overview of rhesus D alloimmunization in pregnancy. UpToDate. http://www.uptodate.com/contents/overview-of-rhesus-d-alloimmunization-in-pregnancy.

Mori, G. F. (2015). *From pregnancy to motherhood: Psychoanalytic aspects of the beginning of the mother-child relationship.* New York: Routledge.

National Association of Certified Professional Midwives. (2015). Vision and purpose. http://nacpm.org/about-nacpm/about-the-organization/vision-and-purpose/.

National Institute on Drug Abuse (NIDA). (2015). What are the unique needs of pregnant women with substance use disorder? http://www.drugabuse.gov/publications/principles-drug-addiction-treatment-research-based-guide-second-edition/frequently-asked-questions/what-are-unique-needs-pregnant-women.

Norwitz, E. R., & Schorge, J. O. (2015). *Obstetrics and gynecology at a glance* (4th ed.). Malden, MA: Blackwell Publishing.

Pavord, S., & Maybury, H. (2015). How I treat postpartum hemorrhage. *Blood, 125*(18), 2759–2770.

Piontelli, A., et al. (2015). Fetal behavioral states. In *Development of normal fetal movements* (pp. 87–98). Milan, Italy: Springer.

Queenan, J. T., Spong, C. Y., & Lockwood, C. J. (2015). *Protocols for high-risk pregnancies: an evidence-based approach* (6th ed.). Hoboken, NJ: John Wiley & Sons.

Raio, L., Bolla, D., & Baumann, M. (2015). Hypertension in pregnancy. *Current Opinion in Cardiology, 30*(4), 411–415.

Rayburn, W. F., Jolley, J. A., & Simpson, L. L. (2015). Advances in ultrasound imaging for congenital malformations during early gestation. *Birth Defects Research. Part A, Clinical and Molecular Teratology, 103*, 260–268.

Reddy, B. S., et al. (2015). Screening, pregnant women, seroprevalence, hepatitis B surface antigen among pregnant women attending antenatal clinics. *Journal of Evolution of Medical and Dental Services, 4*(4), 555–558.

Robeznieks, A. (2016). U.S. has highest maternal death rates among developed countries. Modern healthcare. http://www.modernhealthcare.com/article/20150506/NEWS/150509941.

Rode, J. L., & Kiel, E. J. (2016). The mediated effects of maternal depression and infant temperament on maternal role. *Archives of Women's Mental Health, 19*(1), 133–144.

Ross, C. E., et al. (2015). Screening for human immunodeficiency virus and other sexually transmitted diseases among US women with prenatal care. *Obstetrics and Gynecology, 125*(5), 1211–1216.

Rubin, R. (1967). Attainment of the maternal role. Part I. Processes. *Nursing Research, 16*, 237–245.

Rubin, R. (1972). Fantasy and object constancy in maternal relationships. *Maternal and Child Nursing Journal, 1*(2), 101–111.

Rubin, R. (1977). Bonding in the postpartum period. *Maternal and Child Nursing Journal, 6*, 67–75.

Rubin, R. (1984). *Maternal identity and the maternal experience.* New York: Springer.

Sangkomkamhang, U. S., et al. (2015). Antenatal lower genital tract infection screening and treatment programs for preventing preterm delivery. *The Cochrane Database of Systematic Reviews*, (2), CD006178.

Sawant, V. (2015). Need of moral support during labor and birth. http://www.oratechsolve.com/need-of-moral-support-during-labor-and-birth/.

Silasi, M., et al. (2015). Viral infections during pregnancy. *American Journal of Reproductive Immunology, 73*, 199–213.

Singh, R., & McCloskey, J. (2015). Syphilis in pregnancy. *Venereology, 14*(3), 121–131.

Spencer, L., et al. (2015). The effect of weight management interventions that include a diet component on weight related outcomes in pregnant and postpartum women: A systematic review protocol. *JBI Database of Systematic Reviews and Implementation Reports, 13*(1), 88–98.

Spong, C. Y. (2015). Prevention of the first cesarean delivery. *Obstetrics and Gynecology Clinics of North America, 42*(2), 377–380.

Starling, P., et al. (2015). Fish intake during pregnancy and fetal neurodevelopment—A systematic review of the evidence. *Nutrients, 7*(3), 2001–2014.

Stevenson, D. K., Cohen, R. S., & Sunshine, P. (2015). *Neonatology: Clinical practice and procedures.* Maidenhead, United Kingdom: McGraw-Hill Education.

Stockwell, F. (2015). Maternal-infant bonding. http://www.felicitystockwell.com/the-overview.

Straussner, S. L. A., & Fewell, C. H. (2015). Children of parents who abuse alcohol and other drugs. In *Parental psychiatric disorder: Distressed parents and their families* (3rd ed., pp. 138–153). Cambridge: Cambridge University Press.

Swanson, J. R., & Sinkin, R. A. (2015). Transition from fetus to newborn. *Pediatric Clinics of North America, 62*(2), 329–343.

Tewfik, T. L., Karsan, N., & Kanaan, A. (2015). Cleft lip and palate and mouth and pharynx deformities. Medscape. http://emedicine.medscape.com/article/837347-overview.

Tharpe, N. L., Farley, C. L., & Jordan, R. (2016). *Clinical practice guidelines for midwifery & women's health* (5th ed.). Burlington, MA: Jones & Bartlett Learning.

Tolia, V. N., et al. (2015). Increasing incidence of the neonatal abstinence syndrome in U.S. neonatal ICUs. *The New England Journal of Medicine, 372*, 2118–2126.

Tomson, T., & Klein, P. (2015). Fine-tuning risk assessment with antiepileptic drug use in pregnancy. *Neurology, 84*(4), 339–340.

Tucker, C. M., et al. (2015). Patient-centered, culturally sensitive health care. *American Journal of Lifestyle Medicine, 9*(1), 63–77.

US Department of Agriculture (USDA). (2015). Daily food plan for moms. https://www.choosemyplate.gov/moms-daily-food-plan.

US Department of Health and Human Services (USDHHS). (2010). Healthy People 2020. Washington, DC: US Government Printing Office.

US Department of Health and Human Services (USDHHS), Office of Minority Health. (2015). Infant mortality and African Americans. http://minorityhealth.hhs.gov/omh/browse.aspx?lvl=4&lvlid=23.

US Preventive Services Task Force. (2015a). Final recommendation statements: Behavioral counseling and screening interventions to prevent STIs. http://www.uspreventiveservicestaskforce.org/Announcements/News/Item/final-recommendation-statements-behavioral-counseling-interventions-to-prevent-stis-and-screening-for-chlamydia-and-gonorrhea.

US Preventive Services Task Force. (2015b). Tobacco smoking cessation in adults and pregnant women: Behavioral and pharmacotherapy interventions. http://www.uspreventiveservicestaskforce.org/Page/Document/draft-recommendation-statement147/tobacco-use-in-adults-and-pregnant-women-counseling-and-interventions1.

Villarreal, G. B. (2015). Communicating across cultural differences. In *Communicating with pediatric patients and their families: The Texas Children's Hospital Guide for physicians, nurses and other healthcare professionals* (pp. 227–238). Houston, TX: Texas Children's Hospital.

Viteri, O. A., et al. (2015). Fetal anomalies and long-term effects associated with substance abuse in pregnancy: A literature review. *American Journal of Perinatology, 32*(5), 405–416.

Whitney, E. N., & Rolfes, S. R. (2015). *Understanding nutrition* (14th ed.). Boston: Cengage Learning.

World Health Organization. (2015). Congenital anomalies. http://www.who.int/mediacentre/factsheets/fs370/en/.

World Health Organization. (2016). Zika virus. http://www.who.int/mediacentre/factsheets/zika/en/.

Zakšek, T. Š. (2015). Sexual activity during pregnancy in childbirth and after childbirth. In A. P. Mivsek (Ed.), *Sexology in midwifery* (pp. 87–115). Rijeka, Croatia: InTech.

# 17

# Infant

*Susan Scott Ricci*

## OBJECTIVES

*After completing this chapter, the reader will be able to:*

- Evaluate the infant's health status and give examples of basic growth and developmental principles.
- Analyze the developmental tasks for the infant and the behavior indicating that these tasks are being accomplished.
- Explain the immunization schedule and other safety and health-promotion measures to a parent.
- Detect common parental concerns about infants and describe a model for parent education to allay these concerns.

- Examine accidents that occur during infancy and recommend appropriate counseling for accident prevention and safety.
- Differentiate ways in which nurses can be active in promoting major policies and influencing legislation concerning health.
- Outline governmental strategies to meet the goals of improving infant health.

## KEY TERMS

Active immunization
Birth defect
Body mass index
Infant/child abuse
Growth
Growth index

Oral stage of development
Passive immunization
Paternal engrossment
Poor growth
Reflexes
Sensorimotor period

Sickle cell anemia
Sudden infant death syndrome
Tay-Sachs disease
Trust versus mistrust
Weaning

## ❓ THINK ABOUT IT

### *Car Safety Seats*

Infants are at particular risk in automobile accidents. The proper use of occupant protection systems (infant car safety seats with seat belts) can reduce the risk of death and injury significantly. Although many public service campaigns encourage parents to restrain their infants while riding in automobiles (and all states have laws requiring some type of passenger safety restraint for infants), some parents neglect or remain unaware of the importance of providing safety for their vulnerable infants.

Nurses must have up-to-date knowledge of car occupant protection systems and their proper use to help parents find new products and obtain the most current information available. Parents often rely on the person selling the infant car seat for their information about protection systems and the proper use of

car seats. However, informational brochures and media campaigns fall short because they usually fail to provide explanations or demonstrations. As a result, parents may misinterpret the information that they receive.

- What type of program might you develop to reach and inform parents about the importance of car seat safety?
- In what settings might such a program be implemented?
- How would you modify your teaching plan to meet the needs of illiterate parents?
- How would you modify your program to ensure that parents who come from cultural backgrounds different from your own would respond well to the information?

Infants are recognized as the most vulnerable and dependent members of society, and their well-being is often used to measure the overall health of society. Health is shaped by a broad set of determinants, including socioeconomic status, physical and social environments, genetics and biological influences, and access to health care. Providing a safe and sound source of attachment and interaction is paramount to healthy infant development. Caregiving and mothering activities are the primary ingredients of an infant's preparation for life and ultimate independence. Nurses play a vital role in influencing this positive interaction through health promotion and education.

This chapter focuses on the infant and the infant's family during the infant's developmental period of 1 to 18 months. Because the infant is completely dependent on others, this chapter addresses the infant's parents and significant others as sources of health-promotion activities. The relationship initiated at birth between parents and the infant is the basis for the interdependence that is required for proper psychological and physical infant development. Health care professionals must focus on parent education as a means of fostering healthy, satisfying relationships within the family unit, and promoting the development of healthy future generations.

The principles of normal growth and development are used as a structural framework for this chapter. Understanding these principles helps the nurse identify deviations from the norm and institute appropriate health-promoting interventions.

To promote and maintain health during infancy, a balance between the infant's internal and external environmental forces must be established; any disruption places the infant at risk. Several processes that greatly influence this balance are identified, and appropriate interventions are outlined to assist the nurse in promoting a healthy infant population (American Academy of Pediatrics [AAP], 2015a; Ma et al., 2015) (Box 17-1: *Healthy People 2020*).

 **BOX 17-1   HEALTHY PEOPLE 2020**

### *Selected National Health-Promotion and Disease-Prevention Objectives for Infants*

- MICH-1.3: Reduce the rate of all infant deaths (within 1 year). Target: 6.0 infant deaths per 1000 live births (baseline: 6.7 infant deaths per 1000 live births within first year of life in 2006—10% reduction).
- MICH-1.4: Reduce the rate of neonatal deaths (within the first 28 days of life). Target: 4.1 neonatal deaths per 1000 live births (baseline: 4.5 neonatal deaths per 1000 live births occurred within the first 28 days of life in 2006—10% reduction).
- MICH-1.6: Reduce the rate of infant deaths related to birth defects (all birth defects). Target: 1.3 infant deaths per 1000 live births (baseline: 1.4 infant deaths per 1000 live births were attributed to birth defects [all birth defects] in 2006—10% reduction).
- MICH-1.8: Reduce the rate of infant deaths from SIDS. Target: 0.50 infant deaths per 1000 live births (baseline: 0.55 infant deaths per 1000 live births were attributed to SIDS in 2006—10% reduction).
- MICH-2: Reduce the 1-year mortality rate for infants with Down syndrome. Target: 43.7 deaths within the first year of life per 1000 infants with Down syndrome (baseline: 48.6 deaths within the first year of life per 1000 infants with Down syndrome occurred from 2005 to 2006—10% reduction).
- MICH-20: Increase the proportion of infants who are put to sleep on their backs. Target: 75.9% (baseline: 69.0% of infants were put to sleep on their backs in 2007—10% increase).
- MICH-21: Increase the proportion of infants who are breastfed. Target: 81.9% (baseline: 74.0% of infants born in 2006 were ever breastfed as reported from 2007 to 2009—10% increase).

From US Department of Health and Human Services. (2010). Healthy People 2020. http://www.healthypeople.gov/2020/topicsobjectives2020/objectiveslist.aspx?topicId=26.

## BIOLOGY AND GENETICS

Human development begins when a single sperm penetrates a mature ovum. The changes that follow are undeniable and wondrous. During this early period of growth and development the infant depends completely on others, primarily the parents, to meet all personal needs (Table 17-1). To assist the parents in their understanding of their infant's needs and progress, the nurse must know what behaviors to expect at certain ages. These developmental landmarks serve as a basis for anticipatory guidance (Table 17-2). Parents are aware of age-appropriate behavior to anticipate and facilitate these developmental landmarks. This knowledge, along with the nurse's anticipatory guidance, can also promote closer family relationships. In addition to the growth landmarks, the infant must accomplish developmental tasks to form a healthy personality.

### Developmental Tasks

Infant development begins before birth. A healthy pregnancy and a positive early childhood environment are essential to normal infant physical and mental health. Every infant faces developmental tasks and must accomplish them individually. Different practices in various societies affect the perception and resolution of the tasks, but all must be faced (Berk & Meyers, 2015).

The infant's first and most basic task is survival, which includes the physical tasks of breathing, sucking, eating, digesting, eliminating, and sleeping. Because many of these tasks involve the infant's mouth, this stage of life often is referred to as the **oral stage of development,** reflecting the primary importance of the mouth as the center of pleasure. More developmental tasks that must be accomplished during infancy are listed in Table 17-3. In the first year, infants learn to focus their vision, reach out, explore, and seek out things around them. During this time, infants also develop bonds of love and trust with their caregivers and others as part of their social and emotional development. Nurses can provide the infant's caregivers with guidance to encourage their infant's development by their:

- Talking to their infant, especially in a calming fashion
- Repeating sounds that their infant makes to help the infant learn to use language
- Reading to their infant to help develop and understand language and sounds
- Singing and playing music to help the infant develop a love for music and to help with brain development
- Giving their infant a great deal of loving attention to make the infant feel secure
- Praising their infant when something has been accomplished or learned (Centers for Disease Control and Prevention [CDC], 2015a)

To assist the infant's parents in encouraging achievement of these tasks, the nurse discusses the importance of stimulation and environmental interactions. Many neurological structures are far from completely developed at birth (Feldman, 2015). To continue growing, the brain depends not only on internal, embryological, and maturational forces but also on external stimulation. This external stimulation appears to influence the

TABLE 17-1 **GROWTH AND DEVELOPMENT**

*During Infancy*

**1 Month**
- Follows and fixes on bright object with eyes when it moves within field of vision
- Still has head lag when pulled to sitting position
- Displays tonic neck, grasp, and Moro reflexes
- Turns head when prone, but unable to support it
- Displays sucking and rooting reflexes
- Holds hands in fists
- Looks intently at caregiver when talked to
- Makes small, throaty sounds
- Gains 5 to 7 ounces weekly for 6 months
- Grows 1 inch monthly for 6 months
- Cries when hungry or uncomfortable
- Lifts head momentarily when prone

**2 Months**
- Has closed posterior fontanel
- Listens actively to sounds
- Lifts head almost 45 degrees off table when prone
- Follows moving object with eyes
- Grasp reflex decreases
- Recognizes familiar faces
- Pays attention to speaking voice
- Assumes less flexed position when prone
- Vocalizes; distinct from crying
- Turns from side to back
- Begins to have social smile

**3 Months**
- Visually inspects object and stares at own hand with apparent fascination when either appears in field of vision
- Has longer periods of wakefulness without crying
- Laughs aloud and shows pleasure in vocalization
- Holds head erect and steady; raises chest, usually supported on forearms
- Smiles in response to mother's face
- Recognizes faces, voices, and familiar objects
- Opens and closes hands, shakes toys
- Begins prelanguage vocalizations (coos, babbles, and chuckles)
- Carries hand or object to mouth at will
- Grasp reflex absent
- Follows objects for 180 degrees
- Actively holds rattle, but will not reach for it
- Turns eyes to object placed in field of vision

**4 Months**
- Begins drooling, indicated by appearance of saliva; does not know how to swallow it
- Holds head steady when in sitting position
- Recognizes familiar objects
- Shows almost no head lag when pulled to sitting position
- Rolls from back to side and from abdomen to back
- Inspects and plays with hands; pulls clothing or blanket over face in play
- Begins eye-hand coordination
- Chews and bites
- Enjoys social interaction
- Demands attention by fussing
- Reaches out to people
- Bears some weight on legs when held upright
- Is aware and interested in new environment
- Grasps object with two hands
- Squeals

**5 Months**
- Reaches persistently; grasps with entire hand
- Plays with toes
- Begins to discover parts of his/her body
- Smiles at mirror image
- Begins to postpone gratification
- Shows signs of tooth eruption
- Sleeps through night without food
- Weighs twice the birth weight
- Sits with slight support
- Vocalizes displeasure when desired object is taken away
- Is able to discriminate strangers from family members
- Makes cooing noises
- Squeals with delight
- Looks for object that has fallen
- Rolls from back to stomach or vice versa

**6 Months**
- Gains approximately 3 to 5 ounces weekly during the second 6 months
- Grows approximately 1 inch monthly for 6 months
- Is able to lift cup by handle
- Begins to hitch in locomotion
- Sits in high chair with straight back
- Begins to imitate sounds
- Vocalizes to toys and mirror image
- Recognizes caregivers
- Babbles with one-syllable sounds: "ma, ma, da, da"
- Chewing and biting occur
- Has definite likes and dislikes
- Likes to be picked up
- Plays peek-a-boo
- Makes "guh" and "bah" sounds

**7 Months**
- Has eruption of upper central incisors
- Bears weight when held in standing position
- Sits, leaning forward on both hands
- Fixates on one very small object
- Produces vowel sounds: "ba-ba" and "da-da"
- Shows fear of strangers
- Displays emotional instability by easy and quick changes from crying to laughing
- Repeats activities that are enjoyed
- Bangs objects together
- Develops taste differences
- Transfers objects from one hand to another
- Approaches toy and grasps it with one hand
- Imitates simple acts

**8 Months**
- Feeds self with finger foods
- Sits well alone
- Stretches out arms to be picked up
- Greets strangers with bashful behavior
- Begins to show regular patterns in bladder and bowel elimination
- Responds to "no" but does not obey it
- Makes consonant sounds: t, d, and w
- Dislikes dressing and diaper change
- Releases object at will
- Shows nervousness with strangers
- Pulls toy toward self

*Continued*

## TABLE 17-1 GROWTH AND DEVELOPMENT—cont'd

### During Infancy

**9 Months**
- Creeps and crawls (backward at first)
- Shows good coordination and sits alone
- Responds to adult anger; cries when scolded
- Explores object by sucking, chewing, and biting it
- Responds to simple verbal requests
- Drinks from cup or glass with assistance
- Pulls self to standing position
- Begins to show fears of going to bed and being left alone
- Imitates waving "bye-bye"
- Sits for prolonged periods—10 minutes
- Releases object with flexed wrist
- Repeats facial expressions of adults
- Uses thumb and index finger in pincer grasp

**10 Months**
- Sits by falling down
- Says "da-da" and "ma-ma" with meaning
- Understands "bye-bye"
- Looks at and follows pictures in book
- Object permanence begins to develop
- Plays interactive games such as pat-a-cake
- Crawls and cruises about well
- Pays attention to own name
- Picks up objects fairly well
- Extends toy to another person without releasing
- Pulls self to standing position and stands while holding onto solid object

**11 Months**
- Is able to push toys and place several objects in container
- Attempts to walk without assistance
- Begins to hold spoon
- Explores objects more thoroughly
- Stands erect with help of person's hand
- May have eruption of lower lateral incisors
- Holds crayon to mark on paper
- Acts frustrated when restricted
- Imitates definite speech sounds
- Reacts to restrictions with frustration

**12 Months**
- Loses Babinski sign
- Understands simple verbal commands

- Develops evident hand dominance
- Weighs triple the birth weight
- Has equal circumference of head and chest
- Walks with one hand held
- Knows own name
- Turns pages in book
- Has slow vocabulary growth because of increased interest in walking
- Develops lumbar curve
- Uses spoon in feeding, but often puts it upside down in mouth
- Drops object deliberately for it to be picked up
- Shakes head for "no"
- Plays pat-a-cake
- Recovers balance when falling over
- Tries to follow when being read to
- Does things to attract attention
- Imitates vocalization lead

**15 Months**
- Creeps up stairs
- Uses "da-da" and "ma-ma" labels for correct parents
- Tolerates some separation
- Drinks from cup well, but rotates spoon
- Asks for object by pointing
- Plays interactive games such as peek-a-boo and pat-a-cake
- Expresses emotions; has temper tantrums
- Walks without help

**18 Months**
- Has closed anterior fontanel
- Has long trunk, short and bowed legs, and protruding abdomen
- Walks upstairs with help
- Turns pages of book
- Has short attention span
- Begins to test limits
- Has bowel movements at appropriate time when placed on potty
- Indicates wet pants
- Gets into everything
- Fills and handles spoon without rotating it, but spills frequently
- Runs clumsily and falls often
- Is extremely curious
- Places object in hole or slot
- Becomes communicative, social being
- Imitates behavior of parents, such as mimicking household chores

From Beckett, C., & Taylor, H. (2016). *Human growth and development* (3rd ed.). Los Angeles: Sage Publications; Berk, L. E., & Meyers, A. B. (2015). *Infants, children, and adolescents* (8th ed.). New York: Pearson Education.

internal, anatomical, and maturational processes by different mechanisms (Bhattacharjee, 2015):
- Stimulation favors progressive complex branching of dendrites (the connection between nerve cells).
- Stimulation increases the degree of vascularization of certain anatomical structures of the brain, such as the centers associated with vision.
- Stimulation through social experiences is the portal to linguistic, cognitive, and emotional development in infants.
- Stimulated infants tend to have higher IQs and better memory as they grow older.

- Stimulation increases the process of myelination, which is closely related to the rate of development of a variety of functions. Myelin coats the brain and nerve tissue, which then becomes activated.

When counseling parents, the nurse stresses the importance of a variety of stimuli within the infant's environment. A variety of auditory and visual stimuli should be available, such as colorful mobiles, radio, spoken voice, and toys, to assist the infant in achieving developmental tasks. The sense of touch is an extremely important stimulus, bringing the infant in tune with caregivers in different environments, making it a reality. Ensuring that

## TABLE 17-2  Parenting Tasks for Developmental Landmarks in Infancy

| Age (Months) | Landmark | Parenting Task |
|---|---|---|
| 1 | Lifts head when prone | Place infant in prone position and dangle colorful object above its head |
| 2 | Has social smile | Promote by talking to infant and allowing opportunity for infant to smile |
| 4 | Squeals | Encourage and praise for doing so |
| 5 | Rolls from back to front | Place infant in protected area (crib or playpen) and encourage infant to move by placing toy out of reach |
| 8–9 | Uses pincer grasp to feed self | Make finger foods available |
| 10 | Pulls self to standing position | Provide safe environment; place chair or object of appropriate height within reach |
| 11–12 | Initiates vocalization | Talk to infant frequently and include in family gatherings |
| 12–15 | Walks | Encourage and provide clutter-free, safe walkway; praise infant for attempts |
| 15 | Drinks from cup | Supply cup with appropriate drink; do not scold infant for clumsiness in handling cups or spills |
| 18 | Mimics household chores | Give rags to infant to help with chores and dusting, allow infant to fold clothes, and so on |

From Centers for Disease Control and Prevention. (2016). Developmental milestones. http://www.cdc.gov/ncbddd/actearly/milestones/index.html; The Center for Parenting Education. (2016). Tasks for infants through 18 months. http://centerforparentingeducation.org/library-of-articles/child-development/developmental-tasks/#infants.

## TABLE 17-3  GROWTH AND DEVELOPMENT
### Developmental Tasks Accomplished in Infancy

- Achieves physiological equilibrium after birth
- Establishes self as a dependent person, but separate from others
- Becomes aware of animate versus inanimate objects and familiar versus unfamiliar objects and develops rudimentary social interaction
- Develops a feeling of affection for others and the desire for affection from others
- Manages the changing body and learns new motor skills, develops equilibrium, begins eye-hand coordination, and establishes rest-activity rhythm
- Learns to understand and control the physical world through exploration
- Develops a beginning symbol system, conceptual abilities, and preverbal communication
- Directs emotional expression to indicate needs and wishes

From Centers for Disease Control and Prevention. (2016). Developmental milestones. http://www.cdc.gov/ncbddd/actearly/milestones/index.html; The Center for Parenting Education. (2016). Tasks for infants through 18 months. http://centerforparentingeducation.org/library-of-articles/child-development/developmental-tasks/#infants.

appropriate sensory stimuli are available is vital to the infant's growth and developmental progression (Feldman, 2015).

## Concepts of Infant Development

As infants develop, they go through a series of developmental stages that are important for all aspects of their personhood, including physical, intellectual, emotional, and social aspects. The role of their caretakers is to provide encouragement, support, and access to activities that enable them to master key developmental tasks. The study of how a helpless infant grows and develops into a fully functioning, independent adult has fascinated many researchers. Their theories describe the development of human behavior as overlapping stages that occur in somewhat predictable patterns in an individual's life (Child Development Institute, 2015). Because these developmental theories are presented in Chapter 15, only their specific application to the infant is discussed here.

## Psychosocial Development

Erikson's psychosocial developmental theory is concerned primarily with a series of tasks or crises that each individual must resolve before encountering the next one. The central task during infancy is the development of a sense of trust versus mistrust. This occurs when adults meet an infant's basic needs for survival. The establishment of this basic trust or mistrust determines the manner in which the infant approaches all future stages of growth. The infant develops a sense of trust first in the mother (or other caretaker) and then in other significant people. Trust influences the infant's future relationships, allowing deeper commitment and intimacy. To develop trust the infant requires maximal gratification and minimal frustration to experience a healthy balance between inner needs and outer satisfaction. If the mother or caretaker is consistently responsive to the infant, meeting the physical and psychological needs, the infant will likely learn to trust his or her caretaker, view the world as a safe place, and grow up to be secure, self-reliant, trusting, cooperative, and helpful toward others.

A prompt, skillful, and consistent response to the infant's needs helps foster security and trust because it enables the infant to predict what will happen within the environment. When unpredictability and disorganized routines exist, the infant will develop fear, anger, anxiety, and insecurity, which eventually lead to mistrust. The infant can demonstrate desire by crying but depends on the sensitivity and willingness of others to provide relief. If the most important people fail to do this, the infant has little foundation on which to build faith in others or self in adulthood. If the infant's needs are not met appropriately, the infant will grow up with a sense of mistrust and may view the world as unpredictable.

## Cognitive Development

Piaget's cognitive developmental theory focuses on intellectual changes that occur in a sequential manner as a result of continual interaction between the infant and the environment. The theory is based on the idea that infants actively construct knowledge as they explore and manipulate the world around them (Carey et al., 2015). Piaget's **sensorimotor period** (up to age 18 months) describes the time during which infants develop the coordination to master activities that allow them to interact with the environment. During this period the infant solves problems using sensory systems and motor activity rather than symbolic processes, which develop later.

Fetuses are able to distinguish light from dark, and sight is present at birth. Rod cells in the retina of the eyes, which are responsible for light perception, are functional at birth although the retina (the organ of visual perception) is not fully developed until approximately 4 months of age. However, the infant can perceive color and shape. Infants are startled by loud noises and are soothed by soft voices, indicating that their sense of hearing is functioning. Their hearing can also be tested with audio equipment at birth. Babies cry when pricked with a diaper pin and fuss when too hot or too cold; therefore the senses of pain and temperature are also operative. Touching, stroking, and rocking typically comfort a fussing infant. Infants will also react to odors and tastes.

In addition to perceiving stimulation, the newborn is capable of reflexive behavior. **Reflexes** are responses that are normally exhibited after particular types of new stimulation (Moses, 2015). Because the response occurs after the stimulus, reflexes are unlearned. Some infant reflexes, such as rooting and sucking, have survival value. The rooting reflex, activated by the angle of the lips or cheek being lightly stroked, helps the infant locate the food source. The infant will turn toward the side that is being stroked and will open the lips to suck. The sucking reflex is initiated when an object is placed in the infant's mouth. Together these reflexes ensure that the infant can obtain food. Infants also have reflexes that result in grasping, yawning, hiccoughing, coughing, and sneezing.

Armed with these reflexes and sensory capabilities, the infant is ready to begin interacting with the environment (seeing, hearing, touching, tasting, and smelling) to acquire valuable information.

The infant progresses in various ways between birth and age 18 months, with early capabilities changing and becoming intentional. Piaget outlines five stages within the sensorimotor period that describe the infant's development, from the early reflexive behavior to differentiation between self and the environment (Table 17-4).

The infant in the sensorimotor period uses behavioral strategies to manipulate objects, to learn some of their properties, and to reach goals by combining several behaviors. The infant's behavior is tied to the concrete and the immediate; schemes can be applied only to objects that can be perceived directly.

Knowledge of child developmental theories is extremely valuable to the nurse during interactions with infants. Understanding the infant's level of cognitive thought and emotional and social development helps the nurse decipher a child's communications more meaningfully and interpret behaviors and the processes that motivate the child more accurately. This knowledge can be incorporated in the anticipatory guidance offered to the parents.

### TABLE 17-4  GROWTH AND DEVELOPMENT
**Piaget's Five Stages of Infant Development**

| Stage | Description |
|---|---|
| 1: birth to 1 month | Modification of reflexes<br>Practices and perfects reflexes present at birth<br>Sucking reflex becomes more refined and voluntary |
| 2: 1–4 months | Primary circular reactions<br>Repeats behavior that previously led to an interesting event<br>Only the infant's own body involved in activities |
| 3: 4–10 months | Secondary circular reactions begin<br>Repetitions involve events or objects in the external world<br>Appears to perform actions with a purpose<br>Hand-eye coordination |
| 4: 10–12 months | Coordination of secondary reactions<br>Combines two or more previously acquired strategies to obtain a goal |
| 5: 12–18 months | Tertiary circular reactions<br>Uses active experimentation to achieve previously unattainable goals<br>Infant purposely varies movements to observe results |

From Boundless. (2016). Piaget's stages of cognitive development. *Boundless Psychology.* https://www.boundless.com/psychology/textbooks/boundless-psychology-textbook/human-development-14/theories-of-human-development-70/piaget-s-stages-of-cognitive-development-270-12805/.

The nurse stresses that a variety of sensory and motor stimuli foster learning within the infant's environment.

The Infant Development Inventory is an infant assessment tool that screens children from birth to 18 months. It tracks developmental skills in five areas: social, self-help, gross motor, fine motor, and language. Monthly developmental milestones on the development chart help parents obtain a more comprehensive picture of how infants develop. Parents can also report any questions or concerns about their infant's health, development, or behavior. Parents complete the 60-question survey and the tester scores it. Health care providers may also further assess the infant's development by observing behaviors and recording them on the chart, in which case the baby's progress will be scored "typical," "borderline," or "delayed" in each developmental area.

The infant's growth index—height and weight measurements plotted on a standard growth chart to assess the infant for normal progression—is also important. Physical growth (height and weight) is a valid health status indicator that should be measured during each routine office or clinic visit. During the first year of life, growth is rapid. An infant who is growing properly is at low risk of developing a chronic disease (CDC, 2015b).

The nurse plots the infant's length and weight measurements against exact chronological age on growth grids. In 2009, the World Health Organization (WHO) released new international growth charts for children aged 0 to 59 months. It was recommended by the AAP and CDC that the WHO international growth charts be used for children younger than 24 months and that the CDC growth charts be used for children older than 24 months (CDC, 2015b). **Body mass index (BMI)** is a feature of the new pediatric growth charts that have been released by the CDC. BMI is the individual's weight in kilograms divided by the square of height in meters. In infants and children a high amount of body fat can lead to weight-related diseases and other health issues. A BMI calculator for children and teens can be found on the CDC website: http://nccd.cdc.gov/dnpabmi/Calculator.aspx. Growth charts are not intended to be used as a sole diagnostic instrument. Instead, growth charts are tools that contribute to the formation of an overall clinical impression of the child being measured (CDC, 2015c).

With the addition of body mass index to the charts, the CDC significantly increased the usefulness of this tool as a warning signal for potential obesity as early as 2 years of age. Parents have an opportunity to change their children's eating habits before a weight problem develops. The revised pediatric growth charts more accurately reflect the cultural and racial diversity currently found in the United States and can track children and young people through age 20 years. The growth charts indicate that children are heavier today than in the past, but height has remained virtually unchanged.

An infant's **growth index**, as determined by length and weight, is only one factor used in the assessment of health status. Differences in **growth** curves can influence the diagnosis of undernutrition and overnutrition, and the interpretation of adequate growth following nutritional intervention. The nurse has an overall understanding of growth and developmental principles to counsel parents regarding their infant's progress.

## Sex

The infant's sex is determined at the moment of fertilization. Immediately after childbirth, the parents may ask, "Is it a girl or a boy?" The answer has far-reaching implications for many family units. Sex is one of the many important factors that influence parents' way of relating to the infant.

There are many biological and behavioral differences between male and female infants. Boys are, on average, larger and have proportionately more muscle mass at birth. Girls are generally smaller but physiologically more mature at birth and are less vulnerable to stress. Boys show more motor activity, whereas girls display a greater response to tactile stimulation and pain (Polan & Taylor, 2015). As the infant develops, further differences are noted. By 6 months, girls respond to visual stimulation with longer attention spans and are more socially responsive than are boys; girls also tend to sit up, walk, and crawl earlier than do boys. Girls also learn to communicate with language at an earlier age, whereas male infants use their whole bodies in communicating (Kail & Cavanaugh, 2015).

The sex of the infant, a major concern of many expectant parents, may well influence parental relationships and expectations. The infant's sex can evoke disappointment; in some cases, a woman may feel disappointed in a girl because she knows that her husband wanted a boy. Today, the trend is to want one child of each sex. Because of the availability in America of better forms of contraception and economic factors such as the expense of raising children, most couples are having fewer children today compared with the 1950s. The importance and stress of producing the "right-sex" infant is evident. Being the "wrong sex" can, combined with other factors, place an infant at risk of child abuse. The parents may find fault with and place blame on the infant for not meeting this expectation (Hax, 2015).

Health intervention focuses on the identification of high-risk families and the promotion of positive relationships between infants and parents. The nurse promotes the good health, appearance, and developmental potential of the infant. Increasing the parents' feelings of adequacy and self-esteem will promote their acceptance and care of the infant. Most importantly, follow-up care for these families is a high priority to ensure that adequate support and help are available.

## Race

Race refers to the classification of human beings into groups based on particular physical characteristics, such as skin pigmentation, head form, and stature, attributable to a common inheritance. A range of physical variation exists among people of different races with regard to growth rate, dentition, body structure, blood groups, and susceptibility to certain diseases, as well as a great many other variables.

In assessing an infant, the nurse not only collects data but also compares the data with established norms, such as a standardized growth chart. When the norms chosen are not appropriate for the individual (e.g., an Asian infant's growth is assessed on the basis of norms for white children), the assessment will not be accurate. The nurse who works with families from a variety of racial groups has an understanding of each background and how it relates to health and health care. To facilitate nursing care for a family from a racial group different from that of the health care provider, effective communication must be established. This communication will help foster an understanding of the other's point of view and frame of reference. Each family member is viewed as an individual, as well as a family unit. There is no stereotyping of families within a racial or ethnic group. Despite common language, color, or historical background, not all members of a particular racial group are alike. This diversity presents, without doubt, considerable challenges for nurses who work with families with infants (Simon et al., 2015). Universal norms by which to measure one's growth and skill capacity do not exist. The nurse recognizes the differences and intervenes appropriately. The orientation of health maintenance and disease prevention is basic to good health practices, regardless of racial makeup. This concept is the main focus of all health care. (See Chapter 2 for further details.)

## Genetics

In the past several decades, remarkable progress has been made in our understanding of the structure and function of genes and chromosomes. These advances have been aided by the complete sequencing of human DNA—our genome. This knowledge can now be applied to medical care. The desired and expected outcome of any pregnancy is the birth of a healthy, perfect baby. Parents experience disappointment when they discover that their baby has been born with a defect. A **birth defect** is an abnormality of structure, function, or metabolism as a result of a genetic or environmental influence on the fetus, often a combination of both. Couples may refrain from having another child because they have had one with a serious birth defect and do not want to risk another. In these situations, genetic counseling provides information that is needed to understand a hereditary disorder and its associated risks. The main goal of counseling is to explain birth defects to affected families and to allow prospective parents to make informed decisions about childbearing.

Using the basic laws governing heredity and knowing the frequency of specific birth defects in the population, the genetic counselor can often predict the probability of recurrence of a given abnormality in the same family. An important aspect of primary prevention is identifying families at increased risk and referring them for counseling (Nussbaum et al., 2016). The aspects to be reviewed in the initial interview include the following:

- *Maternal age.* The risk of having a child with Down syndrome increases significantly for the woman older than 35 years. In Down syndrome, there are three chromosomes in the 21 chromosome group (trisomy 21). Characteristic features of Down syndrome include upward-slanting eyes; small, malformed ears; large, protruding tongue; broad hands and feet; and some degree of mental disability.
- *Ethnic background.* Several genetic disorders occur with higher frequency in certain groups. Anyone can be a carrier of Tay-Sachs disease, but the disease is most common among the Ashkenazi Jewish population. The incidence of Tay-Sachs disease in this population is 1 in 3600 people. The carrier frequency for Tay-Sachs disease is 1 in 27 (National Tay-Sachs & Allied Diseases Association, 2015). Abnormal deposits of lipids (fats) in the cells of the cerebral cortex, spleen, liver, and lymph nodes are characteristic of Tay-Sachs disease. Rapid and progressive deterioration of the brain and nervous system ensues, with death typically occurring by age 6 years. An autosomal recessive gene transmits the disease. Blacks have a much greater chance of carrying the sickle cell trait than does the general population. Sickle cell anemia is an autosomal recessive condition that occurs in 1 in 365 black births and causes severe hemolytic anemia crises. Approximately 100,000 Americans have sickle cell disease, which is a lifelong illness. One in 13 black Americans carries the sickle cell trait (National Institutes of Health, 2015).
- *Family history.* Certain diseases, such as Huntington chorea, hemophilia, and mental retardation, are often hereditary. Huntington chorea (an autosomal dominant disease involving the brain) is characterized by deterioration of intellectual functions and involuntary movements of the limbs, face, and trunk. Once symptoms have manifested themselves, a steady deterioration leads to death in approximately 20 years. Hemophilia is a sex-linked recessive coagulation disorder caused by a functional deficiency of a clotting factor; it leads to prolonged bleeding. Hemophilia passes from an unaffected carrier mother to her male offspring. It affects 1 in 5000 male births. Approximately 400 babies are born with hemophilia each year in the United States, with approximately 20,000 people with it in the United States presently (Zaiden et al., 2015).

- *Reproductive history.* Spontaneous abortions, stillbirths, and previous live-born children with birth defects or slow development may indicate an increased risk.
- *Maternal disease.* Several maternal disorders are associated with a higher frequency of birth defects, including diabetes mellitus, seizure disorder, mental disability, and phenylketonuria. Prenatal diagnosis offers the couple the option of aborting a fetus that has certain genetic disorders. For many people, however, this option is unacceptable. Chapter 16 discusses the various tests used for prenatal diagnosis.

The nurse's role throughout the genetic counseling process is to provide the vital link between the counseling team and the high-risk couple. Nurses need to understand not only the foundations of genetics and genomics but also the implications of these sciences for those for whom they provide care. The nurse is involved in case finding, referral, and family education. As a result of the new and expanding technology devoted to genetic and genomic research, a growing number of genetic tests are available for the screening, diagnosis, and treatment of rare and common diseases. All nurses will need to become knowledgeable about the basics of genetics and genomics and their applications to clinical care so that they can provide quality health care that is appropriate to their setting, population, geographical location, access, and coverage. This knowledge will allow nurses to provide appropriate information to care recipients regarding genetic tests that are part of their own health care (Lopes et al., 2015).

# GORDON'S FUNCTIONAL HEALTH PATTERNS

## Health Perception–Health Management Pattern

Health promotion is aimed at assisting the infant and the infant's family to change behavior to produce better physical and emotional health in adulthood. The old saying "an ounce of prevention is worth a pound of cure" has great merit, and if considered, and acted on, this can be very effective in promoting an individual's health. To reach this goal, the nurse encourages childrearing practices that promote normal growth and development, fosters attitudes and values compatible with health, and teaches appropriate use of health services. Health-promotion measures, by nurses, aim to prevent and minimize ill health of all women and their families. Nurses provide a pathway to access health care, engaging them to stay healthy, and share in decision-making concerning their own health, and help families that need to negotiate the health care system (Arnold & Boggs, 2016). The nurse promotes the infant's health through the parents, who determine the care practices for the dependent infant.

Health is largely a subjective judgment. Each person's perception of health is related to physical and mental capabilities, self-concept, relationships with others and the environment, and personal goals and values (Sanders, 2015). With this understanding, the nurse uses every opportunity to convey confidence in the parents' health perception–health management pattern and to improve their ability to implement behaviors that promote the infant's health. When parents learn and adopt behaviors that improve their own health, they are more likely to ensure that the health needs of their infant are met. Parental modeling increases the chances that good health practices will be retained throughout the child's life.

The goals of nursing practice with infants and their families are to promote individual motivation for health, to assist the family to identify health needs, and to develop problem-solving skills within the family unit using the family's own resources. To meet these goals, the nurse identifies the family's perception of good or bad health practices, which greatly influences participation in health-promoting activities. Age, gender, educational level, cultural orientation, financial status, and occupation combine to influence health perception. When parents believe that the infant is more susceptible to a health problem if promotional behavior is not enacted, they become more motivated to adopt the behavior.

The nurse's task helps the parents recognize their infant's susceptibility and the potential consequences when healthy practices are not instituted. The nurse works within the family's health perception framework to become acquainted with the characteristics that influence the infant's health. Unless caregivers meet their own personal needs, they will be unable to meet their infant's developmental needs. The empowerment and growth of mothers is a key element to facilitate the successful development of their infants. Women with higher levels of education have healthier children (US Agency for International Development, 2017). The nurse supports the parents, strengthening their parental confidence and self-esteem, providing information on meeting their infant's needs, and reinforcing their health perception  health management pattern.

## Nutritional-Metabolic Pattern

One of the most important aspects of health promotion in the infant is nutritional status. Many opinions have been expressed about the infant's nutritional needs. As research in this area continues, recommendations and opinions will change; however, some basic facts about nutrition remain fairly consistent. During the infancy period, it is almost all about milk—breast or formula. Milk will provide practically every nutrient the infant needs for the first year of life. Infant nutritional requirements are based on what is considered necessary to support life, provide for growth, and maintain health.

### Essential Nutrients

During infancy, a period of rapid growth, nutrient requirements per pound of body weight are proportionally higher than at any other time in the life cycle. Water, proteins, fats, carbohydrates, vitamins, and minerals are the essential nutrients in any diet. Because the first year of life is a period of rapid growth, nutritional needs during this period are especially important and always changing. Water is vital to survival. A person can live for several weeks without food but can survive only a few days without water. Because the infant's body weight is approximately 75% water, the baby must consume large amounts of fluid to maintain water balance. Under normal circumstances the water requirements of healthy infants who are fed adequate amounts of breast milk or properly reconstituted infant formula are met by the breast milk or infant formula alone. Supplemental water is not necessary, even in hot, dry climates (US Department of Agriculture [USDA], 2015). The sources of water are fluids (primarily milk) and food; most strained foods are 75% to 85% water. Most infant diets, without supplementation, meet the basic water requirement.

The infant must also consume sufficient high-quality protein to facilitate growth and development. The recommended daily protein requirements are 9 g during the first 6 months and 11 g during the second 6 months. No more than 20% of an infant's daily energy requirement should come from protein because infants are not able to process and excrete the excess nitrogen from higher-protein diets (USDA, 2015).

Carbohydrates should supply 30% to 60% of the energy intake during infancy. Approximately 37% of the calories in human milk and 40% to 50% of the calories in commercial formulas are derived from lactose or other carbohydrates. The recommended daily intake of carbohydrates is 60 g for infants up to 6 months of age and 95 g for infants 7 to 12 months old (USDA, 2015).

For infants, 31 g of fats per day for the first 6 months of life and 30 g of fats per day during the second 6 months of life (approximately 40–50% of the calories) are recommended (USDA, 2015). These quantities are present in human milk and in all formulas prepared for infants. Breast milk and formulas provide approximately 50% of their calories as fat. Significantly lower intakes, such as in skim milk feedings, can result in an inadequate energy intake.

Vitamins are essential nutrients in the infant's diet that regulate metabolism and allow more efficient use of carbohydrates, fats, and proteins within the body. Although most infants receive adequate vitamin intake through formula, breast milk, and food, recent research has raised a concern about a vitamin D deficiency in infants who receive only breast milk. Vitamin D deficiency is actually quite common among US infants. The Institute of Medicine (IOM) recently revised the recommended dietary allowances for vitamin D. According to the IOM, nutritional rickets is on the rise in the United States among children with certain risk factors: dark-skinned infants, infants that are breastfed for long periods without receiving any vitamin supplementation, and infants with decreased exposure to sunlight. The IOM (2015) recommends that this population needs vitamin D supplementation of 65 mcg/day from birth to 6 months and 80 mcg/day for the second 6 months of life.

Minerals are found in relatively small amounts in the infant's body but are vital elements in body structure and control of certain body functions. Mineral intake for infants appears to be adequate, except for iron and fluoride.

The full-term infant is born with stores of iron adequate to meet the needs for hemoglobin production for approximately 4 to 6 months. After this time, body stores may need to be replenished. Although iron in human milk is bioavailable, both breastfed and formula-fed infants should receive an additional source of iron by 6 months of age. Iron-fortified formula and cereals are the most commonly used food sources.

Fluoride, concentrated in the bones and teeth, helps reduce dental caries. Although fluoride is important for strong tooth development, it is not recommended during the first 6 months of life. Supplementation is necessary only when the diet contains insufficient fluoridated water.

A review of these requirements shows that milk (breast or formula) meets most of the infant's nutritional needs when consumed in adequate amounts, plus vitamin D supplementation for the high-risk infants. No data support the theory that solid foods are needed to meet these nutritional needs, at least during the first 6 months of life.

If the mother chooses to formula-feed verses breastfeed her infant, the nurse should instruct the mother about safe preparation of infant formula as follows:

- Check the expiration date and condition of each container of formula.
- Wash the top of the container with soap and water before opening it.
- Wash hands thoroughly before preparing infant formula.
- Prepare the bottle by washing it with soap and water or in the dishwasher.
- Follow the manufacturer's instructions for how much water to use.
- Warm the formula by placing it in warm water, never in a microwave oven.
- Shake the bottle well and feed the formula to the infant.
- Store the leftover formula safely in the refrigerator and discard it after 48 hours.

## Food Additives

In addition to their questionable nutritional value, additives in commercial baby food can negatively influence an infant's health status. The purposes of food additives differ, including adding nutritional value; preserving or extending shelf life; facilitating preparation; improving flavor, color, and texture; and keeping flavors and textures consistent (WHO, 2015a).

Commercially prepared baby foods are generally safe, nutritious, and high quality. In response to consumer demand, baby food manufacturers have removed much of the added salt and sugar that their products once contained and have eliminated most food additives.

Nutrition problems include undernutrition, in which infants do not receive an adequate supply of an essential nutrient, and overnutrition, in which they receive more of a certain nutrient than is needed for healthy growth and development (Fildes et al., 2015). For infants in the United States, both of these problems are present. A parent who wants the infant to have family foods rather than commercial baby food can blenderize a small portion of the table food at each meal. This choice necessitates cooking without salt or sugar, which is the practice of baby food manufacturers. Making baby food is easy and economical. Written resources are available for parents who are interested in more details about home food preparation for infants.

Parents should be encouraged to read baby food labels carefully. Nurses can obtain lists of baby foods and their ingredients from the manufacturers. The best overall recommendation that nurses make to parents is to provide their infants with a well-balanced diet and avoid excesses.

## Breastfeeding

An infant's first and preferred source of nutrition should be breast milk. Ongoing evidence-based practice findings strongly indicate that the lifelong health from breastfeeding that is bestowed on the infant also greatly contributes to the health status of the mother, the family, and society at large (Busch et al., 2015). Research throughout the years has demonstrated unequivocally that exclusive breastfeeding is the preferred method of infant feeding for the first 6 months of life and should be continued for at least the first year of life and beyond for as long as mutually desired by the mother and child (AAP, 2015b). Breast milk is often called the perfect food for the infant and for the mother, because of its composition and because it does not have to be purchased, cooked, or stored. Both the American Dietetic Association and the AAP have released position statements in support of breastfeeding. This has influenced a number of health-promotion strategies in the United States. In *Healthy People 2020,* objectives MICH 21 through MICH 24 address breastfeeding. In all objectives the target is to increase these activities by 10% by 2020 (US Department of Health and Human Services [USDHHS], 2010) (Box 17-2: Research for Evidence-Based Practice). The United States breastfeeding initiation rates have risen slowly since the grassroots movement began years ago. The number of mothers still breastfeeding at 6 months is up to 49% and those at 12 months is up to 27% (Lauwers & Swisher, 2016). If the nation is to meet the Surgeon General's goal by the year 2020, efforts to promote breastfeeding must be strengthened in hospitals, health maintenance organizations, private health care offices, and public health clinics. The Affordable Care Act passed in 2010 contains several elements of lactation support. It requires employers to provide a private place for breastfeeding employees to express milk during the work day and also requires health insurance coverage for breastfeeding support, counseling, and equipment (US Congress, 2010).

WHO, the United Nations Children's Fund (UNICEF), and *Healthy People 2020* have adopted the Baby-Friendly Hospital Initiative in an attempt to establish a global effort to increase breastfeeding (WHO, 2015c). To become a baby-friendly health care facility, the 10 steps to successful breastfeeding must be implemented, as shown in Box 17-3.

Women's decisions of whether to breastfeed are influenced by information they receive from their health care providers. The decision to breastfeed is complex and depends on multiple factors—demographic, biological, psychological, social, and educational. Guidance given to mothers on breastfeeding in the postpartum period increases their knowledge of the subject and, consequently, the prevalence of this practice for a longer period. Nurses need to provide mothers with guidance and congruent, sensitive, effective, and beneficial support for them to be successful with the breastfeeding experience (Santos et al., 2015). Low levels of actual or perceived professional support and lack of knowledge, support, and measures needed to cope with breastfeeding difficulties are found to be associated with formula-use decisions. Data suggest inconsistencies between health care provider's perceived support and behaviors, lack of knowledge, and significant lack of skill in the assessment and management of breastfeeding mothers (Radzyminski & Callister, 2015). Because of the important role in the mother's choice of infant feeding, nurses can be instrumental in working toward the national goal to increase breastfeeding

## BOX 17-2  RESEARCH FOR EVIDENCE-BASED PRACTICE

### Trends of US Hospitals Distributing Infant Formula Packs to Breastfeeding Mothers, 2007 to 2013

Objective: Distribution of infant formula samples to new mothers before hospital discharge has been a practice on maternity units since the early 20th century. Although appearing to be innocuous, this practice is viewed as a marketing tactic that adversely affects breastfeeding duration and exclusivity. The purpose of this study was to evaluate trends in the incidence of hospitals and birthing centers still distributing infant formula discharge packs to breastfeeding mothers on their being discharged home in the United States from 2007 to 2013.

Methods: Every 2 years a survey is administered to all hospitals with registered maternity beds in the United States. A Web-based or-paper-based questionnaire was distributed and completed by the person most knowledgeable about breastfeeding-related practices within that facility. The researchers examined the distribution of infant formula discharge packs to breastfeeding mothers from 2007 to 2013 by state and hospital characteristics.

Results: The percentage of hospitals and birthing centers distributing infant formula discharge packs to breastfeeding mothers was approximately 72% in 2007 and 32% in 2013, a decrease of 41% in 6 years. In 2007 there was only one state (Rhode Island) in which less than one-quarter of the hospitals distributed infant formula discharge packs to breastfeeding mothers. By 2013, there were 24 such states with less than 25% distribution. Distribution declined across all hospital characteristics evaluated irrespective of whether they were teaching hospitals or nonteaching hospitals and irrespective of hospital size.

Conclusions: The distribution of infant formula discharge packs to breastfeeding mothers was reduced substantially from 2007 to 2013.

Nursing implications: From results of this study, hospitals are starting to implement optimal, evidence-based maternity care to support mothers who desire to breastfeed by not providing infant formula discharge packs. This trend allows nurses to encourage and support mothers to exclusively breastfeed for the first 6 months of their infant's life and continue to breastfeed for the first year and beyond if they so desire without a "tease" pack available. Nurses play a vital role in preparing, educating, encouraging, and supporting women to breastfeed and are instrumental in facilitating initiation and continuation of breastfeeding.

Modified from Nelson, J. M., Li, R., & Perrine, C. G. (2015). Trends of US hospitals distributing infant formula packs to breastfeeding mothers, 2007 to 2013. *Pediatrics, 135*(6), 1051–1056.

## BOX 17-3  Baby-Friendly Hospital Initiative Breastfeeding Guidelines

- Have a written breastfeeding policy that is communicated routinely to all health care staff.
- Train all health care staff in the skills necessary to implement this policy.
- Inform all pregnant women about the benefits and management of breastfeeding.
- Help the mother initiate breastfeeding within 30 minutes after birth.
- Show mothers how to breastfeed and how to maintain lactation even when they are separated from their infants.
- Give newborn infants no food or drink other than breast milk unless medically indicated.
- Practice rooming-in; allow mothers and infants to remain together 24 hours a day.
- Encourage breastfeeding on demand.
- Do not give pacifiers to breastfeeding infants.
- Foster the establishment of breastfeeding support groups and refer mothers to these groups when they are discharged from the hospital or clinic.

From Baby-Friendly USA. (2016). The guidelines & evaluation criteria. https://www.babyfriendlyusa.org/get-started/the-guidelines-evaluation-criteria.

## BOX 17-4  Advantages of Breastfeeding

### Breast Milk

- Has the correct balance of all essential nutrients for infants
- Is full of immunological agents to protect against disease
- Is easier to digest than is formula
- Contains antiinflammatory properties
- Promotes growth of *Lactobacillus bifidus*
- Reduces risk of childhood obesity, ear infections, and diabetes
- Reduces risk of asthma and respiratory viruses

### Breastfeeding

- Is cheaper and more convenient than formula
- Provides a unique bonding experience for both the infant and the mother
- Assists in the process of uterine involution for the mother
- Decreases postpartum vaginal bleeding
- Reduces childhood obesity
- Strengthens the immune system of infants
- Incidence of pneumonia, colds, and viruses is reduced
- Oxytocin is released, which promotes better healing in the postpartum period
- Protects infants against developing allergies
- Decreases costs for public health programs (e.g., WIC)
- Decreases SIDS rate, overweight, and obesity in adulthood
- Decreases environmental burden for disposal of formula cans and bottles
- Promotes weight reduction for new mother

From Lauwers, J., & Swisher, A. (2016). *Counseling the nursing mother: A lactation consultant's guide* (6th ed.). Burlington, MA: Jones & Bartlett Learning; Mercola, J. (2016). The amazing benefits of breastfeeding. http://articles.mercola.com/sites/articles/archive/2016/01/02/amazing-benefits-breastfeeding.aspx.

by educating all women about the advantages of the practice (Box 17-4). Community nurses who are caring for breastfeeding mothers stress the following tips to increase the duration of this activity:

- Drink 1 quart of fluids daily to produce a sufficient quantity of breast milk.
- Watch the infant, not the clock. Look for early signs of wanting-to-feed behaviors.
- Sunlight is the principle source of vitamin D, so a supplement might be needed.
- Try to rest when the infant sleeps, so you do not become overtired.
- Consume 300 to 400 kcal/day above the prepregnancy energy intake to avoid excessive weight loss.
- Learn the appropriate interventions for engorged breasts, sore nipples, plugged ducts, infection, and leaking nipples.
- Expose nipples to air after each feeding and allow some breast milk to dry on nipples for their lubricating and antiinfective properties.

- Learn about the use of breast pumps and milk storage.
- Join breastfeeding support groups for continued help within the community.
- Learn about the effects of drugs, environmental pollutants, alcohol, and nicotine on breast milk.
- Breastfeeding is more than just supplying nutrients for growth—it contributes to an intimate and special relationship between you and your infant (Lauwers & Swisher, 2016)

## Introduction of Solid Foods

The timing of the first introduction of solid food during infancy may have potential effects on lifelong health. No scientific evidence is available on the best time to introduce solid foods during infancy. At approximately 4 to 6 months of age, the infant is usually physiologically and developmentally ready to have solid foods, either commercial or home-prepared. The infant should be able to do the following developmental tasks before solid foods are introduced: sit with support, have good head and neck control, push up with straight elbows from a lying face-down position, lean forward and open mouth when interested in food, and turn away when not hungry. The AAP and WHO recommend that waiting until the child is 6 months old to introduce solid food decreases the tendency for the child to develop food allergies and reduces the risk of childhood obesity. The introduction of various foods was recommended to supply a more appealing, diversified diet for the infant; supply energy, iron, and vitamins; and provide needed trace elements (Duryea & Fleischer, 2015). The decision to start solid foods at 4 to 6 months of age is based more on neuromuscular and developmental readiness of the infant than on any hard scientific data, but research does validate the lowered risk of developing food allergies if solid foods are not introduced until 6 months of age. It is now thought that early introduction of highly allergenic foods, such as eggs, peanuts, tree nuts, and fish, can actually decrease the risk of allergy (Duryea & Fleischer, 2015).

All infants develop according to their own schedules, and some are ready to start eating solid foods earlier than other infants. The addition of foods should be governed by an infant's nutritional needs and readiness to handle different forms of foods (Brown & Rowan, 2016). The order of food introduction and the specific amounts to be given are based on tradition rather than on scientific fact. No scientific studies have been performed to determine whether a specific order of infant food introduction is necessary or the amounts needed for optimal development. The sequence of solids typically recommended by the AAP is cereal, fruits, vegetables, and meats. Certain foods to avoid for any infant younger than 12 months include whole cow's milk; foods that could cause choking—nuts, grapes, raw carrots, or candy; and honey. Cow's milk is not recommended because it does not contain adequate iron; honey is not recommended because of the potential risk of exposure to a harmful bacteria toxin—botulism poisoning. The typical sequence in which foods are introduced is shown in Box 17-5. A few tips to assist parents in making the introduction of solid foods a smooth transition are listed in Box 17-6. Recommendations for food introduction by age and sequence are given in Table 17-5.

---

> ### BOX 17-5   Solid Food Introduction Sequence
>
> - Cereals, particularly rice because of nonallergenic property
> - Fruits such as peaches, pears, and applesauce
> - Vegetables, with yellow vegetables (squash and carrots) given before green vegetables (peas or beans)
> - Strained meats, such as nonallergenic lamb or veal

From Duryea, T. K., & Fleischer, D. M. (2015). Patient education: Starting solid foods during infancy (beyond the basics). *UpToDate.* http://www.uptodate.com/contents/starting-solid-foods-during-infancy-beyond-the-basics.

---

> ### BOX 17-6   Tips for Introducing Solid Foods
>
> #### *Assess the Infant's Readiness to Consume Solid Foods First*
>
> - The infant can sit up (with support) and can hold her/his head and neck up well.
> - The infant's birth weight has doubled.
> - The infant is interested in what you are eating and may even try to grab food from your plate.
> - The infant can keep food in her/his mouth rather than letting it dribble out.
> - The infant shows signs of being hungry by wanting to nurse more often.
>   If readiness is validated, then begin with the following:
> - The infant's first solid foods should be smooth and runny. Gradually, the infant will be ready to accept a slightly rougher texture.
> - Puréed foods are used until the infant has teeth; chopped foods are used when the infant can chew.
> - Introduce only one new food at a time and in small amounts for 5 to 7 days. When the new food is not tolerated or the infant is allergic to it, the new food can be identified quickly and discontinued.
> - The infant must learn how to handle solid foods. Because infants use sucking movements, part of the food is ejected from the mouth. With time and practice, the infant learns how to take solid food from a spoon.
> - Do not mix solid foods together; the infant should learn to appreciate different tastes and textures.
> - Always feed the infant with the infant in an upright position; do not feed the infant solids from the bottle.
> - Until the infant is 1 year old, feed the infant milk before solid foods.
> - Look at, smile at, and talk to the infant during feeding.
> - Do not give honey to infants younger than 12 months because of the risk of infant botulism.
> - Respect the infant's likes and dislikes; rejected foods may be reintroduced later.
> - Avoid peanuts and peanut butter because of the potential for severe allergic reactions.

From US Department of Agriculture. (2016). Infant feeding guide. https://wicworks.fns.usda.gov/infants/infant-feeding-guide.

## Weaning

**Weaning** is a gradual, caring process that introduces the infant to a cup, which replaces the bottle or breast. The biological norm and desired method for weaning is to allow the infant to self-wean. Weaning should be started when the infant is ready. Developmentally, the infant can usually learn to use a cup by age 5 to 6 months; however, many children continue to nurse after they start using a cup. The infantile extrusion reflex needs to be absent.

| TABLE 17-5 | **First Foods for the Infant** |
| --- | --- |
| **Age (Months)** | **Addition** |
| 4–6 | Iron-fortified rice cereal, followed by other cereals |
| 5–7 | Strained vegetables and fruits and their juices |
| 6–8 | Protein foods (cheese, meat, fish, chicken, and yogurt) |
| 9 | Finely chopped meat, toast, teething crackers |
| 10–12 | Whole egg, whole milk (allergies less likely now) |

From Duryea, T. K., & Fleischer, D. M. (2015). Patient education: Starting solid foods during infancy (beyond the basics). *UpToDate.* http://www.uptodate.com/contents/starting-solid-foods-during-infancy-beyond-the-basics; La Leche League. (2016). First foods for baby. http://www.llli.org/faq/firstfoods.html.

This reflex is present in very young infants and involves the tongue pushing out any material in the mouth not associated with sucking. The safety advantages of this are obvious, but weaning cannot be commenced until the infant has matured sufficiently for the reflex to be absent. In addition, weaning should not be started until the infant can sit only slightly supported and turn away his/her head to indicate food refusal. The AAP recommends breastfeeding for at least the first year of life. WHO and UNICEF suggest that the health benefits of breast milk are important throughout the second and third years of life and that breastfeeding should be continued. However, because breast milk is very low in iron content, there has been concern about the possible impact of this advice on the development of anemia, a condition that if left untreated could cause irreversible developmental delays. The iron in human milk is absorbed more efficiency (60%) than the iron in cow's milk (4%), partly because of the high amount of vitamin C in human milk (Lauwers & Swisher, 2016). Weaning should be started at this age by the infant periodically being offered sips of water or juice. Initially the infant may not be eager to accept these offers but should become accustomed to this new experience fairly quickly (Box 17-7: Quality and Safety Scenario).

Some infants accept the cup readily; other infants are extremely reluctant to give up the bottle, especially the bedtime bottle. Allowing infants to sleep with propped bottles can lead to aspiration if the milk flows too rapidly or the infant becomes too sleepy to coordinate sucking and swallowing. Another potential problem is baby-bottle tooth decay, of all upper teeth and some of the lower posterior teeth, from direct contact with sugar, syrup, honey-sweetened water, or fruit juice. When the infant falls asleep and stops sucking on the bottle, the sugary solution pools around the infant's teeth and remains there for long periods. The carbohydrate in the solution is fermented into organic acids that demineralize the teeth until they decay. By not using the bottle as a pacifier, parents can prevent this condition.

Some additional tips for counseling parents are as follows:

- Keep a calm, relaxed attitude throughout the weaning process.
- Let the child lead the way; it could take days, weeks, or months.
- Anticipate the previous feeding times and offer a cup or snack instead.
- Do not force an infant to use a cup; it is more detrimental to wean an infant sooner than later.
- Introduce the cup for one feeding per day and progress until the breast or bottle is surrendered.
- Drop a feeding out every few days until the evening feeding is the last one left.
- Be sure the infant is getting enough nutrition from other sources.
- Put only purified tap water into the bottle, and give the infant juice and milk from a cup.
- Remember that infants enjoy the accomplishment of using a cup; it is one of their first steps toward independence.
- Make sure to make up the bonding time with your infant by holding and cuddling the infant throughout the day (Williamson & Beatty, 2015).

### Anticipatory Guidance

The infant progresses from a diet of milk alone to a diet of milk and solid foods within a short period. Understanding the infant's nutritional needs and developmental capabilities, the nurse can guide the parents in meeting them and in the process, foster healthy family-infant relationships. The health-promotion activity used in meeting proper infant nutrition focuses on parent education and positive reinforcement of parenting abilities.

## Elimination Pattern

The infant develops an elimination pattern by the second week of life, usually associated with the frequency and amount of feedings. Both breastfed and bottle-fed infants progress to a pattern of fewer stools per day after the first few months of life.

A breastfed infant's stools have a mushy golden-yellow color and seedy, even consistency, with a slightly sour but clean smell, dissimilar to stools passed later in life. A bottle-fed infant's stools are firm, pasty, and smellier and resemble those of an infant eating solid food. The breastfed infant has many daily stools during the first and second months of life, progressing to one stool per day or even one stool every 4 to 5 days in the later months before solid foods are introduced. The bottle-fed infant has two to four stools per day during the first month, tapering to one a day or even fewer at the end of infancy (Polan & Taylor, 2015).

For the first year of life an infant cannot control the bowels. Bowel evacuation remains under involuntary, reflexive control until myelination of the spinal cord is complete, usually by 14 to 18 months of age (Kliegman et al., 2015). Nurses advise overanxious parents to delay toilet training until the infant is developmentally ready. The stress in American culture on daily bowel movements makes many mothers concerned about their infant's elimination patterns. The breastfed infant may go for several days without having a bowel movement, which is usually not a problem. When the infant's behavior and feeding and sleeping patterns are normal, no elimination problem exists. A

## ☑ BOX 17-7 QUALITY AND SAFETY SCENARIO

### How to Hold Your Infant for Feedings

- Sit or lie down comfortably with your back supported.
- Make sure the infant has one arm on either side of your breast as you pull him/her close.
- Use firm pillows or folded blankets under the infant as a means of support during the feeding. As the infant gets older, the extra support will likely be unnecessary.
- Support the infant's back and shoulders firmly.
  - Do not push on the back of the infant's head.
  - Correct positioning enables good attachment.
  - The infant should be at a 90-degree angle, with his/her nose meeting your nipple.
- After the infant's mouth is open wide, pull him/her quickly to your breast.

#### Three Common Breastfeeding Positions
#### Football
- Hold the infant's back and shoulders in the palm of your hand.
- Tuck the infant up under your arm, keeping the infant's ear, shoulder, and hip in a straight line.
- Support the breast. After the infant's mouth is open wide, pull him/her quickly to you.
- Continue to hold your breast until the baby feeds easily.

#### Lying Down
- Lie on your side with a pillow at your back and lay the infant such that you are facing each other.
- To begin, prop yourself up on your elbow and support your breast with that hand.
- Pull the infant close to you, lining up his/her mouth with your nipple.
- After the infant is feeding well, lie back down. Hold your breast with the opposite hand.
- Cradle the infant in the arm closest to the breast with his/her head in the crook of your arm.

- Have the infant's body facing you, tummy to tummy.
- Use your opposite hand to support the breast.

#### Across the Lap
- Lay your infant on firm pillows across your lap.
- Turn the infant, facing you.
- Reach across your lap to support the infant's back and shoulders with the palm of your hand.
- Support your breast from underneath to guide it into his/her mouth.

#### Breastfeeding Is Going Well When...
- Your infant is feeding approximately eight times in 24 hours for 30 to 40 minutes at each feeding. Some infants need to eat more frequently until they learn to breastfeed efficiently. Other infants gain weight although they feed less often.
- At least one breast softens well at each feeding.
- You feel a tug, but not pain, when he/she sucks.
- The infant's arms and shoulders are relaxed during the feeding.
- The infant has bursts of 10 or more sucks and swallows at the beginning of each feeding.
- As your breast softens, the infant slows down to two to three sucks and swallows at a time.
- Your infant is content when you finish breastfeeding.
- By the time the infant is 4 days old, you should see at least six wet diapers and two bowel movements every 24 hours.
- Signs that a good attachment has been made are:
  - The infant's nose is free from the breast.
  - The infant's chin is firmly pressed against the breast.
  - The infant has round cheeks.
- If any areola is visible, it should be more above the top lip versus the bottom lip.

From Lauwers, J., & Swisher, A. (2016). *Counseling the nursing mother: A lactation consultant's guide* (6th ed.). Burlington, MA: Jones & Bartlett Learning.

breastfed infant rarely becomes constipated when consuming adequate amounts of breast milk. Usually the nurse only has to reassure the parents and discuss normal elimination patterns. Urination increases as fluid intake increases. An infant who voids 6 to 12 times a day during the first few months of life is usually healthy and well hydrated. Voiding is involuntary until sometime during the second year of life, when bladder sensation develops. Irregular patterns of voiding characterize the remaining period of infancy.

### Anticipatory Guidance

Anticipatory guidance and health promotion concerning elimination patterns of the infant consist of parental teaching and reassurance, with special emphasis on good hygienic practices. Reassuring the parents about the infant's inability to control elimination is important so that their expectations are realistic.

## Activity-Exercise Pattern

Physical activity and exercise contribute to development and coordination throughout the life span; infants receive their exercise through play. Initially infants engage in play with themselves with their hands or feet, by responding to various sounds, and by rolling and getting into various positions. By manipulating objects and achieving pleasurable sensations, infants learn about themselves and the objects in the environment.

### Activity Through Play

Play is crucial for an infant's social, emotional, physical, and cognitive growth. Exploration is the heart of play, as it is how infants learn about their body and the world around them. Although the word *play* suggests physical activity, the infant's first play is actually an exercise of the senses. The infant's first toys are visual. Through play, infants learn to hone their senses, to exercise their physical abilities, and to relate to other people. Most of the infant's play is solitary and repetitious. As each discovery is made, self-confidence and pride in the achievement are reinforced (as is the skill) through repetition.

As the infant enters the second half of the first year and becomes mobile, the family should provide the infant with increasing opportunities for spontaneous play and exploration. A planned play period in a safe environment should be established.

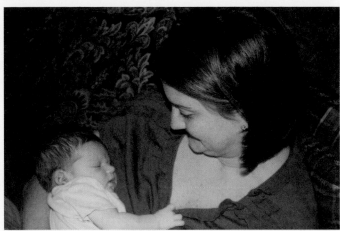

**FIGURE 17-1** The mother provides an infant with comfort by her closeness.

**TABLE 17-6  GROWTH AND DEVELOPMENT**

*Normal Sleep Patterns for Infants*

| Age (Months) | Hours in 24-h Period |
| --- | --- |
| 2–3 | Low: 10<br>Average: 16.5<br>High: 23 |
| 3–4 | Low: 8–10 nightly<br>High: 11–12 nightly (2 or 3 naps daily) |
| 6–12 | 11–12 nightly (2 or 3 naps daily) |
| 12–18 | 8–12 nightly (1 or 2 naps daily) |

From Baby Center. (2016). Establishing good sleep habits: Newborn to three months. http://www.babycentre.co.uk/a7654/establishing-good-sleep-habits-newborn-to-three-months; Stevens, M. S. (2016). Normal sleep, sleep physiology, and sleep deprivation. *Medscape.* http://emedicine.medscape.com/article/1188226-overview.

The infant should have unrestrictive clothing so that movement can be free and unhampered. The caregiver should not interfere directly with the play but should be attentive to the infant's needs.

An important nursing role is assisting parents to promote play, stressing the importance of providing opportunities that are appropriate for the infant's age. Buying expensive toys is unnecessary; common household items, such as pots, pans, lids, and spoons, provide excellent objects for play purposes.

### Activity Through Stimulation

Parental stimulation of the infant is an important developmental technique; the infant needs stimulation to learn about the world. This activity does not require expensive objects, but rather involves experiences in sight, sound, and touch that are free and can be provided by any parent (Figure 17-1). Examples of stimulating experiences for infants include the following:

- Having lullabies sung to them
- Listening to tape recordings of a heartbeat
- Seeing colorful mobiles in the crib
- Being rocked in a rocking chair
- Having a familiar face smiling close by
- Having space to wander when developmentally ready
- Looking at themselves in mirrors
- Listening to music

### Anticipatory Guidance

Knowledge of developmental landmarks allows the nurse to guide parents in proper play and stimulation for infants. Handing a 15-month-old child a ball and placing the child in a fenced-in back yard to play is not enough. These activities must provide interpersonal contact, activity, and exercise. Activity and exercise through stimulation and play are extremely important for adequate and healthy development (Johnson et al., 2015).

### Sleep-Rest Pattern

The amount of sleep that infants need is closely related to their rate of growth. Initially infants sleep approximately 80% of the time, as demanded by their rapid growth. As growth begins to slow toward the middle of the first year of life, less sleep is needed. The 12-month-old infant sleeps for only 12 of 24 hours, a pattern that remains essentially unchanged through the second year. Many new mothers think that there is a link between the amount of food fed to their infant and sleep duration. Recent studies indicate that infants who received more milk or solid feedings during the day were less likely to feed at night, but not less likely to wake (Brown & Harries, 2015). The findings have important implications for nurses who support new mothers with infant sleep and diet in the first year. Increasing infant calories during the day may reduce the likelihood of night feeding but will not reduce the need for mothers to attend to the infant in the night. To assist parents in understanding normal sleep and rest patterns, the nurse stresses that no set schedule exists (Table 17-6).

### Anticipatory Guidance

Infant sleep patterns are a common concern for new parents. Health-promotion activities can also help parents determine the individual needs of their infant. The nurse stresses that longer sleep patterns are signs of maturation and that sleep and rest are recognized as having a significant influence on the infant's growth and development. Sleep problems are highly prevalent in early childhood. Frequently, parents seek professional help when they suspect their child has a sleep problem. The nurse may offer the parents helpful comments for promoting infant sleep patterns, such as the following:

- Provide a quiet room for the infant that is separate from the parents' room.
- Learn behavioral clues that signal that the infant is going to sleep and is not interacting socially.
- Encourage caretakers that periodic, brief arousals at night are normal for infants.
- Encourage the establishment of a bedtime routine and a consistent sleep schedule.
- Learn to become sensitive to sleep cycles and rest periods that the infant is establishing and base care accordingly.

- Attempt to schedule feeding times during wakeful rather than drowsy periods.
- Learn that certain cycles are intrinsic to infants and that each infant is unique.
- Discuss normal development of infants' sleep and napping patterns.
- Review safe sleep practices (sleeping position, surface, environment).
- Perform rituals for the infant, such as rocking or reading a bedtime story, to provide comfort and security and let the infant know the expected behavior (Mindell & Owens, 2015).

If parents express a sleep concern, the nurse assesses their reactions, considers their definition of the concern, assesses the sleep environment, and observes the infant's own unique sleep patterns. Only then can the nurse's health-promotion approach be individualized to assist the family in caring for the infant.

## Sudden Infant Death Syndrome

Sudden infant death syndrome (SIDS) is defined as the sudden death of an infant younger than 1 year old during sleep that is unexpected and unexplained after a thorough postmortem examination including autopsy, a thorough history, and scene evaluation. SIDS is the only cause of death derived by exclusion of other causes. The incidence of SIDS has decreased more than 50% in the past 20 years, largely as a result of the Safe to Sleep campaign. One consequence of the Safe to Sleep campaign is a significant increase in occipital flattening. Infants who develop a flat spot should be placed with the head facing alternative directions each time they are put to bed. Supervised prone

positioning when the infant is awake, avoiding excessive use of carriers, and upright positioning when the infant is awake are also recommended (Horne et al., 2015). Despite declines in prevalence during the past 2 decades, SIDS continues to be one of the leading causes of infant death in the postneonatal period. SIDS is a complex, multifactorial disorder, the cause of which is still not fully understood. Behavioral risk factors identified in epidemiological studies include prone and side sleeping positions, preterm birth and/or infant low birth weight, smoke exposure, soft bedding, bed sharing, not breastfeeding, and overheating. Risk-reducing measures include use of a firm crib mattress, breastfeeding, keeping vaccinations up to date, avoidance of overheating due to overbundling, avoidance of soft bedding and objects in the crib, encouragement of supervised "tummy time" when the infant is awake, and consideration of the use of a pacifier during sleep once breastfeeding is established (Adams et al., 2015) (Box 17-8). These factors may also be associated with sleep disorders in infants, principally with bedtime problems, abnormal night awakenings, and arrhythmic sleep. Although SIDS affects infants from all social strata, lower socioeconomic status, younger maternal age, inadequate prenatal care, and lower maternal education level are consistently associated with SIDS. The incidence of SIDS has varied over time and among nations. SIDS still accounts for 3500 cases of infant death in the United States annually and is the third leading cause of death among infants beyond 1 month of age (CDC, 2015d). By definition, the cause of SIDS is not known.

Parents should be instructed to allow supervised tummy time when the infant is awake and should be cautioned about the

---

### BOX 17-8 Safe to Sleep Public Education Campaign

The Safe to Sleep campaign aims to educate parents, caregivers, and health care providers about ways to reduce the risk of SIDS and other sleep-related causes of infant death.

Safe to Sleep is an expansion of the original Back to Sleep campaign, which started in 1994. Back to Sleep was named for its recommendation to place healthy babies on their backs to sleep, the most effective action that parents and caregivers can take to reduce the risk of SIDS. Since that campaign started, the percentage of infants placed on their backs to sleep has increased dramatically, and the overall SIDS rates have declined by more than 50%.

The expanded Safe to Sleep campaign builds on the success and reach of the Back to Sleep campaign. In addition to strategies for reducing the risk of SIDS, Safe to Sleep also describes actions that parents and caregivers can take to reduce the risk of other sleep-related causes of infant death, such as suffocation.

Safe to Sleep campaign collaborators include the Eunice Kennedy Shriver National Institute of Child Health and Human Development; the Maternal and Child Health Bureau of the Health Resources and Services Administration; the CDC, Division of Reproductive Health; the AAP; the American College of Obstetricians and Gynecologists; First Candle; and the Association of SIDS and Infant Mortality Programs.

The safe sleep strategies outlined in Safe to Sleep materials and publications are based on recommendations defined by the AAP Task Force on SIDS. The Task Force on SIDS released expanded guidelines in October 2011. More information

about these recommendations is available at the Eunice Kennedy Shriver National Institute of Child Health and Human Development website.

On the basis of the AAP Task Force on SIDS recommendations, parents and caregivers can make changes to their babies' sleep environment to make it safer and to reduce the risk of SIDS and other sleep-related causes of infant death.

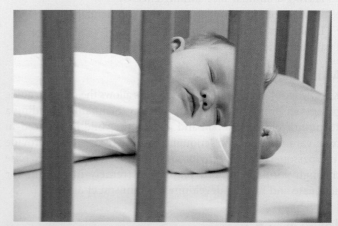

(From Thinkstock.)

From Eunice Kennedy Shriver National Institute of Child Health and Human Development. (2016). Safe to Sleep. https://www.nichd.nih.gov/sts/Pages/default.aspx.

amount of time their infant spends in a car seat. Delayed gross motor development can be prevented by reduction of the amount of time the infant spends in the supine position. Tummy time is the key intervention in preventing gross motor delays in infants. This prone position provides infants with increased physical challenges and gives them a chance to begin developing head control by strengthening neck muscles. Nurses should educate the parents to introduce prone positioning in short periods several times a day. As infants get stronger, they will use arm muscles to lift themselves and aid them to reach for toys or other objects. This strengthening is essential in assisting them in rolling over, crawling, pulling themselves up to stand, and developing fine motor development, including coordination and sensory processing.

Objective MICH 1.8 from *Healthy People 2020* (USDHHS, 2010) is to reduce infant deaths from SIDS from 0.55 per 1000 live births to 0.50 per 1000 live births. Objective MICH 1.9 is to reduce infant deaths from SIDS and other causes (including SIDS, unknown causes, accidental suffocation, and strangulation in bed) from 0.93 per 1000 live births in 2006 to 0.84 per 1000 live births by 2020. Both objectives advocate a 10% reduction in infant deaths.

When an infant dies suddenly, unexpectedly, and for no apparent reason, a family crisis occurs. The parents are devastated and completely unprepared for the shock, reacting with intense guilt, blaming themselves and each other, and agonizing over the part they may have played in the infant's death. Because many unanswered questions remain, these feelings are universal. Parents think there is something they could have done to prevent the tragedy. In most cases, nothing could have been done. Too frequently, the first sign that something was wrong is death. The nurse is in an excellent position to help the family through this crisis. Dealing with the family's grief is very difficult. Many families find strength in their faith to help them through this difficult time. Other family members and close friends can assist the family in their grieving process. Many receive solace and support from talking to other parents who have lost an infant to SIDS. Several parent groups are available from local chapters of the SIDS Foundation; the nurse can refer them to their local chapter.

The nurse's main supportive role for families coping with SIDS is listening and offering compassionate guidance through the weeks and months that follow. The nurse encourages parents to talk about their infant. Too soon, family and friends expect the surviving family to "get over it." A parent, however, is never able to "get over it"; it is only put in perspective and not so near the surface. Nurses need to actively participate in helping parents through their grieving process and remember a standard time frame is not applicable (Andreotta et al., 2015).

Nursing assessment of the infant at risk of SIDS includes observing the infant for apneic episodes. Usually, however, nursing assessment occurs after death and consists of support and providing appropriate resources for the family. Nursing diagnoses for sudden infant death might include the following:

- Spiritual distress related to coping with death
- Ineffective family coping related to the loss of an infant
- Dysfunctional grieving related to the parents' inability to cope

Nurses also discuss with the family feelings about caring for future children. Life can appear out of control, and parents may believe that they cannot care for another infant. These feelings must be resolved before another pregnancy is contemplated. When dealing with the families of SIDS infants, nurses can feel uncomfortable and helpless. As health professionals, they might speak in terms of easing the pain or alleviating the guilt of these families, but many times simple nonverbal human contact is sufficient to express concern and understanding.

## Cognitive-Perceptual Pattern

Cognition is the process by which an individual recognizes, accumulates, and organizes the knowledge of the environment, beginning with the perception or recognition of an event within that environment. Cognitive development is concurrent with biological, adaptive, and psychosocial achievement. The infant's biological and cognitive developmental patterns (Piaget's sensorimotor period) were discussed earlier in this chapter. The focus of this section is on the infant's sensory and language development and the importance of stimulation of both developmental areas. From birth, infants possess sensory capabilities; all sensory organs are well developed and functioning. As the infant is cared for and handled, the special senses become organized neurologically into a pattern of behavior that will greatly influence subsequent development.

### Vision

Sight is the least developed sense at birth. The infant's initial visual impressions are unfocused, bizarre, unfamiliar, and meaningless. The visual system of the newborn infant takes several months to develop. The infant's eyes are not very sensitive to light in the first month of life, so it is okay to leave a light on in the nursery—it will not affect the infant's ability to sleep. Because everything is new and only somewhat significant, visual stimuli must be moving, bright, or flashing to capture the infant's attention. To help stimulate the infant's vision, decorate their room with bright, cheerful colors and also hang a brightly colored mobile above the crib that has a variety of shapes and colors. The infant's eyes are well developed at birth, but the muscles that attach the eyes to their sockets are weak. This weakness may be stressful to parents because the infant's eyes do not appear to function simultaneously. Parents can be assured that most infants coordinate their eye movements by the age of 3 months; by 6 months this function is mature. Table 17-7 summarizes visual developmental milestones.

### Hearing

After the amniotic fluid has drained from the middle ear several days after birth, the infant's hearing becomes acute. Hearing is one of the better-developed senses in the infant; the fetus can even hear in utero and responds to loud sounds (Figure 17-2). The newborn can distinguish sound frequencies and turns toward a voice or another sound. The infant may be familiar with the mother's voice early in life. Sounds gradually gain significance and meaning when they are associated with caregivers, food, and pleasure.

## TABLE 17-7 GROWTH AND DEVELOPMENT
### Visual Development During Infancy

| Age (Months) | Behavior That Indicates Vision |
|---|---|
| 1–3 | Fixes gaze on object 12–24 inches away<br>Takes interest in bright colors and faces<br>Follows objects in field of vision |
| 3–6 | Begins to show interest in hands<br>Follows in range of 90 degrees<br>Recognizes familiar objects<br>Able to see full color by now |
| 6–9 | Visual scanning becomes more integrated<br>Capable of organized depth perception<br>Begins to perceive distances accurately<br>Both eyes should focus equally now |
| 9–12 | Able to look for concealed items<br>Converges on objects in close proximity<br>Peripheral vision is well developed<br>Judges distance well |
| 12–18 | Eye-hand coordination develops<br>Depth perception more refined<br>Ability to identify forms and shapes |

From American Academy of Pediatrics. (2015). Bright futures: Prevention and health promotion for infants, children, adolescents, and their families. https://brightfutures.aap.org/materials-and-tools/Pages/default.aspx; Coats, D. K. (2016). Visual development and vision assessment in infants and children. *UpToDate*. http://www.uptodate.com/contents/visual-development-and-vision-assessment-in-infants-and-children.

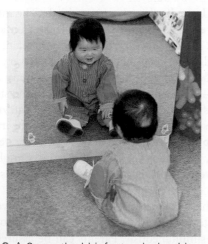

**FIGURE 17-2** A 9-month-old infant enjoying his own image in a mirror. (From Hockenberry, M. J., & Wilson, D. [Eds.] [2013]. *Wong's essentials of pediatric nursing* [9th ed.]. St. Louis: Mosby.)

The ability to listen and discriminate among sounds is an important task during infancy. Caretakers should talk to their infants, sing nursery songs, and make faces so the infants develop language and social skills. The use of baby rattles and musical mobiles is also a good way to stimulate the infant's hearing. The closer the infant is to the sound, the more easily the sound can be discriminated. The groundwork for verbal ability begins to develop long before words appear, and many believe that infants whose mothers talk to them tend to speak earlier than infants who are not exposed to these sounds (Burnham

## TABLE 17-8 GROWTH AND DEVELOPMENT
### Normal Development of Hearing

| Age (Months) | Behavior That Indicates Hearing |
|---|---|
| 1–3 | Is startled by loud noises<br>Stops activity when spoken to |
| 3–6 | Turns eyes and head toward sound<br>Responds to mother's voice<br>Imitates own noises: "ooh" and "ba-ba" |
| 6–9 | Responds to own name<br>Looks toward sounds<br>Recognizes familiar sounds |
| 9–12 | Points to familiar objects or people<br>Imitates simple words and sounds<br>Locates a sound in any direction |
| 12–18 | Follows simple spoken directions<br>Distinguishes between sounds<br>Spoken words are well on their way |

From Delaney, A. M. (2016). Newborn hearing screening. *Medscape*. http://emedicine.medscape.com/article/836646-overview; National Institute on Deafness and Other Communication Disorders. (2016). Your baby's hearing and communicative development checklist. https://www.nidcd.nih.gov/health/your-babys-hearing-and-communicative-development-checklist.

et al., 2015). Table 17-8 summarizes the infant's auditory development.

### Smell

The ability to smell is fully developed at birth. The infant has many receptors in the nose, but it lacks the cilia that line the inside of the adult's nose. As a result, the infant has a keen sense of smell because odors reach the receptor cells easily. Within 2 weeks after birth, an infant can differentiate the odor of the mother's milk from other sources of milk, an ability developed when the infant is held closely (Berk & Meyers, 2015). At this time the infant begins associating the parents with their body odors, a perception that is important for infant-parent bonding.

### Taste

Taste buds in newborns can be found on the tonsils and the back of the throat, as well on the tongue. Infants use their sense of smell from the start and can localize odors by turning their heads in the direction of the odor. The sense of taste is present at birth, and salivation begins at approximately 3 months of age. The four primary sensations are sour, salty, sweet, and bitter. The taste buds for sweet tastes are more abundant during early life than they are in later life, which may account for the preference for sweets that is characteristic of infants and children. An infant's reaction to salty foods does not come until approximately 4 to 5 months of age.

### Touch and Motion

Touch is by far the most developed of all of the infant's senses, as it is the main way in which infants learn about their environment and bond with other people. The skin is the sensory organ for touch. Tactile sensation is well developed at birth, particularly on the lips and tongue. Perceptions of motion and touch are perhaps the most important of all senses. Rocking and other motions are sensations of equilibrium picked up by the middle ear. Skin-to-skin touching should be performed regularly; evidence shows that touch helps relieve the unspent tensions that infants develop and accelerates neuromuscular development (Berk & Meyers, 2015). Infants respond with pleasure to rocking and other motions and to tactile sensations of warmth, closeness, and cuddling.

## Language Development

Language development, an important aspect of the infant's cognitive and perceptual pattern, is affected by development of the intellect, maturation of the central nervous system, development of the organs of speech, and exposure to human verbalization.

As in other areas of development, language acquisition follows a definite sequence. During the first 2 months, most of the infant's sounds are vowels and are made primarily in the front part of the mouth (Fogel, 2015). Crying is the major means of communication during this period. Cooing sounds are heard at approximately 2 to 3 months, usually in response to an adult's voice. By 6 months, babbling sounds are heard, and by 9 to 10 months, the infant forms two-syllable sounds. By 12 months, words such as "ma-ma," "bye-bye," and "da-da" are emerging. From 15 to 18 months, an expressive jargon with rhythmical intonations develops, but words are recognized only rarely. The infant uses jargon along with pointing to express wishes.

## Anticipatory Guidance

The nurse's knowledge and understanding of an infant's cognitive and perceptual behavior facilitates interaction with infants and serves as a guide in parental counseling. The main focus centers on stimulation, because each of the infant's senses is receptive to environmental stimulation. This activity helps the infant learn from the environment. When an infant is exposed to appropriate sensory stimulation, greater curiosity, improved mental capabilities, accelerated neuromuscular growth, enhanced gastrointestinal functioning, quicker weight gain, more rapid language development, and pleasing mother-infant interactions are likely to occur (O'Connor, 2015).

Parents are the primary providers of pleasurable and stimulating experiences for the infant. The nurse assists them by offering suggestions about suitable stimuli for each sensory modality.

## Self-Perception–Self-Concept Pattern

Self-perception has a pervasive influence on all aspects of life. Self-concept consists of a set of attitudes regarding what each person thinks, believes, and feels about the self. These attitudes form a personal self-belief that is an abstraction referred to as "me." Many researchers believe that the infant determines self-existence by first noting that actions such as crying or smiling have an effect on others, which depends on receiving feedback

(Berk & Meyers, 2015). Studies confirm that infants can identify themselves and therefore form a self-concept. Infants at 4 months of age were found to be particularly fascinated with their images in mirrors and smiled more at themselves than they did at pictures of other infants (Fivush & Waters, 2015).

As the infant continues to grow and mature, many circumstances combine to influence self-concept. How others relate to the infant's body and the messages that the infant receives from the body lead to knowledge of a physical self. The ability to use the body to influence others can lead the psychological self to conclude that someone cares about the infant (Feldman, 2015).

The infant's development of body image is gradual. At birth the infant has diffuse feelings of hunger, pain, anger, and comfort, but no body image. Initially, the infant knows only the self and regards the external world as an extension of the self. Only when infants begin to experience the environment through sensory modalities are they able to distinguish their bodies from animate and inanimate objects.

## Nursing Suggestions

The nurse plays a vital role in assisting parents to foster the development of a positive self-concept and a good body image in their infant. Socialization is unique and begins in infancy. Parenting skills and style have a strong influence on outcomes of integrated socialization as infants develop. The nurse first identifies personal self-concept and how it influences individuals (Reed, 2015). The nurse stresses that the way in which parents treat the infant influences the infant's self-concept. Basically, infants and young children incorporate their parents' interactions with them (good or bad) into their own view of self. Parents must understand that their infant's self-concept is an important, continuing event. What the infant knows and later believes about the self will affect all interactions with others, and by influencing what the infant will later attempt, the self-concept may have broad effects on the development of new skills. The mental state or the idea of "me" is that part of the self that makes reference to itself. This mental state develops over the first 2 years of life and is a function of both brain maturation processes and socialization (Reed, 2015).

## Roles-Relationships Pattern

What happens during the first few months of an infant's life matters a great deal because this period of life provides a blueprint for adult well-being and sets the foundation for what follows. Researchers have explored extensively the effect of early bonding between parents and their infants, emphasizing that this initial attraction sets the stage for the later development of love and affiliation. The bonding process has many other implications for the infant's future development as well (Polan & Taylor, 2015).

## Attachment and Bonding

The attachment relationship is a vital bond between the infant and the caregiver that, when secure, facilitates physical and psychological well-being.

Various theories have attempted to explain the basis for attachment behavior. Freudian psychoanalytical theory emphasizes that the bond between the child and the mother develops as a result of the mother's fulfillment of the infant's innate desire to socialize and the physical requirements for survival. Social learning theory contributes the principles of reinforcement to the attachment process; as the mother meets the infant's needs, discomfort is reduced or removed. The infant associates the pleasurable feeling of being satisfied with the mother, who becomes a significant other in the infant's life. The bonding process is the basis for the mother-infant relationship, which, in turn, forms the basis for the interdependence that is necessary for the infant's psychological and physical development. All infants are born with the building blocks that develop into attachment behaviors, and thus all infants have the ability to form an attachment relationship with their primary caregiver (Fivush & Waters, 2015).

Just as the infant's behavior influences attachment, it also continues to influence the evolving maternal-paternal-infant relationship as the infant develops. Studies have shown that if the process of attachment is encumbered, later problems are more likely to occur, such as child abuse, poor growth, formally termed *failure to thrive syndrome,* and behavior problems. Poor growth is a physical sign that an infant is receiving inadequate nutrition for optimal growth and development. Poor growth generally describes an infant whose current weight, or rate of weight gain, is significantly below that expected of similar infants of the same age and sex (Kliegman et al., 2015).

Many factors are present when a relationship is being established and maintained. Most people enter a relationship with unrealistic expectations. Parents are no exception—they are going to be wise, patient, and devoted, and they will nurture their infant. Because the parents' self-esteem is associated closely with their infant's interactions and accomplishments, when parents' self-esteem is low, disappointment, anger, and a disturbance in the relationship with their infant can occur. In some instances this disturbed parent-infant relationship is short-lived and nothing harmful develops. When a disturbed parent-infant relationship continues, however, the infant is at risk of abuse and behavior problems (Box 17-9: Innovative Practice).

Becoming a father and a parent can be a transformational process for a person. When an infant enters a father's life, a new depth of feeling and emotion are awoken within the two of them. The process of bonding is also important for fathers. Fathers do have direct effects on their infants, but their effects also are often indirect, mediated or moderated by their relationship with the infant's mother. Fathers are looking for a psychologically satisfying place within their families (Linton, 2015). Recently, a process called paternal engrossment has been used to describe the behavior pattern of fathers when they interact with their infants. It describes the father's total absorption and preoccupation with the presence of their newborn.

Infant/child abuse has occurred throughout history, yet its prevalence is difficult to estimate, partly because, like an iceberg, it is mostly hidden. Infant/child abuse is an important cause of pediatric morbidity and death and is associated with major physical and mental health problems that can extend into adulthood. Infant and child abuse, as defined by the WHO, constitutes

## BOX 17-9 INNOVATIVE PRACTICE
### The Touchpoints Model

The birth of a baby is a life-changing event for a couple and family. Although most infants develop through predictable yet individual patterns of development, parents, especially first-time parents, are usually unaware of these patterns or have difficulty assessing their infant's progress and problems. All of these processes can be stressful for the parents, the entire family, and the infant.

The Touchpoints Model Program at Children's Hospital in Boston, Massachusetts, delivers a training model for practitioners, emphasizing the building of supportive alliances between parents and professionals around key points in the development of young children. The model is an outgrowth of Brazelton's (2011) book *Touchpoints* and research at Children's Hospital in Boston. The Touchpoints model provides a form of outreach through which multidisciplinary practitioners can engage parents around important, predictable phases of their baby's development. The Touchpoints model stresses preventive health through development of relationships between parents and providers; acknowledges that developing and maintaining relationships is critical to appreciating cultural, religious, and societal family dynamics; and encourages the practitioner to focus on strengths in individuals and families. Touchpoints is not a stand-alone model; it is intended to be integrated into ongoing pediatric, early childhood, and family intervention programs.

**Contact Information**
The Touchpoints Project
Child Development Unit
Children's Hospital
1295 Boylston Street
Boston, MA 02215

Touchpoints has gone on-line. Parents and professionals can get advice and information from Brazelton, T. B. (2011). Brazelton Touchpoints Center. http://www.touchpoints.org; Lester, B. M., & Lester, J. D. (2010). *Nurturing children and families: Building on the legacy of T. Berry Brazelton.* Chichester: Wiley-Blackwell.

all forms of physical and/or emotional ill-treatment, sexual abuse, neglect or negligent treatment, or commercial or other exploitation resulting in actual or potential harm to the infant/child's health, survival, development, or dignity (WHO, 2015b). The family traditionally has been considered a safe place for its members, but many infants are at risk of maltreatment. Infant and child abuse has always been a part of human history. Acceptable behavior toward infants is largely a learned phenomenon; the art of parenting is not instinctively acquired, as many people believe. Abusing parents are seldom "monsters"; they are merely individuals ineffectively coping with the demands of parenthood, for which there is little or no preparation, as well as other life stressors.

The scope of child abuse is extensive: estimates indicate that more than 650,000 infants and children in the United States are victims of abuse annually, and more than 1500 children die of abuse or neglect. Infants from birth to 1 year of age are the most vulnerable to abuse and neglect (CDC, 2015e). Children younger than 3 years of age are the most frequent victims. Women are more frequent abusers than are men, because they are the primary caregivers. Men abuse more severely and commit sexual abuse more frequently. Child abuse does not discriminate among children; it occurs in families of every race, creed, and socioeconomic class.

Child-abuse syndrome is a clinical condition in infants who have suffered serious active or passive abuse at the hands of their parents or other caregivers. Physical trauma is not the only facet, but it is the most overt indicator of a dysfunctional family unit and a disturbed parent-infant relationship (Fanetti et al., 2015).

Active manifestations of abuse include the following:
- Brain injuries, subdural hematomas, and skull fractures
- Soft-tissue injuries, such as bruises, lacerations, or burns
- Fractures of the long bones and ribs; multiple fractures in various stages of healing
- Sexual abuse manifested by genital tissue injury; sexually transmitted infections
- Bullying manifested by intentional, aggressive behaviors toward others

Passive manifestations of abuse include the following:
- Poor nutrition, failure to thrive, and severe malnutrition
- Poor physical condition: neglected safeguards against disease, poor skin condition, and lack of medical attention
- Emotional neglect: rejection, indifference, and deprivation of love
- Moral neglect: allowing the infant or child to remain in an immoral atmosphere
- Spiritual abuse: incorporating religion into abuse of a child (Boy Scouts of America, 2015)

Abusing parents often have common patterns of behavior. As children, their own parents may have abused them. In this way, child abuse is cycled from generation to generation. The development of the maternal role on which the infant depends for health, progress, and survival begins during the mother's early childhood. Unless she received love and proper mothering, she will have difficulty with a relationship that entails the complete dependency of another person. She may find the relationship with her own infant to be unrewarding, threatening, and frustrating. Feelings of inadequacy and guilt in the mother and father roles compound the problems.

Abusing parents are often socially isolated and have few people to whom they can turn during times of crisis; they also cannot support one another emotionally. If parents grew up with harsh methods of discipline, they may be prone to violence with their own children. These parents may view the infant as the person who can provide the love, support, and nurturing that is lacking in their own lives. When the infant does not fulfill their expectations, the risk of abuse increases (Bauer, 2015).

The abused infant or child is frequently singled out as someone who is different. This infant may be chronically ill, may have been born prematurely, may be hyperactive, may have been the product of a difficult and complicated pregnancy, or may have an obvious anomaly. Early bonding disturbances (inadequacies in feeding, holding, and caring for the infant) are characteristic signals.

The long-term effects of child abuse are profound. The victims lack basic trust (a major task of infancy) and confidence and self-worth. These deficits follow the victims into adulthood and parenthood, and the vicious cycle continues. One of the discouraging findings is that infants and children who were abused frequently grow up to be abusing parents (Magana & Kaufhold, 2015).

Across the United States great interest has been generated in attempts to identify parents in the prenatal and perinatal periods who have significant potential for child abuse. Nurses play a critical role in recognizing infants who have been intentionally harmed, because they are often the first to begin taking a history of the infant. The role of the nurse may include identifying abused infants with suspicious injuries who present for care, reporting suspected abuse to the child protection agency for investigation, supporting families who are affected by infant abuse, coordinating with community agencies to provide immediate and long-term care to the victimized infant, providing court testimony when necessary, providing preventive care and anticipatory guidance in the health care setting, and advocating policies that support and protect vulnerable infants (Christian et al., 2015). Nurses work collaboratively with community agencies to provide follow-up care for the infant in danger of continued abuse. Nurses take appropriate action if they suspect an infant is at risk. Some of the biggest challenges of child protection come from our own internal reluctance to act, but doing nothing is not an option. The following measures have been undertaken to help prevent child abuse:
- Predictive questionnaires to be given to parents on postpartum units
- Recognition of parents who have difficulty relating to their infants through body language clues or verbalizations
- Closer follow-up during the postpartum period by the public health nurse
- Crisis hotlines made available to parents in distress

Before focusing on nursing interventions, the nurse makes several observations to assist in identifying a high-risk infant by answering the following questions:
- Does the mother hold the infant close and establish eye contact?
- Does the mother speak negatively about the infant?
- Does the mother intensely dislike the duties of motherhood, such as diapering, feeding, and so on?
- Does the mother expect too much of the infant at a particular stage of development?
- Does the mother focus her attention on the infant rather than on her husband?
- Does the mother have a good support system available?
- Does the mother act overly concerned about the infant's sex?

Most communities are seeking ways in which child abuse can be prevented through educational efforts, improved agency coordination, and development of new collaborative efforts and services for parents and infants. Laws for reporting abuse have been enacted in every state. Reporting all cases of suspected abuse and neglect is mandatory. Everyone must assist in this endeavor to prevent continued abuse. It takes a community effort to address the problem.

## Sexuality-Reproductive Pattern

An infant's identity begins at birth, when the gendered child is identified and caretakers behave a certain way toward the infant because of its sex. The infant's sexuality gives direction to its physical, emotional, social, and intellectual responses throughout life. Infants have a great oral sensitivity, enjoy skin-to-skin contact, and explore their own bodies for pleasure during the first year of life. A healthy, accepting attitude by caretakers is important in an infant's evolving sexual development.

## Coping-Stress Tolerance Pattern

The term *stress* implies intense reaction to an experience and changes in usual behavior. Stress is a normal phenomenon that occurs throughout the life span, as, for example, when an individual experiences a developmental or situational crisis.

### Developmental Crisis

Developmental crises are turning points or periods of great change. Most stressors that an infant experiences are a necessary part of growth and development. For example, learning new skills creates stress. The infant who is unable to move forward while learning to crawl experiences stress. The infant expresses this stress by crying for help. Other stressors are more psychosocial in nature, such as being left with a babysitter or in an unfamiliar place.

### Situational Crisis

Situational crises are not anticipated easily and do not occur necessarily as part of the normal growth and development process. One major situational crisis during infancy is separation from the significant other. The following three distinct phases are evident in the reaction to separation (Coch et al., 2015):

- *Protest.* Infant cries loudly, screams for the mother, and refuses attention of the substitute caregiver.
- *Despair.* Infant stops crying and becomes less active, withdraws, and becomes apathetic.
- *Withdrawal.* Infant takes an interest in the surroundings but tends to ignore or reject the mother when she returns, because she failed to meet the infant's needs.

Initially, with no time framework and no understanding of waiting, the infant has little ability to cope with stress. As maturity and a sense of security provided by the caregiver increase, the infant begins to wait a short time to have its needs met without protest. An infant who experiences stress reacts by crying, the main tool of communication. The infant gradually learns to tolerate greater stress with time.

### Nursing Interventions

Every family needs good information, concrete resources, and consistent support to thrive. Nursing interventions that assist the infant and the infant's family in stressful situations are listed in Box 17-10. By allaying anxiety in the infant's caregiver, the nurse facilitates coping behaviors in the infant. The stressful situation and the problem-solving activities can be turned into growth-producing experiences for the family, with coping capacities strengthened for the future.

## Values-Beliefs Pattern

A value is a standard or principle that reflects a person's judgment on what is important in life. When people communicate, they send both the content message of the spoken words and the

---

### BOX 17-10 Nursing Interventions to Assist in Stressful Situations During Infancy

- Attempt to meet the infant's needs promptly.
- Allow favorite toy or item of security to be present during stressful experiences.
- Allow familiar caregiver to be present to calm the infant.
- Attempt to keep the number of strangers interacting with the infant to a minimum.
- Attempt to provide a warm and accepting environment for the infant.
- Allow freedom of expression (crying) to reduce tension in the infant.
- Identify the infant's established daily routine and try to follow through with it.
- Reinforce the infant's need for expression.
- Establish a trusting relationship with the infant.
- Provide opportunity for play so the infant can vent fears.
- Provide emotional support for the parents so they can, in turn, give support to their infant.
- Try the five "S" system to soothe a crying infant:
  - Swaddling
  - Side/stomach position
  - Shushing sounds
  - Swinging
  - Sucking

From National Fatherhood Initiative. (2016). Preventing child abuse: The crying baby. http://www.fatherhood.org/fatherhood/preventing-child-abuse-the-crying-baby.

---

unspoken message of who they are and what they believe. Values are pervasive and important and give a focus to both individuals and groups within a particular culture. Because values are attitudes learned especially from significant others within the environment, the parents' values-beliefs pattern greatly influences the care and development of the infant.

### Nursing Interventions

By understanding and respecting the parents' value system, the nurse works within their framework of values in the counseling situation. The nurse communicates personal values to the family. To work successfully within a different value system, the nurse incorporates the following attitudes concerning the values-beliefs pattern into the nursing process (Clark, 2014):

- Believe in the ultimate worth of the infant and the family, regardless of their behavior or situation.
- Grant families the freedom to make their own informed choices and to experience the responsibilities and consequences of their decisions.
- Use knowledge of the family's value system in specific ways to reward and reinforce positive health practices.
- Value the growth potential inherent in developmental and situational crisis situations.
- Recognize your own value system and its influence on your behavior.
- Work with families without applying your personal value system in judging their behavior.
- Broaden your value system by accepting lifestyles different from your own.

The nurse influences the behavior of the parents, who have the greatest influence on their infant's values-beliefs pattern. The nurse accomplishes this task by modeling (living congruently with professed values), acting as a consultant by sharing pertinent information with parents, and modifying his or her own values. Nurses can anticipate a family crisis of values and can help to promote positive coping and effective use of social supports (Harkness & DeMarco, 2015).

Modeling can be a potent influence on another individual's behavior. In the counseling situation, the family looks to the nurse for guidance and assistance in promoting healthy childrearing practices. The methods by which the nurse interacts with the infant, listens to the parents' concerns, and demonstrates respect for the family unit are influencing factors in changing behavior.

Second, the nurse acts as a consultant to influence values. Advice on childrearing practices is overwhelming to parents; everyone has opinions. The nurse listens before giving advice to determine whether parents will accept the advice and to allow parents to decide whether the advice can be useful. Repeated attempts to convert parents to the nurse's value system can make them defensive and resistant to the advice.

Third, by expressing values and attitudes, but remaining open to other approaches, the nurse influences the values-beliefs pattern. Parents can realize that they are free to change and are not bound to values that others outside their value system express (Gardner et al., 2016). Communication skills can more effectively promote the health of the infant and the family.

# ENVIRONMENTAL PROCESSES

## Physical Agents

This section discusses various factors within the environment that can affect the infant's health status. The entire realm of accident prevention and safety promotion is applicable here.

According to the CDC (2015f), unintentional injuries, including motor vehicle traffic crashes, falls, poisonings, suffocations, drownings, and fires/burns, are the leading cause of death for people aged 1 to 44 years and the fourth leading cause of death for people of all ages. Beyond the emotional damage that accompanies such tragedies, the American Public Health Association (2015) reports that unintentional injuries cost the United States more than $70 billion per year.

One of the overall goals for the Quality and Safety Education for Nurses (QSEN) project is to meet the challenge of preparing future nurses who will have the knowledge, skills, and attitudes necessary to continuously improve the quality and safety of the health care systems within which they work. One of their competencies promotes safety within the environment.

Some areas applicable to this competency of safety for infants would be the use of flame-retardant sleepwear, car seats, and crib mattresses, and knowledge of measures to promote crib safety and toy safety.

Sleepwear made for infants aged 9 months or younger can be flame resistant or non–flame resistant. Flame-resistant clothing is usually labeled as such, and is either a synthetic fiber or treated cotton. Parents should be advised to select flame-resistant sleepwear for their infant and to follow the laundry instructions carefully to maintain this properly. Sleepwear for infants older than 9 months is required to be either flame resistant or snug fitting. Snug-fitting clothing that conforms to the body has less opportunity to ignite when exposed to a flame than loose-fitting clothing. Smaller sizes are not required to be snug fitting, because a smaller infant is less likely to be mobile enough to expose himself/herself to a fire hazard.

All new cribs are required to meet strict safety standards; however, if parents accept a secondhand crib, they need to be advised to check the following:

- The slats should be no farther than 2.375 inches apart. Wider slats could allow an infant's head to become trapped between them.
- There should be no decorations or projections that could snag an infant's clothes. Avoid cribs with decorative cutouts in the headboard or footboard.
- Some older cribs were painted with lead-based paint, which could poison an infant who mouths or chews the wood. If unsure, strip the old paint and repaint it with new lead-free enamel.
- No screws and bolts that hold the crib together should be missing, and all should be tight. Avoid cribs with drop side rails. If a drop side rail detaches or becomes loose, an infant may become trapped between the mattress and the railing.
- The crib mattress should be firm and should fit very snugly, with no room for the baby to become trapped between the mattress and the crib. Do not cover the mattress with plastic or a quilt, which can suffocate a baby.

Never put an infant to sleep on a waterbed, pillow, quilt, beanbag chair, or sofa. All these surfaces increase the chance that a baby could suffocate or get his/her head or another part of his/her body trapped in the furniture.

Do not put pillows or stuffed animals in an infant's crib, because they can cause suffocation. Crib quilt bumpers also pose a risk for suffocation and should not be used. When your infant learns to sit, lower the mattress so he/she cannot fall out of the crib. Remove mobiles, and make sure draperies and window blind cords are well out of his/her reach.

Anticipatory guidance to promote infant toy safety would include instructions for parents purchasing new toys to follow the age guidelines on the packaging. Infant toys should have no tiny parts that pose choking hazards, and nothing on the toy should be sharp or detachable (Today's Parent, 2016). Infants explore objects with their mouths, so anything they pick up should be too big to swallow. The more chewable and unbreakable a toy is, the safer it will be.

Accidents are always unexpected and, in retrospect, could usually have been prevented. Unintentional injuries are the leading cause of death for children in the United States and globally. Every 1.5 minutes an infant is seen in the emergency department for an unintentional injury (American Public Health Association, 2015). Adults take for granted that they are living in a world designed by adults for adults. They must remind themselves constantly that infants also live in this complex world and that they learn at a remarkable rate, primarily by exploring and playing

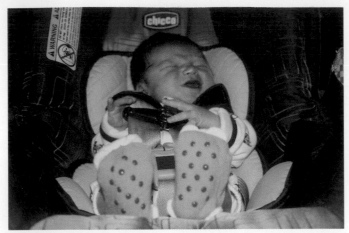

**FIGURE 17-3** Accident prevention for infants in their car seats includes the use of safety belts.

From Remedy's Health Communities. (2017). *Preventing falls in babies.* http://www.healthcommunities.com/infant-safety/children/fall-prevention.shtml

in the environment. These experiences render them extremely vulnerable to accidents, a major problem and a challenging field for preventive measures.

Accidents occur in many situations: in the home, outside, on the playground, and in automobiles. The use of safety belts prevents infant injury (Figure 17-3). Most accidents, however, occur in the home. Their number and seriousness are closely linked to the infant's developmental stage. Accidents tend to increase with the mobility of the infant, but even a 2-month-old infant can wiggle or fall from a high place. Keeping the environment free from hazards and ensuring caregiver supervision are crucial for this age group.

Nurses have the opportunity to help parents and caregivers anticipate and understand the common hazards of early life and provide specific guidance for accident prevention.

## Unintentional Injuries

***Falls.*** Falls are most common after 4 months of age, when the infant has learned to roll over, but they can occur at any age. Falls involving infants happen more often in the home environment, on stairs, from furniture, and out of windows. The best advice is never to place an infant unattended on a raised surface that has no type of guardrails. When in doubt, the safest place is the floor (Gill & Kelly, 2015). Safety tips to assist parents in preventing falls are listed in Box 17-11.

***Burns.*** In the United States, burns are the third leading cause of unintentional injury death in children aged 1 to 14 years, accounting for more than 600 deaths per year in children from birth to 19 years of age. Every day, more than 300 children aged 0 to 19 years are treated in emergency departments for burn-related injuries and two children die as a result of being burned (CDC, 2015g).

Burns are the most frequent and frightening of all accidents during infancy. Most fire deaths occur in the home, and most victims die because of smoke or toxic gases and not because of the burns (CDC, 2015g). Because nearly all burns are preventable, the attendant caregiver can experience severe guilt.

Fire from matches or other sources, hot liquids, ultraviolet light from the sun, electricity or electrical outlets, and heating

### BOX 17-11 Safety Tips to Prevent Falls

- Keep sides up and firmly secured when the infant is in the crib.
- Place the infant seat on a stable surface, preferably the floor. The infant should be strapped in securely.
- Check high chairs, strollers, and carriages for safety, and restrain the infant who is active.
- All windows above the first floor should be locked and have operable window guards.
- Clean up food or liquid spills immediately from the floor.
- Remember that polished floors are hazardous, especially when throw rugs are present.
- Close off stairways with doors or properly installed gates, at the top and bottom.
- To prevent falls, set the crib mattress at the lowest adjustment level after the infant can pull himself/herself up and stand.
- Place furniture away from windows and anchor pieces to the wall.
- Avoid the use of baby walkers.
- Never leave an infant alone on a bed, changing table, or piece of furniture.
- Avoid bringing strollers onto escalators.
- Best fall prevention is to watch, listen, and stay near the infant at all times.

elements such as radiators, registers, and floor heaters can all cause burns.

***Swallowing/choking on foreign objects.*** Choking occurs when a foreign object becomes lodged in the throat, blocking air flow (National Safety Council, 2016). Choking is the leading cause of unintentional death in infants (American Heart Association, 2015). Any small object that an infant puts in the mouth has the potential to be swallowed and choked on. More than 65% of deaths from foreign-body aspiration occur in infants. Liquids are the most common cause of choking in infants, whereas balloons, small objects, and foods are the most common causes of foreign-body airway obstruction in children (American Public Health Association, 2015). Parents should be advised that objects such as safety pins, peanuts, beads, coins, hot dogs, paper clips, nuts, corn, buttons, popcorn, chips, apple with peel, and parts of broken toys are frequently swallowed. Many objects can fit into this category and into the infant's mouth. The carelessness of a caregiver, relative, friend, or babysitter in leaving small objects available and within reach, or giving toys unsuited to the infant's stage of development, frequently causes these accidents.

When choking occurs, the adult should place the infant across the adult's knees and deliver five back blows (slaps) followed by five chest thrusts repeatedly until the object is expelled or the infant becomes unresponsive. Abdominal thrusts are not recommended for infants because thrusts in the abdominal area could potentially damage the relatively large and unprotected liver (American Heart Association, 2015). Cardiopulmonary resuscitation should be performed if the infant becomes unresponsive. The American Heart Association does not recommend use of under-the-diaphragm abdominal thrusts for choking infants younger than 1 year. Prevention of swallowing foreign objects is the best treatment.

## BOX 17-12    Home Childproofing Tips

- Remove any heavy, sharp, or breakable objects from tables and low shelves.
- Bolt bookcases to the wall and remove heavy books to prevent falls.
- Test floor and table lamps to make sure they cannot be pulled over.
- Avoid placing toys, blankets, pillows, or bumper pads in the crib.
- Disconnect unused appliances and wrap up cords.
- Secure all other cords to prevent appliances from being pulled down.
- Safely discard unused and unneeded medicines.
- Avoid referring to medicines as candy.
- Post the National Capital Poison Center telephone number (1-800-222-1222) nearby.
- Store potentially toxic substances out of sight and reach.
- Close reachable outlets with safety covers.
- Avoid leaving an infant unattended in the bathtub, even for a moment.
- Avoid using tablecloths that can be pulled down by a crawling infant.
- Tie drapery and blind cords out of the infant's reach.
- Choose stair gates with openings too small for an infant's head and child-resistant fasteners such as pressure bars.
- Avoid accordion or expandable gates with openings that can trap an infant's head.
- Install smoke detectors and check the batteries at least once a month.
- Use sturdy screens in front of fireplaces.
- Place crib, playpen, and high chair well away from heaters, fans, and electrical outlets.
- Install childproof latches on drawers and cupboards. Store all cleaning compounds and detergents in a high, locked cupboard.
- Keep plants out of an infant's reach, as some are poisonous.
- Buy all medicines in bottles with childproof lids and keep them in their original labeled containers for identification in case of accidental ingestion.
- Install lids on garbage pails and never leave any harmful materials in them, such as sharp can lids or spoiled food.
- Place furniture away from windows and anchor pieces to the wall, such as TVs.
- Check the floor regularly for objects small enough to be swallowed.
- Cut blind cords into two pieces.

From Centers for Disease Control and Prevention. (2016). Safety in the home and community. http://www.cdc.gov/parents/infants/safety.html.

The entire balance of safety for infants depends on allowing them plenty of opportunity to explore and play within the environment while protecting them from harmful agents. According to the AAP, the greatest threat to the health of infants is not illness but injuries, many of which can be prevented. The nurse informs the infant's parents, babysitters, family friends, and day care workers about the need to childproof their environments when an infant is present. The nurse can explain ways to promote the safety of these varied environments (Box 17-12).

## Biological Agents

The fetus is partially protected from some biological agents in the environment by the placental barrier and the mother's defense system. After birth, however, the infant is thrust into an environment that is filled with infectious, disease-causing agents. These bacterial or viral organisms can be found in food, cribs, the air, pets, the parents, and the siblings—literally everywhere (Environmental Protection Agency [EPA], 2015). Even the healthiest environment harbors disease-causing agents. Although the infant cannot escape exposure to these pathogens without being completely isolated, immunizations are given to assist the infant's defense against some communicable diseases.

### Acquired Immunodeficiency Syndrome

Human immunodeficiency virus (HIV) is a retrovirus and can be transmitted vertically, sexually, or via contaminated blood products or intravenous drug abuse. Acquired immunodeficiency syndrome (AIDS) is spread by contact with HIV through blood and body secretions. HIV becomes established in cells of the host's immune system called T cells. The T-helper cells are sometimes referred to as CD4+ cells because they have a glycoprotein on their surfaces. CD4+ helps the T-helper cells recognize HIV, but if the CD4+ T-helper cells are infected with HIV, they cannot coordinate an immune response to the HIV virus. The infant with HIV infection is unable to resist normal infections. Transmission of HIV from mother to infant is the most likely cause of childhood HIV infection. Transmission can occur during pregnancy, at childbirth, or during breastfeeding. For 6 weeks after birth, infants born to HIV-positive women receive the HIV medication zidovudine (Retrovir) to protect them from any infection with any HIV that may have been passed during the birthing process. In addition, because HIV can be spread in breast milk, women with HIV who live in the United States should not breastfeed (AIDS Info, 2015) (see Chapter 16). There is no immunization against HIV infections currently, but frequently preventive options are offered to mothers, and babies are usually delivered by cesarean delivery. Antiretroviral drugs reduce viral replication and can decrease mother-to-child transmission of HIV either by lowering plasma viral load in pregnant women or by providing postexposure prophylaxis in their newborns. In developed countries, highly active antiretroviral therapy (HAART), which usually comprises three drugs from at least two classes, has reduced the mother-to-child transmission rates to approximately 1% to 2%, but HAART is not always available in developing countries (Rivera & Frye, 2015).

Because infants can retain maternal antibodies for HIV infection for as long as 18 months, the diagnosis of HIV infection in an at-risk infant (one whose mother is infected) is extremely difficult. In the last few years, investigators have demonstrated the utility of highly accurate blood tests in diagnosing HIV infection in infants aged 6 months or younger. The standard assay has limited utility in diagnosing HIV reactivity among infants until the age of 18 months, by which time many HIV-infected infants have died. The preferred virological assays for diagnosing HIV infection in infants and children younger than 18 months include HIV branched DNA polymerase chain reaction and HIV RNA assays either by a dried blood spot or by a whole blood sample (Rivera & Frye, 2015). Although signs and symptoms of illness can occur at any time, they usually begin during the first year of life. In infants, the symptoms of the disease include growth failure, oral candidiasis, recurrent bacterial infections, pneumonia, recurrent fungal infections, chronic diarrhea, and delays in reaching important milestones in motor skills and mental development such as crawling, walking, and speaking.

Early recognition and triaging of infants suspected of having HIV infection provide an opportunity for early diagnosis and treatment, which could prevent the adverse impact of rapidly progressive HIV disease (CDC, 2015h).

In response to the urgent need to reduce the number of new HIV infections globally, the WHO and the Joint United Nations Program on HIV/AIDS (UNAIDS) funded research to determine whether male circumcision should be recommended for the prevention of HIV infection (WHO & UNAIDS, 2015). On the basis of the research findings presented, experts recommended that use of condoms and male circumcision be recognized as important interventions to reduce the risk of heterosexually acquired HIV infection in men. There is strong evidence that medical male circumcision reduces the acquisition of HIV in heterosexual men by between 38% and 66% in 24 months. The incidence of adverse events is very low, indicating that male circumcision, when conducted under these conditions, is a safe procedure. Inclusion of male circumcision into current HIV prevention measure guidelines is warranted, with further research required to assess the feasibility, desirability, and cost-effectiveness of implementing the procedure globally. Currently, voluntary medical male circumcisions are being implemented in several sub-Saharan African countries to prevent HIV spread (Wamai et al., 2015). Parents must weigh their decision to circumcise their male infant on the basis of their own values, religious backgrounds, and culture in light of this new information.

Nursing assessment focuses on a careful and complete history of the infant and mother, signs and symptoms of the disease, growth and development history, and psychosocial concerns. Parents are assessed carefully to determine their level of anxiety; knowledge of the disease process, including prognosis, treatment, and transmission; and awareness of resources, support systems, coping strategies, and the infant's needs.

No other disease causes as much public awareness and panic as does AIDS. Part of this behavior is ignorance. Nurses play a major role in educating the public about the disease process, its mode of transmission, and most of all, preventive measures. Preventive education should begin with young children. Most school health programs include information on HIV/AIDS. School nurses can contribute to the success of these programs, as can nurses working in prenatal clinics, to spread the importance of prevention. Nurses in all settings can engage in research related to HIV/AIDS to gather further clarification of this fatal disease.

Although the infant is not an active participant in the spread of HIV, parents should understand the means by which the virus is transmitted and not allow their infant to become a passive participant because of their own high-risk behaviors.

## Immunization

Disease prevention by immunization is a public health priority in *Healthy People 2020* and society as a whole. Progress continues toward the goal of protecting children from serious disease through immunizations. The most recent schedule recommends the rotavirus vaccine in a three-dose schedule at ages 2, 4, and 6 months. The influenza vaccine is now recommended as an annual vaccine for all children aged 6 to 59 months, as well as pregnant women. In addition, varicella vaccines should be administered at age 12 to 15 months, and a newly recommended second dose should be administered at age 4 to 6 years (CDC, 2015i,l). For current-year immunizations, see http://www.cdc.gov/vaccines/schedules/hcp/imz/child-adolescent.html.

The two types of immunization are active and passive immunization. In active immunization, all or part of a disease-causing microorganism or a modified product of that microorganism is injected into the body to make the immune system react defensively. This substance is generally a toxin of the disease organism; depending on the virulence and certain other characteristics of the organism, it is used in the vaccine in a live, killed, or attenuated form (AAP, 2015c). The attenuated form is alive, but its virulence has been reduced significantly by treatment with laboratory procedures that use, for example, heat or chemicals, which reduces the potency of microorganisms. Examples of active immunization include diphtheria, tetanus, and acellular pertussis vaccine; inactivated polio vaccine; and measles, mumps, and rubella vaccine. Active immunity is relatively long lasting, waning over several years if at all.

Passive immunization is accomplished by injection of blood from an actively immunized person or animal. After an individual has been exposed to a disease, a passive immunization is given to prevent the disease from developing. Passive immunizations provide a short immunity, usually 1 to 6 weeks, which will protect the person until the danger of contracting the disease has passed. Passive immunization also helps reduce the severity of the disease when it is contracted. Because of the short duration, active immunization is still needed for a person to remain permanently immune. Passive immunity occurs naturally in newborns when maternal antibodies are passed through the placenta or in breast milk.

The Committee on Infectious Diseases of the AAP and the CDC (2015i) recommend immunization schedules that are revised periodically as new information arises. Table 17-9 lists the current recommendations for healthy infants.

Immunization provides one of the most cost-effective means of preventing infection in infants. Immunizations not only help protect those receiving the vaccinations from developing potentially serious diseases but also help protect entire communities by preventing and reducing the spread of infectious agents. Immunization is additionally important because antibiotics cannot destroy viruses; therefore immunization offers the only means of control. Nurses have a special responsibility to keep informed of the recommendations and document all vaccinations given. Emphasis must be placed on educating parents about the importance of immunization. Children need a series of vaccinations, starting at birth, to be fully protected against potentially serious diseases. To motivate parents to have their infants immunized, the nurse can work toward increasing health education to achieve greater health maintenance knowledge, send reminders for upcoming visits and needed immunizations, vigorously advocate that all infants should receive comprehensive health care, including immunizations, provide health services that make immunizations feasible and available, develop a close relationship with the family, and continue surveillance of the immunization status of every infant in the health care system.

## TABLE 17-9 Recommended Immunization Schedule for Infants

| Age (Months) | Immunization |
|---|---|
| Birth | HepB (first dose) |
| 1 | HepB (second dose) |
| 2 | DTaP (first dose) + Hib (first dose) + PCV (first dose) + PV (first dose) + RV (first dose) |
| 4 | DTaP (second dose) + Hib (second dose) + PV (second dose) + PCV (second dose) + RV (second dose) |
| 6 | HepB (third dose) + DTaP (third dose) + Hib (third dose) + PV (third dose) + PCV (third dose) + RV (third dose) + influenza vaccine (yearly) |
| 12–15 | Hib (fourth dose) + MMR + PCV (fourth dose) + HepA + varicella vaccine |
| 15–18 | DTaP (fourth dose) |

*DTaP,* Diphtheria, tetanus, and acellular pertussis vaccine; *HepA,* hepatitis A vaccine; *HepB,* hepatitis B vaccine; *Hib, Haemophilus influenzae* type b conjugate vaccine; *MMR,* measles, mumps, and rubella vaccine; *PCV,* pneumococcal vaccine; *PV,* polio vaccine; *RV,* rotavirus vaccine.
Modified from Centers for Disease Control and Prevention. (2015). Recommended immunization schedule for birth to 15 months. http://www.cdc.gov/vaccines/schedules/hcp/imz/child-adolescent.html.

## Chemical Agents

### Drugs

Despite advances such as childproof caps on medications, childproof packaging, increased educational efforts, and increased awareness of commonly ingested substances, deaths attributable to unintentional poisonings still occur. Unintentional poisonings are an unfortunate and usually preventable cause of death and disability in infants and children. The very nature of a young child predisposes the child to explore the surrounding environment. As children grow and learn to become independent, they are compelled to investigate new and interesting items, places, and objects, such as medications. On the basis of calls to the US poison control centers, each year more than 1 million children younger than 5 years experience potentially toxic ingestions. More than 90% of poisoning exposures occur in homes (Kelly, 2015).

Ibuprofen is the medicine most commonly ingested, with acetaminophen and vitamins close behind. Ibuprofen and other aspirin substitutes are becoming increasingly popular with parents as antipyretics. Vitamins can be harmful; however, many vitamins contain iron, making them potentially lethal. Infants are frequently attracted to vitamins because of their appealing colors, scents, and flavors, especially children's vitamins.

Recent changes in packaging and limits on the number of tablets contained in each bottle have reduced deaths resulting from overdose. Drug manufacturers are using childproof caps increasingly as a safety measure. Despite a concerted effort by manufacturers, childproof bottle caps differ in effectiveness (Ferguson et al., 2015). Frequently the safety caps are adult proof, although children can readily open bottles with them.

This accessibility points to the dangers of medications, regardless of the bottle. All medications must still be secured in a safe

place when infants are in the home or visiting other homes. Some additional guidelines to help prevent accidents involving drugs include the following:

- Use a prescription drug only for the purpose and the person for whom it is intended. Do not use medication prescribed for someone else for a similar condition in the infant.
- Discard unused drugs by taking them to dump into trash on toxic dump days; many infants have been poisoned by eating tablets found in the trash at home.
- Request safety caps on all prescription drugs.
- Keep all medicines under lock and key.
- Use the dosing device that comes with the medicine.
- Consider products not thought about as medicine—diaper rash remedies, eye drops.
- Have the telephone number of the nearest poison control center readily available.

The main points to be emphasized in giving parents guidance in accident prevention are to eliminate specific environmental hazards, such as drugs, from exploring infants, and to supervise infants while they play, gradually replacing supervision with safety training (Ferguson et al., 2015).

### Plants

Colorful, interesting-looking houseplants add beauty to our homes, but they are often an irresistible attraction to a young infant or child. Infants and small children have a curious nature and cannot keep their hands out of dirt-filled plant pots or resist the temptation of eating leaves from the plant. Houseplants are another source of poison if ingested. Most people fail to think of houseplants as potentially poisonous because people do not consider eating them. However, infants test almost everything by putting things in their mouths, and a number of plants can be deadly when eaten. As a result, plants are one of the leading sources of poisoning of infants, and amateur foragers frequently learn the hard way that not everything that looks good can be eaten. Most plants, however, have an unpleasant taste and therefore are consumed only in small amounts. The effects of unintentional poisonings are typically dose dependent; therefore as children age and their sense of taste becomes more defined, the risk of large-dose unintentional poisonings decreases because they are better able to discriminate the unpleasant taste.

Household plants are frequently placed on the floor, where the leaves or flowers are easy to pull off and taste. The best intervention for plant poisoning is prevention, which, in this case, means previous knowledge. Table 17-10 identifies several common household and garden plants that are poisonous. The nurse must know which plants are harmful when ingested and must inform parents of the potential dangers to infants.

The most prominent groups of plants involved in exposures are those containing oxalates, and the most common symptom is gastroenteritis. The top 12 identified plants (in descending order) nationally were *Spathiphyllum* species (peace lily), *Philodendron* species (philodendron), *Euphorbia pulcherrima* (poinsettia), *Ilex* species (holly), *Phytolacca americana* (pokeweed), *Toxicodendron radicans* (poison ivy), *Capsicum* (pepper), *Ficus* (rubber tree, weeping fig), *Crassula argentea* (jade plant),

## TABLE 17-10 Poisonous Parts of Common Houseplants and Garden Plants

| Plant | Toxic Part | Symptoms |
|---|---|---|
| Apple | Seeds | Release cyanide when ingested in large quantities; can be fatal |
| Azalea | All parts | Nausea, vomiting, dyspnea, paralysis; can be fatal |
| Buttercup | All parts | Inflammation around mouth, stomach pains, vomiting, diarrhea, and convulsions |
| Castor bean | Seeds | Burning of mouth and throat, excessive thirst, and convulsions; one or two seeds are near the lethal dose for adults |
| Croton species | Plant juice | Gastroenteritis |
| Daffodil | Bulb | Nausea, vomiting, and diarrhea; can be fatal |
| Dieffenbachia | All parts | Intensive burning and irritation of the mouth and tongue; death can occur when base of tongue swells enough to occlude air passages |
| English holly | Berries | Nausea, vomiting, diarrhea, central nervous system depression; can be fatal |
| English ivy | Leaves and berries | Dyspnea, vomiting, diarrhea, coma, and death |
| Hyacinth | Bulb | Nausea, vomiting, and diarrhea; can be fatal |
| Iris | Underground stems | Digestive upset |
| Jasmine | All parts | Hallucinations, elevated temperature, tachycardia, and paralysis |
| Lily of the valley | All parts | Arrhythmia, mental confusion, weakness, shock, and death |
| Mistletoe | Berries | Acute stomach and intestinal irritations with diarrhea; can be fatal |
| Oak tree | Acorns | Kidney failure, gastritis |
| Oleander | All parts | Digestive upset, bloody diarrhea, respiratory depression, cardiac arrhythmia, blurred vision, coma, and death |
| Philodendron | All parts | Burning of lips, mouth, and tongue; swelling of tongue; dyspnea; kidney failure; death |
| Poinsettia | Leaves | Severe irritation to mouth, throat, and stomach; can be fatal |
| Potato | All green parts | Cardiac depression; can be fatal |
| Tomato | Green parts | Cardiac depression; can be fatal |
| Violet | Seeds | Taken in quantity, cathartic effects can be serious to infant |
| Yew | Foliage, seeds, bark | Nausea, vomiting, diarrhea, dyspnea, and dilated pupils; death is sudden |

Modified from Chesnut, V. K. (2012). *Principal poisonous plants of the United States*. Ulan Press; and Kinsey, J. (2016). Ten toxic houseplants that are dangerous for children and pets. HubPages. Retrieved from: http://hubpages.com/living/Dangerous-Beauties-Twenty-Toxic-Houseplants-to-Avoid-Around-Children-and-Pets.

*Dieffenbachia* (dumb cane), *Epipremnum aureum* (pothos), and *Schlumbergera bridgesii* (Christmas cactus) (Chesnut, 2012).

The American Association of Poison Control Centers [AAPCC] (2016) lists plants as the third most commonly ingested poison, after aspirin and household cleaning agents. Safety education is stressed at all well-baby visits beginning in the first 6 months of life. Prevention of plant poisoning and other accidents depends on a reciprocal relationship between protection and education that must be related to age. Keep all poisonous substances, medicines, cleaning agents, health and beauty aids, paints, and plants locked in a safe place out of an infant's sight and reach. Find out the names of all the plants in and around the house because if someone ingests one of them, the poison control center will need to know what it is when it is called. Never store poisonous substances in containers other than original ones (e.g., empty jars or soda bottles). Safe behavior is a learned behavior, gradually acquired in a progressive process with increasing age.

When parents are being taught, anticipatory guidance should include ways to prevent ingestions, the phone number for the National Capital Poison Center (800-222-1222), early recognition of common signs and symptoms of poisoning, and the importance of never giving remedies before the poison control center has been contacted. It is also important to discuss with parents and caregivers the importance of storing these medications out of the reach of infants and children, using safety locks on cabinets, and keeping purses (or any other places of storage of these medications) out of the reach of infants and children who are at risk of unintentional poisoning. When parents are provided with anticipatory guidance, particular emphasis must be placed on the prevention of unintentional poisonings. Guidance should be given on the basis of developmental age rather than chronological age (National Capital Poison Center, 2016).

As nurses, part of our role is that of education. Talking with parents outside the health care arena would be a great start. Girl Scout meetings, meetings of parent-teacher associations, church gatherings, day care centers, and other community-based activities can provide a forum for teaching and learning, and such training sessions could also provide an opportunity for questions to be answered.

Box 17-13 lists specific safety measures for parents to prevent plant poisoning of infants (AAPCC, 2016; National Capital Poison Center, 2016).

## BOX 17-13 Nursing Interventions to Prevent Plant Poisoning in Infants

- Keep plants out of reach of infants and young children.
- Never eat any part of a plant except the parts that are grown or sold as food.
- Keep jewelry made from unknown seeds or beans away from exploring infants.
- Learn to identify poisonous plants around your house and garden.
- Do not use unknown plants as medicines or teas.
- Pay close attention to infants at play inside and outside.
- Seek help whenever anyone chews or swallows a poisonous plant.
- Be aware that infants are more susceptible than are adults to the effects of poisonous plants.
- Keep the National Capital Poison Center telephone number handy (1-800-222-1222).

From National Capital Poison Center. (2016). Poison and prevention information by age. http://www.poison.org/by-age.

## Toxins

Susceptibility to environmental toxicants depends on the child's developmental stage and interactions within the physical, biological, and social environment. Infants are at particular risk of exposure to toxic factors in the environment; as dependent, developing organisms, they are inherently vulnerable. Generally, the exposure of infants to potential toxins is quite different from that of adults because of differences in physical environment, activities, and diet. Daily activities of infants, such as proximity to the floor or carpet inside the home and the lawn or soil outside, hand-to-mouth behaviors, and smaller body size and composition, place them at great risk of exposure to environmental toxins. The floor inside the home is an important microenvironment for infants because their breathing zones are low and many chemicals are concentrated near the floor. Ingestion, inhalation, and dermal exposure can occur. Infants are exposed to a host of environmental pollutants on a regular basis. These exposures occur through all possible environmental media: air, water, soil, and food. Infants have a unique exposure pattern and unique vulnerabilities. For example, some studies identify that the infant's oral habits and unique diet (ingesting more fruits, vegetables, and water than do adults) magnify their exposure to certain agents. Finally, because infants have a longer life span, toxins that have a long latency or cumulative toxicity (such as certain carcinogens) pose a greater risk to them than to adults (Falck et al., 2015).

Pesticides are internationally used harmful chemicals that are used to control pest attack on crops. Commonly pesticides are used to kill insects (insecticides), weeds (herbicides), fungi (fungicides), and rodents (rodenticides). Some pesticides that are used to control insects that feed on cereal grains, fruits, and vegetables are notorious for their slow accumulation in human tissue. Produce washes are available now to rid vegetables and fruits of these potential toxins. Over sufficient time, exposure to relatively small amounts of pesticides can result in the buildup of toxic quantities and lead to chronic disease in humans. Pesticides pollute water sources and agricultural products, and consumption of their residues by drinking water or the eating of foods may lead to serious health risks (Hashim, 2015). All pesticides have the ability to harm infants if they are exposed to them. The essence to decreasing the health hazards of pesticides is to limit exposure to them by use of precautionary measures and to have knowledge of their chemistry to decrease their hazards.

Lead is another environmental toxin that has no known physiological role in the human body. Lead exposure is a public health concern, especially in early childhood because young children are more prone to practice hand-to-mouth activity and absorb lead. Lead exposure can slow mental development and cause lower intelligence later in childhood. The effects of lead are more toxic on developing nervous systems of infants and young children than on a mature brain (Sharma et al., 2015). Although lead is essentially a contaminant, most people absorb a certain amount through exposure to lead-based paint in older homes, contaminated soil, household dust, drinking water, lead crystal, and lead-glazed pottery. Before 1950 lead-based paint was used on the inside and outside of most homes. It was used to make several colors, including white, and was known to dry to a hard, durable surface. In 1977 federal regulations banned lead from paint for general use. However, homes built before 1977 are likely to contain lead-based paint. Numerous toys made in China have been recalled and deemed unsafe because they contain lead-based paint. Studies have revealed a high lead content in drinking water, dirt, household dust, and soil. Lead in the air comes primarily from automobile emissions (National Institute of Environmental Health Sciences [NIEHS], 2015a). Absorption of lead is closely related to particle size. Airborne lead of small particle size is readily absorbed through the lungs, whereas larger particles fall to the ground. Lead affects practically all systems within the body. At high levels, lead can cause convulsions, coma, and even death. Lower levels of lead can adversely affect the brain, central nervous system, blood cells, and kidneys.

Infants are vulnerable to lead exposure for several reasons. In proportion to their weight, infants inhale more air and more lead than do adults (EPA, 2015). Additionally, infants breathe closer to the ground, where a higher concentration of lead is located. Their dust-raising play and habit of putting their hands in their mouths add to their lead consumption; they also have a greater rate of gastrointestinal absorption of lead and other chemicals than do adults. Both exercise and blockage of the nasal passages increase mouth breathing, and the mouth is a far less capable filter than the nose. Mouth breathing, coupled with their greater frequency of respiratory tract infections, exposes infants to a greater amount of environmental toxins. The growing prevalence of asthma is also evidence of environmental exposure to lead and other pollutants.

Asthma is an inflammatory disease of the lung. Approximately 7 million children have asthma. Asthma rates have doubled in the last decade, and death rates from asthma have increased in recent years. The reality is that we do not know why asthma is becoming more prevalent, but air pollution is a contributing factor. A few select steps to decrease indoor allergens to prevent asthmatic attacks include vacuuming carpets and upholstered furniture weekly; washing sheets, blankets, and towels in hot water weekly; cockroach elimination; and placing allergen-impermeable covers on pillows, box springs, and mattresses (NIEHS, 2015b).

Human potential and development are clearly important natural resources, and a growing body of evidence now links increased lead exposure to impaired intellectual performance and potential. Clinical lead poisoning affects many children, but it is preventable; excess lead in the infant's environment is made by, and should be eliminated by, human beings. Childhood lead exposure has been linked to numerous health problems, including learning disorders, attention deficit disorder, and hearing loss. Researchers suspect that there is no threshold of exposure to lead for many of these adverse outcomes, especially as a neuro-toxicant (NIEHS, 2015a). Progress has been made in reducing blood lead levels in infants and young children. But still today, more than 300,000 American children remain at risk of lead exposure. Many infants and young children live in poverty and old rented dwellings, which can lead to or exacerbate the effects of lead exposure. The following factors have contributed to the reduction of blood lead levels (USDHHS, 2010):

- Decline in lead used in gasoline
- Decline in manufactured food and soft drink cans containing lead solder
- Ban on leaded paint for residential (indoor) use
- Established standard for lead exposure in industry
- Ban on lead-containing solder in household plumbing
- Implementation of lead poisoning prevention programs
- Ban of toys manufactured in China containing lead-based paint

Parents need education regarding measures that can reduce their infant's exposure to lead:

- Keep areas in which the infant plays as dust-free and clean as possible.
- Do not remove lead paint yourself.
- Do not bring dust into the home.
- If work or a hobby involves lead, change clothes and bathe before entering the environment of infants (e.g., day care centers).
- Do not burn painted wood in a fireplace.
- Eat a balanced diet rich in calcium, iron, and vitamin C.

Infants do not necessarily escape noxious chemicals when they are indoors. The levels of contaminants that cause air pollution are approximately the same indoors as they are outdoors, with perhaps higher indoor concentrations of carbon monoxide, nitrogen dioxide, and various hydrocarbons from tobacco smoke; poorly ventilated heating and cooking equipment; and aerosol sprays. There are radon checks and carbon dioxide detectors that can be used to assess the presence of these contaminants. Many consequences of exposure to air pollution may not be observed during infancy but can surface in problems that affect both physical and mental well-being over a lifetime.

Among the acute illnesses of infancy, respiratory disease is ranked first, representing between 50% and 75% of all childhood diseases (NIEHS, 2015c). In addition to the inconvenience and incapacity induced by respiratory diseases, medical costs are high. Dirty air aggravates and, in some cases, causes nearly all respiratory problems. Infants with chronic respiratory disease can become adults with respiratory problems.

Water pollution can cause gastrointestinal disturbances in the infant. Parents and health care providers are quick to blame food, teething, or a virus for simple diarrhea, when the underlying cause may come from the kitchen tap. Numerous strong chemicals are used today to purify drinking water. These chemicals can irritate the delicate lining of the gastrointestinal tract and cause disturbances. Nurses encourage parents to boil all water for 20 minutes before they give it to their infant to help eliminate any potential problems.

Toxicants are widely dispersed throughout the environment of infants. It is essential for nurses to understand the potential routes of exposure, toxic effects, and strategies for prevention of exposure so as to provide anticipatory guidance to parents and family members.

## Motor Vehicles

This section considers the effects of motion or action of forces on the infant; the focus here is on motor vehicle accidents.

Automobiles present a danger to people of all ages, but especially to infants. Usually an infant is injured because of improper restraint inside the automobile. Many parents have been misled by thinking that it is better to be thrown clear of an accident than it is to be restrained. Many also think that it is safer to hold an infant on the lap in the front seat rather than to have the infant restrained in the back seat. On the contrary, these practices increase the probability of a fatality. A free-moving child not only distracts the driver but also means the child is in a more vulnerable position for being thrown.

Adult seat belts are unsuitable for infants or children younger than 4 years because their pelvic structure is small; the AAP recommends that safety seats for infants be used (USDHHS, 2010). The AAP and the National Highway Traffic Safety Administration recommend four evidence-based sequential steps to properly protect infants and children in passenger vehicles for children from birth through adolescence: rear-facing car safety seats with harnesses for most infants up to 2 years of age; forward-facing car safety seats with harnesses for most children through 4 years of age; belt-positioning booster seats used with a three-point belt restraint for most children through 8 years of age; and lap-and-shoulder seat belts for all who have outgrown booster seats. In addition, a fifth evidence-based recommendation is for all children younger than 13 years to ride in the rear seats of vehicles (Klinich & Manary, 2015). All children should be in the back seat because of the potential danger posed by air bags. Infant safety in motor vehicles depends entirely on the responsible adults.

Each year some infants die of heat stroke after being left unattended in motor vehicles. More than half the deaths are of children younger than 2 years. On days when ambient tempera-tures exceeded 86°F, the internal temperature of a vehicle quickly reaches 120°F to 140°F (Sims, 2015). At those temperatures, children are at great risk (http://pediatrics.about.com/od/summersafety/a/heat_illness.htm) as they can lead to a fever, dehydration, seizures, stroke, and death.

Even at relatively cool ambient temperatures, the temperature can rise inside the vehicle to more than 100°F, which places the infant at risk of hyperthermia. Vehicles heat up rapidly, with most of the temperature rise occurring within the first 15 to 30 minutes. Leaving the windows opened slightly does not

## BOX 17-14 Automobile Safety Precautions

- Be a good role model. Make sure you always wear your seat belt.
- Never leave a child unattended in a parked car or around cars.
- Never hold a child in the lap in the front seat.
- *Look before you lock* the car to make sure no child is left behind.
- Always use an infant car seat that is properly installed by following the manufacturer's instructions.
- Keep car doors and windows locked, even in driveways or garages.
- Use safety restraints for passengers and the driver.
- Do not be distracted by an infant while driving.
- Continue to use car seats as directed by the manufacturer; then use seat belts.
- Never place an infant in a rear-facing car safety seat in the front seat of a vehicle that has a passenger air bag.
- Make sure the seat belt is routed through the correct belt path for adult seat belts.
- Always lock your car and secure the keys so that children cannot access keys.
- Install a trunk release mechanism so that children will not be trapped in the trunk.
- Take the child out of the car seat first, and then worry about getting other items (e.g., groceries) out of the car.
- If you see a child alone in a car, get involved. Call 911 immediately and get the child out of car immediately. It may save the child's life

From American Academy of Pediatrics. (2016). Safety & prevention: Car seats. https://www.healthychildren.org/English/safety-prevention/on-the-go/Pages/Car-Safety-Seats-Information-for-Families.aspx.

significantly slow the heating process or decrease the maximal temperature attained (Kids & Cars, 2015).

Nurses can take the lead in increasing public awareness and improving parental education regarding heat rise in motor vehicles. The take-home message here is to never leave an infant alone in a motor vehicle. Make "look before you leave" a routine whenever you get out of the car. The nurse can also suggest the automobile safety precautions listed in Box 17-14. Much of automobile safety is common sense, but the nurse must cover all areas in anticipatory preventive teaching. The importance of automobile safety cannot be overemphasized.

## Radiation

In its broadest sense, radiation means the transfer of electromagnetic waves or energy through space (CDC, 2015j). Radiation of all types presents a potential hazard in the infant's environment. The risk level depends on the amount of radiation and the length of exposure and on the particular tissues involved. The infant's rapidly growing and immature cells are especially vulnerable.

The infant is exposed to two basic categories of radiation: natural background radiation, which comes from cosmic rays and radioactive material existing naturally in the soil, water, and air; and human-made radiation, which includes X-rays and radiation from nuclear power plants, microwave ovens, and other electronic devices found in the home (USDHHS, 2010). Infants have a developing immune response. As their immune system develops, immunity occurs in response to external factors such as the environment. Their exposure to ultraviolet radiation alters the development of the immune system, leading to long-term implications for suppression of immunity in adulthood (March of Dimes, 2015).

# DETERMINANTS OF HEALTH

## Social Factors and Environment

### Community and Work

As infants grow and develop, their boundaries extend beyond the home environment. Many mothers and fathers of infants return to the workforce, placing the infants in community day care centers. Day care refers to the care provided for infants in a center-based facility. It involves the caring for and supervising of infants by someone other than the parent or guardian.

Today few young families can escape financial burdens. The two-income and single-mother families are ways of life, and the trend will continue. With more than half of all American mothers working outside the home, the need for child care service is growing. This situation is usually an emotional issue for families; the separation process can be traumatic for both the infant and the parent.

Findings from social science research regarding the effects of day care on an infant's development and health can be summarized as follows: little evidence suggests that day care permanently enhances or slows intellectual development; day care can be used, even from earliest infancy, without damaging the mother-infant relationship; and day care can lead to a slight increase in minor illnesses, but excluding ill infants from the center is not an effective means of reducing the spread of illness. The day care environment must promote and positively support the infant's development and the infant's interaction with space, materials, and people (Nefer, 2015).

The question of how old an infant should be before being placed in day care is frequently asked of health professionals. Many experts believe that a mother and infant should have 4 to 6 months together before the mother returns to work. Brazelton and Sparrow (2015) make a good case for the mother and infant transitioning through four stages of attachment together before the mother returns to work:

- In the first stage, which takes 10 to 14 days, the infant learns to be attentive to the mother, and the mother learns cues from the infant about being both ready for and tired of attentiveness.
- The second stage, which lasts 8 weeks, is a stage of playful interaction, when the mother learns how to recognize the infant's nonverbal cues and helps the infant maintain the alert state.
- The third stage, from the 10th week to the fourth month, is when the mother and infant learn to play games together.
- During the fourth stage, which occurs in the fourth month, infants rapidly learn about themselves and their world. A mother, when possible, should spend the first 4 months with her new infant.

A nationwide survey of family day care found that nearly 50% of all infants in day care centers in the United States are cared for in one of three types of arrangements (Clark, 2014):

- Private homes that provide informal day care to infants of relatives, friends, and neighbors

- Regulated independent care licensed by state agencies
- Regulated, sponsored care provided by licensed workers operating as part of home networks under umbrella agencies

The nurse has a vital role in assisting families with infants who need day care. Many factors are reviewed when a family is looking for an appropriate day care program; the nurse can counsel and guide the family in its search. The means by which the nurse counsels and guides the family in selecting a day care center are as follows:

- Promote awareness of the three types of day care available in their local communities.
- Counsel parents on questions to ask employees of a prospective day care facility (AAP, 2015d) (Box 17-15).
- Help parents learn ways to cope with the separation behaviors manifested by their infant:
  - Remain calm in the situation.
  - Attempt to reduce the number of adults who interact with the infant and always introduce them.
  - Instruct parents to ask the question: Where do the infants sleep and are they separate from older children? Exposure to older children increases the risk of infection.
  - Encourage the parents to bring an infant's special cuddly toy from home to the day care facility to promote security.
  - Listen to the parent's understanding of the separation and expected behaviors.
  - Reassure parents that it takes time for the infant to make the transition from the parent to another caregiver and vice versa.

---

### BOX 17-15 Prospective Day Care Facility Questions

- Is the center licensed by the state?
- Is the day care facility open all year?
- Are all children required to have immunizations before they begin?
- What are the qualifications and credentials of the staff here?
- What hours is it open?
- How long has the center been in business?
- What is the center's licensed capacity?
- How flexible are you with pickup and drop-off times?
- How many children are present at the center?
- What is the age range of children at the center?
- What is the teacher-to-child ratio? (For infants, 1:3 is recommended.)
- Describe the day care program.
- What meals are served?
- What is the cost?
- Are there openings?
- Do you have webcam capability so I can view my infant during the day?
- What are the qualifications of the caregivers?
- Are the caregivers happy and interacting with the infant?
- Are infants content?
- What supplies would I need to bring for my infant?
- Are parents welcome to drop in?

From Brightwheel. (2016). What to ask on a daycare center tour. http://mybrightwheel.com/what-to-ask-on-a-daycare-center-tour/; Porpora, T. (2016). Five important questions to ask infant daycare center. *About parenting.* http://workingmoms.about.com/od/childcareissues/a/5-Important-Infant-Daycare-Questions.htm.

- Emphasize that at certain developmental levels stranger anxiety may be heightened (8 months), and separation behaviors of crying and clinging may be repeated.
- Work toward promoting a good relationship among parents, the infant, and the caregiver by providing opportunities for open discussions of concerns.

### Culture and Ethnicity

Culture is defined as a set of learned values, beliefs, attitudes, and practices that are passed from generation to generation (Polan & Taylor, 2015). Culture plays an important role in influencing an infant's development, and what is considered "normal" development differs greatly from one culture to the next. Culture defines how health care information is received, how rights and protections are exercised, what is considered to be a health problem, how symptoms and concerns about the problem are expressed, who should provide treatment for the problem, and what type of treatment should be given. In short, culture is the lens through which one views the world, affecting everything that an individual and that individual's family perceives and does.

The developing infant is subject to the influences of culture from the moment of conception. Partly because of the long dependency period, the family environment is the setting within which the infant experiences overall cultural attitudes. The lives of infants tend to be more under the direct control of parents or other caregivers than the lives of older children, who are often actively involved in selecting their own environments through contacts with peers, teachers, and other adults. The special demands of infancy require extensive and specific caregiving routines across cultures. Effective parenting styles also vary as a function of culture. The parents' perceptions of illness, wellness, roles, childrearing practices, religious values, language, and health practices are all modeled for the infant. In short, culture helps form the infant's view of the world (Boundless, 2015).

The family's ethnicity includes ideas about health, illness, food preferences, moral codes, and family life that persist across generations and survive even the upheaval of coming to a new country. All cultural groups confront repeated challenges as they transfer their families from familiar to unfamiliar surroundings. Infants are exposed to an appropriate mode of behavior that is in accordance with their family's cultural standards. By observing and imitating family members, infants take cues for behavior. These perceptions are then incorporated into their own self-concepts (Calkins, 2015).

In attempting to foster trust with diverse populations, nurses need to help women and their families feel comfortable enough to engage in a dialogue and share information. One approach is being careful not to prejudge as foolish or ill-conceived specific cultural practices and beliefs about health care. For example, a perinatal nurse describes a practice common in Hispanic culture in which an infant who has a sunken fontanel is held upside down by the feet to "fill" the hole. Instead of deeming such a practice foolish and scoffing at it, the nurse should let the families know that a more effective practice is to also "give the infant lots of water, or human milk, or formula, … [and] make sure that the infant gets lots of liquids" (Swota

## BOX 17-16  Factors That Facilitate Multicultural Health Care by Nurses

- Self-exploration of values and beliefs concerning other cultures and their beliefs
- Knowledge of the historical experience, recent and long term, of ethnic groups that live in the community
- Demographic data that include family size, socioeconomic status, and future expectations that are characteristic of diverse ethnic groups
- Understanding and sensitivity to cultural health care practices different from their own
- Recognition of folk beliefs and cultural attitudes toward health and illness
- Awareness of the nature of problems encountered by ethnic group members when they enter the health care system, including fear and distrust of health care professionals, language barriers, and discrimination by caregivers

& Hester, 2011). With such an approach, families are not embarrassed to let nurses know about their traditional cultural practices. This will help bridge the gap and build trust in their relationship.

To assess and plan appropriate interventions for different ethnic groups, nurses must be aware of their own cultural backgrounds. An important consideration is to examine all customs and values in relative terms, seeing none as either good or bad (Box 17-16). Change is inevitable in family life, whether it is resisted or welcomed. An important function of the nurse is to help families monitor the rate of change that is acceptable to various members and reach a consensus.

Culturally competent nursing interventions have been shown to improve outcomes in those seeking care. The need for culturally appropriate nursing care was identified as a key area of intervention by WHO (2015d). Research has identified several strategies that nurses can use that improve communication and reduce stress for culturally diverse populations: answering questions carefully, teaching by demonstration, and "taking time to explain in simple English." In addition, if women felt that the staff truly cared for their infant, this facilitated communication across multiple barriers because they "felt safe to ask questions" or express needs (Lee & Brann, 2015). Thus nurses who are mindful of the specific views of a culture respect the boundaries of the particular cultural perceptions, beliefs, and practices. Culturally competent nurses have achieved efficacy in communication skills and incorporate health care practices and beliefs of a particular culture in health care plans. Furthermore, respect for the individual's cultural values is viewed as essential if the nurse is to successfully help the family achieve a state of health and wellness.

The nurse identifies the power structure within a given cultural group. This knowledge may help dictate which family member to approach with the health teaching. Although the nurse might assume it would be the infant's mother, this may not necessarily be the case. Among some Native American tribes, the grandmother, not the parents, has the authority over the grandchildren. In many Latino cultural groups, the infant's father, not the mother, makes decisions about the infant's welfare (Andrews & Boyle, 2015). The nurse assesses the cultural groups' practices and beliefs before planning interventions. Improving the quality and safety of nursing care for culturally diverse women globally should be

the primary goal of all perinatal nurses. Approaches to infant care practices differ among cultural groups (Box 17-17: Diversity Awareness).

### Language

Language is an important medium for understanding and working together. The nurse may avoid or tend to mumble a person's name when it is foreign; people hesitate to express themselves when the material is unfamiliar. The nurse must consider how the individual who speaks a different language feels about being unable to express thoughts and feelings or to understand what is being said. Both parties may play the avoidance game.

The nurse takes steps to remove communication barriers, including the following:
- Using a professional interpreter to help in the communication process
- Using pictorial flash cards in the individual's native language to assist in explaining instructions
- Sending a health care worker to an educational center or school to learn the basics of the language to help in the interpreting process in the health care facility

Even a person who speaks the nurse's language may not understand and comprehend instructions given by the nurse. The negative impact of poor communication is huge, resulting in poor health outcomes, health disparities, and high health care costs. The importance of good health communication is relevant to all populations seeking care, including those from culturally and linguistically diverse backgrounds (Andrews & Boyle, 2015).

### Religion

In this pluralistic and democratic society, Americans are confronting the ethical and religious values that impinge on health care services. Some providers believe that religion plays no role in individuals' health care practices; therefore they eschew people's religious or ethical concerns and deal mainly with the physical or psychological problems at hand. However, the individual's religious and ethical concerns are generally the major source for human values when health care services are being evaluated.

Religious beliefs can become risk factors when they affect decisions concerning treatment. An example may be the parents who refuse a blood transfusion, surgery, or other medically indicated treatment required to save their infant's life. A court order is needed in many instances to treat these infants. The decision is the parents' responsibility, based on their customs and beliefs, and should be respected. Deciding not to offer an opinion may be extremely difficult, but usually the opinion is unwanted. Religion is often a powerful force, and when the nurse causes conflict and interferes, a gap can be formed. This gap may force the parents to seek nonprofessional health care to help them with their health-related and religious ideas about birth, death, stress, birth control, and other matters. To work successfully with an individual, the person's religious background should be investigated and understood thoroughly. Most nurses recognize that attending to the spiritual needs of families enhances the overall quality of their nursing care and the satisfaction of their care recipients.

---

**⊕ BOX 17-17    DIVERSITY AWARENESS BOX**

## Quick Guide for Cross-Cultural Nursing Care

The dominant American attitudes about infants and approaches to infant care have undergone many changes in the past several years. With the increased numbers of women in the workforce, fathers are becoming more involved in infant care, and day care for infants is increasing. Although children are valued, and raising children within the nuclear family remains a priority, an increasing number of American women are focusing on careers, delaying childbirth, and limiting family size.

Members of some cultures view childbearing and childrearing differently. The birth of a child is crucial for many Hispanic, Navajo, black, Middle Eastern, and Mormon women, whose social role and status are attained through reproduction within the marital relationship. Preference for a male child exists among families of many cultures, particularly Middle Eastern and Asian cultures (Roudsari et al., 2015).

In the dominant American culture, an infant is frequently wrapped warmly in blankets, placed in an infant seat or stroller, and put to sleep in a crib in a room separate from the parents. Mothers from other cultures may choose to carry or wrap their infants differently; women from some cultures carry their infants with them at all times and sleep with them. Southeast Asian infants may be carried in a hip sling or a blanket carrier. Native American infants are often carried in a cradleboard (a wooden frame into which an infant is bundled and tied). The cradleboard is properly blessed before it is used and can be carried, attached to the mother's back, hung from a tree, or propped up to keep the infant comfortable, safe, and secure (Andrews & Boyle, 2015).

Cultural beliefs and practices are continually evolving and changing. Nurses acknowledge and explore their meanings with all the families they meet. Nurses work actively to reduce the experience of culture shock for ethnic minority families, remembering that American medical beliefs and practices may appear strange to others. All behavior must be evaluated from within the context of the family and the family's cultural background and experience.

Nurses must facilitate health-promoting attitudes and practices and show empathic concern and respect for individuals of all cultural backgrounds. By incorporating the assessment of cultural beliefs and practices into the individual's plan of care, nurses can demonstrate respect and take a step forward in developing culturally appropriate patterns of caring.

In American culture the number of women choosing to breastfeed has steadily increased in recent years. Many factors are involved in the decision-making process. Nurses who care for families of newborns are aware of the multiplicity of factors influencing feeding choice and encourage and support parents in their decisions to promote the health of newborns.

The family is the primary health care provider for the infant. The family determines health promotion for the family, including when an infant is ill. Many cultural groups choose between the traditional or folk beliefs that they believe to be appropriate to them and Western medical treatment. The Vietnamese use both. For example, to decrease an infant's high temperature, a basil leaf is tied to the wrist with a piece of cheesecloth. For colic, a silver coin is dipped in wine and rubbed or scratched on the infant's back. Nurses are cautious in imposing their own values, beliefs, and attitudes on others. Rather than judging people, the nurse ascertains how each family's values and beliefs influence health outcomes.

The nurse remembers that all behaviors must be evaluated from within the context of the family's cultural background and experiences. Nurses who strive to foster health-promoting attitudes and behaviors begin at the most basic level: empathic concern and respect for the individual. By incorporating the assessment of cultural beliefs and practices into the infant's plan of care, nurses demonstrate respect, reduce alienation, and take a step toward developing culturally appropriate patterns of health promotion. Respecting another's language and religion is extremely important.

From Andrews, M. M., & Boyle, J. S. (2015). *Transcultural concepts in nursing care* (7th ed.). Philadelphia: Lippincott Williams & Wilkins; Roudsari, R. L., Zakerihamidi, M., & Khoei, E. M. (2015). Socio-cultural beliefs, values and traditions regarding women's preferred mode of birth in the north of Iran. *International Journal of Community Based Nursing and Midwifery, 3*(3), 165.

---

## Levels of Policy Making and Health

### Legislation

Enormous strides have been made in infant health in the past decade: many common, lethal infections have been eradicated (smallpox), malnutrition is seldom seen, and perinatal and infant mortality rates continue to decline. Health and well-being have become generally accepted rights of everyone, without regard to race, gender, age, economic or social status, or creed. The federal government has pledged to promote the general welfare of the United States in the belief that it belongs to everyone.

To fulfill this pledge, several goals were established. One of these concerns is infant health. The goal, as described by the USDHHS (2010), is to "improve the health and well-being of women, infants, children and families."

The infant mortality rate has been on a steady decline since the turn of the century, a result of better infant nutrition, improved technology, improved housing, and improved prenatal, obstetrical, and pediatric care (USDHHS, 2010). To meet the goal of improving infant health, major health problems in this age group must be reduced. A major hazard for infants is low birth weight. To address this problem, factors that increase the

risk of low birth weight in infants must be identified (Johnson et al., 2016).

Many of these factors can be prevented, or risks can be identified early and managed to prevent low-birth-weight infants. The major focus for prevention is prenatal care for all women.

Another major threat to infant survival is congenital disorders, such as malformations of the brain and spine (e.g., microcephaly and myelomeningocele), congenital heart defects (e.g., ventricular septal defects), and combinations of malformations, such as Down syndrome or Tay-Sachs disease. Although some congenital abnormalities cannot be prevented, others can be detected by performing prenatal screening and promoting research to determine their cause.

Other factors identified by the USDHHS (2010) and *Healthy People 2020* that contribute to the high infant mortality rate are injuries at birth, SIDS, accidents, respiratory distress syndrome, and inadequate parenting.

The federal government's plans to attain the goal of healthy infants are as follows:

- Promote family planning services such that all pregnancies are planned and all infants are wanted.

- Provide pregnancy and infant care services through Maternity and Infant Care (MIC) projects to high-risk populations. The Special Supplemental Nutrition Program Women, Infants, and Children (WIC) improves the nutritional status of both the mother and the infant.
- Encourage educational efforts by schools, health providers, and the media to promote prenatal care.
- Promote massive immunization efforts such that each infant is protected from communicable disease.

***Nursing's role.*** Nurses have important roles in promoting change in response to a continually expanding knowledge base, consumer health care needs, and governmental legislation. By actively participating in groups involved with health planning, the nurse helps make governmental policy more responsive to infants' health care needs. Health promotion essentially relates to collective or population well-being, which is wholly compatible with all the nurse's roles. Nurses need to work together with other professionals, agencies, and local people to improve the health and well-being of infants and all people (Christie et al., 2015).

The nurse's role in the development of health care policies has the following three stages: identifying resources for the community to meet its specific needs; planning for resources not available to the community; and coordinating the resources available to the community to promote better use of them.

The nurse can become a member of a health planning council, a concerned citizen's group, or an advisory group to a local legislator or to a state health department grant task force. In this capacity, the nurse's responsibility is to inform the other committee members. Because nurses have firsthand experience with many community needs, they are in a good position to speak out and inform others.

The nurse within the community also has several resources available to assist when a need is identified to promote the infant's health, including resources on the federal level (USDHHS), state level (public health department), local level (MIC clinics and well-baby clinics), and community groups (Parents Anonymous, hotlines, La Leche League, March of Dimes, and SIDS groups).

Coordinating for resources, the nurse actively participates in assessing the availability of services within the community and makes recommendations to consolidate or expand existing services. Increasing public awareness of community resources, their services, and existing needs is the basis of the nurse's role in developing policy.

## Economics

Virtually every major health problem is found more frequently in segments of the population with low income than in high-income groups. The infant mortality rates in low-income families remain significantly higher than those in high-income families, despite an overall decrease in the infant mortality rate nationally (CDC, 2015k; USDHHS, 2010).

In the United States, roughly 45% of children are born into poor or low-income families, and their health suffers when basic needs such as food, housing, and health screening and vaccinations are not met (AAP, 2015e). Parents with low incomes are often unaware of their infant's developmental needs; they are frequently faced with many environmental and social stresses that demand their time, energy, and other resources (Rapaport, 2015). Many parents have so many unfulfilled needs of their own that they cannot meet their infants' needs. In many cases, infants from families in poverty have delayed language development. With limited educational and life experiences, their parents are often unable to be ideal models for language development. Infants learn early language sounds from their parents, but their attempts at language must be reinforced.

Armed with the knowledge of how economics can affect the infant's growth, development, and health status, the nurse, before deciding on interventions, assesses the family situation by performing the following tasks:

- Establish a relationship with the family to obtain pertinent information.
- Evaluate the home environment in which the infant interacts.
- Elicit the parents' health perceptions about their own health and that of the infant.
- Offer assistance for the family to navigate the health care system for their infant
- Complete a thorough physical examination of the infant to identify any problem areas.
- Identify community resources that are available to the low-income family.

The take-home message is that poverty is like any other epidemiological exposure in infants that has health consequences. To the extent that nurses can reach out to these families, they may have a real positive impact on those infants' lives going forward.

## Health Services/Delivery System

The US health care delivery system is diverse and large; many different sectors merge to provide infant care. Within this enormous, multidisciplinary system, the nurse is an advocate who facilitates the family's passage through the many facets of care. Table 17-11 lists a suggested schedule for health-promotion infant care.

The value of health promotion and preventive health care has been validated; it is cost-effective and is here to stay. As nurses' roles continue to expand within the various parts of the health care system, their duty is to keep pace with the needs, concerns, and available strategies (Clark, 2014; Stanhope & Lancaster, 2014). Because many conditions that cause morbidity or death in infants are preventable when health-promotion practices are used, nurses have the mission of working within the health care system to promote infant health (USDHHS, 2010).

## NURSING APPLICATION

Nurses can do more to ensure the health of our youngest and most vulnerable population. It is the responsibility of all nurses to make health-education and health-promotion activities an integral part of their professional role. The primary role of the nurse in promoting the health of an infant is to provide the family with education during the most critical developmental period. Initial health-promotion efforts should focus on the nutritional

| TABLE 17-11 | Suggested Schedule for Health-Promotion Infant Care | | |
|---|---|---|---|
| **Age (Months)** | **Promotional Activity** | **Age (Months)** | **Promotional Activity** |
| 1 | Complete physical assessment: PKU test Immunization: HepB (second dose) **Parent discussion includes:** Basic infant needs: to be touched, held, fondled, rocked, and talked to Appropriate toy: colorful mobile Nutrition: formula or breast milk | 9 | Use of finger foods Playing games with infant: pat-a-cake, peek-a-boo, waving bye-bye, and shaking hands Appropriate toys: blocks, stack toys, and jack-in-the-box Fear of strangers |
| 2 | Complete physical assessment Immunizations: DTaP (first dose), Hib (first dose), PV (first dose), PCV (first dose), RV (first dose) **Parent discussion includes:** Placing infant in prone position to allow lifting of head Need of infant to be exposed to a variety of stimuli within environment Need of infant for change of scenery Colic and other common problems | 12 | Complete physical assessment Immunizations: MMR, PCV (fourth dose), Hib (fourth dose), varicella vaccine, HepA (first dose) Laboratory work: complete blood count **Parent discussion includes:** Accident prevention Getting into things Infant's need to touch and investigate environment, with supervision Parent's need to read, show pictures, and repeat body parts to infant Infant's need for limited independence Sleeping patterns Appropriate toys: sets of measuring cups, nesting toys, pots and pans, and wooden spoons |
| 4 | Complete physical assessment Immunizations: DTaP (second dose), Hib (second dose), PV (second dose), PCV (second dose), RV (second dose) **Parent discussion includes:** Stimulation of infant Providing a mirror in which the infant can see reflection Being talked to and played with Appropriate toy: rattle | 15 | Complete physical assessment Immunization: DTaP (fourth dose) **Parent discussion includes:** Negativism as normal aspect of development Age of curiosity in infant Toys appropriate for age: push-pull toys and ball Accident prevention Elimination patterns Discipline: stress positive aspects of behavior, when possible |
| 6 | Complete physical assessment Immunizations: DTaP (third dose), Hib (third dose), HepB (third dose), PV (third dose), PCV (third dose), RV (third dose), and influenza vaccine Laboratory work: hematocrit level **Parent discussion includes:** Accident prevention Teething and use of cool rings Allowing infant to crawl to explore environment Stranger anxiety | 18 | Complete physical assessment Immunization: HepA (second dose) **Parent discussion includes:** Accident prevention Begin toilet training, if child is ready Encouragement of vocalization Socialization with other small children Importance of reading to child Setting limits on behavior Coping mechanisms of parents |
| 9 | Complete physical assessment **Parent discussion includes:** Accident prevention Dental caries prevention: cleaning teeth with gauze daily Infant's need for space to crawl about Use cup if weaning | | |

*DTaP,* diphtheria, tetanus, and acellular pertussis vaccine; *HepB,* hepatitis B vaccine; *Hib, Haemophilus influenzae* type b conjugate vaccine; *MMR,* measles, mumps, and rubella vaccine; *PCV,* pneumococcal vaccine; *PKU,* phenylketonuria; *PV,* polio vaccine; *RV,* rotavirus vaccine.
From American Academy of Pediatrics. (2016). AAP schedule of well-child care visits. https://www.healthychildren.org/English/family-life/health-management/Pages/Well-Child-Care-A-Check-Up-for-Success.aspx.

needs of the infant during the first 18 months of life. Basic principles of biological growth and development set the stage for appropriate developmental tasks and psychological growth in the coming months. Nurses can make a difference in the lives of infants and their families by encouraging early and adequate prenatal care for the mother, supporting the transition from the hospital to the home, providing increased access to infant care services, and supporting childhood health surveillance.

The nurse promotes the health of the infant through his or her interactions with the parents as the infant is dependent on them for care. The nurse is in a position to encourage practices in the home that create the optimal conditions for normal growth and development. An important starting point for the nurse is to teach new parents about the nutritional value of breastfeeding and to encourage those efforts. Professional support and education play a vital role in increasing the rates of breastfeeding women.

Following a routine immunization and well-child health visit schedule is another aspect of health promotion for the infant. Nurses play a role in this task by educating parents about the importance of immunization. In addition, nurses should remain informed about the immunization recommendations and assist the family in maintaining documentation of vaccines administered. If cost or access to care is a factor, families can be referred to free or low-cost vaccination clinics.

Injuries and accidents are a major concern for the infant population. Accident prevention and safety are topics that should be addressed by the nurse when working with families. Although it is difficult to address the many ways in which an infant can be injured, nurses should be prepared to educate parents about the most common hazards. Some of the educational topics that can be addressed include fall and burn prevention, choking hazards, unintentional poisonings, environmental hazards, and automobile safety. In addition, a significant source of illness in infants and children is associated with infectious diseases from either a bacterial or a viral source. Particularly in younger infants, parents should be taught about the importance of frequent handwashing, avoidance of sick contacts, and signs and symptoms of illness that require immediate medical attention.

Essentially, health promotion should be viewed as an umbrella concept, which encompasses all health-related activities that contribute to the formation of a state of health in that individual or community. It should include education, disease-prevention, and environmental-health promotion-measures. The health-promotion goals of the nurse working with infants are met through the family. The nurse must ascertain the health perceptions and motivation of the family, including the use of good or bad health practices. The family must be motivated to provide good health practices for the infant. As the nurse plans health-promotion activities for families of infants, it is imperative that factors influencing health perception are identified. The ability of the nurse to provide a supportive relationship with the parents is a key element in facilitating successful infant development. The nurse working with this population has a unique opportunity to influence the health status of both the infant and the family for years to come.

The leadership of nurses in collaboration with other health care professionals will be key to improving the health of future generations. Whereas there is still room for improvement in the United States, many of the existing pediatric programs of care offer solutions that improve infants' health. It is essential that nurses continue to support these evidence-based models of care.

## CASE STUDY

### Homelessness: Homeless Minority Infants

As a community health nurse in an inner-city health center, you are increasingly aware that the homeless population in your city appears to be the forgotten aggregate. Your community health center provides primary care to a culturally diverse and indigent population. As a nurse, you believe that the homeless population within your city has numerous health needs. Beyond the basic requirements, many homeless people have mental and substance abuse problems, a deficiency in life skills, and poor family support, and most of all lack access to child health services.

The homeless population has all the usual health problems you would expect in the general population in addition to other problems resulting from their homeless lifestyle. Although there are several glaring concerns, you plan to focus your attention first on securing immunizations for the homeless infants and, second, to obtain formula for them.

#### Reflective Questions

- In planning health services for this special population, what facts do you need to know?
- What barriers to accessing health care for minority infants confront the homeless family?
- How can you overcome some of the barriers in developing your plan for health care?

#### Discussion

- In planning health services for this special population, what facts do you need to know? The following are some of the first questions that should be asked:
  - How many homeless minority infants are in this aggregate?

- Where are they?
- How can they access health care in the city?

To answer these questions, it might be prudent to collaborate and partner with other health and social service agencies, local hospitals, and the state health and human services agency. Collaboration and partnering can bring in additional resources and reduce duplication and gaps in services.

- What barriers to accessing health care for infants confront the homeless family?
  - Lack of transportation
  - Lack of trust in the medical establishment
  - Judgmental care on the part of health care providers and nurses
  - No health insurance to cover medical visits
  - Preventive care, such as immunizations, not a priority when you are hungry
  - No money to get prescriptions filled or transportation to get there
  - Waiting until the condition is serious before seeking treatment
- How can you overcome some of the barriers in developing your plan for health care?
  - Provide health care in the city shelters for use by homeless minority families.
  - Set up a mobile health care team and visit the shelters to provide care.
  - Offer free immunizations for all family members.
  - Establish educational sessions within the shelters to provide information.
  - Stress the importance of preventive measures to reduce illness in infants.
  - Obtain free formula from companies or hospitals to give to homeless infants.
  - Work closely with other health care interests within the community.

## ⊚ CARE PLAN

### *Homelessness: Homeless Minority Infants*

Homelessness is a community dilemma and an example of an economic problem that places infants at risk. Families are the fastest growing group of homeless people. Homeless families do not have health insurance; infants within these families are more likely to lack immunizations, proper nutrition, a safe environment, and a stable family situation. The community health nurse in this chapter's case study wants to address two aspects of homeless infants: immunizations and nutrition.

**\*NURSING DIAGNOSIS: Ineffective health maintenance related to nonadherence to appropriate immunization schedule as manifested by increased incidence of communicable diseases**

**Defining Characteristics**
- History of lack of health-seeking behavior by caregiver
- Lack of financial or other resources
- Reported or observed impairment of personal support systems
- Lack of knowledge regarding health-promotion practices
- Inability to access health care
- Limited basic personal resources

**Related Factors**
- Ineffective family coping
- Perceptual-cognitive impairment
- Lack of material resources
- Ineffective individual coping

**Expected Outcomes**
Caretaker of infant will:
- Begin health-seeking behavior on behalf of the minority infant.
- Increase health-promotion and health-maintenance knowledge.
- Gain access to available health care resources.
- Participate in life change to improve health status; meet goals for health care maintenance.

**Nursing Interventions**
- Assess caretaker's feelings, values, and personal situation.
- Assess the family for family patterns, economic issues, and cultural patterns that influence adherence.
- Assist the caretaker and minority family to access health care resources available to them.

- Refer the caretaker and family to community agencies to address social and economic issues.
- Educate the caretaker and family on the importance of immunizations and disease prevention.
- Provide follow-up care to increase the chance of health status change occurring.

**\*NURSING DIAGNOSIS: Risk of imbalanced nutrition—less than body requirement related factors and socioeconomic factors as manifested by low height and weight measurements for chronological age on growth chart**

**Defining Characteristics**
- Pale conjunctival and mucous membranes
- Poor muscle development
- Inadequate food intake to maintain body weight
- Weight loss, fatigue, frequent irritable, fussy, crying behavior
- Growth and development milestones not met
- Frequent illnesses suggesting depressed immunity

**Related Factors**
- Inability to obtain adequate food or fluid or both to nourish body because of socioeconomic factors

**Expected Outcomes**
Infant will demonstrate the following:
- Progressive weight gains toward desired goal
- Weight within normal range for height and weight
- Minority infant consuming adequate nourishment
- Free of signs of malnutrition

**Nursing Interventions**
- Assess healthy body weight for age and height.
- Observe minority infant's ability to consume food and fluids.
- Monitor food and fluid intake weekly.
- Access nutritional resources for the caretaker or family.
- Refer family to appropriate community agencies to meet needs.
- Assist the caretaker or family to identify area needing change that will make the greatest contribution to improve nutrition.
- Implement instructional dialogue that is appropriate for their level.
- Provide follow-up care to assist them in changing their health status.

\*NANDA Nursing Diagnoses—Herdman T. H., & Kamitsuru, S. (Eds.). Nursing Diagnoses–Definitions and Classification 2015–2017. Copyright © 2014, 1994–2014 NANDA International. Used by arrangement with John Wiley & Sons Limited. In order to make safe and effective judgments using the NANDA-I nursing diagnoses it is essential that nurses refer to the definitions and defining characteristics of the diagnoses listed in this work.

## SUMMARY

Never before has health promotion been more important than it is today. Nurses must have evidence-based understanding of the significant effect that can be made through health-promotion interventions and communicate this understanding to families they care for. Society is changing, as are people's needs and ideas. Families today want more information and knowledge, and they demand that health care professionals be more responsive to their needs. Their demand has been a catalyst for the nurse's expanded health care role and responsibility for health promotion. Nurses have been "touted" as potential major contributors to society's health promotion and illness prevention. Nurses are in

the forefront of the health-promotion movement through their practice. Health promotion by nurses is associated with common universal principles of health education. Nurses should be able to plan, implement, and evaluate health-promotion interventions for infants and their families to improve their health outcomes.

Health-promotion and disease-prevention practices that are applicable during infancy can be used in the nurse's expanded role. A four-pronged approach is stressed:
- Giving anticipatory guidance to the family unit as the infant grows and develops
- Teaching and counseling to ensure the infant's optimal development

- Being a family advocate to ensure the safety and development of the family unit
- Screening infants to identify infants at risk of developing a condition via history gathering, physical examination, observation of parent-child interaction, and laboratory testing

Anticipating potential health problems during infancy and effectively intervening to avert these problems are nursing processes that promote health. Early detection and reduction of risk factors avoid many health problems, such as abuse. By anticipating problems and helping families to avoid them, the nurse promotes health maintenance.

Using the infant's normal growth and development, psychosocial tasks, common health problems, and health maintenance strategies, the nurse assesses the infant, the family, and the infant's developmental status to provide anticipatory guidance.

By teaching (Box 17-18: Genomics), an essential component of the nursing process, the nurse transmits knowledge to families to ensure continuity of care and long-term health maintenance. By counseling, the nurse listens to the identified problem, helps the family to recognize the real issues, and allows the family to make its own decisions regarding health care.

Because the infant is in no position to advocate for itself effectively, the nurse assumes the role of advocate. The ultimate goal of nursing intervention in maintaining the infant's health is future self-care. As the infant grows and matures, well-established family health maintenance habits can only enhance the lives of healthy future generations. The nurse is challenged to join this effort of investment in the future.

## EVOLVE CHAPTER FEATURES

http://evolve.elsevier.com/Edelman/
- Study Questions

## REFERENCES

Adams, S. M., Ward, C. E., & Garcia, K. L. (2015). Sudden infant death syndrome. *American Family Physician*, *91*(11), 778–783.

AIDS Info. (2015). Preventing mother-to-child transmission of HIV after birth. https://aidsinfo.nih.gov/education-materials/fact-sheets/24/71/preventing-mother-to-child-transmission-of-hiv-after-birth.

American Academy of Pediatrics (AAP). (2015a). Bright futures: Prevention and health promotion for infants, children, adolescents, and their families. https://brightfutures.aap.org/materials-and-tools/Pages/default.aspx.

American Academy of Pediatrics (AAP). (2015b). AAP policy on breastfeeding and use of human milk. https://www2.aap.org/breastfeeding/policyOnBreastfeedingAndUseOfHumanMilk.html.

American Academy of Pediatrics (AAP). (2015c). Red book 2015: Committee on infectious diseases. http://redbook.solutions.aap.org/book.aspx?bookid=1484.

American Academy of Pediatrics (AAP). (2015d). Preparing your child for child care. https://www.healthychildren.org/English/family-life/work-play/Pages/Preparing-Your-Child-for-Child-Care.aspx.

American Academy of Pediatrics (AAP). (2015e). Medical legal strategy can improve health care of low-income parents of newborns. https://www.aap.org/en-us/about-the-aap/aap-press-room/pages/Medical-Legal-Strategy-Can-Improve-Healthcare-of-Low-Income-Parents-of-Newborns.aspx.

American Association of Poison Control Centers [AAPCC]. (2016). Baby safety month by raising awareness on the importance of poisoning prevention in the home. http://www.aapcc.org/prevention/home/.

American Heart Association. (2015). Infant CPR. http://www.heart.org/HEARTORG/CPRAndECC/CommunityCPRandFirstAid/CommunityProducts/Infant-CPR-Anytime_UCM_428979_Article.jsp.

American Public Health Association. (2015). Injury and violence prevention. https://www.apha.org/topics-and-issues/injury-and-violence-prevention.

Andreotta, J., et al. (2015). Safe sleep practices and discharge planning. *Journal of Neonatal Nursing*, *21*(5), 195–199.

Andrews, M. M., & Boyle, J. S. (2015). *Transcultural concepts in nursing care* (7th ed.). Philadelphia: Lippincott Williams & Wilkins.

Arnold, E. C., & Boggs, K. U. (2016). *Interpersonal relationships: professional communication skills for nurses* (7th ed.). Philadelphia, PA: Elsevier.

Bauer, M. (2015). What causes parents to abuse their child? Live Strong. http://www.livestrong.com/article/142315-what-causes-parents-to-abuse-their-child/.

Berk, L. E., & Meyers, A. B. (2015). *Infants, children, and adolescents* (8th ed.). New York: Pearson Education.

### BOX 17-18　GENOMICS

Genomic sequencing can identify genetically based conditions that routine blood tests used to screen every newborn baby cannot detect. The standard newborn screening blood tests look for chemical changes and typically screen newborns for a few dozen disorders, such as sickle cell anemia and cystic fibrosis, that are caused by a gene mutation. But researchers have tallied more than 6000 such inherited disorders caused by a single mutated gene. And other genes are associated with higher risks of certain conditions, such as heart disease. Imagine being able to anticipate a child's health all the way to adulthood.

In the next few decades, every infant's genome can be sequenced and used to shape a lifetime of personalized strategies for disease prevention, detection, and treatment.

But this brave new world is fraught with technical and ethical issues that have some scientists questioning whether every infant should have its genome sequenced and what information children and parents should receive about the results.

Every individual's genome is loaded with "variant" genes, and harmful mutations make up just a small fraction of them. Researchers have only begun to catalog which variants cause problems. Questions arise about the wisdom of telling parents and children about conditions for which there is no effective treatment or of letting them know about disorders that will not affect a child until adulthood. Families will need to decide this as this latest technology moves forward.

From Bavley, A. (2016). Genome sequencing hold tremendous promise for infants, but issues abound. *The Kansas City Star*. http://www.kansascity.com/news/business/health-care/article21973176.html; National Human Genome Research Institute. (2016). Newborn screening. https://www.genome.gov/27556918.

Bhattacharjee, Y. (2015). Baby brains: The first year. National Geographic. http://ngm.nationalgeographic.com/2015/01/baby-brains/bhattacharjee-text.

Boundless. (2015). Culture and societal influences on child development. Boundless Psychology. https://www.boundless.com/psychology/textbooks/boundless-psychology-textbook/human-development-14/infancy-and-childhood-72/cultural-and-societal-influences-on-child-development-281-12816/.

Boy Scouts of America. (2015). How to protect your children from child abuse: A parent's guide. http://www.scouting.org/filestore/pdf/100-015(15)_WEB.pdf.

Brazelton, T. B., & Sparrow, J. A. (2015). *Discipline: The Brazelton way* (2nd ed.). Old Saybrook, CN: Tantor Media.

Brown, A., & Harries, V. (2015). Infant sleep and night feeding patterns during later infancy: Association with breastfeeding frequency, daytime complementary food intake, and infant weight. *Breastfeeding Medicine: The Official Journal of the Academy of Breastfeeding Medicine, 10*(5), 246–252.

Brown, A., & Rowan, H. (2016). Maternal and infant factors associated with reasons for introducing solid foods. *Maternal & Child Nutrition, 12*(3), 500–515.

Burnham, E. B., et al. (2015). Phonetic modification of vowel space in storybook speech to infants up to 2 years of age. *Journal of Speech, Language, and Hearing Research: JSLHR, 58*(2), 241–253.

Busch, D., Nassar, L., & Silbert-Flagg, J. (2015). The necessity of breastfeeding–promoting breastfeeding in the primary care setting; A community pilot project applying the tri-core breastfeeding model: Beyond the basics. *Journal of Pregnancy and Child Health, 2*(158), 2–9.

Calkins, S. D. (2015). *Handbook of infant biopsychosocial development.* New York, NY: Guilford Publications, Inc.

Carey, S., Zaitchik, D., & Bascandziev, I. (2015). Theories of development: In dialog with Jean Piaget. *Developmental Review, 38*, 36–54.

Centers for Disease Control and Prevention (CDC). (2015a). Child development: Infants (0–1 year of age). http://www.cdc.gov/ncbddd/childdevelopment/positiveparenting/infants.html.

Centers for Disease Control and Prevention (CDC). (2015b). WHO growth charts for infants and children from 0 to 2 years of age. http://www.cdc.gov/growthcharts/who_charts.htm#TheWHOGrowthCharts.

Centers for Disease Control and Prevention (CDC). (2015c). Infant growth patterns on the WHO and CDC growth charts. http://www.cdc.gov/nccdphp/dnpao/growthcharts/who/using/growth_patterns.htm.

Centers for Disease Control and Prevention (CDC). (2015d). Sudden unexpected infant death and sudden infant death syndrome: Data and statistics. http://www.cdc.gov/sids/data.htm.

Centers for Disease Control and Prevention (CDC). (2015e). Child maltreatment data & statistics. http://www.cdc.gov/violenceprevention/childmaltreatment/.

Centers for Disease Control and Prevention (CDC). (2015f). Accidents or unintentional injuries. http://www.cdc.gov/nchs/fastats/accidental-injury.htm.

Centers for Disease Control and Prevention (CDC). (2015g). Burn prevention. http://www.cdc.gov/safechild/burns/.

Centers for Disease Control and Prevention (CDC). (2015h). HIV among pregnant women, infants and children. http://www.cdc.gov/hiv/group/gender/pregnantwomen/index.html.

Centers for Disease Control and Prevention (CDC). (2015i). Recommended immunization schedule for children and adolescents aged 18 years or younger. http://www.cdc.gov/vaccines/schedules/hcp/imz/child-adolescent.html.

Centers for Disease Control and Prevention (CDC). (2015j). Radiation and your health. http://www.cdc.gov/nceh/radiation/.

Centers for Disease Control & Prevention (CDC). (2015k). FastStats: Infant health. http://www.cdc.gov/nchs/fastats/infant-health.htm.

Centers for Disease Control and Prevention (CDC). (2015l). Recommended immunization schedule for birth to 15 months. http://www.cdc.gov/vaccines/schedules/hcp/imz/child-adolescent.html.

Chesnut, V. K. (2012). *Principal poisonous plants of the United States.* London, England: Ulan Press.

Child Development Institute. (2015). Ages and stages. http://childdevelopmentinfo.com/ages-stages/.

Christian, C. W., et al. (2015). The evaluation of suspected child physical abuse. *Pediatrics, 135*(5), e1337–e1354.

Christie, J., Parkes, J., & Price, J. (2015). The public health practitioner. In J. Hughes & G. Lyte (Eds.), *Developing nursing practice with children and young people* (pp. 87–102). Ames, IA: Blackwell.

Clark, M. J. (2014). *Population and community health nursing* (6th ed.). Upper Saddle River, NJ: Prentice Hall.

Coch, D., Dawson, G., & Fischer, K. W. (2015). *Human behavior, learning, and the developing brain: Typical development.* New York: Guilford Publications.

Duryea, T. K., & Fleischer, D. M. (2015). Patient education: Starting solid foods during infancy (beyond the basics). UpToDate. http://www.uptodate.com/contents/starting-solid-foods-during-infancy-beyond-the-basics.

Environmental Protection Agency (EPA). (2015). Air quality. http://www3.epa.gov/airquality/cleanair.html.

Falck, A. J., et al. (2015). Developmental exposure to environmental toxicants. *Pediatric Clinics of North America, 62*(5), 1173–1197.

Fanetti, M., et al. (2015). Child abuse and neglect. In *Forensic child psychology* (pp. 105–124). Hoboken, NJ: John Wiley & Sons.

Feldman, R. S. (2015). *Child development* (7th ed.). New York: Pearson Education.

Ferguson, R. W., et al. (2015). *Medicine safety for children: An in-depth look at poison center calls.* Washington, DC: Safe Kids Worldwide.

Fildes, A., et al. (2015). Parental control over feeding in infancy. Influence of infant weight, appetite and feeding method. *Appetite, 91*, 101–106.

Fivush, R., & Waters, T. E. A. (2015). Patterns of attachments across the lifespan. In R. A. Scot & S. M. Kosslyn (Eds.), *Emerging trends in the behavioral and social sciences: An interdisciplinary, searchable, and linkable resource* (pp. 1–10). San Francisco: Wiley.

Fogel, A. (2015). *Infant development: A topical approach* (2nd ed.). Cornwell-on-Hudson, NY: Sloan Educational Publishing.

Gardner, S. L., et al. (2016). *Merenstein & Gardner's handbook of neonatal intensive care* (8th ed.). St. Louis: Mosby.

Gill, A. C., & Kelly, N. R. (2015). Prevention of falls in children. UpToDate. http://www.uptodate.com/contents/prevention-of-falls-in-children.

Harkness, G. A., & DeMarco, R. (2015). *Community health and public health nursing: Evidence for practice* (2nd ed.). Philadelphia: Lippincott Williams & Wilkins.

Hashim, M. (2015). Pesticides and drinking water. *Journal of Advanced Botany and Zoology, 3*(1), doi:10.15297/JABZ.V3I1.05. http://www.scienceq.org/archive.php?jname=abz&jid=abz0615394&tit=%20%20%20Pesticides%20and%20Drinking%20Water#div_pdf.

Hax, C. (2015). Baby of 'wrong' gender deserves just as much love. Journal Sentinel. http://www.jsonline.com/features/advice/baby-of-wrong-gender-deserves-just-as-much-love-b99565651z1-324016401.html.

Horne, R. S., Hauck, F. R., & Moon, R. Y. (2015). Sudden infant death syndrome and advice for safe sleeping. *British Medical Journal, 350*, h1989.

Institute of Medicine. (2015). Dietary reference intakes: Estimated average requirements. https://www.nal.usda.gov/sites/default/files/fnic_uploads//recommended_intakes_individuals.pdf.

Johnson, C. D., Jones, S., & Paranjothy, S. (2016). Reducing low birth weight: Prioritizing action to address modifiable risk factors. *Journal of Public Health*, doi:10.1093/pubmed/fdv212.

Johnson, J. E., et al. (2015). *The handbook of the study of play.* Lanham, MD: Rowman & Littlefield Publishing Group.

Kail, R. V., & Cavanaugh, J. C. (2015). *Human development: A life-span view* (7th ed.). Boston, MA: Cengage Learning.

Kelly, N. R. (2015). Prevention of poisoning in children. UpToDate. http://www.uptodate.com/contents/prevention-of-poisoning-in-children.

Kids & Cars. (2015). Child vehicular heat stroke fact sheet. http://www.kidsandcars.org/files/pdfupload/heat-stroke-fact-sheet.pdf.

Kliegman, R. M., et al. (2015). *Nelson textbook of pediatrics* (20th ed.). St. Louis: Elsevier.

Klinich, K. D., & Manary, M. A. (2015). Best practice recommendations for protecting child occupants. In N. Yoganandan, A. M. Nahum, & J. W. Melvin (Eds.), *Accidental injury: Biomechanics & prevention* (pp. 697–719). New York, NY: Springer.

Lauwers, J., & Swisher, A. (2016). *Counseling the nursing mother: A lactation consultant's guide* (6th ed.). Burlington, MA: Jones & Bartlett Learning.

Lee, A., & Brann, L. (2015). Influence of cultural beliefs on infant feeding, postpartum and childcare practices among Chinese-American mothers in New York City. *Journal of Community Health, 40*(3), 476–483.

Linton, B. (2015). Men and fatherhood: Pregnancy and birth. http://www.pregnancy.org/article/men-and-fatherhood-pregnancy-and-birth.

Lopes, L. C., de Omena Bomfim, E., & Flória-Santos, M. (2015). Genomics-based health care: Implications for nursing. *International Journal of Nursing Didactics, 5*(02), 11–15.

Ma, S., et al. (2015). *6 Early childhood health promotion and its life course health consequences. Health and education in early childhood* (pp. 113–144). Cambridge: Cambridge University Press.

Magana, J., & Kaufhold, M. (2015). Child abuse. Medscape. http://emedicine.medscape.com/article/800657-overview.

March of Dimes. (2015). Radiation and pregnancy: Staying safe. http://www.marchofdimes.org/pregnancy/radiation-and-pregnancy.aspx.

Mindell, J. A., & Owens, J. A. (2015). *A clinical guide to pediatric sleep: Diagnosis and management of sleep problems* (3rd ed.). Philadelphia, PA: Wolters Kluwer.

Moses, S. (2015). Newborn reflexes. Family Practice Notebook. http://www.fpnotebook.com/nicu/exam/NwbrnRflxs.htm.

National Capital Poison Center. (2016). Poison & prevention information by age: Infants. http://www.poison.org/by-age/infants.

National Institute of Environmental Health Sciences (NIEHS). (2015a). Lead and your health. http://www.niehs.nih.gov/health/materials/lead_and_your_health_508.pdf.

National Institute of Environmental Health Sciences (NIEHS). (2015b). Asthma and its environmental triggers. http://www.niehs.nih.gov/health/assets/docs_a_e/asthma_and_its_environmental_triggers_508.pdf.

National Institute of Environmental Health Sciences (NIEHS). (2015c). Air pollution. http://www.niehs.nih.gov/research/supported/exposure/air_pollution/index.cfm.

National Institutes of Health. (2015). Who is at risk for sickle cell disease? http://www.nhlbi.nih.gov/health/health-topics/topics/sca/atrisk.

National Safety Council. (2016). Choking prevention and rescue tips. http://www.nsc.org/learn/safety-knowledge/Pages/safety-at-home-choking.aspx.

National Tay-Sachs & Allied Diseases Association. (2015). Tay-Sachs disease. http://www.ntsad.org/index.php/tay-sachs.

Nefer, B. (2015). The effects of child care on infants. LiveStrong. http://www.livestrong.com/article/96488-effects-child-care-infants/.

Nussbaum, R., McInnes, R. R., & Willard, H. F. (2016). *Thompson & Thompson genetics in medicine* (8th ed.). Philadelphia, PA: Elsevier Health Sciences.

O'Connor, A. (2015). All about sensory development. Nursery World, 22–26. http://brightwaltonpreschool.co.uk.

Polan, E., & Taylor, D. (2015). *Journey across the lifespan: Human development and health promotion* (5th ed.). Philadelphia: F.A. Davis.

Radzyminski, S., & Callister, L. C. (2015). Health professionals' attitudes and beliefs about breastfeeding. *The Journal of Perinatal Education, 24*(2), 102–109.

Rapaport, L. (2015). More poor babies get checkups when parents get extra help. Reuters Health. http://www.reuters.com/article/2015/06/03/us-healthcare-poverty-infant-care-idUSKBN0OJ2MP20150603.

Reed, L. (2015). Early socialization. *International Journal of Childbirth Education, 30*(2), 31–34.

Rivera, D. M., & Frye, R. E. (2015). Pediatric HIV infection. Medscape. http://emedicine.medscape.com/article/965086-overview.

Sanders, L. (2015). America: What's your health worth? http://www.foodinsight.org/summer-2015-food-health-survey#sthash.KDIfmxUj.dpbs.

Santos, M., et al. (2015). Parental knowledge on breastfeeding: Contributions to a clinical supervision model in nursing. *International Journal of Information and Education Technology, 5*(1), 10–13.

Sharma, P., Chambial, S., & Shukla, K. K. (2015). Lead and neurotoxicity. *Indian Journal of Clinical Biochemistry, 30*(1), 1–2.

Simon, P., Piché, V., & Gagnon, A. A. (2015). The making of racial and ethnic categories: Official statistics reconsidered. In *Social statistics and ethnic diversity* (pp. 1–14). Cham: Springer International Publishing.

Sims, J. D. (2015). *The no-nonsense guide to heat wave, drought, & hot weather safety* (2nd ed.). North Carolina: Lulu Books & Beyond the Spectrum Books.

Stanhope, M., & Lancaster, J. (2014). *Public health nursing: Population-centered health care in the community* (8th ed.). St. Louis: Mosby.

Swota, A., & Hester, D. (2011). Ethics for the pediatrician: Providing culturally effective health care. *Pediatrics in Review, 32*(3), 39–43.

Today's Parent. (2016). How to prevent choking. http://www.todaysparent.com/toddler/tips-to-prevent-choking/.

US Agency for International Development (USAID). (2017). Gender equality and women's empowerment. https://www.usaid.gov/what-we-do/gender-equality-and-womens-empowerment.

US Congress. (2010). Patient Protection and Affordable Act of 2010 (Sec 4207). https://democrats.senate.gov/2009/12/24/senate-democrats-lead-historic-passage-of-the-patient-protection-and-affordable-care-act/#.WKXqsU0VCM8.

US Department of Agriculture (USDA). (2015). Nutritional needs of infants. http://www.nal.usda.gov/wicworks/Topics/FG/Chapter1_NutritionalNeeds.pdf.

US Department of Health and Human Services (USDHHS). (2010). Healthy People 2020. http://www.healthypeople.gov.

Wamai, R. G., et al. (2015). Male circumcision for protection against HIV infection in sub-Saharan Africa: The evidence in favor justifies the implementation now in progress. *Global Public Health*, *10*(5-6), 639–666.

Williamson, C., & Beatty, C. (2015). Weaning and childhood nutrition. *Education and Inspiration for General Practice*, *8*(3), 141–145.

World Health Organization (WHO). (2015a). Food additives. http://www.who.int/topics/food_additives/en/.

World Health Organization (WHO). (2015b). Child maltreatment. http://www.who.int/topics/child_abuse/en/.

World Health Organization (WHO). (2015c). WHO recommends on health promotion interventions for maternal and newborn health 2015. http://apps.who.int/iris/bitstream/10665/172427/1/9789241508742_report_eng.pdf.

World Health Organization (WHO). (2015d). Health topics: Nursing. http://www.who.int/topics/nursing/en/.

World Health Organization (WHO) and Joint United Nations Program on HIV/AIDS (UNAIDS). (2015). UNFPA, WHO and UNAIDS: Position statement on condoms and circumcision and prevention of HIV. http://www.unaids.org/en/resources/presscentre/featurestories/2015/july/20150702_condoms_prevention.

Zaiden, R. A., et al. (2015). Hemophilia A. http://emedicine.medscape.com/article/779322-overview.

# 18

# Toddler

*Diane Marie Welsh*

## OBJECTIVES

*After completing this chapter, the reader will be able to:*

- Describe the physical growth, developmental, and maturational changes that occur during the toddler period.
- Examine the recommended health-promotion and disease-prevention visits for the toddler with the appropriate topics for anticipatory guidance for the parents.
- Compare and contrast developmentally appropriate approaches to toddlers at different ages.
- Analyze the factors that contribute to the heightened vulnerability of toddlers to injury and abuse.
- Develop a plan to reach the *Healthy People 2020* target objectives specific for toddlers.

## KEY TERMS

Amblyopia
Autism spectrum disorders
Autonomy
CDC growth charts
Child abuse
Conditioned-play audiometry
Doubt
Egocentrism
Lumbar lordosis

Masturbation
Night terrors
Object permanence
Otitis media
Parallel play
Preoperational stage
Rituals
Sensorimotor stage
Shame

Strabismus
Styes
Temperament
Toilet training
Visual-reinforcement audiometry
World Health Organization growth charts

## ? THINK ABOUT IT

### Refraining the Terrible Twos

*A young mother tells the nurse that she is convinced her 22-month-old child, who used to be the sweetest child around, has entered what must be the terrible twos. She reports that her child's favorite words include "mine" and "no," with "no" being the response to every request the mother makes. In addition, the child is becoming increasingly stubborn and just threw her first public temper tantrum. The mother says that she is tired of saying and hearing "no" and turns to the nurse for help.*

- How does the nurse explain the relationship between the child's stage of psychosocial development and meaning behind the child's behaviors?
- What suggestions can the nurse give the mother to respond sensitively to her child's evolving need for independence while balancing her own need to provide for and protect her child?

Having spent their first year of life getting to know and trust their parents and other child care providers and their immediate environments, toddlers' increasing mobility now allows them to begin to expand their worlds, bringing excitement and challenges to both themselves and their parents. Toddlers are ready to develop a sense of self and separate from their parents, and understanding and respecting this evolving independence is a common parental challenge. Their behaviors can be frustrating, but the toddlers' delight in their own emerging competence and achievements can bring a sense of joy and accomplishment to everyone around them (Kochanska et al., 2013).

Nurses explain to parents and other primary care providers the many physical and developmental changes that occur in toddlers and describe how these changes contribute to their vulnerability to injury and overall health, as well as to the health and vulnerability of the family unit (CDC, 2015d). Unfortunately, the recommended schedule for health-promotion and disease-prevention visits for this age group advocates fewer contacts than during infancy. Parents may begin to fall into a pattern of illness care, missing the continued opportunity to receive anticipatory guidance and health-promotion information until they are required by preschool or school prerequisites. The nurse plays an integral role in encouraging health-promotion efforts and behaviors (Hockenberry & Wilson, 2015; Spence et al., 2013).

## BIOLOGY AND GENETICS

The toddler period begins at 12 to 18 months and extends to 3 years of age. The overall growth rate slows significantly, and the increasingly active toddler begins the process of shedding baby fat and straightening his or her posture. Toddlers have a protuberant abdomen, accentuated by a lumbar lordosis, and a characteristic gait, in which their feet are planted wide apart and appear flat because of an extra fat pad in the instep for stability.

A slow, steady growth in height of 2 to 4 inches per year and in weight of 4 to 6 pounds per year occurs during toddlerhood, and growth remains steady until puberty. Birth weight usually quadruples by 2½ years of age, and the toddler's height at age 2 years is approximately 50% of the final adult height (Hockenberry & Wilson, 2015). Growth charts are used to determine the parameters within which an individual toddler's growth lies for head circumference, height, and weight. The Centers for Disease Control and Prevention (CDC) recommends that health care providers use the 2006 World Health Organization growth charts to monitor growth for infants and children up to 2 years of age in the United States, and then use the 2000 revised CDC growth charts for US children aged 2 to 20 years (CDC, 2010; Grummer-Strawn et al., 2010). The toddler's height may be measured with the toddler in a recumbent position for length, as in infancy, or in a standing position for stature. When the CDC growth charts for toddlers aged 2 years or older are being used, measure the height with the toddler in a standing position to obtain the toddler's stature and then use the appropriate chart based on stature.

The nurse continues to measure head circumference throughout the toddler period. The anterior fontanel usually closes by 18 months, the skull begins to thicken, and by 24 months it is 80% of its adult size (Hockenberry & Wilson, 2015).

The kidneys are well differentiated by the toddler years, and specific gravity and other urine findings are similar to those of adults. The daily excretion of urine for the 2-year-old child is 500 to 600 mL, increasing to 750 mL for the 3-year-old. Toddlers empty their bladders less frequently than infants and begin to develop voluntary control of urination. However, full bladder control comes later and begins after 18 to 24 months, when the toddler first becomes physiologically able to control the bladder.

The toddler's gastrointestinal tract also reaches functional maturity, although it continues to grow into adulthood. The toddler tends to need meals and snacks more frequently than an older child or adult. Most toddlers develop sufficient voluntary control of internal and external anal sphincters to accomplish successful bowel training. Bowel control usually occurs before urinary control.

Lung capacity continues to increase as the toddler grows, and the respiratory rate decreases from a mean of 30 breaths per minute at 1 year of age to 25 breaths per minute at 3 years. The diameter of the toddler's upper respiratory tract is small compared with that of an older child or adult, and this may lead to mouth breathing when the nose is obstructed with mucus (Figure 18-1). This small diameter, coupled with the toddler's exploratory nature and lack of judgment in deciding what to place in the mouth,

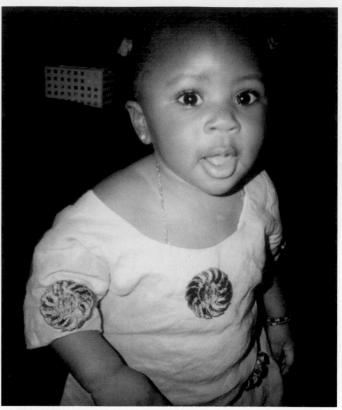

**FIGURE 18-1** Toddler demonstrates mouth breathing.

can result in accidental airway obstruction, which demands emergency action.

The proximal anatomy of the ear, eustachian tube, and nasal pharynx continue to resemble those of the infant more closely than those of the adult, continuing the risk of otitis media. The tonsils and adenoids remain proportionately large during the toddler years (Seidel et al., 2011).

With the exception of reproductive functions, most endocrine organs become functionally mature during the toddler and preschool years, although function continues at a minimum. The production of glucagon and insulin can be limited or labile, producing variations in blood glucose levels throughout early childhood. The production of cortisol, aldosterone, and deoxycorticosterone by the adrenal cortex remains somewhat limited, but they appear to function effectively in protecting the young child from the hazards of fluid and electrolyte imbalance well known in infancy. Secretion of epinephrine and norepinephrine from the adrenal medulla increases sufficiently to perform homeostatic functions of the autonomic nervous system and to mediate certain aspects of increased emotional components of behavior. Regulation of growth during early childhood remains one of the most important functions of the endocrine system.

Changes in the circulatory system include a decrease in heart rate, an increase in blood pressure, and a change in vascular resistance in response to growth in the size of various blood vessel lumens. The toddler's heart rate ranges from 80 to 120 beats per minute, and the mean blood pressure is 90/56 mmHg. Getting the toddler to sit still for a blood pressure reading can be difficult, but it is worth the effort to obtain several baseline readings for future reference.

The capillary beds gradually increase their capacity to respond to heat and cold in the environment, providing the toddler with more effective thermoregulation. Toddlers can also begin to take voluntary measures to relieve the discomfort of heat or cold. For example, the older toddler can put on clothing or move to warmer or cooler areas, assisting physiological efforts to maintain a constant internal thermal environment.

The immune response continues to mature. As toddlers expand their worlds through play groups and day care centers, exposure to new and different organisms is greatly increased. They may experience a period during which they appear to succumb to many minor respiratory tract and gastrointestinal tract infections. As immunity begins to develop against the organisms in their new environments, their resistance similarly increases.

Passive immunity to communicable disease acquired through transfer of maternal antibodies during fetal life has disappeared, and active immunity through the initial immunization series is usually completed by the age of 18 months. The next scheduled immunizations do not occur until age 4 to 6 years, before the toddler enters kindergarten. If a toddler is behind in the initial immunization series, a separate schedule is available that gives catch-up schedules and minimal intervals between doses (CDC, 2015a). For updated CDC immunization schedules and the latest guidance refer to the CDC website at http://www.cdc.gov/vaccines/schedules/.

All 20 primary or deciduous teeth erupt by the end of toddlerhood (Figure 18-2). The timing of these eruptions can differ widely, but a variation in the sequence alerts the nurse to inquire about early trauma to the mouth or familial traits for nonsequential tooth eruption. Application of fluoride varnish to primary teeth is recommended shortly after the teeth erupt through the gum. Important aspects of dental care at this age are included in health teaching and are listed in Box 18-1.

A mature swallowing pattern, using the tongue rather than the cheeks, has not yet developed, and toddlers continue to be at risk of choking. Toddlers who are mouth, rather than nose, breathers because of ongoing respiratory illness or allergies may have an underdeveloped palatal arch. With normal breathing, the tongue rests on and naturally widens the palate; however, when the child is forced to breathe through the mouth, the tongue rests in the lower jaw, not on the palate. This resultant narrowing of the palatal arch predisposes these toddlers to dental crowding when the permanent teeth erupt (Guilleminault et al., 2015).

An increase in the size and strength of muscle fibers continues. During this period, as during infancy, the use of muscle tissues is the primary stimulus for increased size and strength for gross and later fine motor movement. Myelination of the corticospinal tract is functionally sufficient to support most movement, but achievement of full control does not occur until much later in life. Throughout early childhood, voluntary motor movement is often accompanied by involuntary movements on the opposite side of the body. This mirroring of action is more pronounced in children who have some damage to the central nervous system, but the mechanisms by which this occurs are unknown. The toddler generally does not show complete dominance of one side of the body and may still switch hands when eating, throwing a ball, or engaging in other-handed activities.

Genes are passed from each parent to the child, and great similarities may show between the generations. Most genetic syndromes and disease entities are diagnosed either during the prenatal period or during infancy. However, some genetic

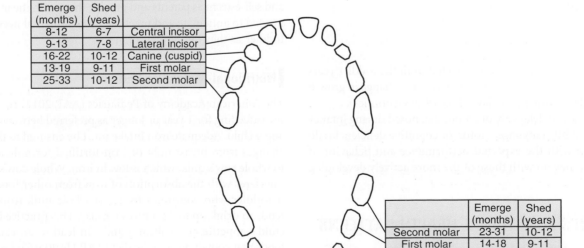

Maxillary (upper) teeth

| Emerge (months) | Shed (years) | |
|---|---|---|
| 8-12 | 6-7 | Central incisor |
| 9-13 | 7-8 | Lateral incisor |
| 16-22 | 10-12 | Canine (cuspid) |
| 13-19 | 9-11 | First molar |
| 25-33 | 10-12 | Second molar |

| | Emerge (months) | Shed (years) |
|---|---|---|
| Second molar | 23-31 | 10-12 |
| First molar | 14-18 | 9-11 |
| Canine (cuspid) | 17-23 | 9-12 |
| Lateral incisor | 10-16 | 7-8 |
| Central incisor | 6-10 | 6-7 |

Mandibular (lower) teeth

**FIGURE 18-2** Eruption (and shedding) of primary teeth.

### BOX 18-1 Nursing Interventions to Promote Dental Health Care for Toddlers

**Brushing**

- When teeth are present, begin to use a soft-bristled brush. The finger-wrapped gauze method used during infancy is no longer adequate because the teeth are too close together to reach all tooth surfaces.
- Introduce only a moist toothbrush at first. After the toddler has accepted the toothbrush, begin using toothpaste. A pea-sized amount is adequate. If the child does not like the taste of the toothpaste, use plain water.
- Toothpaste should contain supplemental fluoride if not in water supply. The US Preventive Services Task Force recommends that primary care clinicians prescribe oral fluoride supplementation starting at age 6 months if the water supply is not fluoridated.
- Toddlers do not have the motor coordination to brush their own teeth. They may enjoy imitating parents and put the toothbrush in their mouths, but an adult should be responsible for the actual brushing.
- Brush daily; for many toddlers, this practice becomes part of the bedtime routine. When the child appears too tired to cooperate in the evening, the parent should choose some other time of day when this important task will not be so difficult.

**Foods**

- Limit intake of foods high in sugar because they contribute to dental caries.
- When the young toddler still drinks from a bottle, only plain water should be given. Milk and juices should be offered by cup. If milk or juice is given in a bottle, this should never be done at naptime or bedtime.

**Visits to the Dentist**

- The first visit to the dentist should occur during the toddler years. Many dentists suggest an introduction-orientation, inspection-consultation type of visit when the child is approximately 18 to 24 months of age. This type of visit provides an early, enjoyable introduction to professional dental health promotion and care.
- Once the primary teeth of infants and children have erupted, the US Preventive Services Task Force recommends the application of fluoride varnish to the primary teeth.

From US Preventive Services Task Force. (2015). Dental caries in children from birth through age 5 years. http://www.uspreventiveservicestaskforce.org.

### BOX 18-2 GENOMICS

***Celiac Disease***

- Immune-mediated disorder that affects those with genetic susceptibility to it. When gluten (a protein found in wheat, barley, and rye) is consumed, the individual gets sick.
- Symptoms include gastrointestinal complications such as constipation, cramping, nausea and vomiting, diarrhea, and weight loss. Nutritional deficiencies may result.
- Affects 0.6% to 1.0% of the population worldwide, with prevalence differing regionally for unknown reasons.
- Certain genes are seen in individuals with celiac disease. Although not causal, it appears that *HLA-DQ2* and *HLA-DQ8* haplotypes are largely expressed in individuals with celiac disease.
- For disease diagnosis, serological testing of antibodies IgA and IgE is performed. Further testing involves biopsies of the intestines, which measures expression of haplotypes *HLA-DQ2* and *HLA-DQ3*.
- Treatment for children with celiac disease is a completely gluten-free diet. As a result of the recent increased awareness around gluten allergies, there are more gluten-free food choices available at the grocery store.

For more information on celiac disease, visit http://www.celiac.org.

syndromes and diseases are not detected until the toddler years or even later. The most common initial sign is a change in growth pattern or developmental delays (Box 18-2: Genomics).

Developmental delays are often not diagnosed during infancy because the subtle language, motor, or cognitive deficiencies do not interfere with the expected performance and behavior of the infant as they do with those of the more actively developing toddler.

## GORDON'S FUNCTIONAL HEALTH PATTERNS

### Health Perception–Health Management Pattern

Toddlers may eventually learn that being sick means feeling bad or having to stay in bed, but they have little, if any, understanding of the meaning of health. They may perform requested health-promotion activities, such as brushing teeth, but they may simply brush their teeth as part of their bedtime ritual and not because they know this activity will prevent dental caries. Toddlers depend on their parents for health management, and their overall health will be greatly influenced by their parents' health perceptions and health-management priorities (Box 18-3: *Healthy People 2020*).

Toddlers identify with parents, caregivers, and other important role models, internalizing a wide range of lifestyle attributes. Parents' and caregivers' health perceptions and health behaviors should model the perceptions and behaviors desired for health promotion. Toddlers whose parents eat a variety of foods are more likely to try new foods. Such modeling increases the chances that good practices will be retained throughout the toddler's life. The nurse's task is to help parents strengthen their confidence and self-esteem as parents and provide them with the information needed to anticipate and meet the developmental needs of their toddler as they develop as a family.

### Nutritional-Metabolic Pattern

The American Academy of Pediatrics (AAP, 2012) recommends breastfeeding for 1 year or longer as preferred between a mother and a child. Adequate iron intake must be ensured as the toddler changes from breast milk or iron-fortified formula and cereal to whole cow's milk, which is low in iron. Whole cow's milk also interferes with the absorption of iron from other food sources. A toddler who continues to ingest whole milk from a bottle tends to drink up to 32 ounces per day. This practice blunts the child's appetite at mealtimes and can lead to an exclusion of foods that contain iron in the diet (AAP, Healthy Children, 2012), requiring iron from fortified foods or supplements. The use of a bottle with milk or juice, especially at bedtime, has also been associated with dental caries (baby bottle tooth decay) because of the high sugar content. If parents want to give a bottle at bedtime, it should contain only water.

### BOX 18-3 HEALTHY PEOPLE 2020

**Selected Health-Promotion and Disease-Prevention Objectives for Toddlers**

- Increase age-appropriate vehicle restraint system use in children aged 1 to 3 years to 79% from the baseline of 72% for children aged 1 to 3 years restrained in front-facing child safety seats in 2008.
- Reduce death among children from child maltreatment for those younger than 18 years from 2.3 deaths per 100,000 children in 2008 to 2.1 deaths per 100,000 children; and reduce unintentional suffocation deaths among infants aged 0 to 12 months from 23.1 deaths per 100,000 infants in 2008 to 20.8 deaths per 100,000 infants.
- Reduce iron deficiency among young children aged 1 to 2 years from 15.9% in 2005 to 2008 to 14.3%, and in children aged 3 to 4 years from 5.3% in 2005 to 2008 to 4.3%.
- Reduce blood lead levels in children aged 1 to 5 years (baseline was 2.5% of children aged 1–5 years had blood lead level of 5.8 mcg/dL in 2005 to 2008, goal is 5.2 mcg/dL by 2020).
- Reduce exposure to selected environmental toxins as measured by blood and urine concentrations of the substances or their metabolites in children aged 1 year or older in 2003 to 2004, especially reduce cadmium, mercury, and lead levels.
- Reduce outpatient visits for ear infections where antibiotics were prescribed to young children, especially for ear infections in those younger than 5 years from 77.8% in 2006 to 2007 to 70%.
- Achieve and maintain effective vaccination coverage levels for universally recommended vaccines among young children aged 19 to 35 months, especially increase the level of four doses of diphtheria, tetanus, and acellular pertussis vaccine from 85% in 2008 to 90%; the level of three doses of *Haemophilus influenzae* type b conjugate vaccine from 57% in 2008 to 90%; the level of four doses of pneumococcal conjugate vaccine from 80% in 2008 to 90%; the

- level of two doses of hepatitis A vaccine from 40% in 2008 to 60%; the level of a birth dose of hepatitis B vaccine from 51% in 2006 and 2008 to 85%; the level of two or more doses of rotavirus vaccine from 38% in 2009 to 80%.
- Increase the proportion of children aged 19 to 35 months who receive the recommended doses of diphtheria, tetanus, and acellular pertussis vaccine, polio vaccine, MMR vaccine, *Haemophilus influenzae* type b conjugate vaccine, hepatitis B vaccine, varicella vaccine, and pneumococcal conjugate vaccine from 68% in 2008 to 80%.
- Reduce invasive pneumococcal infections among children younger than 5 years: reduce new invasive pneumococcal infections from 20.3 cases per 100,000 in 2008 to 12 cases per 100,000; reduce invasive penicillin-resistant pneumococcal infections from 4.3 cases per 100,000 in 2008 to 3 cases per 100,000.
- Increase the proportion of young children screened for an autism spectrum disorder and other developmental delays by 35 months of age from the 2007 baseline of 22.6% of children aged 10 to 36 months to 24.9%.
- Increase the proportion of newborns who are screened for hearing loss by no later than age 1 month from 82% in 2007 to 90.2% in 2020.
- Increase the proportion of newborns who receive audiological evaluation no later than age 3 months for infants who did not pass the hearing screening from 66% in 2007 to 72.6%.
- Increase the proportion of infants with confirmed hearing loss who are enrolled for intervention services no later than age 6 months from the 50% in 2007 rate to 55%.
- Increase the proportion of preschool children aged 5 years or younger who receive vision screening from 40.1% in 2008 to 44.1%

From Borse, N. N., Gilchrist, J., Dellinger, A. M., Rudd, R. A., Ballesteros, M. F., & Sleet, D. A. (2008). CDC childhood injury report: Patterns of unintentional injuries among 0 to 19 year olds in the United States, 2000–2006. Atlanta, GA: National Center for Injury Prevention and Control, Centers for Disease Control and Prevention. http://www.cdc.gov/safechild/images/CDC-childhoodinjury.pdf; Office of Disease Prevention & Health Promotion of the Office of Public Health, US Department of Health and Human Services. (2010). Healthy People 2020: Midcourse review. http://odphp.osophs.dhhs.gov/pubs/.

Fruit juice and other drinks are often overconsumed because they taste good, because they are conveniently packaged and easily carried around by the toddler, and because they are viewed as nutritious. However, the AAP, Healthy Children (2012) cautions parents to use only 100% juice that is pasteurized, that children aged 1 to 6 years have two fruit servings each day, only one of which should be juice, and that consumption of fresh fruit should be encouraged. It further states that 4 to 6 ounces (120 to 180 mL) of fruit juice equals one fruit serving. Fruit juice has no nutritional advantage over whole fruit and in fact lacks the fiber contained in whole fruit (AAP, Healthy Children, 2012, 2015).

A decrease in the growth rate during toddlerhood results in a decrease in appetite. Parents need to be reminded of this if they begin to worry about their toddler's nutritional intake (AAP, 2011). A daily record kept over a 3- to 5-day period presents a better picture of a child's intake and is a useful teaching tool for this age group.

Toddlers often use mealtime as an occasion to assert individuality and control as well as exploration. Families will differ in their expectations of eating behavior and mealtime routines. The nurse's best guide for parents of toddlers is to remind them that parents are in charge of what food is offered, when it is offered,

and where it is offered (Box 18-4: Research for Evidence-Based Practice). Box 18-5 lists some nursing interventions to promote healthy eating in toddlers. However, it is up to the toddler to decide the amount to actually eat. Periodically, a toddler may even refuse a meal altogether. Parents need to be encouraged to offer healthy, age-appropriate food choices (Figure 18-3). Toddlers will eat them, as long as they do not fill up on empty calories from juice and high-carbohydrate snacks that are often given to children "so they eat something." Furthermore, parents should not focus too much attention on food intake or punish children for refusing food. Toddlers may learn how easily parents can be controlled by their behavior around food intake and may then continue the behavior for the attention alone.

Maintaining a record of food intake over time, the nurse can demonstrate the adequacy of the nutrients that the toddler is already receiving during mealtimes and help parents develop a plan to offer more of the essential foods during meals (Holt et al., 2011). Children with inadequate nutrition are predisposed to impaired immune systems, leading to infections and delayed healing and recovery. They are also predisposed to depletion of muscle mass, leading to diminished functional capacity. In addition, although inadequately understood, nutrients

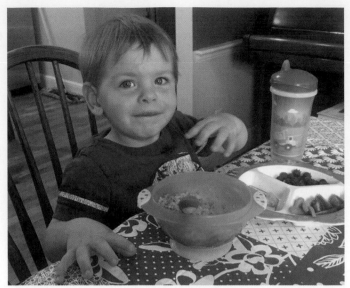

**FIGURE 18-3** Toddlers need healthy, age-appropriate food choices.

and neurotropic factors interact with one another for brain and behavioral development (Ruel & Alderman, 2013).

The family who has a vegetarian or vegan diet may need some assistance from the nurse or a dietitian. Vegetarian and vegan diets differ widely, so it is important to assess precisely the foods that are eaten, the foods that have been eliminated from the diet, and the supplements that are used.

## Elimination Pattern

**Toilet training** is often a major parental concern during toddlerhood. The nurse anticipates this developmental stressor and initiates discussion with the parents to determine their understanding of the child's signs of developmental readiness and their attitude and commitment to establishing a toileting pattern for their toddler. Emotional and physiological readiness for toilet training rarely develops before 18 months of age. Parents who begin before their child is ready usually experience frustration.

### Nursing Interventions

By suggesting the sequence in Box 18-6: Nursing Interventions, the nurse assists parents with toilet training. The parent who can approach toilet training with a relaxed attitude, accepting some delays and frustrations, will have a better chance of success and a more positive outcome for the toddler.

## Activity-Exercise Pattern

Toddlers are always busy—emptying wastebaskets and drawers, building and destroying towers, throwing, kicking, and chasing after balls, or dressing and undressing. Many of their activities are repeated over and over, providing practice opportunities for their newly realized skills. The various toys designed for toddlers capitalize on this ability to explore and imagine with laptop

## BOX 18-5 Nursing Interventions to Promote Healthy Eating in Toddlers

- Routines are important to toddlers. Serve scheduled meals and snacks. Parents are responsible for what, when, and where the toddler eats. The toddler decides whether to eat and how much.
- Schedule meals and sleep periods such that the child is awake and alert during mealtime.
- Turn off the television. Mealtime should be a relaxed and pleasant time, free of distractions.
- Serve small portions and let your toddler ask for more.
- Offer simple, single foods, because mixtures of foods are often rejected.
- Serve your toddler's favorite foods along with new ones. Several introductions may be necessary before the toddler accepts a new food. Make sure you eat it too.
- Encourage the use of utensils, but accept that toddlers still often need to use their fingers.
- Do not use food to bribe, reward, or punish your toddler.
- Avoid foods that may cause choking, such as hard candy, mini marshmallows, popcorn, pretzels, chips, and spoonfuls of peanut butter, nuts, and seeds, large chunks of meat, hot dogs, raw carrots, dried fruits, and whole grapes.
- Drinking more than 24 ounces of milk per day can reduce your child's appetite for other healthy foods. For those younger than 2 years, do not use reduced-fat, low-fat, or fat-free (skim) milk because children younger than 2 years need the extra fat for their developing nervous systems.

## BOX 18-6 Nursing Interventions
### Initiating a Toileting Program for Toddlers

Interest in and awareness of bowel and urinary elimination usually begin by 18 months of age.

- Before beginning toilet training, parents should check their toddlers for the prerequisite skills, which include being able to walk well, stoop and recover, stay dry for at least 2 hours during the day, and communicate sensation before elimination, as well as the discomfort of wet or messy pants and the need for assistance.
- When these prerequisites are present, introduce the child to a potty seat or chair. The potty chair should provide secure seating with the child's feet touching the floor. The potty seat should be used with a small step stool to create the same effect.
- Because of the gastrocolic reflex, bowel elimination is more likely after a meal, so this is a good time to place the toddler on the potty. When a pattern of bowel or urinary elimination is noticed, use this pattern as a guide for placing the child on the potty.
- Encourage the toddler to stay on the chair for 2 to 3 minutes and always explain what to do ("Go potty") rather than what not to do ("Don't wet your pants"). Do not refer to elimination as dirty or yucky. Remember this is your child's first creation.
- Praise the child for desired behavior. Introduce underwear as a badge of success. Ignore undesired behavior and never punish the child by scolding the child, spanking the child, or other punitive measures.

Remember that daytime dryness is usually achieved by 3 years of age and ahead of nighttime dryness, where the need to wear a diaper remains.

trainers, electronic coloring tablets, musical instruments, and books with accompanying audiovisual disks.

During the toddler period, children will advance from taking their first step to running, climbing stairs, and even pedaling a tricycle. They enjoy pushing and pulling, whether it is an unsuspecting laundry basket or a push-pull toy made for the job. They scribble spontaneously, usually with vigor, and will emerge from toddlerhood capable of copying a circle and creating tadpole-like figures. They learn to use a spoon and a fork with fairly good success and to wash their hands. They also advance from being dressed by others to dressing themselves with assistance, although at times they resist it.

Toddlers spend most of their waking hours at play—exploring their expanding environment, imitating others' actions, and creating a safety net of **rituals** around the routines of eating, sleeping, and everything in between. In their enthusiasm to try many activities, toddlers invariably take on tasks that are beyond their abilities, which can result in frustration and an occasional well-known temper tantrum. Their exploratory nature and limited, but advancing, skills also make them vulnerable to injury.

Most toddlers are interested in other children. However, this interest is limited because toddlers, although ready to be with other children, are not ready to share. Successful social encounters with toddlers are best described as **parallel play**, where children play side by side, doing similar things with similar toys, but each working independently (Berger, 2011). Sharing and cooperative play will not develop until well into the preschool age.

### Nursing Interventions

When parents inquire about what toys and activities to provide for their toddler, the following are suggested:

- Provide toys that challenge the child to develop new skills: toys that require skills slightly above the child's present level, but not so advanced that the child cannot achieve some success.
- Provide opportunities for new learning. This may be as basic as a book with pictures of new animals or a walk through the produce section of the grocery store to point out fruits and vegetables.
- Provide opportunities for social encounters with other children, but do not force playing together. Creating separate yet parallel space, with the use of small mats or hula hoops as boundaries, is recommended.
- Follow the child's lead. Let the toddler choose and explore new toys or objects, within safe limits.
- Make sure the toy is safe for the toddler and does not have any parts that can be removed and swallowed, have lead paint, or can cause harm to the curious toddler.

The desire of some parents to raise the smartest, most coordinated, or most musically talented super kids often begins in the toddler period. It is interaction with parents and others in their environment that provides the advantage with cognitive development. The AAP (2013a) recommends no screen time, including television, videos, tablets (iPads), and computers, for children younger than 2 years. For older toddlers, the AAP recommends no more than 1 to 2 hours daily of high-quality screen time with the parent watching too. For interactive computer games that may include touch screens (on smartphones and tablets), the parent needs to be there with the toddler so that two-way conversation occurs. Ideally, children should be allowed to explore their interests, with parents responding to their cues. Past research associated television watching by toddlers with interference at a critical time when language development occurs and suggested that this can cause a delay in that process. Current research indicates that audible television loud enough to decrease the child's exposure to discernible adult speech and decreased child vocalizations also lead to delayed speech development (Pempek et al., 2014). Additionally, the more television shows with advertising watched, the more likely the child will become obese (Zimmerman & Bell, 2010). For more information on helping parents support their toddler's activity, use of technology, and exploration in a safe and educational way, visit the Zero to Three website at http://www.zerotothree.org.

## Sleep-Rest Pattern

Toddlers' need for sleep decreases to 12 hours a day, including one or two naps of shorter duration. One of the naps is usually replaced by quiet time, a brief period to unwind from a busy or noisy activity. Occasionally the parents or caregivers need these rest breaks as much as or more than the toddler. Sitting together in a rocking chair for a soothing song or quiet music or reading side by side or together can be suggested by the nurse.

The toddler may be involved in an activity and not be aware of fatigue, especially when visitors are in the home or some interesting new toys have been discovered. All parents are familiar with the child who is overtired but unable to relax enough to sleep. Parents can potentially avoid this dilemma by scheduling nap and quiet time even when there are house guests or holidays that preempt the toddler's routine.

Rituals are characteristic of this age, and most toddlers have a nap and bedtime ritual. The following might be a typical pattern: eating a nutritious snack, followed by bathing, brushing teeth, listening to a story, getting a kiss, and having overhead lights turned off and the night light turned on. Following this ritual is important because the toddler gets a sense of security when ending the day. Changing this ritual can be upsetting. The nurse encourages parents to establish and follow the bedtime ritual as closely as possible, even when visitors, family illness, or travel makes the routine more difficult. In addition, incorporate rituals as much as possible when the toddler stays outside the home; for instance, staying overnight at their grandparent's house or during a hospitalization.

Many toddlers will try to delay sleep by calling for water, another story, or another kiss, or by making other requests. Parents should be certain that the toddler has ample opportunity for interaction with them during the day, follow the usual bedtime ritual, and be firm and consistent in resisting any requests for attention after the final good nights have been said. Encouraging toddlers to use transition or security objects, such as stuffed animals or blankets, helps them to self-quiet and console themselves both at bedtime and in new situations (Figure 18-4).

**Night terrors** may begin in toddlerhood. Night terrors are different from nightmares, which generally begin at a later age and result in the child awakening and being able to recall the frightening dream. The child who experiences night terrors does not waken completely, but cries out, looks terrified, and cannot be aroused for several minutes. Eventually, usually after 5 to 10 minutes, the child falls back into quiet sleep. Parents need to be reassured that these episodes will become less frequent as the child develops. The parents should talk in a soothing voice but should not try to awaken the child. If the child does waken, the parents should then provide comfort and tuck the child back in bed.

## Cognitive-Perceptual Pattern

Toddlers who experienced the security of a nurturing and reliable source of protection and attachment during infancy have a strong base from which to begin to explore and learn about their expanding world. They begin toddlerhood in Piaget's **sensorimotor stage** of cognitive development and start moving to the **preoperational stage**. Their advancing thought-processing skills and abilities to use the language are heralded by the development of **egocentrism**, an inability to put oneself in another's shoes. Toddlers who come running into a room asking their parents "Where is it?" are confused when parents respond "Where is what?" They assume their parents and all others share their same thoughts and cannot understand why they do not.

Toddlers interpret and learn about objects and events, not in terms of general properties but in terms of their relationship with them or their use to them. Their thoughts are dominated by what they see, hear, or otherwise experience, and they want

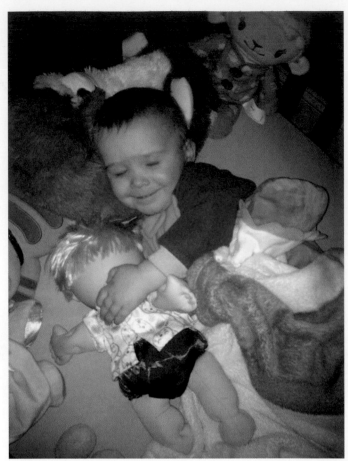

**FIGURE 18-4** Toddlers need adequate sleep for healthy growth, and their stuffed toys can help them feel more secure.

to experience everything. Their two- to three-word phrases are most often related to present events, describing an action, a desire, or a possession (e.g., "Mommy, me up!").

Both receptive and expressive language skills are developing rapidly in toddlers; however, their receptive language skills far outweigh their expressive language ability, and toddlers often use gestures until words are found to represent the meanings already acquired. Toddlers also learn the use of inflection. "Mommy" may mean "Pick me up" on one occasion and "I'm scared" or "Where are you?" on another. Often frustrated by their limited repertoire of expressive language, which usually includes approximately 400 words, young toddlers default to using "no" as a method of gaining control over a situation or expressing themselves (see the Think About It box at the beginning of this chapter).

By age 3 years, children have mastered the basics of language function, form, and content, and these fundamentals will continue to be refined throughout childhood and adolescence. Table 18-1 outlines the landmarks of speech, language, and hearing ability for this age group.

Toddlers have a solid understanding of **object permanence** and are no longer easily distracted when a desired toy, blanket, or parent is not to be found. Many toddlers will sit patiently in front of the washing machine while a favorite blanket is laundered

## TABLE 18-1   GROWTH AND DEVELOPMENT

### Landmarks of Speech, Language, and Hearing Ability During the Toddler Period

| Age (Months) | Receptive Language | Expressive Language | Related Hearing Ability |
|---|---|---|---|
| 18 | Up to 50 words; recognizes between 6 and 12 objects by name, such as *dog, cat, bottle, ball;* identifies three body parts, such as *eyes, nose, mouth;* understands simple, one-step commands such as *give me the doll, open your mouth, stick out your tongue* | Up to 20 words; jargon and echolalia are present; uses names of familiar objects and one-word sentences, such as *go* or *eat;* uses gestures; uses words such as *no, mine, eat, good, bad, hot, cold,* and expressions such as *oh-oh, what's that, all gone;* use of words can be quite inconsistent; 25% of speech intelligible | Has begun to develop gross discrimination by learning to distinguish between highly dissimilar noises, such as doorbell and train, barking dog and automobile horn, or mother's and father's voices |
| 24 | Up to 1200 words; knows *in, on, under;* identifies *dog, ball, engine, bed, doll, scissors, hair, mouth, feet, nose, cup, spoon, car, key;* distinguishes between one and many and formulates a negative judgment (a knife is not a fork); understands simple stories; follows simple, two-step directions; is beginning to make distinctions between *you* and *me* | Up to 270 words; jargon and echolalia almost gone; average 75 words per hour during free play; talks in words, phrases, and two-word to three-word sentences; averages two words per response; first pronouns appear, such as *I, me, mine, it, who, that;* adjectives and adverbs are only beginning to appear; names objects and common pictures; refers to self by name, such as *Katrina go bye-bye;* uses phrases such as *I want, go bye-bye, want cookie, ball all gone;* 60% of speech intelligible | Refinement of gross discriminative skills |
| 30 | Up to 2400 words; identifies action in pictures and objects by use; carries out one-part and two-part commands, such as *pick up your shoe and give it to mommy;* knows what is used to drink liquids, what goes on the feet, what is used to buy candy; understands plurals, questions, difference between boy and girl, the concepts *one, up, down, run, walk, throw, fast, more, my* | Uses up to 425 words; jargon and echolalia no longer exist; averages 140 words per hour; names words such as *chair, can, box, key, door;* repeats two digits from memory; average sentence length is approximately 2.5 words; uses more adjectives and adverbs; demands repetition from others, such as *do it again;* nearly always announces intentions before actions; begins to ask questions of adults; 75% of speech intelligible | — |
| 36 | Up to 3600 words; understands *both, two, not today,* what to do when thirsty (hungry, sleepy), why people have stoves; understands *wait, later, big, new, different, strong, today, another,* and taking turns at play; carries out two-item and some three-item commands, such as *give me the ball, pick up the doll,* and *sit down;* identifies several colors; is aware of past and future | Up to 900 words in simple sentences, averaging three to four words per sentence; averages 170 words per hour; uses words such as *when, time, today, not today, new, different, big, strong, surprise, secret;* can repeat three digits, name one color, say name, give simple account of experiences, and tell stories that can be understood; begins to use more pronouns, adjectives, and adverbs; describes at least one element of a picture; is aware of past and future; uses commands such as *you make it* and expressions such as *I can't, I don't want to;* verbalizes toilet needs; expresses desire to take turns; communication includes criticisms, commands, requests, threats, questions, answers; 85% of speech intelligible | Starts to distinguish dissimilar speech sounds, such as the difference between *ee* and *er,* although there may be some difficulty with the concepts of *same* and *different* |

Modified from Hockenberry, M. J., & Wilson, D. (Eds.). (2015). *Wong's nursing care of infants and children* (9th ed.). St. Louis, MO: Mosby; Ports, N. L., & Mandleco, B. L. (2011). *Pediatric nursing: Caring for children and their families* (3rd ed.). Clifton Park, NY: Thomson Delmar Learning; Quevedo, L. A., Silva, R., Godoy, K., Jansen, M. B., Matos, K.A., Tavares, P., et al. (2011). The impact of maternal post-partum depression on the language development of children at 12 months. *Child: Care, Health and Development, 38*(3), 420–424.

or stare out of a front window awaiting a parent's return. They can inadvertently put themselves in harm's way as they pursue an object or person they sense is just out of view.

The toddler period is dominated by play, but often referred to as "child's work," which is repetitive and ritualistic. When toddlers bounce a ball over and over and over again, they are not trying to drive their parents crazy. They are trying to learn about balls, and repetition is the best teacher. Toddlers' ritualistic behaviors help them master skills and decrease anxiety, and the addition of a seemingly endless string of questions to these behaviors can test the limits of the most patient parents. These queries, however, must be acknowledged and answered in a manner that not only provides solutions but also validates and reinforces the toddler's burgeoning curiosity. The nurse explains the "terrible twos" by teaching parents and caregivers that toddlers might better be viewed as "young scientists" in need of a safe "laboratory" in which to conduct their trial-and-error research. Better now and in parents' close proximity than in adolescence, a developmental period that mirrors and repeats many of the parent-child challenges of toddlerhood.

The AAP has recommended administration of autistic screening at the 18-month preventive care visit (Miller et al., 2011). **Autism spectrum disorders** are defined as pervasive developmental disorders with onset in infancy or childhood and characterized by impaired social interactions, impaired communications, and significantly restricted activities and interests. There is no known cause. The current prevalence is 1 in every 68 American children, and almost 1 in 42 boys versus 1 in 189 girls (CDC, 2014a; Sheldrick et al., 2013). There is not a single treatment that works for all children with autism; however, there are many options available including applied behavior analysis. This involves the principle that positive reinforcement increases the frequency of the desired behavior. It is best to implement treatment early in the child's development. See http://www.autismsociety.org and http://www.myautism.org for more information.

### Hearing

The ability to hear and listen to others is critical for speech and language development. Listening includes attending to what is heard, discriminating among the various qualities of sound, cognitively associating what is heard with previously learned experiences, and remembering what is heard. The quantity and quality of language to which the toddler is exposed is thought to be more important for the development of listening ability and therefore receptive language skills than it is for the development of expressive language skills (Perryman et al., 2013). Toddlers often seek repetition of auditory input, as observed in their seemingly endless repetition of sounds, words, and combinations of words. This repetition is their way of practicing and organizing new language (Neuman & Dickinson, 2011) (see Table 18-1).

Hearing loss is one of the most common conditions present at birth. If undetected during early infancy, even mild hearing loss can impede speech, language, cognitive, and emotional development (Noritz & Murphy, 2013). Health care providers need to continue to monitor, screen, and refer children for formal audiological evaluation if they develop signs of identified risk factors for hearing loss. The timing and number of hearing reevaluations for children with risk factors should be individualized. Infants who pass the neonatal screening but have a risk factor should have at least one diagnostic audiology assessment by 24 to 30 months of age (AAP, 2011a). Early and more frequent assessment may be indicated for children with cytomegalovirus infection, syndromes associated with progressive hearing loss, neurodegenerative disorders, head trauma, or culture-positive postnatal infections associated with sensorineural hearing loss (e.g., herpes viruses); for toddlers who spent more than 5 days in a neonatal intensive care unit at birth or who received extracorporeal membrane oxygenation, exchange transfusions, or chemotherapy; and for caregivers of toddlers who are concerned because there is a family history of hearing loss (AAP, 2007, 2011a).

Younger toddlers are screened with use of **visual-reinforcement audiometry**, in which stimulus tones and visually animated reinforcers (e.g., a lighted toy) are paired and presented together. After the toddler has been conditioned to expect this relationship, the visual reinforcer is withheld, and the sound is presented alone. The toddler looks for the visual reinforcer in response to the sound, and the visual reinforcer is then presented as a reward. **Conditioned-play audiometry** is used for older toddlers and preschool children. The child is first taught to play listening games, using blocks or rings. The child learns to wait and listen for a sound and then perform a motor task (e.g., places a block, a bucket, or a ring on a stacking stick) in response. The motor task is followed by social reinforcement. Noncalibrated toys or noisemakers and signals that lack frequency specificity are inappropriate screening methods and should be used only as gross indicators for monitoring.

**Otitis media**, or middle ear infection, is one of the leading causes of visits to health care providers during the toddler years and the primary reason for which antibiotics are prescribed for these children. Discussing the current literature and evidence-based reports and recommendations often helps parents understand the proper use of antibiotics, which is also imperative in preventing antibiotic resistance. When it is deemed necessary to use an antibiotic, nurses teach how to administer the medication safely and stress the importance of taking the medication at the prescribed time and for the full duration of the course, which is indicated by an empty container of medication, not by the absence of initial symptoms.

### Vision

Toddlers' visual acuity is usually approximately 20/40, although gaining their cooperation for screening is often difficult and not recommended unless parents, caregivers, or health care providers identify a concern. Depth perception is still immature, although more developed than in infancy.

**Amblyopia** is one of the major health care concerns for this age group and occurs in 2 to 3 of every 100 children (National Eye Institute, 2013). It is defined as diminished, or loss of, vision in an eye that has not received adequate use. The eye looks normal, but it is not being used normally. Because the brain favors the other eye, the term "lazy eye" is often used. The most common cause of amblyopia is strabismus, but it may also occur when one eye is more nearsighted, farsighted, or astigmatic than the other. Occasionally amblyopia is caused by other eye conditions such as a cataract.

Amblyopia is preventable and treatable, especially if detected early. The earlier detection of amblyopia will contribute to the greater chance for a complete recovery. The AAP and the American Academy of Ophthalmology strongly recommend that children have their eyes examined at the following times: newborn period, 6 months, 3 years, and before starting school (American Association for Pediatric Ophthalmology and Strabismus, 2015; American Optometric Association, 2015). Management of amblyopia depends on the cause and may include surgery or paralytic, autonomic, and centrally acting pharmacological agents. However, no matter what the cause, management will involve making the child use the lazy eye, the eye with reduced vision. There are two ways to accomplish this: use of atropine eye drops or patching of the stronger eye (American Association for Pediatric Ophthalmology and Strabismus, 2015). If glasses are worn with the patch, the nurse will help the parents secure them with the active toddler. Not all children benefit from eye drop treatment for amblyopia. When the stronger eye is nearsighted, the atropine eye drops may not be as effective (American Association for Pediatric Ophthalmology and Strabismus, 2015) (Box 18-7: Innovative Practice).

Strabismus is a deviation of the line of vision from the midline resulting from extraocular muscle weakness or imbalance and is commonly referred to as crossed eye. One or both eyes may turn in, out, up, or down, and this can be constant or intermittent. Marked or continuous strabismus is usually noticed early by the parents and health care providers and is therefore treated early; the subtler deviations are often unnoticed until older toddlerhood or the preschool years. Every toddler should be screened for strabismus as part of the routine eye examination that is performed by the physician or nurse practitioner during well-child visits.

Other signs of vision problems that the nurse observes or parents report in their toddlers include the following red flags:

- Rubs eyes excessively
- Shuts or covers one eye, tilts head, or looks sideways to view an object
- Has difficulty or is irritable when doing close work
- Blinks, squints, or frowns when viewing objects
- Holds books close to eyes
- Has red, encrusted, or swollen eyelids
- Has red, inflamed, or watery eyes
- Develops recurring styes (swelling at the edge of the eyelid)

### Taste and Smell

Toddlers are beginning to take control of their world and have the capacity to taste and smell, new skills that are rapidly used. Toddlers often refuse to even taste something that looks or smells displeasing to them or eat something that they recall as tasting terrible. They are able to react accurately to a sensation that a taste or smell arouses in them, and they begin to learn conditioned association between certain smells and culturally acceptable values. Foods and smells found in one family or culture become palatable and accepted, and those that are unacceptable become displeasing. Many of our adult eating habits, food likes and dislikes, and visceral responses to odors have their roots in this period.

## Self-Perception–Self-Concept Pattern

According to Erikson (1995, 1998), the developmental task of toddlers is to acquire a sense of autonomy while overcoming a sense of doubt and shame. To exert autonomy, toddlers must relinquish the dependence on others that was enjoyed during infancy. Continued dependency has the potential to create a sense of doubt in toddlers about their ability to take control of, and ultimately take responsibility for, their own actions. Toddlers seem to thrive when parents can accommodate their increasing autonomy yet maintain a strong parenting presence that includes a full measure of patience, enough parental self-confidence to set appropriate limits, and the ability to realize that their toddler's negative behavior is not directed at them and their egocentrism is not a reflection on them.

The toddler must explore the world, not only the physical aspects but also the interpersonal aspects of relationships, to develop a true sense of autonomy. Exploring the physical world involves poking into, climbing onto, crawling under, tasting, smelling, and taking apart the objects encountered. The child explores relationships with others by searching for the limits of the child's power: If a "no" or a temper tantrum means control of another person's behavior, the child learns that one's own self is more powerful than the other person's self. The toddler continually practices separateness to develop a sense of autonomy.

This process can be frustrating and confusing for parents. The toddler may say a vehement "no" when offered a drink and then scream and cry when the drink is taken away; the parents may wonder whether or not the toddler wants the drink. Likely the answer is "yes," but the toddler may also need to express autonomy by refusing it. Occasionally the same toddler who displays a strong need for autonomy spontaneously cuddles or even clings to a parent. These conflicting desires can be confusing to both the parent and the toddler. The toddler's need for more autonomy may conflict with parental expectations, safety limits, or the rights of other children or adults. Any of these conflicts result in feelings of frustration. A typical toddler response to frustration is the well-known temper tantrum.

### Nursing Interventions

The nurse assesses the toddler-parent relationship to determine the following:

- How is the toddler expressing the need for autonomy?
- How do the parents perceive these actions?
- How does the toddler respond to frustration in exploring the environment or controlling personal and others' actions?
- How do the parents respond to the toddler's display of frustration?
- What provisions are the parents making to allow safe choices for the toddler?

The nurse's teaching focuses on the aspects that are troublesome for the toddler-parent relationship. The following examples are some general concepts to include:

- Match the environment to the child's needs and abilities. Childproof the home such that the child can explore safely. Provide toys that the child can master. Give opportunities to play with more challenging toys, but do not make these toys the rule.
- Give advance notice of a change in activity, such as lunch or nap time. Use transition rituals and objects.
- Do not offer a choice if there is not one. For example, rather than ask if the toddler wants to take a bath, say "It is time to take a bath, do you want to take it upstairs or downstairs, or do you want to start at the face and move down to the toes or start with the toes and wash the face last?" This allows the toddler to be in charge and the task of bathing to be achieved.
- Set and enforce consistent limits such that the toddler will come to develop control within these limits.
- To prevent temper tantrums, keep routines simple and consistent, set reasonable limits and give rationales, avoid "head-on clashes," and provide choices.
- If temper tantrums occur, provide a safe environment for the toddler, identify the tantrum's cause, and help the toddler regain control. Do not reason, threaten, promise, hit, or concede. Respond consistently and follow through on discipline free of anger. Overcriticizing and restricting the toddler may dampen enthusiasm and increase feelings of shame and doubt.
- Praise the toddler's skills and abilities. Never miss an opportunity to catch your toddler being good. Be positive. Remember to say "yes" once in a while.

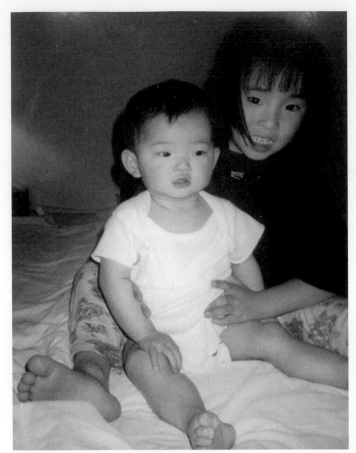

**FIGURE 18-5** It is a big change for a toddler when a new baby is introduced to the family.

## Roles-Relationships Pattern

By toddlerhood, children typically know their mother, father, and older siblings and have established some form of reciprocal relationship with them (Herd et al., 2014). Toddlers' capability for relationships is limited and usually reflects their egocentric approach to everything else. Parents' and siblings' roles are understood, just like everything else in their lives, in terms of how those roles relate to the toddler. One family member may be the fixer of toys or the comforter of bruises, another the troublemaker who takes away toys.

Toddlers are interested in everything, and their parents' and siblings' activities and possessions are often imitated and preferred. Frequently the desire to be like or have something that belongs to a sibling creates sibling rivalry. This happens between toddlers and their older siblings, but even more when a new, younger sibling is introduced (Figure 18-5). A new baby who is often loud, unable to play, unable to be touched or explored too vigorously, and demands and gets too much parental attention quickly becomes a nuisance to toddlers, who have been known to inform their parents that they can "take the new baby back where it came from now." Realizing the new sibling is here to stay, toddlers often regress, reverting to earlier, previously abandoned infantile behavior such as losing toileting skills, wanting to be fed or dressed, or even communicating by "baby talk." They are usually trying to retain or regain a sense of mastery and, once reassured, will progress. This process is not the end of sibling rivalry but only the beginning of what will assume many forms and require ongoing negotiation from all family members. Parents cannot stop sibling fighting by forbidding it, but reasonable limits can be established. One way to deescalate fighting is to remove the reward of the fight. Generally, the desired outcome in the toddler's mind is to see the self-rewarded and the sibling punished. When parents do not reward the toddler or punish the sibling, or when they do not take sides, the gain is missing and fighting becomes less satisfactory. This approach does not mean that all fighting will stop, but the child will look for other ways of getting approval.

Sibling relationships and parent-child relationships can be difficult subjects for parents to discuss. Parents may think that any hint of discord indicates an unhealthy family (Wulff et al., 2015). The nurse includes normal family development and role relationships as part of the anticipatory guidance given during the toddler years (Kochanska et al., 2013). Toddler behaviors are frustrating for all parents, and discipline can often be influenced as much by parental emotions as by parenting knowledge and skill (Gravener et al., 2012). When parental anger, depression (Herd et al., 2014; Sturge-Apple et al., 2012; Wiggins et al., 2014), criticism, and restrictions go unchecked, physical and emotional abuse can occur.

---

### BOX 18-8 Warning Signs of Child Abuse

- Parental delay in seeking help
- Inconsistencies in the history of how the injury occurred
- Injury inconsistent with the history or the child's developmental capability
- Old, unexplained fractures evident on radiographs
- Bruises confined to back surface of the body—neck to knees
- Bare spots and broken hair
- Pattern of injury or bruising descriptive of object used to inflict injury (belt or belt buckle, hand, cigarette, hot water)
- Burns with sharply demarcated edges or circumferential patterns
- Perineal injuries of any kind

For more information about recognizing signs of child abuse, visit the Child Welfare Information Gateway at https://www.childwelfare.gov/pubs/usermanuals/childcare/.

## Child Abuse

Child abuse and maltreatment is not limited to a particular age or particular families (Dodge et al., 2014). However, it is more likely to occur with a major change or turmoil (CDC, 2014b, 2015c; Turner et al., 2012) in the family and when parental role models were abusive. Toddlerhood is a trying time for the most patient of parents, and nurses are alert to family changes and stresses as well as to warning signs of abuse (Box 18-8). Many injuries are difficult to differentiate from accidental injury and, at times, may even be confused with culturally appropriate healing practices (Box 18-9: Diversity Awareness). However, the toddler years have the greatest incidence of child maltreatment, with 27% of nonfatal cases reported for children aged 3 years or younger and 70% of deaths from child maltreatment occurring in children younger than 3 years (CDC, 2014b, 2015c). Nonfatal cases appearing in emergency departments, pediatrician offices, and day care centers may be the only opportunity for health care providers to prevent later death from continued child maltreatment.

Typically, parental responses to childhood injuries include a spontaneous reporting of the details of the illness or injury accompanied by concern, questions about progress and discharge, difficulty in leaving the child, and an attempt to identify with the child's feelings. These parents may also experience guilt for not protecting the child from the accident and may offer gifts to compensate for these feelings of guilt. In contrast, neglectful or abusive parents are often hesitant to provide information about the illness or injury; they may be evasive or even contradict themselves, irritated by the inconvenience of being asked questions. Abusive parents may not exhibit guilt feelings and often contend that the toddler was solely responsible for the injury.

Although these signs of potential abuse are certainly not present in all abusive parents, their presence alerts the nurse to assess and observe further. The nurse also remembers that some of these signs may be found in nonabusive parents, and that the presence of these signs serves only as a cue for further assessment. All nurses are required by law to report any and all suspected child abuse to the local child protective services agency.

---

### 🌐 BOX 18-9 DIVERSITY AWARENESS

#### *Evaluating a Child for Child Abuse With Cultural Sensitivity*

Nurses are required by law to report cases of suspected child abuse to Child Protective Services. The nurse who takes a careful health history may discover that what might appear to be characteristic burns or bruises associated with child abuse may instead be the product of a traditional culturally appropriate healing practice. The following are two examples of healing practices found in the Pacific Islander and Asian populations that might create such confusion.

#### Coining (*Cao Gio*)

Coining is a common healing practice used among Pacific Island and Asian families within the United States. Traditionally, coining is used for conditions associated with "wind" illnesses, as well as a wide variety of febrile illnesses. The lesions seen from coining are produced by rubbing a warm oil or balm on the skin and firmly abrading the skin with a coin or special instrument. The practice produces linear petechiae and ecchymosis on the chest and back that often resemble strap or belt marks. The appearance of the deep red-purple skin color is confirmation that the person had bad wind in the body.

#### Cupping (*Ventouse*)

Cupping involves the creation of a vacuum inside a special cup or glass by burning the oxygen out of it and then promptly placing it on a person's skin surface. Cupping draws blood and lymph to the body surface that is under the cup or glass, increasing local circulation. The purpose for doing this is to remove cold and damp "evils" from the body or to assist blood circulation, or both. The procedure is frequently used to treat lung congestion. The resulting circular ecchymotic marks are approximately 2 inches in diameter and resemble nonaccidental trauma.

---

## Sexuality-Reproductive Pattern

The toileting process, during which attention is focused on the genital area, may precipitate the toddler's curiosity about genital organs. The nurse includes this aspect when teaching about toilet training, giving parents time to consider their feelings and decide on their approach to genital exploratory behavior and masturbation. Some parents accept the child's curiosity, whereas others see this as an opportunity to introduce their own sexual values and taboos (Healthy Children, 2015).

The nurse encourages parents to approach this curiosity and exploration, as well as masturbation, as a normal developmental process. These behaviors provide toddlers with an opportunity to become better acquainted with their bodies. Many parents are uncertain about the vocabulary they should use and often create cute, unrelated words rather than provide the correct anatomical terms. The use of cute alternative words is often a reflection of parental discomfort or embarrassment. Using correct terms will help toddlers develop accurate knowledge about sexuality and communicate more effectively if inappropriate touching by others occurs. For example, a young boy was initially ignored by day care providers because he said an older boy ate his "pickle." After repeated episodes, the parents were contacted because the child seemed so upset (even though day care workers gave him a new pickle to eat). The parents shared that "pickle" was their name for penis.

## Coping–Stress Tolerance Pattern

Perceptions of events and reactions to them are filtered through children's developing cognitive, emotional, and social capacities. The relevance of life events and the child's vulnerability to their impact depend on the given developmental period (see the case study and care plan at the end of this chapter). A child's temperament, which is defined as an individual's style of emotional and behavioral response across situations, especially those involving change or stress, serves as a foundation for coping (Burns et al., 2013). Chess and Thomas (1986) originally described three common temperament patterns that they believe are innate: the easy child; the difficult child; and the slow-to-warm-up child. The easy child is cuddly, affectionate, and easy to manage. Children with a difficult temperament, however, are less adaptable, are more intense and active, and have more negative moods.

Although temperament has generally been accepted as inborn, it is influenced by environmental characteristics and exerts an influence on psychosocial adjustment by way of its effect on parent-child interactions. Nurses assist parents in recognizing their toddler's innate behavioral qualities as expressions of temperament and in developing management strategies. According to the goodness-of-fit interactive model of temperament, adults can accommodate their demands and expectations in ways that match the child's behaviors, including learning strategies to help toddlers adapt positively to social expectations.

Toddlers are developing new ways to cope with the myriad of new stresses that come with being a toddler. As is typical of their stage of development, coping is egocentric and reflective of their need for autonomy. Typical stressors include new siblings, babysitters, day care, toilet training, parental limit setting, and an endless string of tasks involving skills they have yet to develop.

Toddlers often imitate their parents' behavior, and this includes their methods of dealing with stress. They also regress, at times, to earlier infantile behavior when overwhelmed, until they regain some sense of mastery. Parents can help to anticipate and prepare toddlers for stressful experiences before they happen. However, they need to remember that toddlers' sense of time and ability to recall are limited. Preparations should be honest, simple, and focused on what the toddler will experience. Enough time should be allowed for the toddler to rehearse the coping behavior with the parent, but not so early before the event that the toddler forgets.

The nurse helps the parents anticipate developmental stressors and suggests age- and temperament-appropriate coping behaviors for toddlers. Early efforts at dealing with stress are an essential step to more mature coping responses as the child grows (Shonkoff & Garner, 2012).

## Values-Beliefs Pattern

Healthy behaviors are expressions of positive values and beliefs. These values and beliefs are learned, and their recognition and acceptance are fundamental to the integrity of every child. Toddlers believe rules are absolute and behave, according to Kohlberg, out of a fear of punishment. However, toddlers' environments should not only help them become aware of right and wrong but also contribute to their sense of security, belonging, and autonomy. Development of moral integrity is enhanced if toddlers believe they are valued (Arthur et al., 2012).

Because most of toddlers' developing values and beliefs depend on their interactions with parents, the nurse's assessment questions are often directed to or focused on the parent or caregiver. The following are some examples of questions asked by the nurse:
- What are the family's values and beliefs about what is right and wrong?
- How does the parental approach to limit-setting reflect these values and beliefs?
- What religious, spiritual, or cultural traditions and activities do the family have?
- How is the toddler included in these traditions and activities?

Children are exposed to and begin to participate in and imitate their family's religious rituals and practices during toddlerhood. They are often taught prayers and songs with a religious theme that are tied into what the family believes are right and wrong. Toddlers may be able to learn the words to these simple prayers and songs, but parents should be cautioned that knowing the words does not mean that toddlers understand the full meaning of what is said. This early introduction into the family's religious beliefs is important as a socialization factor but should not be assumed to produce a good child.

The creation of values and beliefs in young children is related to their developmental stage and is reflected in their behaviors. An important aspect of teaching young children what is right and wrong involves stating what acceptable behavior is and then reinforcing the behavior when it occurs. Parents often attend to toddlers only when they are misbehaving, leaving them alone when they are being good. In this scenario, toddlers receive no attention for acceptable behavior but gain their parents' attention when they misbehave. The nurse can remind parents to catch their toddlers being good and give them the same or more attention.

# ENVIRONMENTAL PROCESSES

## Physical Agents

### Accidents

*"If a disease were killing our young children in the proportions that injuries are, people would be outraged and demand that this killer be stopped."*

**C. Everett Koop, MD, Former Surgeon General**

Toddlers are at high risk of accidental injury because they lack judgment and experience and have only rudimentary problem-solving skills, limited physical coordination, and a heightened level of curiosity about their environment. There are also behavioral and environmental factors that increase toddlers' risk of injury, such as being in new situations (Kuhn & Damashek, 2015). Most parents think that it is natural for children to get hurt and that childhood injuries are just a part of growing up. However, most injuries are predictable and preventable and can cause disabilities requiring long-term care. Furthermore, they can cause more deaths than all childhood diseases combined.

One in every 10 toddlers who come to the emergency department is treated for accidental injury. Male toddlers tend to have more injuries than their female counterparts, but the overall numbers of accidental injuries peak during toddlerhood for both male and females. A second peak occurs for males during adolescence. Major causes of accidental injury in toddlers involve structural hazards, sports, drowning, burns, motor vehicles, and poisoning.

Recent research indicates that although overall injury rates for young children have decreased in the past 20 years, injury mortality rates remain higher in black American and American Indian/Alaskan Native children. The young children in these groups had higher injury and death risk for residential fires, suffocation, and poisoning. These findings suggest new strategies and approaches are needed to narrow the disparities that continue to exist.

### Structural Hazards

Houses and other buildings can be hazardous for toddlers. Their desire to explore lures them to locations that older children or adults would not consider. The toddler will climb onto furniture or fixtures, out of windows, or into small spaces. Injuries that result from these explorations can range from minor scrapes and bruises to fatal head injuries. Ideally, homes are "baby-proofed" before the infant begins scooting and crawling and toddler-proofed before the toddler becomes increasingly mobile. Parents should reassess the safety of their home as their child acquires new skills. Injuries to toddlers occur most often when they fall from furniture, high chairs, changing tables, stairs, windows, and playground equipment. When the child or family visits the home of a friend or relative, it must be inspected for hazards, or the toddler must be confined to one safe room. Many injuries occur in unfamiliar environments.

Preventive measures for structural hazards include the following:
- Do not leave a toddler unattended.
- Use gates at the top and bottom of stairways, and at doors.
- Keep chairs away from countertops and tables to prevent toddlers from climbing.
- Securely anchor large television screens and other electronic equipment that can fall onto toddlers.
- Lock doors to dangerous areas and use gates and window guards.
- Store guns in a locked, safe area out of reach.

### Toys

Toys commonly found in homes are another source of injury. Parents should inspect not only the toys that are in their own homes but also the toys given to the toddler outside the home by relatives, friends, babysitters, or day care personnel (see the case study and care plan at the end of this chapter). Many toys that are likely to be safe for older children are extremely hazardous for the toddler. Of concern are small, removable parts, magnets and batteries, toxic paint or stuffing, sharp edges, and flammable material.

### Sports

Although sporting and recreational equipment is recognized as a major source of accidents in older children and adolescents, parents and health care personnel occasionally forget that such equipment can also be dangerous to toddlers. Improper storage of this equipment is a primary danger. Firearms that are left loaded and unlocked are deadly hazards, and bodybuilding weights and other heavy equipment easily overwhelm toddlers, who may pull these objects down on themselves. Toddlers should always be supervised closely, especially in new environments or on playground equipment.

As toddlers become more mobile, they are introduced to riding toys, tricycles, and bicycles. Nurses remind parents about the need for, and in most states the requirement of, bicycle helmets that are fitted properly and worn every time the toddler rides or is a passenger on a bicycle.

### Drowning

Children between the ages of 1 and 3 years are at the highest risk of drowning because most do not know how to swim and do not have the skills to keep their heads above water or to get out of the water. Toddlers can drown in water just deep enough to cover their noses and mouths. Although swimming pools and other natural bodies of water are a big part of the problem, even pails of water, toilets, bathtubs, and wading pools are dangerous. When toddlers fall into a pail of water or a toilet, it is hard for them to straighten up because all their weight is forward. Toddlers should never be left unattended—even for a few seconds—near a bathtub, hot tub, wading or swimming pool, toilet, pail of water, or small creek. All swimming pools should be fenced and have self-closing gates and latches. Toddlers must be supervised constantly and competently whenever they are near any body of water regardless of its size and should be fitted properly with personal flotation devices whenever they are on a boat.

### Burns

Each year 28.1% of US children from birth to 5 years of age require emergency department treatment (US Department of Health and Human Services, 2012). Hot tap water, boiling water, coffee, tea, and food are the most common sources of injury resulting in scalds from hot liquids. These very painful and often debilitating injuries often occur as toddlers begin to gain mobility and explore their environments, inadvertently touching hot surfaces or spilling hot liquids on themselves. They may also put their mouths on live electrical cords or their fingers into electrical sockets and become seriously burned, as well as tip their walkers or themselves into fireplaces or woodstoves.

The nurses' role is to educate parents regarding the following:
- Never eat, drink, or carry anything hot while holding a child.
- Lower the water heater temperature to between 120°F and 125°F.
- Never leave hot beverages or foods within a child's reach.
- Put children in a playpen while cooking.
- Never leave a toddler unattended in the bathtub. It takes only a moment to turn on the hot water.
- Put screens around fireplaces or woodstoves.

- Do not let children handle food directly from the microwave oven.
- Use burners at the back of the stove and turn pot handles in toward the stove.
- Install and maintain smoke detectors, replacing batteries annually.

### Motor Vehicles

Motor vehicle–related injuries, which include both passenger and pedestrian injuries, are the primary injury in children from 1 to 4 years of age. For the toddler, passenger injury is more frequent and often involves the lack of use or misuse of child safety seats. Child safety seats, when properly installed and used, have reduced the risk of death and serious injury to children. Unfortunately, improper installation and use of child safety seats are widespread problems, with some experts reporting that more than 72% of them are misused in some way (CDC, 2015b). Certified child passenger safety technicians are trained in installing car safety seats properly and can help parents make sure their children are as safe as possible on the road. To find the closest inspection station, the nurse can visit or direct parents to visit http://www.seatcheck.org or call toll-free 866-SEAT-CHECK (866-732-8243).

The rear-facing child safety seat supports a young child's head, neck, and spine, helping to reduce stress to the neck and spinal cord in a crash. When children reach 2 years and their child safety seat's upper weight or height limit, the nurse confirms with the parents that they can switch to forward-facing child safety seats. All children younger than 12 years should be seated in the rear seat. Rear seat position is safer than the front seat for all child safety seats, and a special warning has been issued that no child should be seated in the front passenger seat if the car has air bags (AAP, 2011b) (http://www.exchange.aaa.com/safety/child-safety/safety-seat-guide).

During the toddler years, it is safest to keep the child in a forward-facing rear seat with a harness until he or she reaches the seat's maximum height or weight (40–65 pounds). Children can use a booster seat when they have outgrown the weight or height limit of their forward-facing harnesses. Children at this stage are not yet ready for adult safety belts and should use belt-positioning booster seats until they are at least 4 feet 9 inches tall and between 8 and 12 years old. Safety belts are designed for 165-pound male adults, so it is no wonder that research shows poorly fitting adult belts can injure children. When a child can sit with his or her back straight against the vehicle seat back cushion and with knees bent over the seat edge without slouching, it is time to switch to an adult safety belt (AAP, 2011b) (http://www.exchange.aaa.com/safety/child-safety/safety-seat-guide). The nurse can provide a list of approved car seats and local retail outlets or agencies that sell, lend, or rent car seats.

Parents should be warned that toddlers may be injured or killed when they are hit by drivers backing up in their own driveways and often by members of their family or nearby neighbors. They are too small to be seen by a driver backing up and are quick to run out after a departing parent or relative who thinks they are still safely inside.

## Biological Agents

### Bioterrorism

Recent events have heightened concern about bioterrorism, and concerns about agents such as *Escherichia coli* (E. coli) are becoming more common questions for health care providers (AAP, 2013b). Other bioterrorism risks that are of concern for children include botulism, salmonellosis, and typhus. Children are especially at risk of these bacterial hazards because of their physiology. Compared with adults, they have a faster respiratory rate, increased skin permeability, higher skin to body mass ratio, and less body fluids (AAP, 2013b). Nurses provide information that can assist parents in dealing with their toddler's and their own fears. Nurses encourage parents to:

- Talk about their fears and worries.
- Stick to family diet routines that help toddlers maintain a varied and nutritious diet.
- Supervise toddlers' television viewing.
- Educate themselves, the best protection against unnecessary fear. Toddlers will be less fearful if they see that their parents are not afraid.

Many parents feel that toddlers, because of their immature immune systems and varied diet, are especially vulnerable to certain agents such as E. coli. Fearful parents might request antibiotics when they hear of an E. coli outbreak, just to be certain their child does not get sick, despite confirmation the child was never exposed to contaminated food. The nurse should reassure parents and explain that giving children antibiotics when they are not needed can do more harm than good. Many antibiotics, especially those identified for E. coli management, have serious side effects, and use of them when they are not needed can lead to the development of drug-resistant forms of bacteria. If this happens, the antibiotics will not be able to kill the resistant bacteria the next time the child needs the same antibiotic to treat common ear, sinus, or other infections.

The AAP website addresses numerous issues related to bioterrorism and children (http://www.aap.org), including the development of a teaching toolkit for parents to use with their children.

## Chemical Agents

### Poisoning

Poisoning happens 10 times more often among young children aged 1 to 4 years than in their older counterparts. Toddlers aged 1 to 2 years are at the greatest risk. They are becoming more mobile, enabling them to explore and discover poisonous substances in the home. These include prescription and over-the-counter medications, alcohol, household products, plants, cosmetics, lead-based paint, and cigarettes (Box 18-10: Quality and Safety Scenario). They are also at risk because they still use their mouths as a way of exploring. Although many parents take precautions against poisoning in their own homes, some forget that toddlers can be poisoned away from the home, while visiting grandparents or other relatives (e.g., see the case study and care plan at the end of this chapter).

The toddler, because of limited experience and cognitive level, is unaware that these items are harmful. Many emergency department

> ### BOX 18-10 QUALITY AND SAFETY SCENARIO
>
> #### Preventing Accidental Poisonings in the Home
>
> - All household, garden, and car products should be kept out of reach.
> - Keep medications out of reach in locked cabinets.
> - Use childproof caps on medication.
> - Keep all products and medication in their original containers for easy identification.
> - No poisonous plants should be kept in the house. A list, which includes poinsettia, amaryllis, aloe vera, English ivy, mistletoe, chrysanthemums, and spider plants, is available from local poison control centers.
> - Avoid outdoor plants and shrubs that are poisonous, including azaleas and chrysanthemums.
> - Supervise the toddler's activity at all times.
> - Post the National Capital Poison Center telephone number (1-800-222-1222) next to every telephone, including your cell phone.

calls and visits are precipitated by a toddler's ingestion of a potentially or actually harmful substance. These incidents are likely to occur in the kitchen, bathroom, bedroom, or work area, and are usually discovered by the parent or caretaker who finds an open or empty container or a half-eaten leaf or other substance.

When parents or caregivers suspect that a toddler has ingested a poisonous substance, they should call the poison control center, even if the child appears perfectly healthy. Each center is part of a nationwide effort to provide immediate information about poisonings. Parents should not attempt to induce vomiting without specific instructions from the center. Vomiting can cause further harm if the child is drowsy, unconscious, or convulsing; or if the substance ingested is corrosive, such as lye or a strong acid. When vomiting is recommended by the poison control center, instructions are often given to use ipecac syrup to stimulate the vomiting rapidly. This medication should be stored as carefully as any other medication or hazardous household product and replaced often because of its short shelf life.

Chronic poisonings, such as lead poisoning, are often undetected until irreversible damage has occurred. Primary prevention involves teaching parents about risk factors and dangers of lead poisoning and the importance of a diet that encourages decreasing fat intake, because lead is retained in fat. Vitamin C, calcium, and iron intake reduce lead levels in the body. Secondary prevention involves performing periodic screening of blood lead levels in all young children identified as at risk. Consumer protection laws in the United States require that all toys and furniture manufactured for small children be free of lead-based paint products. However, imported toys and furniture or antique and older family furniture or paint in older houses may have been painted with a lead-based product.

# DETERMINANTS OF HEALTH

## Social Factors and Environment

### Day Care

During the toddler years many parents return to work or decide that an experience in a group setting would be beneficial for their child. The nurse can provide counseling about the decision to place a child in day care and the resulting emotions, as well as guidelines for selecting a safe child care or day care provider (Dodge et al., 2014).

The US Department of Health and Human Services Administration for Children and Families recommends a four-step approach as a guideline for selecting a child care provider or day care center (see http://www.acf.hhs.gov/programs/occ/parents/index.htm) (see Chapter 17):

- Interview potential child care providers and observe the program or setting.
- Ask about cost; enrollment; ages served; daily activities; accreditation and licensing regulations; caretaker credentials and experience; and policies about visiting, illness, and nutrition.
- Look at provider-child interactions, safety, and the quality of the learning material and toys.
- Check references.
- Talk to parents with children in the center or being cared for by the provider about discipline and responsiveness to parents, and talk to local child care resource or referral agencies and licensing offices.
- Make a decision based on specific criteria.
- Think about safety, values, fit for you and your toddler, and affordability.
- Get and stay involved.
- Talk to the provider regularly about how your child is doing, to your child about what the children are doing each day, and to other parents.
- Visit often, announced and unannounced, and at various times of the day.

Many organizations have developed guidelines and checklists on choosing child care. Child Care Aware (http://www.childcareaware.org or 1-800-424-2246) is a national initiative designed to improve the quality of care and increase the availability of high-quality child care in local communities. Services include helping to find child care and connecting parents with local child care resource and referral agencies. Their brochure, *Give Your Child Something That Will Last a Lifetime—Quality Child Care*, outlines the steps to finding child care and includes an observation checklist.

Regardless of the reasons for the parents wanting or needing day care for their child, the traditional expectation of caring for the young child at home continues to influence the parents' concept of what they should do for their child. Parents must be reassured that a day care environment congruent with the family environment is not detrimental to the child. If a child has been placed in a setting that is detrimental to physical or emotional development, the parent may need assistance in selecting an alternative setting. Changes in caregivers are difficult for toddlers, and regressive behaviors may surface during transition periods.

### Culture and Ethnicity

Culture influences everything we do, know, and believe. Each culture possesses its own values, attitudes, and practices with regard to family and childrearing. Toddlers continue to be shaped by the cultural values and beliefs of their parents and families, the first of many socializing forces they will encounter. As their world expands, other forces and subcultures, including peers, the media, and their schools, will also be encountered.

Unlike older children, toddlers do not question the cultural practices of the family. The toddler who refuses to do certain expected things usually does so out of a need for autonomy and control rather than a questioning of beliefs. However, nurses remind parents of this, because parents may be feeling the pressure of cultural norms and expectations. This is especially true for families who have emigrated recently.

Nurses are prepared to provide culturally sensitive and competent care. Knowledge and respect for various cultural world views, customs, values, and traditions are needed to negotiate different approaches in developing a health-promotion plan with families. Health care practices are culturally influenced. For example, if a culture views immunizations as dangerous or unnecessary, the toddler may be unprotected from certain communicable diseases. Incorporation of knowledge, respect, and negotiation facilitates the development of a therapeutic relationship grounded in trust, as well as effective, high-quality health care outcomes (Burns et al., 2013).

## Levels of Policy Making and Health

A lack or paucity of economic resources is capable of affecting the toddler's health and well-being. According to the Children's Defense Fund (2015), in 2014, more than 15.5 million American children were poor, with the poorest being of color and younger than 6 years (http://www.childrensdefense.org/policy/endingpoverty/). Toddlers who live in poverty have higher mortality rates, poorer health, poorer growth, and more physical morbidity from respiratory tract infections, gastrointestinal tract infections, anemia, asthma, dental caries, otitis media, and visual loss, as well as higher rates of accidental injury and psychological and developmental disorders (Burns et al., 2013).

In 1997, the federal State Children's Health Insurance Program was developed to address this need. Because of this program, the number of uninsured children is at a historical low. Approximately 57% of all children in the United States are enrolled in Medicaid programs, and another 7.3 million are uninsured. Other services that are available to low-income families with toddlers include Temporary Assistance for Needy Families and the Special Supplemental Nutrition Program for Women, Infants, and Children. The nurse can play a critical role in mobilizing these resources for families. The Affordable Care Act has increased access to preventative care for toddlers with private insurance coverage. Private insurance companies are no longer allowed to deny coverage for a preexisting condition. (See more at http://www.childrensdefense.org/policy/health/#sthash.URCLwhGu.dpuf).

### Legislation

Local and state legislation specific to the toddler is directed primarily toward safety and injury prevention. Many states have passed laws requiring the use of child safety seats, bicycle helmets, and temperature limits for household hot water heaters.

Each state has passed laws that provide protection for a child or developmentally disabled adult, define abuse and neglect, require that a report be made to a designated agency in the case of actual or suspected abuse or neglect, and define the responsibility of the protecting agency. These laws also provide for a central registry of reported cases of abuse. Nurses are aware that they are required by law to report suspected child abuse, and should familiarize themselves with the child abuse and neglect laws in their states.

On the basis of current neuroscience and developmental research, as well as "data from a recent 50 state study of current health, child care, and family support policies," Knitzer (2008) proposes five care policy challenges: enacting a national family leave; expanding access to child and family programs such as Early Head Start; providing policy incentives and resources for high-quality infant and toddler child care; strengthening the early identification and treatment for infants and toddlers at risk of poor development; and building a policy framework to support, in every state, an infant and early childhood mental health infrastructure.

Another legislative issue for the toddler is the Education of the Handicapped Act amendment of 1986 (Public Law 99-457). This law creates programs that assist states in planning, developing, and implementing systems within states for handicapped children from birth to 3 years of age. Nurses who work with young children with disabilities need to investigate and familiarize themselves with the programs in their states.

## Health Services/Delivery System

The health of toddlers is significantly affected by the health care delivery system in the place where they live (Burns et al., 2013). Private physicians, nurse practitioners, and public well-child clinics are the most frequently used resources for ongoing health maintenance or illness care for toddlers. Health professionals specializing in pediatrics often coordinate their efforts to provide optimal health care for young children. For young children who do not receive routine health care, some public clinics sponsor special immunization days. Retired health care professionals donate their time at free dental clinics for children.

Each health care visit includes an interval history, assessment of growth and development, physical assessment, discussion of age-appropriate developmental concerns, and anticipatory guidance. Immunizations are given according to the current CDC (2015a) Recommended *Immunizations for Children From Birth Through 6 Years Old*. Both provider and parent schedules are easily found on the CDC website: http://www.cdc.gov/vaccines/schedules. The nurse informs parents that they can anticipate and keep track of their toddler's immunizations with the CDC Childhood Immunization Schedule. Recently, there has been controversy about a possible relationship between childhood immunizations and autism spectrum disorders. Some parents are choosing not to vaccinate their children as recommended by the CDC, which has resulted in multiple measles outbreaks in regions of the United States (Gostin, 2015). Despite what beliefs are held by certain groups of people, researchers have not found anything to indicate that vaccinations contribute to development of autism (Destefano et al., 2013; Larru & Offit, 2014).

Toddlers need to explore their environment to master it, and this is also valid for their health care encounters. They may need to observe and listen as their parents interact with the health care providers, be introduced to and allowed to manipulate examination equipment, and be given simple explanations and choices so that they can maintain some degree of control. Taking the time to enlist the cooperation of a toddler will make the health care visit more productive and conducive to information exchange and health care teaching.

## NURSING APPLICATION

Educating parents about health promotion and disease prevention in the toddler age group is similar to that for the infant. The nurse involved with the family provides education that is focused on the physical and developmental changes that are expected to occur in the toddler stage. This is the period of life from approximately 18 months to 3 years of age.

In addition to educating the parents, the nurse is able to begin to teach some health-promotion activities to the toddler. Examples of this type of toddler education are nutrition and oral hygiene. At this stage of development, it is crucial that caregivers model healthy behaviors and eating patterns. Parents may need education from the nurse on providing age-appropriate food choices while discouraging the intake of empty calories.

The nurse dealing with the toddler and the family can engage in screening activities. Assessments can be performed to evaluate the toddler for hearing loss and vision disturbances. Some conditions associated with vision or hearing can be treated if detected early.

As toddlers begin to explore their autonomy, they become at risk of accidental injury. Parents should be educated about objects on which the child may climb, possibly creating a crush or entrapment injury. They should also be aware of hazardous toys, sports equipment, drowning, burns, poisoning, and motor vehicle safety. In addition to this, medical personnel must remain alert to the potential for child abuse and report any suspicious injuries.

Another important element of health promotion with the toddler age group is educating the parents about routine health examinations and the childhood immunization schedule. Nurses need to remain informed about changes in immunization recommendations and educate families as the changes occur. Nurses working with families need to remain knowledgeable about the resources available in the community that may provide free or low-cost injections.

## CASE STUDY

### *Grandparents Provide Care: Dante*

Maria and Jose are the parents of 18-month-old Dante. They plan to take a week-long vacation while leaving Dante with his grandparents at their house. Because Dante is the first grandchild, the older couple is eager to spend time with him, but they have expressed concern about caring for a toddler.

**Reflective Questions**
- What do the parents need to discuss with the grandparents concerning safety issues?
- What psychosocial issues of a toddler are important for both the parents and the grandparents to consider?
- What resources are available for today's grandparents?

## CARE PLAN

### *Grandparents Provide Care: Dante*

**\*NURSING DIAGNOSIS: At risk of injury related to change in environment and change in primary caregiver(s)**

**Definition**
At risk of injury as a result of environmental conditions interacting with the individual's adaptive and defensive resources

**Related Factors**
- Heightened level of curiosity about environment
- Lack of more mature judgment and experience
- Limited height and physical coordination

**Risk Factors**
- Change in living environment to grandparents' home
- Grandparents home not "childproofed"
- Change in primary caregiver(s) from parents to grandparents
- Grandparents not up-to-date with caregiver/safety knowledge for toddlers

**Expected Outcomes**
- Grandparents will receive instruction regarding toddler care/safety.
- Grandparents will take necessary precautions to childproof their home.
- Grandparents will identify available resources to assist in toddler care/safety.
- Toddler will remain free of injury while in grandparents' care.

**Interventions**
- Surveillance: safety.
- Conduct a safety check in grandparents' home/community.
- Provide a safety checklist for grandparents.
- Assist grandparents in identifying resources/support.
- Contact community groups to emphasize community safety concerns.
- Risk identification.
- Identify potential risk factors in grandparents' home/community.
- Teaching: toddler care/safety.
- Teach grandparents about toddler care/safety issues.

## SUMMARY

This period can be an exciting and challenging time for both toddlers and their parents. Parents who have encouraged their toddlers' desire to explore can now delight in their developing sense of adventure as they enter their preschool years. The world is a wonderful place for the toddler who has known and experienced support, affection, and protection.

## ⓔ EVOLVE CHAPTER FEATURES

http://evolve.elsevier.com/Edelman/
• Study Questions

## REFERENCES

American Academy of Pediatrics (AAP). (2007). 2007 position statement: Principles and guidelines for early hearing detection and intervention programs. Joint Committee on Infant Hearing. *Pediatrics, 120,* 898–921.

American Academy of Pediatrics (AAP). (2011a). Ages & stages: Listen up about why newborn hearing screening is important. https://www.healthychildren.org/English/ages-stages/baby/Pages/Listen-Up-About-Why-Newborn-Hearing-Screening-is-Important.aspx.

American Academy of Pediatrics (AAP). (2011b). Policy statement—child passenger safety. *Pediatrics, 127*(4), 788–793.

American Academy of Pediatrics (AAP). (2012). Policy statement: Breastfeeding and the use of human milk. *Pediatrics, 129*(3), e827–e841.

American Academy of Pediatrics (AAP). (2013a). Policy statement: Children, adolescents, and the media. *Pediatrics, 132*(5), 958–961.

American Academy of Pediatrics (AAP). (2013b). Biological terrorism and agents. https://www.aap.org/en-us/advocacy-and-policy/aap-health-initiatives/Children-and-Disasters/Pages/Biological-Terrorism-and-Agents.aspx.

American Academy of Pediatrics (AAP) & Healthy Children. (2011). Feeding and nutrition: Your two-year-old. https://www.healthychildren.org/English/ages-stages/toddler/nutrition/Pages/Feeding-and-Nutrition-Your-Two-Year-Old.aspx.

American Academy of Pediatrics (AAP) & Healthy Children. (2012). Juice boxes. https://www.healthychildren.org/English/healthy-living/nutrition/Pages/Juice-Boxes.aspx.

American Academy of Pediatric (AAP) & Healthy Children. (2015). Where we stand: Fruit juice. https://www.healthychildren.org/English/healthy-living/nutrition/Pages/Where-We-Stand-Fruit-Juice.aspx.

American Association for Pediatric Ophthalmology and Strabismus. (2015). Amblyopia. http://www.aapos.org/terms/conditions/21.

American Optometric Association. (2015). Children's vision conditions. http://www.aoa.org/patients-and-public/good-vision-throughout-life/childrens-vision?sso=y.

Arthur, J., Powell, S., & Lin, H. (2012). Foundations of character: Methodological aspects of a study of character development in three- to six-year-old children with a focus on sharing behaviours. *European Early Childhood Education Research Journal, 22*(1), 105–122.

Berger, K. S. (2011). *The developing person through the life span* (6th ed.). New York: Worth.

Burns, C. E., et al. (2013). *Pediatric primary care* (5th ed.). Philadelphia: Saunders.

Centers for Disease Control and Prevention (CDC). (2010). Growth charts: CDC and WHO. http://www.cdc.gov/growthcharts.

Centers for Disease Control and Prevention (CDC). (2014a). CDC estimates 1 in 63 children has been identified with autism spectrum disorder. http://www.cdc.gov/media/releases/2014/p0327-autism-spectrum-disorder.html.

Centers for Disease Control and Prevention (CDC). (2014b). Child maltreatment—Facts at a glance. https://www.cdc.gov/violenceprevention/pdf/understanding-cm-factsheet.pdf.

Centers for Disease Control and Prevention (CDC). (2015a). Immunization schedules. http://www.cdc.gov/vaccines/schedules/index.html.

Centers for Disease Control and Prevention (CDC). (2015b). Child passenger safety: Get the facts. http://www.cdc.gov/motorvehiclesafety/child_passenger_safety/cps-factsheet.html.

Centers for Disease Control and Prevention (CDC). (2015c). Child maltreatment: Risk and protective factors.

Centers for Disease Control and Prevention (CDC). (2015d). Learning the signs, act early: Developmental milestones. http://www.cdc.gov/ncbddd/actearly/milestones/index.html.

Chess, S., & Thomas, A. (1986). The New York longitudinal study: From infancy to early adult life. In R. Plomin & J. Dunn (Eds.), *The study of temperament changes, continuities and challenges* (pp. 39–52). Hillsdale, NJ: Lawrence Erlbaum.

Children's Defense Fund. (2015). Children's health coverage in the United States. http://www.childrensdefense.org/policy/health/#sthash.URCLwhGu.dpuf.

Destefano, F., Price, C. S., & Weintraub, E. S. (2013). Increasing exposure to antibody-stimulating proteins and polysaccharides in vaccines is not associated with risk of autism. *The Journal of Pediatrics, 163*(2), 561–567.

Dodge, K. A., et al. (2014). Implementation and randomized controlled trial evaluation of universal postnatal nurse home visiting. *American Journal of Public Health, 104*(1), S136–S143.

Erikson, E. H. (1995). *Childhood & society* (35th anniversary ed.). New York, NY: Norton.

Erikson, E. H. (1998). *The life cycle completed.* New York, NY: Norton.

Gostin, L. O. (2015). Law, ethics, and public health in the vaccination debates. *JAMA: The Journal of the American Medical Association, 313*(11), 1099.

Gravener, J. A., et al. (2012). The relations among maternal depressive disorder, maternal expressed emotion, and toddler behavior problems and attachment. *Journal of Abnormal Child Psychology, 40*(5), 803–813.

Grummer-Strawn, L. M., Reinhold, C., & Krebs, N. F. (2010). Use of World Health Organization and CDC growth charts for children aged 0–59 months in the United States. *Morbidity and Mortality Weekly Report (MMWR), 59*(RR09), 1–15.

Guilleminault, C., et al. (2015). Missing teeth and pediatric sleep apnea. *International Journal of the Science and Practice of Sleep Medicine, 19*(73), 1–8.

Healthy Children. (2015). Common childhood habits. https://www.healthychildren.org/English/family-life/family-dynamics/communication-discipline/Pages/Common-Childhood-Habits.aspx.

Herd, M., et al. (2014). Efficacy of preventative parenting interventions for parents of preterm infants on later child behavior: A systematic review and meta-analysis. *Infant Mental Health Journal, 35*(6), 630–641.

Hockenberry, M. J., & Wilson, D. (Eds.). (2015). *Wong's nursing care of infants and children* (10th ed.). St. Louis, MO: Mosby.

Holt, K., et al. (2011). *Bright futures: Nutrition* (3rd ed.). Elk Grove Village, IL: American Academy of Pediatrics.

Knitzer, J. (2008). Giving infants and toddlers a head start: Getting policies in sync with knowledge. *Infants and Young Children, 21*(1), 18–29.

Kochanska, G., et al. (2013). Promoting toddlers' positive social-emotional outcomes in low-income families: A play-based experimental study. *Journal of Clinical Child & Adolescent Psychology, 42*(5), 700–712.

Kuhn, J., & Damashek, A. (2015). The role of proximal circumstances and child behaviour in toddlers' risk for minor unintentional injuries. *Injury Prevention, 21*(1), 30–34.

Larru, B., & Offit, P. (2014). Communicating vaccine science to the public. *Journal of Infection, 69*(Suppl. 1), S2–S4.

Miller, J. S., et al. (2011). The each child study: Systematic screening for autism spectrum disorders in a pediatric setting. *Pediatrics, 127*(5), 866–871.

National Eye Institute. (2013). Facts about amblyopia. https:// nei.nih.gov/health/amblyopia/amblyopia_guide.

Neuman, S. B., & Dickinson, D. K. (2011). *Handbook of early literacy research* (Vol. 3). New York, NY: Guilford Press.

Noritz, G. H., & Murphy, N. A. (2013). Motor delays: Early identification and evaluation. *Pediatrics, 131*(6), e2016–e2027.

Pempek, T. A., Krikorian, H. L., & Anderson, D. R. (2014). The effects of background television on the quantity and quality of child-directed speech by parents. *Journal of Children and Media, 8*(3), 211–222.

Perryman, T. Y., et al. (2013). Brief report: Parental child-directed speech as a predictor of receptive language in children with autism symptomatology. *Journal of Autism and Developmental Disorders, 43*(8), 1983–1987.

Ruel, M. T., & Alderman, H. (2013). Nutrition-sensitive interventions and programmes: How can they help to accelerate progress in improving maternal and child nutrition? *The Lancet, 383,* 536–551.

Seidel, H. M., et al. (2011). *Mosby's guide to physical examination* (7th ed.). St. Louis: Mosby.

Sheldrick, R. C., et al. (2013). The baby pediatric symptom checklist: Development and initial validation of a new social/emotional screening instrument for very young children. *Academic Pediatrics, 13*(1), 72–80.

Shonkoff, J. P., & Garner, A. S. (2012). The lifelong effects of early childhood adversity and toxic stress. *Pediatrics, 129*(1), e232–e246.

Spence, A. C., et al. (2013). A health promotion intervention can affect diet quality in early childhood. *American Society for Nutrition, 143*(10), 1672–1678.

Sturge-Apple, M. L., Skibo, M. A., & Davies, P. T. (2012). Impact of parental conflict and emotional abuse on children and families. *Partner Abuse, 3*(3), 379–400.

Turner, H. A., et al. (2012). Family context, victimization, and child trauma symptoms: Variations in safe, stable, and nurturing relationships during early and middle childhood. *American Journal of Orthopsychiatry, 82*(2), 209–219.

US Department of Health and Human Services. (2012). Emergency department utilization. http://mchb.hrsa.gov/chusa12/hsfu/pages/edu.html.

Wiggins, J. L., et al. (2014). Developmental trajectories of irritability and bidirectional associations with maternal depression. *Journal of the American Academy of Child & Adolescent Psychiatry, 53*(11), 1191–1205.

Wulff, D., St. George, S., & Tomm, K. (2015). Societal discourses that help in family therapy: A modified situational analysis of the relationships between societal expectations and healing patterns in parent-child conflict. *Journal of Systemic Therapies, 34*(2), 31–44.

Zimmerman, F. J., & Bell, J. F. (2010). Associations of television content type and obesity in children. *American Journal of Public Health, 100*(2), 334–340.

# 19

# Preschool Child

*Susan Ann Denninger, Kristi Coker, and Kevin K. Chui*

## OBJECTIVES

*After completing this chapter, the reader will be able to:*

- Explain the physical and psychosocial changes occurring during the preschool years that influence child and family health needs.
- Discuss the concepts of cognitive development of preschoolers using Piaget's theory.
- Review the *Healthy People 2020* concepts that pertain to preschool children and their families.
- Describe family teaching and nursing support for the typical sleep disturbances of the preschool years.
- Differentiate the nursing roles regarding vision and hearing screening for preschoolers.
- Compare coping skills of preschoolers with those of younger children.
- Outline the primary prevention immunization requirements for preschoolers.
- Identify warning signs of cancer in preschoolers.
- Recognize signs, symptoms, and clinical features of and risk factors for asthma in preschoolers.
- Identify the major causes of injuries during the preschool years.

## KEY TERMS

Acute lymphocytic leukemia
Amblyopia
Ages & Stages Questionnaire
Asthma
Battelle Developmental Inventory
Centering
Chloroma
Deduction
Doll or puppet play
Early and Periodic Screening, Diagnosis, and Treatment
Eccrine sweat gland function
Egocentrism
Expressive language

Heterophoria
Heterotropia
Homeostasis
Induction
Induction explanation
Initiative
Irreversibility
Ishihara test
Lactose intolerance
Mnemonic techniques
Mutual storytelling
Myopic vision
Neuroblastoma
Nightmares

Night terrors
Otitis media
Parental divorce
Parents' Evaluation of Developmental Status
Preoperational stage
Quiet
Receptive language
Refractive errors
Retinoblastoma
Strabismus
Transductive reasoning
Vineland Social Maturity Scale
Wilms' tumor

 **THINK ABOUT IT**

### Aggressive Behavior

Phillip, age 4 years, started preschool 2 weeks ago after spending his early years at home with his mother and his 18-month-old sister. His mother recently returned to her job as an accountant, works 9 hours a day, and is fatigued when she picks up Phillip at 5:00 PM. Phillip's father travels for his job but is home on weekends to spend time with his family. Although Phillip's mother always believed that Phillip was shy because he was quiet, during the last week at child care he started hitting his peers and becoming loudly vocal at story time. His mother,

believing that Phillip's behavior is related to her return to work, feels embarrassed and frustrated by his behavior, especially because she enjoys her new job and the extra income.

- What factors might be contributing to Phillip's changed behavior?
- How might you define Phillip's temperament? Why?
- What discussions might you have with Phillip's parents to help them understand, respond to, and change their son's behavior for the better?

**BOX 19-1  HEALTHY PEOPLE 2020**

*Select National Health-Promotion and Disease-Prevention Objectives for Preschool Children*

- Increase the proportion of children and youth with disabilities who spend at least 80% of their time in regular education programs.
- (Developmental) Increase the proportion of preschool Early Head Start and Head Start programs that provide health education to prevent health problems in the following areas: unintentional injury; violence; tobacco use and addiction; alcohol and drug use; unhealthy dietary patterns; and inadequate physical activity, dental health, and safety.
- Reduce blood lead levels in children.
- Reduce exposure to selected environmental chemicals in the population, as measured by blood and urine concentrations of the substances or their metabolites.
- (Developmental) Increase the proportion of children who are ready for school in all five domains of healthy development: physical development, social-emotional development, approaches to learning, language, and cognitive development.
- Increase the proportion of parents who use positive parenting and communicate with their physicians or other health care professionals about positive parenting.
- (Developmental) Decrease the proportion of children who have poor quality of sleep.
- Reduce infections caused by key pathogens transmitted commonly through food (postdiarrheal hemolytic-uremic syndrome in children younger than 5 years).

- Achieve and maintain effective vaccination coverage levels for universally recommended vaccines among young children.
- Reduce fatal and nonfatal injuries.
- Reduce child maltreatment deaths.
- Increase the proportion of children with special health care needs who receive their care in family-centered, comprehensive, coordinated systems.
- Increase the number of states with nutrition standards for foods and beverages provided to preschool children in child care.
- (Developmental) Prevent inappropriate weight gain in youths and adults (children aged 2–5 years).
- Reduce iron deficiency among young children and females of childbearing age (children aged 1–2 years).
- Reduce the proportion of young children aged 3 to 5 years with experience of dental caries in their primary teeth.
- Increase the proportion of children and adolescents aged 2 years through 12th grade who view television, watch videos, or play video games for no more than 2 hours a day (children aged 2–5 years).
- Reduce asthma deaths (children and adults younger than 35 years).
- Reduce the proportion of nonsmokers exposed to secondhand smoke (children aged 3–11 years).
- Increase the proportion of preschool children aged 5 years or younger who receive vision screening.

From US Department of Health and Human Services. (2011). 2020 topics and objectives. http://www.healthypeople.gov/2020/topicsobjectives2020/default.aspx.

The preschool child (age 3–6 years) has a more developed body structure, an ability to control and use the body, and a facility with language that more closely resembles that of the adult than that of the toddler. The major psychological thrust of this period of development is mastery of self as an independent human being, with a willingness to extend experiences beyond those of the family. Although historically the end of early childhood in the Western world was marked by entrance into the formalized educational system, increasing numbers of children in the United States begin formalized schooling during their preschool years. Box 19-1: *Healthy People 2020* presents objectives related to this developmental stage (US Department of Health and Human Services, 2011).

## BIOLOGY AND GENETICS

The protuberant abdomen of the toddler disappears during the preschool years as the pelvis begins to straighten and the abdominal muscles develop. The hips gradually rotate inward, replacing out-toeing with straight or slight in-toeing. Mild in-toeing (metatarsus adductus) may remain during the preschool years, but anything beyond a mild level should be investigated and treated.

Growth rates remain steady from age 3 to 6 years. Average preschoolers gain approximately 2 kg (4 pounds) of body weight and 7 cm (2 inches) of height each year, whereas head circumference increases by less than 2 cm during the entire preschool period. During early childhood, skin matures in its ability to protect the child from outer invasion and loss of fluids. The

skin's capacity to localize infection increases but remains less than that of a mature person. Negligible secretion of sebum makes the skin fairly dry. **Eccrine sweat gland function,** part of the body's heat-regulation mechanism, gradually matures, but the quantity of eccrine sweat produced in response to heat or emotion remains minimal. Apocrine sweat glands, located primarily in the axillae, areolas of the breast, and the anal area, remain nonsecretory during this period.

The kidneys reach full functional maturity by the end of infancy and early toddlerhood, with only their size changing during the preschool years. By the end of the preschool years, urine excretion ranges from 650 to 1000 mL (19–30 ounces). Under normal homeostatic conditions, the preschooler's renal system conserves water and concentrates urine on a level that approximates adult abilities. Under conditions of stress, however, the kidneys lack the ability to respond fully and to maintain **homeostasis** when compared with the more rapid response of the adult renal system.

Growth of gastrointestinal organs continues through the preschool years without functional changes. Children achieve full voluntary control of elimination. **Lactose intolerance,** intolerance to milk products manifested by diarrhea, often appears during the preschool years. This condition, more common in black, Asian American, and Native American children, can be managed successfully by elimination of lactose from the diet.

Lung capacity continues to increase, with a gradual decrease in respiratory rate. Preschoolers make better decisions than toddlers about objects they place in their mouths, resulting in fewer instances of choking and obstruction. A gradual increase in the size and shape of the ears coincides with decreases in the incidence of otitis media (middle ear infection). Tonsils and adenoids are large compared with their throat, which may contribute to noisy breathing and upper respiratory tract infection in preschoolers.

The cardiovascular system enlarges in proportion to general body growth. Heart rate for preschoolers ranges from 40 to 70 beats per minute, with a mean blood pressure of 100/60 mmHg. Early hypertension develops in some children during the preschool years; therefore routine measurement of blood pressure is indicated, particularly in children with a strong family history of hypertension (see Chapter 20). Preschool children maintain adequate hemoglobin levels when dietary intake is sufficient. Bone marrow of the ribs, the sternum, and the vertebrae become fully established as primary sites for red blood cell formation. The liver and spleen continue to form erythrocytes and granulocytes.

The immune system continues to develop. Preschoolers boost their immune response to common pathogens as exposure occurs. Group activities, such as joining preschool or play groups, increase exposure and subsequently escalate the incidence of common contagious illnesses during the time of exposure, regardless of the child's age. Initial encounters with such group activities usually result in increases in illness. Later these children may be less prone to common contagious diseases because of their early exposure to infectious illnesses and their consequent immunity.

Primary teeth finish erupting by late toddler or early preschool years. Initial permanent teeth generally erupt toward the end of the preschool period. Permanent teeth tend to erupt approximately 6 months earlier in girls than in boys. Older preschoolers usually take responsibility for dental hygiene, although all children need gentle guidance about proper brushing and appropriate nutritional intake for healthy teeth. Parents should continue to assist with brushing and supervise flossing and fluoride intake. Risk of fluorosis exists in children younger than 8 years and is influenced by both the dose and the frequency of exposure to fluoride during tooth development (Wright et al., 2014). Balancing this risk of opacity against the prevention of caries involves assessment of the amounts of fluoride the child receives from various sources. Fluoride sources include public water supply in some regions, foods, drinks, fluoride supplements, and accidentally swallowed toothpaste (Clifton, 2014). Because the preschool period is an age of caries formation, regular dental checkups are essential. The American Academy of Pediatrics recommends use of a smear (the size of a grain of rice) of toothpaste up to age 3 years. After the third birthday, a pea-sized amount may be used. Fluoride varnish is recommended in the primary care setting every 3 to 6 months starting at tooth emergence. Over-the-counter fluoride rinse is not recommended for children younger than 6 years because of the risk of their swallowing higher-than-recommended levels of fluoride (Clark & Slayton, 2014). Nurses assess whether the child is receiving preventive dental care. Parents should be encouraged to begin or maintain this care. Suggestions for promoting good oral hygiene as part of general health-promotion teaching can be found in Chapter 20.

Musculoskeletal and neurological development reaches a level that allows seemingly effortless walking, running, and climbing.

Older preschoolers' ability to copy figures and draw recognizable pictures indicates their advancing fine motor abilities, and they are eager to demonstrate these skills to others. Practice, increases in muscle size, continuing associations among existing neural pathways, and the establishment of new pathways for already accomplished tasks are a few of the many complex factors that contribute to the advances in neurological function observed during early childhood. These advances in fine motor, gross motor, cognitive, communicative, and social-emotional skills are outlined in Table 19-1.

## Gender

Boys tend to experience more childhood illnesses than do girls from 3 to 6 years of age (see Chapter 18). Preschoolers are more aware of their sexual identity than are toddlers and may imitate societal stereotypes more closely. Traditionally boys have been encouraged to take more risks than girls have been and they have more accidents than do preschool girls, who may have been encouraged to choose more sedentary activities. For example, in their study of 476 preschool children (50% male), Brown and colleagues (2009) found that 3-year-old boys were more active than 3-year-old girls. In today's society, boys and girls have more opportunities to choose the same activities, but preschool activities can also be geared to be gender neutral to encourage more female participation. Gender-neutral activities such as tag, hide and seek, kick ball, duck duck goose, red rover, and obstacle courses may encourage physical activity for both boys and girls. It will be interesting to observe whether societal changes or preschool policy changes will reflect accident or obesity statistics in the future.

## Race

Race, with its related economic and cultural issues, can influence health care practices at this age, as is the case at all ages. Cultural preferences and economic issues therefore influence the environments and other health-promoting behaviors, such as nutrition and recreation (Brown et al., 2009; Division of Adolescent and School Health, National Center for Chronic Disease Prevention and Health Promotion, 2011; Dogra et al., 2010; Lee & Im, 2010).

## Genetics

The signs and symptoms of most genetic problems appear during infancy or the toddler years, whereas other genetic problems will be noted during adolescence. Those most likely to appear during the preschool years are cystic fibrosis, Duchenne muscular dystrophy, fragile X syndrome, Williams syndrome, and autism, which is generally considered a genetic disorder with a high degree (90%) of heritability (Freitag et al., 2010). These disorders, characterized by aberrant social interaction, communication, and stereotyped patterns of behavior, affect 0.5% to 1.0% of the population and are often diagnosed or suspected in the preschool years, when social interaction plays a larger role in development (Boyd et al., 2010; Freitag et al., 2010).

Genetic conditions (Box 19-2: Genomics) diagnosed early in life affect the child's health, and nursing strategies focus on continuing parent education, assessing the child's development (including complications), and providing interventions to support family coping (Boyd et al., 2010).

**TABLE 19-1**    **GROWTH AND DEVELOPMENT**

*Developmental and Behavioral Milestones for Preschool Children*

| Age (yr) | Expectations |
|---|---|
| 3 | At this age, the typical child:<br>• Builds a tower of six to eight cubes<br>• Throws ball overhand, rides tricycle, walks up stairs alternating feet<br>• Has self-care skills (self-feeding, self-dressing)<br>• Knows own name, age, and sex<br>• May comprehend cold, tired, hungry; may understand the prepositions over and under; differentiates bigger and smaller; can convey the use of scissors, key, and pencil<br>• Copies a circle, draws a person with two body parts (head and one other part)<br>• Engages in imaginative play that becomes more elaborate with specific themes or story lines demonstrated; enjoys interactive play<br>• Speech is understandable 75% of the time; names a friend; carries a conversation with two or three sentences spoken together<br>• Is toilet trained during the daytime for both bowel and bladder |
| 4 | At this age, the typical child:<br>• Alternates feet when descending stairs; jumps forward; hops on one foot, and can stand on 1 foot for up to 5 sec<br>• Using overhand toss can hit target from 5 feet<br>• Builds a tower of eight blocks<br>• Copies a cross<br>• Holds and uses a pencil with good control<br>• Cuts paper into two pieces<br>• Pours, cuts, and mashes own food<br>• Brushes own teeth<br>• Dresses self, including buttons<br>• Gives first and last name<br>• Engages in conversational give-and-take<br>• Knows what to do if cold, tired, or hungry<br>• Sings a song or says a poem from memory<br>• Talks about daily experiences and things that are used at home (food, appliances)<br>• Can name three or four primary colors<br>• Is aware of sex (of self and others)<br>• Plays board/card games<br>• Draws a person with three parts<br>• Tells you what he/she thinks is going to happen next in a book<br>• Describes features of himself, including sex, age, interests, and strengths<br>• Engages in fantasy play |
| 5 | At this age, the typical child:<br>• May be able to skip; can walk on tiptoes; makes broad jumps<br>• Folds paper parallel; colors between vertical lines<br>• Ties a knot, has mature pencil grasp<br>• Names four or five colors and can identify coins<br>• Tells a simple story and knows several nursery rhymes<br>• Dresses and undresses without supervision<br>• Prints some letters and numbers, is able to copy square and triangle from an illustration<br>• Draws a person with at least six body parts<br>• Begins to understand right and wrong, fair and unfair<br>• Engages in dramatic make-believe and dress-up play during which the child assumes a specific role; engages in domestic role-playing and dressing up<br>• Enjoys the companionship of other children; plays cooperatively<br>• Has good articulation, uses appropriate tenses and pronouns<br>• Can count to 10 |
| 6 | At this age, the typical child:<br>• Bounces a ball four to six times; throws and catches<br>• Skates<br>• Rides a bicycle<br>• Ties shoelaces<br>• Counts up to 10; prints own first name; prints numbers up to 10<br>• Understands right from left<br>• Draws a person with six body parts, with the figure depicted a person wearing clothing |

Modified from American Academy of Pediatrics. (n.d.). Bright Futures. http://brightfutures.aap.org/.

---

**BOX 19-2** **GENOMICS**

The field of cystic fibrosis (CF) has benefited from developments and advancements in genomics in terms of detection, understanding, and monitoring of the disease state. Infants with CF are structurally normal at birth; however, they have an inability to control bacterial infection, which plays a key role in early CF lung disease pathogenesis. Research and application of novel molecular techniques to explore the human microbiome has helped develop an understanding of CF airway microbiology and how it differs from that of those without the disease. The drug ivacaftor was approved by the Food and Drug Administration in 2012 for the treatment of CF patients carrying at least one copy of the G551D mutation in the cystic fibrosis transmembrane conductance regulator gene (*CFTR*). CF is caused by one of several defects in cystic fibrosis transmembrane conductance regulator, which regulates fluid flow within cells and affects the components of sweat, digestive fluids, and mucus. The G551D mutation, in particular, is characterized by a dysfunctional cystic fibrosis transmembrane conductance regulator that cannot transport chloride through the ion channel. Ivacaftor increases the transport of chloride through the ion channel by binding, and thus for the first time is able to treat the underlying cause of CF instead of its symptoms.

From Milla, C. E. (2013). Cystic fibrosis in the era of genomic medicine. *Current Opinion in Pediatrics, 25*(3), 323–328.

## GORDON'S FUNCTIONAL HEALTH PATTERNS

### Health Perception–Health Management Pattern

Preschoolers have a fairly accurate perception of the external parts of their own bodies based on what they can see and do; they may be extremely curious about the body of a member of the opposite sex. Their concepts of what is inside the body and how its internal functions operate are vague and inaccurate. Preschoolers view the internal part of the body as hollow. Most preschoolers can name one or two items inside the body (blood, bones). Many of their questions involve body functions. Anxiety surrounding the body and fear of mutilation and death pervade the children's concerns. Their size as compared with that of adults produces a sense of vulnerability and fear of loss of control (Price & Gwinn, 2008).

By age 4 or 5 years, children have amassed their beliefs about health from the family. They begin to understand that they play a role in their own health. The preschooler often becomes upset over minor injuries. Pain or illness may be viewed as a punishment. The preschooler's declaration "If you don't put your seat belt on you will get in an accident" is a statement that reflects the idea of expected immediate and absolute cause and effect. The preschooler cannot conceive that the purpose of the seat belt is to prevent injury in the event of an accident, not prevention of the accident itself.

Although preschoolers are not completely responsible for their own health management, they certainly contribute by brushing their teeth, taking medication, wearing appropriate clothing for inclement weather, and performing other actions. Preschoolers' memory of these activities can be sporadic, but they are at least beginning to be their own health care agents (Yoo et al., 2010).

Reinforcement of health-promotion activities, which occurs in the home and child care environments, helps to instill behaviors that affect self-esteem, safety, and an individual's overall balance with life. For example, family support for active lifestyles provides one way for parents to assume a positive role to model for children (Division of Adolescent and School Health, National Center for Chronic Disease Prevention and Health Promotion, 2011). The National Association of Pediatric Nurse Practitioners has designed Healthy Eating and Activity Together resources to engage families in health-promoting behaviors (Gance-Cleveland et al., 2009).

In addition, the preschool environment influences health-promotion activities for many children in this age group. For example, when Brown and colleagues (2009) directly observed children in 20 preschool settings, they demonstrated that aspects of the preschool environment affected children's activity levels. Preschool settings with more resources also offered a greater variety of activities. Even these preschools with more resources were well below the physical activity time recommended (120 minutes per day) by the National Association for Sport and Physical Education (2009). Their findings provide further support for those of Bower and colleagues (2008), who demonstrated that in preschool settings, children participated in physical activity for approximately 80 minutes more in settings with more resources than children in settings with fewer resources. These findings indicate a need for health-promotion advocacy and policy development focused on the environment. Many community bookstores carry health-promotion–focused books appropriate to the preschool population; these references provide information for discussion among parents, caregivers, and children on the importance of healthy behaviors for success in life.

### Nutritional-Metabolic Pattern

Establishing healthful nutritional and physical activity behaviors begins during childhood. Children should eat a variety of foods, with at least five servings of fruits and vegetables per day. Children aged 3 to 5 years old should receive 1200 to 1600 calories per day depending on their activity level and sex (US Department of Agriculture & US Department of Health and Human Services, 2010). Preschool children should consume approximately half of their diet in carbohydrates, with the other half consisting of protein ($\approx$5–20%) and fat ($\approx$20–35%) (US Department of Agriculture & US Department of Health and Human Services, 2010). With more than half of the preschool diet consisting of carbohydrates, whole grains and other complex carbohydrates should be plentiful to attain a total fiber intake of 20 to 25 g per day (US Department of Agriculture & US Department of Health and Human Services, 2010). Fat requirements in preschool children are higher than those for older children, but fat consumption should consist primarily of unsaturated fat, with saturated fat, trans fatty acids, and cholesterol intake as low as possible. Guidance for these recommendations along with the types and amounts of foods is depicted in the system called MyPlate (http://www.choosemyplate.gov/). A child-friendly version of MyPlate addresses the special needs of children 6 to 11 years old (Nappo-Dattoma, 2011). Preschoolers need approximately 90 kcal/kg of body weight per day for health maintenance, activity, and growth. MyPlate is used as a guideline for preschool nutrient consumption (Hockenberry & Wilson,

2015). However, because of the unique dietary patterns of preschoolers, the food intake is variable.

Specific issues that impact the preschool age include bone growth, iron-deficiency anemia, milk intake, salt intake, sugar intake, and dentition. For bone growth, children aged 1 to 8 years require a calcium intake of approximately 700 to 1000 mg. Although the frequency of iron-deficiency anemia is decreasing generally, it is more prevalent in vulnerable populations (McCann & Ames, 2007). The studies that have been conducted, although small in number, support the idea that iron deficiency results in behavioral and cognitive deficits (McCann & Ames, 2007). Salt and sugar intake should be moderate. The contribution of sugar intake to caries development is well established. For example, Warren and colleagues (2009) examined factors associated with carcinogenicity in 128 children. Their study suggests that sweetened beverages, in particular, are associated with the development of caries.

Nutrition and dentition impact health at all ages. Pain from dental caries, infection, and poorly maintained teeth affects appetite and chewing ability, with a subsequent impact on future nutritional status. The frequency of dental caries in children has declined dramatically in recent years because of preventive measures, such as use of fluoride toothpaste, fluoridation of community water supplies, implementation of sound dietary practices, and use of dental sealants. Children from low-income families carry the bulk of the burden of these dental caries (Nappo-Dattoma, 2011). Oral health promotion involves self-care and population-based initiatives, along with professional care. The adequacy of professional dental care differs significantly by age, race, educational level, family income, and dental status (Nappo-Dattoma, 2011). Nurses interface with families in a variety of these settings and are therefore in an ideal position to impact dental health promotion.

As early childhood progresses, intense food preferences emerge. This behavior is a natural outgrowth of the increased physical capacity to react to the taste and textures of foods and the realization that expressing an opinion about food is a way to control the environment. Older preschoolers frequently refuse to try new foods. The favorite foods for this age are meat, cereal grains, baked products, fruits, and sweets. Selecting finger foods that facilitate independence helps the preschooler learn to eat without assistance. Examples of appropriate nutritional foods include cheese, crackers, small pieces of meat, and celery stuffed with cheese or peanut butter. Parents' support for food choices has been demonstrated to be an effective strategy to promote healthy food choices in this age group (Marshall et al., 2011). Parents should provide nutritious foods, avoiding salty and sweet foods. Parents should encourage good nutritional habits to help establish healthy eating behaviors. Increased consumption of fats and processed foods along with diminished physical activity has contributed to a significant increase in the frequency of obesity and type 2 diabetes in children and adolescents (Liou et al., 2010; US Department of Agriculture & US Department of Health and Human Services, 2010; US Department of Health and Human Services, 2011). Family tolerance for individual food preferences differs, and children differ in their tendency to develop strong likes and dislikes. When families reach extreme differences over food preferences, major conflicts may arise, requiring insightful counseling to achieve a mutually satisfying solution. For example, some families may institute a "take a little taste before your refuse" standard for foods at the preschool age. Nurses collaborate with families to discover comfortable approaches to maintain nutritional adequacy of foods that children prefer. Community nurses use a variety of approaches and recognize the wide range of possibilities that exist for families of differing cultures.

Preschoolers begin to eat meals away from home more often than toddlers. Minimal standards require licensed child care centers and preschools to serve foods using recommended dietary allowances of basic nutrients. Parents should communicate regularly with agency personnel about foods eaten at home and away from home to provide healthy food variety. Preschoolers in group settings learn both positive and negative eating habits and food preferences from care providers and other children. School settings are ideal for community health nurses to impact the nutritional patterns of the preschool child (Water, 2011). Communication about nutritional intake habits reinforces positive behaviors and discourages negative habits at home (Box 19-3: Innovative Practice).

Preschoolers struggle with the intricacies of using utensils. In the later years of the preschool period, children attain skill

## BOX 19-3   INNOVATIVE PRACTICE
### Healthy Start

Risk factors for cardiovascular diseases are prevalent by 3 years of age, the most common of which are hypercholesterolemia and obesity. Healthy Start, a project located in Valhalla, New York, sponsored by the Child Health Foundation and the American Health Foundation, is a 3-year demonstration and research program to evaluate the effectiveness of interventions for reducing cardiovascular risk factors in preschool centers. Two interventions are recommended. The first is that the preschool food service be designed to reduce the total fat in the preschooler's meals and snacks to less than 30% of calories and to reduce saturated fat to less than 10% of calories. The second intervention is a comprehensive preschool health-education curriculum, which focuses on nutrition and exercise.

The effectiveness of this program is evaluated with use of many components. Changes in the nutritional behaviors (including dietary intake of school snacks and meals of the preschoolers) are being recorded, as are those with regard to snacks and meals consumed at home. Special attention is being given to the intake of total and saturated fat. Additionally, changes in the health knowledge of preschoolers are being assessed to evaluate the education component. Physical examination data include semiannual assessments of growth and body weight and blood lipid levels.

The specific details of the rationale and methods of the randomized controlled trial studies within the Healthy Start project are described at its website: http://www.healthy-start.com.

**Contact Information**
Healthy-Start LLC
Healthy-Start Preschool Education
PO Box 115
Huntington, NY 11743
Telephone: (631) 549-0010
Fax: (631) 824-9182
E-mail: info@healthy-start.com

with spoons, demonstrate fair proficiency with forks, and manage knives for spreading soft foods on bread or crackers. Most preschool children, however, need help cutting meat and pouring liquids from large, heavy containers. Preschoolers enjoy helping to prepare family meals and may be capable of simple tasks, such as washing fruits and vegetables. Involving young children in meal preparation teaches them about healthy nutrition. Sharing important family functions nurtures self-esteem and a sense of value.

The prevalence of food allergy in children in the United States continues to increase, affecting up to 8% of children. Approximately 1 million preschool children are affected, and one-third of these children have the potential for a severe reaction (Fleischer et al., 2012; Gupta et al., 2011). Most allergies develop before the age of 2 years. The foods most likely to cause allergic reactions in the preschool age group include milk, eggs, and peanuts (Fleischer et al., 2012; Gupta et al., 2011). Reactions to peanuts tend to decrease over time; however, children who experience peanut allergy should avoid allergens, and their parents should receive written emergency plans along with instructions for epinephrine injection (Fleischer et al., 2012). Clear food labeling and education are essential for prevention of allergic reactions. Many preschools have banned foods such as peanut products as a precautionary measure. Parents may need help identifying potential hazardous situations and communicating their child's needs to agency personnel. A food allergy action plan that includes a written emergency plan should be developed for parents to use to facilitate communication regarding the child's allergies. Educational resources are available at http://www.cofargroup.org/.

## Elimination Pattern

Toilet training is an important milestone in child development (Kaerts et al., 2012). Older preschool children are capable of and responsible for independent toileting. Their verbal skills have developed to better communicate their needs, they begin to insist on performing independently, and they are proud of their accomplishments (Kaerts et al., 2012). These developmental achievements provide additional signs for independence with elimination patterns. They may forget to flush the toilet or wash their hands when they are rushed, but they have the physical ability to perform the skills. Preschoolers should not be teased or punished when they are unable to perform independently. If their clothing becomes soiled, they should be responsible for changing their clothes and reminded gently and encouragingly of ways to avoid problems in the future. (Enuresis and encopresis are discussed in Chapter 20.)

## Activity-Exercise Pattern

Play continues to be the primary activity for preschoolers as well as for toddlers; however, preschoolers explore intently and demonstrate increased coordination and confidence with motor activities. They venture farther from home than toddlers. Many activities involve other children (Figure 19-1) and involve modeling behavior. Particularly in group care settings, children should be monitored for safe activities that enhance gross and fine motor skills while creating fun in movement.

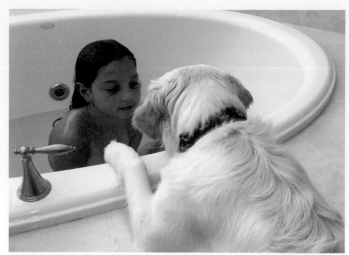

**FIGURE 19-1** Preschool children can enjoy their pet even at bath time.

Most 4-year-old children separate easily from their parents, play simple interactive games, dress themselves, copy a number of basic geometrical figures well, and draw recognizable people. Preschoolers enjoy using language skills to tell stories and ask questions. Their physical abilities include balancing on one foot, jumping, and running (Driscoll & Nagel, 2008). Generally, preschoolers appreciate an audience, enjoy practicing new skills, and demonstrate mastered skills to others. Play constitutes an important role in preschoolers' social and psychological development. Play offers a vehicle that allows them to explore while experimenting with who they are, who they might become, and how they relate to others socially. The drama of play allows preschoolers to view themselves from another perspective. Play often reveals the child's reality and complex perception of the world.

Children mimic the behavior of people familiar to them, expanding their representation beyond self and rehearsing what has been demonstrated to them as appropriate behavior (Driscoll & Nagel, 2008). Young children seldom assume the role of a younger child or infant while playing. They usually assume adult roles and use a doll for the younger child. Through play preschoolers learn to exert control over their own behavior. Assuming an adult role in play allows children to consciously adopt more mature behaviors. Patterns of behavior used in play can be transferred to actual situations. For example, children who express their anger in a play situation aggressively by vocalizing their distress, scolding the offending party, or using withdrawal of attention are likely to respond with aggression or tantrum behavior when facing frustration or anger in real-life situations. Observing children at play, as seen by the study group Brown and colleagues (2009) used in their research, reveals natural physical capacities of children better than observation in an examination or testing environment and provides further evidence of the child's social and inner development for use by practitioners in the field.

Observing symbolic play and imitation play in peer groups helps nurses assess social competency as their perceptions unfold (Driscoll & Nagel, 2008). At first the new child in a peer group may be expected to stand back and observe other children before manipulating a toy. Preschool children engage in more interactive play, particularly dramatic play, than at any other age. Two or more children may become involved in an imaginary plot, especially when toys and equipment support a particular scenario, such as toy kitchen equipment. Patterns emerge in the interactive processes of play: initiating, deciding with whom to play, play themes/roles/rules, and finally enactment or collaborative pretending. These patterns provide opportunities for support to facilitate play initiation and collaborative play (Driscoll & Nagel, 2008). Much of the preschooler's play involves fantasy. The young child frequently invents an imaginary companion who plays, eats, and sleeps with the child. The section entitled cognitive-perceptual pattern addresses more fully the aspects of fantasy during the preschool stage; however, the goal of symbolic or pretend play is to derive meaning from their play experience using their knowledge and skills acquired. The play is a way to integrate previously learned ideas and skills (Driscoll & Nagel, 2008).

Most preschoolers spend some time in a group setting each week. Ground rules at these facilities govern sharing, quiet times, and group activities. Although time orientation remains incompletely developed in preschoolers, they have an idea about past and future. They enjoy planning activities with their parents for the future. Visiting the library to review books about wild animals, packing lunches, and choosing what clothes to wear may preface a trip to the zoo.

The preschooler regulates body activities with more purpose and copes with limit setting better than the toddler, but has much energy and requires outlets for this energy during the day. The young child requires physical activity for energy expenditure. Physical activity, for the developing child, may be more appropriately described as either locomotor play or active play (Pellegrini & Smith, 1998). Active play increases from the toddler to the preschool period, and then declines by approximately 10% for each advancing year of age (Hinkley et al., 2012). Hinkley and colleagues (2012) concluded that efforts to promote children's physical activity should seek to influence children's preference for physical activity, parent rules, and sex-specific strategies. Becker and colleagues (2014) investigated whether active play during recess was associated with self-regulation and academic achievement in prekindergarten children. The results revealed that higher active play was associated with better self-regulation and higher scores on early reading and math assessments. Nurses should encourage parents to engage the preschool child in active, locomotor, and rough-and-tumble play. Parents and child care directors/school administrators should also encourage physical activity and work together to overcome perceived barriers that might limit the young child's ability to access physical activity (Gagne & Harnois, 2014).

Although this age group needs physical activity, many preschoolers spend long periods each day watching television, watching videos, and playing electronic games. Occasionally parents use the electronic diversions inappropriately to entertain the child. Although some excellent television, video, and electronic game programming is available for preschoolers, many electronic entertainment options focus on adult themes and violence. Many experts agree that television, videos, and electronic games disengage the child's mind and support less learning (Frost et al., 2008) (see Chapter 20). Parents should remember that preschoolers who rely on television, videos, and electronic games do not have enough life experiences to interpret many of the issues presented in adult shows (violence, interpersonal relationships, moral decisions); might be missing opportunities for interacting with other children or adults and other opportunities for active learning; and cannot judge which shows are appropriate for them. In addition, these electronic activities usually offer sedentary recreation, hindering the development of an active healthy lifestyle. Parents should choose which electronic devices and activities are appropriate for their child, limiting time and promoting physical activity in lieu of sedentary play. Furthermore, taking time to share activities provides the child with an opportunity for discussion and for the child to ask questions (Frost et al., 2008). Nurses should explain to parents and preschoolers the relationship between watching television/screen time and lack of physical activity that leads to health problems such as obesity (Frost et al., 2008). Family support for engaging in physical activity has been shown to affect children's health-promoting behaviors. In a study of 93 children and their parents, Marshall and colleagues (2011) demonstrated that parental influence shaped children's physical activity and nutritional health-promoting behaviors. The literature review by Kornides and colleagues (2011) also describes factors that influence overweight in Latino children. Their review of 24 studies revealed that parental body mass index (BMI) provided the strongest predictor of BMI in Latino children.

Gordon's health promotion–health maintenance, nutritional-metabolic, and activity-exercise patterns clearly overlap and should be considered together during the assessment phase so as to plan and intervene successfully (Marshall et al., 2011). Resources for these patterns may be used together to provide optimal health promotion. Physical activity in the preschool child is not typically structured exercises. Children do not usually need formal muscle-strengthening programs, such as lifting weights. Younger children usually strengthen their muscles through play activities such as climbing on a jungle gym or trees, riding a tricycle, playing ball, and running/jumping with parents and peers.

## Sleep-Rest Pattern

Most preschoolers sleep from 8 to 12 hours during the night, with wide variation among children (Hoban, 2010). Many children do not receive the recommended number of sleep hours, and sleep problems in preschool children commonly occur (Vriend & Corkum, 2011). For many older preschoolers, a nap is not necessary. By the age of 5 years, most preschoolers no longer regularly nap during the day (National Sleep Foundation, 2011). Quiet time provides a welcome respite for the parent, along with a chance for the active preschooler to relax before afternoon activities. Many child care/preschool environments routinely provide rest periods, enhancing rest and relaxation with soft music and a story. An afternoon rest also gives the young child energy for the evening routine, when family members have other duties beyond work and school.

Sleep time habits, falling asleep, and waking up during the night present challenges for families with preschool children (National Sleep Foundation, 2011). The preschooler's expanded imaginative play and increased physical activity during the day may provoke nighttime fears, nightmares, sleepwalking, and sleep terrors, which are at a peak during this stage of development (National Sleep Foundation, 2011).

## Bedtime Ritual

Preschoolers usually require a ritual of activities at bedtime to move from playing and being with others to being alone and falling asleep. These children prolong bedtime routines more often than the toddler. They insist on sleeping with the light on, take a treasured object to bed, request parental attention after being told good night, and experience delays falling asleep. The bedtime ritual generally lasts 30 minutes or longer. Parents honor reasonable rituals, but repeated requests for attention afterward are handled firmly and consistently. Consistency with the routine helps to ameliorate bedtime battles (Hoban, 2010). Vigorous resistance to bedtime challenges parents more during the preschool period than at any other developmental stage. Behavioral insomnia in children occurs when this resistance is associated with a negative association with sleep (Vriend & Corkum, 2011). Preschoolers learn to use the behaviors that meet their needs and control the family regardless of the disruption created.

## Nursing Interventions

When a demanding bedtime behavior extends beyond 1 year or an episode persists longer than 1 hour, the nurse explores the family situation. A comprehensive assessment in this case includes the following elements:
- Description of early episodes
- The manner in which these early episodes were managed and the progression of events since then
- Current bedtime behaviors of the child and siblings
- Identification of parental temperament and the resulting responses of the parents and family members
- Feelings of the parents and child about each other and about the bedtime situation
- Stressful events and changes that have occurred in the past several years
- Behavior of the child at other times of the day
- Parents' thoughts about the reasons why these episodes continue
- Parents' ideas about strategies to use now

The nurse observes interactions within the family. A home visit at mealtime provides an excellent method to observe active interaction. In the office or clinic setting the nurse can ask a parent to teach the child a task or give directions. The nurse remains as unobtrusive as possible while observing the interaction. The first-hand observation of parent-child interaction, along with the detailed history, usually provides the nurse with adequate baseline information to decide whether to manage the situation in the primary care setting or refer the family to a child behavior specialist. Sharing recent literature about management techniques for children with differing temperaments helps families understand more about the behaviors. For example, the findings from a study of more than 1500 children by Prior and colleagues (2011) support that temperament in children may be somewhat modifiable and that parents may consider strategies to influence their preschooler's behavior that focus on their temperament. Research-based strategies should be used to help parents reach their goals related to managing bedtime concerns.

## Sleep Disturbances

Night terrors and nightmares characterize the nighttime wakening problems that generally occur during the preschool years. Night terrors manifest themselves as frightening dreams that cause the child to sit up in bed, scream, stare at an imaginary object, breathe heavily, perspire, and appear in obvious distress (see Chapter 18). The child, not fully awake, may be inconsolable for 10 minutes or more, before he or she relaxes and returns to a deep sleep. In most cases the child does not recall the dream and in the morning does not remember the incident (Hoban, 2010). These night terrors can start at approximately age 2 years but are more common during the preschool years. Night terrors rarely occur in older children and adults, and only approximately 6% of preschool children have them. Night terrors and nightmares trigger apprehension for the parents (Hoban, 2010).

Nightmares (anxiety dreams) are a more common cause of night wakening. Although infants and toddlers likely have nightmares, their limited verbal skills hinder their relating details of the incidents. After age 3 years, nightmares occur frequently. Approximately 20% of the night is spent dreaming. Dreams frighten preschoolers as they connect to the larger world with their active imaginations and fantastic ideas. These children can waken fully and feel fearful and helpless. Usually they provide vivid descriptions at the time, and they frequently remember the event the following morning. Consolation can be given by a parent who sits with the child, listens to descriptions and fears about the dream, and reminds the child that dreaming is natural and sleep will soon return (Hoban, 2010).

Helping children appreciate the meaning of the words *pretend* and *real* facilitates growth during this phase of childhood. When the parent reads a story to the child or the child tells a make-believe tale, the parents can specify that these are "pretend" and did not really happen. The parent relating a true event can say, "This is real." Children differentiate between the two concepts as they develop cognitively.

## Recommendations

Parents of a preschooler can benefit from knowing the following facts:
- Bedtime rituals of 30 to 45 minutes are common for preschoolers. These rituals, because of their importance to children, are respected within reasonable limits. Maintaining a regular consistent and relaxing routine facilitates sleep (National Sleep Foundation, 2011).
- Night-wakening events are common during the preschool years. A consistent sleep environment with the same bed in a room that is cool, quiet, and dark without a television promotes sleep (National Sleep Foundation, 2011). Children who waken at night are reassured and encouraged to return to sleep.

- Parents have clear rules about children sleeping with them if the children will not stay in their own beds.
- Restricting the watching of frightening television shows and the reading of frightening stories and discussing "real" versus "pretend" ideas and stories can help lessen the incidence of nightmares.

## Cognitive-Perceptual Pattern

During the preschool years, children cultivate their conceptual and cognitive capacities. The quality of the child's care environment enhances these gains. Family and cultural values influence preschoolers' perceptions and their reaction to events (Gonzalez-Mena, 2012). Internalization of family rules has been associated with social competency in this age group (Kochanska et al., 2010). Preschoolers gradually differentiate today from yesterday and define tomorrow and the future more clearly as concepts of time emerge. The child becomes more oriented in space and develops an awareness of the location of the home within the neighborhood. The child also begins to structure daily activities and to value certain activities, objects, and people above others.

### Piaget's Theory

The older toddler enters the first substage of the preoperational stage described by Jean Piaget (see Chapter 18). The hallmark of this preconceptual substage includes the ability to function symbolically using language. The preschool child demonstrates increased symbolic functioning during the intuitive substage, from 4 to 7 years of age. The predominant feature of this and the following period is the concrete thought process, as compared with adult abstract thinking. As they experience symbolic mental representations, preschoolers process mental symbols as though they were actually participating in the event. Adults analyze and synthesize symbolic information without concrete connections between the mental process and the actual event. At this stage, mental abstraction, such as skipping from one part of an operation to another, reversing the operation mentally, or thinking of the whole in relation to the parts, is not feasible.

The egocentrism that is characteristic of the preschool years exemplifies this concept of concrete thinking. At this stage, children concentrate solely on their own perspective. They consider only their own personal meanings for symbols. The preschooler wonders why another person fails to follow these idiosyncratic communications.

Furthermore, attention focuses solely on one part of an object without shifting. This behavior, termed centering by Piaget, illustrates the child's inability to consider more than one factor at a time when solving simple problems. For example, a child can be given two identical cups containing equal amounts of water and asked which cup contains the greater amount of water. During the preoperational stage, the child responds that they contain the same amount of water. The child is then asked to pour the water from each cup into two different containers (one flat and wide, the other tall and narrow). When asked which container has more water, the child always identifies one. The child usually selects the taller, narrower container with water at the higher height. When the water is again transferred to the identical cups and the experiment is repeated, the child returns to the original conclusion that the amounts are equal.

This experiment also illustrates the trait of irreversibility. The child is unable to connect the reversible operation, the transfer of the water back into the original cup, to reach the logical conclusion that the differently shaped containers may hold the same amount of water. The child cannot mentally associate that the transformation from one state to another relates to the shape of the container, not the amount of the water.

Finally, Piaget describes the preoperative stage of thinking as transductive reasoning. The child cannot proceed from general to particular (deduction) or from particular to general (induction); rather, the child moves only from particular to particular in making associations and solving problems. For example, Piaget relates an association made by one of his children between being hunchbacked and being ill. When a hunchbacked neighbor was unable to visit one day because he had a communicable illness, the child understood that the neighbor was ill. However, when the child was told later that the neighbor was better and that she could go see him, her conclusion was that now his hunched back was straight and well. She thought in terms of the man being well or ill, but she placed the man in one or the other category and assumed that he possessed all the attributes and meanings that she linked symbolically with either trait.

The cognitive development of preschoolers is reflected in their symbolic games, which become significantly more orderly and representative of reality (Box 19-4). They begin to incorporate the reality of the world, as it exists outside the self. They increasingly seek play objects that represent models of authentic objects in their environment (Langevin et al., 2009). Preschoolers progressively imitate more social rules in their play. Social interactive play predominates as the young child develops a more secure sense of self.

Preschoolers may have one or more imaginary companions who exist for differing periods. These fantasy companions assume the form of another child, an animal, or some other friendly or fearsome creature. Preschoolers may save special chairs, insist

---

**BOX 19-4  Play as a Method of Learning: Preschool Child**

Throughout life, play develops cognitive, affective, and psychomotor skills that are important for the effective performance of life skills. For the preschool child, the following play activities provide the foundation for later competency and socialization-skill refinement:

- Arts and crafts (jewelry making, painting, drawing, ceramics, printmaking)
- Group sports (softball, volleyball, soccer, swimming)
- Skating, skateboarding
- Bicycling
- Puzzles
- Gymnastics
- Games (board, card, knock-knock jokes, computer)
- Secret clubs
- Imaginary play (being in playhouse productions)
- Horseback riding

that an extra place be set at the table, and talk at length to this companion. Imaginary companions serve an important function; they are controlled totally by the child and are not a threat. In this way the preschooler practices social interactions, controls a fearsome beast, or blames someone for naughty behavior without fear of being scolded, shame, or attack. Imaginary companions do and say only what the child wills.

## Vision

Vision capabilities, which are well developed by 2 years of age, continue to undergo refinement during the early childhood period. By approximately age 6 years, the child should approach a 20/20 visual acuity level. The possibility of developing amblyopia decreases; it appears most frequently during infancy through approximately the fourth year (see Chapter 18). Depth perception and color vision become fully established, and the child recognizes subtle differences in color shading by the sixth year. Maximal visual capability is usually achieved by the end of the preschool years.

Visual capacity throughout the rest of life deteriorates rather than improves. This phenomenon relates partly to changes in the refractive power of the lens and developmental changes that occur in the shape of the eyeball. In the normal sequence of growth, the eyeball becomes increasingly spherical, losing the short shape typical of infancy and progressing to the point at which light converges accurately on the surface of the retina. This change occurs at approximately 6 years of age. When this change occurs before the sixth year, growth continues past the point of ideal light conversion, the eyeball lengthens, and the child may develop early myopic vision, which will progress with age. Glasses are always indicated for the child who develops myopia before approximately age 8 years.

Early detection requires regular screening with standardized tests such as the Denver Eye Screening Test or the Snellen Screening Test. The Snellen Screening Test, when administered under standardized procedures, has the advantage of rendering a reliable estimate of actual visual acuity (Hockenberry & Wilson, 2015). The child must be able to understand the test requirements of either pointing in the direction of the *E* or naming the letters. The Denver Eye Screening Test was designed for preschool children and includes detection of the commonly occurring visual problems, such as refractive errors, strabismus (crossing of the eyes), and amblyopia.

The Prevent Blindness organization recommends regular vision screening of children by health care providers, educators, or public health programs (Prevent Blindness, 2017). In fact, they recommend that parents not take on the role of vision screener. Children who do not pass a vision screen should be taken to an optometrist or ophthalmologist for examination. The pupillary light reflex provides a screening approach for heterotropia, a condition in which the child's eyes do not focus together to transmit effective, coordinated binocular vision. When the child has heterotropia, the light from a penlight held approximately 20 inches from the eyes reflects off the pupil slightly off center. Consistent and observable strabismus may be noted. The cover test provides further evidence of a tendency for the child's eyes to cross, known as heterophoria. The child focuses on a spot

14 inches away, then 20 feet away. As the child gazes at the designated spot, one eye is covered completely for several seconds (the eye and eyelashes must not be touched), and then the cover is removed abruptly. If the covered eye moves from the line of vision of the uncovered eye, that eye has a tendency toward muscle imbalance and must be evaluated further.

Color blindness presents a particular problem for younger children because many cues encountered at school depend on the child's ability to distinguish colors. With early detection the child is able to receive assistance to interpret visual cues, thus minimizing the disadvantage of being color blind. The nurse screens the child for certain types of color discrimination difficulties by asking the child to respond to various colors in the environment; however, accurate testing for all types of color blindness requires a specialized tool, such as the Ishihara test, which uses a series of cards with color-tinted letters and figures.

Preschoolers may be aware of some discomfort or limitations with vision. The nurse gathers the history from the parents, including the questions listed in the Vision section in Chapter 18, about signs of eye problems.

The preschooler is asked questions to elicit information about the following symptoms:

- Itching, burning, or "scratchy" eyes
- Poor vision
- Dizziness, headaches, or nausea after close eye work
- Blurred or double vision

## Hearing

During the preschool years, hearing develops to the level of an adult, when the ability to attend to and interpret what is heard becomes more refined. The 4-year-old preschooler begins to discriminate among remarkably similar speech sounds, such as the difference between sounds made with "f" and "th" or "f" and "s." It is generally accepted that the hearing ability of preschoolers can be hindered by repeated middle ear infections (otitis media). Otitis media with effusion can occasionally result in temporary hearing loss. Parents who notice language delays because of ear infections should be referred to their health care provider for appropriate follow-up care for their children (Hockenberry & Wilson, 2015). Parental reports of difficulty should be taken seriously. Clear evidence supports that effective newborn hearing screening programs correct problems early and often correct developmental delay (Houston et al., 2011). The most effective programs have rigorous evaluation of their policies, procedures, processes, and outcomes (Houston et al., 2011; Yoshinaga-Itano, 2011).

Audiometric methods most accurately measure the child's ability to hear. Preschool children possess the developmental capability to have standard audiometric tests performed on them. The child can follow directions by this age, and most preschoolers enjoy demonstrating their abilities and cooperate easily during vision and hearing screening examinations (Hockenberry & Wilson, 2015). Refractive error can be significant in the preschool child. The prevalence of refractive errors (5–7%) and amblyopia (2–4%) in preschool children places vision loss as an important public health concern; however, some screening tests reveal only refractive errors (O'Donoghue et al., 2012). Children younger than 7 years with amblyopia demonstrate significant improvement in vision when treated, providing a rationale for screening and early recognition programs. The American Academy of Pediatrics on-line resources supply information for nurses and families and can be accessed at http://www.healthychildren.org.

To ensure success, the nurse encourages a positive experience by adhering to the following points:

- Use equipment skillfully.
- Use age-appropriate language. Avoid the word test to limit anxiety or fear of failure.
- Encourage the child to ask questions and scrutinize the equipment.
- Perform screening before other intrusive or painful procedures.
- Perform screening in a quiet, private area without distractions.
- Praise the child for cooperating.
- Allow rest periods when the child becomes distracted or tired.
- Discuss results with the child in age-appropriate language.

## Sensory Perception

Sensory abilities contribute to preschoolers' skill to perceive and interact with the world. Both sensory acuity and sensory perceptual abilities mature during the preschool years. The nature of the visual stimulus determines the response. Preschoolers respond powerfully to visual illusions and have difficulty discriminating right and left mirror images. Confusion commonly occurs with the letters "b," "d," "p," and "q."

## Language

Cognitive and sensory abilities contribute to preschool language development. Toward the end of the preschool period, expressive language rivals that of an adult except for minor deficiencies in refinement, vocabulary, and structure. Language ability depends on aptitude, opportunities to use language, the quality and quantity of language used at home, and the range of experiences. Regardless of expressive capacity, the child develops receptive language during the preschool years that provides a vital foundation for later communication. Throughout early childhood, receptive capacity exceeds expressive capacity. Children comprehend meanings of words and phrases not contained in their expressive vocabulary. Associations between concepts materialize, although the child lacks the ability to explain these concepts. Table 19-2 outlines the receptive and expressive language skills of preschoolers.

During the early childhood years, rhythm develops as an important dimension in speech capacity. Between 3 and 5 years of age, children practice speaking by mimicking adult language patterns. Practice expands neuromotor capacities, and verbal interaction develops vocabulary and sense of grammatical structure. Hesitations, repetitions, and frequent revisions in speech reflect attempts to expand language capacity. Adults may label such preparation as stuttering, but these inaccuracies actually represent normal speech maturation. Stuttering originates during this developmental period, associated with response and reaction from adults and other children to the normal preschool broken speech pattern (Langevin et al., 2009). Reactions of impatience

---

**BOX 19-5  Nursing Suggestions to Encourage Language Development in Preschoolers**

- Read to the child. Encourage the child to be an active listener. Pause during the story to ask questions, such as "What do you think will happen next?" and "Why do you think the boy said that?" and "What would you do now?" Praise the child's storytelling and creativity with stories.
- Always respond to the child's questions. Occasionally a response must be delayed; for example, when the parent is driving in heavy traffic and the child asks a question that requires a complex answer, the parent might say "That's a very good question; let's talk about that as soon as we get home." The parent should remind the child of the question later and respond if the child still expresses interest.
- Never tease or criticize a child about speaking style. If the child speaks so fast as to be fumbling over words, then the parent might say "I can't listen that fast. Slow down a little for me." This is much more encouraging than is the statement "You talk too fast. No one can understand you."
- Play language-focused games, such as naming the colors of houses or kinds of flowers as parent and child walk to the store.

---

while waiting for the child to express thoughts and negative social interactions decrease the child's opportunities to use language. Insisting children use correct speech before capacity for fluent speech develops may hinder normal speech development. As many as 60% of expressive language delays resolve during the preschool years (Conti-Ramsden & Durkin, 2012). As nurses help parents provide anticipatory guidance for language development, they should maintain vigilance to identify those children who are not outgrowing their language difficulties. These children encounter lifelong obstacles with learning and socialization. Suggestions for nurses to assist parents and to facilitate preschoolers' language development are listed in Box 19-5.

## Memory

Memory plays an important role in language development and learning in general (Archibald et al., 2011). Archibald and colleagues (2011) examined 12 preschool students and demonstrated an association between memory and verbal ability. At the preschool level, children label pictures, group objects, and mimic others as ways to aid memory, performing these tasks with less precision than the older child. Younger children benefit from suggestions about how to group items using characteristics to remember. Preschoolers remember pictures better by saying names of pictures rather than simply hearing the name of a picture when it is first shown. Preschoolers do not spontaneously use rehearsal or other mnemonic techniques for remembering, but they do use and benefit from rehearsal when it is suggested. The nurse tests memory by asking the child to repeat an arbitrary sequence of numbers. By approximately age 5 years, children are able to repeat four consecutively named numbers easily.

## Testing of Developmental Level

Parents of preschool children determine their child's readiness for school programs. The child's skill level, the child's and the family's psychosocial status, and the characteristics of the school program under consideration contribute to readiness determination.

## TABLE 19-2 GROWTH AND DEVELOPMENT

*Landmarks of Speech, Language, and Hearing Ability During the Preschool Period*

| Age (Months) | Receptive Language | Expressive Language | Related Hearing Ability |
|---|---|---|---|
| 42 | Up to 4200 words; knows words such as *what, where, how, funny, we, surprise, secret;* knows number concepts to 2; knows how to answer some questions accurately, such as: Do you have a dog? Which is the girl? What toys do you have? | Up to 1200 words in mostly complete sentences averaging 4 to 5 words per sentence; uses all 50 phonemes; 7% of sentences are compound or complex; averages 203 words per hour; rate of speech is accelerating; relates experiences and tells about activities in sequential order; uses words such as *what, where, how, see, little, funny, they, we, he, she, several;* can recite a nursery rhyme; asks permission; 95% of speech is intelligible | |
| 48 | Up to 5600 words; carries out 3-item commands consistently; knows why people have houses, books, umbrella, key; knows nearly all colors; knows words such as *somebody, anybody, even, almost, now, something, like, bigger, too,* full name, one or two songs, number concepts to 4; understands most preschool stories; can complete opposite analogies such as brother is a boy, sister is a girl, and in daytime it is light and at night it is dark | Up to 1500 words in sentences averaging 5 to 6 words per sentence; averages 400 words per hour; counts up to 3, repeats 4 digits, names 3 objects, repeats 9-word sentences from memory; names the primary colors, some coins; relates fanciful tales; enjoys rhyming nonsense words and using exaggerations; demands reasons why and how; questioning is at a peak, up to 500 questions a day; passes judgment on own activity; can recite a poem from memory or sing a song; uses words such as *even, almost, something, like, but;* typical expressions might include "I'm so tired," "You almost hit me," "Now I'll make something else" | Begins to make fine discriminations among similar speech sounds, such as the difference between *f* and *th* or *f* and *s;* has matured enough to be tested with an audiometer; at this age, formal hearing testing can usually be done; not only has hearing developed to its optimal level, but listening has also become considerably refined |
| 54 | Up to 6500 words; knows what materials a house, window, chair, and dress are made of and what people do with eyes and ears; understands differences in texture and composition, such as hard, soft, rough, smooth; begins to name or point to penny, nickel, dime; understands *if, because, why, when* | Up to 1800 words in sentences averaging 5 to 6 words; now averages only 230 words per hour—is satisfied with less verbalization; does little commanding or demanding; likes surprises; approximately 1 in 10 sentences are compound or complex, and only 8% of sentences are incomplete; can define 10 common words and counts up to 20; common expressions are "I don't know," "I said," "tiny," "funny," "because"; asks questions for information and learns to manipulate and control people and situations with language | |
| 60 | Up to 9600 words; knows number concepts to 5; knows and names colors; defines words in terms of use, such as a bike is to ride; defines wind, ball, hat, stove; understands qualifiers such as *if, because, when;* knows purpose of horse, fork, and legs; begins to understand *left* and *right* | Up to 2200 words in sentences averaging 6 words; can define ball, hat, stove, policeman, wind, horse, fork; can count five objects and repeat four or five digits; definitions are in terms of use; can single out a word and ask its meaning; makes serious inquiries—"What is this for?" "How does this work?" "Who made those?" "What does it mean?"; language is now essentially complete in structure and form; uses all types of sentences, clauses, and parts of speech; reads by way of pictures, and prints simple words | |

Modified from Hockenberry, M. J., & Wilson, D. (Eds). (2015). *Wong's nursing care of infants and children* (10th ed.). St. Louis: Mosby.

Early identification of developmental and emotional disorders is critical to the well-being of children and is an integral function and an appropriate responsibility of all pediatric health care professionals.

To obtain a more specific measure of developmental age, the nurse uses one of several screening tools designed for use with the preschool child. These validated instruments help to identify children at risk of developmental delay or disorder. Screening instruments are not diagnostic tools. In the primary care setting, screening for developmental age can be performed through the third edition of the **Ages & Stages Questionnaire (ASQ-3)**, a 30-item parent-report tool for children aged 4 to 60 months. The questionnaire takes caregivers 10 to 15 minutes to complete and takes approximately 2 to 3 minutes to score. ASQ-3 addresses five developmental areas: communication, gross motor, fine motor, problem-solving, and personal-social skills (Schonhaut et al., 2013). The **Battelle Developmental Inventory** is administered by a professional, trained in administering the test, and is designed to screen children from birth to 95 months old for personal-social, adaptive, motor, communication, and cognitive developmental problems. The Battelle Developmental Inventory is commonly used by early intervention programs and also in the primary care setting. The **Parents' Evaluation of Developmental Status** is another parent-completed questionnaire used commonly in the primary medical home setting and preschool setting. It is validated on children aged 0 to 8 years, takes 2 to 10 minutes to complete, and screens children for developmental and behavioral problems.

When a screening tool result is positive/concerning, the nurse should take additional steps to meet the needs of the parent and child. An early return visit should be made to provide additional developmental surveillance as well as anticipatory guidance for the family. Most importantly, the child should be referred for developmental and/or medical evaluations. Early developmental intervention/early childhood services should also be initiated if necessary.

Children who are ready for school demonstrate competencies in areas other than measurable skill performance. Complex home environments with stable caring adults or safe, predictable physical environments with regular, stimulating activities, peers, and materials contribute to readiness. Social norms define expectations; therefore home values that align with school values are more likely to result in children characterized as ready for school. Conversely, when school expectations differ from those at home, children are less likely to be considered ready for school (Conti-Ramsden & Durkin, 2012).

### Autism Spectrum Disorders

Autism statistics from the US Centers for Disease Control and Prevention (CDC; http://www.cdc.gov/) identify approximately 1 in 68 American children as being on the autism spectrum. Autism is 4.5 times more common among boys than girls. Autism has been diagnosed in an estimated 1 in 42 boys and 1 in 189 girls in the United States. Autism spectrum disorder (ASD) is the umbrella diagnosis for all subtypes (autistic disorder, childhood disintegrative disorder, pervasive developmental disorder—not otherwise specified, and Asperger syndrome). For the US population, the prevalence rate for this continuum of conditions increased from 6.7 per 1000 children in 2000 to 9.0 per 1000 children in 2006, and then to 14.6 per 1000 children in 2012 (CDC, 2016a). This corresponds to about 1 in 150 children in 2000, 1 in 110 children in 2006, and 1 in 68 children in 2012 (CDC, 2016a).

These conditions are considered genetically determined disorders and are only rarely associated with nongenetic risk factors, such as maternal valproic acid use during pregnancy, congenital rubella, and cerebral palsy (Freitag et al., 2010). Although the genetic foundation is well recognized, no single gene or gene family is linked to the disorders (LeBlanc & Fagiolini, 2011; Mefford et al., 2012). Chromosome microarray analysis is a promising area for assessment of ASD and currently provides diagnosis 15% to 20% of the time (Mefford et al., 2012).

Multiple studies have linked ASDs with atypical birth weight (high or low), low Apgar scores, hemolytic disease, hyperbilirubinemia (jaundice), respiratory distress, advanced parental age, length of gestation, and environmental factors (viruses), all of which may be subtle and complicated by the genetic influence (May-Benson et al., 2009). In their study of 467 children with ASD, May-Benson and colleagues (2009) provided support for the idea that there is no unique combination of characteristics, but rather a composite of risk factors that provide suspicion for the disorders.

More recently, there has been a question on whether an association between assisted reproductive technology (ART) conception and autism exists. Fountain and colleagues (2015) found in a population-based sample in California that the incidence of autism was twice as high for ART births as for non-ART births. However, they also explain that the association between ART and autism can be primarily explained by adverse prenatal and perinatal outcomes and multiple births. Research is also being performed to look at potential differences in ART procedures and parental infertility diagnoses as they might factor into the incidence of autism in ART-conceived infants. For example, there is a higher incidence of autism during the first 5 years of life when intracytoplasmic sperm injection was used compared with in vitro fertilization and a lower incidence when parents had unexplained infertility (among singletons) or tubal factor infertility (among multiples) compared with other types of infertility (Kissin et al., 2015).

Careful observation is vital during this time of language and communication development to assess children for ASDs because most cases of ASD are diagnosed in children (LeBlanc & Fagiolini, 2011). Most children have symptoms in the first year of life (Shumway et al., 2011); however, a formal diagnosis of autism is typically not made until a child is 2 years old. This assessment includes the family history, clinical history, and physical assessment with a focused neurological examination. Various screening tools exist for the nurse to use to identify children at risk of autism. The Modified Checklist for Autism in Toddlers is a widely used, 23-item, parent-completed screening tool for children aged 16 to 48 months (Chlebowski et al., 2013). For older children, the Childhood Asperger Syndrome Test and the Social Communication Questionnaire are well-developed and validated screening tools.

Manifestations differ considerably (Freitag et al., 2010; May-Benson et al., 2009). Assessment of cognitive and behavioral symptoms is the cornerstone of diagnosis, and early detection may help families address advancing behavioral aberrations sooner (LeBlanc & Fagiolini, 2011). The families of these children manage multiple behavioral and physical challenges early in the child's life; therefore health providers need to remain apprised of current trends in pediatric development connected to the disorders (May-Benson et al., 2009). Providers should consider the prenatal events mentioned earlier in this section along with childhood stressors (e.g., chronic ear infections, sleeping/eating problems, absent/brief crawling phase, language delays, atypical responses to sensory stimulation, lack of separation anxiety, and failure to attain motor skill developmental milestones) as warning signs that warrant further assessment (LeBlanc & Fagiolini, 2011; May-Benson et al., 2009).

In 2016 a population-based ASD surveillance study was published that looked at the characteristics and prevalence of ASD in 4-year-old children (Christensen et al., 2016). The study authors concluded that when compared with diagnosis in 8-year-old children, ASDs were diagnosed in the 4-year-olds approximately 5 months earlier (27 months compared with 32 months respectively) demonstrating improved methods of early identification. They also found that 4-year-old children with ASD were more likely to have intellectual disability than 8-year-old children in the same communities. Lastly, they concluded that among 4-year-old children, girls and white children were more likely to receive their first comprehensive, developmental evaluation by age 3 years compared with boys and black children, demonstrating that although there have been improvements in early diagnosis, at-risk populations still exist for later diagnosis/identification.

It is critical that autism and developmental delay be detected early in an effort to minimize delay and reduce educational costs. Neural circuits, which create the foundation for learning, behavior, and health, have increased plasticity within the first 3 years and become increasingly difficult to change over time. Diagnosis in the preschool child or earlier is imperative. The brain in strengthened by positive early experiences, stable relationships, appropriate nutrition, and supportive environments. High-quality early intervention can change the child's developmental trajectory and improve outcomes for families, children, and communities (Center on the Developing Child at Harvard University, 2010).

## Self-Perception–Self-Concept Pattern

During the preschool years, basic self-concept emerges from the child's personal struggle for autonomy. As children develop beyond the toddler years, they refine their sense of self through both task-oriented and socially oriented experiences. By reinforcing skills and successfully accomplishing tasks, preschoolers build self-esteem, enhancing overall health. Social acceptance helps children feel successful in their role as a child, sibling, and friend. Preschoolers investigate roles through rich imagination. Pretending to be the parent or baby allows preschoolers to imagine experiences and feelings of others (i.e., empathy) and safely experiment with new ideas (Price & Gwinn, 2008).

Preschool children learn about their roles in their child care environments and learn that being dependable within their world is important. When children perceive their value in improving the world in which they live, they experience good feelings about themselves and, ultimately, demonstrate improved mental and physical health. Many simple ways to improve the environment are available, and when children learn ways to contribute to environmental health, they often reinforce these behaviors in their parents (Box 19-6: Quality and Safety Scenario).

### Erikson's Theory

Preschoolers develop a sense of initiative through their vigorous motor activity and active imagination (Figure 19-2). Erikson views this growth as the most central developmental task in the emerging self-concept of the preschool years. By praising preschoolers' efforts and providing opportunities for new experiences, parents promote development of initiative. Rather than requiring a particular behavior, parents should provide avenues for experimentation. Preschoolers then feel mastery, thus encouraging repetition. With mastery, preschoolers become more confident about trying new actions.

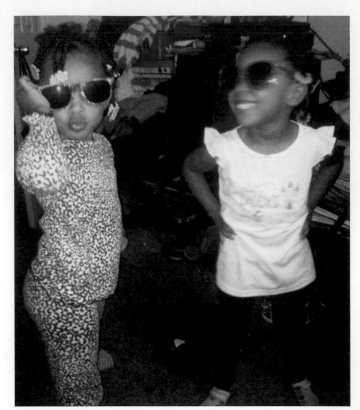

**FIGURE 19-2** Two preschoolers using their imagination in being movie stars.

## Roles-Relationships Pattern

Family members continue to play a vital role in the preschooler's life, but peers become increasingly significant as development progresses. Preschoolers receive ideas and information from peers. They may subsequently question rules or expectations at home, comparing them with their friends' situations. Discussion about family values and behaviors that are acceptable in one place but not another helps them understand differences.

Preschoolers understand sex expectations regarding jobs, activities, and competencies of people in their lives. Ideas about sex differences in work roles or activities are based on models in the home, at child care or preschool centers, and on television. Parents and caregivers should be aware of the powerful influence that the environment has on role perceptions (Bower et al., 2008; Brown et al., 2009; Kochanska et al., 2010). When inaccurate portrayals of male and female roles are depicted, parents and caregivers should discuss more accurate ones with children. Preschoolers experiment through play, including adopting family roles. These roles differ depending on the family structure and function. For example, the role-play for a child of gay or lesbian parents may differ from that of a child of heterosexual parents. As the mother or father in a play situation, the preschooler sets limits, punishes, praises, and makes outlandish demands on the invented child. Play represents an important strategy for preschoolers to use for stress reduction and experimentation with new roles. By playing different roles, children safely experience the effects of their behavior and understand others' roles more

**BOX 19-6 QUALITY AND SAFETY SCENARIO**

**Health Promotion With Preschoolers: Environmental Accountability**

**Rationale for Teaching Preschoolers About Environmental Protection**

- Environmental education at an early age will produce environmental practitioners of the future.
- Preschoolers can learn basic concepts of environmental accountability and gain a sense of empowerment when they perceive that they make a difference to the future world.
- Health care providers, in consultation with child care providers, can promote environmental education that is based on their knowledge of child growth and development and concerns about overall health.

**Basic Ways for Preschoolers to Help the Environment and Promote Overall Societal Health**

- Use water wisely.
- Use electricity only when necessary.
- Recycle.
- Avoid using balloons.
- Plant trees, protect plants, and grow a garden.
- Create a compost pile.
- Care for birds.
- Clean up the neighborhood.
- Decrease the amount of trash; say "no" to Styrofoam and plastic garbage bags, and use paper cups and reusable cloth bags for groceries.
- Recycle old toys by giving them to others.
- Buy and use only Earth-friendly school supplies.
- Walk rather than ride in the car.
- Use live Christmas trees and replant them.

clearly. Parents also better understand the effects of their own actions when they observe the behaviors of their child. Nurses help parents use their observations to improve interactions with their child.

Compared with toddlers, preschoolers relate to older children in the family on a more equal basis. Although their cognitive, motor, and language skills are less refined, preschoolers participate in some activities with their older siblings. Younger children may admire and imitate an older sibling. This behavior flatters the older child initially, but with continued persistence may develop into a source of frustration for the sibling. The older sibling, in a more powerful position, may resort to violence (Phillips et al., 2009).

Social interaction during the preschool period prepares the child for school. Through experience within the family, with peers, and with other adults, the child acquires readiness to interact in group situations, follow directions, take turns, recognize others' rights, channel energy toward an assigned activity, and demonstrate increasing independence. School readiness can be assessed by use of several relevant tests, as discussed in this chapter. The nurse who sees the child repeatedly in an office, clinic, or group care or preschool setting assesses progress as the child develops social competencies. Comparing the preschooler's current, more mature behavior with previous behavior provides

insight into that child's readiness for school. This method of evaluation, however, prevents comparison with other children of the same age. For example, school personnel may view a child who reflects a quiet temperament and is introverted or subdued as overly attached to the mother in comparison with other children the same age. However, if the child's earlier social behavior is known, the behavior may be interpreted as a progression toward independence.

Evidence of social competency can be obtained by discussion and evaluation of the child's family drawings. Children can be given the opportunity to draw pictures while they are waiting for outpatient visits, and the drawings can be used to begin the assessment process. The nurse observes the drawing and responds to any comments or questions volunteered by the child. When asked for advice or assistance, the nurse encourages the child to proceed with drawing. Positive encouragement for the child's efforts may be used, particularly with reluctant children. After the drawing is finished, the nurse discusses the sketch with the child to identify the people and describe individual characteristics. The nurse writes the names of each family member on the picture and documents the perceptions the child describes. Open-ended questions such as "What do you like best about your brother?" or "When do you get angry with your sister?" can be posed to encourage the child to describe the family interaction patterns. When an adult family member is present, the nurse explains the purpose of the drawing and interview and requests that the adult withhold comments or questions until the activity is completed. Any areas of concern or questions should be discussed, assuring the parent that confidentiality will be maintained. The child's perceptions can be verified with the adult at the conclusion of the interview, or further information can be sought to clarify them.

The Vineland Social Maturity Scale provides an objective, standardized estimate of social functioning and social maturity (Scattone et al., 2011). This tool profiles the child's self-help skills, self-direction, locomotion, communication, and social relations. The scoring system seems to be culturally and socioeconomically neutral. The investigator collects data by observing the child's behavior and interviewing the mother or primary caregiver. Designed to measure progression toward independence, this instrument uses direct observation of the child's behavior whenever possible, with the interview data being used only if needed to complete the assessment (Scattone et al., 2011).

These kinds of tools elicit cues indicative of family stress and strain. Parental divorce commonly creates disruption in family relationships. Discussion of the results of the assessment offers the opportunity to discuss family situations that otherwise might have remained unmentioned. Children's responses to changes in family circumstances depend on their developmental stages and their relationships before the change. Divorce represents a final decision, usually culminating from a period of conflict, stress, and changing relationships. Although preschoolers definitely sense stress in the home, they cannot articulate their feelings or determine their origin. Children react to changes in various ways, including regression, confusion, or irritability. Asking the same questions repeatedly—such as "Is Daddy coming home for supper tonight?" or "Why doesn't Daddy stay here anymore?"—can be a child's way of expressing difficulty in coping with or comprehending the situation.

Parents in the midst of marital problems or divorce frequently lack the psychological energy or patience to deal with questions and altered behavior. Nonetheless, their children desperately need closeness, patience, and consistent responses from their parents. Nurses act as advocates for children by helping parents explore ways to address regression and irritability. As parents develop skills to explain situations, they realize children are deeply affected during times of family disruption, regardless of their behavior (Kaakinen et al., 2010). Parents need to connect emotionally with their children to demonstrate that love will continue for the child despite dissolution of the marriage. Books appropriate to the preschooler's cognitive and emotional level can help parents address children's feelings and needs during divorce.

### Child Abuse

The social processes within families and communities that create child abuse are multifaceted and complex. Research focuses on the complexity of the abuse cycle and the challenges involved in resolution. In some communities, hitting children as a form of discipline remains socially acceptable. Parents and caregivers who experience workplace stress, financial worries, and other frustrations may project their anger and abuse toward their children physically, emotionally, or sexually. Effective primary and secondary prevention interventions involve promoting awareness of violence as a social problem, opposing violence to women, and offering community or school programs to teach nonviolent conflict resolution skills to people of all ages. Prevention of child neglect and abuse is the focus of many health-promotion programs. Recognition of signs of child abuse is important, and health care are mandated to report suspected abuse (Moreno, 2014). Although it is important for families to begin to teach children about how to respond to strangers, child abuse in general and sexual abuse in particular occur more often within a family than with a stranger as the perpetrator. Most children suffer the abuse from someone who is familiar to them. The American Psychological Association provides helpful information about abuse for families at http://www.apa.org/pi/families/resources/child-sexual-abuse.aspx.

### Sexuality-Reproductive Pattern

Preschoolers recognize there are two sexes and identify with their own sex. Appropriate and positive representations of both sexes on television and in role models, such as working mothers, allow preschoolers to interpret gender roles broadly and define their own roles more realistically (Hockenberry & Wilson, 2015). Body image, a part of gender identity, also includes perception of sex organs. Preschoolers develop curiosity at this age, including inquisitiveness about bodies and sexual functions of others. Questions should be answered simply and factually. Teasing preschoolers about this interest or implying that sexual information is unacceptable or naughty promotes negativity. Positive feelings about all aspects of the self (including gender role) create positive self-esteem. Many children's books address self-esteem in young children and provide interesting and informative

approaches to nurturing overall health promotion in this age group.

### Coping–Stress Tolerance Pattern

#### Play Approaches

Assessing self-concept in preschool children who struggle to articulate their feelings presents a challenge for the nurse. Play can elicit behaviors that indicate sense of self and self-esteem, future success or failure, sense of acceptance, and competence. **Doll or puppet play** provides valuable insight into a child's sense of self. Dolls or puppets, including those representing a young child of the same sex, race, and cultural background as the preschooler, should be available (Hockenberry & Wilson, 2015). If the child spontaneously begins to engage the dolls or puppets in imaginary activity, no further guidance should be given. With a reluctant child, the nurse begins to pretend, using examples for the child, such as going to the store, moving the dolls through the related activities, and then involving the child. Frequently preschoolers continue the scenario to tell their personal stories.

A related technique is **mutual storytelling**. The nurse begins a story for the child to finish. The nurse might begin with a standard line, such as "Once upon a time there lived a [girl, boy, cow, monkey, etc.] who … ." The nurse then pauses for the child to continue. If the child hesitates, the nurse resumes the story for another sentence or two and asks what the figure in the story is doing. As the child supplies details, the nurse offers encouragement to continue, asking questions such as "And then what happened?" or "How did the child feel?"

The child's inner nature can be explored along several dimensions. The emotional theme of the story is noted and should be congruent with the child's tone and expression. For example, a child who centers on a theme of aggression and destruction but describes the character's anger in a monotone is demonstrating incongruence between content and expression. The child's emotionless response suggests difficulty with expressing feelings. At the conclusion of the story, possible meanings can be revealed by the nurse asking whether the child feels similar to any of the characters or would like to be any of the characters.

Although these dimensions may be explored for meaning, interpretation of a child's behavior in these play situations remains highly speculative. Determining possible themes or estimating the child's self-esteem requires several encounters. Additionally, the nurse's personality and approach influence the child's spontaneity and ability to tell a story. Observed behavior and responses without associated interpretation should be recorded for future reference. Interpretations of the behavior and responses are avoided until validated by a specialist.

#### Coping Mechanisms

Preschoolers use coping mechanisms similar to those of the toddler (separation anxiety, regression, denial, repression, and projection). Protest behavior in the form of temper tantrums normally disappears as a stress response in the older preschooler. Temper tantrums that persist through the fifth year indicate a lack of matured coping responses. The child uses tantrums and continues to gain the desired result.

## BOX 19-7   The Challenge of Temperament and Preschoolers

Temperament describes the way in which an individual behaves or responds to new situations and to life occurrences and has consistently been associated with psychopathology and family function since the early work of Terry Brazelton with maternal attachment in 1978 (Healey et al., 2011; Joosen et al., 2012). Most children can be defined as *easy, difficult,* or *hard to warm up to* on the basis of how they react to their surroundings and to people. Temperament and parental stress are linked; however, multiple other factors influence interactions between the parent and the child, including the child's own temperament (Healey et al., 2011; Prior et al., 2011). For many adults, the challenge in parenting is to learn how to work with a child's temperament, which can differ from the parents' or other children's temperaments, in efforts to attain family happiness. Coping skills and stress management for families, particularly those with children defined as difficult, may improve family function (Healey et al., 2011).

From Healey, D. M., Flory, J. D., Miller, C. J., & Halperin, J. M. (2011). Maternal positive parenting style is associated with better functioning in hyperactive/inattentive preschool children. *Infant & Child Development, 20*(2), 148–161; Joosen, K. J., Mesman, J., Bakermans-Kranenburg, M. J., & van Lizendoorn, M. H. (2012). Maternal sensitivity to infants in various settings predicts harsh discipline in toddlerhood. *Attachment & Human Development, 14*(2), 101–117; Prior, M., Bavin, E., Cini, E., Eadie, P., & Reilly, S. (2011). Relationships between language impairment, temperament, behavioural adjustment and maternal factors in a community sample of preschool children. *International Journal of Language & Communication Disorders, 46*(4), 489–494.

Preschoolers lack the cognitive awareness, social abilities, and motives for communication of adults and older children. They display temperaments and tantrums that appear oppositional to older individuals. Through positive interactions with parents and caregivers, preschoolers frequently learn how to organize their bodies, abilities, and environment to move successfully to the next stage of development (Brown et al., 2009; Luby et al., 2009). A positive relationship between the child's temperament and the demands of the environment (also known as goodness of fit) can be attained by social interaction, which, in turn, prevents the development of problem behaviors later (Box 19-7: The Challenge of Temperament and Preschoolers).

Preschoolers possess a considerable range of experiences and memories; therefore they respond more maturely to stress than do toddlers. Positive coping resources are determined by some of the following variables:

- Availability of emotional comfort and the child's inner resilience
- Ability to work on task
- Availability of play materials and toys
- Opportunity to engage in activities (Kalpidou et al., 2004)

Preschoolers use many of the coping mechanisms developed during their toddler years, but they generally show greater ability to verbalize frustration, have fewer temper tantrums, and display more patience in experimentation to resolve difficulty than the typical toddler. Preschoolers refine their problem-solving skills. Through fantasy play, they investigate solutions or responses to stressful events and find inner control for challenging situations.

Occasionally projection and fantasy lead parents to consider their child dishonest. When faced with the question "Did you break this dish?" the preschooler might respond, "No, Teddy did it." The child might even relate a detailed story of the toy bear mishap. Preschoolers tend to project blame. Active fantasies help tell the story. Parents should not accuse the preschooler of lying, but rather the adult should help the child decide whether the story is pretend or real. The concepts of pretend and real help encourage children to discuss nightmares, television shows, stories, and their own active imaginations (Garrison et al., 2011).

Compared with toddlers, preschoolers better perceive their ability to control and manage situations. Strict adherence to rituals or game rules controls situations. As discussed, preschoolers have longer and more rigid bedtime rituals than those of toddlers. Preschoolers also dislike losing games and may structure the rules to ensure they win. Older children and adults may be able to accept these structures, but these controlling behaviors frustrate other preschoolers because they also need to win. Gentle, consistent direction by parents and caregivers about how to play games fairly and how to move toward positive group outcomes helps preschoolers develop a sense of morality, which is important for later life success and happiness. See the case study and care plan at the end of this chapter for an example of ineffective coping in a preschool child.

## Values-Beliefs Pattern

Preschoolers, like toddlers, lack fully developed consciences; however, at age 4 to 5 years these children do demonstrate some internal controls on their actions. Immaturity limits the consistency and effectiveness of these internal controls. With the child's concrete perspective, the internal controls may be rigid; therefore a preschooler may feel overwhelming guilt when behavior and internal controls conflict. Cognitive developmental level determines, for the most part, preschoolers' maturity and their feelings about their behavioral fluctuations. Cognitive development continues with dramatic transformation during these years, explaining the differences not only among children but also for different times in the same child. Modeling and **induction explanation,** moving from specific to general, influence moral behaviors appreciably. Modeling stems from many sources, not all of which leave positive impressions. Parents affect the availability of models by screening television shows, carefully selecting child care situations, and monitoring play sessions. Responsible parents verify the suitability of the models. More detailed inductive explanations, based on the child's cognitive level, are generally comprehended by the preschool population.

Preschoolers control their behavior to retain parental love and approval. From their perspective, parental disapproval represents a decrease in the child's importance from the parent's viewpoint. The child therefore suffers a decline in self-esteem, which motivates a change in behavior. Guilt results from perceived reduction of self-esteem, a critical step in the development of conscience. Moral actions are demonstrated in simple activities, such as taking turns and sharing. These actions stem from the assumption that other people have rights and desires that are as important as the rights and desires of preschoolers.

Preschoolers frequently express their values by stating who or what they like or what they want to be when they become adults. These values change frequently, even within a few minutes. Preschoolers occasionally use statements of value as punishment for playmates or family members and display insensitivity to the effect of their remarks on others. Preschoolers ask endless questions. When they ask these questions about moral actions or feelings, they may simply be asking "How does this work?" and not questioning the underlying parental value. The same intent exists when the child asks about the spiritual values that the parent may be teaching. Parents may enroll their child in Sunday school or other faith-oriented classes or activities. The preschool child generally enjoys the social aspects of these activities and receives some important modeling of values from the involved adults and from working with peers as they struggle to develop morality (Kochanska et al., 2010).

Life beginnings and death concepts fascinate preschoolers. Because of their limited emotional experiences with death, some ask about dead insects and the process of death with great interest, occasionally with insensitivity. Others become upset with the idea of dying, assuming that when someone becomes angry and wishes them dead, they will cease to exist. Many children worry about who will care for them if their caregivers die, whether pain comes with death, what causes death, and what happens after someone dies. Children who actually lose a loved one to death can experience sleep disturbances and other behavioral changes as part of the grieving process. Parents, on the basis of their own religious and cultural values, should respond to children in a supportive and open manner to provide an accurate interpretation of death. In some cases, counseling may be needed if the parents are unable to cope with their duties or if the child has significant behavioral problems as a result of the family disruption. Assessment using the preschoolers' drawings in such situations provides an accepted method to explore their perceptions about family relationships, death, and the afterlife (Selwyn et al., 2009).

# ENVIRONMENTAL PROCESSES

## Physical Agents

For many children, physiological, psychosocial, and environmental factors create health problems that interfere with physical, social, and educational activities of normal development (Hockenberry & Wilson, 2015). Major disruptions limit fulfillment of the child's potential in adulthood. The environmental processes that affect toddlers also affect preschoolers. Occurrence rates and outcomes of health problems differ in this age group, likely because of developmental differences (US Department of Health and Human Services, 2011). Preschoolers have more refined problem-solving skills, are more coordinated, and have more experience with a variety of situations than do toddlers. Although preschoolers recognize and avoid some environmental hazards, they remain impulsive and immature. Population-based programs ensure that screening occurs at the most developmentally appropriate time (Box 19-8: Research for Evidence-Based Practice).

---

## BOX 19-8 RESEARCH FOR EVIDENCE-BASED PRACTICE

### Effectiveness of Parents' Language Interventions for Preschool Children

Roberts and Kaiser (2011) conducted a systematic meta-analysis of 18 studies with participants aged 18 to 60 months that met the following criteria: used a comparison group, used a parental intervention, and included a child communication component with at least one language outcome measure. Almost half of the studies evaluated used the Hanen Program for parents and focused stimulation. Effect sizes were determined for each study, as well as seven language outcome variables. Intellectual disabilities and parent report versus direct observation measures were also compared. This meta-analysis indicated that parent-implemented language interventions have significant positive influence on both receptive and expressive language skills in preschool children regardless of whether they have intellectual impairment. The findings from this analysis provide evidence to support the use of parent-implemented interventions for preschool children with language impairments.

From Roberts, M. Y., & Kaiser, A. P. (2011). The effectiveness of parent-implemented language interventions. A meta-analysis. *American Journal of Speech-Language Pathology, 20*(3), 180–199.

---

Because many preschoolers attend child care programs, many have been trained to use 911 and can access help in emergencies when this phone code exists. At this age a child needs to know his or her name, address, and how to say "no" to strangers.

## Injuries

Accidents and injuries are often predictable and preventable (CDC, 2007; Ingram et al., 2011). As preschoolers become more independent, causes of injury change; they may chase a ball into a busy street or suffer from sports-related injuries. Preschoolers continue to need supervision to prevent injury related to their developmental age. Nurses guide families to provide a safe environment for preschoolers with opportunities to explore without negative consequences (Box 19-9).

Of all injuries, two-thirds occur in children and adolescents. The rate of death from injuries is decreasing in the United States. On the other hand, death rates continue to be higher than in countries with long-term comprehensive preventive approaches that focus on widespread community change (e.g., Great Britain and Scandinavian countries) (Orton et al., 2012). Although preschoolers have fewer accidents than toddlers, accidental injury continues to be a predominant cause of morbidity in this age group (Orton et al., 2012). Preschoolers are most likely to sustain injuries related to falls, poisonings, and thermal injuries than any other accidental injuries; however, as the child's age increases toward school age, these injuries begin to decline in number (CDC, 2017; Ingram et al., 2011; Orton et al., 2012).

Motor vehicle accidents consistently remain the top-ranked reason for death attributable to injury in the preschool age group (CDC, 2017). Consequently, the *Healthy People* initiative has promoted the use of car seat restraint systems (*Healthy People 2020:* IVP-16.3). An analysis of data from the National Survey of the Use of Booster Seats revealed that unfortunately few children younger than 13 years use the recommended child

## BOX 19-9 Injury Prevention for Preschoolers

A safe and developmental-stimulating environment allows children of all ages to explore without negative consequences. When teaching parents how to modify their homes for preschoolers, the nurse should consider the following requirements for child safety.

### Safe Sleep Environment

Provide beds with guardrails (as needed), soft corners, and appropriate bedding to prevent suffocation.

### Well-Ventilated but Optimal Temperature Environment for Play

Provide safe play areas by using electrical outlet covers, handrails in stairwells, toy boxes with lids that lock securely, nonslip floor materials, well-anchored furniture, and appropriate soft ground coverings and padding for outdoor play equipment.

### Burn Prevention

Use only cool mist humidifier for management of upper respiratory tract infections; dress child only in flame-retardant clothing, particularly at bedtime.

### Appropriate Installation and Use of Emergency Home Equipment

Discuss the importance of properly operating smoke detectors and fire extinguishers, and practice a plan for escape from the home in case of emergency.

### Connection to Emergency Services

Post 911 on all phones; teach the child how to use 911 and how to report the child's name and address over the phone; parents should be trained in cardio-pulmonary resuscitation and the use of abdominal thrusts.

### Prevention of Aspiration

Monitor use of balloons and eating habits of preschoolers.

### Safe Daily Home Environment

Close doors of the dishwasher, oven, washer, and dryer; mark all glass doors with decals to delineate doors; use gates at the top and bottom of stairs for the younger child; set water heater temperature at a maximum of 120°F to avoid burns; store all poisonous substances out of the reach of children; discourage running in the house; avoid using throw rugs on bare floors.

### Prevention, Recognition, and Management of Poison Ingestion or Exposure

Know how to use syrup of ipecac, and have the nearest poison control center phone number within easy access; learn how to evaluate burns or blisters around the mouth, odor of poisons, empty containers around the child, stomach distress, or changes in normal activity level that might indicate poison ingestion.

### Water Safety

Monitor bathtub and pool activity; teach preschooler swimming skills (usually by age 4 years); ensure that all pools are fenced.

### Bicycle Safety

Ensure that the child is riding a developmentally appropriate bicycle with a federally approved safety helmet and is schooled in the rules of riding in the street and interacting with strangers.

### Lead Concerns

Avoid exposure to items with a high lead content in the home (paint, wrapping paper, earthenware, colored newspaper); ensure that children are monitored when lead exposure is a concern.

### Environmental Contaminants Hazardous to the Child's Health

Avoid exposure to tobacco smoke, nitrous oxide from wood-burning stoves, asbestos, pesticides, radiation, and factory-produced irritants.

From Hockenberry, M. J., & Wilson, D. (Eds). (2015). *Wong's nursing care of infants and children* (10th ed.) St. Louis: Mosby.

passenger restraints (Macy & Freed, 2012). The overall critical misuse for child restraints is approximately 73% (Decina & Lococo, 2005). According to the Fatality Analysis Reporting System (a database maintained by the National Highway Transportation Safety Administration), from 2001 to 2010 there were 7625 motor vehicle crash fatalities of children aged 0 to 9 years, of which only half were wearing any child restraint and 20% were sitting in the front seat (Lee et al., 2015). To promote correct car seat use, Weaver and colleagues (2013) recommend conducting meaningful formative research, developing and evaluating injury prevention message strategies, evaluating existing programs and recommendations, conducting transdisciplinary work, and supporting partnerships between manufacturers, retailers, and injury prevention specialists.

As children outgrow a rear-facing car seat at approximately age 2 years, they should move to a forward-facing car seat with a five-point harness. Children should remain in a forward-facing car seat with a harness for as long as possible, up to the highest weight and height allowed by the car seat manufacturer. School-aged children should transition to a booster seat when the weight and/or height are above the forward-facing limit. Children may transition out of a belt-positioning booster seat typically when they have reached 4 feet 9 inches in height and are between 8

and 12 years of age. Federal investigations concluded that children younger than 13 years should ride in the back seat of a motor vehicle, particularly because of potential injury or death from a passenger seat air bag that could inflate in a severe car accident. In 2013 changes were made by car manufacturers regarding the use of LATCH (*Lower Anchors and Tethers for Children*) for older children using child restraints. This is important in the preschooler because per the new guidelines, in general, if the combined weight of the car seat and child is more than 65 pounds, LATCH should not be used. Instead of LATCH, the seat belt should be used. Each car seat and car manufacturer has slightly differing regulations, so parents are encouraged to have a certified car seat technician install their child's seat to ensure proper and safe installation. It is important to note that each state has differing laws regarding child safety restraints. However, these laws are often minimum requirements, not updated often, and not always reflective of best practice.

Nurses actively participate in health-promotion programs in communities and emergency departments that help families use car restraints correctly. Unfortunately, in one study, despite comprehensive nursing education and training programs during the postpartum period, car safety seat misuse was frequent (Rogers et al., 2013). When families have to consider financial constraints to comply with the requirements to restrain their children, nurses are often the first-line of information. Nurses provide information about resources available locally through agencies such as hospitals, physicians' offices, insurance companies, United Way, local Safe Kids coalitions (2015), the fire department, and other community organizations.

Household furniture and fixtures also remain a hazard for preschoolers, as do structural features such as stairs and windows. A meta-analysis found that home safety interventions were effective in significantly increasing the proportion of families with fitted stair gates (Kendrick et al., 2013). Nursery and toy injuries decrease during the preschool years. Sports and recreational injuries increase markedly. This elevated incidence likely reflects a change in many preschoolers being involved in group sports, riding bicycles, and using playground equipment (CDC, 2017). Preschoolers need a broad range of play areas and experiences. Conscientious parents supply age-appropriate limits and supervision (Ingram et al., 2011; Price & Gwinn, 2008). Preschoolers lack the skill or judgment to ride bicycles in the street. They need instruction about safe use of playground equipment. Adult supervision of most preschooler activities, group sports in particular, is required to prevent injury.

Preschoolers begin to safely handle basic tools, kitchen equipment, and cleaning supplies. Children at this age take pride in participating in household projects with a supervising parent. They spend much of their time in the home and in the preschool or child care center. The facilities pose the same potentially harmful environmental conditions as the home, as well as some additional threats to safety (CDC, 2007).

In response to concern about firearm safety in homes with small children, most states have passed child access prevention (CAP) legislation to encourage safe storage of firearms. For young children, CAP results in a decline in the rate of deaths attributable to firearms. The risk of death increases in the mere presence of the firearm. Preschool children are physically capable of pulling a trigger before they are able to cognitively depict the cause and effect of their actions. Even if there is gun safety training, most curious children will handle firearms given the opportunity, which may give families a false sense of security (Children's Defense Fund, 2012).

To appreciate the magnitude of the problem, in 2008 the number of preschoolers killed by firearms (88) was twice that of the number of law enforcement officers killed by firearms (41) (Children's Defense Fund, 2012). A more recent estimate reports 110 unintentional firearm deaths in the United Sates of children aged 0 to 14 years annually from 2005 to 2012 (Hemenway & Solnick, 2015). Most deaths from firearms are preventable when adults take responsibility for minimizing access to and storage of firearms (Faulkenberry & Schaechter, 2015). A recent review of the effectiveness of interventions to promote safe firearm storage found that safe storage device provision, with or without counseling, significantly improved firearm storage practices (Rowhani-Rahbar et al., 2016).

## Burns
Scalds and direct flame burns are major hazards for preschoolers. For many young children, thermal injury results in an emergency department visit or hospital admission (Ingram et al., 2011). Thermal injury (unintentional fire/burn) ranks among the top ten causes of death from injuries in US children from birth to 14 years of age (CDC, 2017). The number of deaths of preschool children in house fires is nearly double that of children of other ages. Children of this age experiment with matches and fire, and they may be unable to escape from a fire once it starts. The measures discussed in Chapter 18 to reduce scald burns in the home apply to this age group as well. Preschoolers should be taught about the dangers of matches, open flames, and hot objects. Parents and caregivers should model appropriate use of active and potentially dangerous burning devices. In a study of five emergency departments, the majority (58%) of thermal injuries were scalds from beverages (49.6%), domestic water (37.6%), and food (12.7%), most frequently caused by pull-down (48%) and spill (32%) mechanisms (Kemp et al., 2014). A meta-analysis found that home safety interventions were effective in significantly increasing the proportion of families with safe hot tap water temperatures, functional smoke alarms, and a fire escape plan (Kendrick et al., 2013).

## Drowning
Children older than 3 years are at lower risk of drowning in the bathtub, but at greater risk of drowning in a swimming pool, than the toddler. Drowning ranks among the top six causes of death from injuries in US children up to 14 years of age (CDC, 2017). Preschool children aged 1 to 4 years are at highest risk of drowning, with two near-drowning episodes for every fatality. Most children are close to safety when drowning occurs. With this in mind, it is important to supervise young children when they are near a body of water, to install fencing to isolate a residential pool from the house, for young children to use personal floatation devices while bathing or playing near a natural body of water, and to teach children how to swim and that swimming alone is unsafe. Preschoolers should receive instruction in water safety and swimming, and should always be supervised by a trained adult or older person. The American Academy of Pediatrics suggests that all children aged 4 years or older should receive swimming lessons (Engel, 2015). Because a good outcome depends on early resuscitation, it is reasonable to encourage parents and pool owners to learn cardiopulmonary resuscitation.

Preschoolers have the cognitive ability to learn water survival. They should always wear a personal flotation device or PFD (i.e., life jacket) when they are on boats, even when they know how to swim, and they must be supervised when near water, even shallow water. The American Academy of Pediatrics recommends the following strategies to prevent drownings: adult supervisor, pool fencing, pool alarms, lifeguards, cardiopulmonary resuscitation training, swimming instructions and water-survival training, and PFDs (Weiss, 2010). Safety campaigns provide one effective measure to prevent unnecessary injury and death (Children's Defense Fund, 2012; Ingram et al., 2011; Orton et al., 2012; US Department of Health and Human Services, 2014). Unfortunately, data from the National Inpatient Sample and Nationwide Emergency Department Sample indicate that despite safety campaigns, the estimated national incidence of nonfatal drowning from 2006 to 2011 was constant at approximately 10 nonfatal drownings annually per 100,000 population (Felton et al., 2015).

## Mechanical Forces

Bicycle accidents become a greater source of injury during the preschool years. Many bicycle accidents involve automobiles, and most of these accidents result from the child's errors. Parents should set reasonable and age-appropriate limits on bicycle use. An epidemiological study of nonfatal bicycle injuries seen by emergency departments (Chen et al., 2013) reported that 5.6% of patients were aged 0 to 4 years (110 injuries per 10,000) and 20.5% were aged 5 to 9 years (389 injuries per 10,000). In children aged 0 to 4 years and children aged 5 to 9 years, 17% and 39% of injuries involved a motor vehicle collision, respectively. For both age groups, in order of incidence, the three most common injured body parts were the face, head, and hands. The two most common locations of the injury were in the street (55.5%) and in the home (28.4%). Most injuries occurred during the summer months (in order of incidence, July, August, June). The transition from tricycle to bicycle provides an excellent time for a child to begin using a helmet. Federally approved bicycle helmets are effective in reducing head trauma, a major cause of death among young children. A study implemented an educational bicycle safety program for kindergarten-aged children and found that they were able to improve their knowledge of appropriate helmet-wearing technique (Cusimano et al., 2013).

Preschoolers, as passengers or pedestrians, are at great risk of an automobile-related accident. At this age, pedestrian injury is more likely to occur than is passenger injury. Preschoolers should be taught proper street-crossing techniques and, generally, should be supervised when crossing streets. Schwebel and colleagues (2012) discuss risk factors for child pedestrian injuries, which include developmental factors (cognitive and perceptual), distraction, temperament and personality, social influences (parents and peers), environmental risks, attention-deficient/hyperactivity disorder, and sleep and fatigue. The prevention strategies reviewed include parental instruction, school-based instruction (including crossing guards), street-side training, technology-based training, and community-based training.

## Biological Agents

Preschoolers seem healthier than toddlers, with fewer illnesses of the respiratory and gastrointestinal tracts. They have developed antibodies to many common organisms through exposure. Children usually become ill more often when they enter their first group situation, where they may be exposed to new organisms. This concerns parents and should be discussed by the nurse before the child begins attending a group setting. Increasingly, child care settings provide instruction to children about appropriate handwashing techniques to decrease disease transmission and provide relevant health-promotion teaching (Rosen et al., 2011).

Immunization recommendations are reviewed annually and updated with professional educational tools and parent-friendly resources. These resources for professionals and families can be found in a variety of formats, in both Spanish and English, at http://www.cdc.gov/vaccines/schedules/index.html. The American Academy of Pediatrics also publishes the most current recommendations annually, with a particular focus on the immunization needs of children. The 2012 recommendations can be found at http://www.healthychildren.org/english/tips-tools/pages/default.aspx#immunization-schedules. The child with a full course of immunizations as an infant receives repeated doses of diphtheria, tetanus, and acellular pertussis; measles, mumps, and rubella; and varicella vaccines between the fourth year and the sixth year (CDC, 2012). Many states require that all children in a school setting be fully immunized. Parents who choose not to immunize their children usually make this choice for religious reasons, but some parents worry about the risk of the immunization itself (Gilmour et al., 2011). Although vaccines provide an extremely safe way to combat communicable disease, issues about safety do arise. Individual health providers should develop their own strategies to impart evidence-based information, and participate in professional and public educational campaigns to disseminate the information widely (Gilmour et al., 2011). Because autism is often diagnosed around the same time a child is vaccinated, some parents have connected the onset of their child's autism with the vaccine. The American Academy of Pediatrics (2013) position statement refutes this association and cites numerous studies that report no link between various vaccinations and autism (for more information see https://www.aap.org/en-us/Documents/immunization_vaccine_studies.pdf).

The risk of consequences of the disease itself far outweighs any vaccine risk, but without first-hand experience with vaccine-preventable diseases such as measles, *Haemophilus influenzae* type b, or polio, families today may minimize their severity (Diekema, 2012). Nurses must remain informed about recommended vaccines, their schedule, and their risks and benefits to provide accurate evidence-based information to families.

Nurses who remain informed about the reasons for avoidance of immunization will be better able to increase parents' understanding of the possible consequences of omitting a dose. Incomplete immunization may also occur as a result of parental forgetfulness or procrastination. Mandatory immunization for school entry provides an effective incentive for these parents. Although immunization rates are increasing, disparities exist in certain regions of the United States (Diekema, 2012). Advances on the horizon include more combination vaccines to decrease the cost of administration. Noninjectable vaccines that could be inhaled or eaten would greatly enhance pediatric immunization programs with ease of administration and simplified storage.

Continued efforts to vaccinate all children are needed, especially children living in poverty, particularly in large cities, where they are traditionally undervaccinated (Diekema, 2012; Gilmour et al., 2011). Nurses use immunization registry programs to consolidate records, to remind parents, to evaluate the person's scheduled program, and to analyze issues for a particular population. Registry programs avoid duplication and are of particular value for the preschool age group that may not be involved in day care or preschool with mandated immunization. The CDC publishes recommendations for individuals who have omitted doses for some reason. These alternative schedules are updated regularly along with the routine schedules and are available at the CDC website (http://www.cdc.gov/vaccines/recs/schedules/child-schedule.htm). When immunizations have been omitted or delayed, the immunization schedule continues from the dose of the last vaccine. Parents should be fully informed about the potential side effects of immunizations. In most office and clinic settings, parents sign state-developed informed consent documents that describe potential side effects.

## Chemical Agents

Preschoolers face exposure to environmental pollutants. The young child's skin area relative to body mass is twice that of an adult's, which increases the risk of toxicity. Environmental exposure has been implicated in the increased prevalence of learning disabilities because of the unique vulnerability of a child's brain to chemicals (Landrigan & Goldman, 2011; Trasande & Liu, 2011; Tucker, 2012). Disparities exist among populations with regard to their risk. Ethnicity, socioeconomic status, and geographical location all have an impact on the risk of exposure (Landrigan & Goldman, 2011).

In particular, lead poisoning and elevated blood lead levels continue to be an ongoing concern in children younger than 5 years. Health care professionals should perform targeted screening for lead poisoning in children who are Medicaid enrolled or Medicaid eligible, foreign born, or identified as high risk by the CDC location-specific recommendations or by a personal risk questionnaire (Box 19-10). A carefully collected finger-stick sample is an acceptable method for measuring blood lead levels. The CDC recommends that the threshold for follow-up and

intervention for lead poisoning be a blood lead level of 10 mcg/dL or higher (Warniment et al., 2010).

Lead is found in products used in folk remedies for many reasons. In the preschool group, lead may be found in products used to treat upset stomach *(empacho)*, constipation, diarrhea, and vomiting. In Hispanic traditional medicine, these products, known as *greta, azarcon, alarcón, coral, luiga, maría luisa,* or *rueda,* may contain extremely high lead contents. Lead has also been found in traditional remedies from cultures other than the Hispanic group. For example, *ghasard,* an Indian traditional tonic, and *ba-baw-san,* a Chinese herbal remedy for colic, have also been found to contain lead. Sources of lead other than those found in traditional medicine include pottery, cosmetics, and food additives.

Chemical agents of concern for toddlers, such as pesticides, lead, and passive smoke, continue to merit consideration in the preschool population. Preschoolers, however, become more independent and understand the concepts of safe and poisonous.

More than 90% of US poisonings occur in the home (McGregor et al., 2009). Even though manufacturers enclose many children's medications in childproof packaging, the product may be administered incorrectly by the caregiver, or the child may experiment with another family member's colorful pills. For example, the medication used to treat attention-deficit/hyperactivity disorder, methylphenidate, poisons many children.

Many household products, drugs, carbon monoxide, pesticides, lead, mercury, polychlorinated biphenyls, ethers, and poisonous plants pose hazards to preschoolers. Secondary smoke and lead exposure represent negative chemical influences on the growing child.

Preschoolers should receive verbal explanations about poisonous or dangerous substances, but parents cannot rely on preschoolers to remember instructions. A poison control program from the University of Pittsburgh introduced a character called Mr. Yuk in 1971, and this symbol has continued to be used to increase awareness and access to poison control centers (http://www.chp.edu/CHP/mryuk). The ability to identify warning symbols such as Mr. Yuk helps preschoolers remain safe. Preschools and child care facilities often incorporate topics about environmental pollutants and dangerous substances into their curricula to promote the health of preschoolers. Information about poison control is widely available on-line (http://www.aapcc.org/dnn/default.aspx). The toll-free National Capital Poison Center number is 1-800-222-1212. From that number the caller is directed to the nearest poison control center.

Parents should teach children about the four forms of poison, which are *solids* (air fresheners, pills, vitamins, aspirin, lipstick), *liquids* (cleaning products, fuel, alcohol), *sprays* (furniture polish, oven cleaner, room deodorizer), and *invisibles* (carbon monoxide, space heater fumes). Communication with parents about environmental dangers remains a major role of the child care provider.

---

### BOX 19-10  Lead Poisoning Screening Criteria

Screen children who meet any of the following criteria:

- All Medicaid-enrolled or Medicaid-eligible children at 1 and 2 years of age
- All children who are identified as being at high risk on the basis of results of a personal risk questionnaire (if one of the following questions is answered "Yes" or "Don't know"):
  - Does your child live in or regularly visit a house that was built before 1950 (this could apply to a home day care center or the home of a babysitter or relative)?
  - Does your child live in or regularly visit a house built before 1978 with recent or ongoing renovations or remodeling (i.e., within the past 6 months)?
  - Does your child have a sibling or playmate who has or has had lead poisoning?
- All refugees, recent immigrants, and international adoptees on arrival in the United States; repeat screening 3 to 6 months later for children 6 months to 6 years of age
- All children who are identified to be at increased risk by the CDC's state or local screening recommendations (i.e., high-risk zip codes)

In the absence of recommendations from the CDC, screen all children at 1 and 2 years of age, and screen children 36 to 72 months of age who have not been previously screened.

Modified from American Academy of Pediatrics Committee on Environmental Health. (2005). Lead exposure in children: Prevention, detection, and management. *Pediatrics, 116*(4), 1036–1046.

---

## Cancer

Cancer mortality in preschool children has declined in the past 20 years; however, disparities attributed to race, ethnicity, poverty, and lack of health insurance exist (Bhatia, 2011). Approximately one-fifth of childhood cancers occur in preschool children (CDC, 2016b). Most cancer deaths annually in children from newborns to 4 years of age are a result primarily of leukemia and brain/central nervous system, endocrine (primarily neuroblastomas), and soft tissue malignancies (National Cancer Institute, n.d.). Even though mortality has decreased, the incidence of brain and other central nervous system tumors has increased (Landrigan & Goldman, 2011). **Acute lymphocytic leukemia,** the most common childhood cancer, accounts for approximately one-third of the cases of cancer in preschool children (CDC, 2016b). Although less common than other solid tumors, **retinoblastoma** merits attention because of the possible loss of vision. Remarkable advances in long-term survival of children with cancer have occurred. Early detection remains the key to successful treatment; therefore early, aggressive efforts have been invested in detection programs. Some of the increases in the rates of diagnosis may be attributed to improved imaging techniques and early detection.

## Leukemia

Leukemia (acute lymphocytic and acute myeloid) accounts for approximately 27% of the deaths in children (CDC, 2016b). The incidence of acute lymphocytic leukemia (ALL) rises from age 2 years, peaks at age 5 years, and diminishes through later childhood and adolescence. The dominant signs and symptoms of ALL appear suddenly, but often the child demonstrates a prodromal period of weakness, malaise, anorexia, fever, and tachycardia. Bone pain, petechiae, and hemorrhages after minor procedures such as dental extractions are encountered frequently. When an unexplained infection does not respond to management, suspicion should arise. Early detection and treatment of ALL has resulted in a marked increase in 5-year survival rates. Survival depends on the age at diagnosis, with the best survival rates occurring when diagnosis occurs during the preschool years (Hockenberry & Wilson, 2015).

With suspected leukemia, the nurse institutes secondary prevention strategies with an assessment that includes the following parameters:

- Examination of the cervical and peripheral lymph nodes
- Palpation and percussion of the liver and spleen
- Inspection of the skin for systemic signs of leukemia, such as pallor, purpura, petechiae, and **chloroma**, which is a localized tumor mass that has a greenish appearance and may be found in the skin, orbits, or other tissues in granulocytic forms of leukemia
- Inspection of the mouth for enlarged tonsils; hyperplasia of the gums; and red, friable gingivae
- Palpation of the sternum, bones, and joints for tenderness and pain

The rate of leukemia is higher in children with Down syndrome; therefore school nurses and public health nurses should monitor these children for early signs of the disease.

## Wilms' Tumor

Most cases of **Wilms' tumor** occur in children younger than 5 years. A strong correlation exists between Wilms' tumor and several congenital malformations. Genetic links may contribute to its occurrence in children with bilateral tumors and those who have family members with the disorder. When Wilms' tumor, aniridia (a congenital malformation of the iris of the eye), genitourinary malformations, and mental retardation occur together, the genetic association strengthens. However, survivors of Wilms' tumor that is unilateral at diagnosis possess a low risk of producing a child who will develop the disease. Information about the risk factors for Wilms' tumor is not definitive. The 5-year survival rates for children with this disease are excellent (Hockenberry & Wilson, 2015).

## Retinoblastoma

Even as the most common intraocular tumor in younger children, retinoblastoma affects only 300 children younger than 20 years each year in the United States. Most of these children are younger than 5 years. Genetic mutations contribute to the incidence of retinoblastoma, usually causing the bilateral form of the disease. Even though the tumor is uncommon, the scientific work surrounding its diagnosis and management has resulted in many of the methods used for treatment of other cancers. Survival rates are excellent (Hockenberry & Wilson, 2015).

The history usually reveals a slow symptom progression. To determine risk factors, the following questions should be asked:
- Do tumors of the eye run in your family?
- If tumors of the eye run in your family, which relatives were affected and how were they treated?
- Have you noticed that your child has eye problems (crossed or lazy eyes or difficulty seeing)?
- Have you noticed any changes in your child's eyes?

Screening eye examinations for high-risk children include the following:
- Visual acuity
- Red reflex, which appears whitish with retinoblastoma (cat's eye reflex)
- Ophthalmoscopic findings
- Lid lag, which is found with exophthalmos
- Strabismus, by doing the cover-uncover test

The cat's eye reflex and strabismus are the most common signs of retinoblastoma. Any suspicious findings indicate referral for further evaluation.

## Neuroblastoma

**Neuroblastoma,** a cancer of the sympathetic nervous system, begins in the abdomen, primarily in the adrenal gland, approximately 70% of the time. The remaining 30% of cases originate in cervical, thoracic, or pelvic areas. Parodi and colleagues (2014) reported a connection between maternal characteristics and perinatal factors in patients with neuroblastoma. More than 90% of diagnoses occur by age 5 years. Unfortunately, many of the children have metastases when the cancer is identified. Frequently, symptoms of secondary distribution bring the child to the health professional. The survival rate for children in whom neuroblastoma is diagnosed during the preschool years is increasing, but in other age groups it has remained static. There is little convincing evidence of specific risk factors. Prenatal exposure to pesticides and hormones and use of certain medications suggest an increased risk (Landrigan & Goldman, 2011).

## BOX 19-11 Warning Signs That May Indicate Childhood Cancer

Cancer remains a leading cause of death in children younger than 15 years, second only to injuries.

**General**
- Continued unexplained weight loss
- Persistent poor appetite
- Tires easily or lack of energy
- Tires constantly
- Noticeably pale

**Leukemia or Lymphomas: "Liquid Tumors" (Cancer of the Blood, Blood-Making System, Lymph Nodes)**
- Persistent fever (more than 2 weeks)
- Bruising without injury and purple or red patches appearing on the skin
- Swollen glands (lymph nodes) unrelated to infection
- Persistent bone pain or limping
- Paleness of the lips, skin, nails, or lining of the eyes

**Brain Tumor**
- Headaches, frequently with early morning vomiting
- Reflection in the pupil of the eye (eye tumor)
- Unexplained, persistent changes in behavior

**Kidney Tumors**
- Lump in the abdomen or abdominal enlargement
- Blood in the urine
- Bulging of the eyes
- Unexplained, persistent cough or chest pain
- A firm mass in the muscles

**Make Bath Time Examination Time**
- These complaints or physical findings should be interpreted only as warnings of possible serious disease. When these warnings are present, you should consult your physician at once.
- Do not forget that your children must be examined by a physician every year. The earlier cancer is detected, the better the chances are for a cure. With current treatment methods of surgery, radiation therapy, and chemotherapy (administration of anticancer drugs), the survival rate of children with certain forms of cancer has increased dramatically.

From Be Child Cancer Aware. (n.d.). Child cancer symptoms. Cancer Association of Greater New Orleans, New Orleans, LA. http://www.bechildcanceraware.org/child-cancer-info/childcancersymptoms.

Cancer in a child can be frightening to parents, particularly if there is a strong family history of cancers of any kind. Early detection continues to be associated with increased survival rates. Secondary prevention programs should include the warning signs of cancer in children. Routine procedures, such as a bath, provide opportunities for parents to examine the child for physical symptoms of disease that are outlined in Box 19-11.

### Asthma

The incidence of **asthma,** a chronic inflammatory disorder of the airways, is rising more rapidly in preschool children than in any other group (US Department of Health and Human Services, 2011). The inflammation in this disorder contributes to a hyperresponsive airway, limited airflow, and respiratory symptoms that include breathlessness, wheezing, cough, and chest tightness. The causes include genetic predisposition, allergens such as animal dander or dust mites, and nonspecific precipitants such as infections, exercise, weather, or stress. The rates for boys exceed those for girls, and the rates in the black and Hispanic populations exceed those in the non-Hispanic white population. Poverty contributes significantly to asthmatic illness, disability, and death (Azad et al., 2012; Tucker, 2012). Multiple factors contribute to exacerbation of asthma symptoms. High levels of exposure to tobacco smoke, pollutants, and allergens contribute. In addition to the generally known allergens of house mite dust and pet and rodent dander, cockroach particles have been implicated. Access to quality medical care, financial resources, and social support to manage the disease on a long-term basis exist in significantly different proportions from one population to another in the United States (US Department of Health and Human Services, 2011).

## DETERMINANTS OF HEALTH

### Social Factors and Environment

Some preschoolers become involved with groups outside their families, such as group child care settings, church groups, or family involvement in other activities, by age 3 years. Other children of the same age experience little outside contact. A preschool setting introduces the child to a wider social arena. Parents learn to release their child to encourage independent activity in a safe, supervised setting. Preschoolers test their independence, interactive skills, and self-discipline as they learn to function in a group. Preschool provides a transition to kindergarten and first grade, where group interaction skills are expected. Parents often select a preschool on the basis of geographical closeness to their home or a friend's recommendation, using the most practical approach (Box 19-12). With many child care facilities and options now available, parents frequently visit and evaluate a number of settings to determine the most appropriate for their needs (Bower et al., 2008).

### Culture and Ethnicity

Family cultural heritage continues to shape preschoolers. Health-promotion assessment should adapt to cultural differences (Box 19-13: Diversity Awareness). For example, a child who has never seen snow may not be able to know that it is cold. Unlike toddlers, preschoolers frequently ask why the family follows certain practices. These young children notice differences from one family to another. Their playmates may celebrate different holidays or practice family rituals different from their own. As preschoolers experience more activities outside their home, differences become more apparent. Discussion about the strength of cultural differences provides an excellent learning opportunity (Andrews & Boyle, 2015).

Preschoolers also notice ethnic differences in appearance and pronounce skin colors, eyes, and hairstyles as "pretty" or "ugly." The socialization process forms presumptions similar to those

BOX 19-12 **Evaluating a Child Care Setting**

Child care that meets the needs and expectations of parents will most likely ensure a happy preschooler as well. The questions that parents should consider in evaluating and choosing a child care setting include the following:

- Will my needs and those of my child be best met with a caregiver in a family home, commercial center, or preschool, or by having a person come to my home to care for my child?
- What kinds of backup plans will I need or will be available if the provider becomes ill?
- What are my standards for nutrition, safety, sanitation, and health, and can these standards be met at the chosen child care facility?
- How important is it to my child to be with other children? How many children would be ideal for my child's socialization needs?
- What personality attributes and educational preparation do I desire in my child's caregivers? What attributes do I dislike, and how will I deal with these attributes to maximize the care given to my child? How important is caregiver stability to me? Can I comfortably communicate with the staff to collaborate with my child's learning?
- What educational philosophy do I want in the setting? What involvement do I wish to have in the educational mission of the facility?
- Do the hours of the facility meet my personal and professional needs? Is close access to my job or home important to me?
- How are the children grouped, and what is the caregiver-to-child ratio?
- Does the cost of the service meet my financial needs? Can I pay part-time fees during vacation or when my child is ill for a lengthy period?
- Is accreditation of the facility mandatory for me to use it?
- What is my internal response or my general feelings about the setting when I visit it before my child's enrollment? Are the caregivers interacting with and responsive to the children? Are the children happy and interactive? Are the children's individual needs addressed appropriately? Is the environment supportive of my child's care? Is discipline appropriate?

BOX 19-13 **DIVERSITY AWARENESS**

*Preschool*

Three groups of 36 Chinese children (each with a mean age of 61 months) were studied to identify cognitive abilities that might distinguish children at risk of dyslexia: teacher- or parent-reported (and health care professional–confirmed) language delay; family history of dyslexia; and not at risk.

The cognitive skills studied included syllable awareness, tone detection, rapid automated naming, visual skill, and morphological awareness. Compared with the control group, the language-delayed group of children scored significantly lower on all measures. Children in the familial risk group performed significantly worse only on tone detection, morphological awareness, and word recognition.

Testing these skills may be important assessment tools for diagnosing the risks of reading problems and may be associated with broader cognitive impairment as found previously in various Indo-European languages.

From McBride-Chang, C., Lam, E., Doo, S., Wong, S. W., & Chow, Y. Y. (2008). Word recognition and cognitive profiles of Chinese pre-school children at risk for dyslexia through language delay or familial history of dyslexia. *Journal of Child Psychology and Psychiatry, 49*(2), 211–218.

of their family or playmates. Parents and caregivers who teach and role model positive behaviors allow children to see differences in others as being positive rather than negative. Mass media influences on physical attractiveness also contribute and become more significant to the adolescent.

Certain cultures apply more pressure for children to assume responsibility for younger siblings or household tasks. Confusion develops in preschoolers when the family's culture differs from that of most playmates. Disciplinary approaches differ from culture to culture. Uncertainty also results when parents integrate their cultural background into the community standards but the grandparents adhere to traditional cultural practices, rituals, and childrearing ideas.

## Levels of Policy Making and Health

Many safety-focused legislative bills have affected preschoolers (see Chapter 18). School issues, as discussed in Chapter 20, also affect this age group. With current concern about health care costs, financial programs that focus on children may lose when competing with the whole of health care. If overall funding for vulnerable populations such as the homeless and the poor decreases, child health care in general in the United States suffers. In the United States, one in every four children younger than 6 years lives in poverty. Poverty is associated with homelessness, which places the child at greater risk of death and less participation in health-promotion and disease-prevention programs (Kerker et al., 2011). In addition, homeless children in the population-based study in New York City by Kerker and colleagues (2011) were less likely to have blood lead levels tested than the comparison populations in outlying metropolitan areas. These children were also more likely than those living outside the city to have high lead levels (>10 mcg/dL). Homeless children had lower blood lead testing rates and a higher proportion of lead levels higher than 10 mcg/dL than did both comparison populations.

### Economics

Poverty influences preschoolers as it does any child. Unlike toddlers, preschoolers become more aware of family economic status. A preschooler may know that the family lacks money for toys but recognizes less the comprehensive limits to resources that influence the family lifestyle. In some cases, the family's financial history prevents attendance at preschool or influences exposure to expanded learning activities. Preschoolers realize money acquires food, toys, and clothes, but they do not yet have a concept of economic values. The child might trade an expensive item for a trinket that looks more interesting. A child who uses the earnings to buy something realizes that more must be earned to buy more things. The child thus begins to learn the concepts of earning and spending.

## Health Services/Delivery System

Access to health care resources for preschoolers is the same as that for toddlers. When preschoolers enter a school setting, admission may require that a health care worker screen them physically and developmentally. For indigent children, **Early and Periodic Screening, Diagnosis, and Treatment** (EPSDT), a Medicaid program, may fund the visit. Screening for individuals younger than 21 years who meet the economic criteria for Medicaid occurs in private offices, local health departments, and community clinics. Medicaid provides one screening examination per year, which includes the following elements:

- Medical history
- Assessment of physical growth, nutritional status, and mental development
- Inspection of ears, eyes, nose, mouth, teeth, and throat
- Vision screening
- Auditory screening
- Screening for cardiac abnormalities
- Screening for anemia
- Screening for the sickle cell trait
- Urine sampling
- Blood pressure reading
- Assessment and updating of immunizations
- Tuberculosis screening, when indicated
- Referral to a dentist for diagnosis and treatment for children aged 3 years or older

Referral for a complete physical examination addresses any health or developmental concerns identified during this screening. Eligible children receive EPSDT as a comprehensive service administered by Medicaid. Enactment of the Affordable Care Act in 2012 ensures health coverage for all children and free immunizations, affecting preschool children's health and health promotion (http://www.healthcare.gov/law/index.html).

## NURSING APPLICATION

Preschoolers show much interest in the tools and procedures of a health screening examination (Price & Gwinn, 2008)

(Box 19-14). These inquisitive children may play with the stethoscope, otoscope, and other diagnostic instruments. The nurse explains the tests in age-appropriate terminology and expects the child to cooperate for most of the visit. Preschoolers may show self-control during injections but definitely need a parent close by to offer support and encouragement. The nurse includes the preschooler in the history by directing questions about dietary intake and health practices, such as tooth brushing, favorite activities, and friends. At this age, children begin taking some interest in health, developing the cognitive maturity to learn many health-promotion skills that they will use for the rest of their lives.

## SUMMARY

Schedules for preventive health care during the preschool years include visits at 4 and 5 years of age. Each visit includes an ongoing history; growth, physical, and developmental assessment; and discussion of age-appropriate developmental concerns.

In addition to the office or clinic contact, the nurse may consult with a preschool nurse or a nurse for a primary school and preschool. Early exposure to and reinforcement of health care information as part of preschool education lays a foundation for later healthy lifestyle habits, which influence overall societal health. Health as a curricular subject during the school-age years continues this focus. The school nurse's role in health promotion and prevention of illness is discussed in Chapter 20.

---

### BOX 19-14   Health-Promotion Screening for Preschool Children

**Annually**
- Health history
- Height and weight
- Blood pressure
- Vision screening (age 3–4 years)
- Developmental and behavioral assessment
- Physical examination

**Periodically**
- Immunizations based on recommended schedule
- Ensure currency
- Diphtheria, tetanus, acellular pertussis
- Oral poliovirus
- Pneumococcal
- Measles, mumps, rubella
- *Haemophilus influenzae* type b
- Hepatitis B
- Varicella
- Hematocrit or hemoglobin level at least once after age 9 months
- Urinalysis at 5 years' old

**Screenings for High-Risk Children**
- Lead
- Tuberculosis
- Cholesterol

**Anticipatory Guidance**
- Injury prevention
- Child safety car seat (age less than 5 years) or seat belt
- Lap and shoulder belt (age 5 years or older)
- Use helmet and avoid traffic when bicycling
- Smoke detectors, flame-retardant sleepwear
- Hot water temperature less than 125°F
- Window and stair guards, pool fence
- Safe storage of drugs, toxic substances, firearms, matches
- Close availability of syrup of ipecac, poison control phone number
- Parents and caretakers trained in cardiopulmonary resuscitation
- Violence prevention
- Nutrition and exercise
- Limit saturated fats; maintain caloric balance; and emphasize grain, fruit, vegetable intake
- Regular fun physical activity
- Tobacco
- Effects of passive smoking
- Antitobacco messages
- Dental health
- Floss, brush with fluoridated toothpaste at least daily
- Regular visits to dentist

## CASE STUDY

### Preschool Child: Ricky

Ricky, age 4 years, arrives in the clinic with his mother. Ricky lives with his mother and father, who both work full-time, and his infant sister. Their extended family lives in a different state more than 100 miles away. Both parents are of average height and in good health. Ricky's mother mentions that Ricky often expresses frustration, particularly in regard to food. Conflict over food occurs every day. Mealtime is a battle to get him to eat, unless his mother feeds him. Ricky's baby sister seems to tolerate all baby foods but requires her mother to spoon-feed. Ricky's mother is quite frustrated and concerned that he will become malnourished.

#### Reflective Questions

- What additional assessment information would you collect?
- What questions would you ask, and how would you further explore this issue with the mother?
- In what ways does the distance of the extended family influence this family's approach to health promotion?
- What factors would you consider to determine whether malnourishment is a factor in this family?

## CARE PLAN

### Ineffective Coping in Preschool Child: Ricky

**\*NURSING DIAGNOSIS: Ineffective coping related to parental feedback for regressive behaviors and lack of consistent limits and fulfillment of appropriate responsibilities**

#### Defining Characteristics

- Parent verbalization of need for help
- Changes in the usual behavior patterns of the child

#### Related Factors

- Inconsistent methods of parental discipline
- Inadequate impulse control
- Lack of social skills

#### Expected Outcomes

- The child will separate from his parents without incident (tantrum, crying).
- The child will join a community or church peer group activity.
- The child will perform one household task (picking up his toys) before bedtime every evening.
- The child will demonstrate independent self-care behaviors (feed himself).
- The parents will have clear, consistent, and age-appropriate expectations for behavior.
- The parents will explain the rationale for limiting a socially unacceptable or unsafe behavior as soon as it is displayed.

#### Interventions

- Discuss with the parents the process of growth and development and the child's need to learn how to compromise, take turns, and channel energy appropriately.
- Use a prescreening developmental questionnaire to validate general assessment data.
- Encourage the parents to leave the child in someone else's care while they go shopping or to see a movie.
- Encourage the mother to formulate a bedtime ritual with the child that does not include her sitting in his room until he falls asleep.

- Discuss with the parents and the child what "jobs" he can do at home and the expectation that they be performed daily.
- Suggest laying out the child's clothes so that he can dress himself. Set a time to be dressed, such as before or after a certain television program.
- Explore with the parents the availability of playgroups or community activities for the child.
- Encourage the parents to take the child to the neighborhood playground so that he can meet and play with other children.
- Have the child help around the house alongside his parents. Specify "work" and "play" times.
- Encourage the parents to praise the child for age-appropriate behaviors, being careful not to bribe him to perform.
- Discuss the principles of discipline consistency, immediacy, realistic expectations, and clear explanations.
- Recognize the parents' frustration and encourage them to try different approaches, such as limited choices, diversion, and incentives ("when you finish your meat, we'll play a game").
- Suggest that the parents keep a diary of how long an approach was tried and how consistently the child responded.
- Discuss the decrease in appetite and reliance of food fads that typify the child's age. Review the principles of nutrition, timing of snacks, and ways of making food attractive to children.
- Refer the parents and the child to a nutritionist for nutrition counseling.

#### Evaluation

- Parents make appropriate verbal, nonverbal, and eye contact.
- Parents demonstrate correct caregiver techniques.
- Parents verbalize intent to maintain relationships.
- Parents attend routine well-child care appointments.
- Parents provide developmentally appropriate play activities.
- Parents describe healthy ways to express frustration.

## ⓔ EVOLVE CHAPTER FEATURES

http://evolve.elsevier.com/Edelman/
• Study Questions

## REFERENCES

American Academy of Pediatrics. (2013). Vaccine Safety: Examine the evidence. https://www.aap.org/en-us/Documents/immunization_vaccine_studies.pdf.

Andrews, M. M., & Boyle, J. S. (2015). *Transcultural concepts in nursing care* (7th ed.). New York, NY: Lippincott.

Archibald, L., Joanisse, M., & Edmunds, A. (2011). Specific language or working memory impairments: A small scale observational study. *Child Language Teaching & Therapy, 27*(3), 294–312.

Azad, M. B., et al. (2012). Influence of socioeconomic status trajectories on innate immune responsiveness in children. *PLoS ONE, 7*(6), e38669.

Becker, D. R., et al. (2014). Physical activity, self-regulation, and early academic achievement in preschool children. *Early Education and Development, 25*(1), 56–70.

Bhatia, S. (2011). Disparities in cancer outcomes: Lessons learned from children with cancer. *Pediatric Blood and Cancer, 56*(6), 994–1002.

Bower, J. K., et al. (2008). The childcare environment and children's physical activity. *American Journal of Preventive Medicine, 34*(1), 23–29.

Boyd, B. A., et al. (2010). Infants and toddlers with autism spectrum disorder: Early identification and early intervention. *Journal of Early Intervention, 32*(2), 75–98.

Brown, W. H., et al. (2009). Social and environmental factors associated with preschoolers' non-sedentary physical activity. *Child Development, 80*(1), 45–58.

Center on the Developing Child at Harvard University. (2010). The foundations of lifelong health are built in early childhood. http://developingchild.harvard.edu/resources/the-foundations-of-lifelong-health-are-built-in-early-childhood/.

Centers for Disease Control and Prevention (CDC). (2007). Surveillance summaries: Fatal injuries among children by race and ethnicity—United States, 1999–2002. *Morbidity and Mortality Weekly Report, 56*(SS-5), 1–20.

Centers for Disease Control and Prevention (CDC). (2012). Recommended immunization schedules for persons aged 0-18 years— United States, 2012. *Morbidity and Mortality Weekly Report, 61*(5), 1–4.

Centers for Disease Control and Prevention (CDC). (2016a). Autism Spectrum Disorder: Data and statistics. https://www.cdc.gov/ncbddd/autism/data.html.

Centers for Disease Control and Prevention (CDC). (2016b). United States cancer statistics: 2013 Childhood cancer by primary site. https://nccd.cdc.gov/uscs/childhoodcancerbyprimarysite.aspx.

Centers for Disease Control and Prevention (CDC). (2017). Injury prevention & control: Data and statistics (web-based injury statistics query and reporting system—WISQRS). https://www.cdc.gov/injury/wisqars/index.html.

Chen, W. S., et al. (2013). Epidemiology of nonfatal bicycle injuries presenting to United States emergency departments, 2001–2008. *Academic Emergency Medicine: Official Journal of the Society for Academic Emergency Medicine, 20*, 570–575.

Children's Defense Fund. (2012). *Protect children not guns 2012.* Washington, DC: Children's Defense Fund.

Chlebowski, C., et al. (2013). Large-scale use of the Modified Checklist for Autism in Toddlers in low-risk toddlers. *Pediatrics, 131*(4), e1121–e1127.

Christensen, D. L., et al. (2016). Prevalence and characteristics of autism spectrum disorder among 4-year-old children in the Autism and Developmental Disabilities Monitoring Network. *Journal of Developmental and Behavioral Pediatrics: JDBP, 37*(1), 1–8.

Clark, M. B., & Slayton, R. L. (2014). Fluoride use in caries prevention in the primary care setting. *Pediatrics, 134,* 626–633.

Clifton, C. (2014). Focus on fluorides: Update on the use of fluoride for the prevention of dental caries. *Journal of Evidenced-Based Dental Practices, 14,* 95–102.

Conti-Ramsden, G., & Durkin, K. (2012). Language development and assessment in the preschool period. *Neuropsychology Review, 22*(7), 1–18.

Cusimano, M. D., et al. (2013). Evaluation of a bicycle helmet safety program for children. *The Canadian Journal of Neurological Sciences, 40,* 710–716.

Decina, L. E., & Lococo, K. H. (2005). Child restraint system use and misuse in six states. *Accid Anal Prev, 37,* 583–590.

Diekema, D. S. (2012). Improving childhood vaccination rates. *New England Journal of Medicine, 366*(5), 391–393.

Division of Adolescent and School Health, National Center for Chronic Disease Prevention and Health Promotion. (2011). School health guidelines to promote healthy eating and physical activity. *MMWR Recommendations & Reports, 60*(5), 1–78.

Dogra, S., Meisner, B. A., & Ardern, C. I. (2010). Variation in mode of physical activity by ethnicity and time since immigration: A cross-sectional analysis. *International Journal of Behavioral Nutrition & Physical Activity, 7*(10), 1–11.

Driscoll, A., & Nagel, N. G. (2008). *Early childhood education: Birth - 8: The world of children, families, and educators* (4th ed.). Upper Saddle River, NJ: Allyn and Bacon.

Engel, S. C. (2015). Drowning episodes: Prevention and resuscitation tips. *The Journal of Family Practice, 64*(2), E1–E6.

Faulkenberry, J. G., & Schaechter, J. (2015). Reporting on pediatric unintentional firearm injury-who's responsible. *The Journal of Trauma and Acute Care Surgery, 79*(3 Suppl. 1), S2–S8.

Felton, H., et al. (2015). Unintentional, non-fatal drowning of children: US trends and racial/ethnic disparities. *BMJ Open, 5*(12), e008444.

Fleischer, D. M., et al. (2012). Allergic reactions to foods in preschool-aged children in a prospective observational food allergy study. *Pediatrics, 130*(1), e25–e32.

Fountain, C., et al. (2015). Association between assisted reproductive technology conception and autism in California, 1997–2007. *American Journal of Public Health, 105*(5), 963–971.

Freitag, C. M., et al. (2010). Genetics of autistic disorders: Review and clinical implications. *European Child & Adolescent Psychiatry, 19*(3), 169–178.

Frost, J. L., Wortham, S. C., & Reifel, S. C. (2008). *Play and child development* (3rd ed.). Upper Saddle River, NJ: Prentice-Hall.

Gagne, C., & Harnois, I. (2014). How to motivate childcare workers to engage preschoolers in physical activity. *Journal of Physical Activity and Health, 11,* 364–375.

Gance-Cleveland, B., et al. (2009). Changes in nurse practitioners' knowledge and behaviors following brief training on the Healthy Eating and Activity Together (HEAT) guidelines. *Journal of Pediatric Health Care, 23*(4), 222–230.

Garrison, M. M., Liekweg, K., & Christakis, D. A. (2011). Media use and child sleep: The impact of content, timing, and environment. *Pediatrics, 128*(1), 29–35.

Gilmour, J., et al. (2011). Childhood immunization: When physicians and parents disagree. *Pediatrics, 128*(Suppl. 4), S167–S174.

Gonzalez-Mena, J. (2012). *Child, family and community, family centered early care and education* (6th ed.). Upper Saddle River, NJ: Prentice-Hall.

Gupta, R. S., et al. (2011). The prevalence, severity, and distribution of childhood food allergy in the United States. *Pediatrics, 128*(1), e9–e17.

Hemenway, D., & Solnick, S. J. (2015). Children and unintentional firearm death. *Injury Epidemiology, 2*(1), 26.

Hinkley, T., et al. (2012). Correlate of preschool children's physical activity. *American Journal of Preventative Medicine, 43*(2), 159–167.

Hoban, T. F. (2010). Sleep disorders in children. *Annals of the New York Academy of Sciences, 1184*(1), 1–14.

Hockenberry, M. J., & Wilson, D. (Eds). (2015). *Wong's nursing care of infants and children* (10th ed.). St. Louis, MO: Mosby.

Houston, K. T., et al. (2011). Newborn hearing screening: An analysis of current practices. *Volta Review, 111*(2), 109–120.

Ingram, J. C., et al. (2011). Identifying facilitators and barriers for home injury prevention interventions for pre-school children: A systematic review of the quantitative literature. *Health Education Research, 27*(2), 258–268.

Kaakinen, J., et al. (2010). *Family nursing: Theory, practice and research* (4th ed.). Philadelphia, PA: F.A. Davis.

Kaerts, N., et al. (2012). Readiness signs used to define the proper moment to start toilet training: A review of the literature. *Neurourology and Urodynamics, 31*(4), 437–440.

Kalpidou, M. D., et al. (2004). Regulation of emotion and behavior among 3- and 5-year-olds. *Journal of General Psychology, 131*(2), 159–178.

Kerker, B. D., et al. (2011). A population-based assessment of the health of homeless families in New York City, 2001–2003. *American Journal of Public Health, 101*(3), 546–553.

Kemp, M. A., Lawson, Z., & Macguire, A. S. (2014). Patterns of burns and scalds in children. *Archives of Disease in Children, 99*(4), 316–321.

Kendrick, D., et al. (2013). Home safety education and provision of safety equipment for injury prevention (review). *Evidence-Based Child Health: A Cochrane Review Journal, 8*(3), 761–939.

Kissin, D. M., et al. (2015). Association of assisted reproductive technology (ART) treatment and parental infertility diagnosis with autism in ART-conceived children. *Human Reproduction, 30*(2), 454–465.

Kochanska, G., et al. (2010). Children's conscience during toddler and preschool years, moral self, and a competent, adaptive developmental trajectory. *Developmental Psychology, 46*(5), 1320–1332.

Kornides, M. L., et al. (2011). Factors associated with obesity in Latino children: A review of the literature. *Hispanic Health Care International, 9*(3), 127–136.

Landrigan, P. J., & Goldman, L. R. (2011). Children's vulnerability to chemicals: A challenge and opportunity to strengthen health and environmental policy. *Health Affairs, 30*(5), 842–850.

Langevin, M., Packman, A., & Onslow, M. (2009). Peer responses to stuttering in the preschool setting. *American Journal of Speech-Language Pathology, 18*(3), 264–276.

LeBlanc, J. J., & Fagiolini, M. (2011). Autism: A "critical period" disorder? *Neural Plasticity, 2011*, 921680.

Lee, L. K., Farrell, C. A., & Mannix, R. (2015). Restraint use in motor vehicle crash fatalities in children 0 year to 9 years old. *The Journal of Trauma and Acute Care Surgery, 79*(3 Suppl. 1), S55–S60.

Lee, S. H., & Im, E. (2010). Ethnic differences in exercise and leisure time physical activity among midlife women. *Journal of Advanced Nursing, 66*(4), 814–827.

Liou, Y. M., Liou, T., & Chang, L. (2010). Obesity among adolescents: Sedentary leisure time and sleeping as determinants. *Journal of Advanced Nursing, 66*(6), 1246–1256.

Luby, J. B., et al. (2009). Shame and guilt in preschool depression: Evidence for elevations in self-conscious emotions in depression as early as age 3. *Journal of Child Psychology & Psychiatry, 50*(9), 1156–1166.

Macy, M. L., & Freed, G. L. (2012). Child passenger safety practices in the U.S.: Disparities in light of updated recommendations. *American Journal of Preventive Medicine, 43*(3), 272–281.

Marshall, S., Golley, R., & Hendrie, G. (2011). Expanding the understanding of how parenting influences the dietary intake and weight status of children: A cross-sectional study. *Nutrition & Dietetics, 68*(2), 127–133.

May-Benson, T. A., Koomar, J. A., & Teasdale, A. (2009). Incidence of pre-, peri-, and post-natal birth and developmental problems of children with sensory processing disorder and children with autism spectrum disorder. *Frontiers in Integrative Neuroscience, 3*, 31.

McCann, J. C., & Ames, B. N. (2007). An overview of evidence for a causal relation between iron deficiency during development and deficits in cognitive or behavioral function. *American Journal of Clinical Nutrition, 85*(4), 931–945.

McGregor, T., Parkar, M., & Rao, S. (2009). Evaluation and management of common childhood poisonings. *American Family Physician, 79*(5), 397–403.

Mefford, H. C., Batshaw, M. L., & Hoffman, E. P. (2012). Genomics, intellectual disability, and autism. *The New England Journal of Medicine, 366*(8), 733–743.

Moreno, A. S. (2014). Examining factors that influence a mandated reporter's decision to report child abuse. http://search.proquest.com/docview/1701636331.

Nappo-Dattoma, L. (2011). Updated dietary standards: The 2010 dietary guidelines for Americans, MyPlate and other nutrition education resources for the oral health professional. *Access, 25*(8), 16–19.

National Association for Sport and Physical Education (2009). *Active start: A statement of physical activity guidelines for children birth to five years* (2nd ed.). Reston, VA: National Association for Sport and Physical Education Publications.

National Cancer Institute. (n.d.). Cancer statistics. http://seer.cancer.gov/statistics/index.html.

National Sleep Foundation. (2011). Children and sleep. http://www.sleepfoundation.org/article/sleep-topics/children-and-sleep.

O'Donoghue, L., et al. (2012). Visual acuity measures do not reliably detect childhood refractive error—An epidemiological study. *PLoS ONE, 7*(3), e34441.

Orton, E., et al. (2012). Independent risk factors for injury in pre-school children: Three population-based nested case-control studies using routine primary care data. *PLoS ONE, 7*(4), e35193.

Parodi, S., et al. (2014). Risk of neuroblastoma, maternal characteristics and perinatal exposures: The SETIL study. *Cancer Epidemiology, 38*(6), 686–694.

Pellegrini, A. D., & Smith, P. K. (1998). The development of play during childhood: Forms and possible functions. *Child and Adolescent Mental Health, 3*(2), 51–57.

Phillips, D. A., et al. (2009). Sibling violence silenced: Rivalry, competition, wrestling, playing, roughhousing, benign. *Advances in Nursing Science, 32*(2), E1–E16.

Prevent Blindness. (2017). Home eye tests for children: Should parents test their child's eyesight at home? http://www .preventblindness.org/home-eye-tests-children.

Price, D. L., & Gwinn, J. F. (2008). *Pediatric nursing.* St. Louis, MO: Saunders.

Prior, M., et al. (2011). Relationships between language impairment, temperament, behavioural adjustment and maternal factors in a community sample of preschool children. *International Journal of Language & Communication Disorders, 46*(4), 489–494.

Rogers, S. C., et al. (2013). Can nurse education in the postpartum period reduce car seat misuse among newborns? *The Journal of Trauma and Acute Care Surgery, 75*(4 Suppl. 3), S319–S323.

Rosen, L., et al. (2011). Enabling hygienic behavior among preschoolers: Improving environmental conditions through a multifaceted intervention. *American Journal of Health Promotion, 25*(4), 248–256.

Rowhani-Rahbar, A., Simonetti, J. A., & Rivara, F. P. (2016). Effectiveness of Interventions to Promote Safe Firearm Storage. *Epidemiologic Reviews,* 1–14.

Safe Kids Worldwide. (2015). Car seat safety tips. http://www.safekids .org/car-seat.

Scattone, D., Raggio, D. J., & May, W. (2011). Comparison of the Vineland adaptive behavior scales, second edition, and the Bayley scales of infant and toddler development, third edition. *Psychological Reports, 109*(2), 626–634.

Schonhaut, L., et al. (2013). Validity of the Ages and Stages Questionnaires in term and preterm infants. *Pediatrics, 131*(5), e1468.

Schwebel, D. C., Davis, A. L., & O'Neal, E. E. (2012). Child pedestrian injury: A review of behavioral risks and preventative strategies. *American Journal of Lifestyle Medicine, 6*(4), 292–302.

Selwyn, N., Boraschi, D., & Ozkula, S. M. (2009). Drawing digital pictures: An investigation of primary pupils' representations of ICT and schools. *British Educational Research Journal, 35*(6), 909–928.

Shumway, S., et al. (2011). Brief report: Symptom onset patterns and functional outcomes in young children with autism spectrum disorders. *Journal of Autism and Developmental Disorders, 41*(12), 1727–1732.

Trasande, L., & Liu, Y. (2011). Reducing the staggering costs of environmental disease in children, estimated at $76.6 billion in 2008. *Health Affairs, 30*(5), 863–870.

Tucker, P. G. (2012). *Principals of pediatric environmental health— Course WB2089.* Washington, DC: US Department of Health and Human Services, Agency for Toxic Substances and Disease Registry. http://www.atsdr.cdc.gov/csem/csem.html.

US Department of Agriculture, & US Department of Health and Human Services (2010). *Dietary guidelines for Americans 2010* (7th ed.). Washington, DC: US Government Printing Office.

US Department of Health and Human Services. (2011). 2020 topics and objectives. http://www.healthypeople.gov/2020/topics -objectives.

US Department of Health and Human Services. (2014) Healthy People 2020. http://www.healthypeople.gov/2020/.

Vriend, J., & Corkum, P. (2011). Clinical management of behavioral insomnia of childhood. *Psychology Research and Behavior Management, 4*(1), 69–79.

Warniment, C., Tsang, K., & Galazka, S. S. (2010). Lead poisoning in children. *American Family Physician, 81*(6), 751–757.

Warren, J. J., et al. (2009). A longitudinal study of dental caries risk among very young low SES children. *Community Dentistry and Oral Epidemiology, 37*(2), 116–122.

Water, T. (2011). Critical moments in preschool obesity: The call for nurses and communities to assess and intervene. *Contemporary Nurse: A Journal for the Australian Nursing Profession, 40*(1), 60–70.

Weaver, N. L., et al. (2013). Promoting correct car seat use in parents of young children: Challenges, recommendations, and implications for health communication. *Health Promotion Practice, 14*(2), 301–307.

Weiss, J. (2010). Prevention of drowning. *Pediatrics, 126*(1), e253–e262.

Wright, J. T., et al. (2014). Fluoride toothpaste efficacy and safety in children younger than 6 years. *Journal of the American Dental Association, 145*(2), 182–189.

Yoo, J., Slack, K. S., & Holl, J. L. (2010). The impact of health-promoting behaviors on low-income children's health: A risk and resilience perspective. *Health & Social Work, 35*(2), 133–143.

Yoshinaga-Itano, C. (2011). Achieving optimal outcomes from EHDI. *ASHA Leader, 16*(11), 14–17.

# 20

# School-Age Child

*Leslie Kennard Scott*

## OBJECTIVES

*After completing this chapter, the reader will be able to:*

- Identify expected physical and developmental changes occurring in the school-age child.
- Explore stages of cognitive development of the school-age child, particularly its relation to academic skills and performance.
- Appraise relevant health-promotion needs and common health risk factors found in the school-age child.
- Analyze cultural, societal, peer influence, and stress on development in the school-age child.
- Describe common developmental problems that occur in the school-age child including ways to assist parents in the management of these common problems.
- Determine strategies for family (parents) to improve child's self-concept, socialization abilities, and stress reduction in the school-age child.

## KEY TERMS

Astigmatism
Asthma
Attention-deficit/hyperactivity disorder (ADHD)
Auditory acuity
Auditory learners
Bullying
Child abuse
Chronic serous otitis media
Classifying and ordering
Concrete operation
Conservation
Coping strategies
Dental caries
Depression
Discipline
Disorders of arousal
Dyslexia
Encopresis
Enuresis
Gastroenteritis
Genomics
*Healthy People 2020* initiatives
Human papilloma virus
Hyperopic (farsighted)
Hypertension

Individualized educational plan
Individuals with Disabilities Education Act (IDEA)
Industry versus inferiority
Intelligence
Intelligence quotient (IQ)
Kinesthetic learners
Latchkey children
Learning disability
Lice
Limit setting
Malocclusion
Menarche
Meningococcal vaccination
Moral development
Myopia (nearsightedness)
No Child Left Behind Act of 2001
Obesity
Orthodontic care
Ossification
Overweight
Pediculosis
Peer groups
Phonics
Preconventional
Puberty

Public Law 94-142 (Education for All Handicapped Children Act)
Punishment
Scabies
Section 504 of the Rehabilitation Act of 1973, Amendment Act of 2008
Self-concept
Self-discovery
Self-esteem
Sexual abuse
Sleep apnea
Sleep talking
Sleepwalking
Snellen chart
Socialization
Somatization
Standardized growth charts
State Children's Health Insurance Program (SCHIP)
Talismans
Tooth eruption
Tympanograms
Visual acuity
Visual learners
Vision screening programs

## THINK ABOUT IT

### School-Age Bullying

Liam is 9 years old and has recently started demonstrating withdrawn behavior. His mother reports "he used to enjoy school." Recently, he has mentioned wanting to stay home from school and has become apathetic regarding participating in school-related activities. Two weeks ago, his mother reports she began driving him to school. "He hasn't wanted to walk to school with his friends lately. I don't understand what is going on; he tells me 'it's nothing.'" He was performing well in school until this most recent grading period. His teacher has voiced concern that Liam seems "distracted" and is not participating in group work conducted in class. Liam's father has voiced frustration that he seems to be "losing" things too. "Earlier this week he lost his backpack. Last week it was a jacket."

- Is Liam's behavior typical for a 9-year-old male child?
- How might a 9-year-old female child's behavior differ from Liam's in this situation?
- As a health care professional, how might you guide this family in finding ways to address Liam's behavior?
- How might you assist/counsel Liam on developing skills associated with resilience?
- Are there any further underlying issues that may be contributing to Liam's behavior?

### TABLE 20-1 GROWTH AND DEVELOPMENT

**Motor Development of the School-Age Child**

| Age (yr) | Gross Motor | Fine Motor |
|---|---|---|
| 5 | Dresses independently<br>Runs well and jumps | Prints letters<br>Ties shoes, buttons<br>Draws triangle, square |
| 6–8 | Balances on one foot for 10 sec<br>Can perform tandem gait<br>Pedals a bicycle<br>Is skilled in physical activities, running, skipping | Spreads with knife<br>Holds pencil with fingertip<br>Draws a person with three to six parts<br>Cuts and pastes<br>Aligns letters horizontally<br>Knows right from left |
| 8–10 | Has good body balance<br>Enjoys vigorous activities<br>Has increased coordination | Spaces words and letters with writing<br>Draws a diamond<br>Has good eye-hand coordination<br>Bathes self<br>Sews and builds models |
| 10–12 | Balances on one foot for 15 sec<br>Catches a fly ball<br>May experience clumsiness from prepubertal growth spurt<br>Possesses all basic motor skills similar to adult | Writes well<br>Has skills similar to those of an adult |

From Ball, J. W., Bindler, R. C., & Cowan, K. J. (2013). *Child health nursing: Partnering with children & families.* Upper Saddle River, NJ: Prentice Hall.

"The school-age years" is a span of time between a child's entrance to kindergarten and the beginning of adolescence, a range from 6 to 10 years of age. During this period observable differences in growth, development, and cognitive ability are prominent. Consider how different the child entering kindergarten is from the preadolescent, particularly the differences in size as well as mental ability. Children grow (physically) much more slowly during this period as compared with growth during infancy and adolescence. Fine and gross motor skills are being perfected, and mental abilities grow tremendously as the child learns to read, write, and compute mathematics, in addition to other topics of interest (Table 20-1). Relationships outside the family, including **peer groups**, are also developing during this phase of growth and development.

Most children are relatively healthy during this period. Health-promotion and health-maintenance strategies are important. During this period of development, children learn to accept personal responsibility and participate in the management of self-care tasks in the areas of personal hygiene, nutrition, physical activity, sleep, and safety. Nurses fill a significant role in the facilitation of parental roles and child roles in meeting growth, developmental, and self-care aspects of the school-age child (Centers for Disease Control and Prevention [CDC], 2015c; Goldfarb et al., 2011).

## BIOLOGY AND GENETICS

A child's growth and development is influenced by genetic inheritance, nutrition, and the physical-sociocultural environments in which the child lives. The school-age child has an overall slimmer appearance as compared with the preschool child. Their legs are longer as compared with the rest of the body, allowing greater strength, balance, coordination, and fluidity of motion

in running, jumping, climbing, throwing, and riding a bicycle (Goldfarb et al., 2011).

Most body systems reach adult level of function during the school-age years. Before 6 years of age, children use the diaphragm as the primary breathing muscle. After 6 years of age, thoracic muscles develop, and the respiratory rate slows to 14 to 24 breaths per minute (Moses, 2015). The school-age child's head circumference continues to grow. However, after age 5 years, head growth slows until **puberty**, at which time the head and brain reach adult circumference measurements (53–54 cm; 21 inches) (Goldfarb et al., 2011). The heart slowly grows in size, and the heart rate slows to an average rate of 60 to 160 beats per minute, approaching that of an adult. Mean blood pressure is lower in this age group than in adults and ranges from 95 to 105 mmHg systolic and from 57 to 71 mmHg diastolic (Moses, 2015). The gastrointestinal system is maturing with increased stomach capacity, resulting in less need for snacks and decreased calorie needs as compared with the preschooler. Bladder capacity increases. The immune system is better able to produce an antibody-antigen response (Durani, 2015). By puberty the endocrine system (with the exception of reproductive function) approaches adult capacity and function.

## Elevated Blood Pressure

The long-term effects of elevated blood pressure, **hypertension**, in adults are well known and documented. The realization that adult hypertension often begins in childhood has encouraged efforts to screen young children for elevated blood pressure. The American Academy of Pediatrics (AAP) and the US Preventive Services Task Force recommend that children have their blood pressure measured annually, beginning at 3 years of age (Moyer, 2013). This recommendation has transpired as a result of concerns of higher blood pressures in children in the past 2 decades, demonstrating risk of cardiovascular disease (Riley & Bluhm, 2012; Rodriguez-Cruz, 2015). Approximately 5 in every 100 children have higher than normal blood pressure (AAP, 2015b). Blood pressure among school-age children may differ greatly depending on the height and weight of the child.

Black American children and Mexican American children should be followed up closely because of earlier onset and end-stage organ damage in those with hypertension as compared with white children (AAP, 2015b; American Heart Association [AHA], 2014b; Riley & Bluhm, 2012; Moyer, 2013). A family history of hypertension or identification of an elevated blood pressure in a child mandates close monitoring and assessment of cardiovascular risk factors at well-child checkups during the school-age years (AAP, 2015b; Moyer, 2013). Differentiation between primary and secondary hypertension should be determined in any school-age child with elevated blood pressure (Moyer, 2013).

## Physical Growth

Although many children have "spurts" of growth alternating with periods of minimal growth, height and weight growth velocities assume a slower and steadier pace as compared with earlier years of growth. The school-age child gains approximately 5 cm (2 inches) in height per year and 2 to 3 kg (4.4–6.6 pounds) in weight per year until puberty, at which time growth rates increase. (Lourenco et al., 2012). Black American children tend to be slightly larger and Asian American children tend to be somewhat smaller than their Caucasian counterparts, as plotted on growth charts that are believed to be standardized for various ethnic groups (World Health Organization, 2015a). Before the onset of puberty there is little difference in size between boys and girls. However, toward the latter part of this developmental stage, girls tend to grow more rapidly in height and weight (Harding, 2015). A preadolescent increase in height and weight tends to occur at approximately 10 years of age in girls and 12 years of age in boys. However, maturation rates differ, resulting in a wide range of sizes in both boys and girls, particularly among those aged 10 to 12 years (Harding, 2015; Lourenco et al., 2012).

Black American and Mexican American children mature earlier than Caucasian children (Bordini & Rosenfield, 2011). Black American children are often taller and heavier than their Caucasian counterparts. They also tend to have longer and denser bones, slimmer hips, more muscle, and less fat on their limbs than on their central body as compared with Caucasian children (Medina-Gomez, et al., 2016). Girls tend to mature, enter puberty, and stop growing earlier than boys. From birth, girls tend to have more fat than boys, and after puberty girls have a greater percentage of body weight derived from fat. Adiposity has a direct correlation to puberty onset in girls, yet conversely relates to a delayed pubertal onset in boys (Bordini & Rosenfield, 2011).

School-age children tend to be concerned about their rate of growth, weight, time of menarche, and final height. These children need to understand that the timing and extent of their physical changes usually reflect their genetic inheritance. When one is assessing a child's height and weight, and before referring to **standardized growth charts**, the height of the child's family must be taken into consideration (CDC, 2010). For more information, see http://www.cdc.gov/growthcharts/. For example, the child whose height is in the third percentile may have parents who are shorter than average. Shorter height can be expected because of the family's genetic composition. Likewise, although the average age of **menarche** is at approximately 12.5 years in Caucasian girls and 12.0 years in black American girls, most girls experience their menarche at approximately the same age their mothers did (Bordini & Rosenfield, 2011). With sufficient body fat to stimulate hormones needed for menses, girls can have their first menstrual period between age 11 years and age 15 years and still be considered normal. As a result of better nutrition and differences in lifestyle, girls appear to experience menarche earlier than did girls of 30 years ago (Harding, 2015). Although the school-age child experiences numerous physical changes before adolescence, changes in three physical areas are of particular interest: oral development, lymphoid tissue, and motor skills development.

## Oral Development

Teeth enable a person to speak, chew, and smile. They also help give the face shape and form. The school-age child appears to be constantly losing or gaining a tooth. Deciduous, or baby, teeth are usually lost in the same order in which they initially erupted. School-age children begin shedding their first teeth when they are approximately 6 to 7 years of age, and the process is complete with the loss of the second molars at 11 to 13 years of age. The first permanent teeth, the 6-year molars, erupt at 6 to 7 years of age and continue to erupt until the third molars (wisdom teeth) appear at approximately 17 to 22 years of age. The child aged between 6 and 13 years loses and gains approximately four teeth per year. A 13-year-old child should have 28 teeth, having lost 20 deciduous teeth (Peristein, 2013). When deciduous teeth erupt, only the crown is lost; the root has been reabsorbed in the developing permanent tooth. As the child's mouth becomes filled with the larger, permanent teeth, the shape of the jaw and the facial appearance normally change. Girls tend to experience earlier permanent **tooth eruption** than do boys (Peristein, 2013).

Dental problems, primarily **dental caries** (cavities), periodontal disease, and **malocclusion**, are among the most common health problems in school-age children today. It remains the most common chronic disease of children 5 to 17 years of age, four times more prevalent than asthma (CDC, 2014a). Present in up to 42% of children 2 to 11 years of age, untreated caries occur more frequently in poor and ethnically diverse children and in those who lack insurance or access to preventive dental care. School dental programs are necessary to educate school-age children on proper care and maintenance of their teeth. School-based oral health education programs and sealant programs are in line with the *Healthy People 2020* initiatives and interventions for reducing dental caries among children (American Academy of Pediatric Dentistry, 2011; US Department of Health and Human Services [USDHHS], 2012a). In the past decade of *Healthy People* initiatives it has been determined that community-based and school-based sealant programs can reduce new cases of tooth decay by up to 60% for 2 to 5 years after a single application in high-risk children (CDC, 2014a). These programs demonstrate an area in which child oral health can be affected to improve the overall health of children in the United States.

The rapid change in the number and type of teeth and the uneven growth in the child's jaw may cause malocclusion, an unacceptable relationship of the teeth in one jaw to those in the other. Dentists evaluate children with overbites, gaps between teeth, and other alignment problems that may influence speech and eating (American Dental Association, 2014). Some children will grow out of these problems, but others may need orthodontic care and appliances (braces) to correct problems or improve their appearance. Peer reaction to braces is addressed as part of the teaching about body changes; this teaching may decrease problems with the child's self-concept or body image as a result of looking different. School dental programs include education about conscientious tooth care for the child who wears braces, because these frequently make brushing and flossing more difficult, especially for the school-age child who lacks manual dexterity.

### Lymph Tissue

Lymph tissue grows rapidly throughout childhood, reaching maximal size before puberty, after which it begins to decrease in size, most likely as a result of changes in the concentrations of sex hormones. The amount of lymphoid tissue of a child up to 10 years of age often exceeds that of an adult (Kanwar, 2015). This is most often reflected in the size of the tonsils. As a result, tonsils that appear pathologically enlarged to a parent can be normal for the child's age. Additional lymphoid tissue during the school-age period generally helps this group to have a stronger immune response than do younger and older children. This is a result of the immune system being activated by environmental antigens and exposure to common organisms (Kanwar, 2015).

### Motor Skills Development

Neurological, skeletal, and muscular changes combine to increase the child's overall motor abilities. With maturation of the nervous system by age 7 or 8 years, the brain's two hemispheres articulate to allow the child more control over and coordination with motor tasks.

The child grows taller because of lengthening of the long bones that continues into adolescence. Ossification, replacement of cartilage with bone, occurs throughout childhood but is not complete until adulthood (National Institute of Arthritis and Musculoskeletal and Skin Disease, 2015). Therefore special attention must be paid to well-fitting shoes, appropriately sized chairs and desks, and backpack loads to avoid strain on an evolving musculoskeletal system (AAP, 2015a). Children at this age also

need protective sports equipment and conditioning exercises before sports to prevent sports fractures (National Institute of Arthritis and Musculoskeletal and Skin Disease, 2015). However, the child builds new bony tissue during the entire period of childhood, which generally allows rapid healing of fractures. Overweight children typically have greater bone density as compared with their normal-weight peers. Although they have greater bone density, this does not translate into reduced risk of fractures and joint pain. Overweight children are more likely to experience bone fractures and have more joint and muscle pain than their normal weight counterparts (National Institute of Arthritis and Musculoskeletal and Skin Disease, 2015). The reason for this finding is not clearly understood at this time.

Muscle mass also increases with muscle strength. During the school-age years, physically active boys are slightly stronger than girls, but this difference is not significant until adolescence. With these changes the child has the potential to perform more complex fine motor and gross motor functions but must practice to perfect these skills. Children willingly exercise their newfound skills and feel pride when others see their improved skill level when bike riding, tying shoes, and engaging in team sports, for example.

## GORDON'S FUNCTIONAL HEALTH PATTERNS

The school nurse can be an integral and influential person for the school-age child. The school nurse provides the infrastructure for the health of the student. Gordan's functional health patterns can be used to comprehensively assess the school-age child.

### Health Perception–Health Management Pattern

The school-age child understands an abstract definition of health and sometimes the factors causing illness, but this understanding differs from that of an adult. Most school-age children perceive symptoms and show an ability to participate in health-promoting behaviors. Health-promoting behaviors taught at school and home must meet the school-age child's cognitive level (concrete operation) and moral level (external rules and forces) to be effective. Teaching strategies using cognitive, psychomotor, and affective senses can help children learn responsibility for their own health (Shroff, 2015). This knowledge provides an excellent foundation for health-promotion behaviors during the school years.

School-age children's understanding of illness is directly correlated with their cognitive development and follows a direct sequence of developmental stages. It is important for nurses to integrate the child's developmental views on illness because this has direct implications for plans related to health education. When specifically asked about their ideas on causes of illness, school-age children usually state the germ theory, the punishment theory, or the external forces theory. Although many younger school-age children know that germs play a role in illness, they have limited understanding of how germs work (Brogan, 2015). They may believe that a misdeed or misbehavior caused their illnesses.

Various cultural influences may also contribute to a child's understanding of illness. Hinduism ascribes to the theory of

BOX 20-1  **HEALTHY PEOPLE 2020 HEALTH OBJECTIVES RELATED TO SCHOOL-AGE CHILDREN**

*Selected National Health-Promotion and Disease-Prevention Objectives for School-Age*

**Oral Health**

- Reduce proportion of children who experience dental caries in their primary or permanent teeth to 49% for all children in 2020. (Baseline is 54% of children aged 6–9 years in 1999–2004; current proportion, 2011–12, is 57.7%.)
- Reduce proportion of children 6 to 9 years of age with untreated dental decay in primary or permanent teeth to 25.9% by 2020. (Baseline is 28.8% of children aged 6–9 years for 1999–2004; current proportion, 2011–12, is 26.5%.)
- Increase proportion of children 6 to 9 years of age who have received dental sealants on one or more permanent teeth to 28.1% by 2020. (Baseline is 25.5% of children aged 6–9 years for 1999–2004; current proportion, 2011–12, is 37.6%.)
- Increase the percentage of school-based health clinics with an oral health component including dental sealants to 26.6% by 2020. (Baseline is 24.1% of schools offered sealants for 2007–08.)
- Increase the percentage of school-based health clinics with a topical fluoride treatment (including fluoride rinse/varnish) program to 32.1% by 2020. (Baseline is 29.2% of schools offered a fluoride program for 2007–08.)

**Respiratory Illness**

- Reduce hospitalizations for asthma among children to 8.6 hospitalizations per 10,000 children younger than 18 years by 2020. (Baseline is 14.9 hospitalizations per 10,000 children in 2007–08.)
- Reduce emergency department visits for asthma among children to 49.1 per 10,000 children by 2020. (Baseline is 56.4 per 10,000 children for 2007–08.)
- Reduce percentage of 5- to 17-year-old children who missed school because of an asthma attack in the previous year to 48.7% by 2020. (Baseline is 58.7% of children 5–17 years of age who had an asthma attack in the previous 12 months missed school in 2008; current proportion, 2011–12, is 59.1%.)

**Injury Prevention**

- Increase percentage of children 8 to 12 years of age who use safety belts to 86% by 2020. (Baseline is 78% of children 8–12 years used safety belt in 2008; current proportion, 2011–12, is 79%.)

- Increase percentage of 6- to 17-year-old children using appropriate protective eye gear to 18.2% by 2020. (Baseline is 16.5% of children wore protective eye gear in 2008.)
- Reduce percentage of children exposed to any form of violence, crime, or abuse to 54.5% by 2020. (Baseline is 60.6% exposed to crime/abuse in 2008; current proportion, 2011–12, is 56.6%.)

**Physical Activity**

- Increase proportion of US public/private elementary schools that require daily physical education for all students to 4.2%. (Baseline of 3.8% schools required physical education in 2006.)
- Increase number of states that require regularly scheduled recess for all students to 17 states by 2020. (Baseline of seven states requiring regularly scheduled recess in 2006.)
- Increase proportion of children from 2 years to twelfth grade who view television or videos or play video games for no more than 2 hours per day to 86.8% by 2020. (Baseline of 78.9% children 6–14 years of age viewed television or videos or played video games for more than 2 hours per day in 2007.)
- Increase proportion of children 5 to 15 years of age who walk to school (up to 1 mile) or bike to school (up to 2 miles). (New objective, no data.)

**Nutrition**

- Reduce the proportion of children and adolescents aged 6 to 11 years who are overweight or obese (defined as at or above sex-specific and age-specific 95th percentile) to 15.7%. (Baseline is 17.4% for 2005 to 2008; current proportion, 2009–12, is 17.9%.)
- Prevent inappropriate weight gain in children 6 to 11 years of age. (New indicator, no data.)
- Eliminate very low food security among children (target 0.2%) by 2020. (Baseline is 1.3% of households with children had very low food security in 2008; current proportion, 2013, is 0.9%.)

From US Department of Health and Human Services. (2015). *Leading health indicators.* https://www.healthypeople.gov.

karma (law of cause and effect). People create their own destiny by thoughts, words, or deeds (Queensland Health, 2014). Illness, accident, or injury results from the karma one creates, and is often seen as a means of purification. Belief in the "evil eye," another cultural influence, occurs in many cultures and manifests itself in slightly different ways depending on where it arises. Most cultures believe that the victims are primarily babies or young children because they are so often praised and commented on by strangers. The evil eye is thought to be based on jealousy, and can have significant implications for the health of the victim (Queensland Health, 2014; Radford, 2013). This belief is strongest in Middle Eastern countries, Asia, Latin America, and Europe. Attempts to ward off the curse have led to the use of a number of talismans within the various cultures. It is important to be aware of such cultural and developmental beliefs of the school-age child when one is defining strategies for teaching health promotion.

School-age children face challenges in meeting health-promotion goals as defined by *Healthy People 2020* (USDHHS,

2012b). The *Healthy People 2020* initiatives present selected objectives related to this age group (Box 20-1: *Healthy People 2020*). However, people in the school-age child's life can facilitate societal attainment of these goals (Inman et al., 2011). Parents, caregivers, school nurses, and teachers teach health-promotion concepts, and they spend time monitoring and reinforcing preventive health practices, such as personal hygiene, dental care, and good nutrition. Role-playing, reading an age-appropriate books, and modeling of health-promotion behaviors (e.g., washing hands) may also help children make the link between behavior and improved health. Unfortunately, by imitating some caregivers, children can become passive health care consumers, asking few questions, doing as they are told, and perpetuating poor choices. These responses may also be caused by children's developmental and cultural obligation to obey authority figures. Parents, caregivers, school nurses, and teachers need to make commitments to demonstrate and teach healthy behaviors at home and in school; this helps children develop health values as part of their educational process toward reaching a healthy adulthood.

Counseling the child and the child's family on a broad definition of health, one that includes personal and environmental health and safety, requires an awareness of the school-age child's normal perceptions of health (Inman et al., 2011). The school nurse, in consultation with teachers, is in a prime position to use such information to present content in a manner beneficial to the school-age child's level of understanding. Topics may include some of the following content areas: cultural difference of causes and management of illnesses, causes of personal and environmental health problems, and critical issues affecting the school-age child's general health (e.g., backpack safety) (AAP, 2015a). All these issues may be integrated into general academic studies to establish a foundation for teaching prevention as well as help the school-age child develop advocacy skills to become an assertive health care consumer.

## Nutritional-Metabolic Pattern

School-age children, like all people, need a well-balanced diet. An average of 1200 to 1600 calories per day is recommended to meet growth requirements (based on sedentary behavior) (AHA, 2015a). Usually these calories are consumed in three daily meals and one or two snacks. School-age children often eat foods low in iron, calcium, and vitamin C, and foods that have a higher fat and sodium content than foods their parents ate when they were this age. There is a disjuncture between current dietary practices and recommended dietary intake of children. These behaviors place children at risk of poor nutritional habits, obesity, iron-deficiency anemia, and chronic illnesses such as diabetes and hypertension (Klish, 2015). The school nurse can be an integral component and assume a leadership role in the education of school-age children on the health and cognitive benefits of consuming nutritional sound foods.

### Factors Influencing Food Intake

Access to food, the influence of mass media, and contemporary busy lifestyles play a role in poor food choices. At the final review of the *Healthy People 2010* initiatives, up to 98% of American households were food secure throughout the year, surpassing the initiative target rate of 94% (USDHHS, 2012c). Federal food assistance programs are in existence to assist in the achievement of these initiative targets.

A multitude of television and billboard messages pressure children to eat certain foods, many of which contain large amounts of salt, sugar, and calories. These messages constitute the bulk of food commercials seen by children. Unfortunately, children are now being exposed to more fast-food commercials than they were in 2003 (Powell et al., 2011). The majority of non–program content time is devoted to food-related advertisements. Frequent and lengthy watching of television and exposure to food-related advertisements have been linked to childhood obesity (Andreyeva et al., 2011; Zimmerman & Bell, 2010). In 2005 American children watched an average of 3 hours 19 minutes of television daily (Powell et al., 2011). In 2010, 50% of meals were eaten away from home, and one in five breakfasts were consumed from McDonald's (AHA, 2015b). These behaviors contribute to more

"fast food" consumption and food of poor nutritional quality. On a typical day, 33% of children consume fast food (Demory-Luce & Motil, 2015). Healthy food often costs more and may be less accessible than unhealthy food (Yukhananov, 2011). Some cultures value food that has high salt and fat content.

Cultural factors, as well as food access, influence poor nutrition among the homeless and children in child care centers and may contribute to the high level of obesity, especially among Hispanic, black American, and Native American children (CDC, 2015d). These groups often lack access to safe and nutritious food. Thus successful interventions for school-age overweight and nutrition must focus on economic, social, and cultural factors that influence access to and use of food. School nurses are in a position to impact intervention strategies because of their familiarity with community needs, local cultural norms, and available resources.

Although some school-age children willingly try new foods, many continue to dislike vegetables, fruits, casseroles, spicy foods, and iron-rich foods and prefer a small range of foods. Some children may eat only raw vegetables and fruits and go through a phase of eating only one food at lunch, such as a peanut butter sandwich. These practices seldom hurt the child nutritionally.

Children frequently make their own after-school snacks and need supervision regarding the content. Daily consumption of foods high in vitamins A and C, fruits, and vegetables should be encouraged. With parental, caregiver, or teacher help and positive reinforcement, school-age children can learn to calculate nutrition needs, plan family meals, and eat better for their overall health. These activities also assist school-age children in developing wise decision-making practices, feelings of empowerment about health, and healthy food habits for the rest of their lives.

American families have such busy lives that they eat few meals together. A positive environment for nutrition and socialization during a shared mealtime is important. Parents encourage positive food habits for each family member, and pressure to eat certain foods is avoided to prevent power struggles between the parent or caregiver and the child. A child's nutritional pattern usually reflects family patterns (Robson et al., 2016). For example, parents who skip breakfast tend to have trouble convincing their children to eat breakfast. Educating children as a group to eat healthy foods can be successful because of the powerful influence of a peer group (people of the same age, experience, and usually sex). The child whose friend is eating a candy bar usually prefers the same rather than an apple for a snack.

### Nutrition Education

Nutrition education incorporated into the general curriculum of school-age children throughout their educational experience is important. Despite evidence that the school can serve as an environment for nutritional health-promotion education, not all schools require nutrition education from kindergarten through 12th grade (Cardoso da Silveria et al., 2013). School nurses and teachers, as part of core concepts usually taught in school, teach students about choices related to weight control and health and help them understand the role of the media and culture in nutritional choices (National Association of School Nurses [NASN], 2013). Teachers and school personnel also serve as role

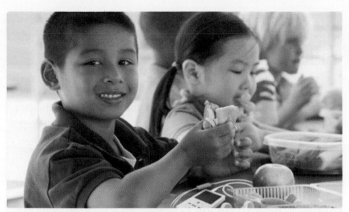

**FIGURE 20-1** Children 9 to 13 years old should eat two or more portions of vegetables and fruit totaling three to four cups daily.

models for optimal eating and exercise habits for children in their charge. Lunch and breakfast programs exist in most schools and meet guidelines established by the US Department of Agriculture (USDA) (2013). Many of these programs continue in after-school programs and during the summer when school is out of session to support needs for quality food intake in 31 million US children (NASN, 2013; USDA, 2013).

The AAP and the AHA have established dietary guidelines for children and adolescents. The daily nutritional needs of a child who is 9 to 14 years old include the following (AHA, 2015a) (Figure 20-1):

- Milk group: 3 cups (24 oz total) of fat-free milk
- Meat group: 5 oz of lean meat or beans, or equivalent combinations of these foods
- Vegetable group: 2 to 2.5 cups of vegetables daily
- Fruit group: 1.5 cups of fruit
- Grains group: 4 to 6 oz daily, of which half should be whole-grain items (AHA, 2015a)

### Overweight and Obesity

Overweight and obesity are major nutritional problems that have reached alarming proportions among adults and children in the United States. The Expert Committee on the Assessment, Prevention, and Treatment of Child & Adolescent Overweight and Obesity lists the following definitions for use in children and adolescents (CDC, 2015d):

- Individuals 2 to 18 years of age with a body mass index (BMI) greater than the 95th percentile for age and sex or a BMI exceeding 30 kg/m$^2$ (whichever is smaller) should be considered obese.
- Individuals with a BMI greater than the 85th percentile, but less than the 95th percentile, should be considered overweight.

The problem of overweight and obesity in children and adolescents has increased significantly in the last 50 years. Childhood obesity is now the number one concern for parents, surpassing drug abuse and smoking. One in three children are now considered overweight or obese (AHA, 2015c). Unfortunately, this demonstrates movement away from the *Healthy People 2010* initiative

target of 15% (Klish, 2015). Evidence suggests that adult obesity begins in infancy or childhood and results from both genetic and environmental factors. For example, a child whose overweight parents constantly use food as a reward faces a greater risk of obesity than does a child of thin parents who do not reward the child with food. Excessive food intake and lack of physical activity also lead to obesity, and once overweight these children tend to exercise even less. Overweight occurs more in black American and Hispanic children than in Caucasian children (35%, 37.9%, and 30% respectively) (AHA, 2015c). These higher overweight and obesity rates may reflect less physical activity of black American and Hispanic children attributable to unhealthy living conditions and an inability to purchase higher-cost healthy food choices (Klish, 2015).

Overweight increases the risk of hypertension, diabetes, sleep apnea, orthopedic problems, and heart disease. Experts believe that overweight and sedentary behaviors are the primary risk factors for the development of insulin resistance, hyperlipidemia, hypertension, type 2 diabetes, and heart disease (AHA, 2015c; Nielson, 2011). There is also evidence that postprandial hyperinsulinemia may result in excessive weight gain (Klish, 2015). In addition, hormones released during the pubertal years make the situation worse in that these hormones cause the body to use insulin less effectively, leading to insulin resistance and thus increasing the risk of development of type 2 diabetes.

Current evidence suggests that overweight is associated with obstructive sleep apnea. Whether each disease state increases the expression of the other is unclear (CDC, 2015d). The potential association between short sleep duration and childhood overweight has been described in the literature (Bonuck et al., 2015; Box 20-2: Research for Evidence-Based Practice). Longer sleep durations are associated with higher degrees of activity, which may assist with weight loss. Recent findings support the proactive approach of ensuring adequate sleep in the prevention of overweight in children.

The overweight and obese child faces ridicule by peers and discrimination later in life. These responses reinforce an already low self-esteem and poor body image and cause a cycle of personal isolation that influences a child's success, current and future (Griffiths et al., 2010, Klish, 2015). Helping the overweight and obese child change lifestyle patterns requires intensive intervention, including the support of parents. Even with these interventions, few overweight children achieve or maintain significant weight loss because of the complexity of factors (environmental, cultural, economic, and psychological) involved. In addition, there are reports that failure to maintain weight loss may be associated with impulsivity behaviors (Van den Berg et al., 2011). Some success has been achieved by programs that include implementation of reasonable caloric restriction; eating a variety of low-fat and low-cholesterol foods; and use of diet support groups, physical exercise, peer counseling groups, and habit changes (AHA, 2015b,c). However, intervention sometimes fails because some school-age children do not show concern about being overweight. Nursing suggestions for parents who are interested in preventing obesity in their school-age children are given in Box 20-3.

## BOX 20-2 RESEARCH FOR EVIDENCE-BASED PRACTICE

### Sleep Duration Relation to Overweight in Children

The purpose of this study was to better describe the association between short sleep duration or sleep problems with childhood overweight. Emerging research has introduced the association between sleep and the regulation of many physiological functions, including energy balance, appetite, and weight maintenance. The researchers sought to determine if the association of short sleep duration and overweight in children existed while controlling the data for measures such as quality of the home environment, parenting, and child behavior problems.

A longitudinal study of 785 children and their parents who were enrolled in the National Institute of Child Health and Human Development Study of Early Childcare and Youth Development was conducted. Data were collected regarding BMI, sex, socioeconomic status, and race in third and sixth grade students. Questionnaires regarding sleep and home environment were completed by the participant's mother at the same time intervals.

The findings revealed an association between short sleep duration in the sixth grade and overweight in the sixth grade. Shorter sleep duration in the third grade was independently associated with overweight in the sixth grade regardless of the child's weight in the third grade. For every additional hour of sleep in the sixth grade, the child was 20% less likely to be overweight in the sixth grade. For every additional hour of sleep in the third grade, the child was 40% less likely to be overweight in the sixth grade. Sleep problems were not associated with overweight in children.

Adequate sleep duration in childhood may offer a protective effect on weight maintenance and overweight risk in children. One preventive approach to overweight in children may simply be to ensure adequate sleep in childhood.

From Lumeng, J., Somashekar, D., Appugliese, D., Kaciroti, N., Corwyn, R., & Bradley, R. (2007). Shorter sleep duration is associated with increased risk for being overweight at ages 9 to 12 years. *Pediatrics, 120*(5), 1020–1029.

## BOX 20-3 Nursing Interventions to Prevent Overweight/Obesity During the School-Age Years

- Incorporate discussion of healthy food intake and daily activity into daily school life.
- Encourage parents to be a role model for their child—be active; plan physically active family outings.
- Make activity fun!
- Limit the amount of time spent watching television, playing video games, and using the computer/Internet.
- Discourage eating while watching television.
- Encourage parent(s) to consider cultural influences on dietary intake. Evaluate snacking habits and food choices. Balance healthy foods with ethnic food choices.
- Encourage the family to assess "fast food" consumption and explore/develop eating habits that support a healthier diet as defined by the food-guide pyramid.
- Encourage child to participate in food/meal selection and preparation.
- Support lunch choices that meet overall healthy nutrition intake.

From American Heart Association. (2015). *Dietary recommendations for healthy children.* http://www.heart.org/HEARTORG/GettingHealthy/Dietary-Recommendations-for-Healthy-Children_UCM_303886_Article.jsp; American Heart Association. (2015). *Healthy eating habits start at home.* http://www.heart.org/HEARTORG/GettingHealthy/NutritionCenter/HealthyEating/Healthy-Eating-Habits-Start-at-Home_UCM_461862_Article.jsp#.VlsKCNKrTIU; American Heart Association. (2015). *Overweight in children.* http:/www.heart.org/HEARTORG/GettingHealthy/Overweight-in-Children_UCM_304054_Article.jsp.

## Elimination Pattern

Most children have full bowel and bladder control by 5 years of age. Control involves the ability to undress and dress, to wipe and flush, and to clean hands. The child's elimination patterns are similar to the adult's, with urination occurring six to eight times a day and bowel movements averaging one or two times a day. For some school-age children, however, elimination continues to be a problem.

### Enuresis

Involuntary urination at an age when control should be present is called enuresis (Kaneshiro, 2016; National Health Service, 2015). Children with primary enuresis have never achieved bladder control, and those with secondary enuresis have periods of dryness and recurrent enuresis. Involuntary nocturnal urination (bedwetting) that occurs at least once a month is defined as nocturnal enuresis, and wetting during the day has been termed diurnal enuresis. Enuresis should be considered not a disease but a variation of normal development. Enuresis affects 7% of boys and 3% of girls at 5 years of age (Goldberg, 2014).

Nocturnal enuresis causes disruption for both the child and the family. The child may frequently experience teasing from classmates and siblings. It can have profound effects on life socially, emotionally, and behaviorally. Although many forms of enuresis do not pose any significant health risk, there are social stressors. A night away from home appears impossible because of fear of wetting. Parents may be angry about the frequent bed changes and laundering and may try punishments, thinking that the child should be able to control the problem. Parental stress places additional pressure on the child, who may already have low self-esteem and lack self-confidence as a result of a perceived inability to control the problem (Pillinger, 2015).

Often because they lack information, frustrated families seek help. Many therapies exist yet require a high degree of motivation from the child and parents. Their views must be taken into consideration when one is considering various treatment options. In addition to providing information, the nurse provides active support to facilitate coping. If a child does not have a urinary tract infection, various forms of management may be considered. These include wet alarm systems, bladder training and retention control, waking schedules, drug therapy, and hormone therapy. Each method has advantages, disadvantages, and cost considerations, but all require consistency and time from the child and parents, as well as positive reinforcement by the parents, to reach a successful outcome (Pillinger, 2015).

Diurnal enuresis is often called daytime dribbling. This term describes a urinary pattern most often seen in school-age girls.

These children demonstrate "holding on" behaviors, including not voiding first thing in the morning, voiding only two or three times a day, and voiding exceptionally quickly (National Institute of Diabetes and Digestive and Kidney Diseases, 2012). It is not clear why children delay urination or empty their bladders only partially, thus promoting overflow incontinence. Evaluation of these children begins with a urine culture to rule out urinary tract infection. If no infection exists or symptoms persist after treatment, then the intervention is focused on increasing fluid intake to prevent "holding" and establishing a voiding routine of every 2 hours, with a conscious effort to empty the bladder completely. The nurse can be instrumental in helping the child and parents understand the problem and its management.

## Encopresis

Another elimination problem that may occur in children is encopresis, defined as the persistent voluntary or involuntary passing of stool into the child's underpants after age 4 years. In most cases the problem has no discernible physiological cause and is not related to laxative use. There may be a history of inconsistent toilet training or early life stress in affected children. Encopresis is a common complication of chronic constipation. More than 90% of children with encopresis have a history of recent constipation and/or painful bowel movements (Barron, 2015). Once children become constipated or have hard and painful stools, they begin to hold their bowel movements to prevent further pain. This creates a cycle that leads to fecal impaction and rectal distention. Stool then begins to leak around the impaction and leaks through the child's rectum, often without the child's knowledge. In most cases, soiling occurs during the day when the child is awake and active. Soiling at night is uncommon.

Encopresis is often associated with recurrent abdominal pain and, for many, enuresis as well. Often these children have emotional difficulties that began before or resulted from encopresis. They experience poor peer relationships and self-esteem, perhaps attributable to their offensive odor. Awareness of this childhood problem is necessary to appropriately identify the affected child, refer the child for treatment, and support the child and the family during a bowel management program and counseling.

## Activity-Exercise Pattern

Physical activity in children is an important aspect of health and an integral component of health promotion. Childhood is considered to be a critical time in which regular physical activity behaviors are acquired and fostered (Figure 20-2). Generally, the school-age child is naturally active, although many do not meet current activity recommendations (CDC, 2015b; Craggs et al., 2011). Boys are typically more active than girls (Figure 20-3). In addition, those who perceive their neighborhood as unsafe or do not have at least one parent who exercises are less likely to exercise themselves. Physical activity and participation in sport activities tends to decrease with age, particularly among girls.

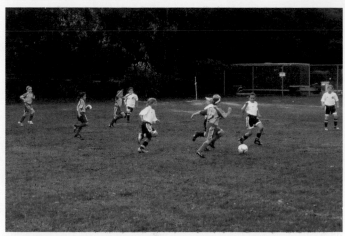

FIGURE 20-2  Peer play is important during the school-age years.

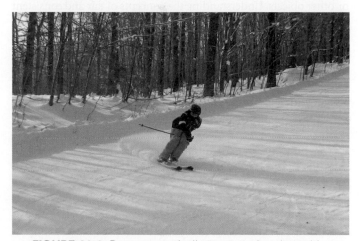

FIGURE 20-3  Boys are typically more active than girls.

As previously discussed, impressive changes in motor skills occur between the age of 6 years and the age of 12 years, allowing the child to engage in many activities that develop strength, balance, and coordination (see Table 20-1). Exercise typically occurs through group activities and organized sports such as Little League baseball and soccer, through individual activities such as gymnastics and ballet, and through unorganized play such as bike riding, sledding, rollerblading, and imaginary play. Play provides important learning and health promotion, and for this reason should be encouraged consistently during the school-age years. For many children, involvement in physical activities is fun and connects them to their peers, family members, and other important people in their lives (Milteer et al., 2012).

Play activities also promote social, personal, and cognitive development. School-age children frequently prefer interacting with peers rather than with the family. This desire for peer interaction, usually with one of the same sex, extends beyond school and carries over to play and outside activities. A child's skill in motor tasks wins the respect of other children and provides a feeling of self-accomplishment (CDC, 2015e). Organized sports such as baseball teach team cooperation, competition, and other social skills. Concerns exist that young children have experienced too much physical and psychological pressure to perform in sports. This has generated a renewed commitment by many parents to focus more on the fun of sports than on the winning of games (Craggs et al., 2011). Organized activities such as Scouts and 4-H clubs teach children about group functioning, processes involved in performing a task, and the power of social relationships to create change. These lessons can prepare them for the discipline needed for a job later in life. Overall, children who perform well in these activities feel good about themselves, their competence, and enhance a sense of industry. Parents and teachers who compliment children when they perform well enhance self-esteem as well.

As part of play, school-age children incorporate new cognitive skills, including the ability to count and sort objects. Children of this age express pleasure in their collections of stamps, rocks, or other objects. Understanding the concepts of fair and consistent rules found in games requires cognitive skills of memory, logical reasoning, and the desire to work with others. Many children like to read, which provides ideas about life and cultures that differ from their own, thereby enhancing their acceptance of human diversity. The nurse helps parents promote healthy play activities for children by encouraging the following (CDC, 2015e):

- Family activities that focus on physical activity and togetherness between parents or caregivers and children
- Use of a library card to encourage reading on a variety of topics and to teach responsibilities involved with borrowing
- Monitoring of daily television and computer use that detracts from physical activity and more active mental activities
- Encouragement of both group and solitary activities to support the child's overall development

## Sleep-Rest Pattern

### Sleep Patterns

Most school-age children have no difficulties with sleep. Generally, their sleep requirements and patterns are more similar to those of an adult than those of a younger child. Individual needs vary on the basis of activity, age, and state of health, but most school-age children sleep between 10 and 12 hours a night without naps during the day (American Academy of Sleep Medicine, 2014; Gupta, 2014). Unlike younger children, school-age children experience few difficulties with going to bed. Most children and parents can agree on a bedtime with some flexibility on nonschool nights and adhere to that agreement. When problems arise regarding bedtime, children may be testing parents who have not been clear and firm about their expectations for their children going to bed or have not been willing to discuss the arrangement with their children (Boyse, 2010). Although most Americans accept the idea that school-age children should sleep in their own beds, some black American, Hispanic, Chinese, and Japanese families may encourage the family or siblings to sleep together (Martin, 2013; Queensland Health, 2014). In the school-age child, bed-sharing does not have any impact on sleep patterns, nor does it show any long-term effects toward health, positive or negative (Boyse, 2010).

### Sleep Disturbances

The most common sleep problems that occur during the preschool and early school-age years are night terrors (see Chapter 19), sleepwalking, sleep talking, and enuresis. As a group, these disturbances have been called disorders of arousal (Boyse, 2010) and share the following characteristics:

- They occur immediately before a rapid eye movement state of sleep.
- Most occur 1 to 2 hours after going to sleep.
- There is a family history of sleep problems; boys experience more sleep problems than girls.
- Problems reflect normal central nervous system immaturity of the child.
- Problems may be influenced by fatigue and stress within the child.
- Problems do not involve the respiratory system.

Approximately one in six children (15%) aged between 5 and 12 years has sleepwalked at least once, but far fewer children walk in their sleep persistently. Sleepwalking is most likely due to the brain's inability to regulate sleep-wake cycles because of immaturity of the central nervous system. It occurs more often in boys and often occurs with enuresis (Gupta, 2014). Shortly after going to sleep, the child may suddenly sit up in bed, make repetitive finger and hand movements, or walk, usually for a short time. In most cases, however, the child stays in bed. The child may mumble when talking to a parent or other person (sleep talking). The words tend to be simple but unclear to the listener. Often the child falls back to sleep quickly after talking or walking (Boyse, 2010; Robinson, 2014).

Parents who are concerned about sleepwalking or sleep talking need to know that most children outgrow these episodes with central nervous system maturation. However, parents should protect their child from injury by placing gates at the top of stairs and removing sharp objects from the child's path. Most parents find that the easiest solution is to direct the sleepwalker back to bed, where the child returns to a normal sleep. Occasionally, parents can intervene effectively by implementing relaxation techniques for their child before bedtime, avoiding stressful and fatiguing situations, and providing consistency with sleep preparation patterns (American Academy of Sleep Medicine, 2014; Boyse, 2010). If a child has many episodes of sleepwalking or sleep talking, or if parents express particular concern, he or she may need further evaluation and treatment by health care professionals.

## Cognitive-Perceptual Pattern

The school-age child spends extensive time in settings that require mastery of new ideas and concepts. The child's basic intelligence, heredity, and environment encourage or discourage learning. Mastery of ideas and learning requires intact senses, such as vision, hearing, language, and memory capabilities that allow cognitive development and acquisition of skills needed for later life success (Goswami, 2015). Unfortunately, many children in society lack these capabilities and will have learning problems if these are not identified early through parental awareness, school observations, or routine health care assessments. For further information about school-age tests or procedural preparations, see http://www.nlm.nih.gov/medlineplus/ency/article/002058.htm (Kaneshiro, 2014).

## Piaget's Theory

Piaget (2001) refers to the age span of 7 to 11 years as the period of concrete operation, a stage when children learn by manipulating concrete objects and lack the ability to perform thinking operations that require abstraction. During this time the child moves from egocentric interactions to more cooperative interactions and increased understanding of many concepts gained through environmental connections (Atherton, 2013). Children increasingly change their reasoning from intuitive to logical or rational operations (rule-governed actions) and engage in serial ordering, addition, subtraction, and other basic mathematical skills. The operations of this period are termed concrete because the child's mental operations or actions still depend on the ability to perceive specific examples of what has happened. Older school-age children use both concrete and recently acquired abstract operations, which add flexibility and control to their thinking and meet developmental needs of adolescence. Unlike the egocentric preschooler, a school-age child begins to take the other person's point of view into account. This trait does not emerge suddenly. The new skill appears occasionally and then more frequently as the child's mental capacity and experience grow.

During the school-age period, the child understands a number of expanding concepts regarding objects, including the concept of conservation of substance (Atherton, 2013). When asked if a difference exists in the amount of liquid poured into two glasses of different shapes, the preschool, preoperational child focuses on the different shapes and says "yes." The concrete operational school-age child realizes that no change has occurred in the amount of the liquid despite the change in shape. Conservation of numbers, weight, volume, and quantity, required to understand basic mathematics, sequentially develops as the school-age child gains chronological age and experience.

The concept of time also develops during this period. Children begin to learn to tell time and understand the passage of time. By age 8 years, most children understand the difference between past and present, and history becomes meaningful. The concept of human aging becomes increasingly understandable, and the child can comprehend the difference between an 18-year-old person and an 80-year-old person.

Two major operations of the school-age period are classifying and ordering. The child classifies or groups objects by their common elements and understands the relationship between groups or classes. For example, when given 12 wooden beads, some brown and some white, the child understands that the beads may be grouped by their color and by their material. Conversely, the preschool child focuses only on one property of the beads, such as color. The newfound ability to classify objects shows in the school-age child's interest in collections, such as stamps or coins (Atherton, 2013). Children in school frequently "order" their world; they line up in school according to height, they repeat numbers and letters in their classic order, and they receive numbers in school to reflect an alphabetized surname. These two operations (classifying and ordering) must exist to learn to read, understand the concepts of numbers, and learn subjects based on relations, such as history (the relation of events in time) and geography (the relation of places in space).

## Vision

The child's sensory abilities continue to develop during the school-age years. Visual capacity should reach optimal function by the sixth or seventh year (Heiting, 2015). Peripheral vision and the ability to discriminate fine color distinctions should be fully developed as well. Although many 4-year-olds have 20/20 vision, a school-age child should have a visual acuity of at least 20/30 in each eye, as measured by the Snellen chart, an assessment tool for children who can read some letters (Segre, 2015).

Physiological changes occur in the eye during the school-age years. Eyes in the preschool years are normally hyperopic (farsighted), a condition in which the visual image of an object falls behind the retina. However, unlike older individuals, preschool children do not need glasses because their eyes normally accommodate by adjusting their lenses. For most children, vision becomes normal as the shape of the eye changes and lengthens with maturation. However, many school-age children need visual correction to prevent academic difficulties and headaches and dizziness when reading or doing close work. The peak incidence of hyperopia diagnosis in school-age children is at approximately 6 years of age (Castagno et al., 2014).

Twenty-five percent of school-age children have visual problems. Unfortunately, only approximately one-third of all states in the United States require children have an eye examination or vision screening before entering school (American Optometric Association, 2015). Vision screening programs for schoolchildren are intended to help identify those children who have or may potentially have a vision problem that may affect physiological or perceptual processes of vision or that could interfere with school performance. Vision screenings are not diagnostic nor do they lead to treatment, but rather only indicate a potential need for further care. The school nurse is in an optimal position to ensure eye screenings are performed, and the nurse encourages parents of children with deficits to seek further optometric care to correct these defects so that these children can learn more effectively.

Two visual problems are common in the age group of the school-age child. Many school-age children inherit myopia (nearsightedness), a condition in which the visual image of an object falls in front of the retina, causing the child to have difficulty seeing distant objects. The other condition, astigmatism, causes blurred vision because the image is focused poorly on the retina because of changes in the surface of the cornea or lens. Eyeglasses correct the defects, but the problem must be identified before it can be solved. For example, a child with myopia may not realize that his visual images are impaired. Children with corrective lenses often express delight and surprise when they first see the fully focused and rich detail of the world after experiencing less refined visual acuity for some time.

### Hearing

The child's hearing ability (**auditory acuity**) is nearly complete by 7 years of age, although some maturation continues into adolescence. Hearing deficits occur less frequently than visual deficits, but hearing loss affects more than 1 million children from birth to age 21 years in the United States (American Academy of Otolaryngology, 2015a). This deficit compromises learning in school and important socialization with peers. **Chronic serous otitis media**, or long-term fluid in the middle ear, remains a common cause of hearing deficit in both the preschool years and the early school-age years (American Academy of Otolaryngology, 2015b). Fortunately, the reduction in the rates of otitis media in children met the *Healthy People 2010* initiative targets (National Institute on Deafness and Other Communication Disorders, 2013). The success of meeting the targets of this initiative has been attributed to the introduction of heptavalent pneumococcal conjugate vaccine in 2000 (National Institute on Deafness and Other Communication Disorders, 2013). New concerns about the potential for long-term hearing loss in children who listen to loud music have been raised.

All school-age children, especially those with a history of recurrent ear infections or fluid behind the eardrum, should have periodic hearing evaluations (National Institute on Deafness and Other Communication Disorders, 2012). These are often performed as part of a health-promotion program in school and as required by many states. Various treatments exist for acute otitis media, including antibiotics and the recent discovery that xylitol gum may be of some preventive benefit (Azarpazhooh et al., 2011). Work continues on a vaccination for prevention of otitis media infections. **Tympanograms**, used to measure the sensitivity of the tympanic membrane to vibrations induced by pressure and sound waves, help detect and monitor this problem as part of well-child and ill-child care (American Academy of Audiology, 2011). By providing education on hearing protection for school-age children, the school nurse plays an important role in the maintenance of this important sense for the future.

### Sensory Perception

Children learn simultaneously through many senses, and most teaching approaches incorporate this concept. For example, young school-age children see a letter, hear its sound, and feel its shape. With this approach, children learn in a number of ways to interpret an event (Willingham et al., 2015). For example, some children learn best by listening (**auditory learners**), others by doing (**kinesthetic learners**), and others by engaging all sensory modalities (auditory, kinesthetic, and **visual learners**). Because no two children have exactly the same sensory acuity, sensitivity, or discrimination, all children build slightly different perceptions and conceptions of the world around them and do not follow the same timetable to grasp concepts. Therefore teaching approaches must be individualized to meet the learning needs of most children.

Of all the senses, visual perception has been studied the most, primarily because of its role in helping children learn to read. Studies have examined children's abilities to discriminate parts of a picture (to see a figure within a picture). Children usually progress from the preschool stage, during which they perceive visual stimuli more as a whole, to the school-age stage, during which they perceive more details, and finally to the point at which they perceive and integrate both. This process helps children recognize letters, the first step needed for reading. Children may first be able to differentiate between obviously different letters, such as "h" and "o," but may have difficulty with letters similar in appearance, such as "b" and "d," until they can distinguish details more effectively.

### Language

Language develops rapidly during the school years. Most school-age children enter this period with an ability to understand and speak a language, but with only a basic knowledge of reading and writing. By the end of the school-age period, most children have acquired at least a functional ability in both areas. Language development mandates that a child have visual perception for reading, auditory acuity and perception for understanding spoken language, and fine motor skills for both articulation and handwriting.

The full capacity to imitate sounds develops during the childhood years. Between 6 and 7 years of age, the child shows the ability to produce proper articulation for most vowel and consonant sounds. However, some have difficulty expressing sounds for "s," "l," "z," "sh," "ch," and "r". By 7 years of age the child should be able to articulate all sounds for speaking, and by age 12 years has a vocabulary of approximately 4000 words. Understanding of the syntax (grammar) and semantics (meaning) of language continues to develop. The child uses more complex sentences and understands multiple meanings for the same word and metaphors. The child should be able to recognize and correct spelling and grammatical errors by 8 or 9 years of age. The capacity to learn foreign languages is at an optimal level at this stage and provides the rationale for foreign language instruction during the school-age years. Foreign language instruction also provides children with information about other cultures and an opportunity to understand people who are different from themselves.

Much of the child's time in school focuses on learning to read and write. Learning to read is a complex process, beginning with letter and sound recognition (AAP, 2015c). Letters combine to form words that the child must learn to decode. Words combine to form sentences, and so on. Most children need help from teachers, peers, parents, or older children to learn to read effectively. Some researchers believe that children learn best by sounding out the individual letters of a word (**phonics**), whereas others think that learning the word as a whole unit is better. Both processes have value, and likely a combination of both is most effective (AAP, 2014). Considering the wide range of processes that support development of reading skills (conceptual, perceptual, verbal, and motor), it is not surprising that most children experience some difficulty in learning to read (AAP, 2014).

Handwriting requires eye-hand coordination, motor control, and perceptual abilities (Harron, 2014). Primarily a motor skill, handwriting does not reflect mental capacity. Many bright children and adults have poor handwriting, and vice versa. Boys tend to have more problems with legible handwriting than do girls. Writing style does not approach adult-level maturity until the end of late childhood, but the handwriting should reflect the child's handedness. No reversal of letter outlines should occur by age 7 or 8 years, and the relative size of letters should be uniform. By age 8 or 9 years, letter strokes should be firm, even, and flow with ease. The individual who has difficulty with handwriting may use a typewriter, computer, or graphics to produce a satisfactory written product. Tutoring by a handwriting specialist can help children with dyslexia, a term defining the tendency to reverse the normal appearance of letters and numbers in writing.

## Memory

Memory abilities, both short term and long term, improve for school-age children. Strategies such as organizing, classifying, and labeling information help them retain information. Rehearsal, repeating an item to be learned, is also a helpful memorization strategy. At age 5 years, children use rehearsal when someone suggests or models it; at age 10 years, they rehearse spontaneously. Memory abilities improve with practice and through various strategies, such as placing the words that need to be remembered in a song or by rhyming words (Raghubar et al., 2010).

## Intelligence

Intelligence tests assess a person's mental abilities and compare them with the abilities of other people through the use of numerical scores. Although the term intelligence is used as if there is agreement on what it means, in reality there is much debate as to how this term should be and has been defined. For example, debate has surrounded whether intelligence should be considered an inherent cognitive capacity, an achieved level of performance, or a qualitative construct that cannot be measured. Psychologists have debated whether intelligence is learned or inherited, culturally specific or universal, or one or several abilities (Kendler et al., 2015). Although these debates are ongoing, evidence is increasing that traditional intelligence tests measure specific forms of cognitive ability that are predictive of school functioning but do not measure the many forms of intelligence that are beyond these more specific skills, such as music, art, and interpersonal and intrapersonal abilities.

The concept of intelligence usually conveys an ability to think and process information learned earlier in life. Scores on an intelligence test should measure the child's basic abilities as compared with those of others of the same age and experience level and, ideally, should predict performance in school or society. However, this is not always the case. Intelligence test scores tend to differ because each test, or each form of the same test, measures slightly different samples of abilities and reflects the test author's philosophy on intelligence. It is important to note that some intelligence tests may be culturally insensitive (123test, 2012). For example, the protectionism of the Asian culture may cause lower test scores on self-help skills and socialization among Asian children, who demonstrate in other ways that they are good students. Furthermore, words on the test may not be part of an ethnic group's usual vocabulary, causing children to miss these items on an intelligence test.

Children also take achievement tests that measure the amount of information learned in a specific area and offer insight into a child's overall intelligence. Although intelligence and achievement tests should measure different issues (basic ability versus learned achievement), their results correlate well. Some researchers believe this correlation exists because both tests actually measure the same thing (achievement, notability).

Reports from intelligence and achievement testing differ. Intelligence tests usually provide a number that represents intelligence quotient (IQ). An IQ of 90 to 110 is considered average (BMJ Best Practice, 2015). Achievement tests compare the child's performance with that of other children and report scores as percentiles. For example, a score in the 20th percentile of a test means the child scored better than only 20% of other children of the same age in that skill. Current beliefs accept that people inherit some of their intelligence but that environmental factors also influence opportunities for learning and overall intelligence. Most likely the greatest environmental influence is socioeconomic, reflected in the correlation in scores: children from low-income families tend to score lower on intelligence tests than do children from middle-income or high-income families. The reason for this probably relates to many subfactors, such as nutrition, language, parental reinforcement and encouragement, and sociocultural environmental stimuli. Social programs such as the federal Special Supplemental Nutrition Program for Women, Infants, and Children and preschool stimulation programs such as Head Start have attempted to address these subfactors to improve the potential of young children from diverse populations. Many people have suggested less focus on IQ tests, primarily because they label children early in life and influence, often negatively, their self-perception and their performance.

## Learning Disabilities

Educators estimate that 10% of children 6 to 17 years of age have a learning disability (Child Development, 2015). Many terms and definitions have been used to describe the impairments of children who have normal or above-normal intelligence and usually do not have visual, hearing, or motor handicaps or emotional problems yet have difficulties in school learning (Disabled World, 2015). Some children have minor, almost unnoticeable difficulties, whereas other children are so impaired that they appear to be mentally retarded until their impairment has been diagnosed and they have been helped. An individual child may have more than one developmental disorder. Some children will develop behavior and self-esteem problems as a response to their inability to function satisfactorily (BMJ Best Practice, 2015).

One well-known condition that causes difficulty in the child's adjustment to the school setting is attention-deficit/hyperactivity disorder (ADHD), a disorder that reflects developmentally inappropriate degrees of inattention, impulsiveness, and hyperactivity (AAP, 2011a). ADHD is the most common neurobehavioral disorder of childhood and among the most prevalent chronic health conditions affecting school-age children. Frequently these children have high energy, intuitiveness, and creativity, personal characteristics that help them succeed in some facets of their lives. Despite diagnostic criteria for ADHD developed by the

## BOX 20-4 Diagnostic Criteria for Attention-Deficit/Hyperactivity Disorder

Consider a criterion is met only if the behavior occurs more frequently than that noted in most people of the same mental age as the child.

- A disturbance of at least 6 months exists during which at least six of the criteria for either inattentive behavior or hyperactivity-impulsivity behavior are met (for specific criteria, see American Psychiatric Association, 2013).
- Some inattentive or hyperactive-impulsive symptoms that caused impairment existed before age 7 years.
- Some impairment for the symptoms exists in two or more settings (at school or at home).
- Clear evidence of clinically significant impairment exists in social or academic functioning.
- The symptoms do not occur only with a pervasive developmental disorder, schizophrenia, or other psychotic disorder and do not support another mental disorder (mood disorder, anxiety disorder, dissociative disorder, and personality disorder).

From American Academy of Pediatrics. (2011). Clinical practice guideline ADHD: Clinical practice guidelines for the diagnosis, evaluation, and treatment of attention-deficit, hyperactivity disorder in children and adolescents. *Pediatrics, 128*(5), 1007–1022; American Psychiatric Association. (2013). *Diagnostic and statistical manual of mental disorders* (5th ed.). Washington, DC: American Psychiatric Association.

American Psychiatric Association (2013), the problem has been difficult to assess, primarily because the child manifests symptoms in varying degrees in different settings and with different people (Box 20-4). Some symptoms associated with ADHD have been identified as changes to the *DRD4* gene (Dadds et al., 2016). Treatment of children with ADHD has been controversial but includes behavior management, family counseling, classroom management, nutrition therapy, and medication (Devore & Schutze, 2015b). These interventions may also be successful in management of ADHD-affected adults. However, with the use of genomics, new treatments and therapies may be developed to better match the needs of the individual with ADHD (Dadds et al., 2016; Box 20-5: Genomics).

The nurse's role with the child who has a learning disability is varied. The nurse may participate in detection of the problem and consultation during evaluations, collaborate with the school administration on implementation of a treatment plan and referral to resources, assist as a liaison between school and home environments, and be a source of instruction for both the child and the family to improve overall development and the family's adaptation to meet the needs of this unique child.

There are two laws protecting children with disabilities, including those with ADHD: the Individuals with Disabilities Education Act (IDEA) of 1997 and Section 504 of the Rehabilitation Act of 1973, Amendment Act of 2008 (Wrightslaw, 2015). The IDEA is a special education law, whereas Section 504 is a civil rights statute. Both guarantee qualified students a free and appropriate public education and instruction in the least restrictive environment. This means that students are to be instructed among those who are not disabled and to the maximal extent appropriate for the student's needs.

## BOX 20-5 GENOMICS
### Medicine in Children

Clinical genome sequencing and exome sequencing technologies are becoming promising tools for determining genetic causality of numerous diseases in children, including cystic fibrosis, asthma, autism spectrum disorders, and childhood cancers. Genomic medicine is looking to find genetic mutations that drive various disease states so as to yield new targets against which novel therapies may be developed (Downing et al., 2012). The next generation of medical treatments and therapies are being designed to better improve outcomes for many childhood conditions. Nurses are well positioned to incorporate genetic and genomic information across all aspects of health care. This translation of clinical, medical research technologies into practice is not without challenges (Thiffault & Lantos, 2016). However, nurses have an opportunity to close the gap between research and therapeutic developments.

From Downing, J. R., Wilson, R. K., Zhang, J., Mardis, E. R., Pui, C. H., Ding, L., et al. (2012). Pediatric Cancer Genome Project. *National Genetics, 44*(6), 619–622; Thiffault, I., and Lantos, J. (2016). The challenge of analyzing the results of next-generation sequencing in children. *Pediatrics, 137*(Supp1), 83–87.

The nurse plays a vital role in promoting the school-age child's overall cognitive and perceptual health, helping to prevent problems in these areas. The nurse must talk to parents and school administration personnel about any child who has language articulation problems beyond 6 or 7 years, because this child should be evaluated by a professional. The nurse helps parents understand their child's level of cognitive and sensory abilities so that learning expectations are realistic. Through educational materials sent to the child's home or provided during school meetings, the nurse may address the socialization needs and development of school-age children. The nurse also needs to help parents understand common tests used for child intelligence and achievement screening (Atherton, 2013). In addition, the nurse helps evaluate a child believed to have a learning disability when the child may actually have a health problem, general immaturity, or an environmental deficit (poverty or divorce; Krause-Parello & Samms, 2010).

## Self-Perception–Self-Concept Pattern

Through each of the developmental processes of physiological growth, cognitive development, and social development, children progressively engage in an important process of self-discovery. Through these processes, children actively build and create their own personalities, develop relationships with others, and expose themselves to a wide range of experiences that influence their behavior, attitudes, and values.

### Erikson's Theory

The stage of personality development described by Erikson for the school-age child is industry versus inferiority. The major task to be accomplished is full mastery of whatever the child is doing (sense of industry). The child focuses on success in personal and social tasks and avoidance of a sense of inferiority. Inferiority occurs with repeated failures at attempted tasks and with little encouragement or trust from people important to the child.

With mastery of the tools of the culture in relation to those of the peer group, a sense of worth and understanding of the self develops (Erikson, 1993, 1994).

## Self-Concept

Self-concept develops over time and through a variety of experiences and relationships. For example, by being responsible for a pet's care and by showing love to this animal, the older school-age child nurtures a positive self-concept. The way in which others, especially peers, view the child influences the sense of self (Ferrer & Fugate, 2014; Sturaro et al., 2011). Increasing cognitive abilities facilitate better understanding of the identifying factors of others (race, ethnicity, disability, or gender) and how those others compare with the child. Self-concept includes self-esteem, sense of control, and body concept.

*Self-esteem.* Self-esteem has been defined as the extent to which an individual believes oneself to be capable, significant, successful, and worthy (AAP, 2015d). The younger school-age child has a limited self-concept, but one that develops with successful completion of the tasks of this period (Erikson's sense of industry). Although engaged in more activities outside the home, the child still depends on the family, as defined by one's culture, to develop high self-esteem. In school, teachers or group leaders frequently reward those who have succeeded in a task with badges, stars, or privileges (tangible objects that validate success).

The peer group's influence on the school-age child's self-esteem is unquestionable. Acceptance by a peer group contributes to feelings of self-worth and a sense of belonging to a desired group. Competition or collaboration with peers in school, clubs, and activities also influences feelings of adequacy and feelings of success (Women's & Children's Health Network, 2013). Parents must be encouraged to expose their school-age children to interesting activities of their choice, involving peers, to nurture their self-esteem and sense of uniqueness.

Concern has been voiced about school-age girls suffering a decline in self-esteem that affects their school achievements. Some research indicates that boys receive more praise in school than do girls, and girls receive criticism on the content of their work, whereas boys receive more criticism on the appearance of their work (Garey, 2015). Girls experience greater competition now than in earlier times, and they face pressures about personal appearance, particularly if they are white. Various authors report that girls need strong adults to support their ways of thinking and behaving in a world often built on "male values." Girls tend to have high self-esteem if they perceive parental harmony that supports perceptions of balance within themselves and promotes their emotional health (Garey, 2015).

In encouraging development of self-esteem in all school-age children, the nurse remembers that a child needs to experience success with tasks, and completely structured activities may not provide this opportunity for some children. A child who succeeds in some things and receives acceptance by peers gains a sense of competence and worth, is self-confident, and has high self-esteem, which are important qualities for life survival.

*Sense of control.* As the school-age child matures and makes choices, a sense of control develops about the self and the environment. Children with an internal locus of control believe they are responsible for their behavior and accomplishments and tend to have higher levels of achievement than do children who believe in an external locus of control. The latter think that fewer reasons exist for them to try hard at a task, because others or fate determines life results. Hispanic and black American cultures may more often support an external locus of control based on a strong belief that God determines one's outcome (Tynan, 2015). Older children and girls tend to have a more internalized locus of control than do younger children and boys.

*Body concept.* The school-age child's concept of the body and its functioning also changes from the preschool period and adds to overall self-concept. By age 8 to 11 years, children know that parts of the body constitute a related whole. The 11-year-old child can name twice the number and functions of internal body structures that a 6-year-old child can and frequently understands the functions of the cardiovascular, musculoskeletal, and nervous systems. For example, the 7-year-old child knows that the heart is important and that it beats, whereas the 13-year-old child knows that the heart pumps blood. Changes or differences in the body may frighten the school-age child until the child understands normal developmental processes, such as losing deciduous teeth. Physical differences, such as freckles, can provoke ridicule and isolation. Children in this age group frequently feel threatened by others with deformities. Children with chronic illness worry that their peer relationships will be negatively influenced if others know about their illness. Children who learn about body differences, by meeting people with chronic health problems as well as by reading and discussion of anxiety about differences, increase their knowledge of the body and ways to maintain health. They also gain an understanding of the value of each person, despite their differences.

## Roles-Relationships Pattern

The family environment provides a sense of security that allows the school-age child to cope with uncertainties in the external environment. Although many live in single, divorced, mixed-race, or same-sex parenting households, the family structure generally encourages a child's cognitive growth through exposure to a variety of experiences that bolster the desire to achieve and develop positive self-esteem.

Parents, caregivers, and children interact in a variety of ways to show love and companionship for each other. Caregivers, such as grandparents or extended family members, protect the dependent child and teach the learning child. The caregiver-child relationship is not equal, primarily because caregivers and parents serve as authority figures that establish the rules needed for the functioning of the family and safe growth of the child. During the school-age years, the child's increasing maturity, independence, and responsibility begin to reduce the amount of parental authority and structure needed. In some cultures, parents set higher standards for child independence than parents of other diverse populations (Women & Children's Health Network, 2013). With increasing independence, the child prioritizes school and peer group relationships to develop socialization skills and understand group social mores (Sturaro et al., 2011). These connections will help prepare the child for future relationships.

School-age children also begin to broaden their interests outside the home, often encouraged by parents. Unfortunately, some older children may become involved in gangs, behavior that causes much stress for both children and their parents. The child's changing world frequently alters family schedules and patterns, supporting studies that have found that parents express the least amount of parental satisfaction when their oldest child is between 6 and 13 years of age. The relationships between siblings differ, depending on birth order, culture, sex, and age differences and perceived power of siblings. Siblings interact with one another in a number of roles, such as playmates, teacher-learner, protector-dependent, and adversaries, based on feelings of jealousy and rivalry that often occur in families. School-age children cope with these feelings better than do preschool children because they have outlets outside the family, including school and friends. Parents can minimize conflicts by recognizing each child's needs and level of maturity and by providing guidance and support.

As children mature, they assume more responsibilities within the family and the community. School-age children learn responsibility for allowance, household chores, self-care, and pets and acquire a sense of empowerment as an integral part of the family. This is the period during which families often give allowances or children earn money through chores or small jobs, such as paper routes. The amount of an allowance may relate to cultural values. In one study, Asian children earned higher allowances than did other children from diverse population groups for completing fewer chores and for meeting higher standards of academic performance (Goldstein & Brooks, 2012). School-age children learn valuable life lessons by earning and spending their allowances.

Children learn socially accepted behaviors when their parents engage in **limit setting** (defining expected behavior and consequences when limits are not honored). Violent behavior must be discouraged, and nonviolent methods to reach resolutions for personal problems should be encouraged (Box 20-6). Parents who express their feelings, explain why things happen, and listen to their children while setting limits encourage the development of self-control and positive self-esteem. Some families with school-age children find it helpful to have periodic family meetings during which everyone discusses family issues, rules, and responsibilities. Behavior contracts between the parent and the child provide direction and may also encourage improved behavior by delineating favorable consequences when the terms of the contract are followed.

Children frequently model their behavior after that of people they love or admire (parents, friends, and other adults). Positive reinforcement (rewards for good behavior) is an effective form of limit setting (i.e., **discipline**), used often by upper-class parents. **Punishment**, a negative reinforcement as reflected in shaming a child in front of the child's community or family (seen with some Asian cultures), may stop an undesired behavior but often only until the child repeats the action and is not caught.

---

**BOX 20-6   The School-Age Child: Points for Effective Discipline**

Effective discipline is essential to family harmony and individual child growth and reflects cultural beliefs. The goal of discipline is to encourage and reinforce positive child behaviors, eliminate inappropriate child behaviors, improve parent-child communication, and meet parental needs. Effective discipline requires these essential components: a positive, supportive, loving relationship between the parent and the child; use of positive reinforcement strategies to increase desired behavior; and removal of reinforcements or application of punishment to reduce/eliminate undesired behaviors.

Specifics of discipline strategies include the following:

- Ignoring the misbehavior and acknowledging the appropriate behavior
- Using distraction or substitution to avoid a problem situation
- Offering choices to prevent inappropriate behavior such as whining or emotional outbursts
- Using humor to decrease the intensity of a situation
- Modeling the appropriate behavior
- Setting age-relevant limits
- Giving specific and clear commands for behavior appropriate to the child's age
- Talking calmly, being a good listener, and encouraging negotiation, perhaps in a family meeting, to promote problem resolution
- Limiting a child's environment (distractions such as music and television)
- Setting clear and consistent consequences for misbehavior (withholding privileges, using contracts)
- Providing one-to-one time, focusing on positive attention
- Taking time for oneself to replenish one's energies as a parent and as an individual

From American Academy of Pediatrics. (2015). *Disciplining your child.* http://www.healthychildren.org/English/family-life/family-dynamics/communication-discipline/pages/Disciplining-Your-Child.aspx.

---

Lower-socioeconomic-class parents tend to use more punishment directed toward misbehavior or failure to adhere to parental values and requirements.

### Child Abuse

**Child abuse** (physical, sexual, or emotional exploitation of children) and neglect (lack of adequate food, shelter, or emotional support) continue to be significant societal problems. According to the USDHHS (2011) and the AAP (2011b), more than 3 million cases of abuse or neglect in children are reported annually in the United States. Abused children have an increased likelihood of becoming violent adults and of abusing their own children. The factors that increase the risk of abuse include family poverty, culture, limited maternal education, needy child syndrome, presence of a stepfather, single-parent status, parental drug addiction, and teenage parenthood (AAP, 2011b). However, child abuse also occurs in families that do not have these risk factors. Cultural factors must be considered in detecting abuse. For example, coin rubbing of the chest (used in the Asian ethnic group for treatment of respiratory tract infections) leaves abrasions that may be perceived as abuse by a nurse assessing an ill child. National governmental agencies and professional organizations require that health care providers report suspected abuse and participate in preventing, assessing, and treating victims.

State nurse practice acts require nurses to report suspected cases of abuse. Ultimately, nurses help interrupt the vicious cycle of abuse by becoming involved in community coalitions and innovative evidence-based programs that prevent and intervene in child and family abuse.

Unfortunately, relationships between children and adults are not always positive. Sexual abuse, use of a child for sexual exploitative purposes, has become a more common but often hidden problem for a variety of reasons (AAP, 2011b; USDHHS, 2011): the child may be too frightened to talk about the situation, families and society do not want to admit its existence, Internet traffic has supported pornography and pedophilia, and fewer agencies exist to respond to these cases. Many victims know their abusers (many are parents), and people in positions of authority (e.g., teachers, coaches, or clergy members) may be abusers. The child may comply for a variety of reasons, such as a need to be good or a need to keep the family together. Emotions are complex and change as the child grows, but they often lead to adult anxiety, depression, and physical symptoms and illnesses. Males less often report sexual abuse but are more likely than girls to suffer negative emotional effects from incest, a form of sexual abuse.

As in any type of suspected abuse, nurses assist these children by recognizing those at risk and those experiencing abuse and referring them to relevant resources. All people who work with young children must acknowledge the warning signs of abuse (Box 20-7). When sexual abuse is suspected, an in-depth interview and examination must be conducted by a specially trained, multidisciplinary team that is sensitive to the needs of the child and can validate the abuse. Most authorities believe that children who describe sexual abuse are telling the truth because the details are usually specific and trauma is evident. Therefore a child's story should be believed unless it is disproved.

---

### BOX 20-7 Warning Signs of Child Abuse

- Physical evidence of abuse or neglect, including previous injuries
- Conflicting stories about the "accident" or injury from the parents or others
- Injury or complaint inconsistent with the child's history or developmental level (e.g., the child received a concussion and broken arm from falling off a bed)
- Signs and symptoms consistent with signs of abuse and inconsistent with history, vague recall of event (e.g., chief complaint is a cold when there is evidence of first-degree and second-degree burns)
- Inappropriate response of caregiver, such as an exaggerated or absent emotional response, refusal to give consent for additional tests or agree to necessary treatment, excessive delay in seeking treatment, or absence of the parents
- Inappropriate response of child, such as little or no response to pain, fear of being touched, excessive or lack of separation anxiety, or indiscriminate friendliness to strangers
- Child's report of physical or sexual abuse
- Previous reports of abuse in the family
- Repeated visits to emergency facilities with injuries

From Smith, M., & Segal, J. (2016). *Child abuse and neglect.* http://www.helpguide.org/articles/abuse/child-abuse-and-neglect.htm.

---

## Sexuality-Reproductive Pattern

The preschool child learns about sex differences and begins to model the general societal behaviors expected of a female or male child. The child enters the school-age years with a strong identification with the parent of the same sex. The child continues to learn the concepts and behavior of the gender role and incorporate these into the self-concept. This challenge is significant for all children, but more so for homosexual children. Societal stereotypes related to gender roles continue to influence the school-age child's ideas of male and female roles. Fortunately, most children receive early teaching about gender roles that emphasizes that sex does not determine one's choices, personality, or behavior. As a result of this teaching, children increasingly choose occupations based on their skills and interests, rather than on what appears appropriate because of their sex.

The school-age child's increasing awareness of the body, its functioning, and a need for sexual identity combine to foster a desire for knowledge about the biological aspects of sexual function. Late in the school-age period, when the physical changes of puberty have begun, concern and curiosity about sexual issues frequently develop. A child may become extremely attached to another of the same sex, and they may explore one another's sexual organs. This is common exploratory behavior and does not reflect true homosexuality, even though parents and children may express concerns about it. With the advent of physical changes of puberty, the school-age child desires more privacy in a bedroom shared with no one. As noted earlier, the physical changes of puberty appear gradually over several years.

Children frequently share questions about sexual matters with their peer group. Parents are often uncomfortable or unsure of what sexual information to give to their children and when to give it. Many health care agencies sponsor short programs to educate parents and older school-age children, in a supportive environment, about body and mental changes during preadolescence and puberty. An increasing number of age-appropriate books that focus on emotional and body changes can be used at home and in school to increase children's understanding. Particularly because menstrual cycles start earlier now than they did 50 years ago, education about body changes and puberty appears appropriate as part of later school-age education.

The nurse plays an important role in sex education in health care and education settings. This professional should be receptive to answering questions in this area and at each health care visit. The nurse employed in the school is in an ideal position to teach group, sex education programs using literature and games. Children at this age appear to respond most favorably with sex-segregated classes because of their general discomfort with sexual topics and unique needs and questions. Some schools appropriately incorporate these classes into school curricula as part of a health-promotion curriculum. Other schools have special programs focused only on sex education based on parental desires or school board policies. Most school-age children have the cognitive skills to respond to programs on responsible sexuality, including discussions on abstinence and condom use, pregnancy, sexually transmitted diseases, and the human immunodeficiency

**TABLE 20-2  The School-Age Child's Coping Strategies and Nursing Interventions to Promote Coping**

| Coping Strategies | Nursing Interventions |
|---|---|
| Use of defense mechanisms (regression, denial, repression, projection, displacement, sublimation) | Accept child's use of defense mechanisms as temporary, healthy coping responses; provide child with options for moving to more age-appropriate ways of responding to stressors |
| Cognitive mastery (problem-solving, communication) | Ask children what they know of the situation and how they might handle it; encourage questions; use diagrams and models to help explain; encourage child to verbalize feelings and use past successful strategies that might help deal with present stressors; try personalized approaches, such as books, puppets, and manipulation of equipment, to increase feelings of control when faced with a stressful situation; encourage praying and other communications to a chosen deity as appropriate |
| Controlling, holding behaviors | Encourage child to participate and to make decisions; accept child's need to direct as appropriate; set consistent age-appropriate limits; respond to signals for help; let child be responsible for self-care |
| Use of repetition | Use books, games, and other communication media to work through feelings; emphasize "ok" for child to continue to ask questions and to receive answers that assist in coping |
| Use of humor | Be a good listener and participate in riddles and jokes used by child; be a good sport with school-age children's desire to play jokes on each other; share stories and cartoons with child |
| Motor activity, aggression, protest behavior | Encourage physical activity to deal with stress; accept appropriate behavior; establish limits on behavior for group safety |
| Withdrawal (resurgence of separation anxiety) | When child is separated from the family, child may have separation anxiety; encourage close emotional contacts between child and significant others (friends, family, church members); allow favorite objects from home to be brought to the hospital or a new environment for child |

virus (Krause-Parello & Samms, 2010). The nurse also wants to include program content specific to disabled children, who face unique body changes and concerns and need to understand ways others can express affection to them without causing accusations of abuse.

## Coping–Stress Tolerance Pattern

The school-age child must learn to cope with stress as part of the developmental process. Through a health-promotion program, children can learn to identify symptoms of stress (pounding heart, stomach "butterflies," and sweaty hands) and ways to cope with these perceived stresses (e.g., deep breathing and walking) before they cause illness. The child actually faces many stressful experiences in life, including competition, homework deadlines, failure at home or school, and decisions whether to cheat, steal, or even join an unpopular peer group. The young school-age child may never have shared his or her life with other children the same age, and cultural values learned earlier in life may not be reflected in school or in peer relationships. Threats to the child's security (e.g., bullying) cause feelings of helplessness and anxiety that may affect the ability to function successfully (Reuschel, 2011). Grief over the death of a loved one, parental divorce, loss of a favorite activity because of misbehavior, or expulsion from a favorite peer group may cause negative behavior. Parents need to provide appropriate discipline in responding to this behavior but should also listen and analyze factors related to the problem so as to increase the child's feelings of control and decrease stress for the family.

Children use a variety of coping strategies, healthy behaviors intended to buffer perceived stressful events. However, in a very stressful situation or many stressful situations, a child may be unable to move beyond the coping behaviors. In conversations with teachers and parents, the nurse may offer a variety of strategies for coping with a school-age child's problems, enabling the child to cope and learn from others (Table 20-2). These strategies may involve role-playing or referral to literature on the problem topic to interrupt the child's negative behavior cycle and improve family health (see Table 20-2). The nurse may also refer a child to relevant religious and spiritual leaders, on the basis of school-age children's belief that prayer will help them cope with an otherwise uncontrollable situation.

### Parental Divorce

More than half of all marriages end in divorce, leaving many school-age children to face stress related to their parents' separation. Often children experience a feeling of loss, although they may hope that their parents will reunite at some point. Box 20-8 discusses the effects of divorce on a school-age child. Children's responses vary with their level of development (Kim, 2011). Factors such as economic security; availability of both of their parents, other family, church, and school supports; and quality of interactions with their parents can influence the child's ability to cope with divorce. Unfortunately, many parents become so immersed in their own feelings that they fail to support their children (Pickhardt, 2011). Conflicts over custody, child support, and visitation rights add to the child's difficulty in coping. Sometimes the school system becomes the child's advocate to encourage the parents to provide a supportive environment during divorce proceedings. Despite this intervention, some children do not cope well with the divorce and have emotional consequences that result in juvenile behavior problems or require long-term counseling (see the case study and care plan at the end of this chapter).

## BOX 20-8   Effects of Divorce on the School-Age Child

School-age children tend to view life in black and white and are likely to blame one parent for the breakup. Boys, especially, mourn the loss of their fathers and frequently express anger at their mothers. Both boys and girls have great difficulty accepting their parents' new dates. Crying, daydreaming, and problems with friends and school are common divorce-related behaviors in children of this age.

Here are some suggestions that might help the school-age child cope with divorce of parents:

- *Discourage reconciliation fantasies.*
  Have parents avoid dinners, outings, or holiday celebrations with the ex-spouse. This only fuels the child's fantasies. Instead, emphasize the finality of divorce.
- *Make sure the child has the phone number of the absent parent.*
  Both parents should encourage easy access and frequent conversations with the noncustodial parent.
- *Do not allow the child to manipulate the parents into buying more possessions.*
  School-age children are likely to feel deprived. Although they may intensify requests for playthings or other possessions, do not try to retain child's affection through material objects. Even children of divorce need to be told "No!"
- *Talk to the child's teachers or school counselors about the divorce.*
  School personnel may better understand possible learning or behavioral problems and will likely offer extra support.

From Pickhardt, C. (2011). *Impact of divorce on young children and adolescents.* http://www.psychologytoday.com/blog/surviving-your-childs-adolescence/201112/the-impact-divorce-young-children-and-adolescents.

## Somatization and Depression

Children, like adults, use defense mechanisms to cope, with various degrees of success. Two strategies used by the school-age child to respond to uncontrollable situations are somatization and depression.

Some children respond to a stressful situation by transferring their feelings to a physical problem (somatization). In this phenomenon, school-age children, unable to discuss their concerns, complain of stomachaches or headaches, symptoms reflective of functional or psychogenic pain. These children may also develop discrete, repetitive movement habits called tics. In many cases the child with these problems must be evaluated to determine whether an underlying physiological cause exists. The child and the family will then need assistance in understanding the child's concerns to define successful ways to cope with the behavior.

Depression occurs in up to 2% of school-age children (AAP, 2015e), and more often in boys than in girls during the school-age period. Depression reflects a disturbance of mood, when a child displays sadness, guilt, or worthlessness, and other unusual behaviors that disengage the child from peers and the family. In defining depression in children, most authors emphasize that they are referring to a more long-term syndrome in which the child's normal development and functioning become impaired, not a periodic sadness that all children occasionally experience. The factors that place a child at risk of depression include

homelessness, death of a parent or significant other, divorce, long-term hospitalization, chronic illness, learning problems, and emotional turmoil at home. Parents and teachers look for symptoms of depression, including anorexia, sleeplessness, lethargy, changed affect, aggressive behavior, frequent crying, and withdrawal from previously enjoyed activities.

Although it has been concluded that there is insufficient evidence to routinely screen all school-age children for depression, the nurse can serve an important role in identifying any child who appears to be depressed and in notifying parents about the need for further assessment. Depending on the child and the situation, differing amounts of counseling and individual child guidance may be required. Nurses in schools and outpatient settings are often the ideal helpers because they have the skills and time needed to help a child cope with a helpless feeling and its cause.

## Values-Beliefs Pattern

Children make decisions related to moral and ethical issues every day. Should they tell the teacher which classmate broke the rule? Should they share their candy with a younger sibling? For these situations, the child makes a decision on the basis of the level of moral development. Moral development involves choosing the most appropriate behavior on the basis of one's values and feelings related to the situation. Environmental factors and culture strongly influence a child's moral development, as do the type of family discipline, role models, people with whom the child identifies, and the child's rehearsal and practice of moral behavior.

### Kohlberg's Theory

Most researchers agree that the younger school-age child is at the preconventional level, a level of moral development characterized by self-interest only. The child continues to do many things simply to avoid getting in trouble and does not understand the reason for rules, but also performs actions that will benefit the self (Kohlberg, 1981). During later childhood (10–13 years) most children progress to the conventional level, a stage of moral development defined by concern about group interests and values. The conventional level of moral judgment involves the child looking to others for approval and to societal authority for a definition of rules. Children aged 10 to 12 years judge a behavior in terms of the intention of the offender, understand the "golden rule" concept, and engage in behavior that maintains a valued relationship. The conventional level coincides with Piaget's cognitive level of concrete operations and the child's increased social involvement with people outside the home (Kohlberg, 1981).

### Moral Behavior Problems

Some moral behavior problems, such as lying, stealing, or cheating, are common during the school-age years. Cultural, religious, and parental values influence a child's moral development, concept of right and wrong, and consequences of not demonstrating moral behavior. Preschool and younger school-age children frequently lie as a result of fantasy, exaggerations, or inaccurate understanding. As children mature, they may use the defense mechanism of denial to block upsetting situations and maintain self-esteem. The lie then becomes an unconscious act. Older children often lie because they fear punishment or ridicule. Children may cheat because of a desire to win, do well in competitive society, or "look good" for their peers. Children usually steal when they think they will not be caught and they think that there is no other way to get what they want (McLeod, 2015). Although these actions can be quite upsetting for parents, they are common developmental behaviors. Parents frequently need reassurance that the child is normal and will probably outgrow the behavior with parental assistance. They may need help in developing fair rules for behavior and communicating their expectations for a child's behavior to meet parental and cultural values. Therefore the nurse encourages the parents to warn the child clearly not to steal, lie, or cheat; offer other, more socially acceptable, ways to cope with the stressor causing the behavior; and then apply appropriate punishment congruent with an understanding of the event.

# ENVIRONMENTAL PROCESSES

## Physical Agents

School-age children, similarly to those of all other age groups, face daily exposure to environmental agents and factors that may cause injury, illness, or death. Many of these agents and factors are harmless if appropriately used or if there is minimal exposure. Examples include physical agents such as fires; mechanical agents such as bicycles, skateboards, and cars; biological agents such as bacteria; chemical agents such as asbestos; and radiological agents such as X-rays. Death rates from these agents differ among ethnic groups because of access to health care and environmental issues. For example, Native Americans and Alaska Natives experience higher death rates from motor vehicle accidents, residential fires, and drowning than do other groups. Black Americans have higher death rates for unintentional injury than do other ethnic group members (USDHHS, 2012b).

## Accidents

Accidents are the leading cause of death in children older than 1 year in the United States (USDHHS, 2013). Most accidents do not result in death, but many serious ones cause significant morbidity and disability. Because of this effect, the nurse has a significant role in educating parents and school personnel on ways to prevent dangers to school-age children and to become involved in public initiatives to create a safer society for them (Safe Kids, 2013).

The agent, host, and environment must be considered when one is developing solutions to decrease the number of accidents. The type of agent varies with the child's age. Most fatal accidents during the school-age period occur from motor vehicle accidents when the child (host) is a passenger or pedestrian (walking or riding a bike). Other fatal accidents occur from fires and burns, riding bicycles, drowning, and use of firearms. Most common nonfatal accidents tend to be caused by simple agents that produce simple injuries. Despite helmet laws in several states, many school-age children continue to experience head injuries related to recreational equipment, such as bicycles, swings, skateboards, and trampolines (CDC, 2014b). Slightly older children have an increased number of accidents from contact sports and cuts, falls, and burns, and injuries from firearms.

Specific accident factors relate to the host—the school-age child (Box 20-9: Quality and Safety Scenario). Children in this age group tend to become hurt because of their carefree attitude, curiosity, love of mimicking older people, and intense oral tendencies. Typically, school-age boys have more accidents than school-age girls, perhaps attributable to differences in personalities, societal expectations, childrearing practices, and increased propensity for risk-taking behaviors. The mechanism differs with the sex of the host. For school-age boys, drowning is the most common fatal accident; for girls, automobile accidents are the most common (AAP, 2012; CDC, 2015a; Daly et al., 2010).

The physical environment of the child dictates the type or frequency of accidents, which occur in the home, neighborhood, and school. Most accidents happen outdoors, which means that school-age children face greater risk of automobile or bicycle accidents than of poisoning or falls, indoor accidents that occur predominantly in younger children. More accidents (drowning and pedestrian-vehicle accidents) occur in the summer than in the winter because of children's outside play. Socioeconomic level affects children's physical environments and access to dangers. For example, space heaters place children of low-income families at risk of burns, whereas skiing places wealthier children at risk of injury.

The social environment, which includes the family, school, and playmates, also plays a role in accidents. Although little research has focused on the physical trauma caused by heavy backpacks that many school-age children use, these bags exert significant pressure against functionally immature muscles of the back and torso. Daily carrying of bulging backpacks causes muscle strain, headaches, improper posture, shoulder slouch, and other physical problems. Additionally, teachers' expectations that all textbooks be available both in the classroom and at home must be considered. At least one study has shown that children will change their backpack-carrying behaviors if they are involved in a school-based program focused on this topic (AAP, 2012).

As part of the social environment, the family may influence the rate of accidents in the school-age child. Chronic familial stress (parental unemployment) or sudden acute stress (parental illness) may contribute to homicide as the third leading cause of death among children aged 5 to 14 years (USDHHS, 2013). Homicide is a more common cause of death among black American and Hispanic children than among white children. Children also face increased risk of accidents when parental supervision is limited, such as during holidays or a move to a new home.

### Drowning

Fewer school-age children than infants and adolescents die of drowning. More black American children of this age drown than do white American children (CDC, 2014e). Water safety measures can help reduce drowning, along with the many other injuries that occur around water, such as falls in slippery areas.

## ☑ BOX 20-9   QUALITY AND SAFETY SCENARIO

### *Safety Concerns Specific to School-Age Children*

Because of increased independence, school-age children face significant exposure to situations threatening their health. Consequently, the parents of these children must be involved in community and legislative activities that provide safe play environments. Additionally, at appropriate health visits, health care workers should provide anticipatory guidance to parents in the following areas:

**Bicycle Safety**

Each child should have a well-maintained bicycle, ride only in safe areas approved by the parents, observe rules for vehicle traffic, ride on the side of the road with traffic, "bike defensively," and use a federally approved riding helmet.

**Street Safety**

Children should look right, left, then right again to check the safety of crossing a street; children should cross only at safe and well-monitored intersections, preferably with an adult present; ensure parental supervision when children play close to streets and heavy traffic areas.

**Motor Vehicle Safety**

Children should wear a seat belt or be in an age-appropriate booster seat as needed; older children should ride with a restraint system and in the back seat until age 12 years.

**Pool Safety**

All children should have swimming lessons and swim with a buddy or adult who swims well; all pools should have drain covers; children should avoid swimming after a heavy meal and avoid "roughhousing" behavior around the pool; children should be monitored by the parents during swimming.

**Firearm Safety**

Adults need to lock away guns and ensure gun safety locks are intact; parents need to educate children *never* to touch guns.

**Playground Safety**

All playground equipment should meet federally approved standards; children should be trained on how to use equipment safely; equipment should be evaluated for safety and repaired before children use it.

**Fire Safety**

Working smoke detectors should be in place in the home and school; the family needs to have a fire evacuation plan and practice it; children need to wear fire-retardant clothing at night; children should not play with matches, open fires, fireworks, or open wires that can cause injury and fire.

**Toxin Safety**

Children should avoid insecticides, radiation sources, inappropriate use of medications, and pollution sources; parents need to store all known toxins, chemicals, and household cleaning agents in an adequately ventilated location that is inaccessible to children.

**Stranger Safety**

Children should play with friends, have a plan for returning home, know the home phone number and address, play in a safe and known area, and report any suspicious activity threatening their safety to an appropriate adult; children should know how to say "no" and how to locate assistance when in an unsafe situation.

**Sports Safety**

Children need to engage in age-appropriate activities and wear protective equipment relevant to the sport; parents need to ensure safety and maintenance of all sports equipment; parents need to caution children against hazardous sports, such as tramlining.

**Animal Safety**

Parents should teach children to avoid strange animals, especially sick or injured ones, and ensure that personal pets receive vaccinations; parents need to teach children not to mistreat pets and not to place their faces close to any animal.

Although nurses offer suggestions to parents to improve their children's play safety, studies have shown that few parents follow these suggestions. The reasons for this behavior include parental difficulty in assessing the safety of and age-appropriateness of play equipment, the amount of effort involved, and a lack of money to create a safe play area. The nurse helps parents respond to these perceived barriers. With more children using skateboards and rollerblades, the nurse also encourages the use of child safety helmets and knee, elbow, and wrist guards to prevent muscle sprains and bone fractures. The school offers an on-site opportunity for teaching children, teachers, and parents about accident prevention. In addition to providing this guidance, nurses can participate in legislative and educational actions to increase community consciousness about child safety.

---

Environment and safety teaching can influence the number of school-age children dying of drowning.

### Burns

Each year many children become victims of house fires, many of which occur during the winter months from Christmas trees, space heaters, and fireplace malfunctions. Many homes lack working smoke detectors because of incorrect installation or inadequate testing. If a fire occurs in a home with a smoke detector, the risk of death is decreased by 40% to 50% (CDC, 2012). Most burned children survive, frequently with various degrees of physical and psychological scars. Children need to learn about fire safety, including the importance of avoiding situations involving fire and practicing fire drills routinely at school and home. The nurse encourages parents to understand other practices to prevent fire-related problems, including parental purchase of flame-retardant sleepwear for children.

### Firearms

People in the United States who use firearms frequently cause fatal injury through homicide, suicide, or accidents. Every 2 hours 45 minutes someone's child dies from a gun accident (USDHHS, 2013). With many US homes containing a handgun and because of recent shootings by adolescents, concern about children's safety remains well-founded. Possibly the best means of preventing accidents with firearms is to ban them from private ownership, as seen in England. However, because handgun ownership is an important individual right in the United States, several states have passed legislation that allows handguns for individual protection. Families with firearms in the home should store them in a locked area apart from ammunition and consider using nonlethal (wax) bullets. All family members should be knowledgeable about gun safety.

Much debate has been raised recently regarding the use of toy guns by children. Unlike video game use, the use of toy guns during childhood does not increase the likelihood of violent or aggressive behavior later in life. Unfortunately, there have been a number of deaths associated with police mistaking a toy gun being used by school-age children for a firearm. These deaths have occurred in spite of mandatory markings on toy handguns.

### Sports and Recreation

Accidents from sports and other recreational activities increase during the school-age years and include lacerations, contusions, hematomas, concussions, sprains, and fractures. Some evidence exists that adolescents now have more musculoskeletal injuries because of involvement in repetitive team sports earlier in their lives. This suggests that society needs to examine the current emphasis on initiating young children with musculoskeletal immaturity into team sports such as football, hockey, soccer, and basketball. Intense social pressure for children to participate in these sports means that parents and school systems must ensure that each child has protective body devices to prevent injuries, as well as psychological support to allow a child to benefit from the team sport. There is a further need to increase safety by ensuring that each child fits the sport, has adequate hydration during the game, and engages in conditioning exercises before and after the game for prevention of injuries. Furthermore, the literature supports societal need to focus more on the collaborative skills children learn by being part of a team, rather than the intense focus on winning philosophy found in many school-age team sports.

Recreation area injuries may be prevented by several measures. The National Bureau of Standards set guidelines in 1976 for home playground equipment, regulating objects such as sharp edges, moving parts, and equipment design. Nurses help prevent accidents by participating in decisions about school playground equipment and counseling families on a variety of issues. Playground safety has become an important issue because 200,000 children need emergency department assessment each year for related injuries (USDHHS, 2013). Girls are slightly more likely to be injured on the playground than boys, and many of these injuries occur in low-income neighborhoods where playgrounds fail to meet safety standards (CDC, 2012).

### Mechanical Forces

Motor vehicles and bicycles are the two most common mechanical agents that cause injury to school-age children.

***Motor vehicles.*** The leading cause of death in the United States in all individuals from age 1 year to age 34 years is motor vehicle accidents (CDC, 2015a). Children die as passengers in cars, as pedestrians, and as bicycle riders. In the United States, more children die from pedestrian-related accidents than from passenger-related accidents (CDC, 2014b). Since 1999, 127 children have died each year in bicycle accidents, 80% of whom did not wear helmets to prevent head injury. Helmet use in

children can reduce the risk of head injury by 45% (USDHHS, 2012b). Although not all accidents result in death, children may also sustain injury that causes permanent disability as a result of motor vehicle accidents.

Automobile passenger injuries can be prevented, or the severity reduced, by alteration of some aspects of the child's environment. Lower speed limits, stricter enforcement of alcohol-related laws, better automobile and highway designs, improved door lock mechanisms, and more effective restraint system requirements in all states have reduced the severity and number of accidents and injuries (USDHHS, 2012b). However, more injuries have been correlated to higher speed limits instituted in the United States several years ago. Furthermore, many children remain at risk of injury because various school districts and states do not require seat belts in buses used to transport students, despite a recommendation by the AAP to do so.

Proper and consistent use of federally approved belt-positioned booster seats for children aged 4 to 7 years decreases the likelihood of child death and serious injury significantly (AAP, 2015a). However, one study showed that only 19% of such children used these seats. Less than 10% of children needing the protection of a booster seat ride in one, and younger, smaller school-age children (shorter than 4 feet 9 inches) often fail to use them correctly (Governors Highway Safety Association, 2015). The reasons given by parents and children for their not using seat belts or booster seats include forgetting to use the device, having difficulty reaching and fastening belts, feeling discomfort from wearing the belt or using the seat, and receiving misinformation about the need for the belt or seat for short trips. Clearly, consistent use of booster seats by young children and seat belts by older children and adults, who model seat belt behavior to their children, will occur only when legal enforcement occurs. Federal government and national professional groups recommend that all children younger than 12 years ride in the automobile's back seat in an appropriate restraint because of the potential for death from an air bag activated in a motor vehicle accident (Daly et al., 2010; Governors Highway Safety Association, 2015). Many families have difficulty meeting this recommendation because of long-term acceptance of older children riding in the front seat after they have outgrown booster seats.

Urban children younger than 15 years old experience more than half of all pedestrian-automobile accidents. These occur when they are using rollerblades, skateboards, and skate scooters and tend to be more severe (head injuries) than passenger injuries. Many factors cause pedestrian accidents: children often have difficulty interpreting traffic signs and judging the speed of cars, and they forget to look carefully before crossing the street. Although overcrowding, poverty, high volume of traffic, stress, and unsafe play areas influence children's street safety, various principles can direct interventions to decrease the number of street dangers.

***Bicycles and motorized vehicles.*** Many accidents occur each year with young children on bicycles, motorized skateboards, and all-terrain vehicles (ATVs). Most of these are not serious, but deaths occur among young children who have suffered head trauma or significant body injury from inappropriate use of this equipment. The AAP (2012) recommends that only people at

## BOX 20-10 Nursing Interventions to Prevent Accidents During the School-Age Period

### Strategies for Counseling

- Discuss accident prevention at optimal times, such as during prenatal visits or well-child visits, after the arrival of a new sibling, or after an accident.
- Rather than discussing all topics at once, pick the main concerns for the developmental level of the child at each well-child visit. For the school-age child, these topics include motor vehicle, water, fire, and bicycle safety.
- Repeat information at other visits to emphasize its importance.

### Community Actions

- Use supplemental materials, such as pamphlets, to reinforce the verbal information.
- Support local and national legislation that sets standards for potentially harmful agents. Mandating standards has been one of the most successful accident preventive strategies, as seen in the Poison Prevention Packaging Act and the Flammable Fabrics Act.
- Encourage children to wear a bicycle helmet and other protective gear when appropriate. Many nurses have been active in lobbying for bicycle helmet requirements in their states.
- Consult with manufacturers on safe designs of materials used by children.
- Report objects that are potentially hazardous.
- Participate in local activities that stress accident prevention, such as those organized by local offices of the National Safety Council.
- Educate groups, such as schoolchildren and parent organizations.

From US Department of Health and Human Services (2012). *An agenda to prevent injuries and promote the safety of children and adolescents in the United States.* http://www.cdc.gov/safechild/pdf/National_Action_Plan_for_Child_Injury_Prevention.pdf

least 16 years old ride ATVs and then only in rural areas with adult supervision. Bicycle accidents occur most frequently near the child's home and during the day, and commonly involve injuries from the spokes when children ride behind the bike seat. More boys than girls experience these injuries from bicycles, motorized skateboards, and ATVs, perhaps because of their greater risk-taking behavior (Daly et al., 2010).

In response to children's developmental behavior related to bicycles, motorized skateboards, and ATVs, the nurse addresses safety issues. Additionally, nurses encourage parents to teach and reinforce safe bicycling habits to their children and should sponsor helmet and bike programs within the school (Box 20-10).

## Biological Agents

School-age children face constant exposure to bacterial, viral, and other biological agents that pose threats to or improve their overall health (e.g., immunizations). Compared with the preschool child, the school-age child has fewer illnesses. The most frequent illness continues to be upper respiratory tract infections (URIs), illnesses shared among schoolchildren who fail to practice good handwashing techniques and avoidance of ill peers. These illnesses cause children to lose school days and learning opportunities. Most URIs result from viruses, but bacteria can play either a primary or a secondary role. Two problems associated with URIs are streptococcal infection ("strep throat") and otitis media.

Strep throat occurs frequently among school-age children. A child with an infection from group A *Streptococcus* may have a severe sore throat, fever, and malaise, or may have only a minor sore throat. A throat culture confirms the diagnosis, and antibiotic treatment typically cures the infection. Children are noninfectious after 24 hours of treatment and may return to school (Wald, 2015). If not treated, the affected child may develop rheumatic fever or acute glomerulonephritis as a secondary infection following the sore throat. Greater transmission of streptococcal infection occurs in areas where there is close personal contact during colder weather. The school nurse's preventive efforts focus on teaching the children good handwashing techniques and identifying children who complain of sore throats. Children with throat infections caused by other strains of *Streptococcus,* such as group B, do not usually require treatment, because these infections generally do not cause the same serious complications.

Otitis media rates have subsided with the integration of the pneumococcal and influenza vaccines into the immunization schedule. Acute otitis media is often self-limiting and can often be regarded as a complication of a preceding or concomitant upper respiratory tract infection. Most cases of otitis media will resolve spontaneously. Without specific treatment, symptoms abate within 24 hours in 60% of children and settle within 3 days in 80% of children (Toll & Nunez, 2012). The nurse is in an integral position to help support the family and educate the family on risk factors associated with otitis media and nonpharmacological therapies that may alleviate symptoms and discomfort during the course of illness.

The school-age child may experience other illnesses. The frequency of gastrointestinal tract infection (**gastroenteritis**) decreases during the school-age years but is still the second most common acute condition of childhood. Usually caused by a virus, gastrointestinal tract infections cause vomiting and diarrhea. Older and larger school-age children have little chance of rapid dehydration; they basically react to the illness the same as do adults and need to be treated similarly. Gastroenteritis is contagious, and therefore the nurse should monitor schoolchildren for symptoms of illness and encourage proper handwashing to prevent transmission of the virus from one child to another.

**Scabies** and **pediculosis** are common skin disorders among school-age children, involving extreme itchiness of either the body (scabies) or the head (pediculosis), and are easily spread to other children (Gupta, 2015). The nurse educates parents to visualize the mites and **lice** or use a lice comb to check their children for mites and lice when they complain of itchiness or seem to be constantly scratching their heads. Previously, children with lice could not come to school until they were lice-free, which isolated students from their peers and influenced state school funding based on student attendance. The AAP now recommends that once children are undergoing treatment for the problem, they should be allowed in school (Devore & Schultz, 2015a).

Most states require that the child's immunizations be current before the child enters kindergarten or the first grade and that additional tetanus immunization be given every 10 years or when an unclean wound is acquired. Other immunizations recommended by the AAP include a meningococcal vaccination at age 11 or 12 years and the series of three injections for hepatitis B and human papilloma virus during the late school-age and early adolescent years (USDHHS, 2012b). If the child has no history of chickenpox, a varicella immunization is also recommended. In many states the school nurse has a responsibility to ensure that all students' immunizations are current, and if they are not current, the nurse informs the parents that the children may not attend school until their immunizations are up-to-date (CDC, 2015f; USDHHS, 2012b). Any child lacking age-appropriate immunizations can "catch up" according to a schedule developed by the AAP. Although 79% of American children receive immunizations by school entrance time, increasing numbers of immigrants and transient workers have deepened concern about exposure of Americans to previously conquered diseases (e.g., tuberculosis). Strides toward meeting the *Healthy People* initiative targets related to immunizations continue to be made according to the midcourse review and the 2020 objectives (CDC, 2015f; USDHHS, 2012b).

## Chemical Agents

A number of potentially toxic chemical agents exist in the environment, and the child is exposed to these through inhalation, ingestion, or direct contact. Children are particularly susceptible to chemical hazards. Food and drugs are two sources of chemicals ingested by children on a regular basis, and some older school-age children ingest tobacco as a result of cigarette smoking. Although normally safe, some foods and drugs can be harmful when used inappropriately. Other environmental hazards include pollution, heavy metals (lead and mercury), and pesticides.

The nutritional needs of the school-age child were discussed earlier in this chapter. As stated, children frequently eat foods with large quantities of sugar, salt, and fat and with chemical additives. The effects of some of these additives have been questioned, and concern has been expressed about the effect of biochemically altered food on children and future generations. On a short-term basis, some foods may cause allergic reactions; on a long-term basis, some may contribute to the development of coronary disease, hypertension, and cancer. Nurses are aware that the child's diet may contribute to future health problems, and therefore assess intake and counsel the child and parents accordingly about ways to improve it.

The incidence of poisoning decreases during the school-age years as children become more aware of the appropriate uses of drugs and other agents. Childproof containers have decreased exposure of children to dangerous poisons and chemicals in the home. However, children continue to face exposure to drugs (alcohol and glue inhalants) because of less monitoring by working parents, and older school-age children face exposure to recreational drugs, primarily through their peers and older children. In the school environment, the nurse and school personnel need to encourage students to engage in wise decision-making about recreational drug use that will affect their future and overall health.

With pressure on older school-age children to smoke cigarettes, attention must be paid to effective strategies to prevent this behavior. Every day, more than 6000 school students try to smoke a cigarette (Tobacco-Free Kids, 2015). Most students who smoke initiate their habit at approximately 11 years of age (AHA, 2014a). White American students start smoking at a younger age than black American students. Males tend to begin smoking earlier than females; however, girls catch up in smoking rates during the middle school years (Tobacco-Free Kids, 2015). The Federal Tobacco Settlement Project provides funds to address the public health problem posed by tobacco smoke in the United States. Although funding for tobacco prevention and cessation programs has reached its highest level in 6 years, many states continue to fall short of the minimal recommendations by the CDC (Tobacco Free Kids, 2015). Attention to smoking as part of a health-promotion program seems merited because so many children begin smoking at a young age; in addition, because nicotine is highly addictive, many believe that this habit leads people to experiment with riskier drugs (cocaine and methamphetamines).

School policies have been instrumental in supporting a tobacco-free environment (Adams et al., 2009). By 2014, 74% of schools had prohibited all tobacco use in all locations (CDC, 2014d). To further assist in health-promotion efforts, many institutions require staff development and education programs related to the effects of tobacco use on health. As of 2014, elementary school students require 3 hours of instruction on tobacco use prevention (CDC, 2014c). There have been various governmental efforts to reduce exposure to environmental tobacco. For example, 40 states and numerous cities nationwide have enacted smoke-free laws (American Nonsmokers' Rights Foundation, 2015).

Pollution has become a fact of life for many Americans and, particularly, for the 25% of urban-dwelling children who must breathe air that exceeds federal government acceptable levels for ozone (Breysse et al., 2010). Air pollution irritates the eyes and the respiratory tract, causing URIs, ear infections, and allergies. More children now experience asthma, and many inner-city children face higher rates of this disease because of poor air quality, including secondary and tertiary smoke. Knowing the negative effects of air pollution and smoking on their health, many school-age children participate in school projects to improve their environmental health.

Children also face exposure to various toxic materials in their environment. Progress has been made in the past decades to reduce children's exposure to chemical hazards. Lead, for example, has been removed from gasoline and paint. This in turn has resulted in significant reductions in children's blood lead levels. Lead exposure continues to exist. Children are exposed to lead through parents' clothes, shoes contacting lead-infused soil, lead in older residential water pipes, traditional medications in some cultures, and in school building structures. Children living in poverty receive high exposure from lead-based paint used on older and less expensive homes. The long-term effects of lead on children remain unclear, but some evidence indicates children suffer neurotoxic effects from this type of exposure. High lead levels in children contribute to dental caries and hearing loss.

Routine use of chemicals to control insects and undesirable weeds in landscaping has led to increasing concerns about children's exposure to these agents. With increased interest in more natural substances to control insects and gardening problems, perhaps less reliance will be placed on chemicals for these problems in the future. Knowing the primary source of exposure to the most hazardous materials and avoiding these materials are often sufficient to accomplish real risk reduction and offer substantial protection within the child's environment (World Health Organization, 2015b). Various behaviors can be implemented to create a safe environment and minimize health risks associated with hazardous chemical exposure. Nurses are instrumental in the assistance and support of parents, schools, and community agencies in the implementation of these behaviors, such as the use of nonhazardous cleaners and pesticide-free foods, and further monitoring of the environment for hazardous materials.

## X-ray Exposure

The child receives exposure from both naturally occurring radiation and human-made ionizing radiation. Exposure occurs in various degrees with radiographic examinations of teeth and bone, from nuclear power plants and explosions, and in the management of many childhood cancers. Children exposed to high levels of radiation risk developing breast or thyroid cancer or leukemia and compromised growth. With little advocacy in this area, nurses and other professionals improve children's health by becoming active in initiatives that focus on prevention of chemical and radiation hazards.

## Cancer

Leukemia is the most common form of childhood cancer. Of those younger than 5 years affected, 90% will be cured with current medical treatment. Among the 12 major types of childhood cancers, leukemia and cancers of the brain and central nervous system (second most common forms of childhood cancers) account for more than 50% of all new cases (National Cancer Institute, 2015). Lymphomas (Hodgkin disease and non-Hodgkin lymphoma) also affect school-age children and adolescents as the third most common group of malignancies. Non-Hodgkin lymphoma is more common during the school-age years, and boys experience this malignancy three times more often than do girls. Mortality rates in the United States tend to be greater in densely populated areas, particularly where the more educated and wealthy live. The most common symptom is abdominal pain caused by intestinal obstruction or organ compression. With effective treatment regimens, children with limited disease may be cured but may experience side effects of treatment later in life (e.g., development of cataracts, dental problems, learning difficulties). Advances are being made with the use of genomic sequencing and the use of genomic medicine to explore novel treatments with the goal of improving childhood cancer outcomes (Downing et al., 2012). Children with cancer present a challenge to the nurse because they are in various stages of recovery, may be developmentally delayed as a result of prolonged periods of absence from peer groups during therapy, and may fear a recurrence of their disease. The nurse provides psychological and emotional support to affected children and their families to help children develop peer relationships and meet developmental goals important to them during the school-age years.

# DETERMINANTS OF HEALTH

The school-age child interacts daily with other children and adults to become more independent by age 12 years. Mutual problem-solving by the child and the parents or friends frequently occurs at this age related to a higher level of maturity in social relationships and concerns. Exposure to a variety of social roles and expectations of others strengthens the process of socialization so that the child develops social competence—the ability and skills to participate effectively in the social interactions of society. Social competence includes both the obvious social behaviors and an inner understanding of the appropriateness of behaviors.

Several elements play a role in the development of the child's social competence. The child's desire for a sense of industry encourages interactions, positive relationships, and accomplishments within society. Cognitive development supports understanding of relationships and effective problem-solving. Moral judgment helps the child understand consequences and fairness in relationships. Understanding and obeying authority help to maintain order in society. Social sensitivity is a result of social interactions and requires the child's ability to perceive the social cues of others, understand the roles of others, and communicate verbally with them. Social behaviors are also a part of social competence; these are learned most frequently through imitation, role-modeling, and reinforcement of others' behaviors. The interaction of all these elements produces a level of social competence and simultaneously plays a role in the child's self-perception. Individuals frequently see themselves as others see them.

## Social Factors and Environment

### Peers

The strongest relationships that school-age children develop outside their families are with their peers (other children encountered in the neighborhood and school). The peer group acts as a new social system, becoming increasingly influential in the child's life. All children continue to be influenced significantly by the family, the culture of the family, and many other environmental factors, but the peer group begins to influence lifestyle, habits, and speech patterns and formulate standards of behavior and performance. The standards of the peer group become vitally important, and children attempt to conform to its rules. Being accepted by the peer group becomes more important than being accepted by anyone else (Ferrer & Fugate, 2014). Conforming to the pressures of peers becomes an issue, especially when it interferes with the parents' expectations. When children realize that their own goals, desires, and aspirations might be quite different from those held by the peer group or the school, they must find ways to cope and perform according to the new standards if they are to succeed. The degree to which children fit in socially, learn to cope, and receive satisfaction from the group is a powerful determinant of healthy socialization.

A child may have one best friend or several important friends and a mutual understanding and willingness to help each other. Friendship groups that form during this age may change and become goal directed, such as groups composing a sports team. These groups frequently have set rules or rituals that connect the members. During the middle school years, friendships often revolve around same-sex relationships, videos, songs, books, and media shared by the group. Later in the school-age years, the development of sexual relationships with the members of the opposite sex occurs during dating and mixed parties.

School-age children also become increasingly involved with adults outside the family, including teachers, coaches, and others who become role models, all of whom influence the child's view of the world and self. Although this influence may not be as significant as that of a child's peers, long-term ideas and beliefs frequently develop from these relationships. Children usually perceive some similarity between themselves and their models, those of the same sex with similar physical or behavior traits. During these years, children may not maintain a strong identification with the parent of the same sex, but they tend to adopt other adult models with whom they can identify.

### Working Parents

Both dual-career couples and single-parent families influence their children's safety when no adult is present to monitor the environment after school. Many **latchkey children** who are left alone until their parents return from work follow directions given by their parents. These directions may include beginning dinner in anticipation of their parents' return or completing homework while remaining inside the home with the doors locked.

Parents and school-age children often disagree about how old is "old enough" to be left at home alone or with an older sibling. Although the school-age child might consider being at home alone to be a real mark of maturity, children who look after themselves after school can become more isolated and miss peer relationships important to their development. Nurses give guidance to families who must cope with the issue of after-school care for school-age children to ensure that relevant and safe decisions are made.

### Culture and Ethnicity

School-age children focus more on the influences of their culture on their lives than do younger children. Aspects of American culture that the child must confront include poverty and affluence, ethnic and racial differences, acceptance of these differences, and the power of media as a cultural phenomenon in American society.

### Ethnic Groups

Preschool children may notice racial and ethnic differences, but school-age children increasingly show evidence of being aware of these differences. This is a time during which attitudes toward race develop on the basis of family and community attitudes. Studies of children aged 5 to 7 years show that most identify

 **BOX 20-11**   **DIVERSITY AWARENESS**

*Expectations for Child Behavior Related to Culture*

**American Indian**
Expect the child to respect elders and take pride in heritage; develop natural talents as the child matures; personal independence must balance with accountability to the family, community, and tribe; help sought from family members, not outsiders.

**Mexican American**
Family environment protects the child; the child is expected to be obedient, respectful, and work hard to reach goals; "next" generation is expected to do better than current generation.

**Filipino**
Family raises the child in a protective environment; expect the child to conform to the values of the culture, and the child shamed if he/she fails to meet expected behaviors; the child is taught to avoid direct confrontation and hide emotions and to be respectful and shy; strong emphasis on education for personal and financial gain.

**Black American**
Children are expected to complete family chores and focus on schooling. Respectful behavior toward adults and elders is expected. Discipline is described as less permissive than for European-decent children.

**Chinese Americans**
The child is highly valued, particularly a male child; the child is expected to honor elders and family needs; high value of education to honor the family and the child.

with and prefer to play with members of their own race. As children get older, they may continue this behavior. Although prejudice exists among some school-age children, they may be encouraged to view people from different cultures and ethnic backgrounds in a positive light. Many schools appropriately focus on the importance of other cultures by having multicultural awareness weeks. During these times, children dress, eat, and live as other cultures do, allowing them to recognize the uniqueness of individual cultural beliefs and values (Box 20-11: Diversity Awareness).

### Television and Video and Computer Games

Television and video and computer games exert a major influence on ideas and behavior in American culture. Unfortunately, many television programs and video and computer games pose harm to children because of their messages and because such activities prevent children from engaging in physical activity. Advances in gaming offer an option for increased activity during gaming activities. Video games and gaming systems have been developed that encourage movement during gaming. Energy expenditure more than doubled when sedentary screen times were converted to active screen time.

Computers connected to the Internet pose a danger unless locking devices have been installed to prevent school-age children from accessing inappropriate websites. Additional concerns have focused on the violent themes of programming, persuasive television commercials, unrealistic depiction of the world, unhealthy food intake, and the passivity of television viewing.

Many times, certain ethnic or racial groups implement the violence in these media sources, leading children to stereotype these groups as the perpetrators of violence. Television facilitates negative attitudes and values among children, increases their aggressive behavior, decreases their emotional sensitivity when aggressive acts occur, and leads them to accept aggressive acts (Adams, 2014). One positive note is that adults who discuss violence with children by pointing out that these acts are unacceptable and cause pain to others can help inhibit some childhood aggression. Discussion of recent acts of violence committed by young people in such a context also helps. Anger control programs, as part of school health-promotion programs, also help decrease societal violence and produce more collaborative workers needed for the future.

The average child views an overwhelming number of television commercials by age 18 years, and these commercials influence daily and future choices and behaviors. Many television commercials focus on sugary foods that cause damage to teeth, diminish overall healthy habits, and lead to increased rates of obesity. Young children cannot always separate the program from the commercials and believe that they must purchase products the television says to buy. Many childhood authorities question the ethics of exposing children to any type of advertising. Although concern about the effect of advertising has led to programming changes during children's watching time, more work is needed to send more socially responsible messages.

The world as presented on many television shows does not accurately reflect the real world. Despite an increasingly diverse and aging population, stereotypes of women and minority groups and a predominance of younger actors continue to make money for the media industry. Parents and health care providers should monitor television viewing to ensure the age appropriateness of the material, respond to television stations about inaccuracies in the content, and write letters to their newspaper or television networks to express concerns about the material presented. Parents may also participate with their children in responding to media presentations on learning and moral themes. Parents should follow recommendations from the AAP—limit television and media viewing to 2 hours per day, have media-free bedrooms, disallow television viewing while eating, and participate in national "Turn Off the Television Week."

Some positive aspects of television viewing exist. A number of children's programs, such as "Sesame Street," "Wishbone," and "Kratt's Creatures" for younger children and "Bill Nye, the Science Guy," "Cyberchase," and "Zoom" for older children, have been deemed developmentally appropriate for children (Public Broadcast Station, 2017). Likewise, there are excellent websites for school-age children that stimulate their learning and promote their health.

Increasingly, parents engage their school-age children in learning and playing on a home computer. Although this technology serves as a good resource for locating information, writing papers, and organizing information, parents must limit the time students spend on computers. Likewise, limitations must be put on use of computer games that detract from socialization with peers and the family and take time away from school work.

## Levels of Policy Making and Health

Throughout this chapter, laws that support the health and well-being of the school-age child have been discussed. These laws include guidelines for the safe use of products, use of flame-retardant clothes, mandates against tobacco advertisements, and nutritional guidelines for federally supported school lunch programs. Another important law is mandatory public education for disabled children. The Individuals with Disabilities Education Act, formally known as Public Law 94-142 (Education for All Handicapped Children Act), established in 1977, states that any child with special needs (disabled) aged 5 to 21 years has the right to free appropriate public education in the least restrictive environment and evaluation by school or health professionals to identify learning needs. Disability includes having a limitation in one or more functional areas (US Department of Education, 2010) and affects as many as 10% of children aged 5 to 17 years.

Many states begin educational services for affected children at 3 years of age based on an individualized educational plan (IEP) for that child and as mandated by law. The school nurse is responsible for collaborating with other school personnel and parents in ensuring that the IEP, including the health care needs of the child and connection to resources addressing the unique learning needs, receives attention. However, some parents have expressed concern that their "normal" or "gifted" child receives less attention in school systems because of the cost and time expenditures associated with implementing IEPs for disabled children. To add further concern, with recent school budgetary shortfalls, people who have received less training than the school nurse often have responsibility for implementing IEPs. Despite these concerns, the value of Public Law 94-142 has been that disabled people have had their problems addressed in the educational arena.

To ensure access to educational opportunities for every individual, the US Department of Education was developed in 1980. Through the US Department of Education, President George W. Bush enacted the No Child Left Behind Act of 2001, aimed at improving the academic achievement of the disadvantaged (US Department of Education, 2010). The No Child Left Behind Act of 2001 intended to help ensure that all children have the opportunity to obtain a high-quality education and reach proficiency on challenging state academic standards and assessments. As a result of the No Child Left Behind Act of 2001, more reading progress was made by 9-year-olds in 5 years than in the previous 28 years combined. Reading and math scores of 9-year-olds and fourth graders have reached all-time highs, and 46 states improved or held steady in all categories of students tested in reading and math (US Department of Education, 2010).

### Poverty

In the United States, more than 22% of children younger than 18 years live in families whose incomes are below the poverty level (National Center for Education Statistics, 2015). Among diverse population groups, 50% of black American, 30% of Hispanic, and an unknown percentage of Native American children live in poor economic conditions that negatively influence their health. These conditions include unemployment, inadequate or crowded housing, poor sanitation, poor nutrition, low educational levels, and limited or sporadic access to health and social services perhaps attributable to lack of health insurance or contextual factors of these people's lives. The number of uninsured children continues to be high and limits the number of children and families receiving primary health care. The lack of primary care among black American, Hispanic, and white American children in rural areas prevents needed asthma management, dictating an expanded role for health care providers to connect families to resources for more effective disease control.

Many homeless children face poor living conditions and high rates of depression related to few friends and poor health status. Migrant children face more disease (e.g., tuberculosis, scabies, and ear infections), injury, and dental caries, and pose treatment challenges because of their transient status. The effects of limited financial resources on children include higher mortality rates at all ages than in those who are not poor or migrant and more school days lost because of illnesses. Numerous problems exist for children in poverty, including greater developmental delay as a result of poor nutrition; increased peer rejection; poorer self-concept; increased risk of accidents, drug abuse, and abuse or neglect by parents; and greater overall poor coping abilities.

Nurses interacting with poor families and their children are familiar with federal health resources, such as the **State Children's Health Insurance Program (SCHIP)**. This program, part of the Balanced Budget Act of 1997 and implemented at the state level, supports comprehensive care for newborns to young adults 18 years of age who do not meet Medicaid criteria but live in families too poor to afford private insurance. This program has advanced children's health by improving access for many groups (SCHIP Information Center, 2010). The nurse improves the overall health of poor children by encouraging relationships with appropriate role models and by reinforcing strong family relationships that help children develop resilient and positive self-images.

Family wealth may have a negative influence on the school-age child if there is frequent substitute caregiving of varying quality attributable to parental absence, extremely high or unreasonable parental expectations, availability of material possessions but little child awareness of relevant responsibilities, and easy access to drugs and alcohol and similar dangers. The nurse reinforces the need in wealthy families for consistent demonstration of parental love and support, firm limits on appropriate behavior, and the value of recognizing the child's unique abilities. The nurse also offers ideas that will help decrease risk-taking behavior (e.g., use of drugs) and increase parent-child connection until a parent is in the home.

When discussing children raised in poverty or affluence, the nurse remembers at least two points. First, many variables affect each child, often in different ways, to influence overall development. Second, although personality and support networks help a child in a socially poor environment to excel later in life, most authorities believe that problems of affluence are easier to overcome than are the all-pervasive problems of poverty.

## Health Services/Delivery System

### Well-Child Care

The AAP recommends that at least every 2 years children 6 years or older have a well-child examination by either a physician or a nurse practitioner. In the ideal situation, the child has a primary health care provider, one person or practice from which the child receives wellness and illness care coordinated by members of a health care team. Unfortunately, many American children still do not have this quality of care (see the Poverty section earlier). With increasing numbers living in poverty because of family violence, single parenthood, and divorce, many lack a primary care provider for their physical and emotional needs often because of a lack of health insurance. In this situation, they often receive emergency care only when they are very ill or injured.

The nurse encourages the school-age child and the parents to be active members of any health evaluation. Children may give some of their own history, answer questions, and discuss their health concerns. During the history, the child's privacy should be respected. Some children in this age group want a parent present during the examination; others do not. When possible, the nurse spends at least some time alone with the child to allow discussions that the child may not feel comfortable with when the parents are present. The examinations can also be a time for education on how the body works and ways to keep it healthy. Preventive information on diet and exercise can be offered relevant to prevention of obesity, cardiovascular disease, and diabetes. Information can also be obtained on school adjustment and performance, particularly because this is a major portion of the child's life. School performance can reflect the child's cognitive and general development. If there are any concerns, the nurse obtains more information through separate testing or discussion with school officials. Health education is directed to both the child and the parents for the best results. Activities that the child performs alone and with the family can give a picture of relationships and adjustments that relate to the child's health (see the care plan at the end of this chapter).

A challenge for nurses who work with school-age children is to maintain their normal healthy status and prevent illness. This task is accomplished through a variety of health-promotion mechanisms, such as examination, guidance, education, and legislation. The success of this health-promotion approach has been illustrated in at least one study in which black American children improved lifestyle choices when engaged in an intervention focused on cardiovascular health. Many professionals have noted that school-age children guided by the nurse generally seek health and use various resources to attain, maintain, or regain optimal health for their future productivity. Aspects of the nursing process are implemented when one is structuring a program to maintain the child's health (such as seen with an assessment of immunization status), promote health habits (seen with teaching bicycle safety), and prevent illness (seen by obtaining throat cultures to detect streptococcal infection).

Nurses have many opportunities and settings to help them implement their interventions as consultants, board members, and active providers of care. For example, nurses and school-age children interact during well-child evaluations and at school. Nurses in other roles, such as in public health positions and in hospitals, also play a role in health promotion, although these nurses must often focus more on helping the child and the family respond to an illness or a crisis. Local and national groups influence the health of children through their activities and regulations. These include organizations such as Boy Scouts and Girl Scouts, Big Brothers and Big Sisters, charities such as the Red Cross, and government agencies such as the Consumer Product Safety Commission.

As an integral part of the community, the school system has the responsibility to provide a healthy school environment and a comprehensive health-education program. In some areas, nurses, physicians, and other health care personnel work as a team in the school health program, which includes health care and maintenance and education. The nurse advocates and searches for resources so that each child has a source of health care, or the nurse is a nurse practitioner who delivers care. School health programs range from an occasional mention of body care and the changes of puberty to a full program that integrates physical and mental health principles into all aspects of the educational experience.

Comprehensive school health services require an interdisciplinary, coordinated effort between health care providers and educators. Recommendations state that each school should have an on-site nurse to conduct and mentor students and faculty in health-promotion areas. Nevertheless, many schools share nurses because of budgetary concerns. However, when available, nurses offer educational and interpersonal skills to initiate health-promotion teaching that improves the overall health of consumers (students, parents, teachers, community). Nurses have a wide scope of practice, including that of referring parents to relevant resources aimed toward activities that improve the school environment and its inhabitants.

The nurse's role in planning health maintenance for children of a school varies, depending on the type of health maintenance program. In one system, the school nurse may refer children to resources available to provide a source of health care, whereas in another system, the school nurse functions as a nurse practitioner. On the basis of the scope of practice and state legal requirements, the school nurse monitors and updates children's immunizations and identifies and intervenes with children who have acute or chronic health care problems, such as scoliosis, strep throat, common cold, or child abuse. Increasingly, school nurses provide sophisticated care according to evidence-based protocols for chronically ill school-age children who have been integrated into the regular academic environment. On the basis of state regulations, the nurse also engages in completing vision, hearing, and scoliosis screening at regular intervals. In most schools the nurse works with the school's physician, community physicians, and parents in meeting children's and community health needs.

For all school-age children, the school nurse plays a role in developing a healthy educational environment through promoting a comprehensive and age-appropriate health-education program focused on children becoming responsible for their own health. A program aimed at accident prevention in and around the school is part of the nurse's role. The program includes assessing the school for pedestrian and automobile traffic patterns, broken playground and classroom equipment, ice and snow dangers, poorly maintained toilet facilities, and inappropriately prepared food. Regular practice drills are held to acquaint teachers and students with emergency procedures (i.e., fire, bomb, or intruder threats or actual events; Box 20-12: Innovative Practice). All people in the school are prepared to respond to chemical hazards. The nurse implements existing school-based programs on drug and alcohol abuse.

It is also important to consider the role of the nurse in fostering a healthy social environment in the school. The nurse examines the social interactions of the children and interacts with them to promote positive relationships. However, social problems continue to constitute a major concern for many children during this time. Children may experience difficulty in making the initial transition away from the family and gaining satisfaction from a group of peers. Children may make the initial adjustment but then have difficulties interacting with others (e.g., bullying). When problems such as these arise, the nurse, parents, and school system determine the reasons for this behavior and intervene appropriately.

## NURSING APPLICATION

The nurse working with the school-age child has a unique and exciting opportunity to engage the child in health-promoting behaviors. Most school-age children are able to participate in the teaching strategies if the strategies are geared toward the child's appropriate cognitive ability. As the age range of the school-age child is from 5 to 12 years, the nurse must consider the mental ability and comprehension of each developmental stage.

Nurses can teach health-promotion behaviors directly to the child through spending time demonstrating, monitoring, and reinforcing preventive health practices such as handwashing, dental hygiene, nutrition, and physical activity. These activities can be taught through age-appropriate reading materials, modeling, and role-playing. Engaging the child in these practices may also help the child conceptualize the link between the behavior and disease prevention. The nurse must partner with parents to model healthy behaviors at home, at school, and in the community settings.

A variety of methods can be used to educate children on health and nutrition. Keeping culture, socioeconomics, and media influences in mind, the nurse should teach children concepts about food choices, exercise habits, and the ways overall health is impacted by those choices. Nutrition education can be individualized to the age of the child through use of games, activities, colorful food guides, and simple cooking activities.

Physical activity in childhood is crucial in promoting healthy behaviors that continue into adulthood. Exercise for this age

**BOX 20-12 INNOVATIVE PRACTICE**

### School Emergency Preparedness

Because children spend a significant portion of their day in school, pediatric emergencies such as exacerbation of a medical condition, behavioral crisis, and accidental/intentional injuries are likely to happen. As a result of the likelihood of such risks, the AAP (2015) and the AHA recommend the implementation of a medical emergency response plan (MERP). The purpose of a MERP is to establish procedures within the school for the administration of emergency first aid services, emergency treatments, and administration of emergency medications for students. A plan helps schools prepare to respond to life-threatening medical emergencies in the first minutes before the arrival of energy medical service (EMS) personnel. All procedures established in the MERP are to be followed during school hours, at school-sponsored activities, and on school buses and other school property.

Because injuries are the most common life-threatening emergency encountered, teachers, trainers, school nurses, and other school personnel should be trained and know the general principles of first aid. Schools now employ fewer nurses, and school nurses often rotate between schools, resulting in many schools being without medical coverage for several hours/days each week. As a result, much of the emergency care is the responsibility of teachers and other school personnel.

The MERP should have the following core elements so as to save the greatest number of lives with the most efficient use of school equipment and personnel:

- Establish an efficient and effective campus-wide communication system for each school.
- Develop a coordinated and practiced MERP with the school nurses, physicians, athletic trainers, and the EMS system, with appropriate evaluation and quality improvement.
- Reduce the risk of life-threatening emergencies by identifying students at risk and ensuring that each has an individual emergency care plan and by reducing the risk of injury and disease triggers at the school.
- Train and equip teachers, staff, and students to provide cardiopulmonary resuscitation and first aid.
- Establish an automated external defibrillator program in schools.

A study assessing school disaster preparedness found only 12 states met the minimal standards of disaster preparedness in 2010 (Save the Children, 2012). School nurses play an important role and should participate in all phases of planning and implementing all emergency preparedness and management plans as they pertain to school health and student safety (National Association of School Nurses, 2011).

Although many schools are in compliance with many of the recommendations for emergency preparedness, specific areas for improvement exist, such as practicing the MERP and ensuring the identification of authorized personnel in the case of an emergency. Preparedness of schools to manage life-threatening emergencies requires the commitment of the entire community. The nurse is in a prime position to facilitate these community efforts and orchestrate partnerships between school officials, local EMS, school personnel, and local pediatricians to ensure the planning and implementation of a disaster plan.

From American Academy of Pediatrics (AAP). (2015). *Children & disasters: Collaborative initiatives.* https://www.aap.org/en-us/advocacy-and-policy/aap-health-initiatives/Children-and-Disasters/Pages/Collaborative-Initiatives.aspx; National Association of School Nurses. (2011). *The preparedness of schools to respond to emergencies in children: A national survey of school nurses. Pediatrics, 116,* e738–e745; Save the Children. (2012). Disaster preparedness for children in the USA. http://www.savethechildren.org.

group is generally provided in group activities and sports. Physical activity provides the school-age child with peer interaction and social relationships. This aspect of health promotion should be encouraged by the nurse as well as the family.

As with younger age groups, health promotion of the school-age child focuses on education about routine health examination and the childhood immunization schedule. The nurse provides the families with immunization recommendations and must remain updated on current guidelines. The nurse also focuses on prevention of childhood injuries by educating them about seat belt and bicycle safety, as well as other things with a potential for causing injury.

Screening for health problems is another aspect of caring for the school-age child. Screenings are generally conducted for problems with vision, hearing, height, weight, and oral health. The nurse may be the first person to identify a potential issue with regard to an acute or chronic condition. At that time, he or she gathers assessment data to determine if the child needs immediate treatment or a referral to another provider. For the nurse working with school-age children and their families, the role is often one of providing education, case management, consulting, counseling, and community outreach.

## CASE STUDY

### Change in Usual Communication Pattern in School: Joey

Joey is an 8-year-old boy in elementary school. His teacher has voiced a growing concern regarding his classroom behavior. In the past 2 months Joey has become more withdrawn from his classmates and rarely participates in class discussion. This is a new behavior in that he "used to talk all the time, and raise his hand to answer questions in class." His teacher reports that they were discussing family and family roles in class this week. Joey became very aggressive and yelled, "My dad isn't at home anymore 'cause of my mom." He went on to say, "I really miss dad. My mom's new boyfriend isn't nice and won't buy me stuff, like my dad does." His teacher determines Joey's parents are divorced. A parent-teacher conference has been scheduled to discuss Joey's behavior because it is now affecting his grades in school.

#### Reflective Questions

- Is Joey's behavior appropriate for his age?
- Joey's parents do not understand his change in behavior. His father yells, "If she would let me spend more time with *my* son, Joey wouldn't be having trouble with school. She doesn't care about *my* son now that *she* has *her* new boyfriend." How might the nurse respond to this situation?
- What interventions might be effective for Joey's parents and teacher in improving his classroom behavior and school performance?

## ⊚ CARE PLAN

### *Change in Usual Communication Pattern in School: Joey*

> **\*NURSING DIAGNOSIS: Ineffective coping related to disruption of home environment**
>
> **Defining Characteristics**
> - Frequent absences from school (1 day per week in the past 2 months)
> - Change in quality of schoolwork: grades have deteriorated in the past month
> - Verbal outbursts in class
>
> **Related Factors**
> - Parents separated 9 months ago
> - Lives with mother; her boyfriend moved into home 2 months ago
> - Mom reports, "He frequently complains of headaches and stomachaches, but his doctor can't find anything wrong." Results in frequent absence
> - Visits father every other weekend
> - No siblings
>
> **Expected Outcomes**
> - Child will decrease number of absences from school related to "headache/stomachache" complaints.
> - Child's grades will improve during the 9-week period.
>
> - Parents will become more involved with the school so as to establish a relationship with the school that addresses the needs of the child related to home and school.
>
> **Interventions (School Nurse)**
> - Assess level of family problems within the home regarding communication between parents and visitation with the child.
> - Assess somatic complaints by the child. Have the child complete a "headache diary"/"stomachache diary" to determine aggravating/alleviating factors. Document the frequency of complaints and discuss/review them with the parents.
> - Meet the child to assess academic and emotional needs as they relate to home and school. Discuss the findings with the child's parents.
> - Meet the parents to develop a plan to help the child meet academic goals and address the emotional needs of the child. Involve the child's teacher in plan development.
> - Offer community resources to address emotional needs of the child such as support groups for children of divorced parents, Boy's Club of America, and peer play groups. Include information for parent support resources as well.
> - Offer after-school tutoring to facilitate the meeting of academic goals as desired.

For further information on developing care plans, see Carpenito-Moyet (2016).
*NANDA Nursing Diagnoses—Herdman T. H. & Kamitsuru, S. (Eds.). Nursing Diagnoses–Definitions and Classification 2015–2017. Copyright © 2014, 1994–2014 NANDA International. Used by arrangement with John Wiley & Sons Limited. In order to make safe and effective judgments using the NANDA-I nursing diagnoses it is essential that nurses refer to the definitions and defining characteristics of the diagnoses listed in this work.

## SUMMARY

Many changes occur in children during the exciting period of the school-age years. The child's development progresses from the immaturity of the preschooler to the beginning of adolescence and eventual adulthood. Cognitive abilities increase dramatically, adding to the desire to master tasks and the ability to develop moral judgment. The child's world expands beyond the family unit as school and peers begin to exert a major influence. Opportunities for nurses during this period occur primarily in ambulatory settings, with the school nurse frequently the most effective and influential health care provider for children of this age group and their families.

## ⓔ EVOLVE CHAPTER FEATURES

http://evolve.elsevier.com/Edelman/
- Study Questions

## REFERENCES

123test. (2012). Culture fair intelligence tests. http://www.123test.com/culture-fair-intelligence-tests/.

Adams, M. L., et al. (2009). Relationship between school policies and youth tobacco use. *Journal of School Health*, 79(1), 17–43.

Adams, N. (2014). How TV violence affects kids. http://www.livestrong.com/article/221006-how-tv-violence-affects-kids/.

American Academy of Audiology. (2011). Childhood hearing screening guidelines. http://www.cdc.gov/ncbddd/hearingloss/documents/AAA_Childhood%20Hearing%20Guidelines_2011.pdf.

American Academy of Otolaryngology. (2015a). Children's hearing health. http://www.entnet.org/HealthInformation/childshearing.cfm.

American Academy of Otolaryngology. (2015b). What is otitis media and ear infection? http://www.entnet.org/HealthInformation/childrensEaraches.cfm.

American Academy of Pediatric Dentistry. (2011). Policy on oral care programs for infants, children, and adolescents. http://www.aapd.org/media/Policies_Guidelines/P_OralHealthCareProg.pdf.

American Academy of Pediatrics (AAP). (2011a). Clinical practice guideline ADHD: Clinical practice guidelines for the diagnosis, evaluation, and treatment of attention-deficit, hyperactivity disorder in children and adolescents. *Pediatrics*, 128(5), 1007–1022.

American Academy of Pediatrics (AAP). (2011b). Child abuse and neglect. http://www2.aap.org/sections/childabuseneglect/.

American Academy of Pediatrics (AAP). (2012). Injuries, manufacturer warnings do not deter ATV use by children under age 16. https://www.aap.org/en-us/about-the-aap/aap-press-room/pages/Injuries-Manufacturer-Warnings-Do-Not-Deter-ATV-Use-by-Children-under-Age-16.aspx.

American Academy of Pediatrics (AAP). (2014). Literacy promotion: An essential component of primary care. *Pediatric Practice*, 134(2), http://pediatrics.aappublications.org/content/pediatrics/early/2014/06/19/peds.2014-1384.full.pdf.

American Academy of Pediatrics (AAP). (2015a). Back to school tips. https://www.aap.org/en-us/about-the-aap/aap-press-room/news-features-and-safety-tips/pages/back-to-school-tips.aspx.

American Academy of Pediatrics (AAP). (2015b). Health issues: High blood pressure in children. https://www.healthychildren.org/English/health-issues/conditions/heart/pages/High-Blood-Pressure-in-Children.aspx?nfstatus=401&nftoken=00000000-0000-0000-0000-000000000000&nfstatusdescription=ERROR%3a+No+local+token.

American Academy of Pediatrics (AAP). (2015c). Helping your child learn to read. https://www.healthychildren.org/english/ages-stages/preschool/Pages/Helping-Your-Child-Learn-to-Read.aspx?nfstatus=401&nftoken=00000000-0000-0000-0000-000000000000&nfstatusdescription=ERROR%3a+No+local+token.

American Academy of Pediatrics (AAP). (2015d). Helping your child develop a healthy sense of self-esteem. https://www.healthychildren.org/English/ages-stages/gradeschool/Pages/Helping-Your-Child-Develop-A-Healthy-Sense-of-Self-Esteem.aspx.

American Academy of Pediatrics (AAP). (2015e). Childhood depression: What can parents do to help. https://www.healthychildren.org/English/health-issues/conditions/emotional-problems/Pages/Childhood-Depression-What-Parents-Can-Do-To-Help.aspx.

American Academy of Sleep Medicine. (2014). Sleep & children. http://yoursleep.aasmnet.org/topic.aspx?id=8.

American Dental Association. (2014). Oral health topics: Braces. http://www.mouthhealthy.org/en/az-topics/b/braces.

American Heart Association (AHA). (2014a). Hey kids, don't smoke, use smokeless tobacco or nicotine products. http://www.heart.org/HEARTORG/GettingHealthy/HealthierKids/LifesSimple7forKids/Hey-Kids-Dont-Smoke-Use-Smokeless-Tobacco-or-Nicotine-Products_UCM_466542_Article.jsp#.Vlke31Qo5jo.

American Heart Association (AHA). (2014b). High blood pressure in children: AHA recommendations. http://www.heart.org/HEARTORG/Conditions/HighBloodPressure/UnderstandYourRiskforHighBloodPressure/High-Blood-Pressure-in-Children_UCM_301868_Article.jsp#.

American Heart Association (AHA). (2015a). Dietary recommendations for healthy children. http://www.heart.org/HEARTORG/GettingHealthy/Dietary-Recommendations-for-Healthy-Children_UCM_303886_Article.jsp.

American Heart Association (AHA). (2015b). Healthy eating habits start at home. http://www.heart.org/HEARTORG/GettingHealthy/NutritionCenter/HealthyEating/Healthy-Eating-Habits-Start-at-Home_UCM_461862_Article.jsp#.VlsKCNKrTIU.

American Heart Association (AHA). (2015c). Overweight in children. http://www.heart.org/HEARTORG/GettingHealthy/Overweight-in-Children_UCM_304054_Article.jsp.

American Nonsmokers' Rights Foundation. (2015). Overview list: How many smoke-free laws? http://www.no-smoke.org/pdf/mediaordlist.pdf.

American Optometric Association. (2015). School-age vision: 6-18 years. http://www.aoa.org/patients-and-public/good-vision-throughout-life/childrens-vision/school-aged-vision-6-to-18-years-of-age?sso=y.

American Psychiatric Association. (2013). *Diagnostic and statistical manual of mental disorders* (5th ed.). Washington, DC: American Psychiatric Association.

Andreyeva, T., Kelly, I. R., & Harris, J. L. (2011). *Exposure to food advertising on television: Associations with children's fast food and soft drink consumption and obesity.* Cambridge, MA: National Bureau of Economic Research.

Atherton, J. S. (2013). Learning and teaching; Piaget's developmental theory. http://doceo.co.uk/learning and teaching/learning/index.htm.

Azarpazhooh, A., et al. (2011). Xylitol prevents acute otitis media in children up to 12 years of age. *The Cochrane Database of Systematic Reviews*, (11), CD007095.

Barron, S. A. (2015). Encopresis (soiling). http://kidshealth.org/parent/emotions/behavior/encopresis.html#.

BMJ Best Practice. (2015). Assessment of learning difficulties and cognitive delay. http://bestpractice.bmj.com/best-practice/monograph/884.html.

Bonuck, K., Chervin, R. D., & Howe, L. D. (2015). Sleep disordered breathing, sleep duration, and childhood overweight: A longitudinal study. *Journal of Pediatrics*, 166(3), 632–639.

Bordini, B., & Rosenfield, R. L. (2011). Normal pubertal development: Part II: Clinical aspects of puberty. *Pediatrics in Review*, 32(7), 281–292.

Boyse, K. (2010). Sleep problems. http://www.med.umich.edu/yourchild/topics/sleep.htm.

Breysse, P. N., et al. (2010). Indoor air pollution and asthma in children. *Proceedings of the American Thoracic Society*, 7(2), 102–106.

Brogan, R. J. (2015). What is a germ? http://kidshealth.org/kid/talk/qa/germs.html#.

Cardoso da Silveria, J. A., et al. (2013). The effect of participation in school-based nutrition education interventions on body mass index: A meta-analysis of randomized, controlled community trials. *Preventive Medicine*, 56(3-4), 237–243.

Carpenito-Moyet, L. J. (2016). *Nursing diagnosis: Application to clinical practice* (15th ed.). Philadelphia, PA: Lippincott Williams & Wilkins.

Castagno, V. D., et al. (2014). Hyperopia: A meta-analysis of prevalence and a review of associated factors among school-age children. *BMC Opthalmology*, 14, 163.

Centers for Disease Control and Prevention (CDC). (2010). National Centers for Health Statistics: Clinical growth charts. http://www.cdc.gov/growthcharts/.

Centers for Disease Control and Prevention (CDC). (2012). Protect the ones you love: Child injuries are preventable. http://www.cdc.gov/safechild/burns/index.html.

Centers for Disease Control and Prevention (CDC). (2014a). Children's oral health. http://www.cdc.gov/oralhealth/children_adults/child.htm.

Centers for Disease Control and Prevention (CDC). (2014b). Pedestrian safety. http://www.cdc.gov/Motorvehiclesafety/Pedestrian_safety/index.html.

Centers for Disease Control and Prevention (CDC). (2014c). School Health Policies and Practice Study: Health education. http://www.cdc.gov/healthyyouth/data/shpps/pdf/2014factsheets/health_education_shpps2014.pdf.

Centers for Disease Control and Prevention (CDC). (2014d). Tobacco use and United States students. http://www.cdc.gov/healthyyouth/data/shpps/pdf/2014factsheets/2014_us_tobacco-compliant.pdf.

Centers for Disease Control and Prevention (CDC). (2014e). Unintentional drowning: Get the facts. http://www.cdc.gov/homeandrecreationalsafety/water-safety/waterinjuries-factsheet.html.

Centers for Disease Control and Prevention (CDC). (2015a). Child passenger safety: Get the facts. http://www.cdc.gov/motorvehiclesafety/child_passenger_safety/cps-factsheet.html.

Centers for Disease Control and Prevention (CDC). (2015b). How much physical activity do children need? http://www.cdc.gov/physicalactivity/basics/children/.

Centers for Disease Control and Prevention (CDC). (2015c). Middle childhood (6–8 years), developmental milestones. http://www.cdc.gov/ncbddd/childdevelopment/positiveparenting/middle.html.

Centers for Disease Control and Prevention (CDC). (2015d). Overweight and obesity: Basics about childhood obesity. http://www.cdc.gov/obesity/childhood/basics.html.

Centers for Disease Control and Prevention (CDC). (2015e). Youth activity guideline toolkit. http://www.cdc.gov/healthyschools/physicalactivity/guidelines.htm.

Centers for Disease Control and Prevention (CDC). (2015f). Immunization schedules. http://www.cdc.gov/vaccines/schedules/hcp/child-adolescent.html.

Child Development Institute (2015). About learning disabilities. http://www.childdevelopmentinfo.com/learning/learning_disabilities.shtml.

Craggs, C., et al. (2011). Determinants of change in physical activity in children and adolescents. *American Journal of Preventive Medicine, 40*(6), 645–658.

Dadds, M. R., et al. (2016). Epigenetic regulation of the DRD4 gene and dimensions of attention-deficit disorder in children. *European Child & Adolescent Psychiatry, 25*(10), 1081–1089.

Daly, L., et al. (2010). Risk of injury to child passengers in sport utility vehicles. *Pediatrics, 117*(1), 9–14.

Demory-Luce, D., & Motil, K. J. (2015). Fast food for children and adolescents. http://www.uptodate.com/contents/fast-food-for-children-and-adolescents.

Devore, C. D., & Schutze, G. E. (2015a). Academy offers guidance on new lice treatments, opposes school bans on infested children. *AAP News, 36*, 5. http://www.aappublications.org/content/36/5/1.3?sso=1&sso_redirect_count=1&nfstatus=401&nftoken=00000000-0000-0000-0000-000000000000&nfstatusdescription=ERROR%3a+No+local+token.

Devore, C. D., & Schutze, G. E. (2015b). Clinical practice guideline: Diagnosis and evaluation of the child with attention-deficit/hyperactivity disorder. *AAP News, 36*, 5.

Disabled World. (2015). Cognitive disabilities: Information on intellectual disabilities. http://www.disabled-world.com/disability/types/cognitive/.

Downing, J. R., et al. (2012). Pediatric Cancer Genome Project. *National Genetics, 44*(6), 619–622.

Durani, Y. (2015). Body basics: The immune system. http://kidshealth.org/en/parents/immune.html#.

Erikson, E. H. (1993). *Childhood and society* (2nd ed., reissued). New York, NY: W.W. Norton.

Erikson, E. H. (1994). *Identity, youth and crisis* (35th ed., reissued). New York, NY: W.W. Norton.

Ferrer, M., & Fugate, A. (2014). The importance of friendship for school-age children. http://edis.ifas.ufl.edu/fy545.

Garey, J. (2015). 13 ways to boost your daughter's self esteem. http://www.childmind.org/en/posts/articles/2012-9-25-13-ways-help-build-your-daughters-self-esteem.

Goldberg, J. (2014). Enuresis in children. http://www.webmd.com/mental-health/enuresis.

Goldfarb, C., et al. (2011). Physical development in school-age children. http://www.aboutkidshealth.ca.

Goldstein, S., & Brooks, R. (2012). Raising resilient children. https://www.psychologytoday.com/blog/raising-resilient-children/201211/giving-children-allowance-nurturing-resilience.

Goswami, U. (2015). Children's cognitive development and learning. http://cprtrust.org.uk/wp-content/uploads/2015/02/COMPLETE-REPORT-Goswami-Childrens-Cognitive-Development-and-Learning.pdf.

Governors Highway Safety Association. (2015). Child passenger safety laws. http://ghsa.org/html/stateinfo/laws/childsafety_laws.html.

Griffiths, L. J., Parsons, T. J., & Hill, A. J. (2010). Self-esteem and quality of life in obese children: A systematic review. *International Journal of Pediatric Obesity, 5*(4), 282–304.

Gupta, R. C. (2014). All about sleep. http://kidshealth.org/parent/general/sleep/sleep.html#.

Gupta, R. C. (2015). Head lice. http://kidshealth.org/parent/infections/common/head_lice.html#.

Harding, M. (2015). Normal and abnormal puberty. http://patient.info/doctor/normal-and-abnormal-puberty.

Harron, W. (2014). Your child's handwriting—Signs of handwriting problems. http://kidshealth.org/parent/positive/learning/handwriting.html#.

Heiting, G. (2015). Eye exams for children. http://www.allaboutvision.com/eye-exam/children.htm.

Inman, D. D., et al. (2011). Evidence-based health promotion programs for schools and communities. *American Journal of Preventive Medicine, 40*(2), 207–219.

Kaneshiro, N. K. (2014). School-age test or procedure preparation. http://www.nlm.nih.gov/medlineplus/ency/article/002058.htm.

Kaneshiro, N. K. (2016). Bedwetting. https://medlineplus.gov/ency/patientinstructions/000703.htm.

Kanwar, V. S. (2015). Lymphadenopathy. http://emedicine.medscape.com/article/956340-overview#showall.

Kendler, K. S., et al. (2015). Family environment and the malleability of cognitive ability: A Swedish National Home-reared and adopted-away cosibling control study. *Proceedings of the National Academy of Sciences of the United States of America, 112*(15), 4612–4617.

Kim, H. S. (2011). Consequences of parental divorce for child development. *American Sociological Review, 76*(3), 487–511.

Klish, W. J. (2015). Comorbidities and complications of obesity in children and adolescents. http://www.uptodate.com/contents/comorbidities-and-complications-of-obesity-in-children-and-adolescents.

Kohlberg, L. (1981). *The philosophy of moral development.* San Francisco, CA: Harper & Row.

Krause-Parello, C. A., & Samms, K. (2010). School nurses in New Jersey: A quantitative inquiry on roles & responsibilities. *Journal for Specialists in Pediatric Nursing, 15*(3), 217–222.

Lourenco, B. H., et al. (2012). Determinants of linear growth. *BMC Public Health, 12*, 265.

Martin, L. (2013). Sleep in different cultures. http://www.howsleepworks.com/anthropology_cultures.html.

McLeod, S. (2015). Piaget's theory of moral development. http://www.simplypsychology.org/piaget-moral.html.

Medina-Gomez, C., et al. (2016). Bone mass and strength in school-age children exhibit sexual dimorphism related to differences in lean mass: The Generation R Study. *Journal of Bone Mineral Research, 31*(5), 1099–1106.

Milteer, R. M., Ginsburg, K. R., & Mulligan, D. A. (2012). The importance of play in promoting healthy child development and maintaining strong parent-child bond: Focus on children in poverty. *Pediatrics, 129*(1), e204–e213.

Moses, S. (2015). Pediatric vital signs. http://www.fpnotebook.com/cv/exam/pdtrcvtlsgns.htm.

Moyer, A. (2013). Screening for primary hypertension in children and adolescents: U.S. Preventive Services Taskforce recommendation statement. *Pediatrics, 132*, 5. http://pediatrics.aappublications.org/content/132/5/907.

National Association of School Nurses. (2013). Overweight and obesity in youth in schools - Role of the school nurse. http://www.nasn.org/PolicyAdvocacy/PositionPapersandReports/NASNPositionStatementsFullView/tabid/462/smid/824/ArticleID/39/Default.aspx.

National Cancer Institute. (2015). Cancer trends progress report. http://progressreport.cancer.gov.

National Center for Education Statistics. (2015). Children living in poverty. https://nces.ed.gov/programs/coe/pdf/coe_cce.pdf.

National Health Service. (2015). Bedwetting. http://www.nhs.uk/Conditions/Bedwetting/Pages/Introduction.aspx.

National Institute of Arthritis and Musculoskeletal and Skin Disease. (2015). Kids and their bones: A parent's guide. http://www.niams.nih.gov/health_info/bone/bone_health/juvenile/default.asp.

National Institute on Deafness and Other Communication Disorders. (2012). Office visits to U.S. physicians resulting in primary diagnosis of otitis media. http://www.nidcd.nih.gov/health/statistics/Pages/officevisits.aspx.

National Institute on Deafness and Other Communication Disorders. (2013). Healthy hearing objectives. http://www.nidcd.nih.gov/health/healthyhearing/what_hh/pages/objectives.aspx.

National Institute of Diabetes and Digestive and Kidney Diseases. (2012). Urinary incontinence in children. http://kidney.niddk.nih.gov/kudiseases/pubs/uichildren/.

Nielson, L. S., Danielson, K. V., & Sorenson, T. I. A. (2011). Short sleep duration as a possible cause of obesity: Critical review analysis of the epidemiological evidence. *Obesity Review, 12*(2), 78–92.

Peristein, D. (2013). My child has a tooth, now what? http://www.medicinenet.com/tooth_eruption_chart/views.htm.

Piaget, J. (2001). *Psychology of intelligence.* Florence, KY: Routledge.

Pickhardt, C. (2011). Impact of divorce on young children and adolescents. http://www.psychologytoday.com/blog/surviving-your-childs-adolescence/201112/the-impact-divorce-young-children-and-adolescents.

Pillinger, J. (2015). Bedwetting (enuresis). http://www.netdoctor.co.uk/diseases/facts/bedwetting.htm.

Powell, L., Szczypka, O., & Chaloupka, E. (2011). Exposure to food advertising on television among US children. *Archives of Pediatric Adolescent Medicine, 161*(6), 553–560.

Public Broadcast Station. (2017). PBS Parents. www.pbs.org/parents.

Queensland Health. (2014). Health care provider's handbook on Hindu patients. https://www.health.qld.gov.au/multicultural/support_tools/hbook-hindu.pdf.

Radford, B. (2013). The evil eye: meaning of the curse & protection against it. http://www.livescience.com/40633-evil-eye.html.

Raghubar, K. P., Barnes, M. A., & Hecht, S. A. (2010). Working memory and mathematics: A review of developmental individual differences and cognitive approach. *Learning and individual differences, 20*(2), 110–122.

Reuschel, L. M. (2011). Generalized anxiety disorder in children and adolescents: Implications for practice. http://www05.casit.ilstu.edu/cc/Comps/Reuschel%20-%20GAD.pdf.

Riley, M., & Bluhn, B. (2012). High blood pressure in children and adolescents. *American Family Physicians, 65*(7), 693–700.

Robinson, J. (2014). Overview of sleepwalking. http://www.webmd.com/sleep-disorders/guide/sleepwalking-causes.

Robson, S. M., et al. (2016). Parent diet and quality and energy intake are related to child diet quality and energy intake. *Journal of the Academy of Nutrition and Dietetics, 116*(6), 984–990.

Rodriguez-Cruz, E. (2015). Pediatric hypertension. http://emedicine.medscape.com/article/889877-overview.

Safe Kids. (2013). Injury trends fact sheet. http://www.safekids.org/sites/default/files/documents/skw_overview_fact_sheet_oct_2013.pdf.

SCHIP Information Center. (2010). SCHIP Information Center. http://www.schip-info.org/1623.html.

Segre, L. (2015). The eye chart and 20/20 vision. http://www.allaboutvision.com/eye-test/.

Shroff, A. (2015). Piaget's levels of learning. http://www.webmd.com/children/piaget-stages-of-development.

Sturaro, C., et al. (2011). The role of peer relationships in the development of early school-age externalizing problems. *Child Development, 82*(3), 758–765.

Tobacco Free Kids. (2015). Tobacco use among youth. http://www.tobaccofreekids.org/research/factsheets/pdf/0002.pdf.

Toll, E. C., & Nunez, D. A. (2012). Diagnosis and treatment of acute otitis media: Review. *Journal of Laryngology and Otology, 126*(10), 976–983.

Tynan, W. D. (2015). Teaching your child self-control. http://kidshealth.org/parent/emotions/behavior/self_control.html#.

US Department of Agriculture. (2013). National School Lunch Program. http://www.fns.usda.gov/cnd/lunch/AboutLunch/NSLPFactSheet.pdf.

US Department of Education. (2010). Laws & guidance: Civil rights. http://www2.ed.gov/policy/elsec/leg/esea02/index.html.

US Department of Health and Human Services (USDHHS). (2011). Child maltreatment 2010. http://www.acf.hhs.gov/programs/cb/pubs/cm10/cm10.pdf#page=31.

US Department of Health and Human Services (USDHHS). (2012a). Oral health. http://healthypeople.gov/2020/topicsobjectives2020/objectiveslist.aspx?topicId=32#186.

US Department of Health and Human Services (USDHHS). (2012b). Leading health indicators. http://healthypeople.gov/2020/LHI/default.aspx.

US Department of Health and Human Services (USDHHS). (2012c). Nutrition and weight status: Healthier food access. https://www.healthypeople.gov/2020/topics-objectives/topic/nutrition-and-weight-status/objectives.

US Department of Health and Human Services (USDHHS). (2013). Injury and violence prevention. https://www.healthypeople.gov/2020/topics-objectives/topic/injury-and-violence-prevention.

Van den Berg, L., et al. (2011). Association between impulsivity, reward responsiveness and BMI in children. *International Journal of Obesity, 35*(10), 1301–1307.

Wald, E. R. (2015). Sore throat overview. http://www.uptodate.com/contents/sore-throat-in-children-beyond-the-basics.

Willingham, D. T., Hughes, E. M., & Doboly, D. G. (2015). Scientific status of learning styles theories. *Teaching Psychology, 42*(3), 266–271.

Women & Children's Health Network. (2013). Self-esteem. http://www.cyh.com/HealthTopics/HealthTopicDetails.aspx?p=114&np=141&id=1702.

World Health Organization. (2015a). Growth reference data for 5-19 years. http://www.who.int/growthref/en/.

World Health Organization. (2015b). Environmental risks. http://www.who.int/ceh/risks/en/.

Wrightslaw. (2015). Discrimination: Sections 504 and ADA. http://www.wrightslaw.com/info/sec504.index.htm.

Yukhananov, A. (2011). Eating healthy food costs more money in the U.S. http://www.reuters.com/article/2011/08/04/us-food-costs-idUSTRE7734L620110804.

Zimmerman, F. J., & Bell, J. F. (2010). Associations of television content type and obesity in children. *American Journal of Public Health, 100*(2), 334–340.

# 21

# Adolescent

*Susan Rowen James*

## OBJECTIVES

*After completing this chapter, the reader will be able to:*

- Summarize the physical growth, developmental, and maturational changes that occur during adolescence.
- Discuss the recommended schedule of health-promotion and preventive health visits for adolescents and the appropriate topics for inclusion during each visit.
- Analyze factors that contribute to risk-taking behaviors and situations during adolescence.
- Develop a health teaching plan addressing some of the physical, emotional, social, and spiritual challenges facing adolescents.

## KEY TERMS

| | | |
|---|---|---|
| Acne | Formal operations | Peer group |
| Adolescence | Gynecomastia | Primary sexual characteristics |
| Anorexia nervosa | Idealism | Puberty |
| Binge eating disorder | Identity | Purge |
| Body image | Introspection | Risk-taking behaviors |
| Bulimia nervosa | Menarche | Role confusion |
| Depression | Menstruation | Scoliosis |
| Egocentrism | Nocturnal emissions | Secondary sexual characteristics |
| Ejaculation | Obesity | Sexually transmitted infection |
| Emancipated minors | Overweight | Tanner staging |

### ❓ THINK ABOUT IT

#### *Risk Behaviors in Adolescents*

*The mortality rate for adolescents (age 15–18 years) is five times higher than it is for school-age children (age 5–14 years). Currently, suicide is the second leading cause of death in adolescents (National Center for Health Statistics, 2014). Thirty-four percent of adolescents in the United States report being currently sexually active, and of those who are sexually active, 14% report not using any method of birth control (Centers for Disease Control and Prevention [CDC], 2014b).*

- *What growth and developmental factors make adolescents susceptible to engaging in risky behaviors?*
- *What anticipatory guidance and strategies might be offered to adolescents and their families to prevent this risky behavior?*

The term *adolescence* is frequently used to describe the transitional stage between childhood and adulthood. The period of adolescence is defined as beginning with the onset of puberty, at approximately age 11 to 13 years. Many researchers and developmental specialists in the United States use the age span from 10 to 24 years as a working definition of adolescence. The term **adolescence** refers to the psychosocial, emotional, cognitive, and moral transition from childhood to young adulthood, whereas **puberty** refers to the development and maturation of the reproductive, endocrine, and structural processes that lead to fertility.

Rapid change in physical, psychosocial, spiritual, moral, and cognitive growth creates an extremely tenuous sense of balance. A pivotal developmental period, adolescence offers health care providers unique opportunities for providing health-promotion and preventive services to adolescents and their families. The CDC (2015a) emphasizes that focusing on adolescent health promotion also includes recognizing and enhancing protective factors against risk. These include positive parenting practices, parental engagement in the adolescent's education, and a strong parent-school connection. The US Department of Health and Human Services (USDHHS), Office of Disease Prevention and Health Promotion (2015) describes two major considerations that should concern health care providers in the upcoming years: practicing "cultural responsiveness" and providing adolescents

## BOX 21-1 HEALTHY PEOPLE 2020

### Selected Health-Promotion and Disease-Prevention Objectives for Adolescents

- Increase the proportion of adolescents who have had a wellness check-up in the past 12 months.
- Increase the proportion of adolescents who participate in extracurricular and out-of-school activities.
- Increase the proportion of adolescents who are connected to a parent or other positive adult caregiver.
- Increase the proportion of schools with a school breakfast program.
- Reduce the proportion of adolescents who have been offered, sold, or given an illegal drug on school property.
- Increase the proportion of middle and high schools that prohibit harassment based on a student's sexual orientation or gender identity.
- Decrease the proportion of public schools with a serious violent incident.
- Reduce adolescent and young adult perpetration of crimes, as well as adolescent and young adult being victims of crimes.
- Reduce the proportion of children and adolescents with untreated dental decay.
- Increase the proportion of adolescents who participate in daily school physical education.
- Increase the proportion of children and adolescents who do not exceed recommended limits for screen time.
- Increase the proportion of students in grades 9 through 12 who get sufficient sleep.
- Reduce the proportion of adolescents who report that they rode, during the previous 30 days, with a driver who had been drinking alcohol.
- Increase the proportion of adolescents never using substances.
- Reduce exposure to violence.
- Reduce suicide risk.
- Reduce suicide attempts by adolescents.
- Reduce the proportion of adolescents who engage in disordered eating behaviors in an attempt to control their weight.
- Reduce the proportion of children and adolescents who are considered obese.
- Increase the proportion of female and male adolescents who have never had sexual intercourse.
- Reduce tobacco use by adolescents.
- Increase educational achievement by adolescents.

From US Department of Health and Human Services. (2015). Healthy People 2020. http://www.healthypeople.gov.

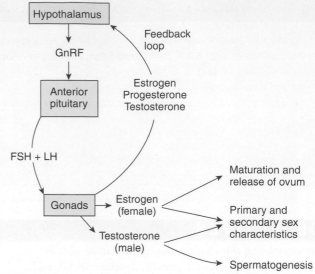

**FIGURE 21-1** Hormonal interaction among hypothalamus, pituitary, and gonads. *FSH,* Follicle-stimulating hormone; *GnRF,* gonadotropin-releasing hormone; *LH,* luteinizing hormone. (From Hockenberry, M. J., & Wilson, D. [2015]. *Wong's nursing care of infants and children* [10th ed.]. St. Louis: Mosby.)

with opportunities to become competent through access to supportive relationships, health resources, and appropriate opportunities for optimal development. *Healthy People 2020* contains specific objectives related to adolescent health (Box 21-1: Healthy People 2020).

## BIOLOGY AND GENETICS

### Sex and Puberty

In contrast to the slow, steady growth of childhood, adolescents experience accelerated physical growth that dramatically alters their body size and proportions. Additionally, adolescents experience the onset of puberty. Changes associated with the onset of puberty occur in a predictable sequence, but the onset and

duration of the sequence differ among individuals. Females usually begin puberty 2 years earlier than males and experience their growth spurt earlier. Demographic studies suggest that racial and ethnic differences in the ages of achieving pubertal milestones differ (Kaplowitz & Bloch, 2016). Biro and colleagues (2013) conducted a 4-year longitudinal study of more than 1200 girls aged 6 to 8 years and found that black girls showed breast development at least 1 year before white or Asian girls and at least 6 months earlier than Hispanic girls. They also found that white females are maturing earlier than in the past, and that body mass index is correlated with earlier onset of puberty. Adolescents who do not follow the normal sequence or who have not begun pubertal development by age 14 years, for males, and age 13 years, for females, should have an endocrine evaluation (American Academy of Pediatrics [AAP], 2015a,b).

The physical changes experienced during adolescence are mediated primarily by the hormonal regulatory systems in the hypothalamus, pituitary gland, gonads, and adrenal glands (Figure 21-1). The hypothalamus releases gonadotropin-releasing hormone (GnRF), which stimulates the anterior pituitary to release the gonadotropin hormones luteinizing hormone (LH) and follicle-stimulating hormone (FSH) (Copstead & Banasik, 2013). In females, this stimulates development of the ovaries and estrogen production. Once sexual maturation is complete, the ongoing release of hormones controls menses, pregnancy, and lactation. In males, luteinizing hormone results in enlargement of the testes and the development of Leydig cells in the testes, which produce testosterone. Follicle-stimulating hormone stimulates the development of the seminiferous tubules of the testes, leading to spermatogenesis and fertility.

During puberty, **primary sexual characteristics** begin to develop and **secondary sexual characteristics** emerge. Primary sexual characteristics involve the organs necessary for reproduction, such as the penis and testes in boys and the vagina and uterus in girls. Secondary sexual characteristics are external features that are not essential for reproduction. Breast development, facial and pubic hair growth, and lowering of the voice are examples of secondary sexual characteristics (Table 21-1). Estrogen produces all secondary sexual characteristics except axillary and pubic hair, which are controlled by adrenal androgens.

Sexual maturity rating, also referred to as Tanner staging, is used widely to assess and monitor the degree of maturation of an adolescent's primary and secondary sexual characteristics. Each of the characteristics, breast, pubic hair, and genitals, is staged separately (from 1 to 5) and compared with the expected sequencing (Figure 21-2).

Breast development is usually confined to females; however, some degree of unilateral or bilateral breast enlargement, termed

## TABLE 21-1 GROWTH AND DEVELOPMENT

### Sexual Maturity Rating, Tanner Stages: Developmental Stages of Secondary Sexual Characteristics

| Stage | Male Genital Development | Pubic Hair Development | Female Breast Development | Other Changes |
|---|---|---|---|---|
| 1 | Prepubertal | No distinction between hair over pubic area and hair over abdomen | | |
| 2 | Initial enlargement of scrotum and testes; reddening and texture changes of scrotum | Sparse growth of long, straight, downy hair at base of penis or along labia | Enlargement of areolar diameter; small area of elevation around papillae (breast bud) | Usual time of peak height velocity for girls |
| 3 | Initial enlargement of penis, mainly in length; further growth of testes and scrotum | Hair becomes dark, coarse, and curly; spreads sparsely over entire pubic area | Further elevation and enlargement of breasts and areolas, with no separation of their contours | Usual time of menarche; facial hair begins to grow on upper lip and voice deepens in boys |
| 4 | Further enlargement of penile diameter, testes, scrotum, and glans | Further spread of hair distribution, not extending to thighs | Areolas and papillae project from breast to form secondary mound | Usual time of peak height velocity for boys; axillary hair begins to grow |
| 5 | Adult in size and contour | Adult in amount and type; spreads to inner surface of thighs | Adult, with projection of papillae only; recession of areolas into general breast contour | |

Modified from Hockenberry, M. J., & Wilson, D. (2015). *Wong's nursing care of infants and children* (10th ed.). St. Louis: Mosby.

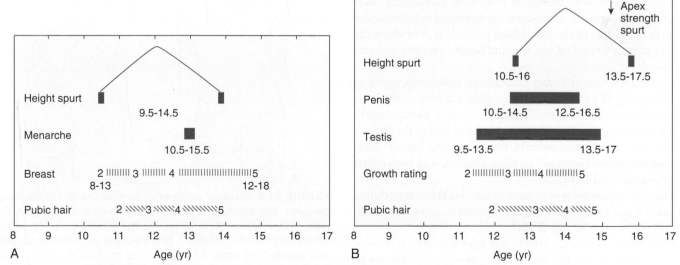

FIGURE 21-2 Sequences of events at adolescence in girls **(A)** and boys **(B)**. Single numbers *(2, 3, 4, 5)* indicate stages of development. The average is represented. A range of ages when each event may begin and end is indicated by inclusive numbers listed below each event. (Modified from Herman-Giddens, M., Slora, E. J., Wasserman, R. C., Bourdony, C. J., Bhapkar, M. V., Koch, G. G., et al. [1997]. Secondary sexual characteristics and menses in young girls seen in office practices: A study from the Pediatric Research in Office Settings Network. *Pediatrics, 99*[4], 505–512; Hockenberry, M., & Wilson, D. [2015]. *Wong's nursing care of infants and children* [10th ed.]. [Figs. 17-2 & 17-5]. St. Louis: Mosby; Marshall, W., & Tanner, J. [1970]. Variations in pattern of pubertal changes in boys. *Archives of Diseases in Childhood, 45*[239], 13–23.)

gynecomastia, may appear early in male puberty, just before the growth spurt. Gynecomastia is usually temporary and typically disappears. However, occasionally it persists and leads to body image problems and can be surgically reduced if psychological assessment warrants it.

The first sign of puberty in males is a thinning of the scrotal sac and enlargement of the testicles. Ejaculation is considered a milestone of male puberty and precedes fertility by several months. Nocturnal emissions, or wet dreams, can concern adolescent males because the events happen beyond their control.

For females, the first sign of puberty is the appearance of breast buds, followed by the growth spurt. The onset of menstruation, or menarche, occurs approximately 2 years after the appearance of the breast buds and near the end of the growth spurt (see Figure 21-2).

Familiarity with the stages of development of sexual characteristics and their expected sequence helps the nurse monitor the adolescent's progression through puberty and detect any variations that might herald an alteration in normal growth and development.

Before the growth spurt, many adolescents experience a transient increase in the amount of body fat or adipose tissue. As puberty progresses the proportion of total body weight composed of fat usually declines, particularly in boys. Body fat begins to accumulate again in both sexes after their growth spurt, but at a slightly higher rate in females.

## Other Physical Changes

The heart grows in size and strength. Blood volume and blood pressure increase, and the heart rate decreases to adult levels. These cardiovascular changes occur earlier in females, corresponding with puberty. Compared with adolescent males, adolescent females also generally have higher pulse rates and slightly lower systolic blood pressure. Adolescents are identified as hypertensive when their systolic or diastolic blood pressure is at or above the 95th percentile (based on age, sex, and height) on three separate occasions.

Respiratory rate decreases throughout childhood, reaching an average rate of 15 to 20 breaths per minute during adolescence. Respiratory volume and vital capacity increase, particularly in males. The larynx and vocal cords grow, producing the characteristic voice changes of puberty. Both male and female voices become deeper, and laryngeal cartilage enlarges, with both effects more pronounced in males.

The gastrointestinal system reaches functional maturity during the school-age years. However, it continues to grow along with the growth spurt (Guyton & Hall, 2011).

Permanent teeth begin erupting at approximately 6 years of age, and all 32, except the third molars, or wisdom teeth, are in place by 13 to 14 years of age. Third molars are often pulled during adolescence to make space for the other permanent teeth. It is not uncommon for one or more of the third molars not to develop, and this lack of development (agenesis) is often familial.

The sweat and sebaceous glands both become more active during adolescence. The sweat glands are located primarily in the axillary, genital, and periumbilical areas and are the primary source of body odor. The sebaceous glands are located primarily on the face, neck, shoulders, upper back, chest, and genitals. They can become clogged and inflamed, leading to the common teenage condition called acne. Acne is seen in nearly all adolescents, and nearly 20% of adolescents experience moderate to severe manifestations. The prevalence is higher in females than in males (Bhate & Williams, 2013).

## Scoliosis

During the growth spurt, adolescents may manifest signs of a common skeletal deformity called scoliosis, which is a lateral S-shaped curvature of the spine (Figure 21-3). The curve is typically convex to the right. Classifications of scoliosis include secondary or functional, congenital, neuromuscular, constitutional, and idiopathic, which has an infantile, juvenile, or adolescent onset. Approximately 10% of all adolescents have a mild truncal asymmetry; however, curves greater than 20 degrees are abnormal and can progress to significant curvature during the growth spurt (Honeyman, 2014; Manworren, 2013). Idiopathic scoliosis is the most common type and is significantly more prevalent in females. Early intervention is important because untreated scoliosis can result in disfigurement, impaired mobility, and cardiopulmonary complications. Evidence shows that early

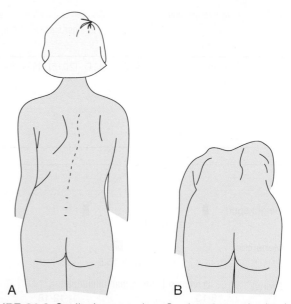

**FIGURE 21-3** Scoliosis screening. So that the entire back can be seen, the adolescent should remove all clothing from the upper body when being assessed for scoliosis. **A,** While the adolescent stands up straight, check for any asymmetry; observe and palpate the body for differences in shoulder or scapular height, prominence of either scapula or hip, waist asymmetry, and misalignment of the spinous processes. Lateral curvature and thoracic convexity of the spine indicate scoliosis. **B,** With feet together, legs straight, and arms hanging freely, the adolescent bends forward until the back is parallel with the floor. Check for prominence of the ribs, or rib hump, on one side only and hip and leg asymmetry. With scoliosis, the chest wall on the side of convexity is prominent, and the scapula on the side of convexity is elevated.

intervention in the form of scoliosis-specific physical therapy exercises or bracing can slow progression of curves and reduce the need for surgery, or, in children with mild scoliosis, reduce the need for bracing (Scoliosis Research Society et al., 2015).

The US Preventive Services Task Force (2015) has issued a statement that routine screening of asymptomatic children for scoliosis is not cost effective. However, the SOS, American Academy of Orthopedic Surgeons, Pediatric Orthopedic Society of America, and AAP (Scoliosis Research Society et al., 2015) support screening by a trained professional provider for girls at ages 10 and 12 years, and for boys at age 13 or 14 years. Referral for orthopedic evaluation occurs when the curvature measures more than 5 to 7 degrees, measured by a scoliometer when the adolescent is in the Adams position (see Figure 21-3, *B*).

## Genetics

Most genetic problems are discovered during infancy and early childhood. Some syndromes, however, may not be diagnosed until adolescence. Turner syndrome in females and Klinefelter syndrome in males result from alterations in the X chromosome. These genetic disorders, which affect both physical and cognitive development, are frequently discovered during the assessment of an adolescent who has delayed or irregular pubertal development, and require referral to an appropriate specialist.

Since the sequencing of the human genome, information on genetic predisposition to disease has expanded exponentially. For example, genomics research has demonstrated a genetic basis for conditions seen during adolescence, such as acne, scoliosis (Box 21-2: Genomics), substance dependence, depression, eating disorders, and autoimmune conditions (e.g., lupus erythematosus and celiac disease) (CDC, 2015b). The risk of conditions of concern to adolescents, such as breast cancer, type 2 diabetes, and cardiovascular disease, can now be identified through genetic testing. Although newborn screening for genetic disease is routinely performed, predictive screening for children and adolescents is not recommended because of unreliable interpretation and ethical considerations (Botkin et al., 2015). The AAP (2013a) has issued a policy statement that genetic testing should not be performed on children or adolescents unless clinically indicated. Predictive genetic testing on adolescents brings up ethical issues, especially regarding disclosure, and testing should be postponed until adulthood (AAP, 2013a; Botkin et al., 2015).

Family history, however, not only can help physicians make a diagnosis if the adolescent shows signs of a disorder but can also help to reveal whether there is an increased risk of a disease for the adolescent (Box 21-3: Innovative Practice).

# GORDON'S FUNCTIONAL HEALTH PATTERNS

## Health Perception–Health Management Pattern

Teens have fewer acute illnesses than younger children and fewer chronic illnesses than adults. They are seen in health care facilities less frequently than younger children and adults, and they rarely are hospitalized. Yet they need to be monitored, because adolescence is a pivotal developmental period with numerous physical, psychosocial, and spiritual changes. Box 21-4 lists interventions recommended for periodic health examinations for adolescents.

A crucial component for understanding adolescent health is an adolescent's own perceptions of health, illness, and health care services. Too often their sense of invincibility and "Peter Pan" ideology couples with typical adolescent experimentation and **risk-taking behaviors** to produce deleterious health care

---

### ⚠ BOX 21-2   GENOMICS

#### *Scoliosis*

For many years the cause of adolescent idiopathic scoliosis (AIS) has been elusive to determine. A body of research reveals that AIS is significantly more prevalent in girls than in boys (up to 10 times more prevalent), that AIS occurs in families, and that the condition is multifactorial. Multifactorial inheritance patterns suggest that a combination of genetics and environment affects the occurrence of a health condition. In the past several years, as genome sequencing has allowed more precise identification of genetic contributions to various diseases, multiple studies have tried to determine an exact genetic inheritance pattern for AIS. Researchers have identified multiple genes that possibly increase susceptibility and are associated with various aspects of spinal development and growth. These genes include those responsible for synthesizing proteins related to ossification, sensory development, collagen, estrogen production, and growth hormone. Unfortunately, researchers have not identified evidence that would suggest a specific genetic pattern, but have concluded that AIS is caused by multiple genes that are modified by environmental influences.

From Janusz, P., Kotwiki, T., Malgorzats, K., & Szulch, A. (2012). Genetic aspects of idiopathic scoliosis – literature review. *Scoliosis*, *7*(Suppl 1), O71.; Krause, L. M., Buchan, J. G., Gurnett, C. A., & Dobbs, M. B. (2012). Polygenic model and sex dimorphisms in adolescent idiopathic scoliosis. *Journal of Bone & Joint Surgery. American Volume, 94*(16), 1485–1491; National Institutes of Health. (2016). Adolescent idiopathic scoliosis. https://ghr.nlm.nih.gov/condition/adolescent-idiopathic-scoliosis.

---

### ✺ BOX 21-3   INNOVATIVE PRACTICE

#### *My Family Health Portrait*

Teens can create a simple family pedigree with the Surgeon General's *My Family Health Portrait* at https://familyhistory.hhs.gov/FHH/html/index.html. *My Family Health Portrait* is a downloadable, Web-based tool for use on a personal computer. It helps individuals create their own family health history and is a part of the National Human Genome Research Institute and the US Surgeon General's Family History Initiative. Because it is Web-based, teens may be the family member best prepared (or most technologically comfortable) to coordinate the input of data. With their family's help, teens gather their family health history and then, using any type of computer, build a drawing of their family tree and a chart of their family health history. Both the chart and the drawing can be printed and shared with other family members and health care providers.

The Surgeon General's Family History Initiative began in 2004. It is suggested that families use holiday gatherings, such as Thanksgiving, when the family is present, to gather and record information for the family health history. In support of the family history initiative, the CDC (2015) has a website with various genomic resources as well (http://www.cdc.gov/genomics/famhistory/index.htm).

Centers for Disease Control and Prevention (CDC). (2015). Genomic tests and family history by level of evidence. http://www.cdc.gov.

---

**BOX 21-4   Interventions Recommended for the Periodic Health Examination: 11 to 21 Years of Age**

**Screening**

- Height, weight, and body mass index
- Blood pressure
- Scoliosis
- Vision and hearing
- Tanner stage
- Anemia
- Hyperlipidemia
- Urinalysis
- Tuberculosis—if at risk
- Eating disorders
- Sports injuries
- Tattoos and piercings
- Substance use assessment*
- Depression screening*
- HIV screening (age 16–18 years)*
- If sexually active, STI screening
- Counseling

**Injury and Violence Prevention**

- Lap and shoulder belts in car
- Bicycle, motorcycle, all-terrain vehicle helmets
- Protective gear for sports, work, and other physical activities
- Learn first aid and cardiopulmonary resuscitation
- Skin cancer, sun exposure (or exposure through tanning beds), sunscreen sun protection factor 15 or higher
- Safe storage and use of firearms

**Substance Use**

- Avoid tobacco, alcohol, and drug use
- Avoid alcohol or drug use while driving, swimming, boating, riding a bike or motorcycle, or operating farm equipment or other machinery
- Do not ride with a driver who has been using alcohol

**Sexual Behavior**

- Abstinence, resisting sexual pressures, saying no
- STI prevention and protection
- Unintended pregnancy, contraception
- Date rape

**Diet and Exercise**

- Choose a variety of healthy foods
- Balance caloric intake and energy expenditure
- Limit fat and cholesterol; emphasize grains, fruits, and vegetables
- Adequate calcium, iron, and folic acid

**Dental Health**

- Regular (every 6 months) visits to dental care provider
- Brush teeth at least twice a day and floss daily
- Avoid tobacco products

**Immunization†**

- Tdap vaccine (tetanus, diphtheria, acellular pertussis) at age 11 to 12 years; Td vaccine (tetanus, diphtheria) every 10 years thereafter
- HPV vaccine; boys and girls at age 11 through 12 years; three-dose series
- Meningococcal vaccine; one dose at age 11 to 12 years, booster dose at age 16 years
- Influenza vaccine yearly
- Catch up vaccines—hepatitis B; measles, mumps, rubella; varicella (two-dose schedule); hepatitis A (if indicated)

*HPV*, Human papillomavirus; *STI*, sexually transmitted infection.

*Recommended additions: American Academy of Pediatrics. (2014). 2014 recommendations for pediatric preventive health care. *Pediatrics, 133*, 568–570.

†Advisory Committee on Immunization Practices. (2016). *Recommended immunization schedule for persons aged 0 through 18 years*. http://www.cdc.gov.

---

choices and outcomes. Caught somewhere between childhood and adulthood, teens may no longer feel as if they are being attended to by pediatricians, pediatric nurse practitioners, and pediatric nurses, yet, at the same time, are often misunderstood by adult health care providers. Health care services for adolescents that are available, visible, confidential, and flexible need to be developed. Recent research (Hargreaves et al., 2015) demonstrates that unmet health care needs during adolescence can result in poor health outcomes during adulthood. The reasons that contribute to unmet health care needs include lack of appropriate access, financial constraints, and adolescent attitudes that health is not important. Whereas adults search for health information using the Internet, adolescents are more likely to use social media (e.g., Facebook, Twitter, on-line blogs) to obtain health information (Korda & Itani, 2013). Because these sites are unmonitored for accuracy, nurses need to advise adolescents and their parents to verify information with their health providers. For information

regarding health care services for adolescents, visit the National Adolescent and Young Adult Health Information Center (NAHIC) at http://nahic.ucsf.edu.

Adolescents are in the process of developing health habits and patterns of problem-solving that are likely to last a lifetime. The cognitive and psychological changes that they experience can affect their adherence to health-promotion and disease-prevention strategies. Teens do not always consider the health risks of their behavior and have an overall sense of invulnerability to illness or injury. Peer influence is primary, and parental input is often rejected. Parents need, however, to be vigilant to recognize when their adolescent needs assistance with avoiding situations that could lead to irreparable harm (AAP, 2015c). Parental monitoring, which involves knowing where the adolescent is, knowing with whom he or she is communicating, setting clear behavioral expectations, and sensitivity to adolescent behavior changes, has been shown to be protective against adolescent risk behavior. Role modeling appropriate health behaviors is also a known protective factor against risk (AAP, 2015c; CDC, 2012). Parents, however, need to guard against overprotection, sometimes known as overparenting, because this behavior can lead to overdependence and lack of confidence as the adolescent transitions to adulthood. Parents who are perceived by their children as being overcontrolling (e.g., give undue advice or assistance, are overly involved with the adolescent's activities, or fail to allow the adolescent to solve problems) can contribute to increased anxiety or stress, decreased self-confidence, and exaggerated egocentric behavior (Segrin et al., 2015). Nurses can advise parents to strike a balance between the desire to overprotect their children and allowing them increasing autonomy as adolescents become increasingly capable of more independent decisions about their health behavior.

Parents, teachers, and health care providers will be more successful in assisting teens to manage their health needs wisely if they treat them as joint partners in planning the care for which the adolescents themselves will assume responsibility. Key components of successful health supervision include gradually facilitating adolescent independence and decision-making, involving parents and schools in a holistic approach to health promotion, and effective communication.

## Nutritional-Metabolic Pattern

Although many adolescents gravitate to low-nutrient, processed foods, it is essential that they consume a well-rounded diet that provides a variety of high-nutrient, low-sugar, and low-fat foods and beverages (USDHHS & US Department of Agriculture [USDA], 2015). Adolescents need to consume daily calorie amounts appropriate for their level of physical exercise (females—1600–1800 calories; males—1800–3200 calories) found primarily in vegetables, fruits, whole grains, fish, and nuts. Nurses need to assist teens with following a healthy diet and educate them about the appropriate nutrients, such as protein (especially for vegetarians), calcium, and iron and folic acid (for females) (USDHHS & USDA, 2015). Recommending regular consumption of milk to prevent later osteoporosis is essential, especially for adolescent girls, as is avoidance of high-sugar and diet beverages. The nurse can encourage adolescents to eat breakfast every day to improve academic performance, or to carry protein snacks. An excellent resource for nurses and adolescents regarding dietary considerations is the MyPlate website: http://www.choosemyplate.gov/teens.

Many teens have concerns about their body, proper nutrition, and exercise. The media not only portray the ideal body as thin, lean, or muscular, but at the same time promote access to unhealthy high-fat, high-sugar, processed foods. Asserting their newfound autonomy, teens may choose dietary intake as a mechanism to gain control over their changing bodies, exert independence, or experiment with a new identity or cause, such as becoming a vegetarian. All of this occurs as their body's nutrient and energy demands increase in preparation for and in response to the adolescent growth spurt. Teen activities, including sports and other vigorous extracurricular physical activity, can further increase these demands. Gymnasts, runners, bodybuilders, rowers,

wrestlers, dancers, and swimmers are particularly vulnerable to eating disorders because their sports necessitate weight restriction. Complicating matters are teens' overwhelming desire to "fit in" with their peers, which often prevails and can lead to unhealthy dietary practices

### Eating Disorders

The occurrence of eating disorders results from a combination of genetic and environmental factors, mediated as well by internal and external factors prevalent during puberty (e.g., family, peer, and media influences) (Kreipe, 2016). In the United States the lifetime prevalence of eating disorders among adolescents is 0.3% (Swanson et al., 2011). Major eating disorders include anorexia nervosa, bulimia nervosa, and binge eating disorder. In general, eating disorders have a higher prevalence in females, but they affect both sexes and people of all cultures (Kreipe, 2016). Most adolescents with an eating disorder experience comorbid psychiatric conditions, such as anxiety, depression, or obsessive-compulsive disorder, and suicide ideation is not uncommon (Kreipe, 2016; Swanson et al., 2011). Adolescents who meet the criteria for eating disorders should be referred to an interdisciplinary team that is experienced and skilled in working with these disorders

At one end of the eating disorder spectrum is anorexia nervosa and bulimia nervosa. At the other end is binge eating disorder and obesity. Adolescents with anorexia nervosa are typically female, perfectionists, and high achievers. Symptoms or warning signs include a relentless pursuit of thinness, self-starving with significant weight loss, lack of menstruation (in females) and decreased sexual interests (in males), compulsive physical activity, preoccupation with food, portioning food carefully, and eating only small amounts of only certain foods.

The adolescent may also have brittle hair and nails; dry, yellowish skin; growth of fine hair over the body; constipation; mild anemia and muscle weakness; and often complains of feeling cold. The severe restriction of food intake eventually contributes to dangerous malnourishment, and, in some cases, death. The onset of anorexia nervosa is typically in response to low self-esteem and real or imagined obesity.

Distorted body image is a hallmark of anorexia nervosa in both males and females. Body image specifically refers to the picture of and feelings about various characteristics of one's body. In females particularly, distorted body image may be related to self-objectification, or judging one's personality or character strictly by one's appearance (Slater & Tiggermann, 2015). Media images and positive or negative comments about appearance from others can contribute to self-objectification (Slater & Tiggerman, 2015).

Bulimia nervosa has symptoms or warning signs that are different from those of anorexia nervosa. Teens with bulimia nervosa typically binge on huge quantities of high-calorie foods and then purge by self-induced vomiting and/or use of laxatives. Binge episodes may alternate with diets, resulting in dramatic weight fluctuations. These teens often try to hide the signs of vomiting by running water as a sound cover. Purging poses serious threats to the teen's health, including dehydration, sometimes fatal electrolyte imbalances, and erosion of tooth enamel.

At the other end of the eating disorder spectrum is binge eating disorder, which can often contribute to obesity. Similarly to the teen with bulimia nervosa, the teen with binge eating disorder frequently consumes large amounts of food while feeling a lack of control over eating. However, this disorder is different from bulimia nervosa because these teens usually do not purge their bodies of the excess food they consume during their binge episodes. Adolescents who are binge eaters experience lack of control over eating, the inability to stop eating when full, social difficulties, altered mood, and decreased self-esteem (Pasold et al., 2014).

The obese adolescent consumes too many calories for the amount of energy expended. Studies have shown a strong correlation between inactivity, such as viewing television, playing computer games, and Internet surfing, and the tendency to be overweight. Other research has identified depression as one of the strongest predictors of adolescent obesity. Obesity can be detrimental to adolescents' self-esteem and social development, because they often become trapped in a vicious cycle of social rejection, isolation, inactivity, and continued obesity. Adolescent obesity has a poor prognosis, with most obese adolescents becoming obese adults. In addition, obesity increases the risk of and occurrence of type 2 diabetes mellitus.

School nurses may be the first to notice a possible eating disorder in students. Questioning students who come to the health office can elicit warning signs (Obadina, 2014). The nurse can ask: Do you have concerns about your weight or think you are fat? How often do you weigh yourself? How often do you exercise? Has your diet changed recently (become more picky with foods, not controlling eating, hiding food, counting calories excessively)? Are you still doing fun activities with friends?

Because of the multiple factors contributing to the occurrence of an eating disorder, there is no one method that can prevent its occurrence. However, when working with families of adolescents, nurses can recommend family members deemphasize the adolescent's body proportions or shape, encourage healthy eating and participation in regular exercise, emphasize the adolescent's positive and unique aspects, and foster the adolescent's self-esteem (Obadina, 2014).

### Obesity, Type 2 Diabetes, and Teens

Soaring obesity rates are making type 2 diabetes, a disease that used to be seen mostly in adults older than 45 years, more common among teens and young people. Diabetes is a group of diseases marked by high levels of glucose in the blood, which, left unattended, lead to blindness, kidney failure, amputations, heart disease, and stroke. Type 2 diabetes, formerly called adult-onset diabetes, is the most common form. People can develop it at any age. However, being overweight and inactive increases one's risk. Teens can access information about weight control with *Take Charge of Your Health! A Guide for Teens* available at http://www.win.niddk.nih.gov/publications/take_charge.htm. Furthermore, the National Diabetes Education Program (NDEP) has now developed a new "Tips for Teens" series that includes a tip sheet on how to lower the risk of type 2 diabetes that is "teen-friendly." Nurses can direct high-risk teens or teens with

type 2 diabetes to visit the NDEP website at http://ndep.nih.gov/teens/LowerYourRisk.aspx.

More than anything, adolescents need reassurance about their bodies. Parents, teachers, and health care providers will be more successful in helping teens assume responsibility and manage their ongoing health needs if they approach and treat them as partners in planning their care. Assessment is of particular importance. Nurses working with adolescents need to be aware of abnormal changes in weight, body image distortion, abnormal food behavior, including thinking about food, and obsessive exercise (Martin & Golden, 2014). Nurses can engage adolescents and help them create an individualized wellness plan that addresses body image, diet, weight concerns, and physical activity.

### Elimination Pattern

The renal and gastrointestinal systems are functionally mature by adolescence, and elimination patterns are consistent with those found in adults. Abnormal variation can occur in teens with eating disorders. It is important to remember that an adolescent's need for privacy or self-protection may inhibit normal elimination in public places, such as schools.

### Activity-Exercise Pattern

During adolescence the alterations in body composition and growth of lean muscle mass allow the teen to experience increased physical strength and endurance. All adolescents should be taught that regular exercise can increase their endurance and improve their appearance and general state of health and that these positive effects can extend into adulthood.

Many teens participate in organized sports, and the preparticipation sports examination is one of the most common reasons adolescents seek primary care (Figure 21-4). This examination offers an opportunity for nurses to identify adolescents at risk, evaluate their general state of health, and promote healthy lifestyle behaviors (Box 21-5). Along with eating disorders related to maintaining or losing weight for sports participation, adolescent athletes are subject to overuse injuries. Often these injuries are related to the specific sport in which the adolescent engages. The sports environment can contribute to or prevent overuse. The factors contributing to injury include environmental temperature (too hot or too cold), type of playing surface, emotional pressure from parents or coaches, inappropriate equipment, and inadequate training of coaches (Kerr et al., 2013). Nurses need to work closely with athletes and coaches to be sure the approach to sports participation is healthy and free of injury potential.

### Sleep-Rest Pattern

During adolescence the amount of time needed each night for sleep declines in comparison with earlier childhood needs. Although their sleep patterns differ greatly, adolescents need at least 9 hours of sleep per night (George & Davis, 2013). Adolescents who are employed, those involved in extracurricular

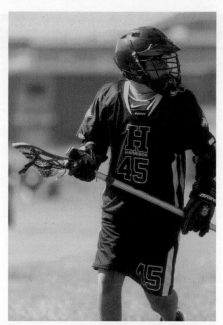

FIGURE 21-4 Adolescents frequently participate in organized activities, especially sports.

---

### BOX 21-5   Adolescent Preparticipation Sports Examination

**Areas for Special Concern**
- Previous trauma, including concussion
- Cardiovascular disease
- Hypertension
- Asthma
- Seizure disorder
- Splenomegaly, or enlarged spleen, often seen with infectious mononucleosis
- HIV infection
- Absence of paired organs: eye, kidney, testicle, or ovary

---

sports, and those who have "too much on their plate" are at increased risk of sleep deprivation. They stay up late and are then forced to wake up before their sleep cycles have finished because the high school day has such an early start. Many adolescents send and receive text messages at bedtime after room lights have been turned off, which can interfere with a good night's sleep. Even a moderate level of nighttime texting can greatly increase the likelihood of having long-term fatigue. Adolescents without sufficient sleep can find it difficult to concentrate and learn, or even stay awake in classes. Too little sleep might also contribute to mood swings and behavioral problems. Adolescents who drive when they are sleep deprived can cause accidents, which could lead to death. Nurses can suggest that adolescents keep their cell phones, computers, and other electronic devices out of their bedrooms at night. Nurses can also suggest strategies for daily living that help adolescents cope with the challenge of balancing their varied responsibilities while preventing exhaustion or burnout.

## Cognitive-Perceptual Pattern

### Piaget's Theory of Cognitive Development

Adolescence is characterized by a shift in cognitive abilities to Piaget's stage of **formal operations** (Piaget, 1969). Piaget's theory used the term *formal* to represent the emergence of ability to focus on the "form" of thoughts, objects, and experiences rather than on the exact content, which in turn lays the groundwork for abstract thinking. These new cognitive abilities are reflected in adolescent behaviors in several ways.

The first change is that, because of their new ability to "think about their thinking," adolescents become highly introspective. As introspection increases, they develop an internalized audience that provides them with a means to evaluate questions such as "Who am I?" "How do others see me?" and "Where am I going?" **Introspection** also combines with a reemergence of **egocentrism**, leading to their sense of being the primary focus—special, unique, and exceptional (Piaget, 1969). Being exceptional adolescents means being the exception, thinking that nothing can happen to them, but only to others. This type of thought can contribute to the risk-taking behaviors for which adolescents are well known:

- I can get drunk on weekends and not develop a drinking problem.
- I won't get pregnant; I've had sex for 6 months and haven't gotten pregnant yet.
- I can take those turns at 60 miles per hour and not lose control.

Another behavioral manifestation of adolescents' formal operations is an intolerance of things as they are. They are able to conceptualize things as they might or could be, rather than how they are, and can think of elaborate means for achieving these changes—now. With this newfound capability, they constantly challenge the ways things are and challenge themselves to consider the way things can or should be. Teens can be vehement in trying to convince others of their viewpoints and untiring in their support of causes that align with them. This **idealism** can lead to a rejection of family beliefs, religion, or social causes, which do not appear to the adolescent to be working fast enough to solve the problems of society. Although this idealism appears to most adults to be a flight from reality, it is a necessary stage in formal thinking. Reality is recognized, but only as a subset of many other possibilities that need to be aligned with their own thinking. Eventually, their thinking becomes less egocentric and omnipotent, giving way to an appreciation of differences in judgment between themselves and others (Piaget, 1969).

### Erikson's Theory of Psychosocial Development

Erikson's theory of psychosocial development describes the central task of adolescence as being the establishment of identity, with the primary risk being **role confusion** (Erikson, 1968). Although it may appear that adolescents are involved in a final rather than a transient or initial stage of development, identity formation in adolescence provides a means of moving into and through what might be termed an identity crisis.

This crisis involves a restaging of each of the previous stages of psychosocial development (Erikson, 1968). Development of trust in self and others, as emphasized in infancy, is encountered again as the adolescent searches for people and ideologies in which to have faith. Toddlerhood, and its search for autonomy, is also revisited as adolescents search for independence from their primary family units. The preschooler's challenge, a sense of initiative rather than guilt, resurfaces as the adolescent searches for direction and purpose. The school-age child's developing sense of industry is carried into the adolescent period also, as teens make choices in social, recreational, volunteer, academic, familial, and occupational activities. The confusion and hesitation in making these choices arise from fears of participating in activities that will not afford them the opportunity to excel or win the approval of their peers.

Erikson (1968) says that the extent to which these earlier tasks were accomplished successfully predicts the success of the current developmental stage, therefore influencing an adolescent's resourcefulness and success in experimenting with the new identity. When the threat of identity confusion is exceedingly great, delinquent behavior and alterations in mental health can occur. This threat is enhanced by conditions of poverty, racism, and other social inequities (see Box 21-13).

The pursuit of a meaningful ideology and an individual identity frequently creates a puzzling combination of shifting interests and sudden extremes in action. Erikson views this behavior as an attempt to try on various roles and to search for some stable principle that might last through the testing of extremes and be carried into adulthood. Reassuring parents that this behavior is normal during adolescence and encouraging them to maintain positive communication with their adolescents is an important nursing function.

### Time Orientation

Adolescents look at time differently than they did as younger children. They realize that the response to a problem can, and sometimes should, be delayed to think through the possibilities for approaching the problem. Additionally, teens develop a future orientation and are able to delay immediate gratification to gain more satisfaction in the future.

### Language

Advances in cognitive skills are reflected in an increased understanding of language. Formal operations and more abstract thought processes require expression in different words than did the more concrete thoughts of younger children. Adolescents give complex definitions, frequently including all possible meanings or uses. Interpretations of pictures or stories are intricate and abstract. Older teens are capable of using and understanding complex sentence structure, although they, like adults, may not use these complex sentences routinely in their speech.

Both receptive and expressive vocabularies increase during adolescence. As with all ages, receptive vocabulary far exceeds expressive vocabulary. The adolescent's vocabulary frequently includes slang. Slang may be centered on topics such as drug use, popular dress, music, and certain peer activities, or it may be more pervasive, in which case adults or "outsiders" may have difficulty following a conversation between two teens. The surge

| TABLE 21-2 | Deciphering and Conversing in the Latest Text Messaging Lingo |
|---|---|
| **Message** | **Meaning** |
| GR8 | Great |
| LOL | Laughing out loud |
| BRB | Be right back |
| AFC/AFK | Away from computer/away from keyboard |
| POS/MOS/DOS | Parent over shoulder/Mom over shoulder/Dad over shoulder |
| 9 | Parent watching |
| 99 | Parent no longer watching |
| CD9 | Code 9: parent watching or in room |
| RUOK | Are you ok? |
| XLNT | Excellent |
| F2F | Face to face |
| Zzz | Sleeping, bored, tired |
| Y | Why |
| B4N | Bye for now |
| YYSSW | Yeah yeah sure sure whatever |
| PCM | Please call me |

in cell phone use, instant and text messaging, and on-line social media has given rise to an entirely new set of communications to decipher (Table 21-2).

## Self-Perception–Self-Concept Pattern

The term *self-perception*, which is often used interchangeably with the terms *self-concept* and *self-esteem*, refers to both the description of the self and to the evaluation of, or feelings about, that description. Tied together and brought to the forefront in adolescence, both self-perception and body image dominate, influence, and are influenced by individual, peer, and societal norms and expectations.

Assessment, anticipatory guidance, education, and counseling are strategies the nurse can use to guide the adolescent in developing a self-perception that incorporates a healthy body image. It is important for parents, teachers, and health care providers to remember to praise adolescents for who they are rather than for what they do, value each of them as unique, demonstrate belief in their abilities to grow and develop, and delight in their discoveries of themselves and their unique means of expressing this.

### Acne

Teenage acne can influence self-perception, as it is a contributor to alterations in appearance. Most adolescents experience some degree of acne, especially during puberty, and they are typically concerned about their skin changes. The sebaceous glands increase production of sebum, a primary factor in the pathogenesis of acne. The sebaceous follicles become clogged with sebum and debris, forming open (blackheads) or closed (whiteheads) comedones. The incidence of acne within families suggests that hereditary factors are involved.

Thorough examination of the adolescent's skin and a discussion of its impact on the overall body image are necessary to determine appropriate management strategies. Intervention should include teaching the individual about the pathophysiological nature of acne. Knowledge allows the adolescent to become instrumental in its management and helps dispel common myths about acne and its care.

The approach to acne management is a stepwise approach according to the severity; all recommended management strategies take between 6 and 8 weeks to be effective (Gailbraith, 2016). Washing the skin with mild soap and water two times a day is the best way to remove surface dirt and oil. Daily topical administration of a retinoid or topical benzoyl peroxide is recommended for all cases of acne. Recent guidelines from the American Academy of Dermatology (AAD) (Zaenglein et al., 2016) suggest that a combination of topical agents (benzoyl peroxide, retinoid, antibiotic) can be used for mild acne. Should the condition worsen, or be more severe than mild acne, management can include adding an oral antibiotic to the topical regimen (Zaenglein et al., 2016). Systemic treatment with isotretinoin is used only for severe or moderate nonresponsive cases (Zaenglein et al., 2016). Vigorous scrubbing should be discouraged because the skin can become irritated, leading to follicular rupture (Well, 2013). The adolescent should not attempt to remove the pustules and papules that form. Squeezing the lesion can result in further irritation of the gland and permanent injury to the tissue. Adolescent females need to be careful when selecting makeup. Most preparations, when applied extensively over the face, prevent adequate exposure to air and light, especially those that have a fat base. Sunlight can have a beneficial effect on acne; however, prolonged exposure should be avoided. Stress can exacerbate acne in some adolescents. In these cases, stress-management techniques should be considered. The effect of diet on acne is a highly controversial issue. Evidence indicates that dietary restrictions specific to acne are unnecessary.

Adolescents with acne need support and understanding. The nurse can help adolescents and their families understand that management does not result in immediate improvement. In fact, topical agents may make acne appear worse initially, with any improvement occurring slowly over several months.

### Body Art and Piercing

Adolescence is a developmental period full of identity experimentation and risk-taking behavior. Body piercing and tattooing have become popular forms of expression of identity, particularly among adolescents, and are intimately related to self-perception. Each carries health risks and potentially fatal complications.

There are very few sites on adolescent bodies that have not been pierced. Ears, nipples, navels, noses, and eyebrows have all succumbed to metallic rings, rods, studs, and barbells. However, relatively frequently, an adolescent who obtains a piercing suffers a complication. Most commonly these include localized infection, bleeding, dermatitis, and possible keloid formation. Intraoral soft tissue piercing of the lips, cheek, uvula, and tongue harbors additional and potentially fatal complications, including a constant risk of aspiration, hemorrhage, and swelling leading to airway compromise, nerve damage, keloid scar formation, abscess, and tetanus. There is also an increased risk of hepatitis and HIV infection, as well as tooth injury, gingival recession, and difficulty with speech, taste, and swallowing.

Tattooing carries similar risks of infection, with a heightened concern for the transmission of blood-borne diseases, including hepatitis and HIV infection, especially with colorful tattoos. Colored ink is expensive and is often reused to cut costs, increasing exposure risks. Tattoos are also permanent markings and do not age well.

Nurses can explore with adolescents the reasons for acquiring body art and explain the potential short-term and long-term consequences to assist with their decision-making. To prevent infection from body piercing, the nurse needs to advise the adolescent to use meticulous handwashing when cleaning piercing sites. The sites should be cleaned with saline or antibacterial soap and protected from injury (AAD, 2015). Adolescents with new tattoos need to avoid sun exposure and apply a moisturizing lotion to the site (AAD, 2016). With both types of body art, adolescents should notify the provider of any signs of infection.

## Roles-Relationships Pattern
### Families

Until adolescence, the younger child is highly dependent on the parents and other adults. Striving for identity and increased independence, the adolescent begins to spend increased time away from the family. Parents sense a narrowing of their influence as their teen not only begins to prefer the company of peers and other adults but also begins to question familial beliefs and values. Parents may respond by setting unreasonably strict limits and asking intrusive questions about their teen's activities, friends, and ideas or decide to drop all rules and limits and assume that the adolescent can now manage alone. Neither of these approaches works well.

Whereas adolescents strive for a sense of identity and independence, their parents try to learn how to let go. Each is temporarily unsure of the relationship with the other, and the family unit may experience more stress than at any previous time. Furthermore, this period is often prolonged because more teens remain financially dependent on their families as they move into young adulthood.

Some families experience better outcomes than do other families. Families in which parents maintain a willingness to listen and demonstrate an ongoing affection for and acceptance of their adolescent yet still maintain some consistent limits experience more constructive, positive outcomes during this period. This situation does not mean that parents necessarily agree with their teen's ideas or actions, but rather that they are willing to hear what the adolescent has to say and to negotiate some limits. Parents may need assistance in determining negotiable versus nonnegotiable rules and in developing ways to voice their concerns in an honest, open way. Even when teens do not want to "discuss" a topic, they need to know why their parents are concerned.

### Peers

Faced with the need to become autonomous, achieve identity, and become productive, the adolescent often turns from the family to the peer group to find a safe psychosocial shelter in which to develop. Belonging to an informally organized clique, crowd, gang, or group is the primary means with which to make the transition from the young child's allegiance to the family to a member of a group. Identification with a group is proclaimed through conformity to standards of clothing, behavior, language, and values. This feature of the adolescent subculture persists despite the strong inclination in society as a whole toward greater levels of individuality.

The **peer group** is a vehicle for disengaging from the family unit and, as such, provides a means of achieving the goals of independence and individualization. Adolescents talk a great deal with their peers. Whether on the phone, on-line, or in person, they can discuss a 10-minute situation for hours on end. This sharing of thoughts and impressions is important. The telephone or computer can provide a "safe" mechanism for the teen to interact with members of the opposite sex as they share intimate ideas and concerns and begin to experience the closeness and caring that develops into the capacity to form a future intimate relationship.

Adolescents in both urban and rural areas can have exposure to, and participate in, gangs. Gangs function as a peer group for adolescents who may feel socially inadequate, have problems at school, or exhibit low self-esteem (Melde & Eskensen, 2014). Feeling unsafe in a community or at school may also be a contributing factor (Lenzi et al., 2015). Not all gangs exhibit delinquent behavior; however, there is a societal perception that violence is part of the gang culture. Nurses can alert parents to the signs that their adolescent may be associating with a gang; these include wearing symbolic clothing, new and extensive body art, secrecy about friends, worsening school performance, and possible substance use (AAP, 2015d). Encouraging strong and positive relationships with friends during adolescence and increased vigilance by parents can be protective against gang membership.

## Sexuality-Reproductive Pattern

### Adolescent Sexual Issues

The emergence of secondary sexual characteristics increases adolescents' awareness of themselves as sexual human beings. They fantasize about relationships and sex and gradually experiment with dating and a myriad of coital and noncoital physical contacts. Adolescents become sexually active for a variety of reasons. They have sex for affection, because of peer pressure, as a symbol of maturity, as spontaneous experimentation, to feel close, or because it feels good or right. Although the prevalence of adolescent sexual activity in the United States has decreased, approximately 34% of teens report being sexually active (CDC, 2014b). At times, they have intercourse without their consent. Approximately 7.3% of adolescents report forced intercourse,

and approximately the same percentage report physical battering by a date (CDC, 2014b). (See the case study and care plan at the end of this chapter).

In the process of establishing a sexual sense of themselves, it is not uncommon for adolescents to question if they are homosexual. Experimenting with same-sex physical intimacy does not necessarily predict future sexual orientation, but feelings associated with the possibility of homosexual identity can give rise to anxiety, mood disorders, and heightened risk of suicide in adolescents, especially if they feel victimized by others (Lim et al., 2013). Approximately 5% to 10% of people in the United States identify themselves as being what may be referred to as "gender nonconforming" (Lim et al., 2014). An important goal stated in *Healthy People 2020* (USDHHS, Office of Disease Prevention and Health Promotion, 2015) is to "improve the health, safety, and well-being of lesbian, gay, bisexual, and transgender (LGBT) individuals." A primary reason for the identification of this goal is the recognition that many health providers, among others, have a negative attitude toward caring for individuals with gender differences (Lim et al., 2013). In addition to emotional issues associated with gender nonconformity, nurses need to educate themselves about health issues associated with adolescents in this population. These include risk of acquiring a **sexually transmitted infection** (STI), increased tobacco use, substance use or abuse, and obesity (Lim et al., 2013, 2014). When providing culturally appropriate care, nurses can create a supportive, nonjudgmental climate that enables disclosure and optimizes social support for both adolescents and their families (Lim et al., 2014).

The technological revolution has opened up a limitless world of unmediated information to adolescents and has led to increased issues of on-line risky behaviors. The use of on-line social networks such as Facebook, Twitter, Instagram, and other messaging sites continues to increase rapidly among all age groups and segments of our society, presenting new opportunities for the exchange of sexual information, as well as for potentially unsafe encounters between predators and the vulnerable or young. Additionally, adolescents who use the Internet to seek sexual information often receive conflicting messages and inaccurate facts. Sexting has been recognized as an increasing occurrence for several years and is a global practice among teens and young adults. Sexting refers to sending a text message with sexually explicit content or a sexually explicit picture. This type of texting can cause emotional pain for the person in the picture, as well as the sender and receiver. Nurses help adolescents understand that text messages should not contain pictures of naked people or of people kissing or touching each other, and that sending such a type of text message is considered a crime in some areas.

Knowing adolescents are heavily invested in these and other sexual issues, nurses are capable of discussing and willing to discuss them with adolescents in a variety of settings, such as physicians' offices, clinics, and schools. Nurses need to be comfortable with their own sexuality; able to discuss the subject of sex and sexual orientation, contraception, and protection against STIs; and be aware of their own limitations, beliefs, and biases. Anticipatory guidance about the decision to become sexually active, to use contraception, and to obtain protection from STIs

## BOX 21-6 QUALITY AND SAFETY SCENARIO

**Performing Breast and Testicular Self-Examination**

Breast self-examination (BSE) or testicular self-examination (TSE) should be performed once a month so that teens become familiar with the usual appearance and feel of their breasts or testicles. This routine makes noticing any changes from one month to another easier. Finding a change from "normal" is the main idea behind regular self-examination. The best time for females to perform a BSE is 2 or 3 days after their period ends, when the breasts are least likely to be tender or swollen. For males, the best time for a TSE is during or immediately after a warm shower.

**Breast Self-Examination**

- Stand in front of a mirror. Inspect both breasts for anything unusual, such as any discharge from the nipples, puckering or dimpling of the skin, or marked asymmetry.
- While watching closely in the mirror, clasp your hands behind your head and press your hands forward, and inspect the breast again.
- Next, press your hands firmly on your hips and bow slightly toward the mirror as you pull your shoulders and elbows forward, and inspect the breast again.
- Next, raise one arm. Use three or four fingers to explore the breast firmly, carefully, and thoroughly. Beginning at the outer edge, press the flat part of

your fingers in small circles, moving the circles slowly around the breast. Gradually work toward the nipple. Be sure to examine the entire breast. Pay special attention to the area between the breast and the armpit, including the armpit itself. Feel the breast for any unusual lump or mass under the skin.
- Gently squeeze the nipple and look for a discharge. Repeat the examination on the other breast.

The last two steps should be repeated lying down. This position flattens the breast and makes examination easier. Some women perform BSE in the shower. Fingers gliding over soapy skin make concentrating on the texture underneath easier.

**Testicular Self-Examination**

- Cup or support the testicles with one hand and feel them with the other.
- Gently roll each testicle between the thumb and fingers. There should not be any pain.
- Feel the testicles for any swelling or hard lumps on the surface of the testicles. Testicles are normally oval, firm, smooth, and rubbery. One may be slightly larger than the other.
- A natural tubelike structure, the epididymis, is along the back of the testicle. Learn what it feels like.

From Lowdermilk, D. L., Perry, S. E., & Cashion, M.C. (2011). *Maternity nursing* (8th ed.). St. Louis: Mosby; Neinstein, L. S., Gordau, C. M., Katzman, D. K., Rosen, D. S., & Woods, E. R. (2008). *Adolescent health care: A practical guide* (5th ed.). Philadelphia; Lippincott Williams & Wilkins.

needs to be provided before adolescents encounter a situation in which they need this information (see Tables 22-2 and 22-3). This is also a good time to introduce the adolescent to breast and testicular self-examinations (Box 21-6: Quality and Safety Scenario).

School nurses are often leaders of, or participants in, school-based sex education programs. Depending on the philosophy of the educational district, sex education programs can be abstinence only or comprehensive, which combines abstinence with discussion of protective measures. Evidence shows that neither of these is totally effective in delaying adolescent sexual intimacy, but both provide straightforward information, which adolescents need (Grossman et al., 2014; Rohrbach et al., 2015). Grossman and colleagues (2014), noting that comprehensive sex education programs have had mixed results on adolescents delaying intimacy, studied the effect of the addition of a parental component to a standard sex education program. Their hypothesis was that this component would facilitate sharing of values between children and parents, as well as increasing the comfort of parents in communicating sexual information to their adolescents. They used a longitudinal study design to follow more than 2400 sixth grade students in 24 schools until they reached eighth grade; schools were randomly assigned to the parent involvement group, and the control group and students were surveyed each year. They found that a higher percentage of students in the experimental group delayed sexual activity, and that the addition of parental involvement enhanced protective effects, especially for middle school boys (Grossman et al., 2014). Nurses need to also consider not only parental beliefs and values regarding the provision of sex education in the schools but also what is the optimal age for introducing information. Children are entering

puberty earlier than in the past, and sex education programs focusing on positive relationships may need to begin at an earlier age than middle school (Jennings, 2015).

### Adolescent Pregnancy

For health care providers, adolescent pregnancy is viewed as a high-risk situation because of the serious health risks and potential complications for both the mother and the infant. For politicians and governmental agencies, it is a social problem that makes overwhelming demands on social and economic resources. For adolescents and their families, it may be seen as positive and normal or the worst disaster imaginable. No matter what the perspective, adolescent pregnancy represents a myriad of concerns with far-reaching social, educational, financial, and emotional effects.

Recent information from the National Center for Health Statistics (Ventura et al., 2014) reveals that births to girls aged 15 to 19 years in the United States number 273,105, or a birth rate of 26.5 per 1000. The overall teen birth rate has dropped dramatically by approximately 57% in the past 2 decades, and this has occurred in all ethnic groups. The birth rate is highest in Hispanic teens, followed by non-Hispanic blacks, American Indian/Alaskan Natives, non-Hispanic whites, and Asian Pacific Islanders.

Adolescent pregnancy has a myriad of negative outcomes for both the mother and the child. For the mother, these include a significant decline in her future prospects, especially educational and economic; single parenthood; reliance on government-sponsored assistance, and poverty (Ng & Kaye, 2012). For the child born to adolescent mothers there is a higher risk of low birth weight. Low birth weight, which may result from disparities

---

**BOX 21-7   Coping Mechanisms of Adolescents**

**Cognitive Mastery**

The adolescent attempts to learn as much as possible about the situation or stressor. This strategy is common for the adolescent with a chronic illness. The nurse can assist by clarifying any misinformation, sharing research findings, and encouraging a discussion of feelings.

**Conformity**

The adolescent attempts to be a mirror image of peers, which includes dress, language, attitudes, and actions. The nurse must respect this need for sameness and can also encourage discussion of feelings about differences among teens.

**Controlling Behavior**

Adolescents must be in charge of some aspects of life and can no longer accept family and school rules without question as they did in the past. This need for

control extends to health care. The nurse cannot simply give directions or instructions, but rather should present the options and allow the adolescent to partner with the nurse to work out an acceptable plan.

**Fantasy**

The adolescent may use fantasy as a way to escape or experiment. The nurse can encourage the teen to use fantasy constructively to develop creative plans to deal with a stressful situation.

**Motor Activity**

Engaging in sports, dancing, running, or other physical activity can be an effective tension-releasing strategy, and can also provide an instant peer group. The nurse can encourage physical activity and offer information about protective gear and injury prevention.

---

in access to prenatal care, is associated with infant death and other health and developmental problems (Ventura et al., 2014). Furthermore, these children often fall victim to abuse and neglect and suffer from poor school performance.

When pregnancy occurs, adolescents and their families deserve honest and sensitive counseling about options available to them, as well as the support systems available for them throughout the pregnancy, birth, and subsequent parenting. Nurses not only need to reinforce reproductive health-education efforts but also need to encourage adolescents to build on the strengths in their lives and opportunities available to them (see Chapter 22 for additional information about pregnancy and contraception).

## Coping–Stress Tolerance Pattern

When all the changes that occur in adolescents are aligned with their need to separate from their parents and gain a sense of their own independence, their ability to cope is put to the test over and over again. Common coping mechanisms, and the strategies the nurse can use to encourage teens to use them in adaptive ways, are listed in Box 21-7.

However, too often adolescents are unable to balance the stresses, lacking the appropriate skills and outlets, adequate support systems, or available mental health intervention. Depression, suicide, and substance abuse emerge as life becomes overwhelming and the future unimaginable.

### Depression

As with many other diseases, the rate of **depression** increases with age, and the incidence continues to increase during adolescence. Approximately 11% of adolescents experience a major depressive disorder by age 18 years, with the prevalence in girls almost twice as high as in boys (Forum on Child and Family Statistics, 2015). The term *depression* includes both major depressive and dysthymic disorders. A major depression is an alteration in mood that is disabling and interferes with normal activities, whereas dysthymia is a depressed or irritable mood that extends for more than 2 years but does not interfere with activities or performance (National Institute of Mental Health, 2011).

Depression is suspected when the adolescent uses words such as down, sad, low, blue, hopeless, worried, bored, or discouraged and exhibits several of the following symptoms:

- Change in weight or appetite
- Insomnia or hypersomnia
- Decreased energy or fatigue
- Loss of interest and pleasure in usual activities
- Out-of-proportion feelings of self-reproach or guilt
- Difficulty concentrating; declining school performance
- Preoccupation with death or suicidal ideation

The AAP has recommended routine screening for mental health disorders in the primary care setting using a reliable and valid assessment instrument (Weitzman & Wegner, 2015). Evidence suggests that when parents complete a mental health screening questionnaire for their children during regular health-promotion visits, referrals for appropriate mental health management increase (Jonovich & Alpert-Gillis, 2014). Nurses need to lead the way in screening and assessing children and teens for mental health problems, including depression. Moreover, nurses may promote mental health promotion in both children and teens by teaching them effective coping skills and stress-reduction techniques.

### Suicide

Adolescence is a period of considerable stress, and when coping mechanisms and social supports are inadequate, suicide may emerge as an outcome. Suicide has become the second leading cause of death among adolescents, aged 15 to 24 years (National Center for Health Statistics, 2014). A national survey revealed that 17% of youths in grades 9 to 12 in the United States reported that they were seriously considering suicide and 8% had attempted suicide during the previous year (CDC, 2014b). These figures might not even reflect the full scope of the problem because many suicides may be classified as accidental deaths. Along with well-known risk factors, such as depression or substance abuse, the risk factors for suicide may be related to physical and cognitive developmental changes. The physical and emotional changes during puberty in younger children evolve into older adolescents achieving a cognitive level that allows them to more carefully solve problems and look at consequences (Fried et al., 2012).

## BOX 21-8 Warning Signs of Suicide Risk in Adolescents

**Behavioral Changes**
- Increased risk taking
- Increased incidence of accidents
- Substance use and abuse
- Physical violence to self, others, or animals
- Decreased appetite
- Alienation from family or peer group
- Giving away personal items
- Writing letters or notes, essays, and poems with suicidal content

**Cognitive and Mood Changes**
- Expression of hopelessness
- Increasing rage or anger
- Dramatic swings in affect
- Sleep disorders
- Preoccupation with death
- Difficulty concentrating
- Hearing voices, seeing things or people
- Newfound interest in religion or cult

Many researchers are convinced that suicide during adolescence is not an impulsive or spontaneous act: it is selected carefully only after other problem-solving methods have failed and suicide is viewed as the only option.

Adolescent suicide can be prevented. Distressed adolescents tend to give clues, both verbally and nonverbally. Any single clue may mean nothing, but when several clues are noted, they should be recognized as important warning signs. Box 21-8 outlines vigilant warning signs for parents, teachers, health care providers, and peers to prevent adolescent suicide. Any signs of suicide or threat to commit suicide should be taken seriously and require immediate intervention and referral. An adult should remain with the adolescent until medical assistance becomes available. Nurses can teach adolescents to be sensitive to the signs that may indicate a friend is suicidal and to seek adult assistance immediately.

## Values-Beliefs Pattern

Values and beliefs are learned phenomena that serve as guides for decision-making and actions. With the development of abstract thought, adolescents begin to expand their understanding of good and bad or right and wrong, to include autonomous moral principles that have validity apart from the authority of a parent or society and instead are based on the individual's beliefs. Their newly discovered maturity in moral reasoning is situational and relational and is often superseded by psychosocial developmental needs and influences. Adolescents may think or feel something is wrong or bad yet may act contrary to that belief because of peer pressure or the need to declare their independence.

Adolescents often align their values and beliefs with a particular religion, philosophical school of thought, social movement or cause, or other formal system, using it to make decisions about what is right or wrong, best or worst, and important or trivial.

During adolescence, these alignments can change drastically and often, causing strife and concern for parents, yet providing the teen with different ranges of experience from which to base eventual and lasting choices.

Kohlberg's theory of moral development (Kohlberg, 1981) demonstrates that the adolescent begins to make the transition to the postconventional stage, equating what is right with the idea of justice and basing actions on the recognition of the universal principles underlying laws and social agreements. Gilligan and colleagues (1990), who developed a parallel theory of moral development for females, proposes that the female adolescent sees "good" as involving self-sacrifice and caring for the relationships in her life. They state that, as moral reasoning matures, the female adolescent learns to achieve a balance between what is good for her and what is good for others in her network of relationships.

As adolescents struggle with their journey to discover who they are, parents, teachers, and health care providers need to provide positive role modeling, reinforce positive behaviors, and remember the difficulty of their own journeys. It is often when we like them the least that they need us the most.

# ENVIRONMENTAL PROCESSES

Because adolescents are in developmental transition, their lifestyle choices may have a significant effect on their current and future health. These choices are particularly sensitive to the immediate physical and social environments. These environmental influences include their family members, friends, community, school, neighborhood, and work environments. Several critical types of adolescent health behaviors—including alcohol and drug use, injury and violence, tobacco use, nutrition, physical activity, and sexual behaviors—have been identified as contributing to the leading causes of death and disability among adults and youth.

## Physical Agents

### Unintentional Injury

Unintentional injury, along with suicide and homicide, continues to be the leading cause of death and injury during adolescence. Approximately 66% of all deaths from unintentional injury among adolescents, aged 15 to 19 years, are attributed to injuries caused by motor vehicle crashes (National Center for Injury Prevention and Control, 2013). Motor vehicle crashes are a significant cause of nonfatal injury as well. Whether drivers, passengers, pedestrians, or cyclists, few adolescents take measures to reduce their risk of injury, with 7.6% rarely or never using a safety belt and 87% rarely or never using a bicycle helmet (CDC, 2014b). Evidence also suggests that distractions, such as talking or texting on cell phones, eating, or playing with the radio, increase teen drivers' risk of being involved in a crash.

Nurses talk to teens about the consequences of texting while driving and encourage teens to wear their safety belts and avoid driving, or riding with someone, under the influence of drugs or alcohol. The tendency to play loud music and change the tune or disc often, as well as the pressure to answer cell phones, can also be distracting, as can a car full of other teens. Recognizing this and that teens have a much higher nighttime crash fatality rate, many states have enacted new driver restrictions and nighttime curfews.

## Sports Injuries

Organized sports in and out of school provide adolescents with experiences in competition, teamwork and effort, and conflict resolution. They also provide a valuable means for adolescents to develop self-esteem. However, adolescents are particularly vulnerable to sports injuries. Their coordination skills are developing, their judgment is often immature and inadequate, their epiphyses have not yet closed, and their extremities are poorly protected by stabilizing musculature. They can also become obsessed or driven to perform beyond their capabilities or to the exclusion of all other activities. The use of performance-enhancing substances, such as steroids, which have been unfortunately modeled by many professional athletes, can create another potential extreme scenario that places the adolescent at risk of injury.

Although traumatic brain injury (concussion) is caused by falls or other mechanical injury, the most frequent contributing factor in children and adolescents is participation in sports (Rivera et al., 2015). Even a minor impact injury to the head or neck, with or without loss of consciousness, can result in long-term physical, emotional, and cognitive effects if it is not appropriately managed (Arbogast et al., 2013). The signs and symptoms of concussion in children include deficits in cognition, altered neurological status, problems concentrating in school, and fatigue. Traumatic brain injury should be managed by a provider who is experienced in recognizing the signs and symptoms and who is experienced in concussion management. Several reliable and valid assessment instruments are available to assist health care providers in diagnosis (Rivera et al., 2015). As a consequence of a body of evidence suggesting that traumatic brain injury effects can be more severe in children and adolescents, many states have enacted "Return to Play" legislation (Rivera et al., 2015), which guides parents, coaches, and health providers in appropriate management. Conservative management is essential and may involve restricting all physical activity and ensuring cognitive rest (no school work; restriction of use of electronic devices, such as television, video games, computers, or phones) until the adolescent is no longer symptomatic (Arbogast et al., 2013; Rivera et al., 2015). Decisions regarding return to activity and school are often based on a stepwise staging system ranging from 1 (no activity until asymptomatic for 24 hours) to 6 (return to full activity with medical clearance) (Rivera et al, 2015).

The nurse advocates the proper use of protective gear during all activities and a thorough preparticipation sports examination, along with concussion training for coaches and parents. The nurse also monitors adolescents for overuse, overexertion, or overinvestment in a sport.

## Violence

Although the rate of adolescent victims of violence has decreased in the past 2 decades, adolescents still experience risk of injury and death from violence in their homes, schools, and communities. In the United States the rate of adolescents, aged 12 to 17 years,

being victims of violent crime is 9 per 1000 adolescents (Forum on Child and Family Statistics, 2015). Adolescents can be perpetrators of violence as well, and homicide is the third leading cause of death in adolescents older than 15 years (National Center for Health Statistics, 2014). Figure 21-5 outlines the interrelationships of internal and external precipitating factors that increase an adolescent's vulnerability to and for violent behaviors. Many teens report carrying weapons to protect themselves or intimidate others. Adolescents often report a fear of violence and try to avoid situations where they might be vulnerable to it, including the home or even the bathroom at school. Victims of violent crime can experience both short-term and long-term physical and psychological health problems.

Becoming increasingly independent, adolescents test the limits of authority, experiment with a variety of roles, question adult values and authority, and look to peers for affirmation. They may feel pressure to join gangs or feel threatened by them. Many studies suggest that witnessing or observing violence, whether in person or projected on the television, video, or movie screen, results in a higher incidence of aggressive or violent behaviors (You, 2014). Graphic violence in the media, current music lyrics, and video gaming has also been implicated in increased violent behavior.

Teenagers may be involved in physical or emotional bullying and/or cyberbullying. Cyberbullying refers to emotional bullying via electronic media, such as harassing texts, e-mails, or instant messages, and social media posts (Carter & Wilson, 2015). A recent study (Carter & Wilson, 2015) of the prevalence of cyberbullying among 367 adolescents shows that 16.9% of them reported being victims of cyberbullying, and 30.1% were victims of traditional bullying. With a significant majority of adolescents having access to technological devices, bullying can occur on a much wider and more destructive scale (Carter & Wilson, 2015). Receiving bullying text messages or being harassed on social media can make a teen feel insecure and may lead to school absences or serious emotional distress, including, in extreme cases, suicide.

Nurses engage adolescents, examining and discussing the messages in videos, songs, movies, games, and television shows. Discussing their developing sense of self, their sense of belonging and where that sense is found, and their fears may help nurses to intercept an adolescent who might otherwise turn to violence. Discussing frightening news events with adolescents in a realistic, contextual way might also help nurses mitigate fear and anxiety. Teens who are valued and nurtured by caring adults have the best chance of emerging from adolescence unscathed. Nurses may also discuss cyberbullying with adolescents; encourage them to talk to a trusted adult if he or she receives harassing text messages and to consider options such as rejecting texts from unknown numbers; and tell them that it is inappropriate to send harassing text messages to others. The warning signs of cyberbullying are similar to those that occur with any type of bullying and include decrease in school performance or reluctance to attend school, increased signs of stress, isolation from friends, and altered sleep or eating patterns (National Society for the Prevention of Cruelty to Children as cited in "Reducing the impact of bullying: Useful resources and guidance," 2015).

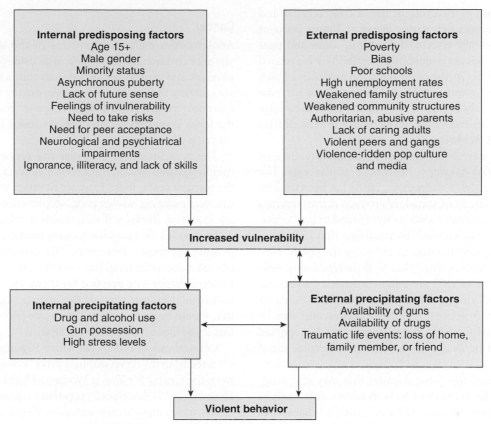

```
┌─────────────────────────────────┐        ┌─────────────────────────────────┐
│   Internal predisposing factors  │        │   External predisposing factors  │
│            Age 15+               │        │            Poverty               │
│          Male gender             │        │             Bias                 │
│         Minority status          │        │          Poor schools            │
│       Asynchronous puberty       │        │    High unemployment rates       │
│      Lack of future sense        │        │    Weakened family structures    │
│    Feelings of invulnerability   │        │  Weakened community structures   │
│        Need to take risks        │        │  Authoritarian, abusive parents  │
│     Need for peer acceptance     │        │      Lack of caring adults       │
│  Neurological and psychiatrical  │        │     Violent peers and gangs      │
│           impairments            │        │   Violence-ridden pop culture    │
│ Ignorance, illiteracy, and lack  │        │           and media              │
│            of skills             │        │                                  │
└─────────────────────────────────┘        └─────────────────────────────────┘
                    │                                        │
                    ▼                                        ▼
              ┌──────────────────────────────────────┐
              │       Increased vulnerability         │
              └──────────────────────────────────────┘
                    ▲                                        ▲
                    │                                        │
┌─────────────────────────────────┐        ┌─────────────────────────────────┐
│   Internal precipitating factors │◄──────►│   External precipitating factors │
│       Drug and alcohol use       │        │       Availability of guns       │
│         Gun possession           │        │       Availability of drugs      │
│        High stress levels        │        │  Traumatic life events: loss of  │
│                                  │        │   home, family member, or friend │
└─────────────────────────────────┘        └─────────────────────────────────┘
                    │                                        │
                    ▼                                        ▼
                          ┌────────────────────────┐
                          │    Violent behavior     │
                          └────────────────────────┘
```

**FIGURE 21-5** Factors contributing to adolescent violence.

Working with parents is essential. Nurses can encourage parents to be vigilant regarding their adolescent's use of electronic media, including restricting use or using parental controls, if necessary. The AAP (2013b) recommends limiting total screen time to no more than 2 hours a day for children of all ages and removing access to all electronic device at bedtime. Parents need to be aware of websites accessed by their adolescent, including YouTube sites, gaming sites, text messaging programs, and social media. Adolescents may be resistant to parental monitoring because of the perception that it invades their privacy; however, nurses can suggest that parents discuss these issues with teens before providing them with electronic access so that adolescents know from the outset that spot checking will occur and the consequences of inappropriate use.

## Biological Agents

### Infection

Infectious mononucleosis is a self-limiting viral infection transmitted by direct contact with oropharyngeal secretions. It is prevalent among adolescents and is often referred to as the "kissing disease"; however, it can occur in younger children. It is caused by Epstein-Barr virus. Typically, adolescents complain of a sore throat, lymph node enlargement, and lethargy. Both splenomegaly and hepatomegaly can occur, creating a risk of injury. The condition is self-limiting and resolves with symptomatic care and appropriate rest.

The rates of meningococcal disease remain highest for infants, but recently rates have increased among adolescents. Reports have identified an increased risk of meningococcal disease among college first-year students who live in dormitories or residence halls, particularly if they are exposed to secondhand smoke. Many colleges now require meningococcal vaccination, along with other vaccinations administered during childhood. Meningococcal vaccine is now being given routinely to adolescents, with a first dose administered when the adolescent is 11 to 12 years old, and a booster dose at age 16 years (Advisory Committee on Immunization Practices [ACIP], 2016).

Adolescents are at the period of life with high sexual energy that may lead to high levels of risk-taking behaviors attributable to an increased sense of invulnerability. As adolescents experiment with and explore their sexual development and emerging independence, they engage in risky sexual behavior and expose themselves to increased risk of acquiring STIs. STIs most commonly include gonorrhea, syphilis, chlamydia, herpes simplex virus infection, human papilloma virus (HPV) infection, trichomoniasis, hepatitis B, and HIV infection. Approximately 50% of the newly diagnosed STI cases in the United States are among adolescents and young adults, and approximately 25% of sexually active girls have an STI, most commonly HPV infection or chlamydia (CDC, 2014b). Minorities, especially black Americans, are disproportionately infected with HIV (CDC, 2015b).

Many contributing factors have been identified and found to negatively impact this significant public and adolescent health problem. Factors such as inconsistent use of contraceptive and protective devices, increasingly earlier age of and more frequent sexual activity, lower self-esteem, depression, social and peer pressure, and an adolescent's sense of invincibility were related to higher risks of STIs. On the other hand, factors such as high self-efficacy, effective parent-child communications, parental monitoring, positive school relationships, and sexual knowledge could be significant protective factors to reduce the risk of STIs in adolescents (AAP, 2015a).

Several theories have been used to guide the practices of preventing sexual risk-taking behaviors in adolescents. The health-promotion model (Pender et al., 2010) has been used by nurses for the development of sexual risk-reduction interventions for adolescents, and these interventions were found to be effective. Most of the cognitive-behavioral interventions that stem from these theories report effectiveness in reducing the risk of HIV infection. Scientific studies show that well-designed and well-implemented HIV infection/STI prevention programs can decrease sexual risk behaviors among adolescents (Box 21-9: Research for Evidence-Based Practice). Although adolescents can be evaluated and treated for STIs, the diseases must be reported and the nurse must be aware of the government rules about reporting.

Nurses are aware of the cultural issues that may play a significant role in the prevention of STIs in adolescents, such as HIV/acquired immunodeficiency syndrome (AIDS). While nurses develop interventions for reducing STI-related sexual risk behaviors, they take adolescents' cultural/ethnic backgrounds into considerations.

---

## BOX 21-9 RESEARCH FOR EVIDENCE-BASED PRACTICE

### An Effective Prevention Program for Adolescents' Sexual Health

Regardless of advances in prevention and treatment, STIs continue to be a significant cause of morbidity and death in the United States. Promoting the ability of children and adolescents to avoid risk-taking sexual behaviors is considered a significant approach to encourage sexual health in adolescents. Standard comprehensive sex education programs have had mixed results in adolescents delaying sexual activity, so Rohrbach et al. (2015) investigated a novel sex education program—a rights-based program. They defined rights-based education as including factual information, along with information about gender and human rights, right to self-determination, and empowerment. Their randomized controlled design compared a standard sex education program with the rights-based program and assessed whether the rights-based program would have long-term results. They surveyed participants before the program initiation and 1 year later and found that the program had a long-lasting positive effect on participants' psychosocial outcomes, but not necessarily on sexual behaviors, although there was an increase in adolescents' use of clinic services for sexual concerns (Rohrbach et al., 2015). Including principles of gender rights and empowerment in a sex education program provides students with additional strategies to determine when they are ready for sexual activity.

From Rohrbach, L. Berglas, N., Jerman, P., Angulo-Olaiz, F., & Chou, C. (2015). A rights-based sexuality education program for adolescents: 1-year outcomes. *Journal of Adolescent Health, 57*(4), 399–405.

---

## Cancer

Adolescents are affected by many of the same cancers as are younger children, such as leukemia, osteogenic sarcoma, lymphomas, and central nervous system tumors. Older adolescents are entering the period of their lives during which cancer of the reproductive and related organs is more common. For females the focus is on cervical and breast cancer; for males, testicular cancer is of concern.

The peak incidence of breast and cervical cancer is during middle age and breast and cervical cancers are actually rare in the teenage years. Risks for later development of these cancers can occur during adolescence, so prevention and surveillance are essential. Breast self-examination, which has been highly recommended for many, has recently been questioned as a routine practice for most adolescents. The extremely small incidence of breast cancer in teens has caused some health care providers to deemphasize this practice for them. However, most still feel that regular examination of the breasts begins a lifelong habit that should begin as soon as the female adolescent develops (see Box 21-6: Quality and Safety Scenario).

Cervical cancer is detected with a Papanicolaou (Pap) smear, obtained from the cervix during a pelvic examination. Information from the Center for Young Women's Health, Boston Children's Hospital (2015) describes factors that increase the risk of cervical cancer, which include early initiation of sexual intercourse, having multiple sexual partners or a sexual partner who has had many partners, any history of STIs in the adolescent or partner, and lack of condom use. Sexually active adolescents should be screened for STIs, which may not require an internal pelvic examination. A pelvic examination with or without a Pap smear is indicated for symptoms of infection or gynecological problems, but no longer routinely; however, all women should have a pelvic examination with a Pap smear beginning at age 21 years (American College of Obstetricians and Gynecologists, 2012).

Administration of a vaccine to prevent cervical cancer and other diseases caused by certain types of genital HPV has been recommended by the ACIP (http://www.cdc.gov/hpv/). An HPV vaccination series is recommended for girls and boys at age 11 or 12 years (ACIP, 2016). The vaccine is also recommended for all adolescent girls and women through age 26 years who did not receive all three doses of the vaccine when they were younger, and for all adolescent boys and men through age 21 years (age 26 years if they are in a sexual relationship with another man) who also did not complete the vaccine series when they were younger (CDC, 2015c). Ideally, females should get the vaccine before they are sexually active. This is because the vaccine is most effective in girls/women who have not yet acquired any of the HPV types covered by the vaccine (CDC, 2015c). Females who are sexually active may also benefit from the vaccine, but they may receive less benefit because the vaccine will have no effect on HPV types they acquired before vaccine administration. The vaccine protects against HPV-related cancers in both boys and girls.

Testicular cancer is the number one cancer in adolescent and young adult males. Adolescent males should learn to perform a testicular self-examination and should continue this practice monthly (see Box 21-6: Quality and Safety Scenario). Nurses introduce and teach methods of self-examination to adolescents, who naturally are interested in their developing bodies.

## Chemical Agents

### Substance Use and Abuse

Adolescents are influenced by a complicated interaction between biological and psychosocial development, environmental messages, and societal attitudes regarding the use of substances such as alcohol, tobacco, or marijuana. Society as a whole is increasingly oriented toward using chemicals such as drugs, alcohol, and tobacco to feel better, look better, act more sociable, stay awake, sleep, be sexy or erect, or lose weight. Some of the most famous music, movie, and sports stars openly model substance use and abuse. It is no surprise that adolescents are making the choice to experiment with and use substances at younger and younger ages.

Alcohol is the substance used most frequently by adolescents (CDC, 2014b), with nearly 35% of adolescents reporting current use in a national survey. Alcohol use is followed by marijuana use (23.4%), use of prescription medications (17.8%), and use of inhalants (e.g., glue or other aerosols; 8.9%). Although overall heroin use has appeared to decrease slightly (2.2%), there are areas of the United States where heroin is readily available and current use would be higher. Heroin is particularly dangerous because it is purer than in the past and also frequently laced with fentanyl, a potent painkiller. The ready availability for sale and consumption of opioid prescription pain medications has led to a nationwide "opioid crisis," which has affected people of all ages but particularly older adolescents and young adults. Opioid overdose is becoming a leading cause of death for people in these age groups (USDHHS, 2016). Evidence suggests that use of prescription pain medications can lead to heroin use (USDHHS, 2016), and many adolescents become addicted through indiscriminate pain management of a musculoskeletal or other injury. Contributing factors to this epidemic include overprescribing, prescribing higher doses than are needed to control the pain, and lack of prescription monitoring, allowing patients to obtain prescriptions from multiple pharmacies (USDHHS, 2016).

Substance use is a precursor to abuse, which emphasizes the need for health care providers to be alert for and screen individuals for its presence. Identifying adolescent substance users or abusers requires a careful nursing assessment that is conducted in an accepting manner (Boxes 21-10 and 21-11) and referral for appropriate management. The AAP (2014) recommends individuals be screened for substance use at every well visit during adolescence using the CRAFFT mnemonic.

Substance use and abuse prevention and management requires a community as well as an individual approach. For adolescent problem drinkers, Alcoholics Anonymous has pamphlets and other resources, including meetings, for young people who are ready to begin recovery. In response to the opioid epidemic, communities have supplied school, police, and emergency personnel with naloxone (Narcan) to be used for treatment of overdoses. Many states are approving legislation directed toward limiting the duration of individual pain medications, instituting

---

### BOX 21-10  Major Signs of Substance Abuse

**Depending on the Substance Used, the Signs Can Include the Following:**

- Agitation
- Altered sleep
- Appetite loss
- Blackouts
- Depression
- Diarrhea
- Distorted perception
- Drowsiness/lethargy
- Dry mucous membranes
- Euphoria
- Hallucinations
- Inability to concentrate or solve problems
- Inability to perform regular work or social activities
- Memory loss
- Nausea
- Poor coordination
- Respiratory depression
- Unintentional injuries
- Weight loss
- Withdrawal

From Substance Abuse and Mental Health Services Administration. (2015). Substance use disorders. https://www.samhsa.gov/disorders/substance-use.

---

### BOX 21-11  CRAFFT: Adolescent Substance Abuse Screening Test

A brief screening test for adolescent substance abuse developed by the Center for Adolescent Substance Abuse Research at the Boston Children's Hospital uses the acronym CRAFFT to guide health care providers when they are interviewing adolescents about substance abuse:

**C**—Have you ever ridden in a CAR driven by someone, including yourself, who was "high" or had been using alcohol or drugs?

**R**—Do you ever use alcohol or drugs to RELAX, feel better about yourself, or fit in?

**A**—Do you ever use alcohol or drugs when you are by yourself, ALONE?

**F**—Do you ever FORGET things you did while using alcohol or drugs?

**F**—Does your family or do your FRIENDS ever tell you that you should cut down on your drinking or drug use?

**T**—Have you gotten into TROUBLE while you were using alcohol or drugs?

Two or more affirmative answers suggest a significant problem and warrant referral and follow-up.

Reprinted with permission from the Center for Adolescent Substance Abuse Research, Boston Children's Hospital ©2009.

---

prescription monitoring programs, and safe disposal of unused medication. Insurance companies are allowing patients to choose to receive fewer doses than prescribed and are increasing coverage for substance abuse treatment. Nurses need to be advocates for these and other approaches to this serious issue.

### Tobacco Use

Although 9.2% of adolescents report beginning smoking at a young age, 5.6% identify themselves as currently frequent smokers. Smoking is more prevalent in white males and females than in black or Hispanic populations (CDC, 2014b). Another form of tobacco use is use of smokeless tobacco, such as chewing tobacco, snuff, or dip. Recently, adolescents have begun using electronic cigarettes (e-cigarettes, vaping). Electronic cigarettes, which are battery operated, vaporize liquid for inhalation through an appliance that resembles a cigarette; there is no smoke involved (Johnson & Pennington, 2015). Flavored liquid in cartridges, either with or without nicotine, is attractive and available to adolescents. Because of the newness of this trend, there is little evidence to determine whether e-cigarette use will contribute to tobacco use. Several states, however, have enacted legislation to regulate the sale and distribution of e-cigarettes to children (Johnson & Pennington, 2015). Adolescents begin using tobacco for a variety of reasons, including wanting to appear older or wanting to imitate their friends, adult role models, or media images. Advertising by the tobacco industry directed at adolescents has been shown to encourage adolescent smoking.

The nurse's primary prevention focus is on keeping nonsmokers from starting smoking and helping smokers to stop. Nurses can become actively involved in smoking-prevention programs through school districts or in the community. The Agency for Healthcare Research and Quality (2012) has published *Five Major Steps to Intervention (the "5 A's")*, which can organize an approach to smokers who are considering quitting soon. These include:

- *Ask* about tobacco use.
- *Advise* to quit.
- *Assess* willingness to attempt quitting.
- *Assist* in quit attempt.
- *Arrange* for follow-up.

# DETERMINANTS OF HEALTH

## Social Factors and Environment

### School

Middle school or junior high and high school bring new social experiences, introducing the adolescent to changing classes, multiple teachers and teaching styles, variable class schedules, homework load, and a variety of peer influences. School populations may be significantly larger than the child has experienced previously, and making and solidifying new friendships may be more difficult. Yet, despite these challenges, these school settings also provide meaningful in-school and after-school learning, peer contact, intellectual stimulation, and social or volunteer community service activities (Figure 21-6).

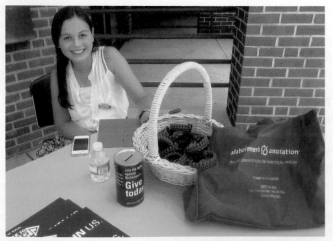

**FIGURE 21-6** Adolescents participate in school-sponsored community service.

Schools and peers, as opposed to home and parents, become the primary setting through which expectations are shared and standards communicated. During health-promotion visits, nurses ask adolescents about school and their friends and how they are doing with both. The nurse can also monitor adolescents as they prepare for and make the transition to their next social arena and role, whether it is college, vocational training, the military, or another career choice.

## Culture and Ethnicity

Cultural and ethnic influences operate throughout childhood and continue into adolescence. The primary difference in adolescence is that teens question, modify, or reject these influences, exchanging them for those of their peers or of the dominant cultural group. First-generation adolescents of immigrant parents have to negotiate two cultures, languages, and sets of expectations. These adolescents often live a double life that might result in increased stress. Adolescents from minority groups, such as black Americans, Hispanics, Asian Americans, Native Americans, Russian Americans, or Arab Americans, might experience discrimination and rejection if they try to fit in to the dominant adolescent culture, which is often middle class, white, and Protestant. Advertising is directed to middle-class or affluent teens, not the economically depressed, and media images might not include attractive ethnic-looking models. Adolescents from different cultures might experience additional stress when their attempts to fit in to the dominant culture are contrary to the values and beliefs of their own culture.

The growing ethnic diversity in the adolescent population influences how adolescent health will be approached. For example, the US Census Bureau reports that the Asian population increased by 43% between 2000 and 2010, growing faster than any other major race group during that period (Humes et al., 2011) (Box 21-12: Diversity Awareness). With fast growth in the numbers of Hispanic and Asian American youth, cultural awareness of health care needs and the highlighted attention to health disparities and academic outcomes, especially among adolescents from racial minorities and ethnic groups, are required. Nurses need to recognize the additional stresses experienced by adolescents and assess them for those stresses as they wrestle not only with their own identities but also with their cultural identities.

## Levels of Policy Making and Health

Many laws and regulations are aimed at adolescents and deal with the minimum age at which they can assume adult responsibilities and decision-making. The rationale for these restrictions is that adolescents, although capable, lack the experience, perspective, and judgment to recognize and avoid choices that might be detrimental to them, so they require protection. A question raised frequently when minimum age is considered is whether strict age criteria are appropriate for any adolescent, particularly because development is variable and experiences are diverse.

The restrictions that have recently been questioned most strongly deal with issues related to sexual activity. The US Supreme Court affirmed the right of all individuals to have equal access to contraceptive service, regardless of age or marital status.

## BOX 21-12 DIVERSITY AWARENESS

**Barriers to Recruiting Chinese American Adolescents for Future Development of HIV Interventional Programs: A Lesson Learned**

It has been suggested that there is an imperative need to deliver culturally sensitive programs for HIV/AIDS prevention. To oppose health disparities in the United States, recruiting participants with an ethnic minority background in health care research is essential. Chinese Americans comprise the largest ethnic group of Asian Americans and have rarely been separated from a combination of various Asian American populations to address issues related to HIV/AIDS prevention. Given that there are many distinct and separate cultures within the Asian American community, this misclassification makes Chinese Americans an underrepresented population in HIV/AIDS research and has resulted in limited public awareness and deprived this population of HIV/AIDS preventive services. It is important for nurses to know about the recruitment strategies or challenges specific to enrolling Chinese Americans so as to have capabilities to efficiently approach Chinese American adolescents and deliver culturally sensitive HIV/AIDS prevention programs.

The purpose of this article was to report identified barriers and challenges experienced in the process of recruiting Chinese American adolescents for a cross-sectional HIV/AIDS-related study. The sexual topic, a taboo in Chinese culture, was the major barrier to recruiting Chinese American adolescents. Barriers to recruitment were also found related to unawareness and denial of HIV/AIDS risks, authoritarian parenting style in Chinese culture, and the required informed consents. The most successful recruitment strategy was found to be associated with the assistance of Chinese American adolescent participants. Providing educational programs targeting Chinese American parents and community leaders to enhance their awareness of the risks and to improve parent-child communication regarding sex-related issues was suggested as the first step to successfully approach and recruit Chinese American adolescents for an HIV/AIDS-related prevention program or research.

From Lee, Y. H., Salman, A., & Wang, F. (2012). Recruiting Chinese-American adolescents to HIV/AIDS related research: A lesson learned from a cross-sectional study. *Applied Nursing Research, 24*(1):40–46.

However, variations occur from state to state, and the nurse must be aware of legal age determinants, as well as variations in definitions of emancipated minors.

The emancipated minor provision of certain laws recognizes that some adolescents become independent from their families at an early age and assume adult responsibilities. An emancipated minor is an adolescent who has not reached the standard legal age for certain activities, such as consenting to marriage or seeking certain kinds of health or illness care, but who is permitted to accept full responsibility for these decisions because the individual is economically and emotionally separate from the family.

Most often confidentiality is the more important issue for adolescents. The nurse can assure them that information shared will be kept confidential unless the teens pose a risk to themselves or others, or state or public health reporting mandates that the information be shared. For example, abuse must be reported, STIs need to be reported, and some states require adolescent sexual activity to be reported if an age difference of 3 years or more exists between the sexual partners.

Nurses need to familiarize themselves with the legal rights of adolescents in their state and the resources available in their community.

## Economics

Identification with peers, the essence of self-image during adolescence, includes dressing alike, having similar possessions, and doing similar activities, all of which require economic resources. This can cause a major conflict between parents and adolescents. Parents may think that they should have the power to decide how their adolescent spends money. Adolescents may believe, just as strongly, that they know the best ways to allocate resources and determine the amount of money they need.

Ideally, parents and adolescents should negotiate economic questions, with the parents becoming less controlling as the teen gains more experience and expertise in these matters. However, the family with limited economic resources has fewer choices, and adolescents from these families may feel trapped by their circumstance. Poverty is particularly hard on children, and as they become adolescents, they often develop a fatalistic view of life.

Some adolescents seek employment to earn their own money and have control over it. Others work because their families need the income. It is important for the nurse to assess the economic resources of each adolescent's family and work within them when partnering with the adolescent in health care planning.

## Health Services/Delivery System

Many health care resources are available to the adolescent. Teens can continue to see their child health care providers in a pediatric center as they did as younger children, but this setting is usually rejected because of the young-child atmosphere.

School-based clinics are frequently available in junior high and high school, and adolescent-focused clinics are available in many communities through both public and private agencies. Each of these clinics serves only adolescents, and the staff is oriented to the needs of this age group. Adolescents frequently have a stronger sense of comfort in these settings than in those in which young children or adults are also served.

Adolescents can also make use of services such as family planning clinics. These settings may designate certain days and hours for teens, whereas other facilities integrate them into the adult-oriented protocols. The pregnant adolescent typically finds prenatal care in an adult-focused setting, although more adolescent-specific programs are being developed. The physical needs of pregnant adolescents may be the same as those of the pregnant adult, but the psychosocial needs are different and should be approached by a professional who has comprehensive knowledge of their development and responses to stress.

The adolescent is a rapidly changing individual. The nurse who works in an adolescent-focused practice is well prepared in adolescent health-promotion strategies. The nurse should have a thorough understanding of adolescent physical and psychosocial growth and development and recognize each teen as a person.

Adolescents not only tend to be fearful about procedures or possible diagnoses but also need to stay in control of the situation. These conflicting feelings can be difficult to manage

(Box 21-13)

---

**BOX 21-13 HEADSSS Assessment**

The HEADSSS assessment provides a mnemonic that guides health care providers through an adolescent's psychosocial assessment. Responses should be interpreted as those that are indicators of strengths or protection from risk and those that are indicators of risky behavior or situations.

**H**ome
**E**ducation, employment, eating
**A**ctivities
**D**rugs
**S**exuality
**S**uicide or depression
**S**afety

From Klein, D., Goldenring, J., & Adelman, W. (2014). HEADSSS 3.0: The psychosocial interview for adolescents updated for a new century fueled by media. http://contemporarypediatrics.modernmedicine.com/contemporary-pediatrics/content/tags/adolescent-medicine/heeadsss-30-psychosocial-interview-adolesce?page=full.

---

simultaneously. By establishing the adolescent as a partner with the health care providers in promoting good health and screening the adolescent for health risks, the nurse facilitates the adolescent's sense of control (Box 21-13).

The adolescent's questions should be answered thoroughly and honestly. In many instances the adolescent is hesitant to voice concerns, so information is offered even when questions are not asked. An effective indirect approach to learning about adolescent concerns, especially about potentially embarrassing or stressful topics, is to say "Many teenagers ask me about [a topic]. Have you ever thought about this?" or "A lot of young people want to know about [a topic]."

Direct questions are also important, even about sensitive topics: "Have you ever thought about suicide?" "Are you depressed?" "Are you sexually active?" "Do you use birth control and/or protection?" However, asking first about friends and the adolescent's feelings about them may be a good lead-in approach: "Are any of your friends doing drugs?" "How do you feel about it?" Vague or circuitous questions may be interpreted as a sign of discomfort or lack of understanding and may cause the adolescent to be equally vague when responding.

Correct anatomical terms and descriptions of laboratory tests, disease processes, and possible outcomes are essential components in treating adolescents as individuals who are capable of being responsible for their own bodies.

# NURSING APPLICATION

Adolescence is a period of rapid growth and development with changes occurring physically and psychosocially. Nurses play a pivotal role in influencing health-promotion, preventive-screening, and disease-prevention activities. The primary responsibility for the nurse dealing with the important period known as the transition from childhood to adulthood is to provide education about some of the expected changes and how to deal with them.

Primary prevention methods are effective when the nurse is able to partner with the adolescent in recognizing his or her health needs. Treating the teen in a respectful manner enables the teen to assume more responsibility. Nurses must remain sensitive to the changes the adolescent is encountering and understand the need for guided independence.

Some important health-education topics for the adolescent population include proper nutrition, exercise, teen pregnancy (National Campaign, 2015), and protection against STIs (CDC, 2014a). Teens are taught about the significance of their lifestyle choices with regard to future health. Drug and alcohol use, injury prevention, violence, and tobacco use are all behaviors that are known to contribute to illness and death among teens. Nurses use educational tools that appeal to the age group by conducting Internet searches for resources. Teens are able to relate to Internet resources, celebrities, and social media sites. Peers have the greatest influence on teenagers.

Nurses need to educate teens in partnership with their parents about the fact that unintentional injuries are the leading cause of death in the adolescent population. Nurses should reinforce research regarding distracted driving, seat belt use, and texting, adjusting the radio, and listening to loud music while driving.

Adolescent girls are educated about breast self-examinations, cervical cancer, and human papilloma virus. Adolescent males are educated about testicular self-examination. Both sexes are encouraged to undergo physical examinations and follow the recommended vaccination schedule.

Various screenings are used by the nurse as a secondary prevention measure for the adolescent. Scoliosis screening is conducted in prepubertal and pubertal adolescents because early identification and treatment is important to prevent long-term disability or disfigurement. Nurses also screen adolescents for hypertension, eating disorders, type 2 diabetes, pregnancy, and STIs.

Adolescents respond better when they feel that they are regarded as young adults and a partner in their health-promotion efforts. The nurse needs to become skilled at discussing difficult or embarrassing topics with teenagers. It is essential that adolescents feel that they are treated with respect and regarded as an individual.

---

**CASE STUDY**

### *Drug-Facilitated Sexual Assault: Jessica*

Sexual assault includes any type of sexual activity to which an individual does not agree. Because of the effects of some drugs, commonly called date rape drugs, victims may be physically helpless, unable to refuse, or even unable to remember what happened.

Jessica, a 16-year-old high school sophomore, expresses concern to the school nurse that she knows someone who might have had sex "without knowing it." How can the nurse answer these common questions?

**Reflective Questions**
- What are date rape drugs and how can a person be unaware that such a drug has been ingested?
- What can you do to protect yourself?
- What do you do if you think you have been sexually assaulted?
- What can you do when someone you care about has been sexually assaulted?

## CARE PLAN

### Drug-Facilitated Sexual Assault: Jessica

**\*NURSING DIAGNOSIS: Risk of powerlessness related to suspected rape/rape trauma syndrome**

**Definition**

At risk of perceived lack of control over a situation and/or one's ability to significantly affect an outcome

**Risk Factors**

- Suspected date rape/rape trauma syndrome
- Acute injury (rape)
- Deficient knowledge
- Disturbed body image
- Situational low self-esteem

**Expected Outcomes**

- Acknowledges personal strength
- Perceived control

- Perceived resources
- Participation in health care decisions
- Increase healthy lifestyle choices
    *Goal:* Increase individual's sense of power over potential/actual situation for self/others.

**Interventions**

- Active listening
- Risk identification
- Health care information exchange
- Support system enhancement
- Rape trauma treatment and referral
- Decision-making support
- Health education

\*NANDA Nursing Diagnoses—Herdman T.H. & Kamitsuru, S. (Eds.). Nursing Diagnoses–Definitions and Classification 2015–2017. Copyright © 2014, 1994–2014 NANDA International. Used by arrangement with John Wiley & Sons Limited. In order to make safe and effective judgments using the NANDA-I nursing diagnoses it is essential that nurses refer to the definitions and defining characteristics of the diagnoses listed in this work.

## SUMMARY

Adolescence is a period of rapid change, when the integration of family, peer, educational, social, cultural, and community experiences begins to take form in the teen's sense of self. Many view adolescence as a construction site in its early stages. Onlookers assume that eventually a recognizable structure will emerge but have no idea what that structure will be. Although many parents, teachers, and health care providers feel that hard hats and steel-reinforced shoes are needed, each is better equipped with an understanding of and respect for the adolescent's developmental struggles with physical and cognitive changes, autonomy, body image, peer relations, and identity. The goal, after all, is for the teen to emerge in young adulthood with a healthy body, mind, and spirit.

## EVOLVE CHAPTER FEATURES

http://evolve.elsevier.com/Edelman/
- Study Questions

## REFERENCES

Advisory Committee on Immunization Practices (ACIP). (2016). Recommended immunization schedules for persons aged 0 through 18 years. http://www.cdc.gov.

Agency for Healthcare Research and Quality. (2012). Five major steps to intervention (the "5 A's"). http://www.ahrq.gov/professionals/clinicians-providers/guidelines-recommendations/tobacco/5steps.html.

American Academy of Dermatology (AAD). (2015). Caring for pierced ears. http://www.aad.org.

American Academy of Dermatology (AAD). (2016). Caring for tattooed skin: Tips from dermatologists. http://www.aad.org.

American Academy of Pediatrics (AAP). (2013a). Ethical and policy issues in genetic testing and screening of children. *Pediatrics, 131,* 620–622.

American Academy of Pediatrics (AAP). (2013b). Policy statement: Children, adolescents and the media. *Pediatrics, 132*(5), 958–961.

American Academy of Pediatrics. (2014). 2014 recommendations for pediatric preventive health care. *Pediatrics, 133,* 568–570.

American Academy of Pediatrics (AAP). (2015a). Delayed puberty in boys. http://www.healthychildren.org.

American Academy of Pediatrics (AAP). (2015b). Delayed puberty in girls. http://www.healthychildren.org.

American Academy of Pediatrics (AAP). (2015c). Independence, one step at a time. http://www.aap.org.

American Academy of Pediatrics (AAP). (2015d). Teenagers and gangs. http://www.healthychildren.org.

American College of Obstetricians and Gynecologists. (2012). Well-woman visit. http://www.acog.org/Resources-And-Publications/Committee-Opinions/Committee-on-Gynecologic-Practice/Well-Woman-Visit.

Arbogast, K., et al. (2013). Cognitive rest and school-based recommendations following pediatric concussion: The need for primary care support tools. *Clinical Pediatrics, 52*(5), 397–402.

Bhate, K., & Williams, H. (2013). Epidemiology of acne vulgaris. *British Journal of Dermatology, 168,* 474–485.

Biro, F., et al. (2013). Onset of breast development in a longitudinal cohort. *Pediatrics, 132*(6), 1019–1027.

Botkin, J., et al. (2015). Points to consider: Ethical, legal, and psychosocial implications of genetic testing in children and adolescents. *American Journal of Human Genetics, 97*(3), 501.

Carter, J. M., & Wilson, F. L. (2015). Cyberbullying: A 21st century health care phenomenon. *Pediatric Nursing, 41*(3), 115–125.

Centers for Disease Control and Prevention (CDC). (2012). Monitoring your teen's activities: What parents and families should know. http://www.cdc.gov.

Centers for Disease Control and Prevention (CDC). (2014a). STDs in adolescents and young adults. http://www.cdc.gov.

Centers for Disease Control and Prevention (CDC). (2014b). Youth risk behavior surveillance – United States 2013. *Morbidity and Mortality Weekly Reports, 63*(4), 1–168.

Centers for Disease Control and Prevention (CDC). (2015a). Adolescent and school health: Protective factors. http://www.cdc.gov/healthyyouth.

Centers for Disease Control and Prevention (CDC). (2015b). HIV surveillance – adolescents and young adults. http://www.cdc.gov/hpv.

Centers for Disease Control and Prevention (CDC). (2015c). Why does my child need HPV vaccine? http://www.cdc.gov.

Center for Young Women's Health, Boston Children's Hospital. (2015). Human papillomavirus. http://www.youngwomenshealth.org.

Copstead, L., & Banasik, J. (2013). *Pathophysiology* (5th ed.). St. Louis: Saunders.

Erikson, E. (1968). *Identity: Youth and crisis*. New York: Norton.

Forum on Child and Family Statistics. (2015). Adolescent depression. America's children: Key national indicators of well-being. http://www.childstats.gov.

Fried, L., et al. (2012). Differences in risk factors for suicide attempts among 9th and 11th grade youth: A longitudinal perspective. *Journal of School Nursing, 29*(2), 113–122.

Gailbraith, S. (2016). Acne vulgaris. In R. Kliegman, et al. (Eds.), *Nelson textbook of pediatrics* (20th ed., pp. 3228–3235). St. Louis: Elsevier.

George, N., & Davis, J. (2013). Assessing sleep in adolescents through a better understanding of sleep physiology. *American Journal of Nursing, 113*(6), 26–31.

Gilligan, C., Lyons, N., & Hanmer, T. (1990). *Making connections: The relational worlds of adolescent girls at Emma Willard School*. Cambridge, MA: Harvard University Press.

Grossman, J., et al. (2014). Protective effects of middle school comprehensive sex education with family involvement. *Journal of School Health, 84*(11), 739–747.

Guyton, A. C., & Hall, J. E. (2011). *Textbook of medical physiology* (12th ed.). Philadelphia: W.B. Saunders.

Hargreaves, D., et al. (2015). Unmet health care needs in the United States. *Pediatrics, 136*(93), 513–520.

Honeyman, C. (2014). Raising awareness of scoliosis among children's nurses. *Nursing of Children and Young People, 26*(5), 30–37.

Humes, K. R., Jones, N. A., & Ramirez, R. R. (2011). Overview of race and Hispanic origin: 2010. *2010 Census Briefs*. http://www.census.gov/prod/cen2010/briefs/c2010br-02.pdf.

Jennings, R. (2015). Too much? Too soon? Or too little? Too late? The case for sex and relationship education in primary schools. *Education and Health, 33*(4), 107–109.

Johnson, M., & Pennington, N. (2015). Adolescent use of electronic cigarettes: An emergent health concern for pediatric patients. *Journal of Pediatric Nursing, 30*, 611–615.

Jonovich, S., & Alpert-Gillis, L. (2014). Impact of pediatric mental health screening on clinical discussion and referral for services. *Clinical Pediatrics, 53*(4), 364–371.

Kaplowitz, P., & Bloch, C. (2016). Evaluation and referral of children with signs of early puberty. *Pediatrics, 137*(1), 1–6.

Kerr, Z., et al. (2013). Prevention and management of physical, social and environmental risk factors for sports-related injuries. *American Journal of Lifestyle Medicine, 96*, 138–153.

Kohlberg, L. (1981). *The philosophy of moral development*. San Francisco, CA: Harper & Row.

Korda, H., & Itani, Z. (2013). Harnessing social media for health promotion and behavior change. *Health Promotion Practice, 14*(1), 15–23.

Kreipe, R. (2016). Eating disorders. In R. Kliegman, et al. (Eds.), *Nelson textbook of pediatrics* (20th ed., Chapter 28). St. Louis: Elsevier.

Lenzi, M., et al. (2015). Adolescent gang involvement: The role of individual, family, peer and school factors in a multilevel perspective. *Aggressive Behavior, 41*(4), 386–397.

Lim, F., Brown, D., & Jones, H. (2013). Lesbian, gay, bisexual and transgender health: Fundamentals for nursing education. *Journal of Nursing Education, 524*, 198–203.

Lim, F., Brown, D., & Kim, S. (2014). Addressing health care disparities in the lesbian, gay, bisexual and transgender population: A review of best practices. *American Journal of Nursing, 114*(6), 24–34.

Manworren, R. (2013). Child with a musculoskeletal alteration. In E. McKinney, et al. (Eds.), *Maternal child nursing* (4th ed., pp. 1353–1356). St. Louis, MO: Saunders.

Martin, S., & Golden, N. (2014). Eating disorders in children, adolescents, and young adults. *Contemporary Pediatrics*, http://contemporarypediatrics.modernmedicine.com.

Melde, C., & Eskensen, F. (2014). The relative impact of gang status transitions: Identifying the mechanisms of change in delinquency. *Journal of Research in Crime and Delinquency, 51*(3), 349–376.

National Center for Health Statistics. (2014). Leading causes of death and number of deaths by age: United States 1980 and 2013. Health United States, 2014. (Table 21). http://www.cdc.gov/nchs.

National Center for Injury Prevention and Control. (2013). Injury mortality. WISQUARS. http://webappa.cdc.gov.

National Institute of Mental Health. (2011). Depression. http://www.nimh.nih.gov.

Ng, A., & Kaye, K. (2012). *Why it matters: Teen childbearing: Education and economic well-being*. Washington, DC: The National Campaign.

Obadina, S. (2014). An overview of anorexia nervosa, bulimia, and binge eating disorder. *British Journal of School Nursing, 9*(9), 441–446.

Pasold, T., McKracken, A., & Ward-Begnoche, W. (2014). Binge eating in adolescents: Emotional and behavioral characteristics and impact on health-related quality of life. *Clinical Child Psychology and Psychiatry, 19*(2), 299–312.

Pender, N. J., Murdaugh, C., & Parsons, M. A. (2010). *Health promotion in nursing practice* (6th ed.). Upper Saddle River, NJ: Prentice-Hall.

Piaget, J. (1969). *The theory of stages in cognitive development*. New York, NY: McGraw-Hill.

Rivera, R., et al. (2015). Concussion evaluation and management in pediatrics. *MCN. The American Journal of Maternal Child Nursing, 40*(2), 76–78.

Reducing the impact of bullying: Useful resources and guidance. (2015). *British Journal of School Nursing, 10*(5), 248–249.

Rohrbach, L., et al. (2015). A rights-based sexuality education program for adolescents: 1-year outcomes from a cluster randomized trial. *Journal of Adolescent Health, 57*(4), 398–405.

Scoliosis Research Society, American Academy of Orthopedic Surgeons, Pediatric Orthopedic Society of America, & American Academy of Pediatrics (AAP). (2015). Position statement – screening for the early detection for idiopathic scoliosis in adolescents. http://www.srs.org.

Segrin, C., et al. (2015). Overparenting is associated with child problems and a critical family environment. *Journal of Child and Family Studies, 24,* 470–479.

Slater, A., & Tiggermann, M. (2015). Media exposure, extracurricular activities and appearance-related comments as predictors of female adolescents' self-objectification. *Psychology of Women Quarterly, 29*(3), 375–389.

Swanson, S., et al. (2011). Prevalence and correlates of eating disorders in adolescents. *JAMA Psychiatry, 68*(7), 714–723.

The National Campaign. (2015). Why it matters: Teen pregnancy and overall child well-being. https://thenationalcampaign.org.

US Department of Health and Human Services (USDHHS). (2016). The U.S. opioid epidemic. http://www.hhs.gov.

US Department of Health and Human Services (USDHHS), & US Department of Agriculture (USDA). (2015). Dietary guidelines for Americans 2015–2020 (8th ed.). http://health.gov/dietaryguidelines/.

US Department of Health and Human Services (USDHHS), Office of Disease Prevention and Health Promotion. (2015). *Healthy People 2020.* Washington, DC: US Department of Health and Human Services, Office of Disease Prevention and Health Promotion.

US Preventive Services Task Force. (2015). Final update summary: Idiopathic scoliosis in adolescents: Screening. http://www.uspreventivetaskforce.org.

Ventura, S., Hamilton, B., & Matthews, T. (2014). National and state patterns of teen births in the United States—1940–2013. *National Vital Statistics Reports, 63*(4), 1–33.

Well, D. (2013). Acne vulgaris: A review of causes and treatment options. *The Nurse Practitioner, 38*(10), 22–31.

Weitzman, C., & Wegner, L. (2015). Promoting optimal development: Screening for behavioral and emotional problems. http://www.aap.org.

You, S. (2014). Impact of violent video games on the social behaviors of adolescents: The mediating role of emotional competence. *School Psychology International, 36*(1), 94–111.

Zaenglein, A. L., et al. (2016). Guidelines of care for the management of acne vulgaris. *Journal of American Academy of Dermatologists, 74*(5), 945–973.

# 22

# Young Adult

*Elizabeth Connelly Kudzma*

## OBJECTIVES

*After completing this chapter, the reader will be able to:*

- Analyze specific health recommendations for the young adult.
- Identify attitudes, behaviors, and habits that compose the lifestyles of young adults.
- Define tasks that are consistent with adult development.
- Describe the nurse's role in reducing the rate of unintentional pregnancies in young adult women.
- Determine occupational hazards that interfere with the young adult's welfare.

- Evaluate strategies that the nurse can use to reduce the risks associated with young adult behaviors.
- Analyze occupational, cultural, and ethnic risk factors that may affect young adults.
- Delineate nursing roles in preventive intervention for healthy young adults in home and community environments.
- Discuss proposed suggestions for preconceptional care.

## KEY TERMS

Achievement-oriented stress
Aerobic exercise
Basal metabolic rate
Binge drinking
Breast self-examination
Congenital defects
Coronary artery disease
Fetal neural tube defects
Genetic impairments

Hepatitis B
Human immunodeficiency virus
Human papilloma virus
Hypertension
Infertility
Intimacy versus isolation
Maternal mortality rate
Metabolic syndrome
Orchitis

Papanicolaou (Pap) smear
Postconventional level of moral reasoning
Sexual consent
Stress
Sun protection factor
Testicular self-examination

### ⚲ THINK ABOUT IT

#### Using Private Information in Shared Living Arrangements

*Young adults in communal living arrangements (college dormitories, the military) are often placed with other individuals who have different cultural, language, or other values. The use of cell phones and computers with video and audio recording capabilities has opened the possibility that private behavior may be recorded without consent and then may be shared through a form of social networking (Facebook, Twitter, instant messaging, apps, and other shared computer sites). There are even instances where recording has occurred in classrooms without the permission of the instructor or others in the class. These situations are expected to become more prevalent.*

- *What are the implications of this for violation of privacy for individuals and even groups (e.g., military, fraternities, sororities)?*
- *What are the legal implications? Some states have laws against unauthorized recording.*
- *How might unauthorized recording alter classroom, dormitory, and communal living dynamics?*

The young adult period encompasses the ages from 18 to 35 years, a time that spans the end of adolescence to the beginning of middle adulthood. Formal education beyond high school to college and graduate school, as well as military experience, and the major milestones of marriage and beginning a family may be included in this phase of development. The major task accomplished in this period is preparing for and assuming full adult responsibilities, rights, and privileges. This is a potentially difficult period as young adults are not totally independent and are learning to separate from the home and their parents (Neinstein, 2013).

## BIOLOGY AND GENOMICS

The young adult period is a time of many physical and emotional changes and is an opportunity for learning by experience and experimentation (Box 22-1: Quality and Safety Scenario). Young adulthood is characterized by greater complexity of thinking,

### ✅ BOX 22-1    QUALITY/SAFETY SCENARIO

#### Topic: Examining Problematic College Drinking Behaviors in Young Adults

A study of 211 college students indicates that 63% of female and 83% of male college-aged students (mean age 20.7 years) engaged in binge drinking. Associated with these intermittent excessive drinking "binges" were various disordered and unhealthy weight-reducing behaviors (skipping meals, fasting, using diet pills, and self-induced vomiting) (Kelly-Weeder, 2011).

You are the clinic director and nurse at a small liberal arts college. Mary, a 19-year-old first-year student, has generally been a good student, easily making the adjustment to living away from home during her first 2 months in the dormitory. She comes to you to talk about an episode that occurred the previous weekend and that frightened her. On Saturday night, she was at a party at a private residence in a rural, wooded setting away from the campus. She remembers consuming five or six alcoholic drinks; however, any memory after midnight is missing. She woke up in a fellow female student's dormitory room without any memory of leaving the party or returning to the dormitory. She was able to piece together information from her friends, who told her that she had consumed at least nine alcoholic drinks that night and that she had left the party with others who were returning to the dormitory, but they were not the friends with whom she had been seen all evening. She is concerned that she may have been drugged or that she may be having memory lapses. Assessment of her previous alcohol use reveals that she can recount at least four occasions during which she drank more than seven drinks at a party or family gathering. She describes her family as "social drinkers." On days that she anticipates drinking, she restricts her caloric intake. Last June, she was involved in a minor car accident that might have been related to her consumption of at least three drinks that afternoon. The road to this rural college has two road side shrines dedicated to students who have died in automobile crashes near the college. To further analyze Mary's situation, you formulate the following questions:

- Do you think that Mary has a problem with drinking? Would you classify her as a binge drinker? How do you clarify what she values?
- Is Mary engaging in risky behavior especially if she drives while drinking?
- What kind of physical assessment might assist you in making a determination that Mary has a drinking problem?
- What kinds of preventive educational programs could you advise?
- What kinds of monitoring and follow-up mechanisms might assist Mary in keeping her safe and in a treatment plan?

From Kelly-Weeder, S. (2011). Binge drinking and disordered eating in college students. *Journal of the American Academy of Nurse Practitioners, 23*(1), 33–41; Quality and Safety Education for Nurses Institute. (2012). http://www.qsen.org; Institute of Medicine. (2003). Health professions education: A bridge to quality. http://www.nationalacademies.org/hmd/Reports/2003/Health-Professions-Education-A-Bridge-to-Quality.aspx

---

further organization of emotional and cognitive development, and decision-making based on the impact on others and future consequences. All phases of young adult development garner considerable interest. Judging by the increase in the number of books on self-development, more young adults are exploring topics in holistic healing and spiritual health and development. Health behaviors, safety practices, diet, exercise, weight control, sexuality, and addictions are widely discussed topics. Preventive health concerns for young adults can be separated into two categories: developing behaviors that promote a healthy lifestyle and decreasing the incidence of accidents, injuries, and acts of violence. In *Healthy People 2020*, it is stated that 72% of all deaths among children and young adults are due to injuries from four causes: motor vehicle crashes (30%), all other unintentional injuries (15%), homicide (15%), and suicide (12%) (US Department of Health and Human Services [USDHHS], 2015).

In 2014, approximately 20.5% of the American population was composed of adults aged 20 to 34 (US Census Bureau, 2014). The young adult population aged 18 to 24 years is projected to be approximately 9.13% of the general population by 2020 and 8.34% by 2035. The percentage of young adults aged 20 to 24 years is expected to decline to 8% in 2060 (US Census Bureau, 2014). A decline in this age group is influenced by birth rates, and the Centers for Disease Control and Prevention (CDC, 2015a) reported that the birth rate per 1000 women of all ages in 2013 was 12.4; this rate has been dropping since 1990, when it was more than 16.7 live births per 1000. Therefore the US Census Bureau projects the young adult population will grow more slowly in future decades as fertility rates decline, and the projections illustrate modest declines in immigration. Health-promotion efforts are particularly important for young adults because health

teaching for this age group has the significant potential to directly influence subsequent generations (Box 22-2: Healthy People 2020).

Young adulthood is generally the healthiest time of life. Physical growth is mostly complete by the age of 20 years; most concerns related to physiological development are focused on ensuring optimal functioning of body systems. The young adult's physical abilities are in peak condition, and compensatory mechanisms operate optimally during illness to provide minimal disruption in health patterns. Nursing goals for individuals of this age group are oriented toward prolonging this period of optimal physical energy; developing the mental, emotional, spiritual, and social potential; encouraging proper health habits; anticipating and screening individuals for the onset of chronic disease and therefore being able to treat it at an early stage; and treating disease when appropriate.

Full adult stature in men is reached at approximately age 21 years; in women, full growth occurs earlier, typically by age 17 years. Optimal muscle strength occurs from age 25 years to age 30 years, and then gradually declines by approximately 10% from age 30 years to age 60 years. Manual dexterity peaks in young adulthood and begins to decline in the mid-30s.

Women have greater longevity than men. Women are considered biologically stronger than men, outlive men, and naturally outnumber men. On average, in the United States women live 5 years longer than men (CDC, 2013a). This statistic may be a result in part of female genetic composition or men's greater exposure to environmental and occupational hazards. Men also seek health care services less frequently than women. Women generally seek preventive care more often than men. Although some of this reflects the inclusion of multiple prenatal visits, it also supports better health practices.

**BOX 22-2** **HEALTHY PEOPLE 2020**

### Selected National Health-Promotion and Disease-Prevention Objectives for the Young Adult

- Increase the proportion of adults who engage in regular aerobic activity of moderate intensity. (In 2013, 49.9% of adults performed the recommended amount of physical activity [150 minutes per week], and the target is 47.9%.)
- Increase the proportion of adults who are at a healthy weight. (From 2009 through 2012, 29.5% of adults aged 20 years or older were at a healthy weight, and the target is 33.9%.)
- Reduce the proportion of adults who are obese. (From 2009 through 2012, 35.3% of adults aged 20 years or older were considered obese, and the target is 30.5%.)
- Reduce the proportion of adults using any illicit drug during the preceding 30 days. (Illicit drug use in adults aged 18 years or older in 2013 was 9.4%, and the target is 7.1%.)
- Reduce the proportion of college students engaging in binge drinking of alcoholic beverages during the past 2 weeks. (In 2012, 37.1% of college students reported binge drinking in the past 2 weeks, and the target is 36.0%.)
- Increase the proportion of females at risk of unintended pregnancy or their partners who used contraception in the most recent sexual intercourse. (From 2011 through 2013, 83% of sexually active females or their partners used contraception, and the target is 91.6%.)
- Increase the proportion of adults aged 18 years or older with major depressive episodes who receive treatment. (In 2013, 68.6% of adults with diagnosed depression received treatment, and the target is 75.9%.)
- Reduce deaths caused by motor vehicle crashes. (In 2012, 10.9 deaths per 100,000 population occurred, and the target is 12.4.)
- Increase the number of states that have adopted a graduated driver licensing model law. (In 2009, 32 states had adopted graduate driver licensing, and the

target is 51 states, including the District of Columbia. There is difficulty in measuring the various components of state laws for graduated licensing.)
- Increase the proportion of motorcycle operators and passengers using helmets. (In 2013, the baseline was 60%, and the target is 73.7%.)
- Reduce sports and recreation injuries. (In 2013, there were 45.6 medically consulted injuries per 1000 population, and the target is 41.9 injuries per 1000 population.)
- Reduce firearm-related deaths. (In 2012, there were 10.5 firearm-related deaths per 100,000 population, and the target is 9.3 per 100,000 population.)
- Increase the proportion of persons with a usual primary care provider. (In 2011, 77% of all individuals had a usual source of health care, and the target is 83.9%, a 10% increase.)
- Increase the proportion of women who receive early and adequate prenatal care. (In 2007, 70.5% received early and adequate prenatal care, and the target is 77.6%.)
- Increase the proportion of adults aged 20 years or older who are aware of the signs of heart attack and the importance of accessing rapid emergency care. (In 2008, 37% of adults were aware of the signs of heart attack and the need for and access to emergency care; the target is 40.9%.)
- Increase the proportion of adults aged 18 years or older who have had their cholesterol level measured in the last 5 years. (In 2008, 74.6% of adults aged 18 years or older had their blood cholesterol level checked, and the target is 82%.)
- Increase the proportion of adults aged 18 years or older who follow protective measures that may reduce the risk of skin cancer. (In 2010, 70% of this population used protective measures, and the target is 73.7%.)

From US Department of Health and Human Services. (2015). *Healthy People 2020*. Washington, DC: US Government Printing Office.

A classic public health indicator of a nation's health resources and services that involves young adults is the **maternal mortality rate**. In 1980 the rate was 9.2 per 100,000 live births, then dropped to 6.6 per 100,000 live births in 1987 and rose to 8.9 per 100,000 live births in 2002. In 2007 the maternal mortality rate was much higher, 12.7 per 100,000 live births (USDHHS, 2015), reflecting inclusion of pregnancy status as a separate item on death certificates in some states. *Healthy People 2020* (USDHHS, 2015) sets a target goal of 11.4 maternal deaths per 100,000 live births, but to reach this goal there is a need for much more national and statewide action to identify gaps in health disparities, early prevention, treatment, and research.

## GORDON'S FUNCTIONAL HEALTH PATTERNS

### Health Perception–Health Management Pattern

Because excellent physical health is frequently taken for granted, concern about health and well-being is relatively low in individuals in their 20s but begins to increase in individuals in their 30s. Monitoring of specific health parameters is both necessary and appropriate to determine health needs and incipient problems. After the mid-30s, an increased sense of the finiteness of life develops with limitations imposed by work choices, well-being, monetary resources, and the deterioration of physical abilities. Specific health care management in the young adult age span is

generally split into health care management for various age groups according to the preventive services that are required.

The assumption that all adults should have an annual physical examination has been supplanted by increased scientifically based information about health screening measures. Screening services provided in a health-monitoring program need to meet effectiveness criteria. Evidence-based practice uses best practices' information for clinical decisions instead of intuition and unmethodical past clinical experience and, as such, forms a basis for the current recommended standard of care. Evidence-based approaches will ultimately determine which screening measures are best supported by scientific data (randomized controlled treatment studies), reduce regional variations in the use of diagnostic and therapeutic modalities, and close the gap between practice and research (Melnyk & Fineout-Overholt, 2014).

### Behavioral Health History

A health history inclusive of behavior is particularly important for young adults. This type of history focuses on risk factors for unintentional injuries, such as accidents, seat belt use, and alcohol consumption, which are major causes of death and disability in this age group. The safety focus of nursing health promotion for the younger adult takes different forms, from the simple—monitoring helmet and seat belt use—to more complex concerns—threats such as bioterrorism and globally spreading infections (USDHHS, 2015). Figure 22-1 lists questions and

**Well Young Adult Behavioral Health History Content**

**Sociodemographic content and questions:**

What organizations (community, church, lodge, social, professional, etc.) are you involved in?_____

_____

How would you describe your community?_____

_____

Hobbies, skills, interests, and recreational activities?_____

Military service? No_____ Yes_____ From _____ to_____

Overseas assignment? No_____ Yes_____

Close friends or immediate family members who have died within the past two years?_____

_____

Names and addresses of relatives or close friends in the area._____

_____

_____

Marital status: S M D W Length of time _____

**Environmental content and questions:**

Do you live alone? No_____ Yes_____

When did you last move?_____

Describe your living situation. _____

Number of years of education completed: _____

Elementary?_____ High school?_____ College?_____

Occupation?_____ Employer?_____

How long have you worked for this employer?_____

Are you satisfied with your work situation? No_____ Yes_____

Do you consider your work risky or dangerous? No_____ Yes_____

Is your work stressful? No_____ Yes_____

Over the past two weeks, have you felt depressed or hopeless? No_____ Yes_____

**Biophysical content questions:**

Have you smoked cigarettes? No_____ Yes_____

How much? Less than ½ pack per day? About one pack per day? More than 1½ packs per day?

Are you smoking now? No_____ Yes_____ Length of time smoking?_____

Have you ever smoked cigars or a pipe? No_____ Yes_____

If yes, how long?_____ Do you smoke cigars or a pipe now? No_____ Yes_____

Do you drink alcohol (wine, beer, or whiskey)? No_____ Yes_____

If you do, how much each day on the average?_____ Each week?_____

Do you consume large amounts occasionally (binge drinking)? No_____ Yes_____

Have you been drunk on work days? No_____ Yes_____

Have you had alcoholic drinks in the morning sometime in the past year? No_____ Yes_____

How much coffee, tea, or cola do you drink?_____

Do you use seat or lap belts? No_____ Yes_____

What type of exercise do you do each week? Describe type and amount. _____

_____

Are you satisfied with your weight? No_____ Yes_____ Body image? No_____ Yes_____

Do you use a bicycle or motorcycle helmet? No_____ Yes_____ Helmet and pads while rollerblading? No_____ Yes_____

How much sleep do you usually get each night?_____

Meals: Do you generally eat: three regular meals per day? two meals per day? irregular meals?

Are you sexually active? No_____ Yes_____

If so, are you aware of the risks of sexually transmitted diseases? No_____ Yes_____

**FIGURE 22-1** Common well young adult behavioral health history content. (From Somers, A. R., & Breslow, L. [1979]. Lifetime health monitoring program. *Nurse Practitioner, 4*[40], 50–54; US Preventive Services Task Force. [2015]. *Published recommendations.* Rockville, MD: Agency for Healthcare Research and Quality.)

**TABLE 22-1   Young Adult Preventive Health Monitoring (Examples)**

| Health Issue | AGE 18–26 YR | |
|---|---|---|
| | Intervention | Frequency |
| Tobacco screening and counseling | History and counseling | Each visit |
| Obesity/nutrition/body mass index | History, weight, and counseling | Each visit |
| Alcohol screening and counseling | History and counseling | At least once |
| Accidental injury, lap and shoulder belts, bicycle or motorcycle helmets, smoke detectors, safe firearm use | History and counseling | At least once |
| Unintended pregnancy | Counseling | At least once |
| Contraception | Counseling | Individually determined |
| Illegal drug use screening | History and counseling | At least once |
| Regular physical activity | History and counseling | At least once |
| Hypertension/blood pressure | Blood pressure measurement | Every 2 yr |
| Tetanus, diphtheria, pertussis | Tdap booster vaccine | Once if 10 yr since last one |
| Hepatitis B | Immunization | If not immunized |
| Diabetes, proteinuria, bacteriuria | Urinalysis | Once |
| Cholesterol levels | Serum cholesterol level determination, triglyceride level | Once |
| Cervical dysplasia | Gynecological examination; Papanicolaou smear | Every 2 yr, start at age 21 yr, or when sexually active |
| STI prevention | Counseling—offer HPV vaccine | Individually determined |
| *Chlamydia* (women) | *Chlamydia* screen | At gynecological examination if sexually active |
| *Gonorrhea* | Vaginal culture | At gynecological examination if sexually active |
| Influenza | Seasonal flu vaccine | Each year |

The ages differ in different publications and sources.

*HPV*, human papilloma virus; *STI*, sexually transmitted infection.

Modified from National Adolescent and Young Adult Health Information Center. (2012). Clinical preventive services for young adults. http://nahic. ucsf.edu/clinical-preventiveservices-for-young-adults/; US National Library of Medicine. (2015). Health screening for women/men ages 18-39. https://medlineplus.gov/ency/article/007462.htm

content that may be appropriately included in a health history for young adults focusing on probable age-specific behaviors.

## Preventive Care

The basic goals of preventive care are to maximize the period of optimal health status and detect incipient health problems. At age 18 years (approximately the time of graduation from high school), a full health appraisal is recommended. Table 22-1 illustrates examples of preventive care that is important during the young adult period, along with the recommended frequency of screening. As a common expectation, the recommendation for most areas is a repeated health history and visit at approximately 2-year intervals. Appropriate intervention is directed toward correcting health issues through history assessment and counseling about avoidance of adverse health behaviors. Subsequent counseling sessions focus on rechecking and updating information gathered in earlier meetings. Young adults are less likely to undergo well visits and ambulatory care visits, leading to lower experience with preventive services (Hing & Albert, 2016; National Adolescent and Young Adult Health Information Center, 2012; Neinstein, 2013).

A physical examination includes measurements of height, weight, body mass index (BMI), and blood pressure, and blood tests, with an emphasis on the need to avoid inactivity and obesity, which are risk factors for many health problems. The US Preventive Services Task Force (USPSTF, 2015) currently recommends against teaching **breast self-examination**, and concludes that the current evidence is insufficient to assess the additional benefits and harm of clinical breast examination beyond screening mammography for women aged 40 years or older. Screening for cervical cancer is strongly recommended in women who have been sexually active (**Papanicolaou [Pap] smear**). **Testicular self-examination** may be taught to men in this age group, although there is little evidence to assess the accuracy, benefits, or effectiveness (USPSTF, 2015) because early testicular cancers often present as benign inflammations (epididymitis or testicular trauma).

The typical young adult health examination also looks for signs of chronic disease. The most common chronic diseases reported by young adults are asthma, arthritis (including rheumatic diseases such as lupus and fibromyalgia), and hypertension (Figure 22-2). Although the percentage of young adults reporting chronic disease is small, more women than men (17.4% versus 12.9%) reported having at least one of the six most highly selected young adult chronic disease conditions (arthritis, asthma, cancer, diabetes, heart disease, and hypertension) (CDC, 2009). Some evidence suggests that young adults do not follow the guidelines

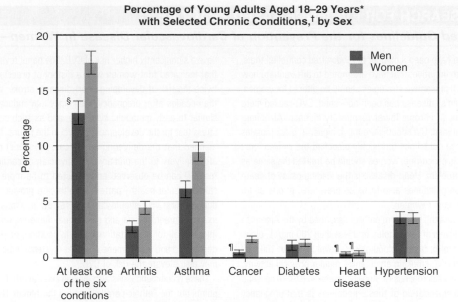

**Percentage of Young Adults Aged 18–29 Years\***
**with Selected Chronic Conditions,† by Sex**

\* Overall respondents: 6898 men and 8532 women

† Estimates are based on household interviews with a sample of the civilian, noninstitutionalized, adult U.S. population. The prevalence of diagnosed chronic conditions was determined by asking respondents if a doctor or other health professional ever told them that they had a specified condition. Asthma estimates are for current asthma and are based on the additional question "Do you still have asthma?" Arthritis includes arthritis, rheumatoid arthritis, gout, lupus, and fibromyalgia. Cancer excludes nonmelanoma skin cancer or skin cancer of unknown type. Diabetes includes all types with the exception of diabetic conditions related to pregnancy. Heart disease includes coronary heart disease, angina or angina pectoris, or heart attack or myocardial infarction. Hypertension is based on respondents indicating that on two or more separate visits they were told by a doctor or health professional that they had hypertension. Young adults who reported more than one condition are counted in each category.

§ 95% confidence interval.

¶ Estimate is statistically unreliable; data have a relative standard error of 20%–30%.

**FIGURE 22-2** Percentage of young adults aged 18 to 29 years with selected chronic conditions, by sex. (From National Health Interview Survey, United States, 2005–07. http://www.cdc.gov/mmwr/preview/mmwrhtml/mm5825a3.htm.)

for prevention of these common chronic diseases, which are the most disabling and costly (McDaniel & Belury, 2012; Neinstein, 2013).

After age 25 years, the preventive emphasis is on modifying coronary disease risk factors. There is evidence that healthy lifestyle changes during young adulthood are associated with decreased cardiovascular risk (Spring et al., 2014). The recommendations for screening for young adults are undergoing revision as more information becomes available about the interactive risks of sedentary lifestyle, high cholesterol levels, familial high lipid levels, diabetes mellitus, and smoking. For men aged 20 to 35 years the USPSTF makes no recommendations for or against routine screening for lipid disorders unless they are at increased risk of coronary disease (USPSTF, 2015). Aging is responsible for some degenerative changes in respiratory and cardiac function, but during the young adult years this decline amounts to less than 1% per year and is largely determined by an individual's fitness level (McCance & Huether, 2015). Cardiovascular

assessment of the young adult includes determination of the presence of hyperlipidemia, hypertension, diabetes, chest pain, or heart disease. A *Healthy People 2020* target is to reduce the mean total blood cholesterol level among adults to 177.9 mg/dL; the baseline between 1988 and 1994 for adults aged 20 years or older was 197.7 mg/dL (USDHHS, 2015). This 2020 target set a goal of 10% reduction. From 2009 to 2012, 12.9% of persons aged 20 years or older had high total blood cholesterol levels (greater than 240 mg/dL); this is appreciably down from 21% for the 1988 to 1994 period. Nurses can assist in gathering a comprehensive health history including pertinent information about hypertension and coronary artery disease in parents and relatives. In women a history of pregnancy-induced hypertension or preeclampsia is important and a risk factor for cardiovascular disease and renal disease (Box 22-3: Research for Evidence-Based Practice).

**Hypertension** results from increases in cardiac output or increases in peripheral resistance, or a combination of both, and

## BOX 22-3 RESEARCH FOR EVIDENCE-BASED PRACTICE

### Effectiveness-Based Guidelines for the Prevention of Cardiovascular Disease in Women—Update

During the last decade there have been a number of randomized controlled trials, such as the Women's Health Initiative, that have attempted to differentiate how cardiovascular disease (CVD) preventive strategies should be altered for women. The myth that CVD is a "man's" disease has been abolished. CVD caused more deaths in women than cancer, chronic lower respiratory disease, Alzheimer disease, and accidents combined. CVD deaths are much higher in black females than in white females. These guidelines thoroughly dispelled the conventional wisdom that as far as CVD is concerned, women should be treated the same as men. This is also a global problem. Heart disease is the leading cause of death in women worldwide. These guidelines also focus on preventive efforts and a long-term risk analysis in younger women.

The "ideal cardiovascular health" long-term pattern described by the American Heart Association includes levels of total cholesterol less than 200 mg/dL, blood pressure less than 120/80 mmHg, fasting blood glucose level less than 100 mg/dL, lean BMI less than 25 kg/m2, smoking abstinence, regular physical activity, and a diet based on the Dietary Approaches to Stop Hypertension (DASH) concept.

An important newer recommendation of these guidelines is that pregnancy history provides the health care professional with a criterion to predict future CVD risk. Women with a history of pregnancy-induced hypertension or preeclampsia have a significantly higher risk of CVD. The panel reviewed a large meta-analysis that indicated that women with a history of preeclampsia have approximately twice the risk of developing heart disease, stroke, and thrombolytic events in the decades after pregnancy. Pregnancy may induce a temporary state that is similar to early metabolic syndrome, and as such could be considered a failed stress test for the development of CVD in the future. Therefore it is highly recommended that the delivering health care personnel refer preeclamptic women after delivery to the primary care physician or cardiologist so that risk factors for CVD can be observed and adjusted to be more in accord with the "ideal cardiovascular health" pattern. Health care providers who are seeing females during a first visit should carefully review previous pregnancy complications, including preeclampsia and gestational diabetes, preterm birth, and birth of an infant small for its gestational age. In addition, other health disorders, such as depression and autoimmune diseases (systemic lupus and rheumatoid arthritis), may also elevate the risk of CVD.

These recommendations also include cultural differences. An interesting finding points out the "ethnic paradox" where the female Hispanic population, despite the stresses of immigration and less access to medical care, has a longer life expectancy than non-Hispanic whites and non-Hispanic blacks.

Guidelines from Mosca, L., Benjamin, E. J., Berra, K., Bezanson, J. L., Dolor, R. J., Lloyd-Jones, D. M., et al. (2011). Effectiveness-based guidelines for the prevention of cardiovascular disease in women—2011 update. *Circulation, 123*(11), 1243–1262. These guidelines have also been published in other journals and at National Institutes of Health Public Access; the guidelines represent the work of many participating organizations and sponsors, including the Nurse Practitioners in Women's Health. Also from Melnyk, B., & Fineout-Overholt, E. (2011). *Evidence-based practice in nursing & healthcare.* Philadelphia: Lippincott Williams & Wilkins.

is the third leading cause of death worldwide. According to a report from the Eighth Joint National Committee (James et al., 2014), the focus of blood pressure assessment is on systolic hypertension and risks from prolonged diastolic hypertension. The risk from diastolic hypertension starts to rise at 75 mmHg. The focus of attention is on lowering blood pressure toward the new lower normal goal of 120/80 mmHg or less (James et al., 2014; USDHHS, 2015). The USPSTF highly recommends (grade A) screening of young adults for hypertension. Increases in blood pressure above 140/90 mmHg in young adults contribute to a consistent rise in the risk of heart attack, stroke, and heart failure. The report from the Eighth Joint National Committee (James et al., 2014) and earlier reports discuss the significance of a new category of "pre-hypertension" to better identify individuals at risk of developing treatable hypertension and to encourage lifestyle changes before vascular disease is fully evident.

There are also noticeable disparities in the development of hypertension in various population subgroups. Data from 2009 to 2012 indicate the Mexican American and the white-only/non-Hispanic populations have the lowest percentage of high blood pressure individuals (27%), and the non-Hispanic/black American population has the highest (42%) level of hypertension (USDHHS, 2015). The prevalence of control of hypertension was also lowest in young adults (39%). This may be related to lack of a usual source of care, but most young adults surveyed had health insurance, so health insurance alone is not sufficient to correlate with better hypertension control (Gillespie et al., 2011). Gillespie and colleagues (2011) also report that adoption of healthy behaviors in young adults, particularly reducing dietary

salt intake from an average of 3400 mg daily to an average of 2300 mg daily, could dramatically reduce the incidence of hypertension.

Although for the entire population deaths attributable to coronary heart disease have declined since the 1960s (CDC, 2011b), the mortality rate remains higher for American Indians/Alaska Natives and blacks. A prevention target of *Healthy People 2020* (USDHHS, 2015) is to increase the proportion of young adults aged 18 years and older with hypertension whose blood pressure is under control from 18% in 1988 to 1994 to 61.2%.

Metabolic syndrome includes a group of cardiovascular risk factors associated with overweight and obesity, particularly abdominal obesity. This syndrome includes the lethal risks of high lipid levels, insulin resistance, and hypertension. Many studies have demonstrated that hyperlipidemia and hypertension in young adults is directly related to later cardiovascular disease (Tran & Zimmerman, 2015). A prominent sign of metabolic syndrome is central or waist-centered obesity. Currently, at least one-fifth of US adults are estimated to have this combination of metabolic risk factors, and the prevalence increases with age. First-step therapy involves lifestyle alterations, including weight management and increase in physical activity.

Diabetes is seventh on the list of leading causes of death in the United States, and it is one of the six major chronic diseases affecting young adults. Currently, 23.6 million Americans have the disease, and it is estimated to be undiagnosed in approximately 25% of Americans with diabetes. Minority populations (black Americans, Native American/Alaska Natives, and Hispanics) are disproportionately affected, with Native American populations experiencing twice the rate for new cases recorded in white non-Hispanic populations (USDHHS, 2015). The incidence of diabetes, especially type 2 diabetes (adult onset), and related complications (cardiovascular disease, blindness, lower limb amputations, and kidney disease) is increasing in the United States (USDHHS, 2015). Of those with diagnosed diabetes, only a few have their blood pressure, glucose levels, and cholesterol levels sufficiently controlled to avoid or delay vascular disease. Diabetes lowers life expectancy by up to 15 years. Because careful control can delay the beginning and progression of long-term complications, nursing efforts directed at early detection and monitoring of diabetes in young adults are important.

### Decision-Making and Risk-Taking

The decision-making of a young adult directly affects health and well-being. Peak physical skills stimulate young adults to be venturesome, daring, enterprising, and aggressive. Young adults have less experience with the death of significant people in their lives, and they may take inordinate risks. The leading causes of death in individuals 15 to 24 years of age combined are unintentional injuries, homicide, and suicide (USDHHS, 2015). The prevalence of adverse behaviors associated with sudden death illustrates a developmental lack of fear in young adults. Bullying, dating violence, and sexual violence are becoming more prevalent. Underuse of seat belts and helmets by motorcyclists and bicyclists is a cause of many accidental injuries and deaths. Some states still do not have laws that require the use of helmets.

### Communicable Diseases and Adult Immunization

Communicable (infectious) diseases affect young adults with differing degrees of severity. Although the increased availability of better drug treatments and/or vaccines, improved hygiene and food handling, and provision of cleaner water supplies have promoted prevention and control of infectious disease, new disease threats are continually emerging. Much of this increase is due to improvements in travel and changes in social, sexual, and other behaviors that expose broader populations of individuals to emerging pathogens.

Current common threats include seasonal influenza, drug-resistant tuberculosis, diarrhea caused by *Escherichia coli* 0157:H7, hepatitis, and meningococcal disease. A more recent goal of *Healthy People 2020* is to increase the percentage of young adults who are vaccinated for seasonal influenza from 14.7% to 19.3% (depends on age group) to 80% (USDHHS, 2015). Even with nurse-staffed flu drives, this goal is difficult to reach in the young adult age group.

Increasingly, new cases of tuberculosis are occurring in foreign-born individuals (USDHHS, 2015), even as the incidence of this disease has declined overall to 3.6 cases per 100,000; the target is 1.0 new case per 100,000 population. An increase in tuberculosis rates, particularly in some minority groups (Asian American/Pacific Islanders, blacks, and Hispanics), illustrates that preventive activities must be reinforced and constant vigilance maintained over monitoring and effectiveness for all communicable diseases. The focus of tuberculosis surveillance is moving toward the tracking of full completion of drug protocols and treatment of drug-resistant types. New infectious agents and

diseases continue to be detected and must be understood in a global context because of increasing travel and migration, importation of foods, agriculture practices, and bioterrorism (USDHHS, 2015).

Cases of acute hepatitis B have declined in young adults because of vaccination programs aimed at children, adolescents, and adults in high-risk groups (USDHHS, 2015). A primary way of achieving high levels of vaccination coverage is to identify settings in which unvaccinated young adults can be vaccinated, such as correctional facilities, drug treatment centers, and clinics treating sexually transmitted infections (STIs) (USDHHS, 2015). An objective of *Healthy People 2020* is to continue to reduce hepatitis B infections in adults aged 19 years or older from 2.0 cases per 100,000 persons in 2007 to a target goal of 1.5 cases per 100,000 persons (USDHHS, 2015).

Another target of *Healthy People 2020* is to keep the incidence of hepatitis C stable at 0.2 new symptomatic cases per 100,000 persons (USDHHS, 2015). Chronic hepatitis became a nationally reportable disease in 2003. The individuals most at risk are those who have injected illicit drugs, are undergoing hemodialysis, are seropositive for human immunodeficiency virus (HIV), or have elevated liver enzyme levels. Recent curative advances in drug treatment for hepatitis C have made better case finding more important (USDHHS, 2015).

Most outbreaks of meningococcal disease are sporadic; however, young adults living in college/university dormitories or crowded conditions may be more susceptible than young adults not living in close settings. Although meningococci are sensitive to penicillin and many antibiotics, the case-fatality rate is high in otherwise healthy adults, and many survivors may have residual neurological disabilities. Those most susceptible are unvaccinated or incompletely vaccinated college first-year students living in dormitories, or military recruits, who have a higher case ratio (CDC, 2013c). Approximately 44% of people aged 13 to 15 years were vaccinated against meningococcal infection, and the *Healthy People 2020* goal is for more comprehensive coverage of 80% (USDHHS, 2015). Specific recommendations are also indicated to control sudden outbreaks of meningococcal disease.

Other viruses, such as human papilloma virus (HPV), commonly affect young adults. HPV is spread through sexual contact, and some forms of the virus in combination with smoking are strongly related to the later development of cervical dysplasia and cancer. The prevalence of HPV infection is highest among 20- to 24-year olds and peaked in the pre-HPV vaccine era (CDC, 2013b). A vaccine to prevent cervical cancer, Gardasil HPV vaccine, is effective against four types of the virus (HPV types 6, 11, 16, and 18); it is available and is recommended for individuals from 9 to 26 years old. *Healthy People 2020* recommends three doses of HPV vaccine for females 13 to 15 years of age. Twenty-eight percent were vaccinated in 2012, and the target is 80% (USDHHS, 2015). Recent study findings report that the rate of HPV infection in younger women has declined as a result of increased HPV testing and vaccine use (Dickson et al., 2015).

Pertussis (whooping cough) vaccination is part of the original vaccine series offered to infants. As it is now known that the antibody titer protection for pertussis diminishes with age, pertussis vaccination is recommended with the 10-year tetanus booster injection. This newly formulated vaccine recommended for adults is known as Tdap (tetanus, diphtheria, acellular pertussis). Adults younger than 65 years who have never received Tdap should substitute it for their next 10-year interval booster dose (http://www.cdc.gov/vaccines/vpd-vac/combo-vaccines/Dtap-Td-DT/tdap.html).

## Nutritional-Metabolic Pattern

Young adults value slimness, defined muscle tone, and athletic ability. Emphasis on body "thinness" can lead to improper eating. Regular physical activity increases muscle and bone strength, decreases body fat, aids in weight control, enhances well-being, and reduces depression. Physical activity levels are positively influenced by structural environmental improvements, such as sidewalks, bike lanes, and parks, and by legislative policies that improve access to physical activity facilities (USDHHS, 2015). An optimally functioning basal metabolic rate in the young adult allows adequate oxygen intake during normal activity and rest periods. A young adult male requires approximately 1600 to 1800 calories a day to meet his body's basal metabolic needs, and a young adult female requires only 1200 to 1450 calories a day. After growth in height stops in the late teens, the basal metabolic rate declines.

During the young adult years, caloric intake increases substantially, particularly in men. Increased caloric intake without a corresponding increase in energy expenditure can lead to obesity, which is a precursor to hypertension, coronary disease, and diabetes. The presence of obesity meets three defining criteria for disease: impairment of function, attributable signs and symptoms, and contribution to bodily harm (Ryan & Urquhart, 2015). According to information from 2009 to 2012, 35.3% of adults aged 20 years or older were at a healthy weight (USDHHS, 2015).

Although trends toward increasing weight occurred in all major racial and ethnic groups, the increase in obesity was more pronounced in the 2009 to 2012 survey period for the Hispanic population (40.5%) and the Mexican American population (42.8%) (USDHHS, 2015). In the same survey period, the prevalence of obesity among men aged 20 years or older was 34.3%, and in women aged 20-years or older it was 36.1% (USDHHS, 2015). To stabilize the trends in increasing weight and obesity, the nurse can be part of education directed toward new lifestyle, nutrition, and physical activity behavior.

For many Americans, food sources are abundant, portion sizes have increased, and lifestyles are becoming increasingly sedentary. More specifically, young adult diets should contain a variety of nutrient-dense foods, especially whole grains, fruits, vegetables, low-fat or fat-free milk, lean meats, and protein sources. Caloric intake and the intake of saturated and trans fats, cholesterol, added sugars, sodium, and alcohol should be limited. Food-label information (now includes trans fats) should be read on all processed and packaged foods. Another challenge is the increasing consumption of food prepared and eaten away from home, which is generally higher in fats, cholesterol, and sodium and lower in fiber and calcium than that prepared in the home (USDHHS, 2015). This suggests that the composition of food prepared outside the home promotes weight gain. Many states have legislation that requires restaurants and fast food outlets to list food composition on menus. There is some evidence that in poor areas with less access to transportation, neighborhood convenience stores stock nutrient-poor snacks, sugar-sweetened drinks, and less fresh fruits and vegetables and that has contributed to lower diet quality (Rummo et al., 2015). Collective national action and community involvement are needed to promote healthful diets among all Americans and to reverse the increasing trend to be overweight and obese. Whereas diet drugs and bariatric surgery may be advised for cases of severe obesity, these treatments must be evaluated for risks and benefits (Burke & Wang, 2011). Young adults, in particular, are influenced by the body shapes of celebrities, and "celebrity worship" may be an important motivator to seeking change in body shape and plastic surgery alternatives (Maltby & Day, 2011).

Nurses with other health providers can investigate weight problems by measuring waist circumference, blood pressure, cholesterol levels, and activity levels rather than using weight alone. Assessments of weight and height are used to calculate BMI. Whereas the BMI may be a good indicator for population screening, it may not be the best measurement for predicting health risks as in each individual person cardiovascular and obesity-related complications must be assessed (Ryan & Urquhart, 2015). Those with a BMI of 25 kg/m2 or less (male waist size of 40 inches or less, female waist size of 35 inches or less) should have weight maintenance teaching. Individuals with a BMI of 30 kg/m2 or greater who have tried diets and exercise may be considered for weight-reducing drugs (CDC, 2010; LeBlanc et al., 2011). A BMI of 35 to 40 kg/m$_2$ or above may meet the criteria for bariatric surgery (CDC, 2010; LeBlanc et al., 2011). However, the focus of nursing advice is conservative at first, recommending lifestyle management, careful diet appraisal, and increase in exercise patterns (Ryan & Urquhart, 2015). Use of activity monitors such as FitBit, heart-rate monitors (Apple watch), and fat/muscle calculators may provide incentives for health eating and exercise patterns. Long-term weight management is a frustrating process. Applying principles of motivational interviewing (collaboration, evocation, autonomy) and addressing the problems of obesity and overweight through use of a chronic care model offers potential for long-range weight management (Apovian & Gordon, 2014; Ryan & Urquhart, 2015). Changing the upward obesity population trend is one of the most difficult goals to achieve (Jiang et al., 2011). The nurse should use people-first and nonjudgmental language that refers to the person before the disability (diabetes) rather than identifying the person on the basis of the disability (diabetic) (Ryan & Urquhart, 2015).

Proper nutrition is particularly necessary for the young adult female during the childbearing years. The factors contributing to iron deficiency in this age group are regular loss of blood (during menses) and pregnancy. The prevalence of anemia in women of childbearing potential was 16.1% in 2003 to 2006, and the 2020 target is 14.5% (USDHHS, 2015) (see the case study and care plan at the end of this chapter). A blood loss of 2 to 4 mL per day (1–2 mg of iron) can cause iron-deficiency anemia; young women who do not eat a healthy diet and have heavy periods or use nonsteroidal antiinflammatory drugs are specifically at risk of iron-deficiency anemia. Iron supplementation is recommended during pregnancy for optimal growth of the fetus and supporting structures (Perry et al., 2013). The CDC and the USDHHS (2015) recommend that all women of childbearing age consume 0.4 mg of folic acid daily to reduce the risk of fetal neural tube defects, including spina bifida. The supplementation period should include at least the month before pregnancy and the first trimester during pregnancy. The CDC and the US Food and Drug Administration (FDA) also recommend folic acid fortification of food to prevent neural tube defects (USDHHS, 2015). In 2007 to 2010, only 22.8% of nonpregnant females aged 15 to 44 years reported a daily intake of folic acid of 400 mcg from fortified foods or dietary supplements; the target for 2020 is 26.2% (USDHHS, 2015). Efforts are also being made to reduce health disparities in neural tube defects, including the use of better communication modalities with the Hispanic population and other population subgroups that have higher rates of neural tube defects (USDHHS, 2015).

Most adolescents and adult women fail to meet their calcium requirements, placing them at risk of osteoporosis and bone fractures in later life. Low calcium intake is a direct result of low milk consumption related to soft drink ingestion. An increase in intake of calcium-containing foods is therefore recommended, particularly for teens and young women (see Chapter 11).

## Elimination Pattern

Patterns of elimination are generally well established by young adulthood. Although eating disorders (anorexia and bulimia) typically begin at an earlier stage of development, they can persist during young adulthood. The fashion industry is widely criticized for using underweight women as young female models, thereby emphasizing excessive thinness as the ideal female standard.

Assessment of young adults is also directed toward teaching about the common complaints of constipation, hemorrhoids, and occasional diarrhea. Although the risk of colon cancer is low in this age group, young adults should be aware that changes in elimination patterns or blood in the stool should be reported to their primary care provider. Nurses can counsel young adults on the benefits of drinking adequate amounts of fluid and eating fruits and vegetables, which are sources of fiber, to promote normal bowel activity.

## Activity-Exercise Pattern

Inactivity is a factor predisposing to cardiovascular disease and obesity; increasing access to and promoting locations for physical activity are increasingly emphasized. A *Healthy People 2020* goal is to reduce the proportion of adults who engage in no leisure-time physical activity. In 2013, 30.5% of adults engaged in no leisure-time physical activity; the target was 32.6%, which was reached, but there is much room for improvement (USDHHS, 2015).

Aerobic exercise, in which oxygen is metabolized to produce energy, develops an optimally functioning cardiorespiratory system. Aerobic conditioning achieves cardiovascular fitness through five periods of moderately intense exercise weekly for approximately 30 minutes or more (USDHHS, 2015) at a heart rate of approximately 220 minus the age of the person multiplied by 65% to 85%. Although this formula is controversial and there

may be individual variations, it seems a reasonable first approach. Young adults are encouraged to engage in fitness activities that increase the heart rate to approximately 150 beats or more per minute. After 5 minutes of activity at this rate, the body is required to make adjustments in cardiovascular capacity by enlarging the lungs and the capillaries in the muscles and the heart. Repeated aerobic exercise, such as swimming, cycling, running, and walking, decreases the likelihood of problems caused by inactivity. Muscle-strengthening activities should also be stressed. Major barriers for young adults are lack of time, lack of access to exercise facilities, and inability to find safe environments in which to exercise.

### Radiation and Excessive Sun Exposure

Nurses need to educate young adults about the risks of sun exposure and tanning, the preventive use of sun-blocking agents, and the awareness of skin symptoms that might indicate cancer. Sun-blocking agents reduce sunburn or other skin damage with the goal of lowering the risk of skin cancer. A number of the agents are rated on the basis of skin type and sensitivity to burning. Many lotions and creams are available with differing radiation protection levels. Sun protection factor (SPF) index is a measure of the effectiveness of various preparations. The agents are rated on a scale by the FDA. For example, a rating of 30 means the sunscreen provides 30 times the protection of unprotected skin. Newer guidelines for sunscreen protection were adopted in June 2012 by the FDA. New sunscreens should provide broad-spectrum protection, SPF of 30 or greater, and water resistance (American Academy of Dermatology, 2011). Women's makeup preparations and moisturizers may include sun-blocking agents. Young adults should avoid sunbathing during the 2-hour period before and after noon, because two-thirds of the day's ultraviolet light comes through Earth's atmosphere during this time. Sunscreens that block both ultraviolet A and ultraviolet B light are more effective in preventing cancer than those that block only ultraviolet B light (American Academy of Dermatology, 2011). The best protection is achieved by application of agents 15 to 30 minutes before exposure and then reapplying every 15 to 30 minutes during exposure to the sun. Further application may be necessary if activities involve swimming, sweating, or rubbing of skin. Sun-protective measures such as use of sunscreen, use of sun-protective clothing, and avoidance of ultraviolet light are an essential part of young adult education. The nurse considers that the most effective skin cancer prevention activities for young adults include primary care counseling, sun protection, and avoidance of the use of tanning beds (DiStefano et al., 2014).

### Sports

Bicycling and motorcycling are encouraged by environmentalists to decrease automobile pollution; this trend is also promoted to relieve traffic congestion, avoid the high costs of fuel and car maintenance, and increase interest in healthy exercise. Cyclists are at risk of being involved in accidents with automobiles. Head injury is responsible for many bicycle-related fatalities. In 2013, 19 states had mandatory helmet requirements for riders younger than 15 years (USDHHS, 2015). Bicycle helmets are believed to be the single most effective preventive measure available to decrease the incidence of brain and head injury (USDHHS, 2015).

Motorcycles have less occupant protection than do automobiles but are appealing to young adults, primarily because they have high-performance and speed capabilities. Use of a motorcycle helmet reduces the chance of dying in an accident. A target of *Healthy People 2020* is to increase the proportion of motorcyclists using helmets from 60% in 2013 to 74% in 2020 (USDHHS, 2015).

Accidental deaths from drowning are also common in young adults. The USDHHS (2015) estimates 1.2 drownings per 100,000 population occurred in 2013. Swimming, boating, and scuba diving are associated with the high number of water-related fatalities. Hang gliding, parachuting, and flying small aircraft are responsible for a large number of outdoor fatalities. Mountain climbing, hiking in poor weather conditions, downhill ski racing, and bobsledding are other hazardous activities. Many so-called accidents are not random, uncontrollable events, but are predictable and preventable if precautions and risks are analyzed (USDHHS, 2015).

Amateur and professional sports activities generally pose few hazards when rules and safety precautions are observed. Relatively few fatalities are associated with the professionally organized contact sports, such as football, hockey, or boxing, but chronic injuries and concussions can cause degenerative brain diseases. In 2013, 45.6 medically consulted injuries occurred per 1000 population, and the target for 2020 is 41.9 per 1000 population (USDHHS, 2015). In addition, pathological investigations by Daniloff (2010) and other Boston University researchers have linked sports-related head injuries to an increase in the incidence of dementia, memory-related diseases, and chronic traumatic encephalopathy (Mez et al., 2016). This has resulted in significant changes in professional football policies and sports concussion protocols. Many of these policy changes have been adopted for college, high school, and amateur sports programs as well (Daniloff, 2010).

A comprehensive history of recreational activities alerts the nurse to specific needs about safety education. Young adults are encouraged to learn and abide by the rules of the sport in which they are engaged. Rules in many sports have evolved from health and safety concerns, enabling the individual to learn the sport well with appropriate instruction.

## Sleep-Rest Pattern

Young adults are subject to fatigue induced by work, **stress**, or inactivity. Changes in activity or stressors can help reduce fatigue. Attempting new and challenging tasks can help reduce mental stress. New physical activities, such as learning a new sport or form of exercise, can also provide stimulation. A number of digital devices now record sleep as well as activity patterns.

## Cognitive-Perceptual Pattern

### Physical and Mental Patterns

Visual acuity is highest at approximately age 20 years and begins to decline at approximately age 40 years, when farsightedness frequently develops. Hearing is also best at age 20 years; the ability to distinguish high-pitched tones decreases with age. The other senses—taste, smell, touch, and awareness of temperature and pain—remain stable until age 45 to 50 years.

Further maturation requires young adults to learn skills and behaviors that increase the performance abilities gained as adolescents. The factors that an individual young adult may perceive as essential to learn will depend on specific goals, values, attitudes, and practices as influenced by intrinsic (constitutional) and extrinsic (environmental or community) factors. Executive decision-making becomes better developed: calculation of risks versus rewards, prioritizing, self-evaluation, self-correction, and long-term planning become more sophisticated. The development of intellectual maturity influences the selection of behaviors and attitudes that affect health and well-being practices.

### Piaget's Theory

Several stage theorists have described the growth of young adult thought and moral development. It is important to note that these stages are fluid, and individual differences occur. Within Piaget's cognitive-developmental theory, formal operational thought evolves from concrete operational thought in adolescence and extends through the reasoning process of young adults (Piaget, 1972). Although more recent developmental theorists dispute Piaget's findings, this scheme of cognitive development assists the nurse in learning about and understanding young adult reasoning (Carey et al., 2015). Achievement of formal operational thinking allows young adults to analyze all combinations of possibilities and construct hypotheses. Young adult thought becomes more perceptive and insightful; issues can therefore be evaluated realistically and objectively. Young adults are energetic and can therefore contribute substantially to social and occupational decision-making. Although they tend to take greater risks, young adults typically demonstrate the use of appropriate reasoning, anticipation, and analytical approaches.

### Intellectual Growth

Organization of information influences memory. Evidence shows that recall performance diminishes with age: at its peak in the 20s, memory starts to diminish during the 30s. Improved strategies for organization of information, however, can enhance recall, and limitation of memory with increasing age is likely a result of retrieval rather than storage mechanisms. Recent evidence from brain development research indicates that during the early years of young adulthood important frontal lobe brain development is still occurring; this is important for control of emotions and later full adult rational decision-making (Neinstein, 2013).

### Erikson's Theory

Erikson (1993), another widely cited psychological theorist, reported that the most important goal for young adults is the development of an increased sense of competency and self-esteem. In developing self-esteem, the young person learns to be truly open and capable of trust through the formation of intimate relationships that are characteristic of this period. This stage is described as a phase of psychosocial development termed **intimacy versus isolation** and loneliness.

Erikson's concept of genuine intimacy extends beyond sexual relations to a broader view of mutual psychosocial intimacy with a spouse or lover, parents, children, and friends. Characterized by the reciprocal expression of affection, intimacy requires mutual trust. These interchanges are spontaneous for the young adult; relationships should be free and allow self-disclosure. Young adults who are unsure of their identity may avoid intimate contact or engage in promiscuous behavior lacking in true intimacy, which can result in isolation and consequent self-absorption. Healthy adults search for continuity, regularity, or unity of meaningful relationships, while avoiding situations of little commitment.

### Moral Development

Young adults who have successfully mastered the previous cognitive, social, and moral stages are usually able to recognize or use principled reasoning. Kohlberg identifies this ability as the **postconventional level of moral reasoning** (Kohlberg & Lickons, 1986). During this phase the individual is able to differentiate the self from the rules and expectations of others and to define principles regarding rights in terms of self-chosen principles. The interests of individuals can be weighed against the needs of society and the state, and violations of law can be justified when individual interests are in accord with principles. Gilligan (1982, 2002, 2013), who studied the development of moral reasoning in women and girls, asserts that their moral judgments reflect less of a "rights" perspective and more of an emphasis on responsibilities in relationships. Newer framing of this theory of women's emotions and relationships is now essential to understanding intelligence and self-awareness (Gilligan, 2013).

Although development of principled moral reasoning is possible during young adulthood, it may never occur if the cognitive and social factors that stimulate higher reasoning are not present. Acts of personal violence representative of lower moral reasoning should not be present; however, such acts do occur during this period, illustrating the need for moral developmental concerns to be addressed at earlier stages of education and socialization.

## Self-Perception–Self-Concept Pattern

In non-Western cultures the entrance to adulthood is generally defined and marked by social events such as marriage. In Western societies, maturation is defined through the individual's achievement of financial and residential independence, and is a more drawn-out, gradual process. There is evidence that young adults have recently been attaining traditional life milestones later; this includes completing school and leaving home, attaining financial independence, marrying, and having the first child (Neinstein, 2013).

Two emotional themes regarding the value of work and financial independence become evident during young adulthood. During their 20s, young adults yearn to explore and experiment, keeping structures temporary and reversible. These individuals may move from job to job and relationship to relationship, remaining in a transient state. At the opposite extreme is the urge to prepare for the future by making firm commitments. During this period, both men and women question their value to society, the merit of their accomplishments, their success as

sexual beings, and the probability of attaining their unfulfilled goals.

The US Census Bureau (2011) reports that more than 74.7% of women aged 25 to 35 years were employed in 2010; this percentage is expected to be approximately the same (74.2%) in 2018. As more mothers enter the labor force, the need for child care increases. The wage gap, or pay differential, between men and women is also significant. Recent legislation signed by President Barack Obama ensures women equal pay in the workforce (Morelli, 2015). Access to insurance and retirement benefits may not be available, especially to high-risk groups such as minorities or people receiving the minimum wage. Even when there is sufficient access to health care, some types of employment expose individuals to occupational risks and hazards.

Many young adults are high achievers and seek opportunities to be challenged. Employment problems are stressful and traumatic to an individual's self-esteem and self-worth, particularly in the current economic environment. The failure to obtain promotions or pay rises can accelerate the degree of stress. Employment is more than a source of income; it provides self-esteem and social interaction. Because the adjustment to the job market influences many other aspects of daily living, young adults frequently require assistance in developing coping mechanisms to manage stress. Properly managing the initial stress prevents further complications that can arise if the young adult uses unhealthy stress relievers such as alcohol or drugs.

Young women have many of the same concerns about employment and success as do young men. Many young women postpone childbearing until they have established their careers; many are absent from the job for only a standard maternity leave. Women who return to work when their children are very young frequently risk the emotional strain caused by guilt feelings and role strain. In addition to helping parents cope with the stress of being absent from their children, nurses can help them identify ways to provide high-quality supervision in their absence, through private babysitters, through day care programs, or through neighbors, friends, and relatives.

The US workforce is changing dramatically as companies merge, restructure, downsize (right size), and shift employees around to meet changing market conditions, company mergers, and buyouts. The nature of work is changing, with a continued trend toward longer hours, increased use of contracted and temporary workers, and increased telecommuting (USDHHS, 2015). There is increasing concern about "globalization," outsourcing, and moving jobs overseas, especially in the industrial centers, the pharmaceutical industry, and the computer industry. Unemployment or underemployment for young adults is a particular concern after recovery from the prolonged recession beginning in 2008 (Rampell, 2011). There is concern that even with better job prospects, this young adult population will be behind in wages for years, and this may impact overall lifetime earnings. Younger hires may start at lower salaries and begin their employed years with firms that pay less or have less potential for advancement. If they have employment within their specific fields, it may come with fewer benefits than for more experienced, older workers (Neinstein, 2013). Nursing activity in occupational and industrial settings can be directed toward improving both working conditions and employer-employee relationships. When nurses advocate healthy work sites, this increases the chance that young adults will have access to comprehensive health-promotion programs.

## Roles-Relationships Pattern

Young adult friendships are more enduring than are earlier relationships. The focus of the relationship is the sharing of feelings or confidences as well as common interests. True friendship is characteristic of a person who wants to give rather than receive. Friendships are necessary in a constantly changing society; they provide a source of emotional support and a basis of stability for developing the self-concept. Social networking sites such as Facebook, MySpace, and Twitter and social apps allow young adults to interact quickly with one another to organize events/ dates and share photos, experiences, thoughts, and perceptions. Young adults use Internet dating services to widen access to potential dating candidates (Murray & Campbell, 2015).

Establishing interpersonal relationships involves agreeable and purposeful interactions with others. Interpersonal relationships can be created with people of the same or the opposite sex. Age is typically a less important factor than it was during adolescence. The formation of intimate relationships develops within or outside a family context, the school setting, or work environment. High-speed cell phone and wireless Internet access facilitate maintenance of relationships from high school and university settings with text messaging, e-mail, and instant messaging.

For some the significant other is a person of the same sex. Among those aged 18 to 44 years, 92.3% of women and 95.1% of men reported they were heterosexual, and 1.3% of women and 1.9% of men stated they were homosexual, gay, or lesbian (Copen et al., 2016). Coming to the realization that a significant other is of the same sex often causes emotional upheaval and distress. Same-sex marriage (also known as gay marriage) legislation has been upheld by the US Supreme Court and applies to all US states; this legislation legitimizes the legal rights of same-sex couples through marriage or civil union statutes. Same-sex marriage supporters argue that civil recognition reduces the legal discrimination involved in such unions. Resistance to legalization of same-sex marriage comes from individuals who note that historically the term "marriage" has been reserved for a religious union between a man and a woman. This issue has been fiercely debated politically in the United States.

Transgender issues and rights have been headlines in the news recently. Transgender issues arise when one's gender identity or expression does not match the individual's assigned sex. Transgender expression is independent of sexual orientation as individuals may be heterosexual, homosexual, or bisexual. This category includes individuals who have reassigned their sexual identity different from that assigned at birth.

In addition to achieving intimacy, the young adult must accomplish other developmental tasks to achieve true psychosocial maturation (Figure 22-3). Decision-making about life and career directions is the developmental milestone that heralds the transition from adolescence to adulthood. Decisions usually entail

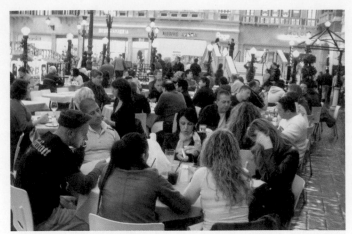

**FIGURE 22-3** Young adults enjoy gathering in a local café to socialize together.

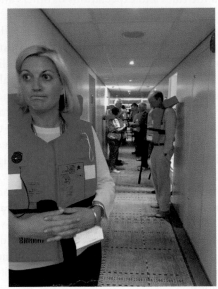

**FIGURE 22-4** Young adults may travel before marriage or beginning a career.

establishing independence from the family of origin. This transition may involve an actual physical move from the parents' home (going away to college, abroad, joining the military, or getting an apartment); however, movement away is not the sole indicator of independence (Figure 22-4). Young adults frequently remain in their parents' home for economic reasons, particularly when life choices involve continued schooling, unemployment, or remaining unmarried. In some cultures, unmarried adults live with their parents until they are married, and newly married young adults share the home of their parents until they begin having their own children.

A greater proportion of young adults are enrolled in higher education than ever before (Pew Research Center, 2012). Many low-income young adults are enrolled at for-profit institutions, which have become the fastest growing sector of US higher education (Institute for Higher Education Policy, 2011). Because college loan repayment typically begins 6 months after graduation, new graduates have to face the harsh realities of trying to find employment and ways to begin loan repayment. Some reports indicate that up to 85% of new college graduates are moving home at least for a short time (Byrne, 2011). Others will start or attend graduate school to obtain better work skills.

Individuals in the later years of this age group typically choose life partners and begin families; they make decisions about childbearing and the number and education of children. Additional consideration must be given to decisions related to childbearing, such as finances, safety, family support, where to live, the relationship with extended family members, and the roles and responsibilities within the nuclear family unit. Young adults who are establishing a family must have open communication about self-development, which includes issues of dual careers, childrearing practices, and domestic duties.

Family harmony and development are major goals for many young adults. Although family size and structure have undergone dramatic changes in recent decades, concern about each member's health and safety continues to be a primary focus. Family life is influenced by the qualities of individual family members. Typically, economic security, status, place in the community, and healthy patterns of living, such as good nutrition, personal hygiene, and physical fitness, are associated with healthy family adjustment.

## Separation and Divorce

Approximately half of marriages end in divorce (US Census Bureau, 2011), and many young adults do not marry but have children. Approximately one-quarter of all children in the United States are living in single-parent, mother-led families, and half of the children affected by divorce frequently never see their fathers again. Although dissatisfaction and unhappiness are frequent precursors to separation and divorce, the decision to dissolve a marriage is not easy. Considerable emotional strain exists for both partners, their children, their families, and their close friends. Divorce requires that young adults reevaluate their basic values, individual personality, spiritual beliefs, and ego strength, job potential, and socioeconomic factors to ensure future security for themselves and their children. Some young adults are unable to adjust to role and status changes and to threats of self-concept. For these reasons, support systems in the form of groups, individual counseling, or special social activities are critical. Nurses can assist young adults to identify sources of assistance (Box 22-4: Innovative Practice). As a result of the dissolution of families or divorce, many women and their young children are forced to seek emergency shelter in publicly operated homes, including welfare hotels and group shelters.

Nursing care and assessment can help to identify the feelings of guilt, grief, and loss that young adults experience during a separation or divorce. Suggesting that young adults read articles or books on issues related to divorce is helpful, because they provide a reference point for their experiences. The nurse recommends marital counseling by a qualified professional; this may be the most beneficial source of support.

## Male and Female Risk of Violence

Violence is a global and national health problem. Violent deaths are intentional deaths that occur from physical force or power exerted against self, others, or a community (CDC, 2011a).

---

### ☀ BOX 22-4  INNOVATIVE PRACTICE

**Social Media and Use of Internet and Cell Phone Delivery Systems for Preventive Health Information**

The use of technology is changing practice patterns and the way that health communications may be transmitted. The transference of technology has often been slowed by the reluctance of policymakers, administrators, providers, advocates, or consumers. Some biomedical innovations for Pap test understanding and prevention of sexually transmitted infections and HIV infection have been adopted (such as use of electronic health records and cell phones/Internet to trace contacts), but full adherence by the person seeking care is often hindered by behavioral factors. Technological interventions allow behavioral supports and educational programs to be delivered with less cost and more convenience. These include STI/HIV testing and partner interventions, behavioral interventions, self-management strategies, and provider care information. These technological interventions have been demonstrated to be as effective as face-to-face interventions. Text messaging is also possible. Smartphones are connecting many individuals domestically and globally. This will allow the dissemination of more active engaging health diagnosis, treatment, and counseling.

From Christensen, S. & Morelli, R. (2012). MyPapp: A mobile app to enhance understanding of Pap testing. *Computers, Informatics and Nursing, 30*(12), 627–631; Swendeman, D., & Rotheram-Borus, M. J. (2010). Innovation in sexually transmitted disease and HIV prevention: Internet and mobile phone delivery vehicles for global diffusion. *Current Opinion in Psychiatry, 23*(2), 139–144.

---

Although the destruction of the World Trade Center in 2001 and violent events in other countries such as France, Belgium, Iraq, Afghanistan, and Syria and ISIS (radical Islamic governance) are examples of organized terrorism, worldwide only approximately one-fifth of violent acts are related to organized events. The overthrow of governments in Egypt and Libya was largely accomplished by young adults. Young adults can be involved as both the agitators and the victims of violence.

In the United States there are approximately 51,000 violent deaths a year, and these deaths affect all Americans not only in emotional terms but also through additional medical costs and lost employment productivity (CDC, 2011a). Domestically, in the United States, the recipients of violence may be older adults, children, and women with whom they are familiar (USDHHS, 2015). Identification of, education about, and strategies to prevent bullying, dating violence, and sexual violence among young adults requires federal and community attention. Homicide (assault) is the second leading cause of death in the 15- to 24-year-old age group and the leading cause of death for black men in the same age category (Neinstein, 2013; US Census Bureau, 2011). Between 1999 and 2008, the homicide rate remained fairly static at approximately 5.4 deaths per 100,000 population; this is a significant decline from the rate seen in the early 1990s, and there are ongoing efforts to understand what has contributed to the reduction (USDHHS, 2015). Firearms are involved in approximately two-thirds of these deaths, and men have twice the risk of dying as do women (US Census Bureau, 2011). When compared with the general population, death rates are higher for men in poorer populations, in urban areas, and with less formal education. Homicide is closely associated with alcohol and drug abuse and is frequently related to other violent acts, such as assaults and robbery. Other risk factors include a history of loss of employment, detention or prison experience, access to firearms, abuse in the home, mental illness, social isolation, and homelessness. The presence of firearms in the home is associated with the increased risk of unintentional and intentional injury to children. A target in *Healthy People 2020* is to reduce firearm-related deaths from 10.5 per 100,000 population in 2012 to 9.3 per 100,000 population and to reduce the number of nonfatal firearm-related injuries from 20.9 per 100,000 in 2010 to 18.6 per 100,000. The firearm-related death rate for young black men and boys was nearly five times the rate for young white men and boys (USDHHS, 2015).

Intimate partner violence has serious health consequences for women and men; however, because of social and legal factors, it is probably the most underreported form of abuse (Box 22-5: Diversity Awareness). Abuse crosses all socioeconomic, racial, ethnic, religious, gender, and age boundaries. Approximately 3 in 10 women and 1 in 10 men during their lifetime report intimate partner violence or abuse. Women report higher lifetime and more recent-year intimate partner violence than men (Black et al., 2011). Nurses and other primary health care providers assist in detecting or treating violence or abuse in an optimal manner; they can help others to understand the cultural background of abuse. However, more efforts must be made to recognize the scope of the problem and to provide appropriate counseling (see Box 22-5: Diversity Awareness). Physical assaults by intimate partners decreased in the last decade; this reduction is attributed to increased economic opportunities for women, increased age at first marriage, and better access to domestic violence services. A target in *Healthy People 2020* is to reduce the rate of physical assault to 19.2 assaults per 1000 from 22 assaults per 1000 recorded in 2012 (USDHHS, 2015).

## Sexuality-Reproductive Pattern

By young adulthood the menstrual cycle is generally well established in the woman. Cyclical hormonal function is responsible for regularity of the cycle and normal functioning of the ovaries and uterus. The normal duration of menses is 4 to 5 days (range of 2–7 days, with a blood loss of 40 mL). Blood loss greater than 80 mL per cycle is abnormal and may lead to anemia. Irregularities such as painful menstruation, premenstrual syndrome, and prolonged or heavy bleeding need further assessment. Although these problems are not always abnormal, the symptoms and the individual's reaction to them can signal functional disorders and the need for further investigation and treatment.

---

### BOX 22-5  DIVERSITY AWARENESS
*Partner and Family Violence: Gender and Culture Differences*

**Assessing the Problem**

Epidemiological researchers have attempted to determine the risks for intimate partner and family violence. Intimate partner violence includes four behaviors: physical violence, sexual violence, threats of physical or sexual violence, and/or emotional abuse. Understanding the roots of partner violence has been more difficult than ascertaining determinants of physical disease. The victims of family violence are usually children, the female spouse, intimate partners, and elderly people (Black et al., 2011). Factors associated with intimate partner violence include young age, low income, pregnancy, mental health problems, separation or divorce, and a history of abuse. The unequal position of women in a relationship and the manner in which conflict is managed, as well as differences in culture, education, and prestige associated with the partners' occupations, are related to the risk of violence. Domestic violence is a problem in all age, ethnic, and religious groups; in some cultures, attitudes toward women even legitimize the practice. Women who have gained positions of respect and power outside the home through activities in their neighborhood or community are less likely to be abused. In men and women, viewing abuse as a child increases the likelihood that abusive behaviors are used by these same individuals as adults (Landenburger & Campbell, 2012).

**Are Nurses Willing to Take Action?**

Some studies indicate that nurses have been reluctant to take action regarding violence against women or men. Some of the traditional reasons for not taking action are based on paternalistic attitudes, in which the victim is blamed for his or her part in the social situation that becomes violent. Nursing's strong advocacy stance and emphasis on the communication of nonjudgmental, genuine concern should provide a strong foundation to avoid blaming the victim and to focus on pathological factors that have been identified by much of the health profession's research in this area.

**How Can Nurses Recognize Abuse?**

Research demonstrates that nurses should be more aware of indicators of partner violence. These include the presence, as revealed by a health history, of separation or divorce, alcoholism, frequent verbal disagreements, and high levels of conflict. Other warning signs include repeated visits to emergency departments, complaints of headaches or backaches, psychiatric illness, and incidents of bruises, sprains, and lacerations. Abusers are more likely to have hostile personality styles with aggressive tendencies. As children, they may have had unattainable goals, and their achievements may have been met with harsh criticism and toxic and depersonalizing behavior (Landenburger & Campbell, 2012). Abusers may also use passive aggressive tactics, turning passive withdrawal and blaming behaviors against the helping individual in an effort to portray the abuser as a victim.

**What Do You Think?**

- Are nurses less than helpful in their detection and management of domestic violence? Why do you think this occurs?
- Are nurses, because of their education and sensitization to people with mental problems, more or less likely than others to experience violence in their own domestic settings? Explain why.

From Black, M. C., Basile, K. C., Breiding, M. J., Smith, S. G., Walters, M. L., Merrick, M. T., et al. (2011). *National Intimate Partner and Sexual Violence Survey (NISVS): 2010 summary report.* Atlanta, GA: National Center for Injury Prevention and Control, Centers for Disease Control and Prevention; Landenburger, K. M., & Campbell, J. C. (2012). Violence and human abuse. In M. Stanhope, & J. Lancaster (Eds.). *Public health nursing: Population-centered health care in the community* (pp. 828–853). St. Louis: Elsevier.

## Reproductive Problems

Infertility is defined as the lack of conception in the presence of unprotected sexual intercourse for at least 12 months. Approximately 10% to 15% of couples of reproductive age in the United States are believed to be infertile (Perry et al., 2013). Infertility has become more of a public issue since the advance of assisted reproductive technologies, such as in vitro fertilization and gamete intrafallopian transfer, which can enable couples with known reproductive problems to conceive children. These technologies frequently create great stress for the couple and often result in marital conflicts and distress. Infertility is not an issue for those in the 18- to 25-year age range as peak fertility is from age 20 years to age 35 years; however, after the age of 30 years, infertility is more common and a more specific diagnostic workup or referral for some type of assisted reproductive strategy may be indicated.

Common problems of the male reproductive system include orchitis, epididymitis, and varicoceles and hydroceles. Mumps in the postpubertal male can cause swelling of the testes, orchitis, and subfertility. Even with appropriate vaccination, mumps cases are becoming more prevalent as the mumps vaccine is not fully effective (Lewis et al., 2015). External conditions such as fungal infections, contact dermatitis, and eczema; parasites such as mites (scabies) and lice; and nonvenereal diseases such as erysipelas, abscesses, and fistulas can occur in the scrotum.

## Unintended Pregnancy

According to the US Census Bureau (2011), the teen birth rate in the United States has been declining since 1990. Improved child health and development is associated with healthy planned pregnancies. Unwanted or unplanned pregnancies can be a considerable source of stress to young adults. Unintended pregnancy is an important public health issue and relates to increased risks of delayed prenatal care, depression, and other personal and relationship problems (USDHHS, 2015). Family planning is one of the biggest public health achievements of the 20th century. Despite the advent of modern contraceptives, unintended pregnancy remains a persistent problem. Approximately half of all pregnancies are intended (USDHHS, 2015); in 2006, 51% of all pregnancies among females aged 15 to 44 years were intended, and the target for intended pregnancies in the United States in 2020 is 56%. Although most young adults consider family planning services as an essential basic health service, health insurance plans historically have attempted to manage and limit such services (USDHHS, 2015). Under the Affordable Care Act, preventive health for women must be covered with no cost sharing. This would include all FDA-approved contraceptive and sterilization methods, in addition to appropriate teaching and counseling (ACA, 2017). The current lower pregnancy rates among teens seem to result from increased involvement in school activities, effective birth control and pregnancy prevention programs, and expanding job opportunities.

College women have high rates of reported sexual violence, STIs, and unintended pregnancy that result most often from the influence of alcohol on risky behavior, lack of negotiation for sexual consent, and haphazard contraceptive use (Fantasia et al.,

2014). First-year students are particularly vulnerable (Demers et al., 2015). To address these problems, colleges and universities have adopted stricter institutional policies and educational programs aimed at making college students fully aware of what an authentic sexual consent entails to protect victims (DeMatteo et al., 2015). The recent reporting on the inadequacies of college/university policies on sexual consent has forced higher education institutions to be more proactive and forthcoming with early incoming student counseling and elaborate policies governing appropriate student campus behavior.

Approximately half of unintended pregnancies are the result of contraceptive failure. Both married and unmarried young adults need information about contraceptives (Table 22-2) to decrease the number of unwanted pregnancies and the need for abortions. The nurse's role in contraceptive counseling involves helping individuals to choose the method most appropriate to their needs. New and improved contraceptive agents are continually becoming available (Nelson, 2015), so the nurse must understand current techniques; for example, two types of intrauterine devices are now available, the ParaGard T 380A (copper) and the Mirena hormonal device (levonorgestrel releasing), and once placed they are highly effective (Eisenberg et al., 2015). Laws and policies in some settings restrict nurses and other health care providers from engaging in certain types of counseling, including providing abortion information. Increasing the services offered by funded planning clinics is also necessary. In 2010, 53.6% of publically funded planning clinics offered the full range of FDA-approved methods, and the target for 2020 is 67% (USDHHS, 2015).

Emergency contraception can reduce the number of unintended pregnancies. In 2010, 81% of family planning clinics offered emergency contraception, and the *Healthy People 2020* target is 87.7%, a 10% increase (USDHHS, 2015). There is a generic two-dose form, Next Choice, and a one-dose form, Plan B One-Step (Teva). The FDA approved over-the-counter use for women of all ages reports that Plan B One-Step is safe and effective. In the United States, progestin-only emergency contraception is available on the shelf without any age restriction (includes Plan B One-Step and generics). Emergency contraception must be started within 3 days of unprotected sex; it works by either altering tubal transport of either sperm or ova, or inhibiting implantation. It will not terminate an existing pregnancy, and it does not provide protection against STIs. The choice to use emergency contraception is frequently made with the partner and may involve complex decision-making centering on responsibility, relationship power, and a woman's right to choose and autonomy over her body (Beaulieu et al., 2011).

## Prenatal Care

Access to prenatal care and financing of sufficient care are critical concerns. High-risk and minority women do not receive sufficient prenatal care. Lack of insurance coverage and less-than-adequate referral mechanisms exist. The well-being of mothers and their infants affects the next generation. Racial and ethnic disparities exist, especially for black American infants (USDHHS, 2015). In 2007 the proportion of mothers receiving care during the first trimester of pregnancy was 70.8%; the target in *Healthy*

**TABLE 22-2 Summary of Risks and Noncontraceptive Benefits of Selected Contraceptive Methods**

| Contraceptive Method | Risks of Use | Noncontraceptive Health Benefits |
|---|---|---|
| Oral contraceptives (various formulations: extended, combined, monophasic, biphasic, triphasic, multiphasic, and progestin only) | Thromboembolic disorders, CVA, coronary artery disease especially with smoking, hypertension, diabetes, breast cancer | Reduced risk of functional pelvic inflammation, endometriosis, uterine fibroids, endometrial cancer, ovarian cancer, iron-deficiency anemia, ectopic pregnancy, irregular cycles |
| Transdermal (contraceptive patch: Ortho Evra) | Similar to oral contraceptives | Easy verification of presence, weekly application |
| Implants (subdermal rod: Nexplanon) | Similar to oral contraceptives, data more limited | Similar to oral contraceptives, data more limited |
| Injectable progestin (Depo-Provera) | Prolonged amenorrhea, venous thrombosis, thromboembolism | Bone loss especially in adolescents, unsure of lifetime risk of osteoporosis |
| Vaginal ring (Nuvaring) | Similar to oral contraceptives, increased risks of cardiovascular events | Vaginal ring hormonal option |
| Intrauterine contraceptive device (IUD: Mirena) | Bleeding, anemia, difficult removal, PID, ectopic pregnancy, cramping | Reduced risk of anemia, low cost for long term |
| Emergency contraception (Next Choice, Plan B One-Step) | Nausea, abdominal pain, delay of menses | Not for routine use |
| Diaphragm | Toxic shock syndrome, allergy to latex or spermicide, urinary tract infection | Reduced risk of vaginitis, cervicitis |
| Condom | Allergy to rubber, latex, or spermicide | Reduced risk of STI and HIV transmission |
| Spermicides* | Sensitivity to agent | Antiviral activity against HPV, decreased activity of other STIs, decreased risk of PID |
| Sponge | Toxic shock syndrome | Decreased activity of STI organisms |
| Female sterilization (tubal ligation) | Anesthesia, infection, hemorrhage | One-time procedure |
| Male sterilization (vasectomy) | Complication rates low, reversal may be difficult | One-time procedure |

*Often used in combination with other methods.
*CVA,* Cerebrovascular accident; *HPV,* human papilloma virus; *PID,* pelvic inflammatory disease; *STI,* sexually transmitted infection.
From Hatcher, R. A., Trussell, J., Nelson, A. L., Cates, W., Kowal, D., & Policar, M. (2012). Contraceptive technology (20th ed.). London: Ardent Media; Nelson, A. (2015). Transdermal contraception methods: Today's patches and new options. *Expert Opinion on Pharmacology, 16*(6), 863–873.

*People 2020* is 77.6% (USDHHS, 2015). The proportion of mothers receiving early prenatal care needs to increase most in American Indian or Alaska Native and black non-Hispanic mothers (USDHHS, 2015). Another target of *Healthy People 2020,* which reviewed both *early* and *adequate* prenatal care, indicated that as of 2007, 70.5% of pregnant females received adequate care, and the 2020 target hopes to raise this to 77.6% (USDHHS, 2015). The reasons why women do not seek early prenatal care are varied but may include the insensitivity and cultural biases of providers.

### Sexually Transmitted Diseases

Young adults aged 20 to 24 years are the group at highest risk of STIs, although the actual rate of infection in this age group has remained fairly stable since 2003 (USDHHS, 2015). Women aged 15 to 19 years and 20 to 24 years have the highest reported rates of chlamydia and gonorrhea respectively (USDHHS, 2015; CDC, 2014). The list of STIs includes HPV infection, *Chlamydia trachomatis* infection, genital herpes, HIV infection, genital mycoplasma infections, cytomegalovirus infection, hepatitis B, and bacterial vaginitis, in addition to the more widely known diseases of syphilis and gonorrhea (Table 22-3). Untreated HPV infection is a risk factor for up to 99% of invasive cervical cancers,

and early recognition of HPV infection has decreased cervical cancer incidence and mortality by 70% (Adams & Carnright, 2013). *Chlamydia trachomatis* is very common, and chlamydia screening efforts should focus on all sexually active nonpregnant and pregnant women aged 24 years or younger (CDC, 2014). The presence of multiple STIs increases the risk of HIV infection. STIs cost billions of dollars in screening, treatment, and reporting. In addition to creating a substantial problem for young adults, STIs impose tremendous demands on health care facilities (USDHHS, 2015). Many cases are unreported and untreated for lack of screening or failure to recognize symptoms. Many young adults do not understand that STIs can be transmitted from oral and anal sex, not just vaginal intercourse. A study sponsored by the CDC found that young adults rarely discussed STIs at home or with partners or close friends; however, young women may look to these intermediary sources if they are worried about having an STI (Friedman & Bloodgood, 2010). Neighborhood structural supports can also be associated with acquisition and incidence of STIs (Ford, 2011; Ford & Browning, 2011). Most of the prevalence statistics on STIs comes from health provider reports; this emphasizes an important nursing role in gathering accurate case information on STIs in the young adult population (Friedman & Bloodgood, 2010).

## TABLE 22-3 Summary of Selected Sexually Transmitted Infections

| Infections | Causative Agent | Diagnostic Methods | Treatment | Risks or Complications | Nursing Teaching |
|---|---|---|---|---|---|
| Viral diseases | Treatment does not eradicate underlying infection | | | | |
| AIDS | HIV | Enzyme immune assay, Western blot, viral tests | Current recommendations | Opportunistic infections, perinatal transmission | Monitor CD4 T lymphocyte analysis and HIV plasma viral load, monitor men who have sex with men, early pregnancy testing strongly recommended |
| Hepatitis B | Hepatitis B virus | Hepatitis B antibody test | No specific therapy available | Perinatal transmission | Routine vaccination or vaccine before pregnancy |
| Genital herpes | Herpes simplex virus | Herpes simplex virus antibody test, culture, viral test | Acyclovir at first diagnosis or episode | Urethral stricture, lymph node enlargement | Examine partners, abstain from sex while symptomatic |
| Genital warts | Human papilloma virus | Clinical inspection, colposcopy, biopsy | Podophyllin, trichloroacetic acid, cryotherapy/laser, valacyclovir, famciclovir | Cervical dysplasia, cervical cancer | Offer Gardasil or Cervarix vaccine and counseling, return for treatment as necessary, treat partner |
| **Bacterial/Other STIs** | | | | | |
| Gonorrhea | *Neisseria gonorrhoeae* | Culture | Ceftriaxone, cefixime, some strains becoming resistant | PID, infertility, ectopic pregnancy | Monitor antibiotic treatment, examine partner, repeat culture, check for chlamydia |
| Syphilis | *Treponema pallidum* | Fluorescent antibody tests of lesion or exudates, VDRL, RPR | Benzathine penicillin G | Secondary/late syphilis | Monitor treatment, test and monitor partner |
| Chlamydia | *Chlamydia trachomatis* | Culture, chlamydia monoclonal antibody test | Azithromycin, doxycycline | Infertility, ectopic pregnancy, urethral scarring, PID, endocervicitis, neonatal infection | Refer partners for evaluation, condoms to prevent future infection |
| Bacterial vaginosis | *Gardnerella vaginalis* | Clinical criteria, wet mount (clue cells) | Metronidazole (Flagyl) | Asymptomatic infection | Sexual transmission not proven |
| Trichomoniasis | *Trichomonas vaginalis* | Trich rapid test, culture (protozoa) | Metronidazole (Flagyl) | Recurrence, excoriation of genital area | Use condoms to prevent new infection |
| Vulvovaginal candidiasis | *Candida albicans,* non–*C. albicans* | Wet mount/potassium hydroxide test (hyphae and spores) | Antifungal medication: butoconazole, miconazole, clotrimazole | Recurrence of disease | Reduce moisture/heat in genital area, recheck in 14 days |

*PID,* pelvic inflammatory disease; *RPR,* rapid plasma reagin test; *VDRL,* Venereal Disease Research Laboratory test.
Based on information from Centers for Disease Control and Prevention. (2010). Sexually transmitted diseases treatment guidelines, 2010. *MMWR. Morbidity and Mortally Weekly Report, 59*(RR-12), 1–116; Hatcher, R. A., Trussell, J., Nelson, A. L., Cates, W., Kowal, D., & Policar, M. (2012). *Contraceptive technology* (20th ed.). London: Ardent Media; Perry, S., Hockenberry, M., Lowdermilk, D., & Wilson, D. (2014). *Maternal-child nursing care* (5th ed.). St. Louis: Elsevier.

## Human Immunodeficiency Virus

More than 1 million people were estimated to have HIV infection in the United States (USDHHS, 2015): improved longevity of infected persons and better treatment have made HIV infection more like a chronic disease. Meeting the treatment or prevention needs of this large group of chronically infected persons, especially HIV-positive low-income Americans, has become a priority. An important challenge is to develop more effective strategies to prevent new infections and improved case finding (USDHHS, 2015). In 2010, the White House published a three-pronged HIV/AIDS strategy to reduce the number infected individuals; increase access and care for affected individuals; and reduce HIV health-related disparities. HIV is transmitted by sexual intercourse (oral, vaginal, anal), shared needles, and infected blood. Another less common source of transmission is from the mother to the baby across the placental barrier or through breast milk. The higher level of worry about contracting HIV and other STIs in young adults is correlated with the implementation of risk-reduction behaviors. The incidence of STIs is greatly reduced with proper use of condoms. In *Healthy People 2020,* use of condoms in various age groups surpassed the targets (USDHHS, 2015), and condom use is considered to be increasing. Prevention education is aimed at all high-risk groups, including heterosexuals and men who have sex with men. All sexually active individuals are counseled on the hazards of unprotected sexual activity and on the effective use and limitations of condoms, stressing that they must be used properly and can fail. Condom failures occur at an estimated rate of 10% to 15%; therefore counseling should stress that condom use is not foolproof. Another success is the decline in perinatal transmission. The rates of HIV perinatal transmission are greatly reduced by drug therapy during pregnancy, changes in obstetric practice, and prohibition of breastfeeding in infected mothers. The US Public Health Service highly recommends voluntary testing for HIV and counseling as a part of basic prenatal care (USPSTF, 2015).

The nurse's role in intervening with regard to STIs includes providing treatment, early diagnosis, and education. When an individual is suspected of having an STI, the nurse obtains a complete history, including sexual history, sexual contacts, previous treatment and test results, any signs or symptoms of a current infection, recent use of antibiotics, and allergic reactions to antibiotics. When treatment is required, the nurse ensures that the person understands the goals of treatment in an attempt to gain cooperation, including follow-up care with partners and adherence to the care plan.

The nurse is an educator not only of the individual but also of the general public (Ford & Browning, 2011). Appropriate health education for the individual with an STI includes the mode of transmission, incubation periods, signs and symptoms, methods of treatment, complications resulting from lack of treatment, and signs of recurrent infections.

## Coping–Stress Tolerance Pattern

### Assessment of Stress Levels

Stress, the result of forces operating on the individual that disrupt physiological or psychological equilibrium, is an integral part of young adulthood; therefore a comprehensive health assessment should include questions to determine stress levels. Anxiety, nervousness, depression, or somatic complaints are indicators of stress, as are events such as divorce, loss of employment, failure to be promoted, or financial difficulties. The role of the nurse is to listen, offer support, and demonstrate concern. The nurse also suggests referrals to appropriate health providers and support groups.

### Achievement-Oriented Stress

Achievement-oriented stress differs from the stress of situational crises in that the stress of an overachiever is derived from internal pressures to succeed as measured by self-defined goals. Among many other stressors, young adults are often engaged in higher education programs at the college or university level. Achievement-oriented stress frequently causes workaholic habits, including loss of sleep and omission of meals. When this behavior becomes extreme, there can be serious physical and emotional consequences, such as nutrition problems or burnout, which, in turn, leads to severe emotional and physical exhaustion. Workaholic behaviors may not be perceived by the individual and may not be apparent until changes in body functions or behavior occur. Young adults are generally health conscious and willing to alter personal lifestyles and behavior patterns to reduce stress and become healthier.

### Suicide and Depression

Suicide is a leading cause of death in the young adult age group. Young adults may be thought of as "young invincibles"; however, they are in an age group exposed to new stressors (Neinstein, 2013). Suicide occurs because many young adults are unable to cope with the pressures of adulthood. For some people, pressure arises when they are dealing with interpersonal conflicts such as marital problems, family discord, or the loss of a close relationship; for others, the precipitating event is a lack of personal resources, unemployment, or dissatisfaction with work or school. Many young adults try to solve their problems before the fatal incident but see no positive solutions; in many cases, a prior suicide attempt was a signal for help.

Suicide rates are higher for men than for women; approximately four to five times as many men as women (18.4 vs. 4.7 deaths per 100,000 population in 2007) take their own lives (US Census Bureau, 2011). However, more women are known to have depressive disorders and to unsuccessfully attempt suicide. Young adults are more likely as a group to attempt suicide than are older individuals, and professionals are more likely to attempt suicide than are nonprofessionals. Suicide is more common among single, widowed, and divorced individuals. Chronically ill young adult males may also be more at risk of depression than young adult females because social support systems are more robust within female relationship networks. Young adults have the lowest rates of health insurance coverage, so a number of these risks can coincide in a "perfect storm" (Neinstein, 2013).

The USPSTF recommends depression screening for adults aged 18 years or older when staff-assisted support is available for adequate diagnosis and treatment. The USPSTF website has a 10-question depression screening survey that includes the following questions: whether in the last month the young adult has been bothered by little interest or pleasure in doing things, and whether the young adult has felt down, depressed, or hopeless in the last month (USPSTF, 2015). A "no" answer to the questions indicates a negative screening result. The USPSTF does not recommend routine screening for suicide or recommend against it because positive research support for routine screening is not clear.

In 2007, approximately 13 per 100,000 population-specific deaths of individuals between the age of 25 years and the age of 34 years were classified as suicides (US Census Bureau, 2011). Nursing interventions are directed toward identifying behaviors in individuals who may be contemplating suicide. Presuicidal individuals also tend to exhibit impaired reality testing; feelings of hopelessness, helplessness, and rejection; impaired judgment and decision-making; anxiety; weight loss; insomnia; or a radically changed affect. In addition to identifying presuicidal behaviors, the nurse also investigates relationship patterns to determine behaviors that are complicated by feelings of worthlessness and defeat. When the nurse identifies a young adult at risk of a suicide attempt, referrals to other professionals are indicated.

If the health care provider becomes more concerned that the young adult may be at risk of suicide, the following two questions may be asked: "What thoughts have you had about hurting yourself or even killing yourself?" To question further the nurse can ask, "Have you actually done anything to hurt yourself?" (Depression Management Tool Kit, 2009; USPSTF, 2015). Even with education of the public and health care providers about the incidence of suicide in the young adult population, suicide continues to be a major health problem, and annual rates, especially for young men, remain high.

## Values-Beliefs Pattern

Young adults enter their 20s with habits, values, and beliefs acquired during childhood and adolescence. Many acquired habits foster continuance of practices that are hazardous to health and well-being in later life. Prevention is directed toward altering value and belief patterns that encourage poor health practices, and reorienting them toward those that support optimal health behaviors. Nursing care is more effective when the nurse can describe, discriminate, identify, and align value and belief patterns consistent with practices known to maximize health.

### Values Involved in Parenting

Parenthood is envisioned as an important developmental stage by most young adults; therefore health-promotion and health-protection activities to ensure healthy offspring are crucial (see the case study and care plan at the end of this chapter). **Genetic impairments**, or **congenital defects** caused by abnormal chromosomes, are responsible for 4% to 6% of perinatal deaths (Perry et al., 2013). Tests are available for approximately 200 genetic diseases (Perry et al., 2013). Most of the genetic testing offered is for single-gene impairment to mothers and fathers who have a family history of genetic disease. Young adults with a genetic disease must make many important decisions; predicting the transmission of the disease to potential offspring is essential to future planning.

### Values Regarding Prenatal Diagnosis and Genetic Impairment

Extensive prenatal diagnostic procedures have been available since the mid-1960s. This capability has enabled the identification of high-risk pregnancies and requires the cooperation and education of childbearing women and their partners, both of whom must provide accurate family health and obstetrical histories and comply with suggested screening and follow-up measures. Decisions about the advisability of reproduction are based on current information on genetics and known deleterious genetic factors.

The finding of a malformed or genetically impaired fetus may result in a parental decision to terminate the pregnancy. Theological and political debates in addition to legislative mandates have greatly influenced family control over many of these decisions. Genetic counseling is an important nursing intervention for young adults. A genetic specialist gives technical explanations of genetic disorders; however, nurses have a strong supportive role in helping young adults decide whether to have children or to carry through a pregnancy that is at risk.

# ENVIRONMENTAL PROCESSES

## Physical Agents

### Ethnicity, Race, and Culture

The young adult whose ethnic background is different from that of the dominant culture may encounter prejudice and discrimination, which can occur because of differences in race, creed, language, attitudes, values, preferences, or behaviors. The young adult is susceptible to these prejudices at work, at school, in health care delivery systems, and in the community.

Race and ethnicity are closely connected to educational and work-related decisions, which subsequently affect the choice of residence. Many minority families live in substandard housing or crowded living spaces. A lifestyle on the margins, when combined with insufficient economic resources, frequently affects health. Poverty is more common among black families, which often leads to unmet basic needs of food, clothing, and housing and, in turn, leads to decreased regard for health needs.

### Accidents

Injuries are the leading cause of death in young adults and individuals younger than 44 years (USDHHS, 2015). Motor vehicle accidents cause more fatalities than all other causes of death combined. Reducing speed limits contributes to lower fatality rates. Most states have seat belt laws, and all states have seat belt requirements for children. All individuals in the car need to use seat belts because an unrestrained occupant can cause harm to another passenger in a crash. In 2013, 87% of motor vehicle drivers and front seat occupants used seat belts, and the target for 2020 is 92.4% (USDHHS, 2015). Distracted driving, texting while driving, and cell phone use are the cause of many motor vehicle crashes. Most states have enacted "hand-free" or Bluetooth wireless audio legislation that limits the use of hand-held car cell phones. The continued high incidence of vehicle accidents in the young adult age group is related to accessibility of cars to young adults and peer pressure on driving behavior; reckless driving and driving under the influence of alcohol and drugs are now viewed as closely connected to violent and abusive behavior. A number of states have specific rules that limit cell phone use by drivers younger than 18 years.

Accident-prevention education, long considered appropriate for young children, is an important part of young adult instruction. Most young licensed drivers have participated in driver education courses, and a number of states have adopted progressive licensing programs. A number of states have "graduated driver licensing" programs (Trust for America's Health & Robert Wood Johnson Foundation, 2015), which have been shown to reduce younger driver crash rates by 8% to 14%. In 2015, 46 states had banned texting while driving, and two additional states ban texting by novice drivers (National Institutes of Health, 2014a). The young adult must understand the potentially fatal consequences of aggressive tendencies or thoughtless risk-taking. When young adults are encouraged to reflect on the consequences of their actions, they tend to be more willing to control and change unsafe driving behaviors.

## Biological Agents

### Noise Pollution

Young adults are exposed to high levels of noise in occupational and recreational settings (concerts and nightclubs). Long-term exposure to loud noise is directly related to impaired hearing and can increase irritability and stress. Young adults can be exposed to noises in the work setting from industrial machinery and equipment. Although industrial exposure can be difficult to mitigate, many young adults worsen the situation through recreational exposure, by listening to music or music videos at excessively high decibel levels. Ear protection is necessary to prevent hearing disability. Recognition of hazards and corresponding appropriate preventive education are early nursing strategies for decreasing excessive noise exposure.

### Air Pollution

Motor vehicles are the largest source of air pollution; vehicles release tons of particles and noxious gases each year, most of which is either carbon monoxide or hydrocarbons. Carbon monoxide in high concentrations is deadly; in lower concentrations, it causes headaches, dizziness, and heart palpitations. In sunlight and low-lying areas, automobile exhaust becomes photochemical smog that contains ozone, which irritates the eyes and the respiratory tract. Although air pollution is not a problem only for young adults, they frequently work in dirty, entry-level jobs in industrial settings and may be among the age group that is most affected.

### Occupational Hazards and Stressors

Occupational hazards pose a threat of illness, injury, or death in all age groups, and occupational safety standards have contributed greatly to the reduction of work-related accidents. The Occupational Safety and Health Act (1970) has resulted in the improvement of work conditions, along with the provision of health care facilities, in many companies.

Young adults should not be allowed to work in certain industrial settings without vocational training to reduce hazards. Young adults frequently want a challenge and high wages; therefore they work in hazardous jobs—for example, on offshore drilling rigs, on high bridges, or in nuclear plants. Because of their age, physical stamina, and agility, young adults are suitable candidates for positions that require extreme physical abilities. Occupational training should include education about personal exposure risks, identification of work-related hazards, and identification of situations in which the severity of accidents is connected to personal behaviors or habits. For example, drivers of heavy construction machinery should be particularly observant, avoid reckless behaviors, and avoid fast driving. Working women who are pregnant can expose their fetuses to industrial chemicals.

Proper evaluation and temporary reassignment may be necessary.

Occupational preventive intervention requires that known work hazards and risks be identified early. Health histories should include questions about the place of work, type of work, and young adults' understanding of the risks associated with their occupations. Occupational risk and health are closely related; stress associated with work, the use of alcohol or drugs, and a negative attitude toward work are predictive of occupational injuries. Job counseling aimed at changing the nature of employment can be an appropriate referral for some people with health conditions. Nurses in occupational settings can provide periodic health assessments, updates of the health history, and counseling.

## Chemical Agents

### Drug Use

Misuse of drugs, a major risk for young adults, is associated with injury, disability, violence, homicide, and suicide and is related to social problems (criminal behaviors and maladjustment to accepted norms) (Neinstein, 2013). Drug abuse, including inappropriate use of prescription drugs (National Institutes of Health, 2014b), may be closely related to an inability to cope appropriately with adult responsibilities. Physical health problems associated with drug misuse account for more than 50% of the major acute and chronic problems of young adults. Heroin users have increased mortality rates because of overdosage or chronic disability associated with hepatitis infections. Drug use is an independent risk factor involved in HIV infections (USDHHS, 2015).

Misuse and overuse of drugs, including prescription drugs and opioids, is widespread. Heroin use more than doubled among young adults aged 18 to 25 years in the past decade, and death from heroin use is now overtaking deaths from motor vehicles in many states (CDC, 2015b; Neinstein, 2013; Trust for America's Health & Robert Wood Johnson Foundation, 2015). Young adults are more likely to use illicit drugs and abuse prescription pain relievers (Neinstein, 2013). In addition, young adult males may also use performance-enhancing drugs such as anabolic steroids. Drug interactions can be fatal. Preventive education should focus on cautious drug use, healthier sports, and exercise. Nursing activities include preventive strategies to curb the problem of drug misuse. Distribution of current drug literature, early treatment of complications, and information regarding drug treatment centers are only part of the answer. Some states have drug monitoring enforcement of prescription drugs by providers, and more widespread legislation is recommended (Trust for America's Health & Robert Wood Johnson Foundation, 2015). Nursing efforts and political activities aimed at increasing personal prescribing awareness and altering drug-taking attitudes and behaviors are of critical importance (Box 22-6: Genomics).

### Alcohol Use

Alcohol-related accidents among individuals aged 15 to 24 years continue to be a leading cause of preventable morbidity, disability, and death. Heavy alcohol use, that is, consumption of five or more drinks on at least one occasion within a month, is more

## BOX 22-6 GENOMICS

### Pharmacogenetics: Genomics and Personalized Medicine

Different genetic types tend to metabolize drugs differently, have different binding receptors, or have different environmental influences that change the utilization and uptake. This field of study is called pharmacogenetics. Early clues to variation in drug response were seen in comparisons of populations from different racial and ethnic backgrounds, so there are important cultural awareness implications of these avenues of study. DNA (nucleotide) gene variations are known as single nucleotide polymorphisms (SNPs) and are caused by the substitution of one nucleotide base for another. When these SNPs direct liver metabolic enzymes, the polymorphism or form of the gene inherited causes differences in drug metabolism.

In many ways, gene selection had positive effects on evolution and favored the chances of a population to survive. For example, sickle cell trait developed through selection factors that favored resistance to malaria. Similarly, gene selection factors also favored the prevalence of glucose 6-phosphate dehydrogenase deficiency, which also provides resistance to malaria but causes drug-related red blood cell hemolysis. In related studies of warfarin response, ethnic differences were shown to affect bioavailability and distribution, which could be controlled through more precise clinical management and dosage regulation. Warfarin dosing is significantly altered by polymorphisms in the liver and enzymes affecting vitamin K synthesis.

In studies of people with hypertension, black individuals responded with a greater decrease in systolic pressure in response to thiazide diuretics (hydrochlorothiazide) and calcium channel blockers. Black individuals have a blunted response to alpha-blockers, which can be increased by addition of a diuretic. Many black individuals have renin sensitivity, which would have favored survival in warmer climates.

The situation in Asians appears to be the exact opposite. In a study of the effectiveness of propranolol in Chinese and white men, the Chinese men had at least twice as much sensitivity as did the white men to propranolol administered at several different dosages. Studies indicate that Asians are more sensitive to alcohol and its drug effects than are whites. The most outstanding difference is in the amount of facial flushing, which was experienced by a substantial percentage of Asians compared with whites. The enzyme alcohol dehydrogenase is reported to be absent in approximately half of Asians.

These examples suggest that nurses should be much more attuned to potential genetic variations that alter drug metabolism and effectiveness. In individuals who do not respond to certain drugs as expected, the nurse may consider whether this might be related to constitutional factors within the person's genomic makeup. Pharmacogenetic research also invites rethinking of managed care practices that restrict diversity of drug use with prescribed drug formulary listings.

From Kudzma, E., & Carey, E. (2009). Pharmacogenomics: Personalizing drug response. *American Journal of Nursing*, *109*(10), 50–58.

common in 18- to 24-year-olds than it is for younger or older adults (Neinstein, 2013; USDHHS, 2015). Raising the legal drinking age to 21 years reduces not only deaths and injuries connected to motor vehicle accidents but also homicides and other violent deaths. All 50 states have now set a maximum blood alcohol concentration of 0.08% for driving while intoxicated enforcement and prosecution. Alcohol abuse is directly related to chronic conditions such as cirrhosis. Modifying alcohol consumption in young adults can decrease the frequency of chronic and disabling conditions in later life.

Binge alcohol consumption is increasing in the young adult population. In 2008, 27% of young adults aged 18 years or older reported that they have engaged in binge drinking in the previous 30 days (USDHHS, 2015). In the 18- to 22-year-old age group, binge drinking is higher among full-time college students than those not enrolled full-time (Neinstein, 2013). In a 2004–2006 study, approximately 7% of young military veterans had a substance abuse problem (USDHHS, 2015). This is important as many young adult men have participated in military operations. Although young adults may drink less frequently than older adults, there is a tendency to consume larger amounts of alcohol at a time; the tendency is toward binge drinking, which causes increased loss of control and is related to an additional risk of automobile crashes. Teens with work schedules of more than 10 hours per week are more often involved in heavy or binge drinking, or both. Working longer hours increases the money available to purchase alcohol and exposes the teen to older adults who drink.

## Tobacco Use

Smoking is a leading cause of preventable death in the United States; therefore smoking cessation is the single most important counseling topic for all people because of its potential to lower the risk of contracting many preventable diseases. More than one-third of current smokers aged 18 to 24 years started smoking before the age of 16 years. Cigarette smoking rates among people aged 18 years or older continued to decline from the 1998 baseline of 24% to a 2013 level of 18.3% (USDHHS, 2015). Whereas general smoking rates are declining, younger adults are more likely than older adults to try or use e-cigarettes; the use of e-cigarettes was highest in current and recent former smokers (Schoenborn & Gindi, 2015). An ancillary goal of *Healthy People 2020* to keep the smoking rate low is to increase tobacco cessation counseling in office-based ambulatory settings and hospital ambulatory settings. To augment antismoking efforts, tobacco advertising and sales have been limited, and the federal excise tax has been increased.

Individuals employed in high-risk occupations (e.g., mining, construction) are informed of the synergistic relationship between smoking and other environmental exposures, including exposure to asbestos, coal dust, and radiation. Fear tactics, nagging, preaching, and threats are generally ineffective in convincing people to stop smoking. A major barrier to smoking cessation is the presence of other smokers, particularly in situations where alcohol is also being consumed.

State enforcement of no-smoking policies is important. Between 2005 and 2009, lung cancer death rates declined in states with strong tobacco control enforcement and increased in states where tobacco control measures were weak. Tobacco control measures are strongly correlated with smoking cessation rates of young adults (Henley, et al., 2014). Nurses are familiar with the antismoking resources in their communities, enabling them to make the appropriate referrals.

## Carcinogens

Young adults can be exposed to environmental carcinogens in their work settings or through unhealthy practices such as having multiple sexual partners. In the work setting, environmental regulations have limited exposure to some hazardous chemicals, but the long-term effects on health of exposure to many industrial chemicals remains unknown. In health care, latex, long considered inert and safe, has now been shown to cause long-term immune system disease in some nurses exposed to it (or the chemicals that bind it) in surgical gloves.

# DETERMINANTS OF HEALTH

## Social Factors and Environment

### Neighborhood Resources

The environment of the community strongly influences the well-being of the young adult and sets the standard for the health of people and families living within a neighborhood. Neighbors can be an excellent source of support, which can be especially important to a young mother who does not have immediate family nearby. Nurses working in community settings facilitate the contact of individuals with common interests through community and religious activities and support groups. Community resources for exercise and recreation can make important contributions to the young adult's physical and emotional health. When these resources are available, the young adult can have the opportunity to exercise and release stress in a positive fashion.

## Levels of Policy Making and Health

Young adults are one of the major political constituencies in the United States, as seen in their involvement in recent presidential elections; they support many causes and have the time and energy to publicize issues related to the common good. Some of these issues involve unemployment, college debt, sustainability, pollution, the environment, nuclear energy, and war. Relative to health, predominant issues have involved housing and health care in neighborhoods and rural areas and health, agricultural, and sanitation concerns in foreign countries. Through these efforts, young adults can influence and improve living conditions for future generations.

One of the young adult's age-related tasks is to choose and develop a lifelong career. This choice is directly related to economic factors; young adults want satisfying occupations that also yield adequate economic returns. To manage financially and maintain a lifestyle in which personal needs can be met, young adults may elect to have fewer children. Caring for aging parents can also cause physical, psychosocial, spiritual, and economic stress.

Although goals differ greatly among young adult couples, they are generally concerned with acquiring material comforts; the desire for housing, transportation, clothing, or recreation generally necessitates that both partners are employed to meet financial obligations. This desire necessitates the changing of roles and the sharing of responsibilities, and open communication becomes a crucial component.

New career opportunities and the economic expansion in the United States during the 1990s allowed young adults obtaining first jobs more career choices. The growing technology industry provided employment in a wide variety of occupations and start-up companies. Work styles within these companies tend to be different from those in the traditional workplace, including an expectation of longer and more fluid workdays. Internet-based companies provide young adults with jobs that have the potential to give them rapid financial rewards at the cost of long-term job stability. Since 2012 the employment rate of young adults aged 18 to 24 years (54%) has been at its lowest since data were collected in 1948. Between 2008–2011, employed young adults also experienced more of a decline in weekly paychecks (decline of 6%) than any other employed age group (Pew Research Center, 2012). Because of the high cost of housing, many young adults have multiple roommates, creating additional demands and health risks. Some continue to live with their parents (Burn & Szoeke, 2016). Some young adults are interested in giving back to society by taking employment at lower salaries in nonprofit agencies involved in education and social issues, such as Habitat for Humanity, and going abroad in the Peace Corps to promote human rights in countries where such rights are nonexistent.

For many young adult couples, problems of unemployment for one or both, different careers, friends, and differing maturity levels place additional strains on their relationship. These circumstances can provide a basis for domestic difficulty. Domestic arguments can precede family disruption, leading to marital separation or divorce. In addition to the emotional strain placed on family members, domestic arguments can result in aggressive acts of abuse and personal injury. Young adults can also be faced with decisions about day care facilities; the couple or mother may need support to resolve guilt feelings related to the separation from the child. Some young adults may also bear responsibilities for caring for aging parents or relatives.

Lifestyles may also include living arrangements with individuals of the same sex or the opposite sex. Although these lifestyles are becoming more acceptable in today's society, attitudes toward varied lifestyles contribute pressures that lead to further stress and uncertainty.

## Health Services/Delivery System

The availability of health services is important. Improving health services generally means finding usual and continuing sources of primary/preventive care. Economic realities, however, influence the effectiveness of resources, particularly for the young adult who lives in an economically depressed area. In some communities, health services are lacking or, when available, are not culturally sensitive or adapted to the customs and beliefs of the people who are served. Access to public transportation can be a critical problem, affecting the ability of the young adult to keep appointments. Young adults have the fewest outpatient health care visits and the highest number of emergency department visits (Neinstein, 2013). Young adults aged 18 to 24 years are the least likely of any age group to have a usual source of care (Hing & Albert, 2016); thus a target of *Healthy People 2020* is to increase the proportion of young adults with a usual primary care provider (USDHHS, 2015). Gaps in health care insurance coverage that occur between the end of schooling and the attainment of full employment can reduce the access of young adults to primary care. The Affordable Care Act, passed in 2010 (https://www.hhs.gov/healthcare/), mandates coverage for young adults up to the age of 26 years within family health insurance coverage. This act has decreased the young adult uninsured rate somewhat from 28% to 24% (Neinstein, 2013) and has maintained millions of young adults insured on the family health plans (Sommers et al., 2013).

Health delivery methods in the United States are based primarily on Western belief systems, which tend to be rigid in their applications. For example, women seeking birth control information and prescriptions are expected to use health clinics and adhere to a set schedule of return visits. The most common insurance claims for young adult women are associated with gynecology and obstetrics (Neinstein, 2013). Because health care provider systems have removed many traditional barriers once assumed to be responsible for poor utilization of services by low-income or minority groups (insurance, location and scheduling), nonattendance at scheduled clinic visits is frequently interpreted as nonadherence. Nurses need to be able to identify health practices and health system gaps that are barriers to care and harmful to people.

Nursing comprises the largest group of professionals within the US health care system. However, nurses may not be able to deliver care optimally within changing health care settings because of barriers to practice and ineffective workforce planning, data, and information infrastructure. A widely circulated report from the Institute of Medicine (2010) noted that the nursing profession cannot contribute optimally unless nurses fully participate in team planning and health care redesign with physicians and other health care professionals. In addition, business, government, health delivery agencies, and the insurance industry must all participate in a newly designed health care system that provides accessible, affordable quality care, leading to increases in measurable health outcomes (Institute of Medicine, 2010) (see the case study and care plan at the end of this chapter).

## NURSING APPLICATION

Young adulthood is generally considered to be the most healthful period of life. In terms of physical changes, growth is complete by this stage. The physical abilities of the young adult are in peak condition, so the goals of the nurse are aimed at maintaining optimal physical condition, encouraging healthy habits, screening individuals for disease, and treating illnesses.

Preventive care is recommended to young adults in the form of screening and preventive care visits (Hing & Albert, 2016). Health examinations at recommended intervals are a crucial component of screening individuals for potential health concerns and providing education about measures to avoid disease and disability. Women are taught about breast self-examinations, whereas testicular self-examinations are taught to men with use of photos, models, and return demonstration.

It is necessary to screen individuals for cardiovascular conditions after the age of 25 years as well as to provide education about risk factor modification. Intervention efforts should reflect diversion of age, sex, ethnicity, and socioeconomic status. As the nurse obtains an assessment of the individual and family history, the necessity of further screening, education, or monitoring is determined. Elements of education include smoking cessation and dietary modifications.

Young adults are encouraged to engage in physical activity and muscle-strengthening exercise. Lack of time or lack of access may be barriers to increased physical activity. The nurse working with the young adult population should consider implementing work site wellness programs. Group fitness or weight loss programs can be an effective means of promoting wellness at work while increasing employee satisfaction and productivity. Some workforce programs use incentive systems where points are awarded for the achievement of particular milestones. Once a set level of points is reached, the employee is given a reward in the form of gift cards or movie tickets. These types of programs are often effective for smoking cessation, weight loss, and exercise. In addition, some companies encourage the formation of facility-sponsored sports teams for charities or sports such as bowling leagues, softball teams, or a running club. This encourages camaraderie among colleagues and increases participation for people who respond well to group motivation. Nonworking young adults looking for a group fitness or sports program should be directed to resources within the community via Internet research.

The nurse working with young adults provides education about skin cancer risk, the need for adequate sunscreen, and signs and symptoms of skin cancer. Safety education is provided about recreational and sports-related injuries and how to prevent them. Additional education is required for young adult females. The nurse may be in a position of providing counseling or referrals for contraception, prenatal care, STIs, and HIV infection. It is imperative that women receive preconceptional and early prenatal care to maintain optimal health for themselves and the unborn child.

The nurse working with the young adult population often becomes a counselor. It is important to assess stressors as prolonged stress, anxiety, or depression can negatively affect the health of the individual. Stressors may be related to relationships, divorce, employment, layoffs, or financial concerns. The nurse listens, offers support and concern, and provides the individual or family with resources or support groups specific to the stressor.

## SUMMARY

Nurses promote health care measures and behaviors at all places where young adults come into contact with the health care delivery system. In community colleges and university settings, efforts can be directed toward health-education curricula with an emphasis on implementation of positive health behaviors, use of appropriate social networking skills, establishment of peer counseling groups, and better utilization of sports and exercise facilities. Workshops on alcoholism, substance abuse, sports or exercise, mental health and self-expression, relationships, and various aspects of sexual care are effective in college and graduate school populations. At the work site, the occupational nurse is involved with employee counseling, blood pressure monitoring and treatment, exercise recommendations, smoking reduction, cafeteria nutrition management, and stress-reduction techniques. Insurance coverage as part of the Affordable Care Act has assisted

## CASE STUDY

### Preparing for Childbearing: Kirsten

Kirsten is a healthy 22-year-old whose favorite sport is running. Most of the time she runs outside, but she also uses gym treadmills. Since this spring, Kirsten has believed that her breathing capacity is diminishing and her levels of energy are decreasing. During her period these symptoms appear to worsen. Last week, while running up a rather steep course, Kirsten became much weaker, dizzier, and more fatigued than usual, and her best friend and running partner recommended that she make a physician's appointment for a physical examination. Kirsten's running partner also noted that she has appeared pale lately.

In the physician's office, Kirsten is noted to have a normal temperature, elevated heart and respiratory rates, and a blood pressure of 90/60 mmHg. Kirsten's description of her period is that it tends to be heavy and has been this way for 5 years. For muscle aches and pains caused by running, she usually takes two aspirin tablets every 3 to 4 hours for as long as 7 days. When her running increases during the summer, she takes aspirin or ibuprofen continually for 2 to 3 months. Diagnostic testing indicates that her hemoglobin level is 7 g/dL, and her red blood cells are pale and small. Kirsten has been in a long-term relationship for several years, her wedding is in several months, and there has been discussion of preconceptional health planning and future children.

### Reflective Questions

- What common health alteration in young adult women is most likely for Kirsten?
- What contributing factors place Kirsten at risk?
- What lifestyle modifications can Kirsten implement to decrease her risk?

## ◎ CARE PLAN

### Preparation for Childbearing: Kirsten

**\*NURSING DIAGNOSIS: Health-seeking behaviors related to preconceptional assessment and preparation for childbearing**

#### Defining Characteristics

- Expressed desire to improve overall health to prepare for childbearing
- Expressed thoughts about planning for pregnancy soon
- Desire to improve nutritional status before childbearing
- Desire to improve nutritional intake of essential vitamins and minerals (iron and calcium)
- Plan to take a multivitamin each day
- Plan to limit consumption of foods high in sodium and fat
- Plan to limit alcohol consumption
- Plan for exercise program to increase stamina and flexibility
- Seeks physical examination to rule out problems that might negatively affect pregnancy
- Seeks information on pregnancy risk factors (biophysical, psychosocial, sociodemographic, and environmental)

#### Related Factors

- Expressed desire to improve the quality of relationship with husband or partner
- Desire to attend education classes to improve knowledge of childbearing and positive health practices
- Plan for room or housing for a young couple that might accommodate children in the future
- Plan for employment arrangements that accommodate child care

#### Expected Outcomes

- Increase in indices of well-being in person
- Healthy pregnancy and future child

- Increase in self-confidence and awareness preparation for childbearing
- Management of pregnancy risk factors before becoming pregnant
- Making the person aware of resources available for pregnancy and child care

#### Interventions

- Assess current level of wellness regarding preparation for childbearing.
- Identify community resources that provide information regarding preconceptional planning and preparation.
- Identify primary health provider, midwife, or obstetrician, and hospitals with delivery services.
- Assess biophysical risk factors (genetic/genomic disorders, nutrition problems, and current medical problems).
- Assess for history of pregnancy loss.
- Test for blood type and Rh factor.
- Screen for STI, tuberculosis, rubella titer, sickle cell trait.
- Review immunization status.
- Assess need to augment diet, particularly to increase intake of calcium and iron.
- Take a multivitamin daily.
- Assess for psychosocial risk factors (mental problems; use of drugs, alcohol, and caffeine; and smoking).
- Counsel to avoid alcohol consumption.
- Assess for possible sociodemographic risk factors (poverty, first pregnancy risks of dystocia or pregnancy-induced hypertension, residence [rural or urban], and ethnicity).
- Assess for environmental risks (exposures to chemicals, drugs, pesticides, pollution, smoke, stress, and radiation).
- Assess current employment situation.
- Identify child care arrangements.

\*NANDA Nursing Diagnoses—Herdman T. H. & Kamitsuru, S. (Eds.). Nursing Diagnoses–Definitions and Classification 2015–2017. Copyright © 2014, 1994–2014 NANDA International. Used by arrangement with John Wiley & Sons Limited. In order to make safe and effective judgments using the NANDA-I nursing diagnoses it is essential that nurses refer to the definitions and defining characteristics of the diagnoses listed in this work.
From Gordon, M. (2016). Manual of nursing diagnosis (13th ed.). Burlington, MA: Jones & Bartlett Learning.

young adults to have significant gains in health insurance and access to care (Sommers et al., 2013). Preventive care, mental health, dental health, and maternity and infertility benefits are being analyzed and increased when necessary. Young adults are generally healthy, which challenges the nurse to be even more creative, sensitive, and insightful in implementing care for individuals within this age group.

## (e) EVOLVE CHAPTER FEATURES

http://evolve.elsevier.com/Edelman/
• Study Questions

## REFERENCES

Adams, H. P., & Carnright, E. L. (2013). HPV infection and cervical cancer prevention. *Clinician Reviews, 23*(9), 42–50.

Affordable Care Act (ACA). (2017). What market place health insurance plans cover. http://www.healthcare.gov/coverage/.

American Academy of Dermatology. (2011). Sunscreens. http://www.aad.org.

Apovian, C., & Gordon, D. (2014). Lifestyle interventions for obesity and weight-related complications. *Clinical Advisor, 17*(9), 47–52.

Beaulieu, R., Kools, S. M., et al. (2011). Young adult couples' decision making regarding emergency contraceptive pills. *Journal of Nursing Scholarship, 43*(1), 41–48.

Black, M. C., Basile, K. C., et al. (2011). *National Intimate Partner and Sexual Violence Survey (NISVS): 2010 summary report.* Atlanta, GA: National Center for Injury Prevention and Control, Centers for Disease Control and Prevention.

Burke, L., & Wang, J. (2011). Treatment strategies for overweight and obesity. *Journal of Nursing Scholarship, 43*(4), 368–375.

Burn, K., & Szoeke, C. (2016). Boomerang families and failure-to-launch: Commentary on adult children living at home. *Maturitas: European Menopause Journal, 83*, 9–12.

Byrne, J. A. (2011). Eighty-five percent of college grads return to nest. *New York Post*, May 9, 2011.

Carey, S., Zaitchik, D., & Bascandziez, I. (2015). Theories of development: In dialog with Jean Piaget. *Developmental Review, 38*, 36–54.

Centers for Disease Control and Prevention (CDC). (2009). QuickStats: Percentage of young adults aged 18-29 years with selected chronic conditions, by sex—National Health Interview Survey, United States, 2005-2007. *MMWR. Morbidity and Mortality Weekly Report, 58*(25), 699.

Centers for Disease Control and Prevention (CDC). (2010). Defining overweight and obesity. https://www.cdc.gov/obesity/adult/defining.html.

Centers for Disease Control and Prevention (CDC). (2011a). Cost of violent deaths in the United States, 2005. http://www.cdc.gov.

Centers for Disease Control and Prevention (CDC). (2011b). Prevalence of coronary heart disease—U.S., 2006–2010. *MMWR. Morbidity and Mortality Weekly Report, 60*(40), 1377–1381.

Centers for Disease Control and Prevention (CDC). (2013a). Mortality data. http://www.cdc.gov.

Centers for Disease Control and Prevention (CDC). (2013b). Other sexually transmitted diseases. http://www.cdc.gov.

Centers for Disease Control and Prevention (CDC). (2013c). Prevention and control of meningococcal disease. Recommendations of the Advisory Committee on Immunization Practices (ACIP). *MMWR. Morbidity and Mortality Weekly Report, 62*(2), 1–25.

Centers for Disease Control and Prevention (CDC). (2014). Chlamydia statistics. http://www.cdc.gov.

Centers for Disease Control and Prevention (CDC). (2015a). Birth data. http://www.cdc.gov.

Centers for Disease Control and Prevention (CDC). (2015b). Today's heroin epidemic. http://www.cdc.gov/vitalsigns/heroin.

Copen, C. E., Chandra, A., & Febo-Vazquez, I. (2016). Sexual behavior, sexual attraction, and sexual orientation among adults aged 18–44 in the US: Data from the 2011–2013 national survey of family growth. *National Health Statistics Reports, 88*, 1–14.

Daniloff, C. (2010). Game changers: How dramatic brain discoveries are influencing American's most popular sport. *Bostonia (Boston, Mass.: 1986), 2010*(3), 24–31.

DeMatteo, D., Galloway, M., et al. (2015). Sexual assault on college campuses: A 50-state survey of criminal sexual assault statutes and their relevance to campus sexual assault. *Psychology, Public Policy, and Law, 21*(3), 227–238.

Demers, J. M., Banyard, V. L., & Pepin, E. (2015). Unwanted sexual experiences: The impact on women's transition to college. *Violence and Gender, 2*(4), 209–213.

Depression Management Tool Kit. (2009). MacArthur initiative on depression and primary care. http://otgateway.com/articles/13macarthurtoolkit.pdf.

Dickson, E. L., Vocel, R. I., et al. (2015). Recent trends in type-specific HPV infection rates in the United States. *Epidemiology and Infection, 143*(5), 1042–1047.

DiStefano, A. D., Sincek, B. L., & Stieler, J. D. (2014). Effective skin cancer prevention methods for young adults (aged 18–30 years). *Journal of the Dermatology Nurses' Association, 6*(4), 171–175.

Eisenberg, D., Schreiber, C. A., et al. (2015). Three-year efficacy and safety of a new 52-mg levonorgestrel-releasing intrauterine system. *Contraception, 92*(1), 10–16.

Erikson, E. H. (1993). *Childhood and society.* New York: W.W. Norton.

Fantasia, H. C., Sutherland, M. A., et al. (2014). Knowledge, attitudes and beliefs about contraceptive and sexual consent negotiation among college women. *Journal of Forensic Nursing, 10*(4), 199–207.

Ford, J. L. (2011). Racial and ethnic disparities in human papillomavirus awareness and vaccination among young adult women. *Public Health Nursing, 28*(6), 485–493.

Ford, J. L., & Browning, C. R. (2011). Neighborhood social disorganization and the acquisition of trichomoniasis among young adults in the United States. *American Journal of Public Health, 101*, 1696–1703.

Friedman, A. L., & Bloodgood, B. (2010). "Something we'd rather not talk about": Findings from CDC exploratory research on sexually transmitted disease communication with girls and women. *Journal of Women's Health, 19*(10), 1823–1831.

Gillespie, C., Kuklina, E. V., et al. (2011). Vital signs: Prevalence, treatment, and control of hypertension—United States, 1999–2002 and 2005–2008. *MMWR. Morbidity and Mortality Weekly Report, 60*(4), 103–108.

Gilligan, C. (1982). *In a different voice.* Cambridge, MA: Harvard University Press.

Gilligan, C. (2002). *The birth of pleasure.* New York: Alfred A. Knopf.

Gilligan, C. (2013). *Joining the resistance.* Malden, MA: Polity Press.

Henley, S. J., Richards, T. B., et al. (2014). Lung cancer incidence trends among men and women-United States, 2005-2009. *MMWR. Morbidity and Mortality Weekly Report, 63*(01), 1–5.

Hing, E., & Albert, M. (2016). *State variation in preventive care visits, by patient characteristics, 2012. NCHS data brief no. 234.* Hyattsville, MD: National Center for Health Statistics.

Institute for Higher Education Policy. (2011). New research shows more low-income young adults begin their higher education experience at for-profit colleges. http://www.ihep.org/press-room/news_release-detail.cfm?id=203.

Institute of Medicine (IOM). (2010). The future of nursing: Leading change, advancing health. http://iom.edu.

James, P. A., Oparil, S., et al. (2014). 2014 evidence-based guidelines for the management of high blood pressure in adults: Report from the panel members appointed to the Eighth Joint National Committee (JNC 8). *JAMA: The Journal of the American Medical Association, 311*(5), 507–520.

Jiang, N., Kolbe, L. J., et al. (2011). Health of adolescents and young adults: Trends in achieving the 21 critical national health objectives by 2010. *Journal of Adolescent Health, 49*(2), 124–132.

Kohlberg, L., & Lickons, T. (1986). *The stages of ethical development: From childhood through old age.* San Francisco, CA: Harper.

LeBlanc, E. S., O'Connor, E., et al. (2011). Effectiveness of primary care-relevant treatments for obesity in adults: A systematic evidence review for the U.S. Preventive Services Task Force. *Annals of Internal Medicine, 155,* 435–447.

Lewis, P., Burnet, D. G., et al. (2015). Measles, mumps, and rubella titers in Air Fore recruits: Below herd immunity thresholds? *American Journal of Preventive Medicine, 49*(5), 757–760.

Maltby, J., & Day, L. (2011). Celebrity worship and incidence of elective cosmetic surgery: Evidence of a link among young adults. *Journal of Adolescent Health, 49*(5), 483–489.

McCance, K. L., & Huether, S. E. (2015). *Pathophysiology, the biologic basis for disease* (7th ed.). St. Louis: Elsevier.

McDaniel, J. C., & Belury, M. A. (2012). Are young adults following the dietary guidelines for Americans. *Nurse Practitioner, 37*(2), 1–9.

Melnyk, B., & Fineout-Overholt, E. (2014). *Evidence-based practice in nursing and healthcare* (3rd ed.). Philadelphia: Lippincott Williams & Wilkins.

Mez, J., Solomon, T. M., et al. (2016). Pathologically confirmed chronic traumatic encephalopathy in a 25-year-old former college football player. *JAMA Neurology, 73*(3), 263–265.

Morelli, C. (2015). Women's issues in the Obama era: Expanding equality and social opportunity under the Obama administration. *Student Pulse, 7*(02), 1–3.

Murray, C. E., & Campbell, E. C. (2015). The pleasures and perils of technology in intimate relationships. *Journal of Couple and Relationship Therapy, 14*(2), 116–140.

National Adolescent and Young Adult Health Information Center. (2012). Clinical preventive services for young adults. http://nahic.ucsf.edu/clinical-preventiveservices-for-young-adults/.

National Institutes of Health. (2014a). Graduated driver licensing programs reduce fatal teen crashes. http://www.nih.gov/news/health/nov2011/nichd-04.htm.

National Institutes on Health. (2014b). Prescription drug abuse: Adolescents and young adults. http://www.drugabuse.gov.

Neinstein, L. (2013). The new adolescents: An analysis of health conditions, behaviors, risks, and access to services among emerging young adults. https://pdfs.semanticsscholar.org.

Nelson, A. (2015). Transdermal contraception methods: today's patches and new options. *Expert Opinion on Pharmacology, 16*(6), 863–873.

Perry, S., Hockenberry, M., et al. (2013). *Maternal-child nursing care* (5th ed.). St. Louis: Elsevier.

Pew Research Center. (2012). Young, underemployed and optimistic: Coming of age, slowly, in a tough economy. http://www.pewsocialtrends.org/2012/02/09/young-underemployed-and-optimistic/.

Piaget, J. (1972). Intellectual evolution from adolescence to adulthood. *Human Development, 15,* 1–12.

Rampell, C. (2011). Many with new college degrees find the job market humbling. *New York Times,* May 18, 2011, A1.

Rummo, P., Meyer, K. A., et al. (2015). Neighborhood availability of convenience stores and diet quality: Findings from 20 years of follow-up in the coronary artery risk development in young adults study. *American Journal of Public Health, 105*(5), e65–e73.

Ryan, D. H., & Urquhart, S. (2015). Scaling up efforts to bring weight down: An update on recommendations, techniques, and pharmacotherapies for adult weight management. *Clinician Reviews, 25*(12), S1–S16.

Schoenborn, D., & Gindi, R. M. (2015). *Electronic cigarette use among adults: US 2014. NCHS data brief no. 217.* Hyattsville, MD: National Center for Health Statistics.

Sommers, B. D., Buchmueller, T., et al. (2013). The Affordable Care Act has led to significant gains in health insurance and access to care for young adults. *Health Affairs, 32*(1), 165–174.

Spring, B., Moller, A. C., et al. (2014). Healthy lifestyle change and subclinical atherosclerosis in young adults: Coronary Artery Risk Development in Young Adults (CARDIA) study. *Circulation, 130,* 10–17.

Trust for America's Health, & Robert Wood Johnson Foundation. (2015). The facts hurt: A state-by-state injury prevention policy report. http://healthyamericans.org/assets/files/TFAH-2015-InjuryRpt-final6.18.pdf.

Tran, D. T., & Zimmerman, L. M. (2015). Cardiovascular risk factors in young adults a literature review. *Journal of Cardiovascular Nursing, 30*(4), 298–310.

US Census Bureau. (2011). *Statistical abstracts of the United States: 2012* (131st ed.). Washington, DC: US Government Printing Office.

US Census Bureau. (2014). *National population projections 2014.* Washington, DC: US Government Printing Office.

US Department of Health and Human Services (USDHHS). (2015). *Healthy People 2020.* Washington, DC: US Department of Health and Human Services. http://www.healthypeople.gov.

US Preventive Services Task Force (USPSTF). (2015). *Published recommendations.* Rockville, MD: Agency for Healthcare Research and Quality.

# 23

# Middle-Aged Adult

*Maureen Murphy*

## OBJECTIVES

*After completing this chapter, the reader will be able to:*

- Name three psychosocial and spiritual changes that frequently occur during middle age.
- Explain the normal biological changes that occur as a result of the aging process.
- Identify the major causes of death in the middle-aged adult.
- Describe frequently occurring health patterns of middle-aged adults.
- Discuss the unique health problems related to the occupations of the adult between age 35 years and age 65 years.
- Analyze the influence of psychosocial stressors on the middle-aged adult and the ways the individual's culture and occupation can affect these stressors.

## KEY TERMS

| | | |
|---|---|---|
| Advance directive | Gingivitis | Osteopenia |
| Body mass index | Glaucoma | Osteoporosis |
| Calcium | Health care agent | Overweight |
| Cardiac output | High blood pressure | Perimenopause |
| Cataract | Kyphosis | Periodontitis |
| Constipation | Living will | Presbycusis |
| Degenerative joint disease | Macular degeneration | Presbyopia |
| Durable power of attorney | Menopause | Sleep disorders |
| Empty nest syndrome | Midlife crisis | Vitamin D |
| Functional aerobic capacity | Obesity | |
| Generativity versus stagnation | Osteoarthritis | |

## ⑦ THINK ABOUT IT

### The "Sandwich Generation"

Charlie Shelton is 48 years old and has been in excellent health. He operates heavy machinery for a construction team that clears environmentally polluted sites in an inner city. These sites are known to be contaminated (lead, mercury, other chemicals), so he visits the occupational health nurse, who supervises intermittent blood testing and physical examinations. He has never smoked and tries to follow the best health advice. He has two children (aged 15 and 18 years). His wife Sarah was working as a licensed practical nurse in a skilled nursing facility until she injured her back and is now receiving disability insurance payments. The elder child plans to enter college next fall, but the Sheltons wonder how they will afford and manage this. Sarah is also the sole caretaker of her mother, who is 80 years old and is in need of increasing assistance. Although Charlie and Sarah worked hard and saved money all their lives, they are worried about college costs, funding an eventual retirement, and the cost of care for Sarah's mother. In addition, Sarah's injury has made them far more conscious about workplace hazards and exposures. The occupational health nurse sees Charlie to assess his physical health; she is also a source for additional referral and support.

- What types of health care providers and referrals are needed by the Sheltons?
- What can health care providers do to guide and support the Sheltons during this stressful time?
- What other health-promotion and wellness strategies might be suggested and implemented to help them?
- What community organizations might the health care provider recommend to meet the needs of this family?
- What responsibilities do health care providers and policymakers have to provide health promotion to middle-aged adults?

An excellent resource for these questions that includes national demonstrations of small work site health programs may be found at CDC Workplace Health Promotion. http://www.cdc.gov/workplacehealthpromotion/.

During their midlife years, many adults experience expanded responsibilities and increased productivity. In most cases, there is a concomitant increased sense of accomplishment. Middle adulthood spans a 30-year interval between 35 and 65 years of age. Within this age interval, significant biological, physiological, social, psychological, and spiritual changes occur. Vital statistics reports published by the Centers for Disease Control and Prevention (CDC) divide the middle-aged adult into three categories for ease of describing mortality and morbidity data. These are 35 to 44 years, 45 to 54 years, and 55 to 65 years. This age group (30-year span) comprises nearly 40% of the population of the United States (US Census Bureau, 2012).

Many changes related to aging and health that occur during this time frame will be discussed in this chapter. Health promotion addresses choices in behavior and practices that optimize health and well-being for the adult in midlife. This concept is the central focus of the presentation of materials and related figures and study aids.

An examination of the gains achieved for *Healthy People 2010* will be compared with the goals and objectives for *Healthy People 2020*. Along with analysis of these findings, the role of nurses will be interwoven throughout the text. Nurses are integral to the health of the American people, and hence to fostering health promotion and health maintenance.

## BIOLOGY AND GENETICS

Although their onset differs, biological changes come to the forefront during the middle years, affecting most body systems. The hair of the adult begins to thin and turn gray. The skin's moisture and turgor decrease, and with the loss of subcutaneous fat, wrinkling occurs. Excessive sun exposure through the years makes some changes more pronounced, especially increased coarseness of facial features.

Fat deposition increases during these years often with concomitant increases in weight. Body height decreases as a result of decreased bone density and mass. This combination of changes results in increased body mass index (BMI). The body contour changes as love handles and saddlebags appear. Sedentary lifestyles and unchanged dietary habits contribute considerably to these changes.

The inactive lifestyle is further compromised by a decrease in energy; "I'm not as young as I used to be" is a common remark. This proclamation is legitimate because the capacity for physical work actually decreases. As functional aerobic capacity decreases, there is a resulting decrease in cardiac output. For individuals who maintain regular exercise programs that provide stretching and strengthening of skeletal muscle, cardiac output remains essentially undiminished for many years.

In the musculoskeletal system, bone density and mass progressively decrease. When 55-year-old adults say that they were 1 inch taller when they were 18 years of age, the observation is likely to be true. A 1- to 4-inch (2.5- to 10-cm) loss in height occurs as a person ages; thinning of the intervertebral disks accounts for approximately 1 inch. However, dramatic losses in height (more than 4 inches) can occur with thoracic kyphosis, an angulation of the posterior spine (commonly known as

*hunchback*). The wear and tear on joints predisposes the adult to degenerative joint disease, deterioration of the joint(s), with more frequent painful backaches. The general decrease in muscle tone, categorized by many as *flab,* reduces physical agility.

Degenerative joint disease, specifically osteoarthritis, has its peak onset in middle age and can greatly influence activity and endurance, which impacts employment. Most frequently the knees and hands, followed by the hips, spine, shoulders, and ankles, are involved. *Healthy People 2010 Final Review* identified two objectives related to arthritis, osteoporosis, and chronic back pain as having moved toward their target attainments: activity limitations attributable to chronic back pain and weight reduction counseling for adults with arthritis. Only one objective exceeded its target by 300%: prevalence of osteoporosis (CDC, 2012).

Osteopenia is a condition of subnormally mineralized bone, usually as a result of a rate of bone lysis that exceeds the rate of bone matrix synthesis. Osteoporosis is a disorder characterized by abnormal loss of bone density and deterioration of bone tissue, with an increased fracture risk. It occurs most frequently in postmenopausal women who have fair complexions and are small, in sedentary individuals, and in people using corticosteroids on a long-term basis. Furthermore, osteoporosis increases with age.

The functional capacity of all organ systems generally decreases. For example, in the gastrointestinal tract, the following chain of events occurs: decreased metabolism leads to less enzyme production, resulting in lower hydrochloric acid levels, which decreases tone in the large intestine. As a result, the middle-aged adult may experience acid indigestion with increased belching.

When the adult leads a sedentary lifestyle, the effects of the diminished motility through the gastrointestinal tract can be more pronounced. It is well known that Americans eat more refined foods (foods that are low in bulk) than residents of third world nations. A low-bulk diet can contribute to the problem of constipation, a change in bowel habits characterized by decreased frequency or passage of hard, drier stools and difficult defecation, and is believed to be a primary contributor to the increased incidence of colon cancer in the United States. Between age 25 years and age 85 years, a 35% loss of nephron units occurs. The remaining nephrons increase in size and undergo degenerative changes. The entire weight of the kidneys decreases. Because blood supply is also diminished, the glomerular filtration rate is decreased by nearly half.

Significant changes occur in the cardiovascular system as the blood vessels lose elasticity and become thicker. This process predisposes middle-aged adults to coronary artery disease, hypertension, myocardial infarctions, and strokes. Heart disease is the second leading cause of death in middle-aged adults (Heron, 2012).

Menopause is the cessation of menses. It is an expected physiological change related to aging, and it marks the end of a woman's reproductive function. Menopause is determined retrospectively after cessation of menses for 12 consecutive months. In North America the median age for menopause is 50.5 to 51.4 years (Palacious et al., 2010). Women now expect to live one-third of their lives after menopause. A great deal more must be learned about what causes many of the symptoms that occur in menopause. Sheehy (1993) conducted interviews of 100 women from their mid-40s to their 60s and also interviewed 75 physicians and other experts. Her analysis showed that many of these people felt there was a renewed sexual vitality and surge of mental energy for menopausal women. She characterized menopause as a gateway to a second adulthood. Northrup (2012) and King and colleagues (2013) propose that many women make menopause a time of personal inventiveness while gradually adapting to the many expected biological, psychological, social, and spiritual changes of menopause. During menopause, production of ovarian estrogen and progesterone ceases; the remaining estrogen is produced by the adrenal glands. As a result of the diminished estrogen level, a woman's secondary sex characteristics regress, evident as, for example, loss of pubic hair and decrease in breast size. The female reproductive organs shrink, and vaginal secretions decrease, requiring additional lubrication.

As men approach the end of the middle years, they experience changes in their sexual response cycle as testosterone levels plateau and then decrease. The testes undergo degenerative changes, the number of viable spermatozoa diminishes, and the volume and viscosity of semen decrease. In men, sexual energy gradually declines; achieving an erection takes longer, but it is sustained longer. Stress, however, can significantly diminish function (Pines, 2011).

## Life Expectancy and Mortality Rates

In the last decade (2001–10), life expectancy increased for all groups of Americans in the middle adult years. Across the 30-year age span, there was a decrease in mortality for all racial and ethnic groups, with the most significant decreases noted between age 35 years and age 44 years. Life expectancies for American men and women are now at record highs: 81.1 years for women and 76.3 years for men (Arias, 2015).

The leading causes of death during middle adulthood are heart disease, cancer, and accidents (National Vital Statistics, 2016). Box 23-1 shows a breakdown for each decile or 10-year interval for the middle-aged adult. Reducing disabilities and deaths from these chronic conditions are national health-promotion and disease-prevention objectives.

The CDC uses a multifaceted approach to mitigate the chronic disease burden: epidemiology and surveillance to monitor trends, environmental strategies to promote healthy behaviors, health system interventions to advance clinical and preventative services, and community resources to improve clinical management of chronic conditions (Bauer et al., 2014). In Box 23-2: *Healthy People 2020*, selected objectives and target goals for the 2020 leading health indicators are outlined to give the reader some perspective of the many tasks and opportunities that lie ahead for Americans. The *Healthy People* initiative was established in 1980 to provide structure for health-promotion and disease-prevention programs. Every 10 years, revised objectives and target goals are established for each leading indicator. For 30 years, Harston (2010) has tracked and disclosed gains made toward meeting the target goals as a result of the influence of the overall health-promotion program. In some cases, progression toward the target goals has been achieved, and in other cases regression has been noted.

Most of the leading indicators identified in *Healthy People 2020* are preventable, or at least modifiable. Knowledge of the direction of the program offers professional nurses an incentive to modify their practice and health-promotion education efforts to best help Americans achieve the target goals specified in the *Healthy People* initiative. Health education, often conducted by professional nurses, has been effective with adults who want to or must change their lifestyle behaviors. Nursing professionals have contributed extensively in helping the nation to meet the target goals for heart disease, stroke, and many types of cancer.

Whereas the data analysis showed some progress toward reaching many of the *Healthy People 2010* target goals, there were a number of areas of backsliding. Most notably, greater proportions of Americans are obese and have symptoms of **high blood pressure** compared with the findings reported for *Healthy People 2000*. Hypertension and obesity are conditions that significantly affect the middle-aged adult. They often lead to heart disease, stroke, and the development of diabetes. Harston (2010) suggests that the 2010 goals were perhaps too ambitious; however, findings of other research positively confirm that more Americans were obese in 2010 than earlier in the decade. The most recent national data from 2011 to 2014 on obesity prevalence indicate obesity was higher among middle-aged adults (40.2%) than among younger (32.3%) or older (37.0%) adults (Ogden et al., 2015).

Areas of improvement in reaching the target goals for *Healthy People 2010* were encouraging. For instance, decreases were noted in the number of cancer deaths and in the number of injuries at work (CDC, 2012). Furthermore, laws that discourage or forbid smoking continue to have a significant impact across populations.

In sum, there was evidence of progress in meeting approximately 670 of 955 leading health indicator target goals. Projecting ahead for 2020, efforts must be directed toward the following: increasing awareness of the *Healthy People 2020* initiative as a tool to improve the overall health of Americans; expanding knowledge of the initiative in schools, tribal communities, and

---

### BOX 23-1  Leading Causes of Death in Middle-Aged Adults

**Age 35 to 44 Years**
- Unintentional injuries (40.2 deaths per 100,000 population)
- Malignant neoplasms (31.9 deaths per 100,000 population)
- Heart disease (28.3 deaths per 100,000 population)

**Age 45 to 54 Years**
- Malignant neoplasms (116.3 deaths per 100,000 population)
- Heart disease (88.0 deaths per 100,000 population)
- Accidents (45.5 deaths per 100,000 population)

**Age 55 to 64 Years**
- Malignant neoplasms (321.2 deaths per 100,000 population)
- Heart disease (207.3 deaths per 100,000 population)
- Bronchitis/emphysema (39.2 deaths per 100,000 population)

BOX 23-2 HEALTHY PEOPLE 2020

### Selected National Health-Promotion and Disease-Prevention Objectives for the Middle-Aged Adult

**Overall Goals**
- Improve access to high-quality health services.
- Improve health and well-being for all age groups.
- Reduce disparities across all racial and ethnic groups of Americans.

**Objectives**
- Increase the proportion of adults who have a specific source of ongoing care. The target is 89.4%, a 10% increase over 2010 expected by 2020. The baseline in 2008 was 81.3% of adults.
- Reduce the proportion of adults aged 18 years or older with physician-diagnosed arthritis who experience a limitation in activity due to arthritis or joint symptoms. The baseline in 2008 was 39.4%. The target is 35.5%.
- Reduce the proportion of adults with osteoporosis. The target is 5.3%, with a baseline of 5.9% of adults aged 50 years or older with osteoporosis in 2005 to 2008.
- Reduce activity limitation due to chronic back conditions. In 2008, 30.7 adults per 1000 population aged 18 years or older experienced activity limitation due to chronic back conditions. The target is 27.6 adults per 1,000 population.
- Reduce the annual number of new cases of diagnosed diabetes to 7.2 per 100,000 population aged 18 to 84 years. The baseline in 2009 (National Health Interview Survey) was 8.0 new cases per 100,000 population.

- Reduce the proportion of persons with diabetes with a hemoglobin $A_{1c}$ value greater than 9%. The baseline was 17.9% in 2005 to 2008. The target is 16.1%.
- Reduce deaths from work-related injuries in all industries. The target is 3.6 deaths per 100,000 full-time equivalent workers. The baseline in 2007 was 4.0 work-related injury deaths per 100,000 full-time equivalent workers.
- Reduce the overall cancer death rate. The target for 2020 is 160.6 per 100,000 population. The baseline was 176.8 per 100,000 population cited in 2007.
- Reduce the proportion of adults with hypertension. The target for 2020 is 26.9%. The baseline was 29.9% in 2005 to 2008.
- Reduce coronary heart disease deaths. The target is 100.8 deaths per 100,000 population. The baseline in 2007 was 126.0 deaths per 100,000 population.
- Reduce the proportion of adults who are obese. The target is 30.6%. The baseline in 2005 to 2008 was 34.0% of persons aged 20 years or older.
- Increase the proportion of adults who engage in aerobic physical activity of moderate intensity on a regular, preferably daily, basis for at least 30 minutes per day to 47.9%. The baseline was 43.5% in 2008.
- Increase recent smoking cessation success for adult smokers. The target is 8.0%, with a baseline of 6.0% of adult smokers aged 18 years or older who last smoked 6 months previously.

local health agencies through the use of public service announcements carried on radio, television, and Internet-based programs; and linking the objectives and goals to preventive health provisions associated with work sites (occupational health programs) and health insurance policies. The good news is the *Healthy People 2020* target goals are more achievable (less ambitious than projected for 2010), and the objectives focus on individuals more than on "big" programs. There are goals that involve health counseling and behavior-modification strategies provided by nurses, advanced practice nurses, and mental health nursing specialists in addition to physicians. In the larger picture, Americans will benefit when nurses, in all roles, incorporate the *Healthy People 2020* objectives into their practice.

### Sex and Marital Status

In the midlife years, the death rate for men is higher. Men are more likely than women to die of heart disease for all age groups (35–44, 45–54, and 55–65 years) and all racial and ethnic groups (*Healthy People 2020*, 2012). Although cardiovascular disease death rates are declining for both sexes, heart disease remains one of the primary causes of death. The risk factors for heart disease include obesity, lack of physical activity, smoking, high total cholesterol level, hypertension, and genetics. Obesity is common, serious, and costly. More than one-third of US adults (36.5%) were reported to be obese in 2011 to 2014. Among American adults, the prevalence of obesity among middle-aged women was higher (38.3%) than in men (34.3%) (Ogden, et al., 2015). (See Chapter 11 for a discussion of overweight, obesity, and *Healthy People 2020* target goals.)

Nearly 60% of adults in the United States are married. The marriage rate for white adults (61%) is higher than that for Hispanic adults (58%) or black adults (38%). Married adults report better health than divorced, widowed, or never-married adults. Findings from the most recent census (2010) show that the number of interracial and interethnic married couples increased by 28% in the preceding decade. Among unmarried, opposite-sex partners, 18% described their union as interracial or interethnic whereas 21% of same-sex couples reported they have an interracial union (US Census Bureau, 2012).

### Race, Sex, and Ethnicity

Black Americans are the second largest racial group in the United States. They constitute 12.6% of the US population (US Census Bureau, 2015). In actual numbers, there are slightly fewer than 40 million black Americans.

Cancer is the leading cause of death for black men and black women (combined incidence rates) in middle age. Findings in recent years show an encouraging decrease in both the incidence and the mortality rate for cancer among black adults since 1993. Black adults are less likely to survive 5 years after diagnosis than white adults. Researchers believe that this disparity is largely related to factors associated with a significantly lower income level than other racial or ethnic groups. Although black Americans constitute 13% of the US population, they represent 25.8% of the nation's poor (Macartney, et al., 2013; US Census Bureau, 2015). Black households have the lowest median income ($34,598), compared with non-Hispanic whites ($58,270), Hispanics ($40,963), and Asians ($67,065) (DeNavas-Walt & Proctor, 2014).

According to the US Census Bureau (2015), Hispanics are the largest ethnic group in the United States, constituting approximately 17.3% of the total population. Data from the National Vital Statistics Reports (2016) indicate accidents (unintentional injuries) are the leading cause of death for 35- to 44-year-old Hispanics; malignant neoplasms rank first among the causes of combined deaths of males and female Latinos aged between 45 and 55 years. Mortality statistics show the set of leading causes of death for white, middle-aged Americans is the same as that for Hispanics.

Individuals who describe their ancestry as Asian/Pacific Islander constitute approximately 5% of Americans. Across all age groups representing "the middle-aged adult," malignant neoplasms and heart disease ranked as the leading causes of death within the Asian/Pacific Islander population. The types of cancer found most often among Asians are liver (including intrahepatic bile duct) and stomach cancer.

American Indians and Alaska Natives represent approximately 1% of the American population. Mortality statistics for both sexes aged 35 to 44 years show accidents to be the leading cause of death; heart disease kills more 45- to 54-year-olds, and in the oldest group (55- to 65-year-olds), malignant neoplasms, notably cancer of the kidney and renal pelvis, cause the greatest number of deaths.

## Access to Health Care

Individuals who are poor, defined as having an annual income less than $20,000 for a family of four, generally have less access to medical care compared with people with a greater income. Driscoll and Bernstein (2012) reported that people who were unemployed self-reported a "poor psychological and physical health status" more often than individuals who were employed. The gravity of the situation increases because of the lost benefits, including health insurance, when individuals become unemployed. Furthermore, government reports indicate that the cost of health insurance premiums has increased and employee medical claims are at an all-time high and continue to rise. Two national initiatives have helped increase access to health care: slow trending increased rates of employment and the Patient Protection and Affordable Care Act, commonly known as the Affordable Care Act (ACA). The employment rate for US adults aged 25 to 65 years was higher in 2014 (72.3%) than it was in 2010 (71.5%) but remained lower than in 2008 (75.5%) or 2000 (77.7%) (National Center for Education Statistics, 2015). Middle-aged adults who remain employed often receive employer-provided health care benefits. Although health care policies vary, guaranteed health insurance significantly reduces the cost of preventative and emergent health care. Furthermore, business leaders across America are offering workplace health programs to help employees adopt healthier lifestyles, lower their risk of developing costly chronic diseases, and curb rising health care costs (CDC, 2016h). On March 23, 2010, the ACA was enacted to increase the quality and affordability of health insurance, lower the uninsured rate by expanding public and private insurance coverage, and reduce the costs of health care. Since the enactment of the ACA, the number of uninsured individuals has continued to decline. The proportion of adults aged 18 to 65 years who were uninsured at the time of interview decreased from 16.3% in 2014 to 13% in the first 3 months of 2015. During this same period, there was a corresponding increase in private health care insurance coverage from 67.3% to 70.4% (Cohen & Martinez, 2015).

Health care insurance coverage, access, and utilization disparities exist. Compared with 2013, the proportion of adults aged 18 to 65 years who were uninsured decreased in 2014: Hispanics 41.1% to 34.1%, non-Hispanic whites 14.5% to 11.5%, non-Hispanic blacks 24.7% to 17.6%, and non-Hispanic Asians 16.1% to 12.2% (Martinez et al., 2015). Because of costs, those without health insurance often forgo needed health care, which can lead to continued compromised health status and potentially to greater medical expenditures in the long term. People 18 to 64 years of age with chronic conditions and without consistent health insurance coverage are much more likely to forgo needed medical care than people with the same conditions and continuous coverage (CDC, 2010b).

The second leading cause of death of non-Hispanic black Americans is heart disease. Of concern is that black Americans are less likely to receive a diagnosis of heart disease, but they are 30% more likely to die of heart disease compared to the population in general. Hypertension and overweight/obesity are risk factors for heart disease and stroke. Black adults are 50% more likely to have hypertension. A higher proportion of black women (77%) than white women (57%) are overweight. Black adults are 50% more likely than white adults to suffer a stroke.

Non-Hispanic black Americans share a disproportionate burden of HIV/AIDS. Black men are eight times more likely than non-Hispanic white men to have HIV/AIDS. Black women are 20 times more likely than non-Hispanic white women and almost five times more likely than Hispanic/Latino women to have HIV/AIDS. In 2010, blacks accounted for 45% of all new HIV infections among US adults despite representing only 12% of the US population (CDC, 2017b).

Latino/Hispanic Americans are the largest ethnic minority group in the United States, constituting 16.3% of the population. Hispanic Americans have the highest uninsured rate of any racial or ethnic group in the United States. From 2004 to 2014, the percentage of uninsured individuals younger than 65 years for whom cost was a reason for not having health insurance coverage decreased from 60.9% to 51.4% among uninsured Hispanics, from 49.5% to 38.0% among non-Hispanic whites, and from 47.4% to 34.0% among non-Hispanic blacks (CDC, 2015c). Cancer is the second leading cause of death for young (35–44 years) middle-aged Hispanics, surpassing unintentional accidents. As the Hispanic population ages (into the 45–65-year age range), neoplasms become the leading cause of death. Breast cancer is the most common type of cancer in Hispanic women. In Hispanic women, breast cancer is less likely to be diagnosed when the disease is localized, before spreading to nearby lymph nodes, tissues, and organs, and they are approximately 20% more likely to die than non-Hispanic white women even when breast cancer is diagnosed in them at a similar age and stage of disease.

Heart disease ranks second as a cause of death among Latino/Hispanics who are 45 to 64 years old. Hispanic adults are less likely to smoke than non-Hispanic white adults, but almost 80% of Mexican Americans are overweight; 42.3% of all Mexican

American women are obese. Mexican Americans constitute approximately 60% of the Hispanic population in the United States. Obesity increases the risk of diabetes, hypertension, heart disease, and premature death (Obesity Society, 2017). Obesity is also associated with increased risk of cancers of the esophagus, pancreas, colon and rectum, breast (after menopause), endometrium (lining of the uterus), kidney, thyroid, and gallbladder (National Institutes of Health [NIH], National Cancer Institute, 2015b).

## Genetics

The middle-aged adult is at greater risk than the young adult of diseases known to be associated with genetics (i.e., familial characteristics). These conditions include diabetes, hypertension, Huntington chorea, arteriosclerosis, gout, obesity, heart disease, and alcoholism. There are some malignancies that are related to genetics; for example, women with a personal or family history of breast cancer are at a higher risk of developing this type of malignancy. In addition, individuals with a family history of colorectal cancer, rectal or colon polyps, or ulcerative colitis have an increased risk of developing this type of cancer (Box 23-3: Genomics).

---

### ⚗ BOX 23-3 GENOMICS
#### *Genotype Targeted Therapies for Lung Cancer*

Lung cancer remains the leading cause of cancer-related deaths worldwide and the second most common cancer among both men and women in the United States. In 2013 (the most recent year numbers are available), 212,584 people in the United States (111,907 men and 100,677 women) were diagnosed with lung cancer and 157,176 people (85,658 men and 70,518 women) died of lung cancer (CDC, 2016b). The number of new lung cancer cases in men is expected to stay the same between 2010 and 2020, but more than 10,000 additional new lung cancer cases are expected to be found in women each year by 2020 (CDC, 2016a). Several types of cancer treatment are available—surgery, radiation therapy, chemotherapy, immunotherapy, hormone therapy, and stem cell transplant—yet the 5-year survival rate has not increased in several decades. Molecular and genomic profiling of lung tumors has revolutionized the treatment of metastatic non–small cell lung cancer (NSCLC). The Adjuvant Lung Cancer Enrichment Marker Identification and Sequencing Trials (ALCHEMIST) involve genetic screening of resected NSCLC specimens (Cardarella & Johnson, 2013). Patients whose tumors test positive for either epidermal growth factor receptor gene (*EGFR*) or anaplastic lymphoma kinase gene (*ALK*) mutations will be referred to the ALCHEMIST for genotype-directed targeted therapies (Govindan et al., 2015; NIH, National Cancer Institute, 2016). Adjuvant targeted therapy, based on tumor mutation genotyping, will likely improve outcomes for all NSCLC patients.

From Cardarella, S., & Johnson, B. E. (2013). The impact of genomic changes on treatment of lung cancer. *American Journal of Respiratory and Critical Care Medicine, 188*(7), 770–775; Centers for Disease Control and Prevention (CDC). (2016a). *Expected new cancer cases and deaths in 2020.* http://www.healthypeople.gov/2020/topics-objectives/topic/hiv; Centers for Disease Control and Prevention (CDC). (2016b). *Lung cancer statistics.* https://www.cdc.gov/cancer/lung/statistics; Govindan, R., Mandrekar, S. J., Gerber, D. E., et al. (2015). ALCHEMIST trials: A golden opportunity to transform outcomes in early-stage non-small cell lung cancer. *Clinical Cancer Research, 24,* 5439–5444; National Institute of Health, National Cancer Institute. (2016). *The ALCHEMIST lung cancer trial.* http://www.cancer.gov/types/lung/research/alchemist.

---

## GORDON'S FUNCTIONAL HEALTH PATTERNS

### Health Perception–Health Management Pattern

To promote health in the middle-aged adult, the nurse performs a health assessment that includes the person's values and beliefs, lifestyle patterns, general perceptions of health, and health practices (Pender et al., 2015).

### Habits

The self-destructive habits of the middle-aged adult that have been practiced for years (cigarette smoking, excessive alcohol use, and overeating) begin to have visible consequences. As pressures increase, adults are tempted to turn to substances such as these as a crutch for coping with stress. Prevention is extremely important, primarily because withdrawal from any of these substances is a difficult process.

### Risk Factors

The major risk factors for adults in the middle years are environmental and behavioral; they can be changed through teaching, counseling, and use of other nursing interventions. Helping adults to take care of themselves and to change, when indicated, can be accomplished on an individual or a group basis.

Some of the health-promotion needs of the middle-aged adult include acceptance of aging, the need to exercise, and weight control. Decreasing or stopping cigarette smoking and alcohol consumption can also be identified needs. Preventive health screening is vital. The adult needs input into and control of as many of these behaviors as possible.

The health risks of middle-aged adults overall are categorized as group risks (age, sex, race) and personal risks. Precritical secondary prevention includes periodic selective screening for the detection of disease before it becomes clinically apparent, such as a breast self-examination. A suggested screening examination appears in Box 23-4.

Chronic conditions are defined as those that last for more than 3 months. The leading chronic diseases found in the middle-aged adult include heart disease, stroke, cancer, diabetes, obesity, arthritis, hepatitis, weak or failing kidney function, and chronic obstructive pulmonary disease, all of which are among the most common, costly, and preventable of all health problems (Lubkin and Larsen, 2013; Ward et al., 2014). As of 2012, nearly half of all American adults (49.8%, 117 million) had at least one chronic condition, of which more than half (approximately 60 million) had multiple chronic conditions: 24.3% had one chronic condition, 13.8% had two chronic conditions, and 11.7% had three or more chronic conditions (Ward et al., 2014). The cost of treating people with chronic diseases accounts for 86% of US health care costs. Two of these chronic diseases—heart disease and cancer—together accounted for nearly 48% of all deaths (CDC, 2016b).

### Nutritional-Metabolic Pattern

Dietary factors are correlated with 5 of the 10 leading causes of death in the United States: coronary heart disease, some cancers,

---

### BOX 23-4  Screening Examination: Age 35 to 65 Years

**Database**
- Health history
- Health hazard appraisal
- Psychological inventories as needed

**Physical Examination Emphasizing**
- Weight and height
- Blood pressure, pulse rate
- Breasts
- Pelvis
- Prostate
- Testicles
- Eyes
- Mouth
- Skin

**Laboratory Procedures**
- Papanicolaou smear and human papilloma virus test: every 5 years
- Hemoccult test: three stools for the Hemoccult test with physical examination after age 50 years
- Colonoscopy or sigmoidoscopy every 5 to 10 years after age 50 years as indicated
- Mammography: initial screening at age 40 years, annually at age 45 to 54 years, then every 2 years at age 55 years or older
- Urinalysis: examined at the time of physical examination

- Lipid profile: all men aged 35 years or older; women aged 20 years or older who have heart disease or risk factors for heart disease
- Chest radiograph with physical examination if heavy smoker
- Tetanus and diphtheria booster every 10 years
- Influenza vaccine: follow current recommendations
- Counseling and testing for HIV as indicated
- Rubella serological test (women of childbearing age)

**Self-Care Education and Counseling**
- With physical examination; individualized according to individual's risk factors
- Injury prevention: seat belts, helmets, firearms, smoke detectors
- Stress reduction
- Exercise
- Diet: cholesterol, fat, sodium, fiber, multivitamins with folic acid (women of childbearing age)
- Calcium
- Breast self-examination
- Testicular self-examination
- Dental care
- Mouth care
- Sexually transmitted diseases
- Contraception
- Skin protection from ultraviolet light
- Alcohol and other substance abuse
- Smoking cessation
- Possible hormone prophylaxis (perimenopausal and postmenopausal women)

From American Cancer Society. (2015). *Guidelines for the early detection of cancer.* http://www.cancer.org/healthy/findcancerearly/cancerscreening guidelines/; Blue Cross Blue Shield of Massachusetts. (2016). *Preventive screening guidelines for healthy adults.* https://www.bluecrossma.com/wps/portal/members/healthier-living/manage-my-health/screening-guidelines-adults/.

---

stroke, non–insulin-dependent diabetes mellitus, and atherosclerosis (CDC, 2010a).

Physical activities and nutritional patterns are frequently correlated. The middle-aged adult typically leads a more sedentary lifestyle than does the young adult primarily because of increased responsibilities at work and home and the many convenience devices that are found in homes and workplaces. Research findings published on the CDC website show that the incidence of obesity is increasing among men and boys compared with women and girls. Linked with less activity is the lack of attention to modification of food intake and calorie consumption, resulting in obesity, one of the major health problems of the middle years.

### Obesity

More than one-third (36.5%) of US adults have obesity (CDC, 2016a). Obesity-related conditions (heart disease, stroke, type 2 diabetes, and certain types of cancer) contribute to the leading causes of preventable death. **Body mass index (BMI)** is used as a screening tool for overweight or obesity. BMI is a person's weight in kilograms divided by the square of height in meters (CDC, 2016b). **Overweight** is defined as having a BMI between 25 < 30. A BMI of 30.0 or greater falls within the obese range. Obesity is frequently subdivided into categories: Class 1 (BMI of 30 to <35), Class 2 (BMI of 35 to <40), and Class 3 (BMI of ≥40) (CDC 2016d). Obesity is more frequent among middle-aged

adults 40 to 59 years old (40.2%) and adults age 60 and older (37%) than among younger adults age 20 to 39 (32.3%) (CDC, 2016b). Of note, the target goal of *Healthy People 2010* of 15% was not attained. The progress report on the *Healthy People 2010* goals indicates that there was an increase in the incidence of obesity to 34% of the adult population compared with 23% in 2008 (CDC, 2012).

Overweight and obesity are major risks factors for preventable, noncommunicable conditions that contribute to increased health costs, morbidity, and death. An increased BMI substantially raises the risk of coronary heart disease, high blood pressure, high cholesterol, stroke, type 2 (non–insulin-dependent) diabetes, gallbladder disease, osteoarthritis, sleep apnea, obesity hypoventilation syndrome, and endometrial, breast, prostate, and colon cancers (CDC, 2012, 2015a; World Health Organization, 2016). Individuals who are obese often suffer from social stigmatization, discrimination, and lowered self-esteem (Hunger & Major, 2015). The US Preventive Services Task Force (2014) recommends all adults be screened for obesity. For patients with a BMI of 30 kg/m², clinicians refer them to a more intensive, multicomponent behavioral interventions.

Women with less education and low incomes and black and Hispanic women are at an increased risk of being overweight. In addition to sex, race, and socioeconomic status, genetics may be a contributing factor. The most significant variables, however, are health behaviors, particularly food intake and exercise and activity patterns. Although an abundance of health information is available, these challenges persist.

As much as 40% of a typical American family's food budget is spent on food in restaurants or for take-out foods, both of which are usually higher in fat (including saturated and trans fats) and salt content than foods prepared at home (Agency for Healthcare Research and Quality, 2012). Losing weight and maintaining weight loss may require an individual to change eating and activity behaviors, but the social, food preparation, and consumption behaviors of the family must change as well.

Prevention of obesity is the goal of weight management during the middle years. When the adult is obese, a clear-cut history of the onset is imperative. A lifelong history of obesity is significantly more arduous to alter than that of adult-onset obesity. A decrease in calories should be accompanied by at least 30 minutes of exercise five times a week. When calories are reduced and exercise is increased, weight loss is achieved and maintained.

The weight-management resources available to the adult are plentiful. Weight-management programs using behavior modification can be found in various settings, such as universities and work sites, Weight Watchers, Overeaters Anonymous, and Take Off Pounds Sensibly. If the nurse identifies a need for weight management and no program is available, a self-help group can be started. A suggested list of topics generated by the group is assembled. A discussion of basic nutrition with appropriate handouts is a good place to start. Having adults record their individual goals and keep a 1-week diet log is nonthreatening and helpful for future planning; it also gives the participants some responsibility in the program. Intake food journals assist the individuals in maintaining weight loss outcomes.

### High Saturated Fat Diet

Lipid levels and ratios have a significant influence on cardiovascular and cerebrovascular morbidity and mortality rates. The National Heart, Lung, and Blood Institute considers a total blood cholesterol level less than 200 mg/dL as desirable. The mean total blood cholesterol levels for adults in the United States declined by 3.9% from 1988–94 to 2005–08, from 206 to 198 mg/dL, exceeding the 2010 target of 199 mg/dL. During the same time frame, the proportion of adults with high blood cholesterol levels fell by 28.6%, from 21% to 15%, also exceeding the 2010 target of 17% (CDC, 2012).

Much of this success is attributed to the use of statin drugs that lower the level of low-density lipoproteins in the blood. Some studies demonstrate the beneficial effects of estrogen administration on heart health (Mikkola, et al. 2015). The reference Coronary Primary Prevention Trial demonstrates that men at high risk of coronary heart disease are able to reduce the risk by approximately 2% for every 1% lower blood cholesterol level. Before using medication to reduce cholesterol level, individuals with high cholesterol levels are advised to reduce their intakes of saturated fat, total fat, and dietary cholesterol; normalize their weight; and increase their level of physical activity. If lifestyle changes are not successful, medication is often advised.

### Calcium and Vitamin D

Adequate calcium intake is essential for developing and maintaining bone mass. Additionally, calcium is needed for other physiological processes, including muscle contraction and blood pressure regulation. Men and women need a minimal daily intake of 1000 mg of calcium. Pregnant and nursing women need 1200 mg, and postmenopausal women need either 1000 mg (when taking estrogen) or 1500 mg (when not taking estrogen). When daily intake of calcium is less than adequate, the serum calcium level will be maintained by leaching calcium from bone, resulting in osteoporosis. Weight-bearing exercise contributes to bone mass by increasing mechanical stress on the bones, whereas vitamin D promotes calcium absorption and regulates serum calcium and phosphate concentrations to maintain bone health (Heaney, 2013). Together with calcium, vitamin D helps to protect older adults from osteoporosis.

Vitamin D also plays an important role in overall health and the prevention of chronic diseases. Emerging studies suggest an association between inadequate levels of vitamin D and an increased risk of chronic diseases, such as in osteoporosis, diabetes, heart disease, hypertension, cancers, obesity, depression, cognitive decline, fractures and falls, and autoimmunity (LaFevre, 2015; Nair & Maseeh, 2012). Worldwide, across all ethnic, sex, and age groups, an estimated 1 billion people have inadequate levels of vitamin D (Holick, 2012; Lips, 2010). Possible causes of vitamin D deficiency include an insufficient consumption of vitamin D–fortified foods, lack of dietary supplements, and limited exposure to sunlight. It is very difficult to achieve sufficient vitamin D intake through dietary sources alone as few foods naturally contain vitamin D. The food sources that provide vitamin D include fatty fish, dairy products, liver, and fortified cereals and beverages. The best way to ensure adequate vitamin D serum levels is through supplementation (NIH, Office of Dietary Supplements, 2016).

Vitamin D is unique because it can be synthesized endogenously when the skin is exposed to ultraviolet B radiation. Many factors can interfere with ultraviolet B exposure and the body's ability to synthesize vitamin D from sunlight: seasons, time of day, length of day, location, cloud cover, smog, skin melanin content, and use of sunscreen (Nair & Maseeh, 2012). Aging may also impede cutaneous synthesis of vitamin D. As people age the skin cannot synthesize vitamin D as efficiently as when they are younger. Older adults are also more likely to spend more time indoors (homebound or occupations that limit sun exposure). Prolonged sun exposure to prevent vitamin D deficiency is not generally recommended because exposure to ultraviolet radiation increases the risk of skin cancer. The exact definition of a low vitamin D level is not well established. Daily vitamin D intake of 600 IU in adults aged 18 to 70 years and 800 IU in adults older than 70 years will meet the needs of most adults (Institute of Medicine, 2011) (Table 23-1).

### Caffeine

Caffeine is a popular stimulant found in coffee, tea, and some soft drinks, such as colas. Caffeine prolongs the amount of time that physical work can be performed and appears to decrease

| TABLE 23-1 | Dietary Reference Intake for Calcium and Vitamin D |

**DIETARY REFERENCE INTAKES FOR CALCIUM AND VITAMIN D**

| | CALCIUM | | | VITAMIN D | | |
|---|---|---|---|---|---|---|
| List Stage Group | Estimated Average Requirement (mg/day) | Recommended Dietary Allowance (mg/day) | Upper Level Intake (mg/day) | Estimated Average Requirement (IU/day) | Recommended Dietary Allowance (IU/day) | Upper Level Intake (IU/day) |
| Infants 0 to 6 months | * | * | 1000 | ** | ** | 1000 |
| Infants 6 to 12 months | * | * | 1500 | ** | ** | 1500 |
| 1–3 years old | 500 | 700 | 2500 | 400 | 600 | 2500 |
| 4–8 years old | 800 | 1000 | 2500 | 400 | 600 | 3000 |
| 9–13 years old | 1100 | 1300 | 3000 | 400 | 600 | 4000 |
| 14–18 years old | 1100 | 1300 | 3000 | 400 | 600 | 4000 |
| 19–30 years old | 800 | 1000 | 2500 | 400 | 600 | 4000 |
| 31–50 years old | 800 | 1000 | 2500 | 400 | 600 | 4000 |
| 51–70 year old males | 800 | 1000 | 2000 | 400 | 600 | 4000 |
| 51–70 year old females | 1000 | 1200 | 2000 | 400 | 600 | 4000 |
| >70 years old | 1000 | 1200 | 2000 | 400 | 800 | 4000 |
| 14–18 years old, pregnant/lactating | 1100 | 1300 | 3000 | 400 | 600 | 4000 |
| 19–50 years old, pregnant/lactating | 800 | 1000 | 2500 | 400 | 600 | 4000 |

*For infants. Adequate intake is 200 mg/day for 0 to 6 months of age and 260 mg/day for 6 to 12 months of age.
**For infants. Adequate intake is 400 IU/day for 0 to 6 months of age and 400 IU/day for 6 to 12 months of age.
From The National Academies of Sciences, Engineering, and Medicine, Health and Medicine Division. (2010). Dietary reference intakes for calcium and vitamin D as recommended by the Institutes of medicine. http://www.nationalacademies.org/hmd/Reports/2010/Dietary-Reference-Intakes-for-Calcium-and-Vitamin-D.aspx.

boredom and increase attention span. On the negative side, coffee has recently been the subject of significant scrutiny from the media, with reports of a link between cancer of the pancreas and coffee consumption. There is controversy regarding whether daily moderate intake of caffeine has any detrimental effects.

Like alcohol and nicotine, caffeine is readily available and has become an accepted part of daily living. Because caffeine is a strong stimulant with effects that are typically taken for granted, its importance as an addictive substance must be emphasized. Ingestion of 0.5 g of caffeine (three to four cups of coffee) can increase the basal metabolic rate by an average of 10%, and possibly as much as 25% for some people.

Long-term stimulation of the central nervous system results in restlessness, sleep disturbances, cardiac stimulation, and withdrawal effects. Nurses' assessment should screen individuals for stimulating and addictive substances that may be producing these symptoms.

### High-Sodium Diet

High-sodium diets play a significant role in hypertension, especially when consumed over many years. The result may be an increase in the amount of total body fluids, which increases peripheral vascular resistance. Salt contains approximately 40% sodium and is a contributing factor for hypertension in the 10% to 20% of Americans who are at risk. On average, Americans consume 4 to 5 g of sodium per day. A major contributor to dietary sodium is the salt found in processed foods.

In the past 3 decades, many clinical studies have demonstrated the effectiveness of lowering blood pressure by lowering dietary sodium intake. Other studies have described the relationships between urinary and sodium excretion and the change of blood pressure with age (Pöss et al., 2015).

### Alcohol Abuse

Substance abuse can be a devastating habit. Many adults abuse prescription and illicit drugs and, especially, alcohol. Alcohol is frequently treated as a nondrug, but alcohol addiction is second only to nicotine addiction. Alcohol is readily available, reasonably inexpensive, and considered a part of social exchange; its long-range physiological and psychological effects are well documented. It is estimated that 16.6 million adults in the United States struggle with alcohol use disorders. These affect men (9.8 million) nearly twice as often as women (5.8 million). In 2013, approximately 1.3 million adults received treatment for an alcohol use disorder at a specialized facility (7.8% of adults who needed treatment). This included 898,000 men (8.8% of men in need) and 417,000 women (7.5% of women who needed treatment) (USDHHS, NIH, NIAAA, 2015b).

The *Dietary Guidelines for Americans,* issued jointly by the US Department of Agriculture and the USDHHS (http://www.nutrition.gov), defines moderate drinking as no more than one drink a day for women and no more than two drinks a day for men. Women are more vulnerable than men to the effects of alcohol because, pound for pound, women have less water in their bodies, and they tend to weigh less than men. This means that identical doses of alcohol per kilogram of body weight will result in significantly higher blood alcohol levels in women. A woman's brain and other organs are exposed to more alcohol and to the toxic by-products of alcohol as it is metabolized. A woman is more likely to drink excessively if her parents, siblings, or other blood relatives have problems with alcohol; if she was abused physically or sexually as a child; if her partner drinks heavily; if she is experiencing difficulties with intimate and close relationships; or if she has a history of depression. (USDHHS, NIH, NIAAA, 2015a). Research also suggests that a woman's heavy drinking patterns may be associated with posttraumatic stress disorder, eating disorders, and suicidality although causality in the associations remains unclear (Wilsnack et al., 2014).

Alcohol use disorders are associated with motor vehicle accidents, violence, homicides, suicides, drownings, heart disease, strokes, liver disease, pancreatitis, and fetal alcohol syndrome. Fetal alcohol syndrome is the most common known preventable cause of mental impairment. The brain damage that occurs with fetal alcohol syndrome can result in lifelong problems with learning, memory, attention, and problem-solving (USDHHS, NIH, NIAAA, 2015a).

Initially, alcohol appears to be a stimulant, but it is actually a central nervous system depressant and anesthetic. Long-term alcohol use produces tolerance, thereby necessitating a gradual increase in dose to achieve the same effect. Alcohol contributes to problems with safety because of decreased reaction time and depression of the central nervous system. Those experiencing alcohol use disorders may report symptoms such as heartburn and gas, stomach distention, poor eating habits, nausea and vomiting, gastric pain, right upper quadrant pain, and irritation of the mouth, throat, and esophagus. Two additional subtle findings are spider angiomata and palmar erythema.

Primary prevention for substance and alcohol abuse is complex, especially because adults consume these agents for many reasons, including peer pressure, loneliness, alienation, frustration, anxiety, and low self-esteem. Heavy drinkers may also be following the example established by influential people in their lives. Merely telling people about the potential physical, emotional, and legal hazards appears to have little effect as a preventive measure. Promotion of more realistic portrayals of substance abuse through the media is difficult to implement. Although techniques such as assertiveness training and teaching adults to resist persuasion are helpful, more useful approaches might include helping them learn to manage anxiety and increase their self-esteem. Less anxious and more confident people have greater skills in resisting peer influences to participate in substance abuse; they also are more likely to have fewer episodes of isolation and loneliness.

Early detection and intervention can decrease ongoing and future physical and psychosocial problems resulting from alcohol abuse. Nurses use a variety of screening strategies to identify individuals' perceptions and consequences of drinking. The CAGE questionnaire is one of the most popular screening tools used in primary care. The Michigan Alcohol Screening Test (http://counselingresource.com/quizzes/alcohol/-mast/index.html) and the Alcohol Use Disorders Identification Test (https://

www.drugabuse.gov/sites/default/files/files/AUDIT.pdf) are examples of other screening instruments.

Abnormal laboratory test results, including elevations in aspartate aminotransferase level, erythrocyte mean corpuscular volume, and serum glutamyltransferase level, are not adequately sensitive and specific enough to detect alcohol use disorders as these may be a result of other causes, including trauma, disease, and medications.

A variety of treatments are known to be effective, but no single "best" intervention has been identified. Effective treatments may be to address other problems with use of interventions such as pharmacological agents, stress management, acupuncture, individual and family therapy, and supportive environments.

### Oral Health

***Gingivitis.*** Gingivitis is found commonly among adults who fail to brush their teeth and use dental floss regularly. Redness and swelling develop around the teeth. Bleeding of the gums, while the teeth are being brushed, is an early sign of gingivitis. The gums may or may not be tender. When inflammation is not adequately treated and controlled, periodontitis, involving bone destruction, can develop in addition to tooth loss.

***Dental hygiene and decay.*** Dental health is essential to overall health. Brushing the teeth and flossing after eating, receiving routine dental checkups, and consuming fewer carbohydrates (especially simple sugars) are important interventions to prevent dental caries. Adults in the middle years have responsibility not only for their own regular dental care but also for the care of their children and parents. Fluoridation of water (versus bottled or tap water) and use of applied sealants are additional health choices that support prevention of dental caries and, possibly, tooth loss.

Dental health is one of the leading indicators identified in *Healthy People 2020*. There is increasing evidence to show that periodontal, or gum disease, is closely linked to diabetes, heart disease, and stroke. For the middle-aged woman, poor oral health can cause premature births and low-birth-weight infants (Bensley et al., 2011).

There are many conditions that begin with changes in the oropharyngeal mucosa, such as cancer of the mouth and esophageal cancer. Consequently, annual dental checkups are important because dental professionals (dentists or dental hygienists) may be the first to detect a symptom or irregularity that points to a potentially dangerous condition.

Findings described on the *Healthy People 2020* oral health webpage indicate that approximately 41.2% of Americans representing all racial and ethnic groups receive annual health care by a dentist. The target goals for oral health services use (OH-7 outlined in the objectives for *Healthy People 2020*) indicate an expectation of a 10% increase in the proportion of adults and children aged 2 or older who receive dental care annually. The target goal is 49.0% of the population seeking dental care on an annual basis compared with the baseline of 41.2% reported in 2012.

People who are in vulnerable populations (individuals whose annual income is below the poverty line, others who are chronically ill or disabled, or still others whose medical or psychiatric treatment plans are very complicated) may not receive adequate or proper oral health care. The Surgeon General commented that, whereas there is evidence of progress being made to increase access to oral health services for a greater proportion of the population, those who are vulnerable because of their illness, such as people with HIV/AIDS, still find difficulty in obtaining proper and adequate oral health care (Benjamin, 2012). The Oral Health Care Initiative will help address the multilayered complexities that people with HIV/AIDS face. The factors that frequently deter oral health care in this population include lack of dental insurance, lack of transportation, limitations of disability, increasing costs of treatment, inability to afford the cost of oral health care, and discrimination on the part of dental health care providers. In sum, "the lack of dental care for individuals with HIV and AIDS undermines their treatment and diminishes their quality of life which in turn, can affect the overall outcomes of their overall treatment regimen" (USDHHS, 2010).

National data also indicate that the cost of dental care is a major deterrent to sustained oral health. Findings from the Healthy People Final Review (CDC, 2012) indicate that 16% of dentate adults aged 18 to 64 years reported an unmet dental need because of cost in the previous 12 months. Among adults aged 18 to 64 years, the main reason to forgo a dental visit for an oral health problem in the previous 6 months was cost; 42% could not afford treatment or did not have insurance.

Tobacco use in any form (cigarettes, pipes, and smokeless [spit] tobacco) raises the risk of gum disease. Findings from Bloom et al., 2012 indicate that dental health is often poor among smokers (currently smoking) compared with former smokers and with those who have never smoked. Smokers who were interviewed said that they had three or more dental problems. In addition, current smokers reported infrequent visits to their dentist (in some cases, more than 5 years) or never seeing a dentist. Research findings indicate the prevalence of gum disease is two times greater in individuals who smoke cigarettes compared with individuals who have never smoked (CDC, 2017f).

In summary, oral disease is preventable. Regularly scheduled dental care with a dentist and dental hygienist is highly recommended for good dental hygiene and early treatment of dental decay and periodontal diseases, such as gingivitis. In addition, dentists can provide screening for oropharyngeal cancer. Oral health is essential in the overall digestive and elimination processes.

## Elimination Pattern

Aging brings a gradual decrease of tone in the large intestine. This change, accompanied by a sedentary lifestyle, lack of fiber in the diet, and inadequate fluid intake, can predispose the adult to constipation. Advertising on television and other forms of media present strong arguments that encourage individuals to rely on external controls rather than on exercise and dietary means to solve this problem. Consequently, many adults are dependent on taking fiber products, as well as laxatives, for regular bowel movements.

In the kidneys, degenerative changes in the nephron units gradually increase during the middle years. In most cases, adults do not have any appreciable alteration in kidney function unless the person has experienced repeated infections, trauma, or the long-term effects of diabetes mellitus or hypertension.

Alteration in bladder control (incontinence) can occur in both women and men because of weakening of the muscles of the pelvic floor or damage to pelvic nerves. Urinary incontinence is problematic in women who have experienced multiple births. In men, urinary incontinence frequently occurs as a complication of surgery for prostate cancer. Incontinence can be socially embarrassing, but the condition can be relieved with Kegel exercises (Santacreu & Fernández-Ballesteros, 2011; Siegel, 2014).

## Activity-Exercise Pattern

Regular physical activity increases life expectancy and the quality of life. Exercise helps to prevent coronary heart disease, hypertension, diabetes, osteoporosis, and depression. Research findings show there is a strong correlation between physical exercise and lower rates of osteoporosis (National Osteoporosis Foundation, 2014), back injury, stroke, and colon cancer. Weight loss programs that incorporate physical activities also make significant contributions to health promotion as evidenced by increased life expectancy and quality of life.

One of the objectives of *Healthy People 2020* is to continue to decrease deaths related to heart disease. Evidence suggests that a significant percentage of Americans in the middle-aged adult bracket do not engage in regular moderate physical activity for at least 30 minutes on five or more days a week. Only a fraction of adults perform the recommended level. The proportion of adults who did not participate in any form of leisure-time physical activity (objective 22-1) decreased by 9% between 1997 and 2008, from 40% to 36%, moving toward the 2010 target of 20% (CDC, 2012). Sedentary behavior increases with aging. This finding may be due to the onset of conditions that affect mobility and strength.

Continuous, rhythmic exercise maintained for a period sufficient to stress the cardiac system (increase heart rate and blood pressure) is desirable. Some suggested activities include brisk walking, jogging, swimming, bicycling, and skipping rope, as well as walking or biking to work. Activities that focus on skill and coordination should be attempted by the adult older than 40 years rather than activities necessitating speed and strength. Moderation is key for all groups of individuals. Caution is recommended for adults nearing age 65 years to prevent muscle strains and/or falls. Overexertion, as evidenced by dizziness, chest pressure or chest pain, and unresolved shortness of breath, should be avoided. Additionally, in hot weather, strenuous exercise should be balanced with rest periods and increased intake of fluids to prevent heat stroke.

Nurses play significant roles in assessing, teaching, and evaluating individuals relative to activity-exercise programs. Advanced practice nurses are often instrumental in creating and guiding weight loss programs; nurses working in the community may see local citizens at health fairs or health-promotion events; and other nurses or therapists visit individuals at home for care following hospitalization for surgery or acute illness as home health professionals. Activity programs are initiated to restore health (following heart attack) or to improve cardiac function (such as cardiac and pulmonary rehabilitation), and in some cases to control blood glucose levels. A thorough assessment, including a cardiac stress test, is necessary when an individual has not exercised regularly in the past. Parameters for heart rate, blood pressure, and length and frequency of exercise sessions are set in advance by a cardiologist. Nurses support and guide individuals by helping them determine program goals, by monitoring their progress, and by teaching individuals how to modify lifestyle behaviors to obtain particular objectives.

To achieve maximal effectiveness, physical exercise should involve as many muscles as possible and be performed on a regular basis. Adults should spend 30 minutes or more in brisk physical activity every day for a total of 3 to 4 hours per week. The optimal performance level differs for each individual and should be based on parameters set by the individual's physician in advance of the individual starting a fitness program. The following formula to calculate the target heart rate is shown on the American Heart Association (2012) website. Begin by subtracting one's age from 220 and then multiply this number by 0.75 to determine a heart rate that is within safe limits. For example, for an individual who is 50 years old, $(220 - 50) = 170$; $170 \times 0.75 = 127.5$ (or 128 beats per minute) for the optimal heart rate. Comparatively, the cardiac muscle capacity of a person younger than 50 years would be greater than 128 beats per minute; and as the functional aerobic capacity is increased, the target heart rate required to tone the cardiac muscle will increase.

To summarize, routine exercise is essential to the health of the heart and overall muscle strength. The type of activity and style is an individual choice. Program goals are achieved more readily when exercise is incorporated into leisure activities or is a part of a group activity.

## Sleep-Rest Pattern

Middle-aged Americans may not get as much sleep as young adults because of increased demands in their lives. Caring for immediate family, children, and sometimes parents, as well as employment responsibilities, consume most of a 24-hour period.

Insomnia is a common finding in this age category. It may be the result of overstimulation resulting from drinking too many caffeinated beverages, strenuous exercise within 2 hours of bedtime, or failure to have a regular sleep-wake schedule in a 24-hour period (National Sleep Foundation, 2017). Frequently occurring insomnia can lead to distractibility, irritability, and fatigue during the daytime hours.

Sleep apnea is a common disorder during which normal breathing is disrupted by breathing pauses or shallow breaths. Breathing pauses may occur 30 times or more each hour and may last from a few seconds to minutes. Because of collapsed or blocked airways, a loud snorting or snoring sound is produced when normal breathing resumes. This pattern of pauses and shallow breathing is typical for the most common type of sleep apnea: obstructive sleep apnea. Although obstructive sleep apnea may be experienced by all, this type of sleep apnea commonly affects obese adults. Central sleep apnea is the less common type of sleep apnea. It occurs because of a disruption of central nerve

signals to the diaphragm resulting in brief periods of not breathing while asleep.

Sleep apnea is a chronic condition and may increase the risk of myocardial infarction, stroke, arrhythmias, and heart failure. Treatments include lifestyle changes such as weight loss, continuous positive airway pressure therapy, the use of mouthpieces, or surgical intervention (USDHHS, NIH, National Heart, Lung, and Blood Institute, 2012).

Rest is essential to allow restorative functions of the body to occur. The effects of insomnia can be counteracted by regularly scheduled, high-quality sleep, and occasional napping when fatigued. If insomnia becomes a chronic problem, cognitive-behavioral therapy has also been demonstrated to be an effective treatment option (Kaldo et al., 2015). The National Sleep Foundation (http://www.nationalsleepfoundation.org) offers detailed information about treating insomnia and other sleep disorders with medications if that modality is indicated.

## Cognitive-Perceptual Pattern

Learning is a phenomenon that occurs across the life span. The need to increase knowledge or information and the need to acquire new skills are constants as adults develop through a variety of experiences. Employment demands or new roles in life, such as becoming a parent or suddenly needing to care for an elderly family member, thrust the middle-aged adult into numerous different learning situations. The ability to learn a range of skills or to acquire knowledge through observing, performing, or participating in play activities begins in childhood as described by Gardner (1983, 1993) and extends into the middle years and beyond. The capacity to perform intellectually (i.e., reason through critical thinking, use/increase vocabulary, and apply spatial perception skills) stays constant through the 35- to 65-year-old age range. However, some decreases in reaction time and cognitive flexibility become more apparent as age increases.

### Intellectual Ability

The ability to acquire new knowledge or skills, or "learning intelligence," accumulates through formal education and life experiences and continues to increase throughout life. The evidence of this phenomenon is demonstrated by the many scholars and artists who become more productive in their middle years than when they were young adults. Some individuals discover "new talents" later in life because they have more leisure time or motivation to explore new areas or interests.

The theories of Piaget (1970), Bloom (1984), and Havighurst and Orr (1956) are relevant to the middle-aged adult. These theorists conclude that the prime time to be in the learner role is when the developmental task for that role is to be accomplished. The adult in the middle years as the learner-performer is a case in point. For example, to balance the responsibilities of caring for children and parents and being employed outside the home, the adult may explore new career options or creative endeavors.

Havighurst and Orr (1956) defines developmental tasks as the basic tasks of living that must be achieved for the adult to live successfully. These tasks are dictated by the expectations of

> ### BOX 23-5  Developmental Tasks of Middle Age
>
> - Helping children become responsible, happy adults
> - Rediscovering or developing new satisfaction in the relationship with one's spouse (for the single adult, this can occur in a relationship with a sibling or significant other)
> - Developing an affectionate, but independent, relationship with aging parents
> - Reaching the peak in one's career
> - Achieving mature social and civic responsibility
> - Accepting and adapting to biological changes
> - Maintaining or developing friendships
> - Developing leisure-time activities

society, the physiological changes of the body throughout life, and the individual's own value system and goals. Although initially described in 1956, Havighurst and Orr's developmental tasks of middle age remain timely (Box 23-5).

If career goals have been previously identified, then attaining them can be highly rewarding, both psychologically and financially. In addition to career activities, the mature adult has an increased social awareness and often assumes more civic responsibility.

Piaget's theory of cognitive development, formal operations are the highest or most complex level. This stage begins at approximately age 12 years and continues throughout life. Piaget describes the thoughts of adults as being both flexible and effective. The adult can deal efficiently with complex problems of reasoning, including hypothesis testing (Piaget, 1970).

Bloom (1984) developed a hierarchy of cognitive levels in the adult learner. Knowledge is the simplest or most basic cognitive level. Knowledge is the acquisition of information. The adult learner defines "high blood pressure" in lay terms.

Comprehension is the second level, as indicated by the learner grasping the meaning of the communicated message and relating the term(s) to other material. For example, the individual can state one way that obesity influences high blood pressure.

The third level is application of knowledge. At this level the learner demonstrates an understanding of ideas and concepts by extending them to describe or relate them to real-life situations. For example, the individual with hypertension becomes involved in an exercise program.

The fourth level is analysis. At this level, all aspects of learning are united in thought, and the individual is cognizant of the relationships and interactions of all the parts. For example, the individual considers his or her values and life goals when making decisions about taking action in regard to understanding health care needs.

The highest order of learning involves synthesis and evaluation. The person is able to combine various elements to form a plan and then is able to judge the extent to which the actions and results satisfy the original objectives. For example, people may develop plans to improve their health status and increase their disease self-management responsibilities. The next step is to validate the results of ongoing health care programs in relation to their projected expectations. Genetic and personality factors, in combination with environmental conditions and lifestyle

practices, account for the large difference in the ways in which individuals maintain mental abilities. Schaie and Willis (2005) have identified seven factors that maintain cognitive function in later life:

- Absence of chronic diseases
- Living with favorable socioeconomic factors, including maximal occupational complexity, a low degree of routine, and an intact family
- Involvement in complex social activities
- Flexible personality style
- Marriage to a spouse with high cognitive function
- Maintaining high levels of performance speed
- Personal satisfaction with accomplishments in midlife and early old age (see Box 23-5)

## Perceptual Changes

Presbyopia (farsightedness) is common in middle-aged adults, even in individuals who have had no previous problems with their vision. This condition occurs because of the loss of elasticity in the lens of the eye so that the adult cannot focus on objects that are in close range, such as reading without using prescription lenses.

Presbyopia is corrected with prescription lenses, which may be needed only for reading or for close work. LASIK surgery, a surgical intervention to correct refraction, is currently widely used and is favored by individuals who do not want to use standard eyeglasses.

Other visual conditions that may not be as easily corrected include decreased peripheral vision and decreased visual sensitivity in the dark. Both conditions are slow and insidious in their development and occur as the cornea becomes less transparent. Because all these conditions are not readily detected by the individual, middle-aged adults should undergo a routine professional eye examination every year.

Glaucoma occurs as a result of increased intraocular pressure, which can damage the optic nerve, resulting in vision loss and blindness (CDC, 2017a). Loss of peripheral vision, or tunnel vision, is a common condition associated with glaucoma. Damage to the optic nerve is irreversible, but visual loss can be prevented if damage is identified early and treatment is initiated. Information available at http://www.aao.org/eyecare-america shows that glaucoma is the leading cause of blindness among black Americans in the United States. A current estimate is three times the number of black Americans compared with white Americans have glaucoma; also in addition, the rate of blindness attributable to glaucoma is four times greater in black Americans relative to white Americans. The importance of regular eye examinations by an ophthalmologist cannot be underestimated.

A cataract, opacity of the lens, can develop and cloud the vision in the later years of middle age. Often cataracts develop in people who have diabetes. Another disorder, diabetic retinopathy, gradually causes rupture of vessels in the retina, which leak into the eye causing lack of color differentiation and central vision changes.

Macular degeneration is often referred to as age-related macular degeneration (AMD). This age-related disorder is a progressive deterioration of the maculae of the retina and choroid structures of the eye and results in damaged sharp and central vision. Approximately 1.8 million Americans aged 40 years or older are affected by AMD, and the number of people with AMD is estimated to reach 2.95 million by 2020 (CDC, 2015b). This condition is very serious because it represents the effects of several disorders. Once a diagnosis of macular degeneration has been made, retinal ophthalmologists should be involved in the care of the individual.

Another common perceptual change in middle age is **presbycusis** (impaired auditory acuity). The first sounds to be lost are higher frequencies, such as a woman's voice. This is important in the work environment and situations that require social interaction. Because this process is subtle, middle age is a time for auditory evaluations as a part of routine examinations.

Beginning in the middle years, the sense of taste diminishes in a progressive and predictable manner. The taste buds located more anteriorly on the tongue are the first to be affected, causing an inability to detect sweet and salt. When the effectiveness of the posterior taste buds declines, detection of bitter and sour flavors is lost. Consequently, this change can alter a person's food preferences and present problems for people who insist on adding salt to compensate for the deficit. Nurses involved in the care of the middle-aged adult, perhaps in the community or in home health, can show the individual how the use of various herbs and spices can enhance flavor.

## Self-Perception–Self-Concept Pattern

### Levinson's Theory

In Levinson's research on men (Levinson, 1986a,b) and women (Levinson, 1996), a theory on "individual life structures" is posed. Levinson describes age-associated seasons or eras. The midlife transition, beginning at age 38 to 40 years, appears to include reappraising one's life, integrating the polarities, and modifying one's life structure toward being who one wants to be. Middle-aged adults struggle with meaning, value, and direction of their lives.

### Erikson's Theory

In Erikson's eight stages of the life cycle (Erikson & Erikson, 1998), the last three stages are related to adulthood. Stage 7, generativity versus stagnation or self-absorption, is most frequently associated with the middle years.

Erikson identifies generativity as the primary task to achieve during adulthood. Generativity includes a sense of productivity and creativity as evidenced by reaching previously established goals versus stagnation, the failure to achieve lifelong goals (Hornstein, 1986; Reifman et al., 1991; Thomas, 1995). Generativity also encompasses a desire to care for others versus self-absorption, the tendency to direct most of one's interest and attention to oneself thereby excluding others.

Middle age is a time of critical self-review. For some, this review may prompt sadness, disappointment, self-doubt, and regret if the desired and expected life goals have not been met. Both women and men question their value to society, the merit of their accomplishments, their success as sexual beings, and the probability of attaining yet unfilled life goals. Women generally

make this life assessment between 35 and 50 years or age, whereas men do not usually begin until approximately age 40 years. Women typically begin earlier to look for changes they may want to make in their lives (Apter, 1995), whereas men remain content with the status quo. Because the male life assessment tends to begin later, there is potential for couples of approximately the same age to experience conflict within the relationship. This type of self-review and lack of effective communication of personal needs with a spouse or life partner is a threat to marital stability (Erikson & Erikson, 1998; Vaillant & Vaillant, 1990).

### Physiological Changes

The effect of physiological changes on mental health is nearly as critical during the middle years as it is during adolescence. Some of the most obvious changes that influence self-esteem are graying hair, an increase in the number of wrinkles, decreased visual and auditory acuity, and changes in body shape. The extent to which these changes are tolerated depends largely on the person's level of self-satisfaction and acceptance. Some people try to "hold on" to youth by dressing as more youthful counterparts dress, whereas others adapt their attire to their age and position in life.

Before 2002, hormone therapy (estrogen alone or estrogen and progesterone) was given to millions of postmenopausal women. Estrogen is still the only therapy approved by the Food and Drug Administration for the treatment of hot flashes associated with menopause. Millions of women took hormone therapy not only to relieve hot flashes but also in the hope that it might prevent heart disease, the number one cause of death in postmenopausal women. All of that changed in 2002, however, when data from the Women's Health Initiative (WHI) showed that postmenopausal women who took estrogen and progesterone actually had higher rates of heart attacks and other health problems, including stroke, blood clots, and breast cancer.

Follow-up analysis of the WHI data showed that the effects of hormone therapy depend on a woman's age and the length of time since menopause. In younger postmenopausal women, between 50 and 59 years of age, hormone use did not increase the risk of cardiac events, as it did in older women. There is new evidence that hormone therapy may actually be beneficial for younger postmenopausal women, but for now, hormone therapy is not recommended for the prevention of heart disease (Whayne & Mukherjee, 2015).

Health benefits of hormone therapy include decreased risk of osteoporosis and decreased rates of colorectal cancer (American Cancer Society, 2015; Whayne & Mukherjee, 2015). Research is ongoing regarding the risks and benefits of hormone therapy. Currently, the only approved indication for postmenopausal hormone therapy is for the relief of moderate to severe vasomotor symptoms (hot flashes). Only short-term use is advised (1–3 years) (Lowdermilk & Perry, 2012).

Increasing numbers of women are now looking for non-hormonal ways to treat hot flashes and other symptoms associated with menopause. The law passed in 1994 to regulate dietary supplements provides some oversight for natural health products but does not require manufacturers to prove that dietary supplements are either safe or effective (AACE Menopause Guidelines Revision Task Force, 2011).

Because there are few scientific data, many midlife women find it difficult to make decisions about using alternative products. Black cohosh, soy, and vitamin E are just a few of the products marketed to women. Even if these products are effective, women must be cautious about drug interactions that may occur. The use of prescription medication increases with age. The benefits of using alternative therapy may outweigh the risks, but more research is needed on the safety profile of natural remedies (AACE Menopause Guidelines Revision Task Force, 2011).

It is difficult to separate menopause from the physical and psychological changes that women experience as they age. The stressors common to women in their 40s and 50s include raising a family, helping parents as they age, coping with divorce or death of a spouse, retirement, and financial insecurity. Menopause happens in the midst of this. All the events in a woman's life influence her experience of menopause and the **perimenopause**, a period that precedes menopause and lasts approximately 4 years. Symptoms such as mood swings, nervousness, agitation, fatigue, and depression are often ascribed to the decline in estrogen levels that occurs during this time. The physiological changes are important, but a woman's experience in menopause is profoundly affected by all the events in her life (Lowdermilk & Perry, 2012).

Men also experience physical and psychological reactions to middle age. The hormonal changes in men are gradual, typically beginning between 40 and 55 years of age. The symptoms are similar to those experienced by women with the emotional effects related to other life events, past coping patterns, and general feelings of self-esteem.

## Roles-Relationships Pattern

Middle age is frequently a time of reassessment, turmoil, and change. This time has been called "**midlife crisis**." The turning point occurs for several reasons. Over time, middle-aged adults become aware of subtle and compromising changes in physical, cognitive, and emotional agility. Furthermore, the inevitability of one's own death is recognized, perhaps for the first time. Middle-aged adults must accept that lifestyle choices have been made, unintended consequences may have lasting repercussions, and the opportunity to amend prior decisions may no longer be possible. Alternatively, middle-aged adults may be quite satisfied with prior life choices and the resultant personal satisfaction and contentment (Box 23-6: Research for Evidence-based Practice).

### Family

Duvall and Miller (1985) delineate eight stages of the family life cycle, with stages 5, 6, and 7 in the middle years (see Chapter 7):
- Stage 5: Families with children, with the oldest child aged 13 to 20 years; lasts approximately 7 years
- Stage 6: Families launching young adults, from the first leaving until the last; lasts approximately 8 years

### BOX 23-6 RESEARCH FOR EVIDENCE-BASED PRACTICE

#### *"Regrets are the natural property of grey hairs"—Charles Dickens*

Disappointment and regret are common emotions experienced across all ages. Life-span theorists suggest that regret-producing consequences are associated with low levels of life satisfaction, low levels of subjective well-being, and high levels of biological age-related changes among midlife and older adults more often than among younger adults (Wrosch et al., 2005). Time lived was understood to intensify the degree of angst associated with perceived regrettable situations because middle-aged and older adults have less time to take corrective action or make amends.

The latest research suggests that middle-aged and older adults are less likely to engage in remorseful rumination than are younger adults (Brassen et al., 2012; Charles, 2010; Mather, 2012). Despite normative age-related physical decline, middle-aged and older adults typically report greater life satisfaction and remarkably higher levels of emotional well-being than young adults, including a decline in their experience of negative emotions (Chowdhury et al., 2014). Even in the presence of physical comorbidities, decreased cognitive agility, a diminishing social circle, and perhaps the death of a spouse, family member, or close friends, middle-aged and older adults have harnessed strategies that preserve emotional well-being, even as they continue to age (Mather, 2012). According to Mather (2012), age-related emotional processing has a biological basis that helps explains why patterns of coping with regret differ between young adults and those in the middle years and beyond.

From Brassen, S., Gamer, M., Peters, J., et al. (2012). Don't look back in anger! Responsiveness to missed changes in successful and nonsuccessful aging. *Science, 336*(6081), 612–614; Charles, S. T. (2010). Strength and vulnerability integration: A model of emotional well-being across adulthood. *Psychol Bull, 136*(6), 1068–1091; Chowdhury, R., Sharot, T., Wolfe, T., et al. (2014). Optimistic update bias increases in older age. *Psychological Medicine, 44*(9), 2003–2012; Mather, M. (2012). The emotion paradox in the aging brain. *Annals of the New York Academy of Sciences, 1251*(1), 33–49; Wrosch, C., Bauer, I., & Scheier, M. F. (2005). Regret and quality of life across the adult life span: The influence of disengagement and available future goals. *Psychology and Aging, 20*(4), 657–670.

- Stage 7: Families from empty nest to retirement; lasts approximately 15 years

The developmental tasks identified for the families in stages 6 and 7 are similar to those described by Havighurst and Orr (1956); they focus on changes from a nuclear family to a marital couple with other responsibilities. For example, in stage 6, the parents who are helping their children become independent may also be caring for their aging parents. Additionally, middle-aged adults fulfill multiple complex responsibilities within a variety of career, social, and civic positions.

These transitions can be even more challenging for the family headed by a single parent. Approximately 21 million children, approximately 28% of children in the United States, lived with one parent in 2012, most typically the mother. The single most significant health risk in families headed by a single mother is poverty. In 2012, nearly one in two children whose mother was the sole head of the household were found to be living below the poverty level. Comparatively, 70% of children who lived with two married parents were in households that were at least 200% above the poverty level (US Census Bureau, 2013). Inadequate resources make it extremely difficult for middle-aged mothers, who are frequently raising grandchildren as well, to fulfill their responsibilities.

Families with young adolescent or young adult children have been described in research studies as both *postparental* and *launching families.* In contrast, criticism of this emphasis on the separation of children (regardless of age) from their families is increasing. Gilligan (1982) criticizes the work of many human development theorists who identify human development in terms of separation from the family. Apter (1990) also challenges the conventional view that adolescent girls must reject their mothers as part of a healthy development. Middle-aged parents are encouraged to continue to care for and nurture their adolescent and adult children while recognizing the increasing interdependence of their relationships.

By supporting their children's efforts, parents can increase the self-esteem of their children while being effective role models. The parent assumes less of a parent-child relationship while interacting more on an adult-to-adult level. As the children are "launched," the parents may have uninterrupted time alone and time to share activities. Family life may also be threatened by older children living at home, opposition to a child's partner, or the inability to establish satisfactory relationships with potential or actual partners or sons-in-law and daughters-in-law. For many parents, the idea of their children leaving home is anticipated with relief that the heavy care responsibilities of parenting are over or with dread over having to fill the void of time and inactivity. The empty nest syndrome may be exacerbated if the husband and wife have never learned to communicate effectively and to enjoy each other's company without the children.

At the other end of the family spectrum, aging parents can place demands on the adult child primarily because older adults are frequently beset with health problems. A caring relationship is in order, in which the aging parent's need for independence is recognized.

Because of society's emphasis on youth, the middle-aged adult must associate feelings of self-worth with personal integrity rather than with body appearance or physical prowess. Friends of both sexes can provide invaluable support systems. With the newly found free time after children have left home, the middle-aged adult can share favorite activities and learn new ones. Middle-aged adults should remind themselves how much and how well they are doing, especially considering the complexity of the demands placed on them. Never before in history have families pursued such varied and individual-oriented goals as they do today.

Although for many Americans the concept of family remains of major importance, the perceptions are different from those held by previous generations. Parents and children in most families are involved in numerous activities, as evidenced by a "let's-hurry-or-we'll-be-late" orientation. Even younger children frequently have schedules that must be met if they are to get to their dance, drama, play, or enrichment classes. None of these activities necessarily have a negative effect, but the cumulative influence places heavy demands on all family members. Additionally, many activities in which both children and adults are involved

have a certain degree of competitiveness. For example, parents frequently become emotionally involved in the athletic activities of their children to the extent that the failure of a 6-year-old to play a winning softball game causes a great deal of parental anguish. One only has to listen to the cheering of parents at a Little League baseball game to note whose self-esteem is at stake. Shouts of "Kill her," "Grab the third baseman," and so on do not tend to engender feelings of team spirit or a notion of playing for the sake of having a good time (Erikson & Erikson, 1998).

## Work

Perhaps the most common role that middle-aged adults share is that of a worker. Much of their pride and sense of satisfaction is derived from their work. Work is equated with being "grown up." One can easily recall the "What do you want to be when you grow up?" questioning of youth. Success and achievement are evaluated in terms of careers and family life. The work ethic still persists, especially for individuals born during the Great Depression and for many of their offspring as well. Much of their conversation evolves from what they do, such as "My name is Leslie Smith. I am a real estate agent." To be mature is to be a responsible, hard-working individual (Erikson & Erikson, 1998). Research has shown that middle-aged adults are more satisfied with their jobs than are younger adults.

Middle-aged adults constitute most of the American workforce. For many, vocations play a major role in defining personal levels of wellness. There were approximately 2.9 million nonfatal workplace injuries and illnesses in 2015. The 2015 rate continues a pattern of annual decline over the last 13 years. Employers reported nearly 48,000 fewer nonfatal injury and illness cases in 2015 compared to 2014 (US Department of Labor, Occupational Safety and Health Administration, 2016b). The highest rates of nonfatal injuries occur in construction, manufacturing, and health services. Thirty percent of nonfatal injuries and illnesses requiring days away from work continue to be due to overexertion and repetitive motion (Nicholson, 2011).

A total of 4836 workers died from a work-related injury in the US during 2015, the highest annual figure since 2008. Nearly 20% of the fatally-injured workers were employed in the private construction industry (US Department of Labor, Occupational Safety and Health Administration, 2016a). More than 22% of workplace fatal injuries involved motor vehicles; other causes included falls, nonvehicular injuries, blows, and electrocutions. In decreasing order, workers in mining, agriculture, forestry, fishing, construction, and transportation are at an increased risk of dying from a work-related injury (Nicholson, 2011; US Department of Labor, Occupational Safety and Health Administration, 2010). Poor housekeeping and poor design predispose workers to falls and other accidents; exposure to noise and toxic chemicals also make employees susceptible to injury and illness. Many injuries that contribute significantly to the morbidity and mortality of adults can be prevented. Fixing faulty steps, repairing faulty electrical wires, and securing carpets are only a few of the many preventive measures.

Accidents are twice as common among smokers than among nonsmokers. Possible explanations include the loss of attention, the use of one hand for smoking, and irritation of the eyes.

## BOX 23-7  QUALITY AND SAFETY SCENARIO

### Lifetime Prevention of Cardiovascular Disease in Women

- **Eat a healthy diet** with fruits, vegetables, whole grains, and fat-free or low-fat milk and milk products. Choose foods low in saturated fats, cholesterol, salt (sodium), and added sugars.
- **Exercise regularly.** Adults need 2 hours and 30 minutes (or 150 minutes total) of exercise each week. You can spread your activity out during the week, and can break it up into smaller chunks of time during the day.
- **Be smoke-free.** If you are ready to quit, call 1-800-QUIT-NOW (1-800-784-8669) or 1-855-DÉJELO-YA (1-855-335-3569 for Spanish speakers) for free resources, including free quit coaching, a free quit plan, free educational materials, and referrals to other resources where you live.
- **Limit alcohol use,** which can lead to long-term health problems, including heart disease and cancer. If you do choose to drink, do so in moderation, which is no more than one drink a day for women. Do not drink at all if you are pregnant.
- **Know your family history.** There may be factors that could increase your risk for heart disease and stroke.
- **Manage any medical condition** you might have. Learn the **ABCS** of heart health. Keep them in mind every day and especially when you talk to your health provider:
  - **Appropriate aspirin therapy** for those who need it.
  - **Blood pressure control**
  - **Cholesterol management**
  - **Smoking cessation**

From Centers for Disease Control (CDC). (2017). *Lower your risk for the number 1 killer of women.* https://www.cdc.gov/features/wearred/index.html.

Other work-related problems include exposure to harmful substances resulting in lung diseases, cancers, and workplace violence (Box 23-7: Quality and Safety Scenario).

The effect of life events on mental health depends on the personal strength of the individual, the availability of supports, and the nature and number of events and their significance for the person. Three common examples of life events with potential disruptive effects are marital separation or divorce, having two or more jobs, and caring for aging parents. Their negative effects may be alleviated if assistance is provided early in the process of a change. In some organizations, resources for managing problems of addiction, life transitions, emotional issues, financial problems, stress reduction, and grief counseling are available off-site to all employees. These resources are offered without cost to the individual and, in some cases, to their family members or support persons.

### Two-or-More-Job Family: Family and Work Responsibilities

More and more women are in the workforce for their own financial well-being or that of their family, especially with the increased cost of living, health care insurance, and college expenses and the decreased availability of employer-sponsored pension. Other women, who are postmenopausal and have launched their last child, have a newfound freedom and begin to rediscover themselves, sometimes through a new career. The husband may be a support person in this venture or he may feel threatened by his wife's new pursuits. These role changes and life transitions can be stressors to the family.

The balance between marital status, with or without children at home, caring for older parents, and employment obligations can significantly affect the psychological well-being of the woman in her middle years. In recent years, changes in family patterns with adult children moving back into their parents' home, sometimes with their offspring, bring new challenges to relationships, resources, and responsibilities within the home.

Historically, women worked with their husbands within the family farm or business. Only in the few decades immediately after World War II did many middle class white women stay at home while their husbands went to work. Currently, women make up a significant portion of the workforce. Additionally, many women have become highly educated and motivated to pursue careers. Both men and women are increasingly taking jobs that do not end at 5:00 p.m. The problems and challenges of the workplace are experienced at home as adults bring projects and problems home with them.

Job-related travel has also increased during the last few years for both men and women. Travel by either partner means additional responsibilities for the one who remains at home. Additionally, if one spouse travels far more than the other travels, feelings of resentment may develop, or the common ground for discussion of work events may be altered. The one who stays at home may feel "put upon" when the spouse is perceived as having fun. In contrast, travel is tiring and is not usually as exciting as it appears to observers. The traveling spouse can come home tired and irritable and desire peace and quiet, which may conflict with the expectations of other family members.

Men may feel threatened by highly successful and visible women. For some families the post–World War II prototype was for the husband to support the family financially and gain status through achievements of work outside the home. As women gain recognition and acclaim for their career accomplishments, even the most "enlightened" man may experience twinges of envy and discomfort. Men have few role models to learn how best to be a participant in a successful two-career family. Men may need as much, if not more, support than women in adapting to contemporary family styles. Opportunities to discuss what it means to be a man in today's society can be helpful, such as in support groups with volunteers or professionals who provide services to various agencies and community resources.

In addition to the changes in women and the effect on families of each adult working at one or more jobs, the nature of the parental work environment is critical to family coping ability. Work that is emotionally draining, particularly when it is filled with conflict, poses special threats to family stability. When parents come home tired, angry, or frustrated from their experiences at work, they likely have limited emotional support to share with other family members. When people gain self-esteem from their jobs and generally enjoy going to work, they tend to experience less frustration and dissatisfaction with themselves and their positions, enabling them to give more of themselves to other members of the family.

Middle age is important when one is looking at the career clock. Issues that need to be considered include midcareer changes and preretirement planning. Retirement is a major turning point; to many people, it is the transition from middle age to old age and the period of work to the period of leisure or different work.

Adults are working up to and beyond the age of retirement. Many are entering new careers later in life because they are living longer and are in need of more financial resources to successfully enter the older adult years. As adults progress through the middle years, they become increasingly aware of the time remaining until retirement: "Can I readjust my goals?" "Is there disparity between where I am in my career and where I would like to be?" An example might be the 60-year-old veteran nightclub singer whose goal to record a solo album remains to be achieved. The heightened awareness of age and the decreased likelihood of finding another suitable job can precipitate increased anxiety or depression in this singer.

Comprehensive health-promotion programs at the work site contain these elements: "health education that focuses on skill development and lifestyle behavior change in addition to information dissemination and awareness building, preferably tailored to employees' interests and needs; supportive social and physical work environments, including established norms for healthy behavior and policies that promote health and reduce the risk of disease, such as work site smoking policies, healthy nutrition alternatives in the cafeteria and vending services, and opportunities for obtaining regular physical activity; integration of the work site program into the organization's administrative structure; related programs, such as employee assistance programs; and screening programs, preferably linked to health care service delivery to ensure follow-up and appropriate treatment as necessary and to encourage adherence. Optimally, these efforts should be part of a comprehensive occupational health and safety program" (US Department of Labor, Occupational Safety and Health Administration, 2010).

### Caring for Aging Parents

The needs of aging parents and of the middle-aged adult's own children can create additional demands during the middle years (Figure 23-1). The middle-aged adult can feel caught between the children and the parents. Both children and older parents can present unrealistic, excessive demands and be difficult to please.

Middle-aged adults may be faced with having frail and ill parents live within their own family unit or placing them in a nursing home. These dilemmas are complicated by the reality that their parents are growing older and may not have long to live. The recognition of the parents' impending death heightens middle-aged adults' awareness of their own aging and mortality.

Difficulties in caring for older parents can be somewhat lessened when potential situations are discussed before a crisis arises. This is particularly true when all members of the middle-aged adult family are working, space in their home is limited, and the community has few resources for the well or ill older adults. Although institutionalization is undesirable to many families, the care of ill, older parents may eventually require it. By anticipating these needs and preparing for them, middle-aged adults and their parents can develop further meaningful relationships with one another.

### Divorce

Divorce is a major disruption to the marriage and family and to each individual's short-term and long-term health. As the divorce rate has risen in recent years, individuals and families have been challenged to find solutions to new and multiple problems. When a divorce occurs, each family member must confront the necessity to examine and, in many cases, modify an accustomed style of living and adapting.

In the early 1970s, Wallerstein and colleagues (2000) began a longitudinal study of 131 children of divorced parents through extensive interviews with the children and their parents. The children are now adults with families of their own. The most significant findings of this ongoing study are the long-lasting, cumulative, and demonstrative effects of divorce, which continue for decades. Although Wallerstein found healing in adults is more or less complete 3 years after divorce, this is not so for the children, who experience the divorce differently from their parents.

Some of the limitations of Wallerstein's research are anecdotal methods versus double-blind interviews; the children are primarily white, educated, and upper middle class; and the findings are not differentiated from those of high-conflict families, nor are distinctions made between the influences of conflict that caused the divorce and the actual divorce itself. Continuing research is being done to illuminate these initial findings on the long-term effects of divorce. Sumnera (2013) suggests that parental midlife divorce also impacts children who are adults at the time of parental separation. Therapeutic interventions that assist adult children of divorced parents to reconcile the divorce experience of their parents should be offered and available.

### Death

Similarly to divorce, death of a spouse can result in grieving for the loss of companionship and the loss of an anticipated future free from the responsibilities of work and children. The surviving spouse may be unprepared to be single again, to be the only parent, or to live alone. The loneliness may be exacerbated by

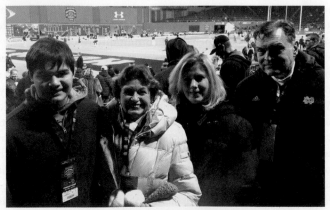

**FIGURE 23-1** Middle-aged adults, young adults, and older adults can enjoy meaningful relationships with one another.

ill or dying peers or parents. Middle-aged adults become increasingly aware of the finite nature of life, thinking not only of the number of years since birth but also of the number of years left to live. The midlife review is a common outcome of this recognition.

## Sexuality-Reproductive Pattern

Research suggests that a high proportion of men and women remain sexually active well into later life (Lochlainn & Kenny, 2013). Men and women can continue to have a satisfactory pattern of sexual functioning throughout the middle and older adult years. As they would in any other developmental phase, middle-aged adults may need counseling to make health-promoting decisions about their sexual and reproductive behaviors and health.

Unintended pregnancies are high across all ages of American women but are highest (77% of all pregnancies) in middle-aged women. Fertility begins to decline for women between 35 and 40 years of age; however, perimenopausal women are still at risk of an unintended pregnancy (Nelson, 2011). Nearly 30% of pregnancies in women older than 35 years are unintended (Godfrey et al., 2011). Upson and colleagues (2010) found that 14% of women aged between 35 and 44 years failed to use a contraceptive at the last sexual intercourse and that the rate of unprotected intercourse nearly doubled for women aged between 40 and 44 years. In contrast, women planning to have children during the fourth and fifth decades of life should know that fertility rates decrease and infant mortality rates increase, especially when mothers are aged 45 years or older. In 2013, fetal mortality rates for women aged 45 years or older were more than twice the rate for women aged 25 to 29 years (MacDorman & Gregory, 2015).

The pregnancy-related mortality rate for all women in the United States was 17.8 deaths per 100,000 live births in 2011 as compared with 7.2 deaths per 100,000 live births in 1987. Research indicates that an increasing number of pregnant women in the United States have chronic health conditions such as hypertension, diabetes, and chronic heart disease that increase the risk of complications. Considerable racial disparities in pregnancy-related mortality exist. In 2011, the pregnancy-related mortality rates were 12.5 deaths per 100,000 live births for white women, 42.8 deaths per 100,000 live births for black women, and 17.3 deaths per 100,000 live births for women of other races (MacDorman & Gregory, 2015). Achieving the *Healthy People 2020* target goal of reducing maternal deaths will require that national, state, and local policies address women's needs before and during pregnancy, and that gaps in research and prevention programs be identified through improved monitoring.

Changes in the reproductive systems of men and women result in changes in sexual function throughout adulthood. During middle adulthood, sexual arousal is slower, orgasms are less intense, and a return to pre-arousal levels is more rapid, with men having longer refractory periods between erection and ejaculation. When a person continues to be sexually active, these functional changes occur over decades and are minimally noticeable until later in adulthood, unless external factors are present,

such as the negative effects of some antihypertensive and antidepressant agents.

After menopause, many women enjoy sex more, especially because the risk of pregnancy no longer exists. Conversely, menopause can bring many challenges to a woman. American culture values women largely for their youth, beauty, and childbearing ability. Middle-aged women may confront their own aging for the first time and may be perplexed as to the symptomatic factors and possibly changing roles. Women can experience vaginal dryness, difficulty finding a partner, less interest in initiating sex, and longer times to reach orgasm. However, perceived emotional closeness during sex was found to be associated with more frequent arousal, lubrication, and orgasm (Trompeter et al., 2012).

Although men and women frequently enjoy satisfactory sexual relationships throughout the middle adult years, men in their middle age are more vulnerable to sexual dysfunction than are women. Erectile dysfunction, the inability to attain or maintain an erection sufficient enough for sexual activity, is a common disorder among older men. The gradual decline of age-related physiological function combined with chronic comorbidities may impair erectile function (Hockenberry & Masson, 2015). Common disorders related to erectile dysfunction include cardiovascular disease, diabetes, lower urinary tract symptoms, and depression—all of which should be considered by health care providers when assessing middle-aged men experiencing erectile dysfunction. Several readily available, nonsurgical treatments for erectile dysfunction exist: medications, supplements, hormonal therapy, penile injection, and external vacuum devices. The successful treatment of erectile dysfunction has the potential to increase sexual performance satisfaction, intimacy between partners, and overall quality and satisfaction with life. Although the risk of pregnancy is no longer a concern for middle-aged consenting adults, improved sexual function may increase the frequency of sexual activity and perhaps with more than one partner. Health care providers should not hesitate to initiate a sexual wellness assessment with middle-aged adults. Discussions should include specific sexual wellness strategies designed to prevent sexually transmitted infections.

Abnormal genital bleeding and secondary amenorrhea are common gynecological conditions that indicate serious physical problems. Abnormal genital bleeding is the most common reason for gynecological office visits by adult women. Although pregnancy and menopause are the most common causes of secondary amenorrhea, other conditions related to abnormal pregnancy, functional disorders, physiological changes, and pathological factors must be considered (Eliopoulos, 2010).

As for adolescents and young adults, sexually transmitted diseases continue to be a major public health problem for middle-aged adults. Women and children bear an inordinate share of the burden: sterility, ectopic pregnancy, fetal and infant deaths, birth defects, and mental retardation. Virtually all cases of cervical cancer are caused by human papilloma virus (HPV), and just two HPV types, 16 and 18, are responsible for approximately 70% of all cases (NIH, National Cancer Institute, 2015a). As with many other health behaviors and diseases, the full effect on the life of an individual and the family may not be realized until middle age.

Adults in middle age have many of the same HIV/AIDS risk factors as younger people, but they may be less aware of their risk. In 2014, people aged 50 years or older accounted for 17% (7391) of an estimated 44,073 HIV diagnoses in the United States. Of these, 44% (3242) were among those aged 50 to 54 years (CDC, 2017d). More than 50% of new HIV infections occur as a result of people who have HIV but do not know it (CDC, 2016e). The actual numbers may be higher because HIV/AIDS is often misdiagnosed, underreported, and undertested in this population. Middle-aged Americans are more likely to receive a diagnosis of HIV infection later in the course of their disease, which can lead to a poorer prognosis and shorter survival after an HIV infection diagnosis (CDC, 2017d).

Nearly three-fourths of all people currently with HIV/AIDS in the United States are men. In 2015, gay and bisexual men accounted for 82% of the estimated HIV diagnoses among men and 67% of the estimated AIDS diagnoses in the United States (CDC, 2016f). Among all gay and bisexual men who received an HIV diagnoses in the United States in 2015, African American accounted for the highest number (10,315; 39%), followed by whites (7,570; 29%) and Hispanics/Latinos (7013; 27%) (CDC, 2017c). Transgender women who have sex with men are among the groups at highest risk of HIV infection, followed by injection drug users, who remain at significant risk of getting HIV. The US Preventive Services Task Force now recommends HIV screening for adolescents and adults between 15 and 64 years, those who engage in risky behaviors, and all pregnant women, including those who present in labor whose HIV status is unknown (USPSTF, 2013).

## Coping–Stress Tolerance Pattern

Kobasa (1979) was the first to investigate the concept of stress hardiness. She identified hardiness as an aspect of personality which included control, commitment, and challenge. Her theory is clinically relevant because it suggests hardiness acts as a mediator between perceived stress and self-efficacy across many dimensions: physical, psychological, mental, and emotional. According to Kobasa, individuals who demonstrate hardiness, across the health continuum, appear to be more resistant to the effects of stress.

Stress is an unavoidable human life experience that triggers a reactive physiological response often derived from perceived psychological stressors. The many negative effects of perceived stress on physical health are well documented. Physiologically, stress causes the hormones cortisol, epinephrine, and norepinephrine to activate or exacerbate a number of conditions, including chronic physical, mental, and comorbid health conditions (Manchanda & Madan, 2014; Vranceanu et al., 2014). Stress tolerance is a learned behavior. More than 35 years ago, Benson first described the "relaxation response" as a reproducible state of deep rest (Benson & Klipper, 1975). The immediate and long-lasting effects of stress can be mitigated with effective coping skills including holistic mind-body interventions such as meditation, yoga, tai chi, and deep breathing (Manchanda & Madan, 2014; Wang et al. 2014). Evidence-based research demonstrates

how the mind-body connection helps individuals to cope with a wide range of illnesses and stressful life events (Box 23-8: Innovative Practice).

In a 45-year longitudinal study of 173 men, Vaillant and his colleagues (Vaillant, 2003; Vaillant & Vaillant, 1990) found that the extent of tranquilizer use before age 50 years was the most powerful negative predictor of both mental and physical health outcomes at age 65 years. Another important predictor for health outcomes was the maturity of defenses against stress such as sublimation, anticipation, altruism, and humor.

### Stress and Heart Disease

As reiterated throughout this chapter, heart disease is the second leading cause of death in the middle-aged adult. In landmark studies, Haynes and colleagues (1978, 1980) described the relationship of psychosocial factors to coronary heart disease using the Framingham study. In the study, 24 measures of psychosocial stress were used. In men, aging worries correlated significantly with systolic and diastolic blood pressure. Marital disagreement and personal worries correlated significantly with diastolic blood pressure. Both diastolic and systolic pressure correlated significantly with work changes and anxiety in employed women between 45 and 64 years of age. Anger suppressed, anger discussed, tension, and anger symptoms correlated significantly with diastolic blood pressure in this age group.

Among white-collar men in this age group, the Framingham type A and ambitiousness scales also correlated significantly with elevated diastolic blood pressure. The correlation of anger symptoms and anger discussed with diastolic pressures was significant for white-collar women aged between 45 and 65 years. The initial findings of Haynes and her colleagues have been supported by many other studies, including those of Spielberger and colleagues (1983), Kawachi and colleagues (1996), Williams and colleagues (2000), and Sanchez-Gonzalez and colleagues (2015).

The death of a parent enhances awareness of one's vulnerability to illness and death. The more opportunities and time people have to prepare for these stressful events, the more likely they will be to feel in control and the less likely they will be to feel anxious and helpless. When individuals assume more responsibility for their life, decisions lead to concrete behaviors, such as drafting a will, developing an advance directive (which includes **living will**, **health care agent**, and granting a durable power of attorney), and making funeral prearrangements. An **advance directive** is a legal document prepared when an individual is alive, competent, and able to make decisions to provide guidelines for health care providers in the future, when the individual is not able to make decisions because of physical disability (being unconscious) or mental incompetence. By granting a **durable power of attorney**, the individual designates another person (spouse, son, daughter, or friend) to make health care decisions (especially about how aggressive treatment should be in forestalling death) when an individual becomes unable to make such decisions. The nurse helps middle-aged adults anticipate stressors so that they are better prepared to cope with and to prevent additional physical, psychosocial, and spiritual stressors, thereby optimizing their health.

## ✳ BOX 23-8  INNOVATIVE PRACTICE

### *Benson-Henry Mind Body Institute of Massachusetts General Hospital, Harvard Medical School Mind/Body Medical Symptom Reduction Programs*

Research demonstrates that 60% to 90% of health care visits are for symptoms such as headaches, insomnia, weakness or fatigue, and gastrointestinal symptoms, all of which are frequently stress related. The Mind/Body Medical Symptom Reduction Programs are designed to help individuals who have chronic illnesses (including life-threatening illnesses) or stress-related symptoms to better manage their health problems and optimize their quality of life. The interventions combine conventional medical care with knowledge of the effects of behaviors and attitudes on health. The following are included in the biopsychosocial-spiritual approach of the assessment and treatment plans:

- Eliciting the relaxation response, a state of deep rest that changes responses to stress (decreases vital signs and muscle tenseness, increased mindfulness)
- Enhancing coping skills through cognitive-behavioral strategies
- Encouraging exercise or physical activity
- Providing nutritional counseling
- Monitoring and adjusting medication, when necessary, in consultation with the physician

Insurance claims for these outpatient visits are submitted directly to each person's insurance carrier. Because health insurance policies differ, coverage and reimbursement differ. An advocate helps persons seeking care research their specific health insurance coverage and billing requirements. Research demonstrates the following results may occur after these interventions:

- Persons with pain reduced their number of physician visits by 36%.
- Visits to a health maintenance organization were reduced by approximately 50% after a relaxation response–based intervention, resulting in significant cost savings.
- Blood pressure was lowered and use of medications decreased in 80% of hypertensive persons; 16% were able to discontinue all of their medications.
- Sleep patterns were improved for 100% of persons with insomnia; 90% reduced or eliminated the use of sleep medication.
- Infertile women reported decreased levels of depression, anxiety, and anger, along with a 35% conception rate.
- Women with severe premenstrual syndrome experienced a 57% reduction in physical and psychological symptoms.
- Health-promoting behaviors, such as nutrition, social supports, self-esteem, health responsibility, and exercise, increased after the program and were maintained by the 6-month follow-up visit.
- Six months after the program, 80% of persons continued to experience reduction of their physical symptoms.
- Anxiety and depression normalized for most participants and were maintained for 6 months following the program.
- Women with menopause reported fewer hot flashes, lower blood pressure, improved sleep, and decreased depression, anxiety, and anger.

## ▌Values-Beliefs Pattern

When adults make decisions affecting their lives, this is usually the result of a personal, complex pattern of values and beliefs. Much of what people value or believe to be true is formed early in life and can be the most difficult to alter. Usually, people do not spend a great deal of conscious thought on abstract explanations of the meaning of life and why certain things are valued. However, during times of illness or crisis, most people will take time to review their value systems and seek meaning about what is important.

A crisis at any age can be a turning point during which both increased vulnerability and increased potential are present. When the crisis is managed successfully, a virtue or strength will evolve. Erikson and Erikson (1998) identified *caring* as a middle-aged adult virtue that is often developed during times of crisis.

Committed responsibilities for the care and welfare of others promote moral development. When middle age is lived with generativity, many opportunities are afforded to live life by one's higher principles. The middle-aged adult can differentiate among personal wants and needs, duties demanded by society, and principles by which to live. Kohlberg's work on moral development delineated these phases as conventional and postconventional. His studies of men described stage 3 as an interpersonal definition of morality, whereas stage 4 is a societal definition based on law and order. Kohlberg concludes that most American adults are in these phases of moral development. In contrast, stage 5 is the concern and willingness to sacrifice oneself for the well-being of others (Kohlberg & Lickona, 1986). Subsequent studies by Gilligan (1982) on moral development in women and men demonstrate sex differences when describing high morality. Women discussed issues of selfishness versus responsibility, of exercising care with decision-making, and avoiding hurting others. Men described terms of *justice, fairness,* and *rights of individuals.* Gilligan (1982, 1990) concluded that women possess a process of moral development different from that of men.

Valuing others, having relationships, and being responsible to others enable middle-aged adults to make the transitions of moral development. This process is accomplished through raising children, developing more junior employees, and serving the community. As people fulfill these commitments, they increasingly treat others as equals and gradually develop a sensitivity and desire to change barriers to human worth and equality such as racial prejudice, homelessness, inadequate access to health care, and the availability of stockpiles of weapons.

## ▌ENVIRONMENTAL PROCESSES

Environmental factors are significant variables in health promotion. Cleanliness in home, work, and school environments helps control the spread of infectious diseases such as influenza. The effect of handwashing in controlling illness cannot be overstated. In a larger context, continued efforts at improving sanitation and controlling pollution (air, water, noise) will result in a reduction of health problems such as lung disease, transmission of bacterial and viral infections, and hearing loss.

Because there are approximately 100 million workers in the United States, occupational hazards are a serious threat to national health. Exposures to toxic chemicals, asbestos, coal dust, cotton fiber, ionizing radiation, physical hazards, excessive noise, and stress can precipitate numerous health problems (USDL, 2012). For the middle-aged worker, these problems include cancers, lung and heart diseases, decreased hearing, physical injuries, and mental health problems (USDL, 2010).

## Physical Agents

Ionizing radiation is a physical agent that can cause cancer. One example of this is cancer caused by medical procedures that include the use of diagnostic radiography and therapeutic radiation.

Water pollution has become another major concern. Many industrial and agricultural wastes, such as benzene and chlordane, have been recovered in rivers and lakes from which drinking water is obtained. These substances can potentially lead to carcinomas and other health problems.

Air pollution from automobile emissions, burning fuels, and industrial incineration has warranted smog alerts and air pollution indices. This issue is especially important to the individual with chronic respiratory or cardiovascular disease (USDL, 2010).

Noise pollution in industry is a potential problem for the middle-aged adult worker. Hearing loss is the most common occupational disease, but it can be prevented if federal guidelines are followed with regard to noise exposure levels and hearing conservation programs, especially prevention activities aimed at miners and construction workers, for whom hearing loss is a major problem. Exposure to excessive noise, radon, radiation, sunlight, and vibration can produce problems such as chronic obstructive lung disease, cancer, and degenerative diseases (Nissenbaum et al., 2012).

## Biological Agents

As noted throughout this text, health and disease are influenced by the interactions among the agent, host, and environment. Agent factors can be biological, physical, chemical, or psychological. The biological causes of diseases include bacteria, viruses, rickettsiae, fungi, parasites, and food poisoning. Because these causes are often limited to identifiable occupations, they can be readily diagnosed, treated, and prevented. Many of these agents are transmitted through the air or by contact with certain media, such as water, food, blood, or feces.

Hepatitis A is caused by viral infection, with transmission occurring primarily through the fecal-oral route. This host-agent interaction typically occurs in the middle-aged adult living in an environment with poor sanitation and having close contact with an infected person. The person may also be exposed through contaminated food and water. The Hepatitis B viral agent is transmitted primarily in the blood or plasma of the infected individuals, which is particularly significant for the adult who is employed in a health care setting. Among medical and dental personnel (with surgeons, oral surgeons, and pathologists at the highest risk), the risk of contracting hepatitis B is six times higher than that of the general population.

There are two other infections that are of particular concern for middle-aged adults: pneumonia and varicella/herpes zoster ("shingles"). Both can be prevented through vaccinations, which adults aged 60 years or older are advised to receive (CDC, 2017e).

## Chemical Agents

Chemicals include a wide variety of substances that increase the risk of morbidity and death in the middle-aged adult. When a home is located near an industry, there is the risk of exposure to toxic chemicals that pollute the air. Contaminants can also be carried home on the clothing from the workplace.

Workers at increased risk include coal miners, wood handlers, and those who work with asbestos and coke. Pneumoconiosis is found in approximately 15% of coal miners, with "black lung disease" implicated in 2430 deaths in 2005 (the *Healthy People 2020* target is a 10% reduction). Wood handlers have increased risk of certain cancers. The asbestos worker has an increased risk of mesothelioma and asbestosis. Approximately 2 million workers each year are exposed to benzene and vinyl chloride, which may be carcinogens. Among American industrial workers, 9 in 10 may be inadequately protected from exposure to at least 10 of the 163 most common hazardous chemicals. More than 2000 of the 50,000 chemicals found in the workplace are suspected human carcinogens (USDL, 2012).

### Tobacco

Cigarette smoking is the leading cause of preventable death, disease, and disability in the United States. In 2014 an estimated 40 million adults in the United States smoked cigarettes. Currently, 18.8% of men and 14.8% of women in the United States smoke. Adult smoking rates differ across the Unites States, but the states with the most smokers are in the Midwest and Southeast (CDC, 2016c). Among Americans, cigarette smoking, and exposure to second hand smoke, is responsible for more than 480,000 premature deaths annually: 278,544 deaths annually among men and 201,773 deaths annually among women (CDC, 2016g). Smoke recipients are at increased risks of heart disease as well as colds, chronic bronchitis, emphysema, and cancers of the mouth, lungs, esophagus, pancreas, and bladder. Many 50-year-old adults have a 30-plus-year history of cigarette smoking. The life expectancy for smokers is at least 10 years less than that of nonsmokers; however, quitting smoking before the age of 40 years reduces the risk of dying of smoking-related disease by approximately 90% (CDC, 2016g).

Few smokers realize that cigarettes contain 2000 known chemicals, including tar, nicotine, hydrogen cyanide, formaldehyde, and ammonia. Cigarette smoking is, for most smokers, an addiction to nicotine, which is absorbed into the bloodstream. Nicotine acts on the two divisions of the nervous system: central (brain and the spinal cord) and peripheral (autonomic nervous system and motor and sensory fibers to the arms and legs). The effects of nicotine stimulation can be observed both in electroencephalographic changes and in hand tremors. Nicotine also stimulates the heart, leading to an increased pulse rate and elevated blood pressure. Although smokers frequently believe that cigarettes have a calming effect, this notion is misleading. Nicotine stimulates the body, whereas carbon monoxide causes lethargy. Smokers may feel calm, although they are actually having their sensations dulled by carbon monoxide. Additive effects such as those from chlorine, cotton dust, and γ-radiation can lower midexpiratory flow values. Profound effects can also be observed with asbestos interaction.

## DETERMINANTS OF HEALTH

### Social Factors and Environment

Culture is a set of beliefs, practices, norms, customs, rituals, and assumptions about life that are first learned from one's parents and extended family during the early years of socialization (Spector, 2012). Spector further relates the ways in which one's cultural background is a component of one's ethnic background.

Nurses understand the potential influences their own ethnic cultures have on those of others. The middle-aged adult may not interpret dizziness as a possible symptom of hypertension; for example, it may be described simply as a spell. The black adult's definition of health may be completely different from that of the white health care provider or the Asian person. The obese adult who has received positive reinforcement throughout life for being pleasingly plump is less motivated to lose weight than is the adult who defines health as being svelte.

The health problems of middle-aged adults, even within major ethnic groups, are varied. Recent immigrants who live in crowded urban areas have higher mortality rates than do earlier immigrants of the same cultural group who live in healthier environments. Immigrants' working conditions continue to be poor, with long hours and minimal wages. Modern preventive health care is difficult, if not impossible, to obtain.

Poverty rates are important indicators of community well-being and the health status of community members. According to the 2007 to 2011 American Community Survey, 42.7 million people, or 14.3% of the US population, had income below the poverty level. By race, the highest national poverty rates were for American Indians and Alaska Natives (27.0%), followed by blacks (25.8%). The poverty level for whites was 11.6% (US Census Bureau, 2013). Economic adversity, disproportionate access to health services, and cultural differences may contribute to lower life expectancy and the disproportionate disease burden for American Indians and Alaska Natives. The American Indian life expectancy (73.7 years) is still more than 4 years less than that for the US general population (78.1 years). Death rates are significantly higher in many areas for American Indians compared with the US general population, including those for chronic liver disease and cirrhosis, diabetes mellitus, unintentional injuries, assault/homicide, intentional self-harm/suicide, and chronic lower respiratory disease (USDHHS, Indian Health Service, 2015).

Culture also determines acceptable gender-specific and age-specific attitudes and behaviors. Accepted gender-specific attitudes and behaviors associated with life-defining rituals (birth, marriage, illness, and death) are particularly important for stabilizing and preserving one's culture. Aging confers vast decline and compromise for both sexes. Middle-aged adults who conform to stereotypical patterns of expected role behaviors often receive continued communal support and reverence even as their health

---

### BOX 23-9 DIVERSITY AWARENESS

**Health Care for Middle-Aged Gypsies**

Culturally competent and effective health care is imperative for all, especially people with several comorbid conditions who do not have a consistent primary care provider or clinic. Middle-aged gypsies, or Roma, are in need of consistent health care. The Roma are a large vulnerable population in Europe. However, because they tend to travel from one place to another and do not put down roots, health providers need to understand their beliefs so the episodic interactions will be most productive. Barriers to adequate care delivery include affordability of care, lower self-reported health, and higher death risks. The Roma population is very distinctive in its use of language, community, family, and cultural traditions. It is important to realize the Roma prefer to involve their family when it comes to their health. Hence a family member should be allowed to participate in each interaction with a health provider. Involvement of the family will increase the person's adherence to the health regimen.

From Cook, B., Wayne, G. F., Valentine, A., Lessios, A., & Yeh, E. (2013). Revisiting the evidence on health and health care disparities among the Roma: A systematic review 2003–2012. *International Journal of Public Health, 58,* 885–991.

---

status and abilities decline. Conversely, those who choose not to conform to expected changes in behaviors and roles risk exclusion, isolation, loneliness, and compromised health. Nurses who have attained cultural competency can ensure that appropriate health promotion is provided, especially for vulnerable populations and those individuals, families, and communities who have special health care needs (Box 23-9: Diversity Awareness).

### Levels of Policy Making and Health

Adults in the middle years are frequently at the peak of their careers. Although their net income may be greater than it was during early adulthood, they frequently have significant additional financial obligations. For many individuals in their late 50s or early 60s, retirement is a life stage they have dreamt about and anticipated for years (Figure 23-2). Leaving full-time employment for a less strenuous daily routine may not be possible for many middle-aged adults. A number of reasons are offered to account for this relatively new trend:

- The high quality of health care in the United States provides technological advances that extend the limits for life expectancy. Individuals are living longer than previous generations, and therefore they cannot "afford" to retire in their mid-50s to early 60s because they have a financial need to "fund" another 25 to 30 years of life.
- Quality health care is expensive. The costs of health care are mounting because research and development expenses associated with medical treatments, including pharmaceuticals, are escalating. When an illness has been diagnosed, individuals expect "the best" type of care and interventions, which, in turn, influences the financial burden borne by almost all Americans.
- Changes in the American economy in the past 10 years have necessitated significant changes in family patterns. Increasingly, more than one generation lives together in the same home

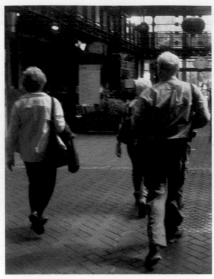

**FIGURE 23-2** Middle-aged adults may enjoy travel after retirement.

so as to afford the rising costs of commodities that have been taken for granted. For example, the costs of a college education funded by middle-aged adults are not necessarily balanced by a full-time position at the end of the 4 or 5 years needed to obtain a college degree. Young adults are not leaving home at 22 or 23 years of age. Consequently, their parents, if still employed, must continue to work to support adult children and also to pay the debt of the college educational experience.

- Individuals may have accrued increasing debt to pay for health insurance that is becoming more costly. As people develop health conditions that are related to accumulated stress and the aging process, they require more use of their benefits from their health insurance companies. In addition, they may be supporting elderly parents, whose health conditions have consumed their savings and home investment to pay for their parents' medications, hospitalizations, and/or nursing home expenses. When the adult or family members have ongoing health problems, the economic status of the family can be compromised further (see Box 23-9: Diversity Awareness).

- Unemployment statistics show an increasing rate of unemployment across the United States. When people lose their jobs, they are often without health insurance, and when they develop illness or conditions that are associated with the middle years, they rely on their savings or must resort to less expensive housing. Such changes can cause extreme mental strain and possibly lead to mental health problems. The individual's economic status plays a role in the incidence of mental illness, with higher rates of anxiety, depression, and phobias evident in adults at the lower socioeconomic level.

- Technological changes have opened opportunities for individuals to work at home and/or remote sites. These extensions of the workplace often necessitate individuals to change their routines, and to take educational courses to keep current with job requirements, or to be competent to take on more

responsibilities. Training to increase skills or knowledge can be expensive and often must be funded by the individual.

## Health Services/Delivery System

Numerous agencies are geared to providing information and other resources for the middle-aged adult. These can be categorized as official, voluntary, and service agencies. Councils of community services frequently publish a directory. Official agencies include those that are state and federally funded, such as public health departments and drug treatment centers. Voluntary agencies include the American Heart Association, the American Cancer Society, the American Lung Association, and Alcoholics Anonymous. Many educational and self-help programs are sponsored by these organizations. The American Lung Association sponsors a "Stop Smoking" program, which can be conducted on a group basis in a work or community setting. Service agencies include professional organizations, such as state nurses' associations, the American Medical Association (sponsor of the Tel-Med program), bar associations, Young Men's Christian Association (YMCA), hospice programs, and the Women's Occupational Health Resource Center. The Affordable Care Act of 2010 is a law with provisions (Internal Revenue Service, 2012) that meet one of the primary objectives of *Healthy People 2020;* that is, increasing access to health care for all Americans. The implications of this statute are most significant for middle-aged adults who are currently uninsured and/or have preexisting health conditions. Preventive screening will allow individuals to receive testing for the detection of cancer and other conditions that can influence initiation of treatment at an earlier stage of illness. Thus the financial expense of treatment will potentially be less and the stresses on the individual and family considerably eased. In addition, costs for unemployment benefits where individuals work will be reduced.

From another perspective, the Affordable Care Act has already expanded coverage for individuals younger than 26 years who are still carried on the health insurance policy held by their parents. This provision is particularly relevant for young adults who are still in college or who have not found employment after college graduation. The economic impact of unemployment among this age group on families with middle-aged parents described in the previous section cannot be understated (Jarrett, 2012). Specific details of the Affordable Care Act of 2010 may be found at http://www.irs.gov/newsroom/article.

## NURSING APPLICATION

Interventions focused on health promotion span the gamut for nurses working in the community or on location at work sites. Consequently, there are many ways nurses interact with middle-aged adults.

Individuals in this middle-age range will likely need the services of a professional nurse *several times* before they reach their 60s. They may meet a nurse when seeking care for themselves in a physician's office or primary care center. As a parent, they are likely to accompany their school-age child or their own elderly parent to the emergency department to obtain care for a sports-related injury or trauma following a fall. In the employment realm, some individuals will have their initial experience with a nurse through a pre-employment evaluation visit. As a company employee, the same person may receive first aid for a minor injury or have his or her blood pressure monitored periodically by a nurse working in the occupational health department.

If the individual needs surgery or hospitalization, they may meet a home health nurse after discharge. Nurses are also available in rehabilitation settings to instruct and coach people regarding lifestyle changes following a heart attack or other acute events. Community health nurses provide health-promotion activities such as senior health fairs that include "flu clinics" where adults are vaccinated against influenza. Life events such as the death of a partner, sudden unemployment, or disability may cause anxiety, depression, or other stress-related symptoms. Nurses who specialize in mental health can provide counseling and other forms of treatment for grief support or mental disorders resulting from trauma or sudden losses.

In a variety of settings, nurses are health educators. For example, the nurse who works in the community or in occupational health initiates events that raise awareness to identify health risks among middle-aged adults. She teaches strategies for controlling symptoms and accepting responsibility for changing potentially dangerous health habits. These interventions can be provided on a one-to-one or group basis or as a lecture presented in a health seminar.

The target groups identified by occupational health nurses frequently have common needs for information, interventions, and periodic monitoring. The following are common concerns in the workplace: exposure to chemical or toxic substances, tobacco and substance abuse and addiction, and ongoing problems with fatigue attributable to frequent changes in scheduled shifts.

The occupational health nurse has a wide range of responsibilities. For example, he or she may evaluate patterns of absenteeism to identify a source for infection that is affecting a group of employees. The nurse participates in policy development focused on preventing or reducing the incidence of work site injuries or incidents. In another instance, the nurse provides clarification of Occupational Safety and Health Administration (OSHA) regulations when new machinery is incorporated into operation. The nurse is wise to invite a broad spectrum of employee participants to join a company safety committee. Their primary purpose is focused on keeping the work site safe for employees. Strategies to achieve that objective include determining health hazards that exist in each department of the company and developing or refining procedures that promote safety, such as creating policies that address infection control or procedures for fire drills. If the nurse has certification from the American Heart Association, he or she can offer classes in cardiopulmonary resuscitation and use of the automated external defibrillator.

The scope of practice for community health nurses (CHNs) differs from state to state. They may be employed by a city or town, or derive their authority through the state health department. The role of the CHN focuses on health promotion and disease prevention for a population living in a specific area. The CHN interfaces with nurses working in the municipality and surrounding areas such as in medical offices, state health department offices, hospitals, urgent care clinics, schools, emergency services, YMCA/Young Women's Christian Association (YWCA), and local businesses. Frequently, lectures or demonstrations are sponsored by the CHN at the request of service organizations in communities such as the Lions or Kiwanis Club. The CHN may combine efforts with nurses who volunteer as parish nurses. Together they may present an annual health fair or senior health fair to serve a broad scope of health-information needs of the local community. The features of the fair would include 15 to 20 displays that offer some of the following—all on a single occasion: demonstrations in the use of car seats and seat belts; short presentations on fall prevention; screening measures to identify risk factors for heart disease, cancer, and diabetes; town planning guides for emergency preparedness; massage therapy for stress reduction; informational guides for the regional poison control center; and "flu shots" against influenza for anyone who desires one. Such events allow the CHN to generate interest and enthusiasm among people who are interested in improving the health and well-being of residents living in their local community.

Health-promotion strategies will become more widely recognized as the objectives and target goals of *Healthy People 2020* are incorporated into health plans supported by health insurance policies, employers, wellness programs, and health care providers. With the passage of the Affordable Care Act in 2010, accessibility and utilization of health care services, especially for minorities, are expected to increase. Nurses will be in leadership roles to organize and implement early detection and screening programs. They will survey communities and identify needs of the specific populations, and evaluate the effectiveness of public health measures already in place. They will be called on to develop educational programs and create on-line information sites that disseminate current medical research findings to the public showing how changes in lifestyle behaviors can positively influence health outcomes. Progress toward the target goals of *Healthy People 2020* can be incorporated in these websites or blogs so that the American people can see, and learn first-hand, how important changes in their own lifestyle will affect the overall health of the United States.

In summary, better health and enhanced well-being of the American people are expected outcomes of health promotion. The *Healthy People 2020* objectives and target goals provide the framework and direction for improving health awareness and practices among US residents.

In this chapter, health needs and potential diseases and conditions relevant to middle-aged adults have been addressed along with strategies to mitigate symptoms, prevent complications, and foster well-being. Normal changes expected with the aging process were also presented. Selected objectives and target goals of *Healthy People 2020* were compared with findings published for outcomes of *Healthy People 2010*. In addition, the impact of social processes, such as relationships, family, work, values and belief systems, disability and death, and finances, completed the discussion.

Nurses provide important strategies for fostering health promotion. They are employed in most settings where middle-aged adults live, work, play, and raise their families. Because of this integral position in society, nurses are highly influential in identifying health concerns, organizing interventions, and evaluating the effectiveness of program outcomes. *Healthy People 2020* is presented as one approach for health professionals to use in their mission to improve the health and well-being of the American people.

The Occupational Safety and Health Administration (OSHA) mandates that the employee have a healthy and safe work environment. Therefore a complete health history is essential. Is there a history of hypertension, arthritis, cancer, or hernia? Is there significant family history? Is the person a smoker? How many packs per day are smoked? Does the person take medications? Medical limitations must be addressed; for example, decreased visual acuity means no driving, and dermatitis means no skin exposure to oils, chemicals, or solvents. Removing a worker from a particular job may be indicated if the worker might endanger coworkers, if the worker has a disease condition that might be aggravated by the job, or if the worker is taking prescribed medications with potentially harmful side effects.

The nurse in the community and in industry should reiterate key safety directives to the middle-aged adult. For example, wear seat belts and observe speed limits, use only hands-free phone communication, and avoid texting while driving. The middle-aged adult's reaction time is also decreasing, which reinforces the need for periodic driving testing as recommended by the National Highway Traffic Safety Administration.

With an increase in leisure time, the middle-aged adult is at greater risk of recreational accidents. As noted, moderation should be stressed. Alcohol is a depressant and should be avoided in activities that require attentiveness.

Protection from burns is essential; 56% of fatal residential fires are directly related to cigarette smoking while in bed. Falls can occur at any age; safety measures should be considered for the entire family, including specific preparatory planning for the very young and aging parents. A few suggestions to the middle-aged adult might be to avoid highly waxed floors, correct poor environmental lighting, avoid high beds, and avoid bathtubs lacking nonslip bottoms.

Handgun availability is controversial at best; however, approximately 20% of American households have handguns. When the person believes strongly that it is necessary to have a firearm, safety measures to avoid accidental injury should be discussed, such as security locks and proper storage.

The Occupational Safety and Health Act (1970) was designed to ensure that workers are employed under safe and healthy working conditions. The act is applicable to every employer who is engaged in a business that affects commerce. The employer must ascertain that the workplace is free from recognized hazards and must comply with the act. The OSHA has offices in most major cities and can provide recommended standards for occupational agents.

Nurses can participate actively in the safety committee of the industry in which they are employed. When no such committee exists, many protection measures will fall on the nurse. The following are some suggestions:

- Tour the facilities on a regular basis. Be familiar with resource books, laws, and codes.
- Develop a toxicology chart with symptoms of overexposure and recommended treatment. Update this chart frequently.
- Be a role model in safety issues; wear safety glasses, protective footwear, and gloves; and do not smoke.
- Discuss the pre-employment physical examination with the employee, with an emphasis on risk factors. Monitor health problems and exposure levels in the work setting.

The worker must be aware of the protective clothing that should be worn, sanitation measures for the work environment, general hygiene measures, and proper immunization. The food handler, for instance, should have an annual tuberculosis skin test, wear clean clothing and appropriate hair protection, and use good handwashing techniques. The nurse should not assume that workers know how to protect themselves and others.

Since 1996, the National Occupational Research Agenda has become the research framework for the National Institute for Occupational Safety and Health and the nation. Partners work together to identify, research, and address the most critical issues in workplace safety (http://cdc.gov/niosh/about.html).

A major challenge for the nurse is to encourage workers to assume responsibility for protecting their own health. Increasingly, organizations are interested in promoting the health of their employees for many reasons, including enhancing their recruiting efforts and minimizing lateness, absenteeism, turnover, physical and emotional inability to work, disability costs, and health and life insurance costs. Health-promotion programs are increasingly recognized for their vital contributions to the financial viability of organizations.

Health-promotion programs within an organizational setting can be categorized in one of three levels: awareness, lifestyle change, and supportive environment. The goal of a health program, at the level of awareness, is to increase the individual's knowledge or interest in a particular health issue, such as smoking cessation. Examples of awareness programs include special events, flyers, lunch seminars, meetings, and newsletters. Changing health behaviors or status is not the goal of awareness programs, but is the goal of lifestyle change programs.

Lifestyle change programs last at least 8 to 12 weeks and include assessment, education, and evaluation components to help individuals implement long-term modifications in health behavior and experience the results of their instituted changes. To maintain these long-term changes and to develop a healthy lifestyle, a supportive organizational environment is needed. This type of environment may include health-promoting physical settings, corporate policies and culture, ongoing programs, and employee ownership of programs.

## SUMMARY

Nurses help middle-aged adults improve their quality of life, both for the present and for the future, through the identification of risk factors, health promotion, and other nursing interventions. Nurses work in a variety of health care settings available to middle-aged adults: outpatient clinics, occupational health clinics, and private practice.

Health promotion and disease prevention are aimed at the personal habits and lifestyles of adults to improve their biological, spiritual, and psychosocial development. The strategies to help an adult achieve a higher level of health include individual and group counseling based on identified risk factors, providing self-help information that is most relevant to the middle-aged adult, and describing available resources. Using these strategies, the nurse can motivate middle-aged adults to prioritize their own health and quality of life for the individual middle-aged adult, including it as a prerequisite for their own present and future health and particularly preceding the responsibilities in promoting the health and quality of life of younger and older generations. After years of poor health practices, adults can make changes that reduce their risk of disability from chronic disease and promote functioning and quality of life.

## CASE STUDY

### Caregiver Role Strain: Ms. Sandra A.

Sandra, a 47-year-old divorced woman, received a diagnosis of stage 3 ovarian cancer 4 years ago, for which she had a total hysterectomy, bilateral salpingo-oophorectomy, omentectomy, lymphadenectomy, and tumor debulking followed by chemotherapy, consisting of cisplatin (Platinol), paclitaxel (Taxol), and doxorubicin (Adriamycin). She did well for 2 years and then moved back to her hometown near her family and underwent three more rounds of second-line chemotherapy. She accepted a less stressful job, bought a house, renewed old friendships, and became more involved with her two sisters and their families.

Sandra developed several complications, including metastasis to the lungs. Then she could no longer work, drive, or care for herself. She had been told by her oncologist that there was nothing else that could be done and that she should consider entering a hospice. She met her attorney and prepared an advance directive and completed her will. She decided to have hospice care at home and, with the help of her family, set up her first floor as a living and sleeping area. She was cared for by family members around the clock for approximately 3 days.

Sandra observed that she was tiring everyone out so much that they could not really enjoy each other's company. At this time, she contacted the Visiting Nurse Association (VNA) to seek assistance. Her plan was to try to enjoy her family and friend's visits. After assessment, the VNA nurse prioritized her problems to include fatigue and caregiver role strain. Other potential problem areas that may need to be incorporated into the care plan include anticipatory grieving and impaired comfort.

#### Reflective Questions

- What are some of the stresses on Sandra's middle-aged sisters and their families?
- What resources are available to manage these stresses and support the sisters while caring for their dying sister Sandra?
- Describe Sandra's feelings about dependency and loss of autonomy because she is unable to do her own activities of daily living any longer.

## ◎ CARE PLAN

### Caregiver Role Strain: Ms. Sandra A.

**\*NURSING DIAGNOSIS: Risk of caregiver role strain related to sister's terminal cancer**

#### Defining Characteristics
- Sandra's sisters are weary from doing all of the daily care for Sandra.
- Sandra and her family are at a point where they are accepting her terminal status.
- Sandra and her family want to prepare for a death at home.

#### Related Factors
- The sisters are missing work and neglecting their own families.
- The sisters need assistance to care for Sandra as she continues to become compromised.

#### Expected Outcomes
- Sandra and her sisters will contact the VNA to assist in planning daily hospice care at home.

- The VNA and the family will plan realistic care.
- Sandra will have quality time with her sisters and friends as her condition allows.
- The sisters will be able to voice their grief and anger about Sandra's upcoming death.

#### Interventions
- Home health aides are scheduled for 24 hours a day.
- A psychiatric nurse practitioner will meet Sandra and her family to schedule therapy time for anticipatory grieving.
- The sisters will attend a support group for families involved in hospice care at home.
- A schedule will be made to allow each sister time at home, one-on-one time with Sandra, and time for rest.

## ⓔ EVOLVE CHAPTER FEATURES

http://evolve.elsevier.com/Edelman/
• Study Questions

## REFERENCES

AACE Menopause Guidelines Revision Task Force. (2011). American Association of Clinical Endocrinologists medical guidelines for clinical practice for the diagnosis and treatment of menopause. *Endocrine Practice*, *17*(6), 1–25.

Agency for Healthcare Research and Quality. (2012). Closing the quality gap: A critical analysis of QI strategies: volume 3 – Hypertension care. AHRQ publication no.12 EHC003. http://www.effectivehealthcare.ahrq.gov/.

American Cancer Society. (2015). Menopausal hormone therapy and cancer risk. http://www.cancer.org/cancer/cancercauses/othercarcinogens/medicaltreatments/menopausal-hormone-replacement-therapy-and-cancer-risk.

American Heart Association. (2012). Calculating target heart rate. http://www.americanheartassociation.org.

Apter, T. (1990). *Altered loves: Mothers and daughters during adolescence*. New York: Ballantine Books.

Apter, T. (1995). *Secret paths: Women in the new midlife*. New York: Norton.

Arias, E. (2015). United States life tables, 2011. *National vital statistics reports*, *64*(11), https://www.cdc.gov/nchs/data/nvsr/nvsr64/nvsr64_11.pdf.

Bauer, U. E., et al. (2014). Prevention of chronic disease in the 21st century: Elimination of the leading preventable causes of premature death and disability in the USA. *The Lancet*, *384*(9937), 45–52.

Benjamin, R. M. (2012). Oral health care for persons living with HIV/AIDS. *Public Health Reports*, *127*(Suppl. 2), 1–2.

Bensley, L., Van Eehwyk, J., & Ossiander, E. M. (2011). Association of self-reported periodontal disease with metabolic syndrome and a number of self-reported chronic conditions. *Prevention of Chronic Disease*, *8*(30), A50.

Benson, H., & Klipper, M. Z. (1975). *The relaxation response*. New York: Hapertorch.

Bloom, B. S. (1984). *Taxonomy of educational objectives: Handbook 1, cognitive domain*. New York: Longman.

Bloom, B., et al. (2012). Oral health status and access to oral health care for U.S. adults aged 18-64: National health Interview Survey, 2008, National Center for health statistics. *Vital Health Statistics*, *10*(253), 1–22.

Centers for Disease Control and Prevention (CDC). (2010a). Health, United States, 2010 with special features on death and dying. http://www.cdc.gov/nchs/data/hus/hus10.pdf.

Centers for Disease Control and Prevention (CDC). (2010b). Vital signs: Health insurance coverage and health care utilization— United States, 2006–2009 and January–March 2010. *MMWR. Morbidity and Mortality Weekly Report*, *59*(44), 1448–1454.

Centers for Disease Control and Prevention (CDC). (2012). Healthy People 2010 final review. https://www.cdc.gov/nchs/data/hpdata2010/hp2010_final_review.pdf.

Centers for Disease Control and Prevention (CDC). (2015a). Adult obesity facts. http://www.cdc.gov/obesity/data/adult.html.

Centers for Disease Control and Prevention (CDC). (2015b). Common eye disorders. https://www.cdc.gov/visionhealth/basics/ced/index.html.

Centers for Disease Control and Prevention (CDC). (2015c). QuickStats: Percentage of uninsured persons aged <65 years with no health insurance coverage because of cost, by race/ethnicity – National Health Interview Survey, United States, 2004 and 2014. *MMWR. Morbidity and Mortality Weekly Report*, *64*(47), 1320.

Centers for Disease Control and Prevention (CDC). (2016a). Adult obesity facts. https://www.cdc.gov/obesity/data/adult.html.

Centers for Disease Control and Prevention (CDC). (2016b). Chronic disease overview. http://www.cdc.gov/chronicdisease/overview.

Centers for Disease Control and Prevention (CDC). (2016c). Current cigarette smoking among adults in the United States. https://www.cdc.gov/tobacco/data_statistics/fact_sheets/adult_data/cig_smoking/.

Centers for Disease Control and Prevention (CDC). (2016d). Defining adult overweight and obesity. http://www.cdc.gov/obesity/data/adult.html.

Centers for Disease Control and Prevention (CDC). (2016e). HIV. http://www.healthypeople.gov/2020/topics-objectives/topic/hiv.

Centers for Disease Control and Prevention (CDC). (2016f). HIV in the United States: At a glance. https://www.cdc.gov/hiv/statistics/overview/ataglance.html.

Centers for Disease Control and Prevention (CDC). (2016g). Tobacco-related mortality. https://www.cdc.gov/tobacco/data_statistics/fact_sheets/health_effects/tobacco_related_mortality/.

Centers for Disease Control and Prevention (CDC). (2016h). Workplace health promotion. http://www.cdc.gov/workplacehealthpromotion/index.html.

Centers for Disease Control and Prevention (CDC). (2017a). Don't let glaucoma steal your sight! https://www.cdc.gov/features/glaucoma-awareness/index.html.

Centers for Disease Control and Prevention (CDC). (2017b). HIV among African Americans. https://www.cdc.gov/hiv/group/racialethnic/africanamericans/index.html.

Centers for Disease Control and Prevention (CDC). (2017c). HIV among African American gay and bisexual men. https://www.cdc.gov/hiv/group/msm/index.html.

Centers for Disease Control and Prevention (CDC). (2017d). HIV among people aged 50 and over. http://www.cdc.gov/hiv/group/age/olderamericans/index.html.

Centers for Disease Control and Prevention (CDC). (2017e). Recommended immunizations for adults: By health condition. https://www.cdc.gov/vaccines/schedules/downloads/adult/adult-schedule-easy-read.pdf.

Centers for Disease Control and Prevention (CDC). (2017f). Smoking, gum disease, and tooth loss. https://www.cdc.gov/tobacco/campaign/tips/diseases/periodontal-gum-disease.html.

Cohen, R., & Martinez, M. (2015). Health insurance coverage: Early release of estimates from the National Health Interview Survey, January–March 2015. http://www.cdc.gov/nchs/nhis/earlyrelease/insur201508.pdf.

DeNavas-Walt, C., & Proctor, B. D. (2014). *U.S. Census Bureau, current population reports, P60-249, income and poverty in the United States: 2013*. Washington, DC: US Government Printing Office.

Driscoll, A. K., & Bernstein, A. B. (2012). Health access to care among employed and unemployed adults: United States 2009-2010. NCHS data brief no. 83. https://www.cdc.gov/nchs/products/databriefs/db83.htm.

Duvall, E. M., & Miller, B. (1985). *Marriage and family development* (6th ed.). New York: Harper Collins.

Eliopoulos, C. (2010). *Gerontological nursing: Common aging changes.* Philadelphia: Wolters Kluwer.

Erikson, E. H., & Erikson, G. M. (1998). *Life cycle completed.* New York: W.W. Norton.

Gardner, H. (1983). *Frames of mind: The theory of multiple intelligences.* New York: Basic Books.

Gardner, H. (1993). *Multiple intelligences: The theory in practice.* New York: Basic Books.

Gilligan, C. (1982). *A different voice: Psychological theory and women's development.* Cambridge, MA: Harvard University Press.

Gilligan, C. (1990). *Mapping the moral domain.* Cambridge, MA: Harvard University Press.

Godfrey, E. M., et al. (2011). Contraceptive methods and use by women aged 35 and over: A qualitative study of perspectives. *BMC Women's Health, 11,* 5.

Harston, B. (2010). A look at Healthy People 2010: How did Americans fare? http://www.healthypeople2010.us.

Havighurst, R. I., & Orr, B. (1956). *Adult education and adult needs.* Chicago: Center for Study of Liberal Education for Adults.

Haynes, S. G., et al. (1978). The relationship of psychosocial factors to coronary heart disease in the Framingham Study. I. Methods and risk factors. *American Journal of Epidemiology, 107*(5), 362–383.

Haynes, S. G., Feinleib, M., & Kannel, W. B. (1980). The relationship of psychosocial factors to coronary heart disease in the Framingham Study. III. Eight-year incidence of coronary heart disease. *American Journal of Epidemiology, 111*(1), 37–58.

Healthy People 2020. (2012). *A closer look: Health disparities.* Washington, DC: U.S. Department of Health and Human Services. https://www.HealthyPeople.gov/.

Heaney, R. B. (2013). Vitamin D and calcium absorption: Toward a new model. In P. Burckhardt, B. Dawson-Hughes, & C. M. Weaver (Eds.), *Nutritional influences on bone health* (pp. 261–272). London: Springer.

Heron, M. (2012). Deaths: Leading causes for 2008. *National Vital Statistics Reports, 60*(6), 1–95.

Hockenberry, M. S., & Masson, P. (2015). Erectile dysfunction in the elderly. *Geriatric Urology, 4*(1), 33–43.

Holick, M. F. (2012). Vitamin D: Extraskeletal health. *Rheumatic Diseases Clinics of North America, 38*(1), 141–160.

Hornstein, G. (1986). The structuring of identity among midlife women as a function of their degree of involvement in employment. *Journal of Personality, 54,* 551–575.

Hunger, J. M., & Major, B. (2015). Weight stigma mediates the association between BMI and self-reported health. *Health Psychology, 34*(2), 172–175.

Institute of Medicine (US) Committee to Review Dietary Reference Intakes for Vitamin D and Calcium. (2011). A. C. Ross, et al. (Eds.), *Dietary Reference Intakes for Calcium and Vitamin D.* Washington, DC: National Academies Press (US). doi:10.17226/13050. https://www.ncbi.nlm.nih.gov/books/NBK56070/.

Internal Revenue Service. (2012). Affordable Care Act tax provisions. https://www.irs.gov/affordable-care-act/affordable-care-act-tax-provisions.

Jarrett, V. (2012). Affordable Care Act: Making a difference. *St. Louis American.* http://www.stlamerican.com/news/columnists/affordable-care-act-making-a-difference/article_48a153c4-8f40-11e1-9990-001a4bcf887a.html.

Kaldo, V., et al. (2015). Guided internet cognitive behavioral therapy for insomnia compared to a control treatment – A randomized trial. *Behaviour Research and Therapy, 71,* 90–100.

Kawachi, I., et al. (1996). A prospective study of anger and coronary heart disease: The Normative Aging Study. *Circulation, 94,* 2090–2095.

King, D. E., et al. (2013). *Dealing with the psychological and spiritual aspects of menopause: Finding hope in the midlife.* New York: Routledge.

Kobasa, S. (1979). Stressful life events, personality and health: An inquiry into hardiness. *Journal of Personality and Social Psychology, 37,* 1–11.

Kohlberg, L., & Lickona, T. (1986). *The stages of ethical development: From childhood through old age.* New York: Harper Collins.

Lafevre, M. L. (2015). Screening for vitamin D deficiency in adults: US Preventive Services Task Force Recommendation statement. *Annals of Internal Medicine, 162*(2), 133–140.

Levinson, D. (1986a). A conception of adult development. *American Psychologist, 41,* 3–13.

Levinson, D. (1986b). *The seasons of a man's life.* New York: Ballantine.

Levinson, D. (1996). *The seasons of a woman's life.* New York: Knopf.

Lips, P. (2010). Worldwide status of vitamin D nutrition. *The Journal of Steroid Biochemistry and Molecular Biology, 121,* 297–300.

Lochlainn, M. N., & Kenny, R. A. (2013). Sexual activity and aging. *Journal of the American Medical Directors Association, 14*(8), 565–572.

Lowdermilk, D., & Perry, S. (2012). *Reproductive system concerns. Maternity and women's health care* (10th ed.). St. Louis: Mosby.

Lubkin, I. M., & Larsen, P. D. (2013). *Chronic illness: Impact and intervention* (8th ed.). Burlington, MA: Jones & Bartlett.

Macartney, S., Bishaw, A., & Fontenot, K. (2013). Poverty rates for selected detailed race and Hispanic groups by state and place: 2007–2011. American Community Survey Briefs. http://www.census.gov/prod/2013pubs/acsbr11-17.pdf.

MacDorman, M. F., & Gregory, E. C. W. (2015). Fetal and perinatal mortality: United States, 2013. *National Vital Statistics Reports, 64*(8), https://www.cdc.gov/nchs/data/nvsr/nvsr64/nvsr64_08.pdf.

Manchanda, S. C., & Madan, K. (2014). Yoga and meditation in cardiovascular disease. *Clinical Research in Cardiology, 103*(9), 675–680. https://www.cdc.gov/nchs/data/nvsr/nvsr64/nvsr64_08.pdf.

Martinez, M. E., Ward, B. W., & Adams, P. F. (2015). *Health care access and utilization among adults aged 18–64, by race and Hispanic origin: United States, 2013 and 2014. NCHS data brief, no. 208.* Hyattsville, MD: National Center for Health Statistics.

Mikkola, T. S., et al. (2015). Estradiol-based postmenopausal hormone therapy and risk of cardiovascular and all-cause mortality. *Menopause (New York, N.Y.), 22*(9), 976–983.

Nair, R., & Maseeh, A. (2012). Vitamin D: The "sunshine" vitamin. *Journal of Pharmacology and Pharmacotherapeutics, 3*(2), 118–126.

National Center for Education Statistics. (2015). Employment rates and unemployment rates by educational attainment. http://nces.ed.gov/programs/coe/indicator_cbc.asp.

National Institutes of Health (NIH), National Cancer Institute. (2015a). HPV and cancer. http://www.cancer.gov/about-cancer/causes-prevention/risk/infectious-agents/hpv-fact-sheet#r7.

National Institutes of Health (NIH), National Cancer Institute. (2015b). Obesity and cancer. http://www.cancer.gov/about-cancer/causes-prevention/risk/obesity/obesity-fact-sheet#q3.

National Institutes of Health (NIH), Office of Dietary Supplements. (2016). Vitamin D fact sheets for health professionals. https://ods.od.nih.gov/factsheets/VitaminD-Health Professionals.

National Osteoporosis Foundation. (2014). *Healthy bones for life. Patient's guide.* Washington, DC: National Osteoporosis Foundation. http://nof.org/files/nof/public/content/resource/4029/files/1032.pdf.

National Sleep Foundation. (2017). What to do when you can't sleep. https://sleepfoundation.org/insomnia/content/what-do-when-you-cant-sleep.

National Vital Statistics Reports. (2016). Deaths: Leading causes for 2014. https://www.cdc.gov/nchs/data/nvsr/nvsr65/nvsr65-05.pdf.

Nelson, A. L. (2011). Perimenopause, menopause, and postmenopause: Health promotion strategies. In R. A. Hatcher, et al. (Eds.), *Contraceptive technology* (20th ed., pp. 737–777). New York: Ardent Media.

Nicholson, J. (2011). Five leading causes of workplace injury. http://www.ehow.com/info_7933497.

Nissenbaum, M. A., Aramini, J. J., & Hanning, C. D. (2012). Effects of industrial wind turbine noise on sleep and health. *Noise and Health, 60,* 237–243.

Northrup, C. (2012). *The wisdom of menopause: Creating physical and emotional health during the change.* New York: Random House.

Obesity Society. (2017). Why treat obesity as a disease? http://www.obesity.org/obesity/resources/facts-about-obesity/why-treat-as-disease.

Ogden, C. L., et al. (2015). *Prevalence of obesity among adults and youth: United States, 2011–2014. NCHS data brief, no 219.* Hyattsville, MD: National Center for Health Statistics. https://www.cdc.gov/nchs/data/databriefs/db219.pdf.

Palacious, S., et al. (2010). Age of menopause and impact of climacteric symptoms by geographical region. *Climacteric: The Journal of the International Menopause Society, 13*(5), 419–428.

Pender, N., Murdaugh, C. L., & Parsons, M. A. (2015). *Health promotion in nursing practice* (7th ed.). Upper Saddle River, NJ: Pearson.

Piaget, J. (1970). *Structuralism.* New York: Basic Books.

Pines, A. (2011). Male menopause: Is it a real clinical syndrome? *Climacteric: The Journal of the International Menopause Society, 14*(1), 15–17.

Pöss, J., et al. (2015). Effects of renal sympathetic denervation on urinary sodium excretion in patients with resistant hypertension. *Clinical Research in Cardiology, 104*(8), 672–678.

Reifman, A., Biernat, M., & Lang, E. (1991). Stress, social support, and health in married professional women with small children. *Psychology of Women Quarterly, 15,* 431–445.

Sanchez-Gonzalez, M. A., et al. (2015). Impact of negative affectivity and trait forgiveness on aortic blood pressure and coronary circulation. *Psychophysiology, 52*(2), 296–303.

Santacreu, M., & Fernández-Ballesteros, R. (2011). Evaluation of a behavioral treatment for female urinary incontinence. *Journal of Clinical Interventions in Aging, 6,* 133–139.

Schaie, K. W., & Willis, S. L. (2005). *Intellectual functioning in adulthood: Growth, maintenance, decline, and modifiability.* Philadelphia: American Society on Aging.

Sheehy, G. (1993). *Menopause: The silent passage.* New York: Random House.

Siegel, A. L. (2014). Pelvic floor muscle training in males: Practical applications. *Urology, 84*(1), 1–7.

Spector, R. E. (2012). *Cultural diversity in health and illness* (8th ed.). Upper Saddle River, NJ: Prentice Hall.

Spielberger, C. D., et al. (1983). Assessment of anger: The state-trait anger scale. In J. N. Butcher & C. D. Spielberger (Eds.), *Advances in personality assessment* (Vol. 2). Hillsdale, NJ: Lawrence Erlbaum Associates.

Sumnera, C. C. (2013). Adult children of divorce: Awareness and intervention. *Journal of Divorce and Remarriage, 54*(4), 271–281.

Thomas, S. P. (1995). Psychosocial correlates of women's health in middle adulthood. *Issues in Mental Health Nursing, 16,* 285–314.

Trompeter, S. E., Bettencourt, R., & Barrett-Connor, E. (2012). Sexual activity and satisfaction in healthy community-dwelling older women. *The American Journal of Medicine, 125*(1), 37–43.

Upson, K., et al. (2010). Factors associated with contraceptive nonuse among US women ages 35–44 years at risk of unwanted pregnancy. *An International Reproductive Health Journal Contraception, 81*(5), 427–434.

US Census Bureau. (2012). Age and sex composition: 2010 census. https://www.census.gov/prod/cen2010/briefs/c2010br-03.pdf.

US Census Bureau. (2013). Poverty rates for selected detailed race and Hispanic groups by state and place: 2007–2011. http://www.census.gov/prod/2013pubs/acsbr11-17.pdf.

US Census Bureau. (2015). Quick facts - USA people. https://www.census.gov/quickfacts/table/PST045216/00.

US Department of Health and Human Services (USDHHS). (2010). *Reports of the Surgeon General, U.S. Public Health Service Oral Health Initiative.* Washington, DC: US Department of Health and Human Services.

US Department of Health and Human Services (USDHHS), Indian Health Service. (2015). The Federal Health Program for American Indians and Alaska Natives. Disparities. https://www.ihs.gov/newsroom/index.cfm/factsheets/disparities/.

US Department of Human Health and Services (USDHHS), National Institutes of Health (NIH), National Heart, Lung, and Blood Institute. (2012). What is sleep apnea? http://www.nhlbi.nih.gov/health/health-topics/topics/sleepapnea.

US Department of Health and Human Services (USDHHS), National Institutes of Health (NIH), National Institute on Alcohol Abuse and Alcoholism (NIAAA). (2015a). Alcohol: A Women's health issue. https://pubs.niaaa.nih.gov/publications/brochurewomen/Woman_English.pdf.

US Department of Health and Human Services (USDHHS), National Institutes of Health (NIH), National Institute on Alcohol Abuse and Alcoholism (NIAAA). (2015b). Alcohol facts and statistics. http://pubs.niaaa.nih.gov/publications/AlcoholFacts&Stats/AlcoholFacts&Stats.pdf.

US Department of Labor, Occupational Safety and Health Administration. (2010). *You have a right to a safe workplace.* Washington, DC: Occupational Safety and Health Administration.

US Department of Labor, Occupational Safety and Health Administration. (2012). *Toxic and hazardous substances.* Washington, DC: Occupational Safety and Health Administration.

US Department of Labor, Occupational Safety and Health Administration. (2016a). *Employer-reported workplace injuries and illnesses-2015.* Washington, DC: Occupational Safety and Health Administration. https://www.bls.gov/news.release/pdf/osh.pdf.

US Department of Labor, Occupational Safety and Health Administration. (2016b). *National Census of fatal occupational injuries-2015.* Washington, DC: Occupational Safety and Health Administration. https://www.bls.gov/news.release/pdf/cfoi.pdf.

US Preventative Services Task Force (USPSTF). (2013). Final recommendation statement: Human Immunodeficiency virus (HIV) infection: Screening https://www.uspreventiveservicestaskforce.org/Page/Document/RecommendationStatementFinal/human-immunodeficiency-virus-hiv-infection-screening.

US Preventive Services Task Force (USPSTF). (2014). U.S. final recommendation statement: Obesity in adults: Screening and management. http://www.uspreventiveservicestaskforce.org/Page/Document/RecommendationStatementFinal/obesity-in-adults-screening-and-management.

Vaillant, G. (2003). *Aging well: Surprising guideposts to a happier life from the landmark Harvard Study of Adult Development.* New York: Little, Brown.

Vaillant, G., & Vaillant, C. (1990). Natural history of male psychological health, XII: A 45-year study of predictors of successful aging at age 65. *The American Journal of Psychiatry,* *147*(1), 31–37.

Vranceanu, A. M., et al. (2014). Exploring the effectiveness of a modified comprehensive mind-body intervention for medical and psychologic symptom relief. *Psychosomatics,* *55*(4), 386–391.

Wallerstein, J. S., Lewis, J., & Blakeslee, S. (2000). *The unexpected legacy of divorce: A 25 year landmark study.* New York: Hyperion.

Wang, F., et al. (2014). The effects of tai chi on depression, anxiety, and psychological well-being: A systematic review and meta-analysis. *International Journal of Behavioral Medicine,* *21*(4), 605–617.

Ward, B. W., Schiller, J. S., & Goodman, R. A. (2014). Multiple chronic conditions among US adults: A 2012 update. *Preventing Chronic Disease,* *11,* 130389.

Whayne, T. F., & Mukherjee, D. (2015). Women, the menopause, hormone replacement therapy and coronary heart disease. *Current Opinion in Cardiology,* *30*(4), 432–438.

Williams, J., et al. (2000). Anger proneness predicts coronary heart disease risk: Prospective analysis from the Atherosclerosis Risk in Communities (ARIC) study. *Circulation,* *101*(17), 2034–2039.

Wilsnack, S. C., Wilsnack, R. W., & Kantor, L. W. (2014). Focus on: Women and the costs of alcohol use. *Alcohol Research: Current Reviews,* *35*(2), 219–228.

World Health Organization. (2016). Obesity and overweight. http://www.who.int/mediacentre/factsheets/fs311/en/.

# 24

# Older Adult

*Jeanne Merkle Sorrell*

## ❓ THINK ABOUT IT

### *Older Adult Smokers*

*You are the director of a senior center in which 10 of your 40 members smoke. Several of the smoking individuals currently experience health problems. One older woman has chronic obstructive pulmonary disease and avoids using her oxygen because she is not supposed to smoke while the oxygen tank is in the room. One older man has high blood pressure; lung cancer has been diagnosed in another one of the smokers. As director of the center, you would like to help these older adults to stop smoking. You have referred them to their physicians to obtain assistance with smoking cessation. All involved are on limited incomes and cannot afford to pay the charge for either a behavior-management class or nicotine-replacement therapy.*

- What additional information do you need to determine the potential efficacy of a smoking cessation program in your center?
- What types of resources are available to help you obtain the necessary assistance for these smokers?
- What provisions are available under Medicare and the Affordable Care Act of 2010 to assist a person with smoking cessation?
- What policy changes might be instituted within the senior center to prevent secondhand smoke from harming the residents in the center's care?

There is a popular poster featuring an older man with an impressive muscular physique that is obviously the result of hours and hours of working out. The poster's title carries a strong message: "Aging is not for sissies." Because older adults are living longer and healthier as a result of health-promotion and technological advances, health care professionals often enjoy the gift of caring for older adults who are active and still making important contributions to society. To be caring for a group of human beings that was virtually nonexistent 100 years ago is truly extraordinary. It is important to help ensure, however, that these individuals are not only living longer but also that their lives are fulfilling and lived in dignity with as much independence as possible.

Who is the older adult today? Older adults are living longer and working longer. In 2014, 23% of men and approximately 15% of women 65 years or older were still working (Mather, 2016). According to preliminary data from the US Census Bureau, an individual who was 65 years of age in 2010 could expect to live 19.2 years more, for a total of 84.2 years. Individuals aged 85 years in 2010 could expect to live an average of 6.6 years more, for a total of 91.6 years (Murphy et al., 2012).

The older adult population is also becoming more racially and ethnically diverse. The percentage of white Americans in the population of adults aged 65 years or older is expected to decrease during the next 30 years, whereas the percentages of black Americans, Hispanics, and Asian Americans will continue to rise. By 2044, it is projected that more than half of Americans will belong to a minority group, with almost one in five being foreign born (US Census Bureau, 2015b). Considering this shift in population characteristics, nurses need to develop an awareness of the cultural diversity of this population and identify the cultural beliefs that influence their health care decisions.

There are many positive changes for older adults today. This share of the population is much better educated and more proficient in using technology than in the past. In 1965 only 5% of older adults had completed a bachelor's or higher degree, and by 2014 this had increased to 25% (Mather, 2016). Also, the gap in life expectancy of the sexes is narrowing, with the gap between men and women decreasing from 7 years to less than 5 years between 1990 and 2013 (Mather, 2016). The poverty rate for older adult Americans has also decreased significantly from approximately 30% in 1966 to 10% today (Mather, 2016). More older adults are "aging in place" in the community, with new living options that include retirement communities and independent living facilities or assisted living facilities, as well as skilled care institutions.

On the other hand, there are new challenges for health promotion in older adults. Obesity rates are increasing, and there are widening economic disparities across minority groups. In 2014 the percentage of Latino and black American older adults who lived in poverty was more than double the percentage of non-Hispanic whites (Mather, 2016). There has also been an increase in divorce rates, and more women are living alone. Forty-two percent of women aged between 75 and 84 years are living alone; the proportion jumps to 56% for women aged 85 years or older (Mather, 2016). All these changes have implications for health-promotion planning and interventions.

In 2013, approximately 44.7 million Americans (14.1% of the population) were 65 years or older (US Census Bureau, 2015a). By 2060 the number of adults aged 65 years or older is expected to be 98.2 million, with 19.7 million aged 85 years or older (US Census Bureau, 2015b). The 65 years or older population is expected to increase from 15% today to 24% by 2060 (Mather, 2016). Adults aged 85 years or older are the fastest-growing group within the older adult population, which means that nurses in the community, acute care settings, and long-term facilities will increasingly be caring for these individuals. Women comprise approximately four-fifths of the centenarians (Health Editor, 2016). Many factors have come together to help older adults live longer and healthier. These include continued vaccination development, injury prevention, decrease in smoking, less air pollution, and health-promotion activities (Health Editor, 2016).

During the past few decades, older adults have used the most health care dollars in the last 7 years of their lives, tending to wait until they became sick before seeking health care. Health care providers focused more on illness care than wellness care, resulting in a high prevalence of illness and limited health-promotion interventions. Misconceptions surrounding health promotion for older adults can impede the ability of nurses and other health providers to provide care that will enhance healthy aging. These misconceptions need to be overcome so that older adults receive health-promotion interventions that help to keep them active and healthy.

Health promotion is as important in later adulthood as it is in childhood. Older adults derive the same benefits from health-promotion activities as do their younger counterparts; they are not "too old" to stop smoking, start exercising, change their diet, or relinquish other bad health habits. Specific health-promotion strategies may differ for the young old (55–75 years), the middle old (75–85 years) and the very old, or oldest old (85 years or older). For example, strength training may be very appropriate for the young and middle old groups but may not be feasible for the oldest old. Balance exercises need to be addressed especially for those in the older two age groups. The potential for improvement with all groups is great, and nurses have a key role in changing common societal misconceptions and in creating new understandings regarding health promotion for older adults.

The diversity of cultural backgrounds in the United States influences the many biological, psychological, social, and economic changes as well as the spiritual and life transitions associated with aging that will be discussed in this chapter. Older adults who have immigrated to the United States have brought with them different languages, spiritual and cultural beliefs, eating preferences, and views about health and illness that may seem strange to younger Americans. Furthermore, people of different cultures may value older adults differently on the basis of their cultural perspective. Many cultures view older adults as a source of family and cultural history and wisdom. Throughout this chapter, cultural norms and behaviors will be discussed within each functional health pattern.

## HEALTHY PEOPLE 2020

In 2005, halfway through the *Healthy People 2010* project period, a midcourse review of the status of the national objectives was conducted. Data were collected to measure the progress of the goals and to revise and reword the goals to make sure they were accurate and scientifically relevant. Through this process it was determined that many goals focusing on older adults were being met. Importantly, the life expectancy continues to increase and the quality of life continues to improve throughout the nation. The number of years in good or better health and the number of years free of activity limitations and chronic illness have also increased slightly. At the same time, it was determined that new goals, topic areas, and topic-specific objectives needed to be developed. In December 2010 the US Department of Health and Human Services (USDHHS, 2010) released *Healthy People 2020.* The overall goals of *Healthy People 2020* expanded on previous goals and are to:

- Attain high-quality, longer lives free of preventable disease, disability, injury, and premature death.
- Achieve health equity, eliminate disparities, and improve the health of all groups.
- Create social and physical environments that promote good health for all.
- Promote quality of life, healthy development, and healthy behaviors across all life stages.

As part of the development of *Healthy People 2020,* several new topic areas were added, several of which focus on the health and wellness of older adults. These new topic areas are dementias, including Alzheimer disease; health-related quality of life and well-being; health care–associated infections; sleep health; and a unique category—older adults—which recognizes the special needs of this population. Selected national health-promotion and disease-prevention objectives for the older adult are listed in Box 24-1: *Healthy People 2020.* These objectives focus on increasing health-promotion programs and decreasing morbidity and mortality related to various disease states. In addition, other specific topic areas provide objectives that address the needs of older adults. Some of these will be addressed later in this chapter.

As the population of older adults continues to increase, the cultural diversity within this population will also increase. Cultural background and race have an effect on the prevalence of disease in the United States. A 2011 National Healthcare Quality and Disparities Report noted that despite some improvements, inequities persist among racial and ethnic minority groups (Agency for Healthcare Research and Quality, 2012). Researchers found a serious disparity in health care quality for blacks (41%), Hispanics (39%), and Asians (30%) as compared with whites. Language barriers are also associated with decreased quality of care, as well as decreased safety. The report emphasized the need to step up measures to increase quality and access to health care so as to achieve equitable health care for all.

## BIOLOGY AND GENETICS

Although there is a serious need to promote the health of the older population, there are numerous challenges in meeting this need. One of the great challenges to health promotion for older adults lies in the misconceptions about the benefits of disease prevention and health promotion. Another challenge relates to the difficulty in separating normal changes of aging from pathological processes and illness. Age-related changes are frequently regarded as inevitable and irreversible. However, there is a large amount of variability in age-related changes within each individual. Environmental, economic, physiological, genetic, psychological, social, and cultural factors combine to influence the aging process. Many older adults have an interest in learning about their genetic makeup and how this may influence their aging process and development of disease. Box 24-2: Personal Genomic Testing provides information about personal genomic testing.

Most researchers agree that biological changes show that growth and development peak during early adulthood, with subsequent linear decline until death. These normal changes must be distinguished from pathological changes to focus health-promotion interventions on behaviors that can be changed. For example, it is normal for older adults to experience a decline in their respiratory vital capacity. Therefore when nurses are recommending exercise programs, older people must start gradually, allowing them to experience the exercise free from respiratory distress. Selected changes will be discussed specifically in the Gordon's Functional Health Patterns section.

Another challenge in promoting the health of older adults relates to the prevalence of chronic illness and multiple health problems. Although chronic illness is not a normal part of aging, years of environmental assault, poor health behaviors, and stress have placed older adults at a high risk of developing these illnesses. Table 24-1 lists the percentage of older adults with chronic conditions. Illness influences the older adult's capacity and motivation to learn new behaviors, so health-promotion activities need to be individualized to fit functional abilities. According to the Centers for Disease Control and Prevention (CDC, 2014a), in 2013 61.1% of adults aged 65 years or older had difficulty in performing at least one basic action or had a complex activity limitation. Most of these limitations are associated with physical changes of aging and chronic disease such as arthritis, heart disease, stroke, and respiratory disease. The prevalence of preventable illness and the concomitant physical limitations associated with chronic disease clearly indicate that there is a great need for health-promotion and disease/injury-prevention activities in this population. It is important to note that health-promotion practices among older adults may vary because of the individual's self-perception of health status and the individual's economic and cultural background (Box 24-3: Diversity Awareness).

### Theories of Aging

The study of how and why people age has continued over many years and has been the source of a great deal of debate. For many years, the cause of death on many older adults' death certificates was listed simply as "old age." At the 55th Annual Meeting of the Gerontological Society of America, Butler and Olshansky (2002) explored this mind-set in a presentation entitled "Has Anyone Ever Died of Old Age?" As the specialization of gerontology has progressed, researchers have clarified the physiological, social, and psychological reasons related to why people die.

BOX 24-1 **HEALTHY PEOPLE 2020**

*Selected National Health-Promotion and Disease-Prevention Topics and Objectives Relevant for Older Adults*

**Older Adult**

- Increase the proportion of older adults who are up-to-date on a core set of clinical preventive services.
- Increase the proportion of older adults with one or more chronic health conditions who report confidence in managing their conditions.
- Increase the proportion of older adults who receive diabetes self-management benefits.
- Reduce the proportion of older adults who have moderate to severe functional limitations.
- Increase the proportion of older adults who engage in light, moderate, or vigorous leisure-time activities.
- Increase the proportion of the health care workforce with geriatric certification.
- Reduce the proportion of noninstitutionalized older adults with disabilities who have an unmet need for long-term services and supports.
- Reduce the proportion of unpaid caregivers of older adults who report an unmet need for caregiver support services.
- Reduce the rate of pressure ulcer–related hospitalizations among older adults.
- Reduce the rate of emergency department visits attributable to falls among older adults.
- Increase the number of states, including the District of Columbia, and tribes that collect and make publicly available information on the characteristics of victims, perpetrators, and cases of elder abuse, neglect, and exploitation.

**Dementias, Including Alzheimer Disease**

- Increase the proportion of persons with diagnosed Alzheimer disease and other dementias, or their caregivers, who are aware of the diagnosis.
- Reduce the proportion of preventable hospitalizations in persons with diagnosed Alzheimer disease and other dementias.

**Hearing and Other Sensory Communication Disorders**

- Reduce the proportion of adults who have elevated hearing thresholds, or audiometric notches, in high frequencies (3, 4, or 6 kHz) in both ears, signifying noise-induced hearing loss.
- Increase the proportion of adults bothered by tinnitus who have seen a physician or other health care professionals.
- Increase the proportion of adults for whom tinnitus is a moderate to severe problem who have tried appropriate treatments.

- Increase the proportion of adults with balance or dizziness problems in the past 12 months who have ever seen a health care provider about their balance or dizziness problems.
- Increase the proportion of adults with moderate to severe balance or dizziness problems who have seen or been referred to a health care specialist for evaluation or treatment.
- Reduce the proportion of adults with chemosensory (smell or taste) disorders who as a result have experienced a negative impact on their general health status, work, or quality of life in the past 12 months.
- Increase the proportion of persons with communication disorders of voice, swallowing, speech, or language who have seen a speech-language pathologist for evaluation or treatment.
- Increase the proportion of persons with communication disorders of voice, swallowing, speech, or language who have participated in rehabilitation services.

**Sleep Health**

- Increase the proportion of adults who get sufficient sleep.

**Respiratory Diseases**

- Reduce activity limitations among adults with chronic obstructive pulmonary disease.
- Reduce deaths from chronic obstructive pulmonary disease among adults.
- Reduce hospitalizations for chronic obstructive pulmonary disease.
- Reduce hospital emergency department visits for chronic obstructive pulmonary disease.
- Increase the proportion of adults with abnormal lung function whose underlying obstructive disease has been diagnosed.

**Vision**

- Reduce visual impairment.
- Increase the use of personal protective eyewear in recreational activities and hazardous situations around the home.
- Increase vision rehabilitation.
- (Developmental) Increase the proportion of federally qualified health centers that provide comprehensive vision health services.

From US Department of Health and Human Services. (2012). 2020 topics & objectives. http://www.healthypeople.gov/2020/topicsobjectives2020/default.aspx.

There is no formula to predict how a person will age or how long that individual will live. Many **theories of aging** continue to be examined today, including those regarding metabolism, free radicals, stress, the role of the immune system, genetics, epigenetics (the blending of nature/genetics and nurture/environment), and diet. It is postulated that genetic markers may predict the development of disease and play a large role in determining how a person will age and how long the person will live. In addition, researchers report that calorie-restricted diets have resulted in an increase in longevity in animals; however, there is debate regarding whether calorie restriction alone or calorie restriction in the presence of genetic markers increases longevity. The role of antioxidants in binding free radicals is

also being researched as an important influence on increasing longevity. Although no consensus has yet been reached that describes the entire aging process, exciting theories continue to be forthcoming (National Institute on Aging, 2011). Some of the theories used to explain aging are briefly described in Box 24-4.

# GORDON'S FUNCTIONAL HEALTH PATTERNS

## Health Perception–Health Management Pattern

Motivation is an important factor in maintaining health. Nurses who care for older adults know that the best nursing in the world

## BOX 24-2   GENOMICS

### Personal Testing

Older adults are increasingly interested in learning about their own DNA to find clues about their heritage and about factors that may affect their future health. With technological developments in recent years, it is now possible to purchase low-cost genetic kits for as little as $100. Do the results of these tests prompt older adults to change their habits to more healthy lifestyles?

In the United States, three companies have dominated the market for do-it-yourself, direct-to-consumer (DTC) genetic kits that allow consumers to bypass medical intermediaries: 23andMe, Navigenics, and DeCODEme. These genetic tests offer a wide array of information about ancestry, physical traits, and health information. (Ancestry.com does not provide health information at this time). Health-related genetic tests include predictive tests for alterations in genes known to be strongly associated with disease onset (e.g., Alzheimer disease and several cancer syndromes), along with susceptibility tests that give feedback of much lower increased risk of developing common health conditions (e.g., type 2 diabetes).

Bioethicists and health researchers have raised concern about the health-risk genre of these tests, and the Food and Drug Administration asked 23andMe to stop marketing the health tests until it could provide evidence that their results are reliable. Those who favor DTC health-related testing argue that direct access to personal genetic information is a fundamental right and helps to preserve autonomy and privacy by eliminating health care intermediaries. Others argue that providing genetic information directly to consumers without health professional

support to explain the information could result in numerous harms, in that consumers may not have adequate information to make determinations about the meaning of the results. There is concern that individuals who are told they carry genetic risk variants may have harmful psychological responses, such as feeling fatalistic about their potential to reduce their risk of health problems. Early users of the DTC kits, however, have not reported strong emotional response to test results, regardless of whether or not the findings show increased risk.

An important advantage of DTC testing is the potential that the results could motivate consumers to make lifestyle changes to reduce their disease risk. Consumers state that genetic susceptibility tests for conditions such as obesity would motivate them to adopt a healthier lifestyle and could also provide information that could help their primary care provider monitor their health.

Very few studies have evaluated whether individuals change their lifestyle after receiving genetic risk results. Early evidence suggests, however, that thus far genetic test results have not had a demoralizing effect on consumers' efforts or desire to change health habits. There is mixed evidence on how susceptibility testing may influence use of health services. The bottom line is that when consumers receive the results of their testing, they often find that their personalized risk results are matched with the same health recommendations they already know. Most experts believe that potential breakthroughs that could enable genomic risk information to be used routinely to prevent disease and foster healthy aging are still in the future.

From McBride, C. (2015). Personal genomic tests for healthy aging: Neither feast nor foul. *Generations. Journal of the American Society on Aging.* http://www.asaging.org/blog/personal-genomic-tests-healthy-aging-neither-feast-nor-foul.

### TABLE 24-1   Average Percentage of People Aged 65 Years or Older Who Have Chronic Health Conditions

| Chronic Condition | Age 65–74 yr | Age ≥75 yr |
|---|---|---|
| Hypertension | 54.2 | 57.3 |
| Arthritis | 49.0 | 54.1 |
| Heart disease | 16.5 | 25.8 |
| Cancer | 20.4 | 27.2 |
| Diabetes | 22.0 | 21.7 |
| Asthma | 8.7 | 7.4 |
| Chronic bronchitis or emphysema | 11.4 | 12.6 |
| Stroke | 6.1 | 10.7 |

From Centers for Disease Control and Prevention, National Center for Health Statistics. (2010). Summary health statistics for U.S. adults: National Health Interview Survey 2010. http://www.cdc.gov/nchs/data/series/sr_10/sr10_252.pdf.

cannot make an individual do something he or she believes to be unnecessary. A primary factor in the older adult's motivation to promote personal health is the perception of health and its subsequent management. For older adults who have always been healthy and then receive a diagnosis of a serious disease, it is important that they find ways to promote health while living with the disease. For example, new research shows that many of the debilitating aspects of Parkinson disease can be minimized through active exercise, including bicycling (Paddock, 2012). Older adults with a diagnosis of spinal stenosis or back pain

that prevents them from walking long distances may think they can no longer travel. New mobile devices such as scooters, which allow the person to ride through the airport and then check the scooter at the gate, help to make travel to visit friends or family or dreamed-of adventures possible. These devices also provide independence for older adults to go out in their neighborhood to socialize (Figure 24-1).

Nurses can be very helpful in talking with older adults to learn their goals for health and what motivates them. If a person dislikes group activity, it may not be effective to encourage him or her to take exercise or nutrition classes. Suggesting an exercise DVD that can be used at home or reading about nutrition may be more helpful. It is important not to underestimate older adults' abilities; many older adults continue to actively participate in competitive sports. Even chronic illnesses do not need to prevent health-promotion activities. Older adults should be encouraged to continue with self-care activities rather than to relinquish them to caregivers. Because some memory impairment may be present in cognitively healthy older adults, memory aids and familiar environments should be encouraged so that they keep their minds active, continue learning, and maintain their self-confidence.

A variety of activities promote health and prevent frailty. These include maintaining healthy weight and diet; staying active; practicing fall prevention; maintaining relationships; and keeping regular medical appointments. Additionally, the CDC (2011a) recommends clinical preventive services for older adults that include immunizations (influenza and pneumococcal) and screenings for early detection of breast cancer, colorectal cancer, diabetes, lipid disorders, and osteoporosis; and smoking cessation

## 🌐 BOX 24-3 DIVERSITY AWARENESS

### Perceptions of Health Status, Need for Assistance With Routine Needs, and Need for Assistance With Activities of Daily Living Related to Race

Data from the National Health Interview Survey conducted by the CDC in 2010 (CDC, National Center for Health Statistics, 2010) provide interesting information about the perceptions of Hispanic, non-Hispanic black, and non-Hispanic white older adults regarding their health status, their need for assistance with routine activities, and their need for assistance with activities of daily living.

When asked about health status, 42.7% of white adults 65 years or older stated that their health was excellent or very good, 34% described their health as good, and 22.9% described their health as fair or poor; 44% of Asian American older adults reported their health as excellent or very good, 34.4% stated their health was good, and 21.6% stated their health was fair or poor. In contrast, 25.3% of black older adults reported their health as excellent or very good, 36.4% stated their health was good, and 38.2% stated that their health was fair or poor. Of Hispanic older adults, 28.1% reported that their health was excellent or very good, 33.8% reported their health as good, and 38.2% stated their health was fair or poor. In all groups, those who described their health as fair or poor were also more likely to be financially poor, with 40% of white older adults, 51.6% of black older adults, 53.4% of Hispanic older adults, and 45.6% of Asian American older adults who reported their health status as fair or poor also being financially poor.

Respondents were also asked about their need for assistance with activities of daily living, such as bathing, showering, dressing, eating, getting in and out of the bed or chair, using the toilet, or getting around inside the home; and their need for assistance with routine activities, such as performing everyday household chores, doing necessary business, shopping, and getting around for other purposes outside the home. The results indicated that 11.2% of non-Hispanic white older adults reported needing assistance with routine needs, 18.1% of Hispanic and 17.1% of non-Hispanic black older adults reported needing assistance, and 6.2% of non-Hispanic white older adults reported needing assistance with activities of daily living, whereas 11.5% of both Hispanic and non-Hispanic black older adults reported needing assistance.

Nurses must be aware of racial disparities in the incidence of chronic disease, perceived health status, and perceived need for assistance with activities of daily living and routine tasks in the people for whom they provide care. Assessing older adults holistically and planning interventions that focus on health promotion, illness and injury prevention, and effective management of chronic illness will help to ensure improved quality of life for all older adults.

From Centers for Disease Control and Prevention, National Center for Health Statistics. (2010). Summary health statistics for U.S. adults: National Health Interview Survey 2010. http://www.cdc.gov/nchs/data/series/sr_10/sr10_252.pdf.

## BOX 24-4 Theories of Aging

### Biological Theories of Aging

- Programmed theories of aging: Aging is the result of predictable cellular death.
  - Immunity theory: Aging is a programmed accumulation of damage and decline in the function of the immune system resulting from oxidative stress.
  - Neuroendocrine control/pacemaker theory: Aging is a programmed decline in the functioning of the nervous, endocrine, and immune systems. The cells lose their ability to reproduce.
  - Gene theory: Longevity may be associated with a genetic trait or a "longevity gene," "juvenescent" genes mediate youthful vigor and mature adult well-being, "senescent" genes promote functional decline and structural deterioration.
- Error theories of aging: Aging is the result of an accumulation of random errors in the synthesis of cellular DNA and RNA.
  - Oxidative stress theory (free radical theory): Errors are a result of random damage from free radicals.
  - Cross-linkage theory: Aging is a product of accumulated damage from errors associated with cross-linked proteins where cross-linked proteins become stiff and thick.
  - Wear-and-tear theory: Cellular errors are the result of deterioration over time because of continued use.
- Calorie restriction theory: In animal models, calorie restriction increased the life span and the health of the animals.

### Sociological Theories of Aging

- Activity theory: Continued activity is an indicator of successful aging.
- Disengagement theory: In the course of aging, the individual slowly withdraws from former roles and activities.

- Role theory: The ability of an individual to adapt to changing roles throughout life is predictive of adjustment to the changing roles associated with aging.
- Continuity theory: In normal aging, personality remains consistent. Personality influences role activity and life satisfaction.
- Age stratification theory: Focuses on the relationship between age as an element of social structure and aging people as a cohort.
- Subculture theory: Older people have their own norms, habits, and beliefs and interact better among age peers than with other age groups.

### Developmental Theories of Aging

- Erikson's developmental theory: There is a predetermined order of development, and specific tasks are associated with specific periods in a person's life. For older adults, the developmental stage is integrity versus despair.
- Peck's developmental theory: This theory expanded on Erikson's theory with identification of discrete tasks of late life that when accomplished together result in ego integrity.
- Havighurst's developmental theory: There are specific tasks associated with aging, including adjusting to the losses of aging (e.g., health, income, death of spouse and age peers), adapting to change and new roles, and accepting life's experiences.
- Tornstam's theory of gerotranscendence: Aging is viewed as the movement from birth to death and maturation toward wisdom. Gerotranscendence involves achieving wisdom through personal transformation.

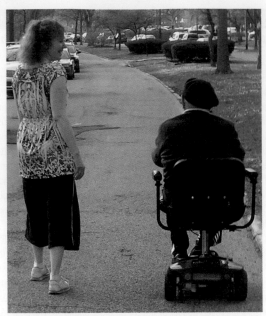

**FIGURE 24-1** Mobile devices such as scooters provide independence for older adults with limited mobility.

counseling for those who smoke. Under the Affordable Care Act of 2010, many of these services are provided at no cost to older adults who have Medicare. SilverSneakers is a popular exercise program that is available at no cost to many older adults through their Medicare or private insurance plan (Healthways, 2014). There are also many different on-line and mobile applications that aid in monitoring exercise and may be fun for older adults to use. Helping an older adult to understand the importance of learning or maintaining healthy behaviors is an essential nursing role.

Health-maintenance behaviors include exercise, good nutrition, sexual safety, and appropriate sleep-rest patterns. Health-maintenance practices also include regular health care checkups, which will provide early detection and management of disease. Although these behaviors are important for all older adults, the perception of these activities and the ability to practice good health behaviors differ by cultural group. It is essential that nurses are culturally competent and understand the cultural values that guide behavior. In so doing, the nurse will be most effective in helping the older adult form a positive health perception and practice good health behaviors (Box 24-5 Innovative Practice).

---

### ✳ BOX 24-5   INNOVATIVE PRACTICE

#### *Geriatric Assessment*

The health care system, with its emphasis on acute care, busy office schedules, and fragmented delivery systems, often frustrates older people and their families. The very old or frail person's health problems are often overlooked, ignored, or only partially treated. Many communities have a health care service that uses a team approach to meet the special needs of older adults. This service is known as geriatric assessment.

#### Goals of Geriatric Assessment
- Maintain health and health maintenance practices.
  - Promote disease prevention through routine immunizations and health screenings.
  - Implement fall prevention strategies to decrease the incidence of falls and fall-related injuries.
- Minimize hospitalizations.
- Establish complete diagnoses that are often missed or overlooked, including hearing impairment, vision deficits, early dementia, depression, and poor nutrition.
- Decrease overprescription and misuse of medications, including prescription medications, over-the-counter medications, vitamins/minerals/supplements, and herbal remedies.

Geriatric assessment uses an interdisciplinary team consisting of a geriatric nurse practitioner, a physical therapist, and a social worker. Each member of the team evaluates the person from a health care, functional, cognitive, or psychosocial perspective. Additional members of the team might include a geriatric psychiatrist, geriatrician, nutritionist, pharmacist, dentist, or podiatrist. The program team evaluates the home environment, risk of falls, incontinence, vision and hearing impairments, memory loss, depression and anxiety, functional decline, physical deconditioning, caregiver stress, economic resources, advance directives, and quality-of-life issues. The team is coordinated by the geriatric nurse practitioner.

Geriatric assessment is not meant for all older people. The people who benefit are those who are frail. An older person who might benefit from geriatric assessment is one who:
- Is older than 80 years
- Has a history of frequent falls
- Is losing weight
- Is depressed
- Has mild memory loss
- Has been hospitalized three times in 2 months
- Takes more than five medications regularly and frequently gets them confused
- Has no close family or other support persons in the community
- Is in need of health teaching

Geriatric assessment usually identifies the strengths and weaknesses of the older adult and evaluates that person's situation, including family and other social support. Following the assessment, the geriatric nurse practitioner begins developing a care plan to incorporate usable strengths and assist with weaknesses.

The primary care physician, family physician, internist, geriatrician, or geriatric nurse practitioner is a key link between the geriatric assessment team and the individual, primarily because this provider carries out the team's recommendation and monitors the person's progress. In most cases the nurse practitioner coordinates between the team and the person's primary physician and family.

Geriatric assessment clinics are available in many larger cities. As the US health care system changes from its costly system of treating acute health problems with frequent office and hospital visits to a more cost-controlled, coordinated, comprehensive health management system, geriatric assessment will play a key role in identifying individual strengths, correcting problems, and maintaining the health and quality of life of older citizens.

## Nutritional-Metabolic Pattern

Proper nutrition helps prevent cancer, obesity, and gastrointestinal disorders and provides older adults with the energy required to function in all activities of daily living. One can measure good nutrition by determining whether the individual is meeting the recommended daily allowance (RDA) for caloric intake. The US Department of Agriculture (2010) established the RDA of 2000 to 2800 calories for men aged 51 years or older: 2000 to 2200 calories for sedentary men, 2200 to 2400 calories for moderately active men, and 2400 to 2800 calories for active men. The range for women aged 51 years or older is 1600 to 2200 calories—1600 calories for sedentary women, 1800 calories for moderately active women, and 2000 to 2200 calories for active women.

Poor nutrition in older adults not only affects their overall health but also contributes to higher health care costs. Specific nutritional risk factors for US older adults include solitary living, being of a particular race/ethnicity, low income, social isolation, and low social support (Tyler et al., 2014). The National Resource Center on Nutrition, Physical Activity & Aging (2012) stated that between 35% and 50% of older residents living in long-term care facilities are malnourished and approximately 65% of older adults in hospitals may be malnourished. These data underscore the problems of maintaining good nutrition. For independent seniors, the barriers that may interfere with the ability to obtain adequate and nutritional food include limited transportation, income, and social support resources.

Problems with access to food are compounded by the effect of normal changes of aging. Declines in gastrointestinal organ function can lead to changes in digestive metabolism and the absorption and elimination of nutrients. A deterioration of the smell, vision, and taste senses and the high frequency of dental and swallowing problems make maintaining adequate daily nutrition even more difficult. Additionally, side effects of required medications may affect appetite. Cultural food preferences and lifelong eating habits, such as diets high in fat and cholesterol, are other obstacles to maintaining optimal nutrition.

Because of physiological and metabolic changes associated with aging, nutritional problems are more difficult to quantify and evaluate in older adults (Mueller, 2015). A nutritional assessment for an older adult entails a comprehensive approach that includes a health history, physical examination, laboratory data, dietary data, and measurement of functional status. Initial nutritional screening, however, is more straightforward. Nutritional screening evaluates the risk of malnutrition and may identify the need for a more formal nutrition assessment. There are a variety of tools, such as the Mini Nutritional Assessment (MNA), that can be used for nutritional screening in older adults. The MNA contains an initial set of questions that if scored below 11 indicates risk of malnutrition and requires the completion of additional questions to confirm the likelihood of malnutrition (Mueller, 2015). The MNA and other screening tools can identify the risk of malnutrition, but a formal nutritional assessment is needed to establish a diagnosis of malnutrition and appropriate interventions.

The living environment further affects nutritional status. Community-dwelling seniors are at high risk of nutritional disorders because access to food may be limited. Older adults in long-term care facilities do not have a problem with availability of food, but the meals may contain excessive fat, cholesterol, or salt, and may lack sufficient fiber. Additionally, fresh fruit and vegetables are less available. Institutional food may be unappealing, and institutions may not be able to adapt their meals to the cultural and religious preferences of their residents. Encouraging family members to bring in special foods that the resident enjoys is helpful. Nurses who work in institutional settings make an important difference for older adults by assessing the person's food preferences and any difficulties in eating, followed by careful planning of an appropriate menu, to encourage healthy eating.

A pleasant setting with social interaction enhances the desire to eat. In one study an expert panel of nutrition practitioners concluded that the two most important enablers of healthy eating among older adults are accessibility and social support (Tyler et al., 2014). Many older adults want to age in their own home without having to relocate to a long-term care facility. Research suggests that nutritional supports play a critical role in older adults' ability to remain in their homes (Tyler et al., 2014). Food assistance from friends and family in the form of cooking or food sharing is an important facilitator of nutritional health and being able to age in place. One study focused on how social lives and community environmental supports and barriers affected older adults' nutritional health (Tyler et al., 2014). The researchers conducted 29 focus group discussions with 144 residents of one of the largest retirement communities in the United States. The findings revealed that the high social connectedness of residents was associated with both positive and negative influences. The high degree of social support in the retirement community positively influenced the nutritional health of the participants. Social gatherings, however, also appeared to encourage residents to eat more than they would by themselves and to eat less nutritious foods. The findings also suggested that friends and neighbors provide an excellent point of entry for nutritional interventions such as information about food assistance strategies and other types of educational programs for health promotion.

Anorexia, or lack of appetite, can accompany disease. Medications, poor dentition, difficulty swallowing, or a lack of dentures can also cause older people to eat less than is optimal. Those in acute care hospitals or long-term care facilities may experience a lack of appetite as a result of illness. The hospital stay is a time during which good nutrition is most important to heal wounds and to restore energy; however, a lack of interest in or energy for eating during hospitalization places the older adult at a high risk of developing nutritional disorders.

Obesity is also a problem for older adults. Ogden and colleagues (2012) reported that 39.7% of adults aged 60 years or older are obese, with older women having a greater incidence of obesity (42.3%) than older men (36.6%). Obesity is associated with several chronic health conditions, including hypertension, diabetes, and heart disease. It is important to recognize, however, that scientists have described a phenomenon called "the obesity paradox," in which obesity in older adults, unlike in younger individuals, does not appear to be clearly associated with a shorter life span. Some studies have suggested that the "ideal" protective weight might be higher in the older population (Pietrzykowska, 2016). There is still much debate about this, however, and because obesity is clearly linked to a lesser quality of life, it is important to discuss options for weight reduction. During weight loss, muscle is lost, as well as fat. This is an important consideration when one is planning a weight loss program for older adults because, as a result of normal aging and often deconditioning, they are likely to have less muscle mass and more fat than when they were younger. Studies have found, however, that a moderate weight loss of 5% to 10% results in significant health benefits and that even a weight loss of 3% in older adults significantly reduces inflammation, blood pressure, cholesterol levels, and blood glucose levels (Pietrzykowska, 2016). For nurses working with older adults who are trying to lose weight, it is important to recognize that these individuals may have struggled with trying to lose weight for years and may be very frustrated with their unsuccessful efforts to achieve an ideal weight. Factors such as living alone and not wanting to cook for one person, the expense and short shelf life of fresh fruits and vegetables, medications, fast food, lack of motivation, and difficulty exercising make losing weight difficult. Nurses can help empower older adults by identifying realistic strategies for them to attain and maintain a healthy weight.

Nurses assist older adults in maintaining the highest possible nutritional level by teaching them about the food needed to maintain optimal nutritional status and by providing information about resources to help purchase food. One important resource is the federal Supplemental Nutrition Assistance Program (SNAP), formerly known as the Food Stamps program. SNAP is available to those who meet certain economic criteria, and can help older adults obtain nutritious food at participating markets without them depleting their limited budgets. When the economy declines, there is an increase in unemployment and poverty, and more people need help buying nutritious food. SNAP can provide needed help, but many people who are eligible for SNAP benefits, including 67% of struggling older adults, do not apply (Squires, 2014). Only three in five older adults who qualify for SNAP actually use it, which means that 5.2 million seniors are missing out on benefits of the program (National Council on Aging, n.d.). Some older adults are too embarrassed to apply, and others think it is too difficult to apply or do not even know the program exists. Yet for years they have paid taxes that help to support the program. The American Association of Retired Persons (AARP) has implemented initiatives to encourage more older adults to participate in SNAP. As a result of the AARP's work, in collaboration with other organizations, 20,000 new SNAP applications were submitted in 2013 (Squires, 2014).

In addition to SNAP, there are other federally supported nutrition assistance programs available to older adults, including the Commodity Supplemental Food Program, the Child and Adult Care Food Program, older adult nutrition program ("meals on wheels"), and the Emergency Food Assistance Program. The Older Adults Nutrition Services Program, which includes meals on wheels, provides nutritional services specifically to older adults. Detailed information about this program, as well as other important nutritional information related to older adults, is given in Chapter 11.

## Elimination Pattern

Bowel and bladder functions in the older adult are altered by normal changes of aging. The bladder retains its tonus, but its capacity decreases. Gastrointestinal motility decreases as people age. In addition to some of the normal changes of aging, diet plays a significant role in problems with intestinal motility and constipation. Decreased intake of fluids and fiber contribute in large part to constipation. Many medications taken by older adults also cause elimination concerns. Lack of physical activity and changes in the environment that decrease privacy also contribute to elimination problems. Many older adults may believe elimination problems are a necessary part of aging and may be embarrassed to mention their concerns to health care providers. It is important to reassure them that through diet and exercise they can gain control of most elimination problems.

Constipation is often a major problem for older adults and has far-reaching effects on their quality of life. There are several bowel elimination problems that are described by people as constipation: hard stools, infrequent stools, the need for excessive straining, and a feeling of incomplete bowel evacuation often associated with abdominal cramping or feeling bloated. Although inadequate diet and inactivity are common causes of constipation, it is important to consider whether constipation is related to metabolic disease such as hypothyroidism, neurological disease such as Parkinson disease, psychological illness such as depression, or medications. Nurses can assess the cause of constipation and develop an appropriate plan of care. Encouraging older adults to exercise and increase their fluid intake helps reduce the incidence of constipation. Integrating more fiber into the diet and eating prunes each day can also be very effective for preventing constipation.

Urinary incontinence affects approximately 50% of older adults who live at home or in long-term care facilities (Gorina et al., 2014). Incontinence is classified as either acute (transient) or chronic (established) (Touhy & Jett, 2012). Acute incontinence has a sudden onset, has been present for less than 6 months, and is usually secondary to a treatable condition. Chronic incontinence has either a sudden or a gradual onset and is categorized into four major types: stress incontinence, which is the most common and occurs during exercise, laughing, coughing, or sneezing; urge incontinence, or the inability to delay voiding after the bladder is full; urge, mixed, or stress urinary incontinence with high postvoid residual incontinence, which occurs when the bladder does not empty completely and becomes overdistended, which may be caused by an obstruction in the urinary elimination tract, such as that caused by an enlarged prostate gland; and functional incontinence, which is associated with environmental barriers, physical limitations, or cognitive impairment where the person is unable to reach the toilet.

Incontinence results in threats to both psychological and physical health, including depression, urinary tract infections, skin breakdown, and falls. Nurses can help older adults to understand incontinence as a manageable problem. Implementing appropriate management is important for the older adult's continued good health and self-esteem. Pelvic floor or Kegel exercises can be taught to strengthen the musculature of the urinary system (Mayo Clinic, 2015a,b). Pilates exercises have also been demonstrated to be effective in treating incontinence (Crawford, 2013). Management programs may include scheduling regular times to void, improving access to toileting facilities, management of diet and fluids, and the use of disposable absorbent undergarments. Voiding schedules are most effective when the person selects specific times during the day for urination. Eliminating dietary caffeine helps people with urge incontinence and increasing fiber in the diet helps those whose incontinence is related to constipation.

## Activity-Exercise Pattern

It is estimated that only 20% of American adults meet the aerobic and muscle-strengthening components of federal physical activity recommendations, and studies show that older adults get even less activity (CDC, 2013b). Men are more likely to meet the guidelines than women, and white older adults are more likely to meet them than black or Hispanic older adults. The benefits of regular exercise in promoting health and preventing disease are widely accepted. The overwhelming evidence of the positive effects of exercise has led the USDHHS to develop within its *Healthy People 2020* program national objectives for increasing the percentage of adults who exercise regularly. Regular physical activity helps and may even prevent many chronic health problems associated with aging, including hypertension, obesity, diabetes, and depression. Regular physical activity can increase both the years of life and the quality of those years. Strength training can improve balance and reduce the risk of falls, strengthen bones, and reduce blood glucose levels. Normal changes of aging, pathological conditions, and environmental deterrents do not need to prevent the older adult from exercising (Figure 24-2).

The CDC (2011b) recommends a combination of aerobic exercise and muscle-strengthening activities every week. Aerobic exercise may range from moderate intensity to vigorous intensity depending on the older person's level of fitness, and muscle-strengthening activities can include exercises that work all major muscle groups. Teaching the many benefits of exercise is the first lesson in motivating older adults to engage. With respect to the role that culture plays on the value of exercise, individual counseling is needed to identify exercises that can be enjoyed and continued (Figure 24-3). The nurse or physical therapist assists in designing an appropriate exercise program that will help to maintain strength, flexibility, and balance. Walking, which can be done in both community settings and health care facilities, is a popular form of exercise among older adults.

Other popular activities for older adults include swimming, weight-bearing exercises, and aquatic exercises. Weight-bearing and muscle-building exercises help to maintain functional mobility, promote independence, and prevent falls. Weight-bearing exercises are shown to be highly effective in reducing bone wasting associated with osteoporosis. Regular exercise promotes maintenance of bone mineral density in older adults. People with conditions such as spinal stenosis and arthritis often find that they can exercise in a swimming pool without pain, so this is an important way for them to maintain an exercise plan and increase their functional ability. Box 24-6 lists many benefits that can be derived from participation in an exercise program.

Before beginning any exercise program, an older person who has not been exercising should consult a physician or nurse practitioner. After the program begins, activity levels can be increased gradually. Adherence to an exercise program is a major problem for all populations. The best strategies to encourage continued exercise among older adults are to communicate the importance of exercise in maintaining quality of life and to help them choose an exercise that they enjoy and is easily accessible. Exercising with a family member or friend is also helpful in motivating older adults to exercise.

## Sleep-Rest Pattern

Inability to sleep is a frequent concern of older adults. Neikrug and Ancoli-Israel (2010) reported that approximately 50% of older adults state that they have difficulty sleeping. Sleep difficulties may include sleep apnea, the inability to fall asleep, the inability to stay asleep, the inability to fall back to sleep when awakening in the night, or the feeling of not being refreshed when awakening in the morning. Sleep-disordered breathing, or sleep apnea, may affect 20% to 40% of older adults and is associated with increased risk of stroke and death (Redline et al., 2010). Restless legs syndrome, characterized by unpleasant throbbing, pulling, or creeping sensations in the legs and an almost uncontrollable urge to move the legs, is a neurological disorder that affects many older adults (National Institute of Neurological Disorders and Stroke, 2015). As the sensations are worse when the person is lying down and trying to sleep, the disorder can seriously limit sleep quality. Older adults are more likely to report excessive daytime sleepiness, which means that they find it difficult to remain awake or alert at appropriate times during the day (Chervin, 2015). The high prevalence of sleep disorders in older adults indicates that it is an important area for health care providers to address.

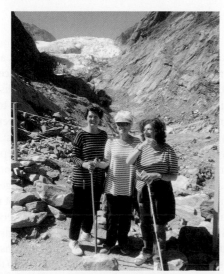

**FIGURE 24-2** Normal changes of aging and environmental deterrents do not prevent older adults from exercising.

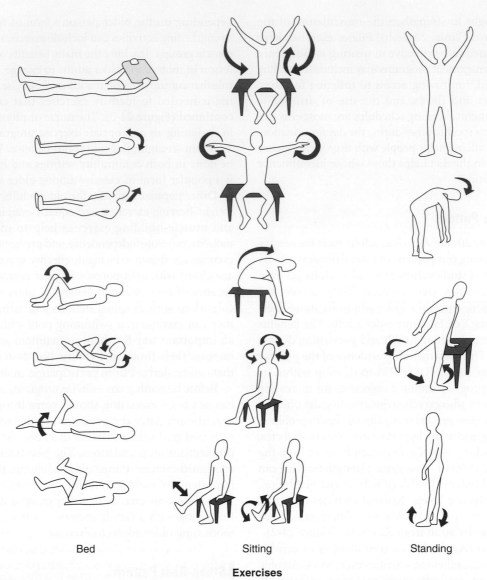

Bed      Sitting      Standing

**Exercises**

**FIGURE 24-3** Bed-lying, sitting, and standing exercises. (Redrawn from Ebersole, P., & Hess, P. [1998]. *Toward healthy aging: Human need and nursing response* [3rd ed.]. St. Louis: Mosby.)

---

### BOX 24-6 Benefits of Exercise in the Older Adult

- Better sleep
- Reduced constipation
- Lower cholesterol level
- Lower blood pressure
- Better digestion
- Weight loss
- Socializing opportunities
- Greater sense of well-being

---

The benefits of a good night's sleep are numerous. Quality sleep results in overall increases in energy, motivation to continue a high quality of life, and improved immune function. Because of the problem with sleep, *Healthy People 2020* added a new topic related to sleep health with the goal to "increase public knowledge of how adequate sleep and treatment of sleep disorders improve health, productivity, wellness, quality of life, and safety." Nurses assist older adults in achieving a good night's sleep through assessment that might reveal possible causes of sleep disturbances. The Pittsburgh Sleep Quality Index is a subjective tool that is helpful in assessing the quality and patterns of sleep in older adults (Smyth, 2012). The tool measures seven areas: subjective sleep quality, sleep latency, sleep duration, habitual sleep efficiency, sleep disturbances, use of sleeping medication, and daytime dysfunction. Teaching older adults about normal changes reassures them that their sleep patterns have changed but are not necessarily harmful. Having this information may decrease anxiety. Identifying normal bedtime rituals, such as drinking a glass of milk, taking a relaxing bath, reading, or meditating, and ensuring that the person is able to continue these practices may help to establish normal sleep routines. Increasing physical activity during the day also helps them fall asleep more readily at night. Taking pain medication or using alternative pain-relief methods before going to bed can help those who suffer from painful conditions obtain better rest at night.

Residents of nursing facilities or people in acute care facilities may have difficulty adjusting to the environment at night. Adjustments in noise and lighting help these individuals sleep better. Emotional disorders frequently interfering with sleep can be identified, and therapy and medication can be administered during the day to help people experiencing these problems sleep peacefully at night. Although a nap may be beneficial, it is important to ensure that daytime napping is not interfering with nighttime sleep (Box 24-7: Innovative Practice).

Sleep medications may be helpful for short-term use; however, the American Geriatrics Society (2015) Beers criteria recommend avoidance of long-term use of benzodiazepines, barbiturates, and chloral hydrate for treatment of insomnia in older adults because of older adults' increased sensitivity to these drugs and increased risk of dependency, and the decreased metabolism of long-term agents, resulting in an increased risk of cognitive impairment, falls, and overdose.

---

### ✸ BOX 24-7  INNOVATIVE PRACTICE

#### *Measures to Promote Sleep*

Sleep problems can be caused by many things, including stress; medications; medical conditions such as angina, asthma, anxiety, or depression; poor sleeping habits; and sleep disorders. The following are some suggestions to improve sleep in older adults.

**Do**
- Plan a regular bedtime and wake-up schedule.
- Participate in exercise, hobbies, and other activities during the day.
- Develop specific bedtime rituals, such as reading, meditating, drinking a glass of milk, or taking a warm bath. These tell the body it is almost time for sleep.
- Ensure a comfortable and quiet sleep environment, which is dark except for night safety lights.
- Sleep on a comfortably firm mattress with comfortable pillows and bedclothes.
- Use the bed only for sleep and sexual activities.
- Check with a physician about prescription and over-the-counter medications that may interfere with sleep.

**Avoid**
- Long daytime naps that may interfere with nighttime sleep
- Exercise or vigorous activity immediately before bedtime
- Caffeine after mid-morning
- Drinking alcohol before going to bed
- Sleep medications
- Tobacco products
- Driving when tired or sleepy

**When Sleep Problems Persist**
- Keep a sleep log, recording times and duration of sleep throughout the 24-hour period for at least 1 week.
- Ask sleep companion about sleep habits, such as snoring or restlessness.
- See health care provider.

---

## Cognitive-Perceptual Pattern

### Cognition

Thinking processes (cognition) in old age have been the subject of intensive study in the past few decades. Brain weight decreases with aging, and a shift occurs in the proportion of gray matter to white matter. The ways in which these changes are manifested in individuals differ because of culture, heredity, lifestyle, environmental exposures, and many other factors. Obesity affects cognition, which includes the processing of information, memory, comprehension, problem-solving, and decisions. It is important to think about how even subtle changes in cognition may affect older adults in their day-to-day activities. For example, older adults are often targeted by scams that ask them to send money or personally identifiable information to callers who appeal to their sense of fear or the promise of a reward.

There is a common belief that most older adults will eventually develop dementia; however, cognitive problems are not a normal change of aging, and many individuals live well into old age without ever experiencing dementia. It is important to be cautious in assessing older people who present with confusion, because confusion is not always indicative of dementia, but can be the result of many treatable health problems, including electrolyte imbalances, diabetic ketoacidosis, and hypoxia. **Mild cognitive impairment** is a pathological collection of symptoms that results in memory loss, language difficulties, and impairments in judgment and reasoning. A review of **instrumental activities of daily living** will help identify changes in higher executive functions, such as paying bills, taking medications as ordered, using the phone, and driving safely.

A condition that is receiving increased attention in older adults is **postoperative cognitive dysfunction** (POCD). POCD is a temporary deterioration in cognition that is associated with surgery and anesthesia (Sorrell, 2014). As the population of older adults has increased dramatically in recent years, surgery is more common at advanced ages. Individuals with POCD experience postoperative cognitive changes that may include anxiety, blurred vision, inability to sleep, hallucinations, and depression. POCD is not the same as **delirium**, which is a short-term change in cognition that may develop in the immediate postoperative period. Cognitive changes in POCD are more subtle and extend over a longer period—sometimes for months after discharge from the hospital. These changes can be very distressing to the older adult and the older adult's family. POCD is thought to be related to the type or amount of anesthesia administered during surgery, but more research needs to be done to establish the cause of POCD and how to prevent it. It is important for nurses in all health care contexts to be aware of the possibility of POCD in older adults and to identify ways in which they can intervene. Because there is no specific treatment for POCD, nurses need to anticipate the needs of both older adults and their family. Educating the older adult and the family about POCD and emphasizing that it is usually temporary helps to decrease anxiety.

**Dementia** is not accepted as a normal change of aging. Dementia is an umbrella term for a group of cognitive disorders that affect memory and lead to difficulty in areas of language, motor activity, object recognition, and ability to plan and organize.

---

**Mini Mental Status Examination Sample Items**

**Orientation to Time**

"What is the date?"

**Registration**

"Listen carefully,

I am going to say three words.

You say them back after I stop.

Ready? Here they are...

HOUSE (pause), CAR (pause), LAKE (pause).

Now repeat those words back to me."

[Repeat up to 5 times, but score only the first trial.]

**Naming**

"What is this?"

[Point to a pencil or pen.]

**Reading**

"Please read this and do what it says."

[Show examinee the words on the stimulus form.]

CLOSE YOUR EYES

---

**FIGURE 24-4** Mini-Mental State Examination sample items. (Reproduced by permission of Psychological Assessment Resources, Inc., Lutz, FL, from the Mini-Mental State Examination, by Marshal Folstein and Susan Folstein, Copyright 1975, 1998 by Mini Mental LLC, Inc. Published 2001 by Psychological Assessment Resources, Inc. Further reproduction is prohibited without permission of Psychological Assessment Resources, Inc. The Mini-Mental State Examination can be purchased from Psychological Assessment Resources, Inc., by calling 800-331-8378 or 813-968-3003.)

The high incidence of dementia and Alzheimer disease in older adults prompted the USDHHS to add *dementia, including Alzheimer disease,* as a new topic in *Healthy People 2020* with a goal to decrease morbidity and costs associated with dementia and maintain or enhance the quality of life for people with these cognitive disorders.

Dementias include Alzheimer disease, the most common dementia, as well as Parkinson-related dementia, Huntington disease, Creutzfeldt-Jakob disease, Pick disease, and Lewy body dementia. The Alzheimer's Association estimates that approximately 5.1 million Americans older than 65 years have Alzheimer disease and approximately 81% of individuals with Alzheimer disease are 75 years or older (Alzheimer's Association, 2015).

The symptoms of dementia include forgetfulness, inattentiveness, disorganized thinking, altered levels of consciousness, perceptual disturbances, sleep-wake disorders, psychomotor disturbances, and disorientation. Assessment for dementia can be made part of the routine assessment of older adults, especially if any of these symptoms arise. One tool that has been used successfully to screen older adults for cognitive impairments is the Mini-Mental State Examination (MMSE) (Folstein et al., 1975; Yellowlees, 2015) (Figure 24-4).

The MMSE was developed to assess the baseline mental status of older adults and to evaluate change or decline in mental functioning. The instrument is based on a 30-point scale that measures the level of awareness and orientation, appearance and behavior, speech and communication, mood and affect, disturbances in thinking, problems with perception, and abstract thinking and judgment. The higher the older adult scores on the examination, the more intact the mental status is presumed to be. When the result of the examination is 23 or lower, the individual is determined to have a problem with cognition. It is important to note that this instrument has been criticized for its cultural insensitivity, and it is difficult to use among individuals who speak languages other than English and among those with visual impairment and low literacy.

The MMSE is relatively easy to perform after a little practice and has been used for initial and subsequent evaluation of older adults in a variety of settings. The most effective way to perform the assessment is to make the person comfortable and establish a rapport. Eliminating extraneous noise and promoting attention and concentration will allow individuals to answer questions to the best of their ability. After the examination the score can be computed and used as a basis for care planning and further evaluation.

There is no cure for Alzheimer disease (CDC, 2015a). Treatment of Alzheimer disease includes the use of medications for memory loss, including cholinesterase inhibitors and memantine, treatments for behavioral changes associated with Alzheimer disease, and treatment for sleep changes. Medications to treat Alzheimer disease are known as cholinesterase inhibitors. These medications are most effective during the early stages of the disease and act by increasing the levels of acetylcholine in the brain to prevent further loss of cognition and improve cognitive status.

Nonpharmacological techniques for managing the problems associated with dementia include developing and keeping routines; working in a calm, gentle, and unhurried manner; encouraging self-care activity; and reducing sensory overload. Interventions to keep the older adult safe include curtailing wandering behavior and preventing falls and other injury.

## Sensory Factors

Older adults experience age-related changes in vision, hearing, taste, smell, and touch sensation. Because of the normal changes and potential pathological changes associated with the senses, older adults of all cultural backgrounds and in all settings benefit from routine assessment and appropriate nursing interventions. Safety, particularly while driving, is a concern for older adults and society. Sensory changes affect a person's ability to drive safely. Nurses can encourage older adults to take senior driving classes to learn how to become safer drivers as these changes occur.

A variety of structural changes cause visual acuity to decrease, color discrimination to become less acute, pupil size and constriction ability to decrease, and peripheral vision to diminish. Presbyopia is a loss of accommodation that occurs as people age and results in the inability to maintain focus on objects close to the eye. The lens of the eye thickens and becomes yellow and predisposes the older adult to cataracts. The older adult is also at increased risk of glaucoma, a group of eye disorders characterized by increased intraocular pressure. Because of the normal changes in the aging eye and the high risk of disease, a baseline eye assessment should be done to identify age-related changes and any disease processes. Follow-up eye appointments should be scheduled annually.

The nurse routinely assesses the older adult for the accumulation of cerumen (earwax) to ensure optimal hearing (see the case study and care plan at the end of this chapter). Hearing deficits are common in old age, resulting from inner ear atrophy or sclerosis of the tympanic membrane. The inner ear also undergoes a number of changes, including those that are cell degenerative and nerve related. Presbycusis is a progressive sensorineural hearing loss associated with aging, and results in difficulty filtering background noise and understanding higher-pitched voices. Sound threshold changes, with an associated difficulty in understanding what others are saying. Similarly to

the changes of the eye, changes in hearing and the increased risk of pathological conditions indicate that older adults should have ear and hearing screening. Hearing loss occurs in approximately one in three persons aged between 65 and 74 years and in almost half of those older than 74 years (National Institute on Deafness and Other Communication Disorders, 2015). Loss of hearing can result in decreased quality of life, as it may lead to miscommunication, loss of self-esteem, depression, falls, safety risks, and cognitive decline. Hearing aids assist those with hearing loss to communicate more effectively.

Taste changes with aging because of a loss of taste buds. The flavors of sweet, sour, salty, and bitter become blurred with this loss. The sensations brought about by touch may also diminish with the decrease in sensory nerve endings, especially in the presence of debilitating diseases such as diabetes, stroke, or Parkinson disease. The ability to smell and the acuity of the olfactory nerve also decrease with age. Because of the loss of smell and taste sensations, older adults have the tendency to increase the amounts of salt and sugar in their food, possibly negatively affecting chronic health conditions. Teaching older adults about safe cooking and the use of alternative seasonings in food may be helpful in helping them adjust to these sensory changes. Additionally, the sense of smell is impaired, which may result in the inability to sense common warning signals such as smoke or rotten food. It is helpful to teach older adults to check the dates on their food packages frequently and to be attentive when cooking and preparing meals so as to ensure safety.

The decline in taste and smell sensations, combined with problems of obtaining adequate nutrition, makes dental care of vital importance to this population. Lack of fluoridated water and preventive dentistry during the developmental years may have led to tooth and periodontal problems in the older population. Periodontitis, or gum disease leading to tooth loss, is a common contributor to decreased taste sensation and poor nutrition. *Healthy People 2020* established oral health objective OH-4-2 to reduce the proportion of older adults aged 65 to 74 years who have lost all their natural teeth and oral health objective OH-5 to reduce the proportion of adults aged 45 to 74 years with moderate or severe periodontitis (USDHHS, 2012a). The inability to chew and swallow food in a comfortable manner works synergistically with decreased smell and taste sensations and other problems that inhibit proper nutrition. The American Dental Association recommends that adults be seen for oral hygiene checks and counseling at least twice a year. During the initial evaluation, follow-up visits are scheduled to ensure that teeth and gums remain in good condition and that appropriate dental care devices are being used.

The skin of the older adult changes, becoming thinner, less elastic, wrinkled, and more fragile. Although sweating decreases and injuries take longer to heal, the skin remains capable of sensing and performing its protective role. Chronic disease, however, can place an individual at risk of decreased sensation throughout the body. Cerebrovascular accidents (strokes) and neuropathies resulting from diabetes are two examples of diseases that disrupt the ability to feel pain and pressure through the skin. This lack of sensation can threaten safety. Older adults benefit from information about safety when cooking on a hot stove and the appropriate temperature for bathing and showering to prevent burns.

Nurses should perform frequent skin assessments to detect alterations in skin integrity at an early stage and implement appropriate interventions. The potential for skin impairment is common for those who have sensory impairment from physical disease or dementia. A pressure sore (decubitus ulcer) is a localized area of tissue necrosis that develops when soft tissue is compressed between two bony prominences or between a bony prominence and an external surface for a prolonged period. In addition to prolonged pressure on the skin, friction, moisture, shearing, and inadequate nutrition place the older adult at risk of developing a decubitus ulcer, which is difficult to treat. Preventing the ulcer is the best method for maintaining intact skin. People at risk of decubitus ulcers should change their position at least every 2 hours to redistribute pressure appropriately throughout all areas of the skin. Elevating the lower extremities and maintaining proper body alignment are imperative to prevent decubitus ulcers. Specialty beds are readily available in most care settings to decrease pressure and assist in positioning individuals who are at risk. Positioning pillows and other orthopedic devices provide ways to help maintain the proper support of body parts and body alignment. Proper nutrition, including adequate amounts of zinc and vitamins C and E, will help prevent this skin problem.

## Self-Perception–Self-Concept Pattern

The variability of self-concept in the older adult is similar to the variability that is seen in the general population. As in all aspects of health, culture, environment, family, lifestyle factors, and heredity combine to form self-concept. Self-concept includes an individual's attitudes, perception of abilities (cognitive, affective, or physical), body image, identity, general sense of worth, and general emotional pattern. Personality traits tend to remain constant throughout life.

### Developmental Theories of Aging

Many believe that adults no longer grow emotionally or physically in their later years. In truth, although the rate of physical decline exceeds the rate of physical growth, no evidence was found that emotional growth declines in any way. One need only view the classic film *Driving Miss Daisy* to understand that older adults go through many developmental changes in the 30 to 40 years that often make up older adulthood. Erikson's (1982) theory of development asserts that older adults must pass through developmental stages as do infants, children, and younger adults. As in all stages of psychosocial development, unsuccessful passage through a stage can result in psychological illness, and successful passage through the stage promotes health (Erikson, 1982).

Ego integrity versus despair is the developmental stage of older adults (Erikson, 1982). The quality associated with successful passage of this stage is to achieve a balance between integrity and despair. "The process of bringing into balance feelings of integrity and despair involves a review of and a coming to terms with the life one has lived thus far" (Erikson et al., 1986). On the basis of the increasing life span, this stage of development

was expanded into three additional stages: ego differentiation versus work role preoccupation, which involves achieving identity apart from work; body transcendence versus body preoccupation, which focuses on adjusting to normal aging changes; and ego transcendence versus ego preoccupation, which involves accepting death (Erikson, 1997).

Other developmental theorists have built upon Erikson's work. Some of these are included in Box 24-4: Theories of Aging. Levinson moved away from Erikson's focus on the role of tensions that emerge during successive stages and instead emphasized that major life transitions are influenced by evolving physiological, psychological, and role-oriented life changes (Agronin, 2013). Vaillant also moved from an emphasis on "stages" to focus on developmental tasks of life. Vaillant theorized that generativity grows out of one's career. His studies suggested that successful generativity tripled the chances for a person to experience more joy than despair in their 70s (Agronin, 2013). Gilligan criticized Erikson, Levinson, and Vaillant for proposing theories that addressed only male development and focused her work primarily on the unique role of interpersonal connections in female development (Agronin, 2013).

Cohen is considered a founding father of geriatric psychiatry, bringing forth a modern conception of old age. He focused on the continued potential for growth that occurs not in spite of old age but because of it. His work demonstrated how the brain continually resculpts itself in response to experience and learning. Cohen also emphasized the role of creativity, which he believed persisted and even increased in old age. He proposed that older adults can develop a social portfolio to enhance moving through various phases. The social portfolio comprises individualized lists of vital activities that a person can engage in through an active review of lifelong personal assets. The social portfolio should include vital activities than a person can engage in even when faced with serious disability or loss (Agronin, 2013).

Nurses working in all settings are charged with helping older adults accomplish the task of balancing ego integrity and despair. Two successful methods of support for older adults at all cognitive levels are reminiscence and life review. An increasing number of researchers have found that there are substantial psychosocial health benefits for older adults who participate in reminiscence programs, with beneficial outcomes of enhanced mood, increased socialization, improved cognitive functioning, and enhanced well-being (Chippendale & Bear-Lehman, 2012; Smiraglia, 2015). There are many different types of reminiscence programs that are designed to engage participants in discussing their memories, sometimes with reflection prompts such as food or objects from the person's past. Life review is a more formal therapy technique taking the person through his or her life in a structured and chronological order. Both of these therapeutic approaches can be done individually or in groups, orally or through writing.

## Roles-Relationships Pattern

Although the general framework of self-perception remains constant throughout the life span, the source of an individual's self-perception often changes with older adulthood. The formation of the self that has focused on a person's role in the family

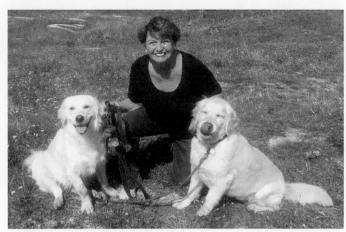

**FIGURE 24-5** Loss of some roles can provide an opportunity for new roles. As family members grow up and move away, the older adult may decide to devote time to training dogs to be pet therapy dogs.

changes when one's children become independent or a spouse dies. Roles such as daughter, son, sister, brother, wife, or husband may be lost because of death or illness. The loss of these roles can result in grieving, sadness, and potentially depression in the older adult. In contrast with the loss of these roles, however, new roles, such as grandparenting, evolve (Figure 24-5).

In the United States in 2012, 7 million grandparents (10%) lived with at least one grandchild (US Census Bureau, 2014). The role of grandparent frequently brings great joy and happiness at a time when the older adult feels loss; however, grandparents who rear grandchildren encounter both emotional and physical stress. Their new role as grandparent-caregiver may lead to role confusion and increased health-related problems (Bundy-Fazioli et al., 2013). Researchers have also found, however, that these grandparents may show positive levels of physical activity and self-care, especially if they do not perceive the caretaking responsibility as highly stressful (Bundy-Fazioli et al., 2013). Thus it is important for nurses to explore with these individuals what activities may help to reduce stress. Coping strategies such as accepting responsibility, self-control, positive reappraisal, planned problem-solving, and distancing may be helpful. Support groups, counseling, and education to help them manage stress more effectively are other resources that should be explored. Encouraging and supporting older adults in their caregiving role is important to help them ease the stress and strain of changes that come with the caregiving experience.

With the average life span increasing, older adults can spend many more years in retirement than previous generations. There were approximately 54 million Social Security beneficiaries at the end of 2010 (Social Security Administration, 2012). Hooyman and Kiyak (2011) noted a variety of factors that were predictors of satisfaction with retirement. Those factors included good health and functional ability, adequate income, a suitable living environment, a strong social support system, and a positive outlook. An important factor was the autonomy of the retiree in choosing retirement and the preparation for the retirement while still working. For married retirees, having a good marital relationship and sharing similar interests with the spouse supported satisfaction with retirement. Having retirement activities that provide an opportunity to feel useful, to learn and grow, and to enjoy oneself are important. Many retirees enjoy sports and hobbies developed during their working years, whereas others become actively involved in volunteerism and other community and civic activities.

Volunteering can be an effective method for older adults to continue to feel engaged in the community as a productive, contributing member of society. Older adults who volunteer have an external incentive for getting dressed and going out of the house in the morning; they take a great amount of pride in their work. Filling a volunteer position provides a feeling of self-worth and helps to change negative feelings about retirement and other role changes. It also makes important contributions to society.

Federal and state funding has created a number of subsidized work programs for older adults. With the assistance of this funding through private agencies and local Area Agencies on Aging, older adults are given the opportunity to work for pay. Although the pay may not be comparable to that earned before retirement, the earnings can be a necessary supplement to Social Security benefits. These programs allow older adults to work in programs such as those involving children in day care centers and disabled and ill older adults at home and in administrative positions. Nurses can provide interested individuals with information about these programs.

Downsizing from the family home to a smaller residence, widowhood, retirement, and relocation can elicit profound feelings of loss. Older adults who remain engaged in a variety of activities and relationships are happier and healthier. Personality, and its expression over time, is considered a major determinant of how engaged or active a person will be late in life. Other variables such as culture, health, bereavement, and habit affect activity as well.

Health-promotion activities center on an understanding of the individual's usual behavior and any unexpected or unexplained deviation from that behavior. Nurses can help older adults identify the meaning of their lost roles and the results of those losses, and work through reactions to the losses. In more traumatic cases, support groups, such as bereavement groups, can be helpful. The nurse supports people going through role changes by eliciting reactions and facilitating communication about these reactions. Significant others, such as children, neighbors, and friends, can provide important support. The nurse is integral in helping older adults develop and explore their new roles in their older years.

## Sexuality-Reproductive Pattern

The World Health Organization defines sexual health as "a state of physical, emotional, mental and social well-being in relation to sexuality" (CDC, 2014b). In older adults, as in all adults, sexual health is characterized by an approach to sexual relationships that is positive and respectful. There has been much debate regarding the presence or absence of sexual desire among older adults, and many assume that older adults do not participate in sexual relationships. According to the AARP (2012), myths regarding sexual activity among older adults include the following: most older men have erectile dysfunction (**impotence**) and are unable to have sexual intercourse; after menopause, older women no longer have sexual desire; physical and psychological impediments in older adults make them unable to have sexual intercourse; an aging body is not sexy; and older people should not have sex. It is important to realize that sex does not belong solely to the young and that sexual contact correlates with enhanced health, positive relationships, and improved stress management (AARP, 2012).

Older adults who are not heterosexual may experience health disparities as a result of their gender orientation. There are an estimated 1.5 million older adults in the United States who self-identify as gay, lesbian, bisexual, or transgender (LGBT), and this number is expected to double by 2030 (Zelle & Arms, 2015). Although *Healthy People 2020* includes goals to achieve health equity and improve the health, safety, and well-being of LGBT individuals, research suggests that these individuals continue to face health disparities linked to social stigma, discrimination, and denial of their civil and human rights (Office of Disease Prevention and Health Promotion, 2014). The LBGT older adult population is more likely to delay seeking treatment for health problems and has a higher incidence of psychosocial problems. Nurses who use a nonjudgmental approach and open-ended questions related to marital status and sexual orientation can be very supportive in encouraging LGBT individuals to openly express their concerns about their health and well-being.

The most accurate predictor of sexual interest in older adulthood is the enjoyment and frequency of sex at a younger age. No data were found to show that men or women lose interest in sexual activity as they age. Older adults also need to fulfill the human need for intimacy and love, and to touch and be touched. Touch is an overt expression of closeness and an integral part of sexuality. Although the need to express sexuality continues, older adults are susceptible to many chronic medical conditions, such as cardiac problems, arthritis, and normal aging changes that can make sexual intercourse difficult. In both sexes, reduced availability of sex hormones results in less rapid and less extreme vascular responses to sexual arousal. The lack of circulating hormones in both men and women results in changes in four areas of the sexual system: arousal, orgasm, postorgasm, and extragenital changes. In women the vagina becomes narrower, shorter, and thinner, and there is less natural lubrication. Men experience less intense and slower erections, increased difficulty regaining an erection, decreased force of ejaculation, and an extended refractory time. Medications and other measures to manage medical conditions can also hinder sexual response.

Nurses are in an ideal position to help older adults find ways to fulfill their sexual desires by compensating for normal aging changes and chronic medical conditions and medications. Knowledge is essential to the successful fulfillment of sexuality needs. After making a sexual assessment, nurses can intervene to prevent or correct problems, but they frequently choose not to consider sexuality when planning care. One of the reasons for this is that nurses may believe the societal myths about older adults' sexuality. With proper education and experience, they may be sufficiently confident to venture into this delicate area.

One way in which nurses can gain knowledge of the sexual needs of older adults is through a staff development program using role play to discuss and process feelings associated with an older person's limitations in fulfilling intimate and sexual relationships. The expression of intimacy and sexuality among older adults results in a higher quality of life achieved through fulfilling a natural desire. In long-term care facilities, the need to address sexual needs of residents is great because of difficulties related to their chronic illnesses and because of a lack of resident privacy to engage in intimate and sexual relationships. Long-term care facilities can develop policies to assist residents in effectively fulfilling the need for intimacy and sexuality.

Many nurses believe that acquired immunodeficiency syndrome (AIDS) and other sexually transmitted infections (STIs) are not problems for older adults. However, the number of cases of human immunodeficiency virus (HIV) infection and AIDS in older adults continues to increase because greater numbers of older adults are becoming newly infected with HIV and an increasing proportion of those who have HIV are reaching their older years (CDC, 2017). Two areas that are so important for successful aging—cognition and social engagement—are of particular concern for those aging with HIV, as declines in both of these areas have been observed in this population (Vance, 2013). Approximately 50% of individuals with HIV experience cognitive problems, and as people age they may be at increased risk of developing cognitive changes. Social support and engagement often decline for many older adults and may be exacerbated by stigma and depression in older adults with HIV (Vance, 2013). It is important for nurses to suggest ways to promote social engagement, as this may help to improve both mood and cognitive functioning.

Older adults are just as susceptible to STI as younger adults. Yet one survey showed that only 5.1% of men older than 61 years had used a condom in recent sex (Esposito, 2016). There seems to be a lack of awareness in the older adult population about the risks of STIs in their sexual relationships. Esposito (2016) noted that if you go into an STI clinic and look at the brochures about AIDS or STIs, you do not see people with wrinkles and gray hair on the front of those brochures. It is important that older adults become more aware of risks in their sexual relationships and follow the safer sex guidelines recommended by the CDC (2013a).

## Coping–Stress Tolerance Pattern

An individual's ability to cope with the common stresses of older adulthood is a key factor in maintaining self-concept. As people age, they tend to encounter many losses, such as the loss of a home, spouses, friends, siblings, and even children. They also experience declines in income and in health and physical functioning. The nurse who cares for the older adult can provide support during the coping process related to these losses. Trying to find the positive and developmental benefits of losses is preferable to continually thinking about a loss or bad event. Negative associations have been found between depressive symptoms and rumination, catastrophizing, and self-blame. After assessing the most appropriate way in which the individual desires to cope with a situation, the nurse may help create a suitable environment for coping.

The spirituality of older adults is also an important consideration in helping them cope with stressful situations. Spirituality is very individual and may be exercised privately or through a religious framework. However, the impact of spirituality on quality of life has been well documented among older adults and often has a strong relationship with older adults' ability to cope with the changes and losses of aging.

## Depression

Among older adults, depression may mainly affect those with chronic illnesses and cognitive impairment and result in suffering, family disruption, and disability. Depression can worsen the outcomes of many illnesses and increase mortality. Aging-related and disease-related processes, including arteriosclerosis and endocrine and immune system changes, compromise the integrity of frontostriatal pathways, the amygdala, and the hippocampus, and increase vulnerability to depression. Heredity factors may also play a part. Psychosocial adversity—economic impoverishment, disability, isolation, relocation, caregiving, and bereavement—contributes to physiological changes, further increasing susceptibility to depression or triggering depression in already vulnerable older individuals.

It is important to know that most older adults are *not* depressed. Estimates of major depression in community-dwelling older adults range from less than 1% to 5%, but these percentages rise to 13.5% in those who need home health care (CDC, 2015b). The National Institute of Mental Health (n.d.) noted that the risk of depression increases in older adults as they experience chronic illnesses and when their ability to function becomes impaired. The numerous losses experienced by older people may be partly to blame. Depression is also caused by physiological changes in the aging body. Although depression appears to affect older adults in much the same way that it affects younger individuals, certain patterns of symptoms and older adults' overall susceptibility are different from those of younger counterparts.

Nurses are integral in helping to diagnose and manage depression in older adults. Depression can be found in all care environments. Some common behaviors include sullen affect, lack of appetite and weight loss, sleep disorders, fatigue, decreased ability to think or concentrate, psychomotor agitation, decreased participation in daily living and social activities, social withdrawal, and suicidal ideation. Many instruments are available to assist nurses in assessing older adults for this commonly occurring disorder. The Geriatric Depression Scale (Yesavage et al., 1983) is available in several formats, with 30, 15, 5, or 1 question, and is easily administered. Positive results on the screening examinations require referral to social services for a diagnostic workup. After depression has been diagnosed, successful management may include implementation of antidepressant medications and psychosocial therapy.

## Suicide

The suicide rate for older Americans is disproportionally high in the American population. The suicide rate for men is highest in those who are 75 years or older, 36.1 per 100,000. Non-Hispanic white men aged 85 years or older were the most likely to die by suicide, with a rate of 49.8 per 100,000 (National Institute of Mental Health, n.d.). Firearms, poison, overdose of pills, gas, and suffocation are common methods of suicide used by older adults.

The reason for the high number of suicides in the older adult population continues to be explored. The elevated rate of depression helps the medical community understand the motive of many older adults. Many older adults have serious medical illnesses that provide an explanation for wanting to die. Risk factors for suicide include social isolation, alcohol and substance abuse, psychosis, bereavement, and serious medical illness. Many who committed suicide were found to have alcohol and/or pain-killing drugs in their bodies on autopsy.

The importance of different aspects of life also differs by culture. Some older adults may visit a health care provider with a somatic problem before the suicide attempt as, perhaps, a final call for help. Nurses working with older adults must be aware of the high rate of suicide in this age group and be alert for the risk factors. Older adults exhibiting signs of depression must be asked about possible suicidal thoughts. Suicide threats must be taken seriously and appropriate interventions implemented to keep the older adult safe.

The incidence of chronic illness that frequently accompanies old age raises a concern for ethical care. Many members of society believe that with the increased life span, individuals may be subjected to more suffering. A solution to ending the suffering of those with chronic illness has been euthanasia, or physician-assisted suicide. In many states, people are lobbying to legalize physician-assisted suicide. Nurses help society to understand the many benefits of older adulthood and celebrate the extended life span rather than deeming it wasteful. Nurses caring for chronically ill older adults have the added responsibility of determining who is at risk of wanting physician-assisted suicide and helping them to be as comfortable as possible and free of pain through the use of pharmacological and nonpharmacological interventions. Nurses are instrumental in ensuring that the older person experiences a pain-free death by advocating an appropriate pain-management program and working with other health care professionals toward this goal.

## Values-Beliefs Pattern

Every person who nurses care for will have a different sense of spirituality, which will have an influence on the way the person chooses to live and the decisions made by the person about health care. Hodge and colleagues (2010) found that most older adults describe themselves as both spiritual and religious. The life of the spirit may help older adults to overcome the pain and suffering of chronic health and psychosocial problems encountered in their later years.

Nurses may find themselves in the providential but difficult position of attempting to promote the spiritual health of individuals. One reason for this perceived difficulty may be the nurse's discomfort with the person's belief system. Spirituality plays a significant role in meaning-making in relation to attitudes and beliefs about the world, self, and others.

There may be as many different spiritual values and beliefs as there are individuals. Differing spiritual values make helping older adults actualize their spirituality, and thus acquire a high quality of life, difficult for nurses. Because of the highly personal quality of spirituality, an unobtrusive and sensitive presence by the nurse is needed to allow the person in any setting to achieve spiritual health. Spiritual assessment tools are available to guide nurses with questions to better understand the person's spirituality. Open-ended questions such as "What is your perception of a higher being and spirituality?" encourage discussions about the person's innermost spirituality. The nurse can provide an environment that is supportive to the practice of the person's spirituality. Assisting older persons to actualize their spirituality can provide great comfort to the person and lead nurses to a deeper understanding of their own spirituality.

# ENVIRONMENTAL PROCESSES

## Physical Agents

### Accidents

*Healthy People 2020* identifies a goal of preventing unintentional injuries and violence, as well as reducing the consequences of these problems (USDHHS, 2015). One important focus for injury prevention in older adults is falls. Falls are a leading cause of morbidity and death among older adults. One in three older adults fall each year, and one in five falls result in a serious injury, such as a fracture or head injury (CDC, 2015c). Each year 2.5 million older adults are treated for fall injuries in emergency departments. More than 95% of hip fractures are caused by falls, and each year 250,000 older adults are hospitalized for a hip fracture. It is essential that nurses are knowledgeable about interventions for prevention (Box 24-8: Quality and Safety Scenario).

Some of the causes of falls in older adults are neuromuscular dysfunction, osteoporosis, stroke, and sensory impairment. Falls can result in decreased mobility, decreased ability to live independently, and increased risk of an early death. Although a fall in a younger individual may not be problematic, a fall in an older adult can have devastating consequences. Falls account for 40% of admissions to nursing homes each year. Even if the person is not injured in a fall, he or she may develop a fear of falling, and therefore limit his or her activities and increase his or her risk of future falls.

Because of the higher risk of osteoporosis in the older population, a fall can result in a fracture. Osteoporosis is a disease of bone loss common to women aged 70 years or older and men aged 80 years or older. The disease develops six times more frequently in women than it does in men. The rapid decline in estrogen secretion at the onset of menopause signals the calcium in the bones to move into the bloodstream, which causes the bones to become weak and brittle. Because of this weakness, falls in older adults with osteoporosis frequently result in fractures, which place these individuals in a spiral of iatrogenic risk, beginning with weeks of decreased mobility and possibly resulting in

---

**☑ BOX 24-8  QUALITY AND SAFETY SCENARIO**

### Fall Prevention for Older Adults in the Community

Falls in community-dwelling older adults are a critical problem for nurses to address, as falls are the leading cause of injury in older adults. Between 30% and 40% of community-dwelling adults aged 65 years or older fall at least once per year. The US Preventive Services Task Force (USPSTF) makes and periodically updates recommendations about the effectiveness of specific clinical preventive services for older adults. The recommendations are based on the evidence of both the benefits and harms of the service. These recommendations are intended to provide helpful information for clinicians, but the USPSTF emphasizes that clinical decisions involve more considerations than evidence alone and clinicians need to individualize decision-making for a specific client.

The USPSTF notes that various approaches to identify people at increased risk are helpful. There is no single evidence-based instrument that accurately identifies older adults at increased risk of falling. Clinicians need to assess risk on the basis of a variety of factors, such as a history of falls and impaired mobility and balance. Early intervention is important for people assessed to be at risk, as these interventions can prevent serious injury.

The USPSTF states that more research is needed for clinical validation of tools to identify older adults at risk of falling. It also recommends efficacy trials for interventions related to vision correction, medication withdrawal, protein supplementation, education or counseling, and home hazard modification.

Summary of Recommendations:

Exercise or physical therapy and vitamin D supplementation are recommended to prevent falls in community-dwelling adults aged 65 years or older who are at increased risk of falls.

The USPSTF does not recommend a routine in-depth multifactorial risk assessment in conjunction with comprehensive management of identified risks to prevent falls because the likelihood of benefit is small.

From US Preventive Services Task Force. (2012). Falls prevention in older adults: Counseling and preventive medication. http://www.uspreventiveservicestaskforce.org/Page/Document/Recommendation StatementFinal/falls-prevention-in-older-adults-counseling-and-preventive-medication.

---

decubitus ulcers, psychological trauma, pneumonia, and even death.

The risk factors for osteoporosis include a small, thin frame; white or Asian ancestry; family history of osteoporosis; excessive thyroid medication or high doses of cortisone-like drugs for treatment of asthma, arthritis, or cancer; a diet low in dairy products and other sources of calcium; physical inactivity; smoking cigarettes; and drinking alcohol. Osteoporosis is typically diagnosed after an older adult sustains a fracture. However, bone density testing is readily available to determine individuals at risk before a fracture occurs. Sufficient calcium intake remains vitally important and will continue to reduce the normal bone loss of aging. Health care providers frequently monitor calcium and vitamin D levels as a part of wellness care in older adults. Most women need 1000 mg daily before menopause and 1500 mg daily after menopause. Consuming this amount of calcium from today's average diet is difficult; therefore a calcium supplement is essential. Vitamin D is also essential for bone health. Although one can obtain adequate vitamin D by daily exposure to the sun, because of concerns about the amount of sun exposure necessary, 400 to 800 IU of vitamin D supplements is usually recommended in conjunction with calcium. For the prevention of osteoporosis and the optimal maintenance of both psychological and physical well-being in the older adult, regular physical activity is necessary.

Governmental concern about falls among older adults has resulted in a *Healthy People 2020* objective to prevent an increase in the rate of fall-related deaths (USDHHS, 2012b). Less than half of older adults tell their physician about a fall, so it is important for nurses to inquire about falls. Because many factors contribute to falls, risk assessment is essential. If a fall has been sustained, the older adult is at increased risk of falling again, and fall-prevention strategies must be implemented. Several fall risk assessment tools have been developed, but more research is needed to validate their use in different settings. By identifying the risks of falls and assessing an older adult's vision, hearing, medication use, blood pressure, mobility, and other factors, nurses can predict and prevent many falls.

Table 24-2 lists frequent causes of accidents that occur in the home and nursing interventions to prevent them. Home care nurses are in an ideal position to prevent injuries. During the initial and subsequent assessments, the nurse can evaluate individuals' homes for common factors leading to fires, poisoning, and falls, such as frayed wires on electrical appliances that can produce sparks and start fires, improperly labeled cleaning products that can be accidentally ingested, loose rugs on the floor, absence of handrails on stairs or in bathrooms, and poor lighting that can cause falls. Appropriate health teaching incorporates the concept of accident prevention for all older adults living not only in the community but also in acute care facilities and long-term care facilities.

The older adult's ability to feel changes in heat and cold may be impaired as a result of normal and pathological changes of aging. This process can cause older adults to die of the effects of excessive heat or cold. During periods of high temperature and humidity, older people should increase fluid and salt intake, stay in a cool and shaded environment, remain calm, have more rest periods, and refrain from going outdoors when the temperature is higher than 90°F. Sweating, which is reduced in older adults, can be accommodated by the wearing of light-colored, lightweight cotton clothing. If sweating ceases or is inadequate, the older person is at risk of heat stroke. Heat stroke can contribute to sepsis, myocardial infarction, and cerebrovascular accidents, particularly in people with diabetes. Reduced body heat can also present problems in the older adult. Symptoms of and interventions for hypothermia are listed in Box 24-9.

## Preventing Injury

Falls and fires are leading causes of unintentional injury and death in people 65 years or older. Other unintentional injuries and deaths in older adults are caused by motor vehicle accidents, suffocation, and poisoning. Because of normal age-related changes and the increased incidence of chronic illness, older adults can experience decreased muscle strength and delayed reaction time and subsequently become more vulnerable to environmental

| TABLE 24-2 | Safety Risk Areas and Related Interventions |
|---|---|
| **Area of Attention** | **Intervention** |
| Stairways | Secure handrails |
| | Illuminate stairways with light switches at both top and bottom |
| | Eliminate clutter on all steps and stair landings |
| | Use nonskid treads on steps |
| Bedroom | Use nightlights |
| | Tack down carpet |
| | Discourage use of throw rugs |
| | Arrange furniture so that it will not obstruct clear pathways |
| | Secure extension cords and telephone wires and remove them from walking areas |
| | For smokers, never smoke in bed |
| Bathroom | Use handrails near tub and toilet |
| | Use nonskid mats in tub area and on floor |
| | Use a bath thermometer to measure hot water in tub |
| | Use nightlights |
| Kitchen | Wear nonflammable, lightweight clothing when cooking |
| | Place dishes and cooking utensils at reasonable heights |
| | Use stepstools with a handrail according to specifications and only when not alone |
| | Keep off wet floor and refrain from using slippery wax |
| | Never climb on chairs |
| | Keep emergency numbers near the telephone |
| | Ensure locks can be easily opened in times of emergency |
| | Cook at front of the stove rather than at the back |
| | Do not use electrical appliances with frayed cords |
| Living room | Use furniture that is easy to get in and out of |
| | Eliminate clutter on all floor areas |
| | Install fire detectors at appropriate places |
| Outdoors | Make sure stairs are free of breaks and cracks, and clear of snow and ice |
| | Use safe handrails |
| | Provide good lighting for stairs and walkways |

hazards. Decreased sensory acuity and impaired balance further diminish their ability to interpret the environment.

As the percentage of older adults living in the United States increases, the number of older drivers also increases. The CDC (2015d) reported that in 2012 there were approximately 36 million licensed drivers 65 years of age or older. Each day an average of 586 older adults experience an injury from a car crash. Age-related changes in vision, joint mobility, and cognitive changes may affect the older person's ability to drive. Because of these changes, older adults often avoid driving at night, in bad weather, in heavy traffic, on long trips, or on highways or high-speed roads.

Older individuals are at increased risk of severe injury resulting in hospitalization, disability, or death from motor vehicle injuries because of the many changes in their neuromuscular and sensory abilities, which slow response time in emergency situations. In 2008 more than 5500 older adults were killed and more than 183,000 were injured in motor vehicle crashes; older men had a substantially higher death rate than older women. Most traffic

---

**BOX 24-9   Nursing Interventions for Hypothermia**

**Symptoms**
- Cold to touch
- Slow respiration
- Bradycardia
- Low blood pressure
- Slurred speech
- Drowsiness
- Temperature 95°F rectally

**Interventions**
- Warm hands and feet
- Cover with blanket
- Set room temperature to 70°F
- Wear cap to bed at night
- Wear socks to bed at night
- Wear several layers of clothing
- Increase activity
- Decrease alcohol intake
- Use extreme caution with space heaters, heating pads, or electric blankets

---

**BOX 24-10   When to Stop Driving**

Poor driving skills that are warning signs of unsafe driving include:
- Not using turn signals correctly or not using them at all.
- Having trouble making turns.
- Having difficulty moving into or maintaining the correct lane of traffic.
- Having trouble judging the space between vehicles in traffic on highway entrance or exit ramps.
- Parking inappropriately.
- Hitting curbs when making right turns or backing up.
- Unpredictable stopping in traffic.
- Driving too slowly; other drivers often honk horns.
- Failing to stop at stop signs or stop lights.
- Failing to notice important activity on the side of the road.

From American Association of Retired Persons. (2010). 10 signs that it's time to limit or stop driving. http://www.aarp.org/home-garden/transportation/info-05-2010/Warning_Signs_Stopping.html.

---

fatalities involving older adults occur during the daytime and involve other vehicles. In two-vehicle fatal crashes involving both older and younger drivers, the older driver's vehicle was more than twice as likely to be struck than the younger person's, indicating a decline in defensive driving as opposed to an increase in aggressive driving among older adults. Older drivers involved in fatal automobile accidents, however, had the lowest blood alcohol level.

Older adults are encouraged to take a seniors' driving safety course to learn how aging changes can affect their driving and strategies for safer driving. Nurses working in the community may encourage older drivers to contact the AARP or the American Automobile Association for driving classes designed to meet their needs. In addition, attending these classes often provides savings on vehicle insurance. At some point, it may be better for older adults to stop driving. Box 24-10 offers warning signs that suggest when an older adult should limit or stop driving. Older adults are often highly resistant to requests to stop driving however, as being able to drive is an important sign of independence. Many families find out only after a car accident that the older adult has not heeded their warning and has been driving without their knowledge. In the case of an older adult with dementia, health care providers may need to talk with family members to find a way to prevent the person from driving. If an older adult has been found to be an unsafe driver and refuses to stop driving, a family member may take away the car keys or mechanically disable the car so that it cannot be driven. It is important, however, to find ways for the older adult to continue to participate in pleasurable activities and not to become isolated. For example, a loss of spiritual connections may occur when older adults can no longer drive to their place of worship. In rural areas, there are many older adults managing farms and dependent on being able to drive to obtain needed supplies and

services. Family members or friends may be able to set up a schedule to alternate driving the person to the grocery store, church, and other places. This can also help to provide important social interactions.

### Elder Mistreatment

Elder abuse (elder mistreatment) refers to intentional or neglectful acts by a caregiver or "trusted" person that results in, or may lead to, harm of a vulnerable elder. The National Center on Elder Abuse (n.d.) lists the following forms of elder abuse and mistreatment: physical abuse, neglect, emotional or psychological abuse, verbal abuse and threats, financial abuse and exploitation, sexual abuse, and abandonment. In many states, self-neglect is also considered mistreatment. *Women's Health USA 2010* (USDHHS, Health Resources and Services Administration, Maternal and Child Health Bureau, 2010) reported that in 2004 caregiver neglect accounted for 20.4% of elder abuse and self-neglect account for 37.2%. Emotional or psychological abuse—described as threats or other verbal attacks, isolation, rejection, or denigrating acts that cause or could cause mental anguish, pain, or distress—accounted for 14.8%; financial abuse and exploitation, including theft, fraud, misuse or neglect of authority, and use of undue influence to gain control over an older person's money or property accounted for 14.7%; physical abuse, including the use of physical force that may result in injury, physical pain, or impairment, accounted for 10.7%; and sexual abuse, which includes any type of nonconsensual sexual contact with an elderly person, including those who cannot give consent, accounted for 1.0%.

Victims of elder abuse are more likely to be single women older than 75 years who are dependent on the caregiver for food and shelter. They are more likely to be frail, to be incontinent, or to have mental disability. The abuser is usually the adult son or daughter of the victim, who has poor impulse control and low self-esteem (Nies & McEwan, 2011). Nurses have a responsibility to identify abuse, provide appropriate care for injuries, and report suspected abuse to appropriate state agencies or law enforcement personnel. The nurse may consult social services to find a more suitable living arrangement for the victim. The most important consideration is to provide a safe environment for the older adult who is in immediate danger.

## Biological Agents

Because of decreased immune system response, older adults are susceptible to bacterial and viral disease. In many cases, older adults have not received primary immunization against diphtheria and tetanus. A large emphasis is placed on immunizing young children against communicable disease; however, older adults can also be protected by commonly available vaccines that have been shown to lower both morbidity and mortality. Influenza and pneumonia are two disease processes that are associated with higher mortality and morbidity.

### Influenza

Influenza has been a significant cause of morbidity and death in older adults. In 2009, there were 638 deaths from influenza and 42,831 deaths from pneumonia in people aged 65 years or older (CDC, 2011c). In 2010, the hospitalization rate for influenza among older adults 65 years of age or older was 62.1 per 100,000. The CDC reported that influenza vaccination levels among older adults was 65% to 70% in 2011–12 (Lu et al, 2013), but this was less than the *Healthy People 2010* target of 90%. The vaccine, composed of inactivated whole virus or viral subunits grown in chick embryo cells, is given annually to older adults, especially those with chronic conditions such as pulmonary or cardiac problems and those in long-term care facilities. Vaccination is contraindicated in people who have experienced a reaction to the vaccine, and caution must be exercised in administering the vaccine to people who have allergies to eggs. A *Healthy People 2020* objective (IID-12-7 and IID-4-2) is "to increase the percentage of older adults who are vaccinated annually against influenza and to decrease the incidence of pneumococcal infections among older adults to 31 new cases per 100,000" (USDHHS, 2012c).

### Pneumococcal Infections

Deaths from pneumococcal infections declined in previous years, indicating the value of public health initiatives to make information widespread about the importance of immunization against pneumonia and influenza. Implementation of immunization programs in public places such as supermarkets and drugstores, in addition to physicians' offices and clinics, has enhanced access to this preventive measure. Nevertheless, many older adults remain unvaccinated. The CDC recommends that adults aged 65 years or older receive the pneumococcal vaccination. It is important that nurses inform the public about the importance of immunizations and counteract the myth that receiving the vaccination will result in the disease, which often prevents older adults from receiving immunization.

### Cancer

Cancer rates for older adults are disproportionately high in the United States. Although only 12% of the population are considered older adults, more than 50% of all diagnosed cancers are found in this population, and the death rate for cancer is highest among adults aged 65 years or older. The reason for the large proportion

| TABLE 24-3   2010 Estimated US Cancer Deaths | | |
|---|---|---|
| | **Men (N/%)** | **Women (N/%)** |
| All causes | 299,490 | 270,290 |
| Oral cavity and pharynx | 5430/0.018 | 2450/0.009 |
| Digestive system | 79,010/0.263 | 60,570/0.224 |
| Respiratory system | 89,550/0.299 | 72,120/0.266 |
| Bones and joints | 830/0.002 | 630/0.002 |
| Soft tissue including heart | 2020/0.006 | 1900/0.007 |
| Skin | 7910/0.026 | 3880/0.014 |
| Breast | 390/0.001 | 39,840/0.147 |
| Genital system | 32,710/0.109 | 27,710/0.103 |
| Urinary system | 19,110/0.063 | 9440/0.035 |
| Brain | 7120/0.023 | 5720/0.021 |
| Endocrine system | 1140/0.003 | 1430/0.005 |
| Lymphoma | 1140/0.003 | 10,080/0.037 |
| Myeloma | 5760/0.019 | 4890/0.002 |
| Leukemia | 12,660/0.042 | 9180/0.034 |
| Other | 23,690/0.079 | 20,340/0.075 |

From American Cancer Society. (2010). Cancer facts & figures 2010. Atlanta, GA: American Cancer Society. http://www.cancer.org/acs/groups/content/@epidemiologysurveilance/documents/document/acspc-026238.pdf; Murphy, S. L, Xu, J., & Kochanek, K. D. (2012). Deaths: Preliminary data for 2010. *National Vital Statistics Reports, 60*(4). http://www.cdc.gov/nchs/data/nvsr/nvsr60/nvsr60_04.pdf.

of cancer in the United States is unknown. Theories include longer exposure to carcinogens, increased susceptibility to cancer in the older body, decreased cellular healing ability, loss of tumor-suppressing genes, and decreased immune function. Although the exact cause cannot be determined, cancer is a significant problem for older adults in the United States.

The types of cancer common to older adults are listed by sex in Table 24-3. Prostate cancer is the leading cancer among men of all races and ages and is clearly the most common male cancer and the second leading cause of death from cancer in men in the United States. It is estimated that 8% of all men in the United States will receive a diagnosis of prostate cancer during their lifetime. Early detection of prostate cancer allows treatment while it is still localized in the prostate gland and highly curable. Evidence suggests that by use of a combination of screening techniques, more cases of prostate cancer can be detected earlier. There are three key components of an appropriate prostate screen: symptomatology, prostate-specific antigen level measurement, and a digital rectal examination. The four major treatment options for prostate cancer are surgery, radiation therapy, watchful waiting, and hormone therapy.

Breast cancer is the most common cancer in women of all ages and races in the United States. It is surpassed only by lung cancer as the cause of death in women. Reports suggest that one in nine women will develop breast cancer in their lifetime. Three-quarters of all breast cancers occur in women older than 50 years. The risk is increased in women whose close female relatives (mothers or sisters) have had the disease. Women who have never had children or who had their first child after age 30 years appear to have an increased risk. The causes of breast cancer remain unclear. The best protection is early detection and prompt treatment. New guidelines from the American Cancer Society (2015) recommend that women aged 55 years or older have mammograms every 2 years, although they may continue to have annual screening if they wish.

Nurses help older adults change the habits that place them at high risk of developing cancer. Following nutritional guidelines (as suggested earlier in this chapter), reducing stress, adopting a program of regular exercise, and stopping smoking and other use of tobacco products are a few of the approaches that nurses can advise to promote individual wellness. Periodic monitoring and screening in the form of regular visits to a primary health care provider or community screening can alert older adults to early signs and symptoms of cancers that occur during the later years.

## Chemical Agents

Chemical agents can be both therapeutic and harmful depending on their use. The increased use of prescription and over-the-counter medications can result in increased adverse drug events. The use of alcohol and tobacco products can be especially harmful for older adults.

### Drug Use

Normal changes of aging have a significant effect on the pharmacodynamics of drugs in older adults. The ways in which medications are absorbed, distributed, metabolized, and excreted from the body are affected by normal physiological changes and by illness. Even when medications are taken as prescribed, age-related changes and disease increase the risk of undesirable side effects. Older adults are more likely to take multiple medications, resulting in increased risk of serious drug interactions. In addition to potential adverse effects caused by prescription drugs, older adults take many types of nonprescription substances, including over-the-counter medications; vitamins, minerals, and supplements; herbal remedies; and foods and other traditional remedies used to resolve common ailments. Polypharmacy, or the use of multiple medications for the same or for different health problems, is a major concern for older adults. Approximately one-third of older adults in the United States take five or more prescription drugs (Brookes & Scott, 2015). The higher rate of polypharmacy in older adults as compared with younger groups is related to increased health problems in older adults and new medications that effectively treat these conditions. The Beers criteria (American Geriatric Society, 2015), developed from the Health Care Financing Administration *Guidelines for Potentially Inappropriate Medications in the Elderly,* present medications known to place older adults at risk of adverse reactions.

Many older adults who reside at home take their medications independently. Although self-medication with prescription and nonprescription substances is an effective method of disease management, little is known about the process of taking medications after the person leaves the health care practice or facility. Although it is generally assumed that medications are taken as prescribed, sensory disturbances; lack of knowledge; and alternative drug, alcohol, and nutrition practices may present challenges to medication self-administration that interfere with medical management of health problems. Nurses should take a thorough medication history to assess the individual for past drug reactions and identify all currently prescribed and nonprescription substances taken. New medications should be started at their lowest effective dose, and the dose should be increased slowly as necessary.

One of the major barriers to drug adherence in the older adult is affordability. Medicare provides prescription drug coverage to everyone eligible for Medicare under Medicare Part D. One can get Medicare drug coverage in one of two ways: a Medicare Prescription Drug Plan (PDP) or a Medicare Advantage Plan (preferred provider organization [PPO] or health maintenance organization [HMO]). For poor older adults, assistance for the purchase of prescription drugs is available in several ways: switching coverage to a less costly drug plan; or applying for assistance to pharmaceutical company assistance programs, state pharmaceutical assistance programs, national- and community-based charitable programs, and the Extra Help program through Medicare and Social Security.

### Alcohol and Drug Abuse

Substance abuse among Americans aged 60 years or older, including misuse of prescription drugs, is estimated to affect approximately 17% of older adults (Hazelden Betty Ford Foundation, 2015). By 2020 it is anticipated that the number of older adults with substance abuse problems will double. Forty percent of adults aged 65 years or older drink alcohol (National Institute on Alcohol Abuse and Alcoholism, n.d.). Alcohol and drug abuse problems among older adults have been underestimated. In Americans aged 65 years or older, excessive alcohol use, including binge drinking, accounts for more than 21,000 deaths each year (Rubin, 2014). Older adults may be classified as moderate drinkers but frequently consume large amounts of alcohol at a time.

Alcohol and drug abuse in older adults is often unreported and unnoticed because the symptoms can be similar to those of other common problems of aging, and health care providers often do not ask people about alcohol or nonprescription drug use. The longer the problem remains undetected, the greater it becomes and the more the potential harm related to other chronic health problems.

Older adults are more vulnerable to the effects of alcohol and illicit drugs because their detoxification and excretion systems are not as efficient as those of younger people. Alcoholism and drug abuse predispose older adults to accidents and injury, cognitive decline, physical debility, nutritional deficiencies, disease, and decreased function. Additionally, alcohol use while taking medications can interfere with the desired effect of the medication.

### Tobacco Use

Tobacco use includes cigarette smoking, cigar smoking, pipe smoking, and chewing tobacco. Use of tobacco products is associated with cardiovascular disease, several types of cancer, and chronic lung disease (CDC, 2015e). Some older men and women today may be the first generation to have smoked throughout their lives, starting in their teens or 20s when smoking seemed fashionable. The results of smoking occur slowly over time, and problems are usually not experienced until signs and symptoms of smoking-related health problems occur. Because smoking can initiate and promote disease processes, it is one of the most important negative predictors of longevity. Smoking is a particular problem for older adults because of the large number of medications they take and the potential for drug interactions. Nicotine-drug interactions can potentiate or interfere with a desired drug effect.

Older adults can experience the benefits of smoking cessation even after the age of 65 years. These people may be more motivated to quit smoking than when they were younger, because they are likely to see some of the damage that smoking has caused and anticipate that smoking cessation will restore or improve their health. Nurses can assist older adults in making the commitment to quit smoking through education and referral to smoking cessation programs.

# DETERMINANTS OF HEALTH

## Social Factors and Environment

The incidence of chronic and acute illnesses, the subsequent decline in functional status, changes in economic status, and changes in family structure frequently place older adults in situations for which they are admitted to acute care facilities or must make a temporary or permanent move into a residential facility or a long-term care facility. When providing health-promotion services to older adults, nurses must take into account the type of setting in which the person lives. Box 24-11: Research For Evidence-Based Practice provides helpful information about transitional care for older adults with chronic illness, as well as their caregivers.

When older adults leave their homes, they may enter a continuum of care extending from an independent living center and assisted living facilities to skilled care facilities or nursing homes, with possible short-term stays in acute care settings. Nurses who work in each of the settings on the continuum can promote health to this population in many ways. From the acute care setting through each stage of the continuum, opportunities are available for nurses to introduce older adults and their families to community resources (Table 24-4). The acute care nurse has the opportunity to present health-promotion strategies at a time during which individuals may perceive the greatest need to change their lifestyle behaviors so that they can return to an improved health state. In most cases an acute care admission is an opportunity to introduce health-promotion teaching. However, the acute care nurse may feel frustrated by the inability to see the results of this teaching and may therefore give it a low priority in the care plan.

Some older adults will rapidly grasp material that they believe will prevent future hospital admissions and restore their health. Home health nursing appointments, transportation services, housekeeping services, adult day care, and assistance with grocery shopping or home-delivered meals will help older adults return to the home environment better prepared to recover from the illness. Helping older adults and their families locate adult day care programs, smoking-cessation programs, stress-management workshops, or weight-loss and exercise programs before leaving the hospital will encourage older adults to enter these programs immediately after discharge, while they are motivated.

Long-term care nurses are able to locate and plan community resources during the resident's stay. Some community services will enable an older person to return home to an environment in which active health promotion continues. Community resources that may help older adults who are discharged from long-term care facilities include adult day care programs, support groups and medical resources, telephone and Internet information, and referral services. In addition to their role in individual care planning, long-term care nurses can be more involved in institutional policy changes. Recommendations about smoking policies, healthy diets, and exercise programs may prompt interdisciplinary changes that will result in improved health for the entire institution.

## BOX 24-11  RESEARCH FOR EVIDENCE-BASED PRACTICE

### Evidence-Based Transitional Care for Chronically Ill Older Adults and Their Caregivers

Unplanned readmissions within 30 days of discharge are estimated to be at 90%. A multidisciplinary research team developed a transitional care model (TCM) to focus on the needs of very high risk chronically ill older adults who are transitioning from the hospital to the home following an acute illness. The TCM is led by an advanced practice nurse (APN) using a holistic person-centered and family care–centered approach. The APN acts as the "point person" throughout the episode of care, facilitating timely exchange of information across all settings. The criteria identified to determine high-risk persons include those who are 80 years or older, those who have moderate to severe functional deficits, and those who are unable to complete self-care or manage daily tasks.

The tools used to assess potentially affected persons include the Hospital Admission Risk Profile, the Katz Index of Independence in Activities of Daily Living or the Lawton Instrumental Activities of Daily Living Scale, and the Mental Status Assessment of Older Adults (Mini-Cog). Potentially affected persons are also screened with use of the Geriatric Depression Scale—Short Form to assess symptoms of depression. The following risks associated with readmission have been identified: having four or more active coexisting health problems, being treated with six or more prescribed standing medications, having two or more hospitalizations within the previous 6 months, being hospitalized within the previous 30 days, having been hospitalized with baseline dementia, being treated for delirium, lacking formal or informal family caregiver support, and having low health literacy.

With APN services under the TCM, mutual goals are developed, there is improved communication and collaboration among health care providers, there is improved medication and dietary adherence, there are decreased numbers of rehospitalizations during the 52 weeks of follow-up, and there is high person, caregiver, and physician satisfaction. The barriers to widespread adoption of the TCM identified include the organization of current systems of care, barriers of regulation, lack of quality and financial incentives, and culture of care issues.

From Bixby, M. B. (2011). Evidence-based transitional care for chronically ill older adults and their caregivers. *Journal of Geriatric Care Management, 21*(2), 20–24.

## TABLE 24-4 Long-Term Care Housing and Assessment Continuum

| | Independent Living | Retirement Community | Assisted Living | Nursing Facility |
|---|---|---|---|---|
| Description | Covers a broad range of housing options (residential houses, apartments, condominiums, townhouses, subsidized senior housing) for older people who are functionally and socially independent | Provides a living arrangement that integrates shelter and services for older people who do not need 24-h protective oversight | Provides a living arrangement that integrates shelter and services for frail older people who are functionally and/or socially impaired and require 24-h protective oversight | Provides a living arrangement that integrates shelter with medical, nursing, psychosocial, and rehabilitation services for older people who require 24-h nursing supervision |
| Primary services | **A** Environmental security Possibly coordination of resident services (transportation, activities, housekeeping) Or no services are available | **B** A plus: Meals (one to three per day) Transportation Activities Housekeeping assistance Assistance with coordination of community-based services | **C** A and B plus: Assistance with activities of daily living Medication monitoring, 24-h protective oversight | **D** A, B, and C plus: Medication administration, 24-h nursing supervision |
| Mobility | Capable of moving about independently OR ambulatory with cane or walker Independent with wheelchair, but needs help in an emergency | Capable of moving about independently Able to seek and follow directions Able to evacuate independently in emergency OR ambulatory with cane or walker Independent with wheelchair, but needs help in an emergency | Mobile, but may require escort or assistance resulting from confusion, poor vision, weakness, or poor motivation OR requires occasional assistance to move about, but is usually independent | May require assistance with transfers from bed, chair, and toilet OR requires transfer and transport assistance Requires turning and positioning in bed and wheelchair |
| Nutrition | Able to prepare own meals; eats without assistance | Able to prepare own meals; eats without assistance. Generally, a minimum of one meal a day is available | All meals and snacks are provided. May require assistance getting to dining room or requires minimal assistance (opening cartons or other packages, cutting food, or preparing trays) | May be unable or unwilling to go to dining room. May be dependent on staff for eating or feeding needs OR may be fully dependent on staff for nourishment (includes reminders to eat) |
| Hygiene | Independent in all care, including bathing | Independent in all care, including bathing and personal laundry | May require assistance with bathing or hygiene OR may require assistance, initiation, structure, or reminders. Resident may be able to complete tasks | May be dependent on staff for all personal hygiene |
| Housekeeping | Independent in performing housekeeping functions (includes making bed, vacuuming, cleaning, and laundry) | Independent in performing housekeeping functions (includes making bed, vacuuming, cleaning, and laundry) OR may need assistance with heavy housekeeping, vacuuming, laundry, and linens | Housekeeping and laundry services provided | Housekeeping and laundry services provided |
| Dressing | Independent and dresses appropriately | Independent and dresses appropriately | May require occasional assistance with shoelaces, zippers, or medical appliances or garments OR may require reminders, initiation, or motivation | May be dependent on staff for dressing |
| Toileting | Independent and continent | Independent and completely continent OR may have incontinence, colostomy, or catheter, but independent in caring for self through proper use of supplies | Same as for retirement community OR may have occasional problem with incontinence, colostomy, or catheter and may require assistance in caring for self through proper use of supplies | May have problem with incontinence, colostomy, or catheter and requires assistance OR may be dependent and unable to communicate needs |

## TABLE 24-4 Long-Term Care Housing and Assessment Continuum—cont'd

|  | Independent Living | Retirement Community | Assisted Living | Nursing Facility |
|---|---|---|---|---|
| Medications | Responsible for self-administration of all medications | Responsible for self-administration of all medications *OR* may arrange for family or home health agency to establish a medication administration system | Able to self-administer medications *OR* facility staff may remind the person about or monitor the actual process *OR* facility staffed by registered nurses or licensed practical nurses who administer medications | Medications administered by staff personnel or self if assessed as capable |
| Mental status | Oriented to person, place, and time<br>Memory intact, but has occasional forgetfulness *AND* able to reason and plan and organize daily events. Mentally capable of identifying needs and meeting them | Oriented to person, place, and time *AND* memory is intact, but has occasional forgetfulness without consistent pattern of memory loss *AND* is able to reason and plan and organize daily events. Mentally capable of identifying environmental needs and meeting them | May require occasional direction or guidance in getting from place to place *OR* may have difficulty with occasional confusion that may result in anxiety, social withdrawal, or depression *OR* orientation to time or place or person may be impaired | Judgment can be poor and may attempt tasks that are not within capabilities *OR* may require strong orientation and reminder program. May need guidance in getting from place to place *OR* disoriented to time, place, and person *OR* memory is severely impaired |
| Behavioral status | Deals appropriately with emotions and uses available resources to cope with inner stress | Deals appropriately with emotions and uses available resources to cope with inner stress *AND* deals appropriately with other residents and staff *OR* may require periodic intervention from staff to resolve conflicts with others to cope with situational stress | May require periodic intervention from staff to facilitate expression of feelings to cope with inner stress *OR* may require periodic intervention from staff to resolve conflicts with others to cope with situational stress | May require regular intervention from staff to facilitate expression of feelings and to deal with periodic outbursts of anxiety or agitation *OR* maximal staff intervention is required to manage behavior |

The geriatric care manager who visits older adults in their homes or in other residential facilities may be charged with individual health-promotion planning. Home care nurses provide health care information and services to individuals and their families. The resources available to community health nurses are frequently rich and enable the nurses to draw on a variety of sources to assist in promoting the health of community-dwelling older adults. Transportation options, home-delivered meals, assistance with housekeeping, socialization activities, exercise programs, and self-help groups are only a few of the health-promotion resources available within the community. Nurses in all settings can consult a social worker or contact the community older adult services office for information on available resources.

It is important for the nurse to consider the health literacy level of the older adult and their family when providing information and health teaching. The USDHHS (n.d.) defines health literacy as "the degree to which individuals have the capacity to obtain, process, and understand basic health information needed to make appropriate health decisions and services needed to prevent or treat illness." People who are at risk of low health literacy are the elderly, minorities, people of low socioeconomic level, and the medically underserved. Older adults with low health literacy may have difficulty finding appropriate health care providers, seeking preventive health care, filling out health forms, managing chronic illness, following directions, understanding the relationship between risk behaviors and health problems, and following medication and treatment plans. It is important for nurses to identify older adults who have low health literacy and develop instructional materials that use simple language and short sentences, avoiding or defining technical terms. Nurses can provide assistance for older adults who have difficulty completing forms. For older adults who have limited English skills, written and oral instruction can be provided in their native language.

In recent years there has been a substantial increase in the use of palliative and hospice care by older adults. Palliative care is provided for people with a serious illness who will continue to receive curative treatment and symptom relief. Whereas palliative care is available to anyone with a serious illness, hospice care requires a terminal prognosis with an expected death within 6 months. Once the person is placed in hospice care, treatment to relieve pain and other symptoms is continued but the person and his or her physician have decided to end all curative treatment. In 2011 approximately 1.65 million persons received hospice care (National Hospice and Palliative Care Organization, 2012). In 2010 there were 5150 hospice providers in the United States. Of approximately 2.5 million deaths in the United States in 2010, slightly more than 1 million, or 42%, died under hospice care. Most hospice care provided in 2010 was in the person's home (41.1%), followed by a hospice inpatient facility (21.9%), nursing home (18%), and acute care hospital (11.4%). Most hospice care recipients were female (56.1%), white (77.3%), and 65 years or older (82.7%). Hospice services provided include direct clinical care for individuals and bereavement services for the person and the family (National Hospice and Palliative Care Organization, 2012).

People in a hospice are empowered to live with dignity, alert and free of pain. The goal of hospice care is to facilitate a "good death" for individuals. Families and loved ones are consistently engaged in caregiving for the dying and helping them maintain the highest possible quality of life. The hospice environment promotes quality of life within the context of differing cultural and spiritual values and beliefs. Nurses in all settings may identify and refer individuals for palliative or hospice care and facilitate use of these services to promote wellness during serious or terminal illness.

Older adults can be overwhelmed with the amount of advertising that is directed at them about such "necessities" as nutritional supplements, drugs, hearing aids, alarms to use if they fall, phones, Internet sites, and digital devices. Nurses can help them sort out the confusion related to this advertising and direct them to reliable sources of information. The AARP provides many services to people older than 50 years, including excellent educational materials and community program packages. The topics reflect a broad range of concerns and are generally presented in a self-help manner. Among the topics covered are smoking, exercise, nutrition, and wellness. Each program serves as a guide to negotiate a system or learn more about a health problem. These topics are written in lay terms (in easily understood language) and are printed in large print to accommodate vision changes. This self-help method is especially important for those who feel uncomfortable addressing questions on finances or sexuality to nurses and physicians.

The National Institute for Aging (http://www.nia.nih.gov) conducts research to examine many aspects of aging so as to improve the quantity and quality of life in older years. It provides free educational publications called *Age Pages* that can be given to older adults to help them adapt safely and successfully to the many changes and concerns encountered as a person ages. *Age Pages* are easily accessed on the Internet and are written in large font and language easily understandable to the lay public.

Two additional environments of care emerged in the United States in the second half of the 20th century: continuing care retirement communities (CCRCs) and assisted living facilities (ALFs). CCRCs are full-service communities offering long-term contracts that provide older adults with a continuum of care, extending from retirement services through assisted living to skilled nursing, all in one location. The mission behind CCRCs is "aging in place." CCRCs are expensive and require an entrance fee and a monthly payment. Residence in a CCRC requires commitment to a long-term contract that specifies the housing, services, and nursing care provided. ALFs are defined as homelike settings that promote resident autonomy, privacy, independence, dignity, and respect while providing necessary support. The lower cost of ALFs in comparison with skilled nursing facilities and the greater emphasis on functional autonomy make these facilities appealing to older consumers and their families. Although residents of ALFs have many long-term health care needs, it is important to understand that the role and availability of nurses in these facilities differ greatly by state guidelines.

One additional social factor should be considered—that of age discrimination. Even today when many older adults are active contributors to society, they experience discrimination in seeking employment and in many other areas. Older adults have described situations where they seek medical care and instead of health care providers speaking directly to them, they direct their inquiries to a family member who is present. Many of these older adults are highly educated, cognitively aware, and perfectly capable of implementing advice from health care providers to maintain their health. Getting old should not carry a stigma. Older adults are in a position to enrich the lives of others through the wealth of knowledge and experience that they have accumulated through the years.

## Diversity Awareness

The percentage of white older adults is expected to decrease from 1990 to 2030, whereas the percentages of black, Asian, and Hispanic older adults are expected to increase. These changes in the diversity of the United States bring unprecedented challenges to the US health care delivery system. Challenges will continue to present themselves in the way that each culture perceives the status of the older person within society, the way health is maintained or improved, the causes and meanings of disease throughout life, and the ways in which disease and injury are managed from the cultural perspective versus how they are managed according to the health care system.

Nurses must be aware of the cultural diversity of older adults for whom they care and the cultural beliefs that influence health care decisions of older adults. Cultural competence refers to the ability of nurses to understand and accept the cultural backgrounds of individuals and provide care that best meets the persons' needs, not the nurses' needs. To develop cultural competence, the first step is to examine personal beliefs and the effect of these beliefs on professional behavior. Nurses may best accomplish this by conducting personal cultural assessments. After identifying personal cultural biases that influence care, nurses must bracket these beliefs to make sure they do not affect delivery of care. After this step has been accomplished, it is important to increase understanding about population-specific health-related cultural values, beliefs, and behaviors. It is important to remember that although an older person may be part of a cultural group, the individual may have become acculturated while living in the United States. A cultural history is therefore an essential first step in determining the person's health care beliefs and practices. When conducting cultural assessments, the nurse must remember that some of the standardized assessment tools, such as the Geriatric Depression Scale and the MMSE, are available in languages other than English. Caution must be taken in interpreting a tool that has not been formally translated, because the meanings of many words and phrases may not have an appropriate translation. The nurse must also be cautious when using assessment tools that have not been tested and validated with people of different cultures and nationalities.

The final stage in attaining cultural competence is to develop skills for working with culturally diverse populations.

This entails the development of knowledge in working with culturally diverse populations and consistently using those skills with older adults. Conducting cultural assessments, using translation services, and providing culturally competent care are integral components to developing culturally competent institutions and improving care.

## Levels of Policy Making and Health

This chapter has attempted to emphasize the need for health-promotion services for older adults. Governmental efforts to improve health promotion and illness/injury prevention continue. The Affordable Care Act of 2010 (http://www.healthcare.gov) strengthens Medicare by providing important new benefits, including free or low-cost preventive services, free annual wellness visits, and a discount on prescription drugs for Medicare recipients in the "donut hole." Older adults continue to be able to choose their own physician. Preventive immunizations include those for influenza, pneumonia, and hepatitis B. Preventive screening examinations include those for diabetes, cholesterol and cardiovascular diseases, colorectal cancer, breast cancer, cervical cancer, and prostate cancer. Counseling services for smoking cessation and for medical nutrition therapy for those with diabetes or kidney disease are also provided.

Medicare and other federal expenditures for older adults (direct or indirect) constitute a large part of the federal budget. Most goes to old age and retirement programs, disability programs, and Medicaid. Because of the large percentage of the federal budget consumed by Medicare, this insurance program is undergoing much scrutiny. Legislation to more effectively manage or cut the Medicare budget is under review. Lawmakers anticipate that approximately $49 billion in savings could come from more effective use of health maintenance organizations and prospective payment systems instituted in the home. Regardless of the nature of funding cuts, illness and injury prevention contributes to financial stability of the older adult. Nurses continue to play a key role during the years of Medicare reform in promoting health not only to prevent illness and injury but also to prevent older adults from losing all their savings and becoming impoverished.

Medigap policies have been promoted to pay for the health care coverage not afforded by Medicare. The various policies provide differing levels of coverage. Choices about whether to purchase coverage for durable health care supplies, prescription medications, and other medical charges must be made to select the most appropriate policy. The charge for the policy varies according to the level of coverage selected.

Nongovernmental organizations also influence policy decisions affecting older adults and health. Professional health care provider organizations such as the American Nurses Association, the National Gerontological Nurses Association, and the American Medical Association conduct research to determine best practices in elder care and to provide information to policymakers. The ARAP and the Gray Panthers are examples of two consumer organizations that gather information, fund research related to issues of older adults, and act as advocates for older adults in policy making organizations.

## Health Services/Delivery Systems

Unfortunately, many people are not financially prepared for older adulthood. Although some individuals receive supplemental income from pensions or individual retirement accounts, many do not, and the amount of income from these sources is often very limited. Most older adults live on limited incomes. Several resources are available to help those with limited finances live quality lives. Medicaid, authorized by Title 19 of the Social Security Act, is designed to help older adults who are receiving public assistance pay for medical expenses. Both federal and state governments fund the Medicaid program. To qualify for Medicaid, an individual must have limited income and assets. The coverage afforded by Medicaid is more extensive than that of Medicare. For example, Medicaid covers stays in long-term care facilities, transportation for health care visits, and prescription drug services. Medicare covers these services in limited and medically acute situations. Frequently older adults and their caretakers desire the more extensive coverage provided by Medicaid. These individuals are required to "spend down" their assets to be eligible.

Careful financial planning before the onset of illness is ideal to avoid the need to spend down assets and to help the older adult live at a desirable income level. This task can be accomplished through meetings with lawyers and financial planners as early in life as 30 years of age. Completing advance directives, including naming a conservator in advance of illness, assists caregivers, physicians, clergy, and the family in making difficult decisions at the end of life, when the affected person is no longer able to make them. The better prepared the older adult is, the easier it is to receive appropriate care and treatment during times of illness. Reverse annuity mortgages are one option for increased income during the later years. A reverse annuity mortgage is obtained when a bank or private business purchases the home of an older adult. The bank pays the person a set amount of money each month until the house is paid for in its entirety. The older adult continues to live in the home. This approach provides the person with necessary funds and negates the need to move and sell the house if an illness arises. When the older adult (mortgagee) dies, the bank or mortgager then owns the property.

Long-term care insurance is an option for those planning for the possibility of long-term care. As with other insurance programs, younger adults can purchase a policy, now widely available from insurance agents. A premium is paid each month that entitles the beneficiary to receive long-term care benefits at home, in an assisted living facility, in a day care facility, or in a long-term care facility. Older individuals are cautioned to explore the many options available for this type of insurance. The benefits and coverage differ, and exclusions are frequently written into the contract to prevent care in certain situations. An important feature of these policies is the option to hire a personal caregiver if the need arises.

Because population shifts have created a large number of older adults in the United States, political movements toward protecting the rights of older adults are abundant and strong. Nowhere is there more political activity than among the groups responsible for social policy and aging. However, this has created problems of consistency, equity, and authority. Several large programs, including those directed by the Social Security Administration, the Health Care Financing Administration, and the Department of Veterans Affairs, have coordination problems because of their size and the large number of cases they handle.

The nurse who specializes in the care of older adults helps a great deal to promote their health and well-being through education, research, and practice. Educational curricula must be evaluated continually to ensure that content is appropriate and accurate with respect to aging. The quality of care depends on the clinician's knowledge base. Education for the older person is equally important and begins with an assessment of the individual's level of understanding of health-promotion activities.

Health-promotion and illness/injury-prevention research for this population is only beginning. Much more remains to be done in exploring the concepts of health promotion, relating these concepts, and developing and testing hypotheses. Research is needed to debunk commonly held beliefs, myths, and stereotypes about aging. Defining some of the concepts of health promotion, such as quality of life and functional ability, will yield immeasurable amounts of information that can be tested. Eventually, with the commitment of qualified nurses, health promotion will be respected for the integral role it plays in the quality of life of older adults.

## NURSING APPLICATION

Nurses in a position of providing care to older adults focus on promoting quality of life, promoting the health of the population, maintaining self-care, and preventing disease and its complications. Nursing activities with the older adult often focus on the management of chronic conditions. While concentrating on healing, the nurse delivers care in a holistic manner that addresses the functional and psychosocial needs of the older adult.

Nurses assist older adults by engaging them in health-promotion activities. Some of the major areas of focus are healthy weight and diet, activity, fall prevention and home safety, and medical appointments for screening. Pneumococcal and seasonal influenza immunizations are extremely important for the older adult. Additionally, the older adult is educated about cancer screenings and other screenings aimed at detecting diabetes,

late-onset heart disease, osteoporosis, and hypertension. An effective method of ensuring that older adults participate in screenings is to coordinate health fairs in senior centers. The nurse is able to provide a common location where the older adult can obtain vaccinations, necessary education, blood pressure checks, and fingerstick glucose monitoring. The nurse offers counseling as needed and refers the older adult to his or her primary care provider for follow-up.

## SUMMARY

Life expectancy is now beyond 75 years for both men and women, with the fastest-growing age group being those older than 85 years. This phenomenon is indeed wonderful. However, as noted at the beginning of this chapter, aging is not for sissies. The aging process causes physiological changes in many body functions, and older adults have a higher frequency of illness than the younger population. The many physical, emotional, and role changes of aging are complicated by the increased diversity in cultural and spiritual backgrounds. Older adults who have immigrated to the United States have brought with them different languages, values and beliefs, spiritual patterns, eating habits, views toward modern medicine, and other customs foreign to US culture. Culturally competent health-promotion services are integral to helping older adults lead high-quality lives throughout their extended life spans.

Some of the dysfunctional aspects of aging have extrinsic causes, such as environmental pollution. Older adults are as susceptible as any age group to society's problems, such as homelessness, mistreatment, and drug and alcohol abuse. In conjunction with physiological and pathological changes, multiple acute and chronic diseases can result. Internal and public policy changes will continue to help older adults live in a world in which old age can be the most rewarding stage of life.

Many problems of old age are related to lifestyle. Changes in nutritional needs, sleep patterns, and activity level are required to adapt to normal and pathological processes. Psychological health depends on reassessing spirituality, self-concept, and role functions. Change and adaptation are possible. Aging healthfully is hard work, but with the assistance of nurses and other health care professionals, older adults can be empowered to live their final years with a sense of peace in their life review of happy memories and accomplishments.

## CASE STUDY

### *Unsafe Driving: Larry Johnson*

Larry Johnson, a healthy 75-year-old man, lives in his own apartment and is completely independent in activities of daily living and instrumental activities of daily living. Last Friday morning, Larry left his apartment complex at 8:00 AM to go to the store. While backing out of his driveway, he failed to see a school bus passing on the intersecting street, and his car struck the bus. Although no one was injured, this incident indicated the need for a sensory and neurological assessment. The assessment revealed both hearing and visual deficits.

**Reflective Questions**
- What would the nurse do to help with the results of the assessment?
- Should this person undergo further neuropsychological tests?
- How best can the nurse support this person during this difficult time in his life?
- In what ways might the family be helpful in this situation?

## CARE PLAN

### Unsafe Driving: Larry Johnson

**\*NURSING DIAGNOSIS: Risk of injury related to unsafe driving**

**Defining Characteristics**
- Altered response time
- Change in vision or hearing

**Related Factors**
- Past accident
- Stressful life events
- Receipt of traffic tickets
- Witnessed poor driving

**Expected Outcomes**
- Person will have realistic expectations of ability to drive.
- Person and nurse will set appropriate limitations on driving.

- Person will take a driver refresher course.
- Family will help to monitor driving competencies.
- Person will have no further accidents.

**Interventions**
- Assist Larry in registering for a renewal driving program.
- Meet Larry and a family member to discuss ways to ensure consistent safe driving.
- Assist Larry in finding alternative modes of transportation until visual and hearing alterations are corrected and instead of driving in the evening.
- Schedule hearing and vision appointments for Larry and assist in transportation to appointments.

*NANDA Nursing Diagnoses—Herdman T. H. & Kamitsuru, S. (Eds.). Nursing Diagnoses–Definitions and Classification 2015–2017. Copyright © 2014, 1994–2014 NANDA International. Used by arrangement with John Wiley & Sons Limited. In order to make safe and effective judgments using the NANDA-I nursing diagnoses it is essential that nurses refer to the definitions and defining characteristics of the diagnoses listed in this work.

## EVOLVE CHAPTER FEATURES

http://evolve.elsevier.com/Edelman/
- Study Questions

## REFERENCES

Agency for Healthcare Research and Quality. (2012). Racial and ethnic groups. Selected findings from the 2011 National Healthcare Quality and Disparities Reports. http://archive.ahrq .gov/research/findings/nhqrdr/nhqrdr11/minority.pdf.

Agronin, M. E. (2013). From Cicero to Cohen: Developmental theories of aging, from antiquity to the present. *The Gerontologist*, 54(1), 30–39.

Alzheimer's Association. (2015). 2015 Alzheimer's disease facts and figures. https://www.alz.org/facts/downloads/facts_figures_2015 .pdf.

American Association of Retired Persons (AARP). (2012). 5 myths about sex and aging. http://www.aarp.org/relationships/love-sex/ info-05-2011/sex-myths.print.html.

American Cancer Society. (2015). American Cancer Society guidelines for the early detection of cancer. http://www.cancer.org/healthy/ findcancerearly/cancerscreeningguidelines/american-cancer-society -guidelines-for-the-early-detection-of-cancer.

American Geriatric Society. (2015). Expanded AGS Beers criteria offer new guidance, tools for safer medication use among older adults. http://www.americangeriatrics.org/press/ id:5907.

Brookes, L., & Scott, I. A. (2015). Deprescribing in clinical practice: Reducing polypharmacy in older patients. Medscape Multispecialty. http://www.medscape.com/viewarticle/814861_2.

Bundy-Fazioli, K., Fruhauf, C. A., & Miller, J. L. (2013). Grandparents caregivers' perceptions of emotional stress and well-being. *Journal of Family Social Work*, 16, 447–462.

Butler, R., & Olshansky, S. J. (2002). Has anybody ever died of old age? *The Gerontologist*, 42(Special1), 285–286.

Centers for Disease Control and Prevention (CDC). (2011a). Enhancing use of clinical preventive services among older adults—Closing the gap. http://www.cdc.gov/aging/pdf/Clinical_ Preventive_Services_Closing_the_Gap_Report.pdf.

Centers for Disease Control and Prevention (CDC). (2011b). How much physical activity do older adults need? http://www.cdc.gov/ physicalactivity/everyone/guidelines/olderadults.html.

Centers for Disease Control and Prevention (CDC). (2011c). Update: Influenza activity—United States, 2010–11 season, and composition of the 2011–12 influenza vaccine. *MMWR. Morbidity and Mortality Weekly Report*, 60(21), 708–711.

Centers for Disease Control and Prevention (CDC). (2013a). Compendium of evidence-based interventions and best practices for HIV prevention. Retrieved November 28, 2015 from http:// www.cdc.gov/hiv/prevention/research/compendium/rr/ safersex.html.

Centers for Disease Control and Prevention (CDC). (2013b). One in five adults meet overall physical guidelines recommendations. http://www.cdc.gov/media/releases/2013/p0502-physical-activity .html.

Centers for Disease Control and Prevention (CDC). (2014a). Disability and functioning (noninstitutionalized adults 18 years and over). http://www.cdc.gov/nchs/fastats/disability.htm.

Centers for Disease Control and Prevention (CDC). (2014b). Sexual health. http://www.cdc.gov/sexualhealth/default.html# who.

Centers for Disease Control and Prevention (CDC). (2015a). Alzheimer's disease. http://www.cdc.gov/aging/aginginfo/ alzheimers.htm.

Centers for Disease Control and Prevention (CDC). (2015b). Depression is not a normal part of growing older. http:// www.cdc.gov/aging/mentalhealth/depression.htm.

Centers for Disease Control and Prevention (CDC). (2015c). Home and recreational safety. http://www.cdc.gov/HomeandRecreational Safety/Falls/adultfalls.html.

Centers for Disease Control and Prevention (CDC). (2015d). Older adult drivers. http://www.cdc.gov.

Centers for Disease Control and Prevention (CDC). (2015e). Health effects of cigarette smoking. http://www.cdc.gov/tobacco/data_statistics/fact_sheets/health_effects/effects_cig_smoking/index.htm.

Centers for Disease Control and Prevention (CDC). (2017). HIV among people aged 50 and over. https://www.cdc.gov/hiv/group/age/olderamericans/index.html.

Chervin, R. D. (2015). Approach to the patient with excessive daytime sleepiness. http://www.uptodate.com/contents/approach-to-the-patient-with-excessive-daytime-sleepiness.

Chippendale, T., & Bear-Lehman, J. (2012). Effect of life review writing on depressive symptoms in older adults: A randomized controlled trial. *The American Journal of Occupational Therapy*, 66, 438–446.

Crawford, B. (2013). Pilates and the pelvic floor. *Advance Healthcare Network*, 24(16), 25.

Erikson, E. H. (1982). *Life cycle completed: A review*. New York: W. W. Norton.

Erikson, E. H. (1997). *The life cycle completed*. New York: W.W. Norton.

Erikson, E. H., Erikson, J. H., & Kivnick, H. Q. (1986). *Vital involvement in old age: The experience of old age in our time*. New York: W.W. Norton.

Esposito, L. (2016). Seniors and sexual health: What older adults should know. U.S. News and World Report. Health. http://health.usnews.com/health-news/patient-advice/articles/2016-03-16/seniors-and-sexual-health-what-older-adults-should-know.

Folstein, M. E., Folstein, S. E., & McHugh, P. (1975). "Mini-mental state." A practical method for grading the cognitive state of patients for the clinician. *Journal of Psychiatric Research*, 12, 189–198.

Gorina, Y., et al. (2014). Prevalence of incontinence among older Americans. Vital Health Statistics. Series 3, no. 36. Hyattsville, MD: National Center for Health Statistics. http://www.cdc.gov/nchs/data/series/sr_03/sr03_036.pdf.

Hazelden Betty Ford Foundation. (2015). Substance abuse among the elderly. http://www.hazeldenbettyford.org/articles/substance-abuse-among-the-elderly-a-growing-problem.

Health Editor. (2016). This is why more Americans are living to age 100 (and beyond). HealthDay News. http://news.health.com/2016/01/22/americans-100-and-older-are-living-even-longer-now/.

Healthways. (2014). Learn more about SilverSneakers. https://www.silversneakers.com/about.

Hodge, D., Bonifas, R., & Chou, R. (2010). Spirituality and older adults: Ethical guidelines to enhance service provision. *Advances in Social Work*, 11, 1.

Hooyman, N., & Kiyak, H. (2011). *Social gerontology: A multidisciplinary perspective* (9th ed.). Boston, MA: Allyn & Bacon.

Lu, P., et al. (2013). Surveillance of influenza vaccination coverage — United States, 2007–08 through 2011–12 influenza seasons. *MMWR. Surveillance summaries*, 62(ss04), 1–29. https://www.cdc.gov/mmwr/preview/mmwrhtml/ss6204a1.htm.

Mather, M. (2016). Fact sheet: Aging in the United States. Washington, DC: Population Reference Bureau. http://www.prb.org/Publications/Media-Guides/2016/aging-unitedstates-fact-sheet.aspx.

Mayo Clinic. (2015a). Kegel exercises: A how-to guide for women. http://www.mayoclinic.org/healthy-lifestyle/womens-health/in-depth/kegel-exercises/art-20045283?pg=1.

Mayo Clinic. (2015b). Kegel exercises for men: Understand the benefits. http://www.mayoclinic.org/healthy-lifestyle/mens-health/in-depth/kegel-exercises-for-men/art-20045074.

Mueller, C. M. (2015). Nutrition assessment in older adults. *Topics in Clinical Nutrition*, 30(1), 94–102.

Murphy, S. L., Xu, J., & Kochanek, K. D. (2012). Deaths: Preliminary data for 2010. *National Vital Statistics Reports*, 60(4), http://www.cdc.gov/nchs/data/nvsr/nvsr60/nvsr60_04.pdf.

National Center on Elder Abuse. (n.d.). Why should I care about elder abuse? http://www.communitysolutions.com/assets/2011_Institute_Presentations/whyshouldicareaboutelderabuse033111.pdf.

National Council on Aging. (n.d.). Senior hunger. https://www.ncoa.org/resources/senior-hunger-and-snap-fact-sheet/.

National Hospice and Palliative Care Organization. (2012). NHPCO facts and figures: Hospice care in America. http://www.nhpco.org/sites/default/files/public/Statistics_Research/2012_Facts_Figures.pdf.

National Institute of Mental Health. (n.d.). Older adults, depression and suicide facts. http://www.wvdhhr.org/bhhftest/ScienceOnOurMinds/NIMH%20PDFs/12%20Old%20Adults.pdf.

National Institute of Neurological Disorders and Stroke. (2015). Restless legs syndrome fact sheet. http://www.ninds.nih.gov/disorders/restless_legs/detail_restless_legs.htm.

National Institute on Aging. (2011). Biology of aging: Research today for a healthier tomorrow. http://www.nia.nih.gov/sites/default/files/biology_of_aging.pdf.

National Institute on Alcohol Abuse and Alcoholism. (n.d.). Older adults. http://www.niaaa.nih.gov/alcohol-health/special-populations-co-occurring-disorders/older-adults.

National Institute on Deafness and Other Communication Disorders. (2015). Hearing loss and older adults. http://www.nidcd.nih.gov/health/hearing/pages/older.aspx.

National Resource Center on Nutrition, Physical Activity & Aging. (2012). Malnutrition and older Americans. http://nutritionandaging.fiu.edu/aging_network/malfact2.asp.

Neikrug, A. B., & Ancoli-Israel, S. (2010). Sleep disorders in the older adult—A mini review. *Gerontology*, 56(2), 181–189.

Nies, M. A., & McEwan, M. (2011). *Community/Public health nursing: Promoting the health of populations* (6th ed.). Philadelphia: Saunders.

Office of Disease Prevention and Health Promotion. (2014). Lesbian, gay, bisexual, and transgender health. http://www.healthypeople.gov/2020/topics-objectives/topic/lesbian-gay-bisexual-and-transgender-health.

Ogden, C. L., et al. (2012). Prevalence of obesity in the United States, 2009–10. NCHS data brief no. 82. http://www.cdc.gov/nchs/data/databriefs/db82.htm.

Paddock, C. (2012). Fast cycling benefits Parkinson's patients. Medical News Today. http://www.medicalnewstoday.com/articles/253197.php.

Pietrzykowska, N. B. (2016). Obesity in the elderly. Obesity Action Coalition. http://www.obesityaction.org/educational-resources/resource-articles-2/general-articles/obesity-in-the-elderly.

Redline, S., et al. (2010). Obstructive sleep apnea hypopnea and incident stroke: The sleep heart health study. *American Journal of Respiratory and Critical Care Medicine*, 182(2), 269–277.

Rubin, R. (2014). America's surprising binge drinkers: People over 65. http://www.nextavenue.org/americas-surprising-binge-drinkers-people-over-65/.

Smiraglia, C. (2015). Qualities of the participant experience in an object-based museum outreach program to retirement communities. *Educational Gerontology, 41*(3), 238–248.

Smyth, C. A. (2012). The Pittsburgh Sleep Quality Index (PSQI). http://consultgerirn.org/uploads/File/trythis/try_this_6_1.pdf.

Social Security Administration. (2012). Annual statistical supplement to the Social Security Bulletin, 2011. http://www.ssa.gov/policy/docs/statcomps/supplement/2011/supplement11.pdf.

Sorrell, J. M. (2014). Postoperative cognitive dysfunction in older adults. A call for nursing involvement. *Journal of Psychosocial Nursing and Mental Health Services, 52*(11), 17–20.

Squires, B. (2014). Why are we encouraging struggling seniors to enroll in SNAP? AARP Foundation. http://www.aarp.org/aarp-foundation/our-work/hunger/info-2012/snap-food-benefits-help-seniors-enroll.html.

Touhy, T., & Jett, K. (2012). *Toward healthy aging: Human needs & nursing response* (8th ed.). St. Louis: Mosby.

Tyler, S., et al. (2014). "You can't get a side of willpower": Nutritional supports and barriers in The Villages, Florida. *Journal of Nutrition in Gerontology and Geriatrics, 33*, 108–125.

US Census Bureau. (2014). 10 percent of grandparents live with a grandchild, Census Bureau reports. http://www.census.gov/newsroom/press-releases/2014/cb14-194.html.

US Census Bureau. (2015a). FFF: Older Americans month: May 2015. https://www.census.gov/newsroom/facts-for-features/2015/cb15-ff09.html.

US Census Bureau. (2015b). Projections of the size and composition of the U.S. population: 2014 to 2060. https://www.census.gov/content/dam/Census/library/publications/2015/demo/p25-1143.pdf.

US Department of Agriculture. (2010). Dietary guidelines for Americans 2010. http://www.health.gov/dietaryguidelines/dga2010/DietaryGuidelines2010.pdf.

US Department of Health and Human Services (USDHHS). (n.d.). Quick guide to health literacy. https://health.gov/communication/literacy/quickguide/quickguide.pdf.

US Department of Health and Human Services (USDHHS). (2010). HHS announces the nation's new health promotion and disease prevention agenda. HHS News. https://www.healthypeople.gov/sites/default/files/DefaultPressRelease_1.pdf.

US Department of Health and Human Services (USDHHS). (2012a). Oral health. http://www.healthypeople.gov/2020/topicsobjectives2020/objectiveslist.aspx?topicId=32.

US Department of Health and Human Services (USDHHS). (2012b). Older adults. http://www.healthypeople.gov/2020/topics-objectives/topic/older-adults.

US Department of Health and Human Services (USDHHS). (2012c). Immunization and infectious diseases. https://www.healthypeople.gov/2020/topics-objectives/topic/immunization-and-infectious-diseases/objectives.

US Department of Health and Human Services (USDHHS). (2015). Injury and violence prevention. http://healthypeople.gov/2020/topicsobjectives2020/objectiveslist.aspx?topicId=24.

US Department of Health and Human Services (USDHHS), Health Resources and Services Administration, Maternal and Child Health Bureau. (2010). Injury and abuse. http://mchb.hrsa.gov/whusa10/hstat/wa/pages/243ia.html.

Vance, D. (2013). The cognitive consequences of stigma, social withdrawal, and depression in adults aging with HIV. *Journal of Psychosocial Nursing and Mental Health Services, 51*(5), 18–20.

Yesavage, J., et al. (1983). Development and validation of a geriatric depression screening scale: A preliminary report. *Journal of Psychiatric Research, 17*, 37–49.

Yellowlees, P. M. (2015). The value of the Mini-Mental State Exam. http://www.medscape.com/viewarticle/844603.

Zelle, A., & Arms, A. (2015). Psychosocial effects of health disparities of lesbian, gay, bisexual, and transgender older adults. *Journal of Psychosocial Nursing and Mental Health Services, 53*(7), 25–30.

# 25

# Health Promotion for the 21st Century: Throughout the Life Span and Throughout the World

*Ratchneewan Ross and Rosanna F. Hess*

## OBJECTIVES

*After completing this chapter, the reader will be able to:*

- Identify global trends and directions for health promotion and disease prevention including immunization programs.
- Discuss recent and emerging infectious disease including Ebola virus disease, Zika virus disease, human papilloma virus and cervical cancer, and methicillin-resistant *Staphylococcus aureus* infection.
- Describe problems and implications related to HIV/AIDS.
- Discuss problems and implications related to violence.
- Discuss problems and implications related to bioterrorism and terrorism.

## KEY TERMS

Anthrax (*Bacillus anthracis*)
Bioterrorism
Botulism
Ebola virus
Essential public health services
Human immunodeficiency virus

Human papilloma virus
Malnutrition
Methicillin-resistant *Staphylococcus aureus*
Plague
Self-abuse

Smallpox (*Variola major*)
Suicide
Terrorism
Violence
World Health Organization
Zika virus

 **THINK ABOUT IT**

### Human Papilloma Virus Infection and Cultural Practices

- *Adila lives in Ghana, West Africa, with her husband and her two daughters, aged 13 and 10 years. Adila learned 6 weeks ago that she has cervical cancer. When Adila told her husband that she had cervical cancer and needed treatment, he accused her of having sexual relations with another man and refused to give her money. He also refused to have his daughters vaccinated against human papilloma virus (HPV), which would prevent them from contracting cervical cancer. He said that this immunization would make them more sexually promiscuous as teenagers.*
- What kind of problems would you anticipate that Adila will encounter if she does not have treatment for her cervical cancer?

- How could Adila's husband be encouraged and educated to change his mind about his wife and daughters?
- What do you think could be done in this Ghanaian village to prevent further HPV infections *in addition* to an immunization campaign?

Visit the World Health Organization website (http://www.who.org) to identify the incidence and prevalence of HPV and cervical cancer in West African countries.

In the new millennium, the gap in life expectancies between people in developed and developing cultures has been widening. In many developed nations, such as Japan, France, Monaco, and the United States, people have a life expectancy at birth ranging from 80 to 89 years, whereas residents of some countries, such as Chad, Guinea-Bissau, and Afghanistan, can have a life expectancy as low as 49 to 50 years (Central Intelligence Agency [CIA], 2015a), attributable primarily to political instability and a high level of poverty, high rates of **human immunodeficiency virus (HIV)** infections, and low quality of life (CIA, 2015a,b; Joint United Nations Programme on HIV/AIDS [UNAIDS], 2014).

In 2012 there were 56 million deaths worldwide; 68% were due to noncommunicable diseases (cardiovascular diseases, cancer, respiratory diseases, and diabetes); more than 48% occurred in low- to middle-income countries, with a disproportionate rise in low-income countries. Almost 10 million children younger than 5 years died in 2015, a steady decline since 2000, but still a rate of 16,000 per day (WHO, 2015a). The mortality rate of children younger than 5 years was 11 times higher in low-income countries than the average rate in high-income countries (WHO, 2015a). On the basis of WHOs 2012 statistics, lower respiratory tract infections, HIV/AIDS, diarrheal diseases, and stroke were the leading causes of death for people in low-income countries, whereas ischemic heart disease and stroke were the leading causes of deaths in lower-middle-income, upper-middle-income, and high-income countries (WHO, 2015b) (Box 25-1: Quality and Safety Scenario).

Approximately 10.9% of the world's population, or 795 million of 7.3 billion, are chronically undernourished, and all but 10% of them are in developing countries (Food and Agriculture Organization of the United Nations et al., 2015). Annually, more than 3 million children die of starvation (Food and Agriculture Organization of the United Nations et al., 2015). Undernutrition heightens the effect of every disease. (Figure 25-1). At the other end of the spectrum, obesity is a rising cause of health problems in both medium- and high-income countries. The number of the world population with obesity more than doubled from 1980 to 2008, and almost 43 million children 5 years or younger were obese in 2008 (WHO, 2012a). Whereas urgent interventions to combat hunger and infectious diseases (such as HIV infection and diarrheal diseases) are needed in many developing countries, behavioral interventions to fight cardiovascular disorders and obesity are crucial in medium-income and high-income countries.

Emerging infections, various forms of intercultural and interpersonal violence, terrorism, and bioterrorism also pose great threats and risks to the world. This chapter presents information on malnutrition, **Ebola virus** disease (EVD), **Zika virus** disease (ZVD), **methicillin-resistant *Staphylococcus aureus*** (MRSA), HIV, and HPV infections, violence, bioterrorism, and terrorism, followed by discussion of their important implications for the future.

## MALNUTRITION

WHO (2000) defines **malnutrition** as "bad nourishment" that can be associated with "either too much or too little food intake and [is] not limited to the wrong types of food." Malnutrition is characterized by "inadequate or excess intake of protein, energy, and micronutrients such as vitamins." In general, malnutrition can be classified into three categories: protein-energy malnutrition, micronutrient deficiencies, and obesity (WHO, 2000). This chapter will address only protein-energy malnutrition because it is the most serious among the three types (WHO, 2000).

### Protein-Energy Malnutrition

Protein-energy malnutrition, a lack of calories and protein, is widespread in low-income countries and is the most lethal form

---

### ☑ BOX 25-1  QUALITY AND SAFETY SCENARIO

#### *HIV Education for Migrants From Russia*

A study examined male migrant workers' sexual behavior in St. Petersburg, Russia (*n* = 499), and revealed that 30% of these migrants reported having multiple female partners in the last 3 months. Condom use with their partners was reported to range from 35% to 52%. When asked about their knowledge of health risks in three major areas, central European migrant workers had the lowest levels of AIDS knowledge, followed by knowledge of the dangers of substance use, and the risks of unhealthy sexual activity. This group also reported high levels of depression and poor social support. In contrast, eastern European migrant workers reported higher levels for the same three areas of knowledge. More education about HIV is needed to prevent its transmission among these immigrants.

When one educates migrants from Russia as a health care professional, questions concerning the following should be included as part of an HIV educational session:

- The region in Russia from which the migrant emigrated
- The migrant's knowledge of HIV/AIDS and any unhealthy sexual activity
- The migrant's social support network

From Amirkhanian, Y. A., Kuznetsova, A. V., Kelly, J. A., Difranceisco, W. J., Musatov, V. B., Avsukevich, N. A., et al. (2010). Male labor migrants in Russia: HIV risk behavior levels, contextual factors, and prevention needs. *Journal of Immigrant Minority Health, 13*, 918–928.

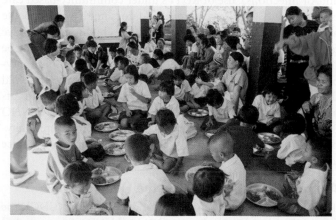

**FIGURE 25-1** Lunchtime for schoolchildren in a remote area of Thailand. The food was made possible through donations from health care providers.

of malnutrition/hunger (World Hunger Education Service, 2012). Humans convert food into energy, and the energy contained in food is measured in calories. Protein is necessary for key body functions, including provision of essential amino acids and development and maintenance of muscles (WHO & United Nations Children's Fund, [UNICEF], 2009). Protein-energy malnutrition can be severely harmful to the mental and physical development of individuals, especially children younger than 5 years (WHO, 2016h). Worldwide, one in two deaths among children younger than 5 years old stem from protein-energy malnutrition (WHO, 2016h). One in four children are underweight, and one in three children are stunted (WHO, 2016h).

## Severe Acute Malnutrition

WHO defines severe acute malnutrition as the presence of serious wasting and/or edema (WHO & UNICEF, 2009). Severe wasting is defined as the weight of a child being less than 70% (or less than three standard deviations) of the median weight for height (WHO, 2011) and/or having a mid-upper arm circumference less than 115 mm—a new cutoff (WHO & UNICEF, 2009). Children with severe acute malnutrition require immediate treatment because they have a higher risk of death than children without severe acute malnutrition (WHO & UNICEF, 2009). Severe wasting is caused by loss of subcutaneous fat and skeletal muscle and is highly noticeable because of underdeveloped buttocks, thighs, and upper arms. It is also characterized by sunken eyes, visible ribs, and protruding shoulder blades (WHO, 2004). Children with severe wasting usually have a distended abdomen and a general overall appearance in some way similar to that of an older adult. In general, these children are irritable, anxious, and cry easily; yet they will often have an absence of tears while crying because of lacrimal gland atrophy (WHO, 2004).

Treating children with severe acute malnutrition involves providing special therapeutic, milk-based foods called ready-to-use therapeutic foods (RUTFs), which are soft, crushable, and tasty, nutrient- and energy-rich foods that can be consumed by children 6 months of age or older (WHO & UNICEF, 2009). When a child has a good appetite with no medical conditions (e.g., hypoglycemia, hypothermia, dehydration, electrolyte imbalance, and/or infections), use of RUTFs under community-based care is appropriate. However, when a child does not have an appetite and/or medical conditions are present, the child needs to receive facility-based care (WHO & UNICEF, 2009). The child may be transferred from a facility-based care setting to a community-based setting when the following conditions are met: the child does not have bilateral edema, regains a good appetite, and eats at least 75% of his/her calculated RUTF ration for the day (WHO & UNICEF, 2009). The child can be discharged from a community-based care setting when he or she has a weight gain of 15% since admission (WHO & UNICEF, 2009) (Figure 25-2).

## Addressing Malnutrition at the Global Level

The Centers for Disease Control and Prevention (CDC), the World Health Organization (WHO), and UNICEF have worked collaboratively to create several initiatives to address the malnutrition issue. These include the Baby Friendly Hospital Initiative

programs to manage nutrition needs during emergencies, global nutrition data banks, a global network of collaborating centers in nutrition (UNICEF, 2012), and the International Micronutrient Malnutrition Prevention and Control (IMMPaCt) program (CDC, 2012a).

The Baby Friendly Hospital Initiative, launched in 1991 by UNICEF and WHO, has as its goal to promote exclusive breastfeeding during the first 4 months of life when it is most required by the infant (UNICEF, 2012). The program involves at least 170 countries and more than 16,000 hospitals (UNICEF, 2012). Through the initiative a mother starts breastfeeding as soon as her child is born and continues to breastfeed her child exclusively, unless medically otherwise indicated or until the child is 4 months old. This includes avoiding supplemental food and drink until the older child is ready for such intake (UNICEF, 2012).

The IMMPaCt program, established in 2000 by the CDC, works with global partners such as WHO, UNICEF, and the US Agency for International Development to provide its skills and resources to eradicate vitamin and mineral deficiencies around the globe (CDC, 2012a). The IMMPaCt program's activities include conducting surveys; providing micronutrients to infants, young children, and women of childbearing age; and monitoring and evaluating intervention systems (CDC, 2012a). Since its establishment, the IMMPaCt program has provided assistance and/or training in more than 70 countries around the world.

## EMERGING INFECTIONS

### Ebola Virus Disease

EVD (originally known as Ebola hemorrhagic fever) emerged on to the world scene of deadly infections in the mid-1970s in the African countries of the Democratic Republic of Congo and what is now known as South Sudan. The most recent major outbreak occurred in three countries in West Africa: Guinea, Sierra Leone, and Liberia. Case-fatality rates for EVD average approximately 50%, with deaths in some outbreaks as high as 90%. The virus spreads by human-to-human contact from an index case infected by contaminated blood, secretions, or bodily organs of a wild animal such as a fruit bat or monkey. Humans can be infected by contact with bedding and clothing of an infected person (CDC, 2016a; WHO, 2016a). The risk of transmission by sexual contact is an important concern, and research is ongoing (Fischer & Wohl, 2016). Current recommendations include abstinence from sexual intercourse for 3 months after development of symptoms or use of condoms if abstinence is not feasible (Rogstad & Tunbridge, 2015).

Currently there are no vaccines available to protect people from Ebola virus; therefore community involvement is vital for the prevention and control of an outbreak. Control measures include careful case management, contact tracing, a viable laboratory service, safe internment of deceased persons, and risk reduction for spread of the virus. See the section entitled "Prevention and control" in WHO (2016a) for details on these measures. Cultural practices differ greatly from country to country, region to region, and even village to village. The diversity of cultures must be taken into consideration when one is expecting a public

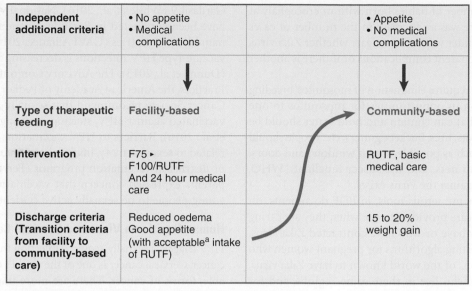

| Independent additional criteria | • No appetite<br>• Medical complications | | • Appetite<br>• No medical complications |
|---|---|---|---|
| Type of therapeutic feeding | Facility-based | | Community-based |
| Intervention | F75 ►<br>F100/RUTF<br>And 24 hour medical care | | RUTF, basic medical care |
| Discharge criteria (Transition criteria from facility to community-based care) | Reduced oedema<br>Good appetite<br>(with acceptableᵃ intake of RUTF) | | 15 to 20% weight gain |

aChild eats at least 75% of their calculated RUTF ration for the day

**FIGURE 25-2** Severe acute malnutrition management. *RUTF,* Ready-to-use therapeutic food. (Reprinted with permission from World Health Organization. [2011]. The WHO child growth standards. http://www.who.int/childgrowth/standards/en/.)

health response (Alexander et al., 2015). Burial practices, bushmeat consumption, use of traditional medicines, beliefs about modern medicine and health care interventions, and stigmatization of Ebola survivors are topics to include (Alexander et al., 2015). Ways to modify practices particularly related to the preparation of a dead body for burial must be found to curtail the spread of Ebola virus. This must be done in conjunction with an understanding of other nonpharmaceutical interventions (Pandey et al., 2014).

The prevention of the spread of infection in the health care setting must start with standard precautions when any patient is being cared for: basic hand hygiene, personal protective equipment, and respiratory hygiene. If EVD is suspected, health care workers must add extra protective measures to avoid contact with all bodily fluids and contaminated surfaces during direct patient care (Lupton, 2015; Marion et al., 2016). Protective clothing must include a face shield of some type, long-sleeved gown, and gloves. Laboratory workers must follow strict protection protocols. In the community, safe burial practices using the same techniques health care workers have instituted are essential.

Follow-up of EVD survivors is important for surveillance and treatment of long-term complications. Tiffany and colleagues (2016) found that 57% of EVD survivors followed up in Sierra Leone developed ocular complications. Others complications included arthralgia, fatigue, headaches, abdominal pains, and anemia. Even more difficult for survivors is the stigmatization they experience when discharged from the hospital. In a study of 81 EVD survivors in Sierra Leone (Nanyonga et al., 2016), 96% reported being rejected by their communities, leading to fear and anxiety about returning home. Economic hardships accompanied the physical and psychosocial sequelae. A full range of services are needed to care for these survivors.

## Zika Virus Disease

ZVD burst onto the global scene in 2015 with reports of hundreds of children in Brazil born with microcephaly to mothers who had been ill because of this virus. Zika virus was actually identified in the 1940s. The main vector is *Aedes* mosquitos known to live in Africa, the Americas, Asia, and the Pacific. Classic transmission is from the bite of an infected mosquito to a human. It is also now known that Zika virus can be transmitted from men who are infected with the virus during sexual contact. As the virus can stay in semen longer than it can in blood, the virus can be transmitted before a man develops symptoms, during the symptom phase, and even after symptoms have disappeared. Though transmission of Zika virus from male to female sexual partners in more likely (Coelho et al., 2016), reports confirm that female to male transmission is also possible (CDC, 2016c). For couples in which the woman could get pregnant, a condom should be used during every sexual contact or the couple should abstain from sexual relations to prevent infection with Zika virus for at least 6 months after symptoms appeared. If there were no symptoms but the man has traveled to a Zika virus–infested region, the couple should use a condom or abstain from sex for 8 weeks after the man returns (CDC, 2016c,d).

Most people infected with Zika virus will not exhibit symptoms. If symptoms appear, they are usually mild and can last up to 1 week. The symptoms include fever, joint and muscle pain, headache, and a rash. The virus can be detected by laboratory testing confirming its presence in blood, urine, and/or saliva. The incubation period is not yet well established but is believed to be a few days from bite to symptoms.

In 2015, public health officials in Brazil observed an increase in the number of patients with Guillain-Barré syndrome and an increase in the number of babies born with microcephaly at the same time as there was an increase in the number of cases of ZVD. Research is under way to investigate whether Zika virus is the cause of these apparent complications or if there is another reason.

Prevention of ZVD requires elimination of mosquitos' breeding sources and reduction in opportunities for mosquitos to bite people. Any objects that can contain and hold water should be removed or cleaned: pots, tires, buckets, gutters, etc. People should cover their skin as much as possible, screen windows and doors, sleep under mosquito nets, and use insect repellant (WHO, 2016b). No vaccine against the virus exists.

The CDC provides numerous tools, in PDF documents, on its website for health care providers to use when they are caring for patients who may have or who have contracted Zika virus. These tools include testing algorithms for pregnant women who have traveled to regions of the world known to have Zika virus, for pregnant women who live in these same regions, and for infants whose mothers reside in or traveled to Zika virus–infested areas of the world. Other tools include one to measure an infant's head circumference, fact sheets on testing for the virus, and preconception counseling (CDC, 2016b). There is also a page on the CDC website with details about a US Zika Pregnancy Registry. This page includes links to fact sheets for health care providers in general, one specific to pediatric health care providers, and one for pregnant women (CDC, 2016o). Interim guidelines are also available on this website.

## Human Papilloma Virus Infection

**Human papilloma virus (HPV)** is a group of approximately 150 related viruses, each with an assigned number. HPV is named for the warts it causes called papillomas. Almost 80 million people in the United States are infected with HPV, the most common sexually transmitted infection (CDC, 2016n). HPV is transmitted by intimate vaginal, anal, or oral contacts, even if the person is asymptomatic. Most HPV infections are asymptomatic and disappear without causing any problems; persistent ones, however, may lead to precancerous lesions, progressing years later to cervical cancer. HPV infections occur in men and women. Most HPV infections are acquired shortly after a person becomes sexually active with a person or persons infected with the virus. Abstinence, delay in becoming sexually active, use of condoms, limits on the number of sexual partners, and vaccination against HPV should slow down the increase in the number of people who carry and propagate HPV (WHO, 2015c).

### Vaccination

WHO 2014 guidelines included the following elements: vaccination of all girls aged 9 to 13 years with two doses of the HPV vaccine; screen women with HPV tests; and promote screening to a larger audience (WHO, 2014). Men should be included in any screening awareness efforts because without their support women in many cultures will not participate in screening practices (Learmonth et al., 2015; Lim & Ojo, 2016; Modibbo et al., 2016; William et al., 2014).

The HPV vaccine was introduced in 2006. The current FDA-approved vaccines against HPV are Gardasil, Cervarix, and Gardasil 9 (White et al., 2016). National vaccination programs have been conducted in Rwanda, Uganda, and Uzbekistan, to name a few countries (GAVI Alliance, 2014). The prevalence of vaccine-type HPV infections is decreasing in US vaccinated girls (Dunne et al., 2015). The Advisory Committee on Immunization Practices, the American Academy of Pediatrics, and the American Cancer Society recommend that sexually active young men be vaccinated against HPV, starting at the age of 11 years (White et al., 2016). Barriers to HPV vaccination include social norms related to sexual activity, financial constraints, and levels of trust or distrust in vaccination programs (Ferrer et al., 2014). Some parents expressed concern that vaccination would encourage young people to be sexually active (Griebeler et al., 2012).

### Human Papilloma Virus and Cervical Cancer

HPV triggers a sexually acquired infection that may lead to cervical cancer. Cervical cancer is one of the world's deadliest, but preventable, forms of cancer. There are more than 500,000 new cases each year (International Agency for Research on Cancer, 2013; WHO, 2015c). Approximately 85% of the approximately 270,000 annual deaths occur in the developing world. Cervical cancer incidence rates in sub-Saharan Africa are the highest in the world (De Vuyst et al., 2013). The risk factors for persistent HPV infection and progression to cervical cancer include early first sexual intercourse, multiple sexual partners, and a compromised immune system (WHO, 2015c). Lack of access to effective screening and to services that promote early detection and treatment may explain the dramatic differences in prevalence.

### Screening and Testing

Screening recommendations in the United States are set by the American Cancer Society, the American College of Obstetricians & Gynecologists, and the US Preventive Services Task Force. The current recommendations for routine cervical screening are as follows (CDC, 2015b): start at age 21 years and continue through to age 65 years; conventional or liquid-based cytological tests (Papanicolaou test) for women younger than 30 years; for women 30 years or older, include oncogenic or high-risk HPV tests; every 3 years for women 21 to 29 years of age perform a Pap test; for women aged 30 to 65 years, perform co-testing; if the results of both tests are negative, screening is not recommended again for 5 years; the testing recommendations are the same for women regardless of whether they have been vaccinated against HPV or not; refer women with abnormal test results to an appropriate provider for follow-up. Barriers to cervical screening include fear of diagnosis, lack of access, lack of spousal support, lack of finances, cultural modesty (only wanting a female provider), not knowing about cervical cancer, and not seeing self as having risk factors (Compaore et al., 2015; Lim & Ojo, 2016). A promising screening test is careHPV (Bansil et al., 2014; Jeronimo et al., 2014).

Health care professionals have an important role to play in the promotion of vaccinations against HPV and screening for HPV and cervical cancer. Studies have noted that when health care providers, particularly nurses, educate women and recommend the vaccine, immunization rates increase (Lau et al., 2012). Fact sheets, continuing education courses, and vaccination schedules and recommendations for use by health care providers in combating HPV infections and subsequent cancer risks can be found on the CDC website (CDC, 2016n).

## Methicillin-Resistant *Staphylococcus aureus* Infection

Colonization of *S. aureus* in the nasal area is common and asymptomatic in one in three healthy individuals (CDC, 2011; Perencevich & Diekema, 2010). On the other hand, MRSA, a form of staphylococcus bacteria that causes skin/soft tissue infections, is estimated to be colonized in only 1% of healthy individuals (CDC, 2011). It is resistant to β-lactams (e.g., methicillin, oxacillin, penicillin, and amoxicillin) (CDC, 2012b).

Health care–associated MRSA (HA-MRSA) infection may occur in hospitalized individuals who undergo medical or surgical procedures, such as administration of ventilation apparatus or introduction of a nasogastric tube or catheter (particularly in those with minimized immune functions), and can lead to life-threatening infections, such as pneumonia and bacteremia. However, a study that reviewed 82% of all MRSA cases in the United States from 2005 through 2008 showed that life-threatening HA-MRSA infections dropped by 28% (Kallen et al., 2010). Factors related to the decline were not reported.

In the community setting, community-associated MRSA (CA-MRSA) strains have emerged as serious threats in the past 2 decades and can cause dermatitis and soft tissue infections (CDC, 2010, 2012b), with the ability to also cause fatal infections in the lungs (e.g., necrotizing pneumonia, purpura fulminans, and postviral toxic shock syndrome) (Schlievert et al., 2010). Most CA-MRSA cases are mild and include a skin or soft tissue infection (i.e., a boil or abscess). Usually, the infected area resembles a red, swollen, and painful "spider bite" (CDC, 2010). Pus or other drainage may be present. If the infection is limited to the skin, it can be difficult to distinguish CA-MRSA from HA-MRSA (CDC, 2010).

Among severely CA-MRSA-infected people, complications may include serious necrotizing infection, septicemia, pneumonia, and death (CDC, 2010).

CA-MRSA cases have been reported by emergency departments, day care centers, schools, correctional facilities, sports facilities, dormitories, and military stations (CDC, 2011; Sedighi et al., 2011). People who are generally healthy can contract the bacteria through close skin-to-skin contact, cuts in or abrasions of the skin, crowded conditions, shared utilities (e.g., clothing items and towels), and poor hygiene (CDC, 2011; Kirkland & Adams, 2008). In addition, those who are taking or have previously received antibiotic therapy have a greater risk of infections than those who do not have a history of antibiotic intake (Fekete, 2007).

The most up-to-date clinical guidelines for CA-MRSA management were published in 2011 by Liu and colleagues (2011). The guidelines suggest that CA-MRSA skin infections, such as boils or abscesses, may be treated by incision and drainage. Antibiotic regimens guided by sensitivity test results should be administered to infected individuals. Intravenous antibiotic treatment should be considered among hospitalized individuals who show signs of oral therapy nonadherence. Oral antibiotics may include sulfamethoxazole-trimethoprim, clindamycin, doxycycline, minocycline, and linezolid.

Knowledge of this disease is essential to enable health care professionals to initiate appropriate infection control. In general, CA-MRSA spreads more easily, has higher recurrence rates, and causes more skin problems and serious damage than the traditional HA-MRSA found in hospital settings (CDC, 2012b). Standard precautions—a combination and expansion of universal precautions and body substance isolation—are required among health care professionals to prevent cross-contamination (CDC, 2011). Meticulous hand washing has been found to be important and is recommended as a cost-effective everyday practice; see CDC (2006) for more details. Current recommendations by the CDC for various sectors of the community are on the CDC website at http://www.cdc.gov/mrsa/community/index.html.

## Human Immunodeficiency Virus/Acquired Immunodeficiency Syndrome

Approximately 36 million people worldwide are infected with HIV, with 25 million in sub-Saharan Africa, 3.9 million in South/Southeast Asia, 1.5 million in Latin America, 1.3 million in eastern Europe and Central Asia, 1.3 million in North America, 860,000 in western/central Europe, 880,000 in East Asia, 260,000 in the Middle East/North Africa, 250,000 in the Caribbean, and 51,000 in Oceania (UNAIDS, 2017).

Although the number of newly infected people continues to decline each year, approximately 2.5 million people were infected in 2012. During the same year, there were 1.6 million AIDS-related deaths (CDC, 2016p). Overall, the number of people living with HIV reflects the fact that people receiving antiretroviral therapies are living longer (CDC, 2016p).

In some low-income countries, HIV prevalence rates in the adult population are higher than those in high-income countries. For instance, the 2014 rate was 27.73% in Swaziland and 25.16% in Botswana (CIA, 2015b). The rate is approximately 0.18% in Sweden and 0.33% in the United Kingdom (CIA, 2015b). Although economic level is sometimes negatively associated with HIV rates, evidence also shows that cultural beliefs and practices are significant factors contributing to HIV infections.

The modes of HIV transmission include sexual contact with persons of the opposite sex, sexual contact with persons of the same sex, from mother to baby at birth or through breast milk, contact with objects contaminated with HIV such as needles, syringes, and knives, and through blood transfusions of HIV-infected blood. In east and southern Africa, 60% to 95% of the new infections are occurring among the heterosexual population, people with multiple sex partners, their usual partners, and couples in a mutually faithful discordant relationship. (*Discordant relationship* in this context is defined as one partner infected with HIV and the other partner HIV negative.) In Caribbean and Latin American countries, the largest group of new infections is in men who have sex with men, although there are sizeable new infections also among sex workers and their clientele, and in the general heterosexual population. In Eastern Europe, newly infected individuals are mostly those who are intravenous drug users and their sexual partners. In Asia, male risk behaviors dominate the transmission methods (Gouws & Guchi, 2015).

Clearly, the challenges of reducing HIV/AIDS rates are complex and the solutions require multidisciplinary and multidimensional approaches. Ordinary people, community leaders, health care professionals, and organizations at all levels must work collaboratively. Together, we can consider gender/social inequalities and cultural/religious beliefs and practices as we work to identify barriers to understanding and facilitate the reduction of HIV infections (Box 25-2). Support from all parties will enable us to set priorities and fight HIV/AIDS more effectively at the global level. UNAIDS (2011) is working collaboratively with its partner organizations, such as UNICEF, UNESCO, WHO, and the World Bank. The ambitious visions of UNAIDS include zero new HIV infections, zero AIDS-related deaths, and zero discrimination; the commitment is that everyone globally should have universal access to HIV prevention, treatment, care, and support (UNAIDS, 2011). To reach these optimal goals, UNAIDS has outlined three strategic directions: revolutionizing HIV prevention; catalyzing the next generation for treatment, care, and support; and advancing human rights and gender equality in responses to HIV (UNAIDS, 2011).

*Revolutionizing HIV prevention* means that the focus is shifted from HIV rates of "prevalence" to "incidence" (UNAIDS, 2011). "Incidence" deals with the number of new HIV infections in a particular population during a certain period, whereas HIV "prevalence" is the percentage of all cases (new and old) of HIV infections at a certain time point (AVERT, 2012). In this focus, hot spot transmissions need to be identified, and empowerment (especially among young people) needs to be encouraged so that all people involved will adopt more proactive behaviors to decrease the number of new HIV infections. UNAIDS (2011) has announced its support of political change in terms of HIV, new approaches to technology, the reduction of stigma and discrimination associated with HIV, and comprehensive sex education for HIV-positive individuals, networks, and related key populations.

*Catalyzing the next generation of treatment, care, and support* involves universal access to antiretroviral treatment for all HIV-positive individuals who need medication (Box 25-3: Research for Evidence-Based Practice). UNAIDS (2011) expects that all HIV-positive individuals and their families will have access to essential care and support. UNAIDS (2011) will act with each nation to make it possible that simpler, more effective, and more affordable therapy will be universally accessible so that HIV deaths related to tuberculosis infection will be minimized.

*Advancing human rights and gender equality for the HIV response* means working toward the day when gender inequality, violence against women and girls, and stigmatization and discrimination related to HIV will be eradicated (UNAIDS, 2011).

Punitive laws and practices against HIV-positive individuals need to be eliminated. UNAIDS (2011) will work with each government to reinforce the rights of HIV-positive individuals and to better educate infected individuals about their rights. UNAIDS proposes to accelerate the full implementation of these goals within countries by building synergies with communities and other organizations.

## Nongovernmental Organizations

UNAIDS has recognized the importance of the inclusion of nongovernmental organizations (NGOs) in the worldwide fight against the spread of HIV/AIDS. The UNAIDS Programme Coordinating Board has as its nonvoting members representatives from three NGOs from developing countries and two NGOs from developed countries. "The NGO representatives actively seek input from their respective communities on key issues related to UNAIDS policies and programs, and advocate with Members States (governments) and Cosponsoring organizations (the ten United Nations organizations that make up the UNAIDS Joint Programme) for meaningful improvements in the implementation and evaluation of AIDS policies and programmes" (UNAIDS, 2007).

## VIOLENCE

**Violence** can happen to individuals anywhere, regardless of gender, age, or nationality, and is among the leading causes of physical, sexual, reproductive, and mental health problems worldwide. Each year, violence has been estimated to cause the loss of 1.6 million lives globally. In addition, violence costs nations immeasurable amounts of money in terms of health care, law enforcement, and loss of productivity. The cost of violence containment to the world economy was approximately US$9.46 trillion in 2012 (Dickenson-Jones et al., 2014).

## Definition of Violence

Violence is defined differently in different parts of the world, depending on people's beliefs and cultures. The definition proposed by WHO is used in this chapter. According to WHO (2012b), violence is defined as "intentional use of physical force or power, threatened or actual, against oneself, another person, or against a group or community, that either results in or has a high likelihood of resulting in injury, death, psychological harm, maldevelopment or deprivation."

In response to violence, WHO has proposed the four-step public health approach that includes the following steps: defining the problem; identifying risks and protective factors; devising and testing means of dealing with violence; and applying successful means on a large scale (CDC, 2012c). Successful response prevention of violence should be based on rigorous research and collaboration among health care professionals and other experts in areas such as epidemiology, criminology, education, and economics.

The CDC is an example of an organization in the United States that is applying the preceding four-step public health model. Activities, projects, and funding supported by the CDC are outlined in the following sections as an exemplar.

### Defining the Problem

To understand the magnitude of violence in the United States, different data sources are needed. Such sources may include police reports, medical examiner files, vital records, medical records, population-based surveys, and research results. Extrapolation of the data from these sources can help us to learn about violence frequencies, places, trends, and perpetrators. The CDC has provided funding to studies deemed to be helpful in defining violence problems. The National Violent Death Reporting System is an example of a project funded by the CDC to ensure that timely, complete, and accurate data are collected about violent deaths for different states in the United States. It is hoped that the data will enable each state to gain a clearer picture of violence so as to respond more effectively (CDC, 2012b).

### Identifying Risk and Protective Factors

A "risk factor" is defined as "a characteristic that increases the likelihood of a person becoming a victim or perpetrator of violence," and a "protective factor" is defined as "a characteristic that decreases the likelihood of a person becoming a victim or perpetrator of violence" (CDC, 2015a). Knowing risk and protective factors can help responsible organizations and personnel to estimate violence magnitudes and devise appropriate prevention measures. It is important to note that the identification of risk factors should be used not to blame victims of violence but rather as a focus for intervention.

### Devising and Testing Means for Dealing With Violence

In this step, data on violence from all available sources are extrapolated and assessed. On the basis of the evidence, programs and interventions are planned. Such programs and interventions are then implemented, tested, and rigorously evaluated to determine their effectiveness. An example of step 3 activities is the Choose Respect project—a communication initiative for sixth grade to eighth grade students to guide adolescents in forming healthy relationships so as to prevent dating violence (CDC, 2012b). Technology also plays a role in protecting violence victims. The MyPlan app is a web-based safety planning tool that helps violence victims to respond to dating violence. It enhances victims' decisional conflict and safety behavior (Glass et al., 2015).

### Applying Successful Means on a Large Scale

After a program has been tested successfully for its effectiveness, large-scale dissemination should occur. At this stage, communities are encouraged to adopt a program tailored to their own problems and needs. The program should be evaluated in each community. Training, networking, technical assistance, and process evaluations are to be supported by all parties involved. An example of step 4 activities initiated by the CDC is the National Youth Violence Prevention Resource Center with its goal to prevent youth violence and suicide. In this project, a website, toll-free hotline, and fax-on-demand service were created as helpful resources for youth. Any interested community can request more information from the CDC.

## Forms and Context of Violence

WHO (2016c) classifies violence into three major categories: interpersonal, self-directed, and collective.

### Interpersonal Violence

Interpersonal violence (IPV) is violence committed by an individual or a small group of people in a wide range of acts and behaviors (emotional, physical, sexual, and psychological). The violence could happen to people of any age (adolescents, children, and older adults). It could also occur anywhere, including the home, workplace, neighborhood, and unfamiliar places.

Whereas violence in the community (e.g., youth violence or crimes) is highly visible, violence in the home is usually hidden. The impact of such hidden violence is complicated by the fact that authorities or health personnel are less willing or prepared to deal with it (Koistinen & Holma, 2015).

The risk factors for IPV include a victim's low self-esteem, low self-control, and personality/conduct disorders (CDC, 2015a). Other risk factors are reported to be lack of social support, dysfunctional family structure, family history of violence, and drug and alcohol abuse (Ross et al., 2015; Sullivan, 2013). Alcohol intoxication may increase violent actions by impairing the drinker's cognitive functions and processes through alterations of social cue perceptions and inhibitions (Bernardin et al., 2014). According to the Department of Justice, 37% of convicted offenders were drinking at the time of their arrest (National Council on Alcoholism and Drug Dependence, 2015).

In addition, four subtypes of male perpetrators are reported as the mentally ill, undercontrolled/dysregulated, chronic batterer, and overcontrolled/catathymic subtypes (Koistinen & Holma, 2015). Shared characteristics were found among the four subtypes of male perpetrators. For example, most of them were abused as children, tend to be in their mid-30s to late 30s, and tend to show pathology (Koistinen & Holma, 2015).

Mothers who are victims of violence along with their children who witness such violence are at risk of physical, emotional, psychological, and developmental damage (McFarlane et al., 2014). A study in New York revealed that IPV is a primary cause for seeking treatment at the emergency department because of the different injuries (Gilbert et al., 2012). In the Latino population, help-seeking action is increased among children who witness IPV episodes as they call 911 for help (Falconier et al., 2013).

Culture and gender inequality are also significant factors in IPV. Evidence shows that women in countries where gender equality is emphasized experience violence less than those in countries with gender inequality (Fulu et al., 2013). Fulu and colleagues (2013) reported that that the highest rate of physical and/or sexual violence among women was in Papua New Guinea (80.0%), whereas a rate of 25% was reported in Indonesia.

A study among 245 women in Thailand revealed that the rate of emotional abuse was 88.2%, that of physical abuse was 59.2%, and that of sexual abuse was 23.9% (Ross et al., 2015). Predictors of emotional abuse included partner's drug use and gambling behavior. The predictor of physical abuse was drug abuse. No predictor was found for sexual abuse. Violence in this study was found to be associated with depression and physical problems (Ross et al., 2015). This result aligns with a study that summarizes the literature concerning history of childhood sexual abuse and depression or depressive symptoms among pregnant and post-partum women, which revealed that women who were abused reported higher rates of postpartum depression than those who did not experience abuse (Wosu et al., 2015). Social support was found to mediate the effects of IPV on depression and physical health in the Thai study (Ross et al., 2015).

It is important for health care providers to understand the seriously negative impact that IPV can have on individuals. They should be able to identify such violence and be aware of helpful resources for people affected by violence, as well as their children. Local domestic violence crisis contact information (i.e., numbers and counseling services) should be readily provided to these people. A sexual violence assessment and care guide as proposed by Ross and colleagues (2009) is a helpful resource for health care professionals who work with female care recipients, especially for those who feel uncomfortable mentioning the subject (Ross et al., 2010). This tool has been used successfully by community health nurses in Thailand (Sawangchareon et al., 2013).

## Self-Directed Violence

Self-directed violence is defined by WHO (2016c) as "violence in which the perpetrator and the victim are the same individual and is subdivided into self-abuse and suicide." It is estimated that almost 1 million individuals die by suicide annually (a person commits suicide every 40 seconds) (WHO, 2012d). Previously, suicide rates had been highest among the male older adult.

However, the rates among young people aged 15 to 24 years have been increasing to such an extent that suicide is the second leading cause of death in this age group in some developed and developing countries (WHO, 2012d). Although the major factors contributing to suicide in Europe and North America include mental disorders, especially depression, and alcohol use disorders, impulsiveness is found to be a major factor in Asian countries (WHO, 2012c).

WHO (2012c) recommends that effective suicide prevention interventions should include restriction of access to common methods of suicide where possible or when prudent, along with effective prevention and treatment of depression and alcohol and substance abuse. However, there are clearly challenges to such interventions. In many countries, for example, a lack of awareness about suicide and the taboo to discuss suicide openly exist. Many countries will need to initiate training for prevention of suicide, including appropriate certification for health care personnel, and to seek the involvement of individuals from sectors other than health care, including education, labor, law, politics, police, justice, religion, and the media.

## Collective Violence

Collective violence is defined as the instrumental use of violence by a particular group of people for specific political, economic, or social objectives. Such violence may include armed conflicts within or between states or nations, genocide, terrorism, repression, and other abuses of human rights (WHO, 2012d) (Figure 25-3).

In the 20th century, it is estimated that 191 million people lost their lives as a result of armed conflict. More than half of these people were civilians. In 2000, more than 300,000 people died because of collective violence. Most victims lived in the poorer regions of the world (WHO, 2012d). Besides death, the aftermath of collective violence includes physical and psychological disabilities that exert burdens on families, communities, and nations. Young children and refugees are usually among the most vulnerable to the aftermaths of disease and posttraumatic stress disorders (PTSDs) related to violence (WHO, 2012b).

WHO (2012b) is committed to working with its partners at the regional, national, and international levels to prevent collective violence. Its goal is to identify and implement preventive strategies. Data collection systems are used to support and evaluate the

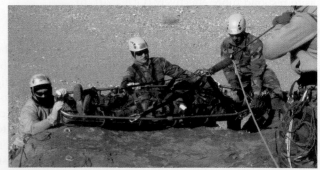

**FIGURE 25-3** Armed conflicts can be within or between states and nations.

success of the strategies. In this effort, political commitment and momentum are required from a wide variety of concerned parties to strengthen and increase violence prevention endeavors in the next 5 years (WHO, 2012b).

## TERRORISM

The threat of terrorism—whether homegrown or international—creates a unique brand of fear among individuals and communities within our increasingly interconnected global cultures (Braithwaite, 2013). Moreover, the need to be able to respond to terrorism—potential or actual—poses important challenges to health care professionals and community planners at all levels of our society (Figure 25-4). The International Council for Nurses describes its position on the role of nursing concerning disaster preparedness to include risk assessment as well as management strategies bridging multiple disciplines and system levels.

Nursing plays a key role in responding to the short-, medium-, and long-term requirements of populations stricken by disaster. The establishment of a set of tailor-made disaster nursing core competencies for the community and the development of a comprehensive curriculum for public health will help nurses plan for and streamline health care responses to such mass events internationally (Loke & Fung, 2014). Much work in laying the foundations for such a broader, more global preparedness has already been started.

Research on the surgical responses to the 2008 terrorist attacks in Mumbai, India, reveals the importance of an initial disaster management plan to treat casualties. The earliest victims of firearm and blast trauma were received in a primary triage zone and then sent to different stations for further treatment. The study concluded that onsite triage—established as soon as a site

is found to be safe—optimizes the treatment of bullet and blast injuries (Bhandarwar et al., 2012). Another study examined the effectiveness of including a pediatric trauma center (PTC) in responding to victims of a disaster surge. This study added a hypothetical PTC to the response of the Israeli Defense Forces field hospital to the Haiti earthquake in 2010 and measured its effectiveness mathematically, concluding that "aggressive inclusion of PTCs in planning for disasters by public health agencies" (Barthel et al., 2011) can significantly increase overall rates of admission and greatly reduce treatment times (Barthel et al., 2011). Regarding the responses of health care providers to the repercussions of mass disasters, the results from the literature are sometimes conflicting. In the United Sates, studies among victims of the World Trade Center disaster in terms of PTSD suggest that early and brief interventions at the work site were most effective in responding to PTSD, and that informal support from family, friends, and spiritual communities was also beneficial. Conversely, more extensive postdisaster psychotherapy was not found to be beneficial and sometimes led to worse outcomes (Boscarino & Adams, 2008). Mental resilience following the World Trade Center disaster tended to be linked with victims who had higher self-esteem and more social support, whereas victims who experienced "delayed" PTSD following the attacks tended to be "non-native born, or to have recently experienced lower self-esteem and/or negative life events" (Boscarino, 2011). In Thailand, cognitive-behavioral therapy as a means to treat PTSD was studied in a randomized controlled effectiveness trial. The researchers found that cognitive-behavioral therapy can successfully treat PTSD, even "in settings where very regular [terrorist] attacks are made upon communities in which the patient lives" (Bryant et al., 2011).

Among its overarching influences, one must also weigh terrorism's negative consequences for economies around the world. These include changes in "variables such as Gross Domestic Product (GDP), unemployment, foreign direct investment (FDI), and the tourism industry" (Waxman, 2011). Such economic changes affect the lives of everyday people and, in turn, their health. The threat of terrorism is thus real, and its actual and potential negative effects are pervasive and far-reaching, spanning cultures and ranging from the concrete and immediate to the psychosocial and lasting. Nurses and health care professionals must be among the front lines of response.

### Bioterrorism

*A bioterrorism attack is the deliberate release of viruses, bacteria, or other germs (agents) used to cause illness or death in people, animals, or plants. These agents are typically found in nature, but it is possible that they could be changed to increase their ability to cause disease, make them resistant to current medicines, or to increase their ability to be spread into the environment. Biological agents can be spread through the air, through water, or in food. Terrorists may use biological agents because they can be extremely difficult to detect and do not cause illness for several hours to several days. Some bioterrorism agents, like the smallpox virus, can be spread from person to person and some, like anthrax, cannot.*

*(CDC, 2016e)*

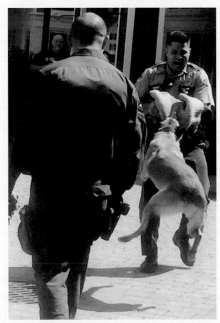

**FIGURE 25-4** The need to be able to respond to terrorism poses important challenges to all.

The preceding definition reflects what many people in different nations may feel or know about bioterrorism. As health care professionals, we are required to be knowledgeable about possible diseases/agents that could be used for bioterrorism and the proper responses we should make to an act of bioterrorism.

Bioterrorism is classified by the CDC (2016e) into three different categories: A, B, and C. These categories are based on the ease with which the disease or agent might be spread; the potential negative impact it could have on public health; the extent to which it could cause public panic or social disruption; and the degree to which it would require the public to prepare for an attack.

## Category A Diseases/Agents

Category A diseases/agents include various biological agents and pathogens that are not usually seen in the United States and pose the highest risks and have the highest priority. They include anthrax, botulism, plague, smallpox, tularemia, and viral hemorrhagic fevers.

**Anthrax (Bacillus anthracis).** Since the anthrax (*Bacillus anthracis*) mailing attacks on a few recipients in the United States in 2001, no other attacks have been reported (CDC, 2016g). These unfortunate mail recipients contracted the bacillus either cutaneously or inhalationally. Cutaneous anthrax contractors developed erythema (red, inflamed area similar to cellulitis) on exposed areas of the hands, arms, or face that later transformed into painful vesicles and then necrotic painless, depressed, black eschar. Inhalation anthrax contractors had fever, dyspnea, cough, and chest discomfort (CDC, 2016h). Usually, respiratory failure and hemodynamic collapse will follow. Other symptoms may include lymphangitis and painful lymphadenopathy. It is recommended that individuals receive a complete treatment of ciprofloxacin, levofloxacin, doxycycline, or penicillin for 60 days (Hendricks et al., 2014). Vaccines against anthrax have been developed, and evidence shows that they can be effective in preventing the disease (Wright et al., 2014). The CDC (2016i) and its partners are working collaboratively to develop more effective anthrax vaccines. Questions and answers about anthrax vaccines can be found at http://www.cdc.gov/vaccines/hcp/vis/vis-statements/anthrax.pdf.

**Smallpox (Variola major).** It is believed that smallpox (*Variola major*) was eradicated in 1977. However, there are fears that a strain kept in a laboratory could be used as a bioweapon. According to the CDC (2016j), however, the United States has enough vaccines for everyone if needed. The side effects from smallpox vaccination mostly involve a mild fever, soreness in the injection area, and enlarged glands in the armpit (CDC, 2016k). In rare circumstances, severe side effects may occur and need medical attention. To learn more about potentially serious and life-threatening side effects, visit https://www.cdc.gov/smallpox/vaccine-basics/vaccination-effects.html.

Smallpox symptoms usually resemble influenza symptoms, which include fever and myalgias, followed by a rash. Rashes in smallpox can be differentiated from those of chickenpox (varicella). A rash from smallpox is most prominent on the face and extremities with the same stage of lesion development. A rash from chickenpox is more prominent on the trunk, with different stages of lesion development and resolution. The CDC (2016l) provides an acute, generalized vesicular or pustular rash illness testing protocol in the United States. The CDC (2016q) also provides an on-line assessment of a rash as a way to identify whether or not the rash is an indicator of a smallpox infection.

## Category B Diseases/Agents

Category B diseases/agents are those that pose the second highest risks for world and national security. They include brucellosis; food safety threats (e.g., *Salmonella* sp., *Escherichia coli* O157:H7, *Shigella*); glanders; melioidosis; psittacosis; Q fever; ricin toxin; staphylococcal enterotoxin B; typhus fever; viral encephalitis; and water safety threats (e.g., *Vibrio cholerae*, *Cryptosporidium parvum*).

## Category C Diseases/Agents

Category C diseases/agents are emerging pathogens that could be reproduced for mass dissemination. They include emerging infectious diseases such as Nipah virus and hantavirus.

## Epidemic and Pandemic Alert and Response

The CDC has created a public health emergency response guide to help public health professionals at the state, local, and tribal levels respond to an emergency in the first 24 hours. Health care providers should be alerted to any unusual symptoms indicative of an infectious outbreak related to bioterrorism. In turn, if a bioterrorist action is suspected, health care providers should report it to their local or state health department. According to the CDC (2016f), indications of bioterrorism include "an unusual temporal or geographic clustering of illness (e.g., persons who attended the same public event or gathering) or individuals presenting with clinical signs and symptoms that suggest an infectious disease outbreak (e.g., more than two persons presenting with an unexplained febrile illness associated with sepsis, pneumonia, respiratory failure, or rash or a botulism-like syndrome with flaccid muscle paralysis, especially if occurring in otherwise healthy persons); an unusual age distribution for common diseases (e.g., an increase in what appears to be a chickenpox-like illness among adult persons, but which might be smallpox); and a large number of cases of acute flaccid paralysis with prominent bulbar palsies, suggestive of a release of *botulinum* toxin." To learn more about clinical diagnosis, management, and responses to bioterrorism, refer to the CDC website at https://emergency.cdc.gov/bioterrorism/ and http://www.cdc.gov/mmwr/preview/mmwrhtml/mm5041a2.htm.

At the international level, responses to bioterrorism have also been prepared. WHO is a core organization responding to the needs for such preparation at this level. WHO works collaboratively with agencies in many countries to gather reports of suspected outbreaks and rumors regarding bioterrorism through advanced technologies from all sources available, both formally and informally.

The Global Public Health Intelligence Network, a significant source of informal information related to outbreaks, was also collaboratively established by Health Canada and WHO. Its multilingual capabilities are Internet based, constantly searching data worldwide to identify information regarding disease outbreaks that can place international public health sectors at risk (WHO, 2016d).

The 2005 International Health Regulations—legally-binding regulations across countries led by WHO—are embraced by most nations throughout the world. Their mission is to provide legal frameworks to ensure health security among nations without unnecessary international traffic and trade interference (WHO, 2016e). To learn more about the International Health Regulations, see WHO (2016e).

## NATURAL DISASTERS

Natural disasters have existed since Earth was formed. They are phenomena that occur through natural forces involving land, air, or water, and they often have large-scale negative impacts on humans who live in the affected areas. Examples of natural disasters include tsunamis, earthquakes, floods, landslides, mudslides, tornadoes, hurricanes, cyclones, typhoons, wildfires, volcano eruptions, extreme heat, and winter weather (CDC, 2016m). Natural disasters in recent decades have been reported to cause more harm in developing countries than developed countries, attributable in part to deforestation and inadequate warning and emergency management systems (Cameron & Shah, 2015). Health care professionals should be aware of recent large-scale natural disasters and be familiar with their negative impact on human well-being. Critically, lessons learned from the successful or unsuccessful management of these disasters should be shared among health care professionals so as to appropriately address and minimize the effects of future disasters.

### Effects of Natural Disasters on Human Well-Being

All humans are affected by natural disasters economically, physically, and psychologically. In 2014, 317 natural disasters were reported around the world, which affected 94 countries. This means 107 people were affected by disasters around the world, and 8186 deaths were caused by these disasters. For example, 58 million people were affected by floods and storms in China (International Federation of Red Cross and Red Crescent Societies, 2015).

Concerning the physical effects of natural disasters, victims tend to have limited access to essential infrastructures for survival related to food, water, shelter, and sanitation. These deficiencies can lead to infections and undernutrition (Kouadio et al., 2012). Undernutrition, in turn, can lead to malnutrition and starvation—especially among infants and children in low-resource countries (Food & Agriculture Organization, 2016). Infection outbreaks commonly diagnosed after natural disasters during the period from 2000 to 2011 included diarrhea, acute respiratory tract infections, viral hepatitis, and snail and trematode infections (Kouadio et al., 2012)

In terms of the psychological impact of natural disasters, PTSD is a classic negative effect that occurs among victims of all ages. Natural disasters can cause a significant amount of stress, especially from the loss of loved ones (Bread, 2014). A survey of flood victims in 2000 in Hunan province, China, showed that PTSD among the victims still existed 13 years later. No relationship was found between demographic characteristics and the recovery from PTSD (Hu et al., 2015). A follow-up study in China among 1573 adolescent survivors at 6, 12, 18, and 24 months after an earthquake found that negative life events, less social support, and less positive coping were common predictors of poor recovery (Fan et al., 2015). A cross-sectional study of 350 survivors from the Mount Merapi volcanic eruption in Indonesia reported that female adults aged between 18 and 59 years, and individuals who owned their own home experienced the highest levels of negative psychosocial impact (Warsini et al., 2015). In conclusion, psychological trauma has been reported as a result of natural disasters regardless of age or country of residence.

### Natural Disaster Responses and Preparedness

In general, immediate medical care and rapid emergency response are important to address natural disasters, especially among children and women. Unfortunately, such care and response are reported to be inadequate regardless of the country type. However, the inadequacy of emergency care is heightened in developing nations (Zhong et al., 2014). For example, with the 2010 earthquake in Haiti, more than 200,000 people lost their lives, with 1.5 million people losing shelter (Thomson Reuters Foundation, 2015). As the poorest country in the Western world, Haiti already had limited resources before the earthquake. As many as 40% of rural Haitians did not have access to primary health care before the disaster, and 70% of health provisions in Haiti overall before the disaster were offered by NGOs (Gelting et al., 2013). Although psychiatric mental health needs surged after the earthquake, existing mental health services in Haiti were damaged by the two crumpled, understaffed psychiatric hospitals as a consequence of the earthquake.

The psychiatrist-to-person ratio was 0.2 to 100,000 before the earthquake, and this ratio became worse when some health care workers were among the injured (WHO, 2016f). Vodou, a common belief about magic and illness in Haiti, is deemed by some to function as the main Haitian health care system (McAlister, 2016). Vodou beliefs might be considered by some professionals as a hindrance to modern mental health acquisition. Yet evidence shows that if a strong collaboration is established between traditional healers and health care providers, mental health services can be enhanced in the process (Khoury et al., 2012).

### International Standard Guidelines for Emergency Mental Health Response

Before 2007, there was a lack of consensual international guidelines for emergency mental health response (WHO, 2016g). However, after the Asian tsunami in 2004, a taskforce was established composed of both governmental and nongovernmental experts from more than 100 various organizations and 27 different countries (WHO, 2016g). This taskforce, the Inter-Agency Standing Committee (IASC), developed the 2007 "IASC Guidelines on Mental Health and Psychosocial Support in Emergency Settings," reflecting standards for appropriate emergency mental health care for victims around the world (WHO, 2016g). The IASC guidelines are consistent with WHOs recommendations for emergencies among developing nations in that all victims and affected families should have access to emergency assistance with equality and dignity, and that helping people to remain resilient after a disaster is important. Besides these general principles, the minimum response for primary care clinics to help victims with severe psychological needs is outlined by the IASC and includes 10 major tenets (WHO, 2016g):

- Each victim is assessed holistically.
- Each victim will have access to essential psychiatric drugs.
- At least one emergency primary health care (PHC) professional is available to tend to victims' mental health in the affected area.
- The care provided by the PHC professional is adequately supervised.
- PHC professionals will be assigned to specific trainings and will not be overwhelmed by unnecessary training sessions.
- Additional mental health service points will be established for victims' accessibility.
- Unnecessary duplicating services should be avoided.
- All people affected by a disaster are informed about available mental health services.
- Primary care clinics should work collaboratively with local community agencies to discover, visit, and help the target population.
- Primary care clinics should have a major role in collaboration with other mental health agencies.

To learn more about the IASC's guidelines and related work, see WHO (2016g).

### Emergency Management for Infants in Developed Countries

Most infants in developing countries are breastfed. Thus when natural disasters occur, they tend to do better than infants in developed countries because their mothers have mobile fresh milk supplies for them as long as they are with their mothers during the disaster (Gribble & Berry, 2011). Infants in developed countries whose primary food is based on formula feeding can be vulnerable because of a lack of supplies during a disaster (Gribble & Berry, 2011). Therefore emergency preparedness for these infants should be in place. In general, it is recommended that a week's supply of necessary items is available for infants. For exclusively breastfed infants, 100 diapers and 200 wipes are the only items needed. For bottle-fed infants, more items are recommended for their survival (Gribble & Berry, 2011). Mothers of infants with ready-to-use formula will need the following items: 56 single servings of the formula, 84 L of drinking water, 56 feeding bottles or cups, 56 zip-lock plastic bags, a large storage container, a small bowl, a metal knife, 120 antiseptic wipes, detergent, 200 sheets of paper towels, 100 diapers, and 200 wipes (Gribble & Berry, 2011). Mothers of infants with powdered infant formula will need the following items: 2 cans of infant formula, 170 L of drinking water, a feeding cup, a large storage container, a measuring cup, a large cooking pot with a lid, a kettle, a gas stove, a box of matches/lighters, 14 kg of liquid cooking gas, a metal knife, a pair of metal tongs, 120 antiseptic wipes, detergent, 300 sheets of paper towels, 100 diapers, and 200 wipes (Gribble & Berry, 2011). Health care professionals who care for mothers with their infants should be trained to provide appropriate information to the mothers based on their feeding strategy.

The Office of Public Health Preparedness and Response provides very helpful information about the steps and types of emergency responses on the CDC website (CDC, 2012d).

## IMPLICATIONS

The health-promotion and disease-prevention priorities that have been outlined in this chapter present challenges and opportunities for health care providers—as individuals and as a collective profession—to play key roles in emerging systems emphasizing health promotion and disease prevention. The goals for optimal health of individuals include greater longevity and quality of life, while decreasing sex, racial, and ethnic disparities (Purnell, 2008). The principles of primary prevention, health care policies, cultural diversity, cultural competency, and multidisciplinary teamwork in health promotion are critical to a new era that strives to achieve dramatic changes in health care delivery (Purnell, 2008). Through a perspective on the development of community-based, health-promotion programs, health care professionals can bring a balance to decisions that will be made about the appropriate use of traditional and newer health care resources (Box 25-4: *Healthy People 2020*).

Ten essential public health services as proposed by the CDC (2014) were developed in 1994 by the Core Public Health Functions Steering Committee, comprising representatives from various US Public Health Service agencies and other key public health organizations. This framework can be instrumental for health care professionals in various fields and can be applied at all levels, ranging from local to international. The 10 essentials include:

- Monitoring the health status of individuals and communities so as to address identified health problems
- Diagnosing and investigating health problems and health hazards among individuals in the community
- Informing, educating, and empowering people with regard to health problems and various ways to address the problems, including applying strengths found in the community
- Mobilizing community partnerships and community actions so that health problems can be identified and addressed
- Developing policies and plans that will assist individuals and their communities to address identified problems
- Enforcing laws and regulations to provide and protect the safety and health of individuals and communities
- Linking people to appropriate health services to ensure accessible health care
- Ensuring proficient personal and public health care workforces
- Evaluating the accessibility, effectiveness, and quality of health services
- Searching for innovative ideas and solutions to identified health problems

For more information about the 10 essentials, see CDC (2014). These 10 essentials—along with an awareness of human rights, empowerment, cultural diversity, and cultural competence (Box 25-5: Diversity Awareness)—can help health care professionals effectively deliver care to individuals and communities. It is important, moreover, to help individuals, families, and communities become active participants in defining their own health needs, in making informed decisions to meet those needs, and, ultimately, in bringing about real improvements in their own health status and quality of life.

An increasing demand for primary health care providers will continue to spur the need for more advanced practice

**BOX 25-4 HEALTHY PEOPLE 2020**

**Topic Area: Genomics**

- To increase the proportion of women with a family history of breast and/or ovarian cancer who receive genetic counseling. (In 2005, 23.3% of US females with such a history obtained genetic counseling. The target for 2020 is 25.6%.)
- To increase the proportion of individuals with newly diagnosed colorectal cancer who receive genetic testing to identify Lynch syndrome (or familial colorectal cancer syndromes).

**Topic Area: Global Health**

- To reduce the number of cases of malaria reported in the United States. (In 2008, 1298 new cases of malaria were reported in the United States. The target for 2020 is 999 new cases.)
- To decrease the tuberculosis (TB) case rate for foreign-born individuals living in the United States. (In 2008, 20.2 cases of TB per 100,000 population were reported for foreign-born individuals living in the United States. The target for 2020 is 14.0 cases per 100,000 population.)
- To increase the number of global disease detection regional centers (GDDRCs) worldwide to detect and contain emerging health threats. (In 2009, seven GDDRCS were active. The target for 2020 is to have 13 active GDDRCs.)
- To increase the number of public health professionals (PHPs) trained by global disease detection (GDD) programs worldwide. (In 2009, 37,132 PHPs were trained by GDD programs. The target for 2020 is to have 144,132 trained by GDD programs.)
- To increase diagnostic testing capacity in host countries and regionally through the GDDRCs. (In 2009, 154 tests were established or substantially improved by GDD programs. The target for 2020 is 264 established/substantially improved tests.)

**Topic Area: Health Care–Associated Infections**

- To reduce central line–associated bloodstream infections. (In 2006–08, a standardized infection ratio of 1.00 was reported. The target for 2020 is a standardized infection ratio of 0.25, a 75% reduction.)
- To reduce invasive HA-MRSA infections. (In 2007–08, 26.24 infections per 100,000 persons were reported. The target for 2020 is 6.56 infections per 100,000 persons, a 75% reduction.

**Topic Area: (Selected) Health Communication and Health IT**

- To increase the proportion of individuals who report that their health care professional (HCP) always listened carefully to them. (In 2007, 59% of individuals reported that their HCP always listened carefully to them. The target for 2020 is 65%.)
- To increase the proportion of individuals who report that their HCP always explained things so they could understand them. (In 2007, 60% of individuals reported that their HCP always explained things so they could understand them. The target for 2020 is 66%.)
- To increase the proportion of individuals who report that their HCPs always involved them in decisions about their health care as much as they wanted. (In 2007, 51.6% of individuals reported that their HCPs always involved them

in decisions about their health care as much as they wanted. The target for 2020 is 56.8%.)

- To increase the proportion of individuals who use the Internet to keep track of personal health information, such as care received, test results, or upcoming medical appointments. (In 2007, 14.3% of individuals reported using the Internet to keep track of personal health information, such as care received, test results, or upcoming medical appointments. The target for 2020 is 15.7%.)
- To increase the proportion of individuals who use the Internet to communicate with their provider. (In 2007, 13.6% of individuals reported using the Internet to communicate with their provider. The target for 2020 is 15.0%.)
- To increase the proportion of individuals with access to the Internet. (In 2007, 68.5% of individuals reported having access to the Internet. The target for 2020 is 75.4%.)
- To increase the proportion of individuals with broadband access to the Internet. (In 2007, 75.6% of individuals reported having broadband access to the Internet. The target for 2020 is 83.2%.)
- To increase the proportion of individuals who use mobile devices. (In 2007, 6.7% of individuals reported using mobile devices. The target for 2020 is 7.7%.)
- To increase the proportion of adults who report having friends or family members with whom they talk about their health. (In 2007, 79.5% of adults reported having friends or family members that they talk to about their health. The target for 2020 is 87.5%.)
- To increase the proportion of on-line health information seekers who report easily accessing health information. (In 2007, 37.3% of on-line health information seekers reported easily accessing health information. The target for 2020 is 41.0%.)
- To increase the proportion of medical practices that use electronic health records. (In 2007, 25.0% of medical practices reported using electronic health records. The target for 2020 is 27.5%.)

**Topic Area: Selected Preparedness**

- To reduce the time necessary to activate designated personnel in response to a public health emergency. (In 2009, 66 minutes was needed for designated personnel to report for immediate duty with no advance notice. The target for 2020 is 60 minutes.)
- To increase the proportion of Laboratory Response Network (LRN) biological laboratories that meet the proficiency standards for category A and category B threat agents.
- To increase the proportion of LRN chemical laboratories that meet the proficiency standards for chemical threat agents. (In 2008, 92% of LRN chemical laboratories met the proficiency standards for chemical threat agents. The target for 2020 is 95%.)
- To reduce the time for state public health agencies to establish after-action reports and improvement plans following responses to public health emergencies and exercises. (In 2009, 46 days were required for state public health agencies to establish such reports and plans. The target for 2020 is 41 days.)

From US Department of Health and Human Services. (2010). *Healthy People 2020*. Washington, DC: US Government Printing Office.

nurses, including nurses with degrees of doctor of nursing practice and doctor of philosophy. This demand can be met if undergraduate students are introduced early to concepts of health promotion and disease prevention with an emphasis on evidence-based practice, human rights, cultural diversity, and cultural competency, and with a global perspective (Purnell, 2008). In this way, health promotion, quality of life, and socioeconomic justice might become increasingly valued in cultures throughout the world.

In addition, health care educational programs in culturally diverse global frameworks that teach about malnutrition, emerging diseases, HIV/AIDS, bioterrorism, violence, and other contemporary challenges will help nurses and other professionals play innovative roles in health care and maximize the quality of life around the world. Faculty and students will ideally increase their work together in interdisciplinary teams, using an expanding variety of health-promotion services and guided by national and international standards. Given the increasing focus on cultural

## 🌐 BOX 25-5 DIVERSITY AWARENESS

### Health and Health Promotion in a Native American Tribe: The Navajo

The Navajo people of the *Dine Bikeyah* live on a vast land in which the four states of Arizona, Utah, New Mexico, and Colorado intersect. The Navajo hold this land as sacred and as an integral part of their lives. They believe that health is a part of the *hozho'*, which is a personal sense of well-being and rightness with the world and is all-inclusive. For the Navajo, health is not separate from the overall state of balance among the body, mind, spirit, and the surrounding environment. When one of these is out of balance, *hozho'* is not achieved. *Hozho'* is everything that a Navajo thinks of as being good, in terms of good and evil or favorable and unfavorable. The Navajo strive to maintain *hozho'* and to live in harmony with all things that surround them. The goal of Navajo life in this world is to live to attain maturity with *hozho'* and to die of old age, the result of which incorporates beauty, harmony, and happiness or *sa'ah naagh"ii bik'eh hozho'*. When the body, spirit, or mind fall out of *hozho'*, a traditional healer or medicine man is sought. In many instances, the medicine man recommends that the individual seek both Western medicine and the traditional ways to cure the problem.

Since 1955, trends in Navajo health have demonstrated a progressive improvement, particularly in the areas of maternal and infant mortality. However, on the increase are lifestyle-related diseases and premature deaths, for which health-promotion activities can have an effect. Among these lifestyle-related diseases are adult-onset diabetes, AIDS, and alcohol and substance abuse. Health care providers who work with the Navajo must address all health-promotion and disease-prevention activities in terms of an appreciation for the cultural and economic realities and the needs of this community.

From The Official Navajo Nation Visitor Guide. (2017). Navajo cultural history and legends; Anonymous. (n.d.). Navajo land. http://www.discovernavajo.com.

diversity and self-care in disease prevention and health promotion, nurses can respond directly to the health needs of individuals, families, communities, and groups by focusing on health promotion and disease prevention tailored to particular cultures and spiritual beliefs and by supporting new ways to work and live.

In the area of research, understanding health care practices and the impact of culture on people from different nations will enable health care professionals to create appropriate health-promotion and disease-prevention interventions. Thus international collaborative research is important. Sex and age disaggregated data quantitative and qualitative analysis needs to be used more widely in research so that data can be categorized by sex and age/age group, which will allow examination and identification of needs that are specific to each sex and age group (Mazurana et al., 2011). Sex and age disaggregated data could be especially beneficial in the assessment of crisis situations such as bioterrorism and terrorism because they help to identify the immediate needs of particular groups, the reasons they need immediate help, and the resources that can be most helpful (Inter-Agency Standing Committee Gender Sub-Working Group, 2009).

To be advocates for newly emerging priorities for disease prevention and health promotion, nurses in the 21st century need to engage in the following:

- Participate in policy development for health promotion as the health care of individuals in acute settings shifts from hospitals to home and community settings. Thus the attention to health-promoting behaviors in home and community environments provides an entry point for the development of models of primary care that emphasize both health promotion and disease prevention in communities.

- Influence public expectations about health promotion. Presentations and other forms of public dialogue and education will help raise awareness of the value of individual and community health promotion. Nurses have the collective capacity to change the philosophy of the system from selling health care in the marketplace to creating a milieu for changing health behaviors. Encouraging meaningful community participation in addressing health issues provides a significant opportunity to narrow the gap between what is possible in terms of health promotion in each country and what is reality. As mentioned earlier, violence and emerging diseases are among the challenges today that require heightened public awareness.

- Promote equitable access to preventive health care. Given the higher rates of preventable conditions among populations in resource-poor countries, a need to promote the justified distribution and utilization of preventive health services is apparent. Community-based efforts that combine public and private resources should be targeted to those most in need of health care. Delivery models that focus on integrating preventive and primary care should be expanded.

Preventive health care delivery should be based on broad research agendas that encompass multiple health and social science perspectives. Health care providers should participate in areas of research that will cost-effectively influence both personal and community health. Service delivery can also benefit from expanded health service research agendas that foster collaboration among disciplines and countries. Most important, preventive health care should be adapted to the health and social problems of specific groups and cultures. Alternative approaches to health-promotion and preventive service delivery should be used where they are most effective to meet new international health challenges, including mobile vans, school and work site clinics, and other community-based, collaborative actions (Box 25-6: Innovative Practice).

## SUMMARY

This chapter has presented priority issues and future directions for health professions in the areas of health promotion and disease prevention from a world perspective. Current emerging health care reform efforts pose significant challenges and opportunities for health care providers, educators, and researchers, with the emphasis on human rights, cultural diversity, and cultural sensitivity; health promotion and disease prevention; evidence-based practice and advanced technology; and global perspectives. Nurses in the new millennium are required to have sufficient vision, expertise, and the ability to truly make a difference in the health of the people for whom they care at individual, local community, national, and international levels. Through leadership, creativity, and determination, nurses and other health care providers can establish a healthier future for people around the globe with a respect for human needs, cultural diversity, and human rights.

### Haitian Health Foundation: A Charitable Outreach to Neighbors in Need

A volunteer effort of health professionals initiated in Haiti in 1982 by Dr. Jeremiah Lowney and his wife, Virginia, has grown into an outpatient health care facility supported by a nondenominational foundation called the Haitian Health Foundation (HHF). In 1985, after working for 4 years in Port au Prince, HHF moved its outreach to Jeremie, Haiti, at the suggestion of Mother Teresa of Calcutta, to bring health care, hope, and opportunity to this especially poor and remote area. The clinic at Jeremie employs 105 people, including 2 full-time physicians, 1 full-time dentist, 10 registered nurses, 2 licensed professional nurses, a medical technician, a dental assistant, and 70 to 80 auxiliary personnel (all Haitians). The clinic provides health care to more than 120,000 Haitians yearly (Haitian Health Foundation, 2016).

The Haitian Agents de Sante program currently employs villagers in 936 villages surrounding Jeremie. This program was initiated by a nurse who enlisted an individual who had a seventh grade education in each village. After being educated in health promotion, the person became the health agent of that village. These health agents are trained by HHF to provide preventive and basic health care and education. Many villages have also begun mothers' groups, by which women can share experiences and knowledge relating to nutrition, health care, and other topics that have an effect on their quality of life. Breastfeeding classes and immunization programs are available.

Another program was begun by the building of a food distribution pavilion. This building will be used to store and distribute food to more than 1000 children and pregnant women three times a week. The pavilion will also be used to educate participants in nutrition and preventive health care. Much of the education in these programs is accomplished through song, primarily because this approach appears to enable the Haitians to remember what is being taught.

For more than 8 years, another education program has provided access to schools for poor children in a country in which education is neither free nor mandatory. In 2016, almost 3300 students attended school through this program. Tuition, uniforms, books, and shoes are provided by HHF funds or through the Save-a-Family Plan.

HHF relies heavily on the generosity of donors and the many volunteers who donate their time and talents to supplement the staff in Haiti. Volunteers travel to Jeremie at their own expense from the United States, Canada, and Europe to share their skills and resources with the poor. These volunteers include health care providers, electricians, plumbers, teachers, clergy, and students.

These programs are only a few examples of the health-promotion programs sponsored by HHF. These efforts show how dedicated professionals can make a difference, even in third world countries in which health care resources are rare.

Courtesy Jeremiah Lowney. (2016). *Our impact*. Haitian Health Foundation. http://www.haitianhealthfoundation.org/our-impact/

---

## CASE STUDY

### Nutrition: Don

Don is a 4-year-old boy who is brought to a rural health department clinic by his grandmother. Don and his family are recent immigrants from Laos and have lived in this area for less than 1 year. This is Don's first visit to the clinic. Don looks weak, with sunken eyes and a dry mouth. His weight is less than 70% (or less than three standard deviations) of the median weight for height, and he has underdeveloped buttocks, thighs, and upper arms. Through a translator, Don's grandmother tells the community health nurse that Don has had diarrhea for more than 2 days and that the family can barely "make ends meet." Don's parents are seasonal farmworkers and are at work today.

**Reflective Questions**
- Who is Don's caretaker during the day?
- How can the nurse help Don's family learn about the resources available in their community?
- Where does the nurse direct Don's family for immediate help?
- How would the nurse follow up with the family to prevent further problems with this child?

---

## ◎ CARE PLAN

### Nutrition: Don

**\*NURSING DIAGNOSIS: Imbalanced nutrition—less than body requirement related to inadequate food intake and diarrhea as evidenced by a weight of less than 70% (or less than three standard deviations) of the median weight for height; underdeveloped buttocks, thighs, and upper arms; and sunken eyes and dry mouth**

**Defining Characteristics**
- A weight of less than 70% (or less than three standard deviations) of the median weight for height
- Underdeveloped buttocks, thighs, and upper arms
- Sunken eyes, dry mouth, and a history of diarrhea

**Related Factors**
- Poverty, lack of knowledge about available resources

**Short-Term Expected Outcomes**
The grandmother will:
- Increase health-promotion and health-maintenance knowledge regarding Don's nutrition
- Increase health-promotion and health-maintenance practices regarding Don's nutrition

- Gain access to available resources, such as Food Stamps and the Special Supplemental Nutrition Program for Women, Infants, and Children

**Long-Term Expected Outcome**
- Don will show no signs of malnutrition.

**Interventions**
- Give Don fluids/food per protocol.
- Observe Don's fluid/food intake and monitor his signs and symptoms.
- If necessary, refer Don to an appropriate health setting.
- Assess the grandmother's knowledge and practices regarding Don's nutrition.
- Educate the grandmother about the negative effects of malnutrition on Don's growth and development.
- Educate the grandmother about appropriate food choices for Don.
- Assist the family to access and connect with available nutrition community resources.
- Assist Don's parents to access the community career center.
- Provide follow-ups to monitor Don's physical progress (body weight for age and height) and family's access to available resources.

\*NANDA Nursing Diagnoses—Herdman T. H. & Kamitsuru, S. (Eds.). Nursing Diagnoses–Definitions and Classification 2015–2017. Copyright © 2014, 1994–2014 NANDA International. Used by arrangement with John Wiley & Sons Limited. In order to make safe and effective judgments using the NANDA-I nursing diagnoses it is essential that nurses refer to the definitions and defining characteristics of the diagnoses listed in this work.

## ⓔ EVOLVE CHAPTER FEATURES

http://evolve.elsevier.com/Edelman/
- Study Questions

## REFERENCES

Alexander, K. A., et al. (2015). What factors might have led to the emergence of Ebola in West Africa? *PLoS Neglected Tropical Diseases, 9*(6), e0003652.

AVERT. (2012). Understanding HIV and AIDS statistics. http://www.avert.org/statistics.htm.

Bansil, P., et al. (2014). Acceptability of self-collection sampling for HPV-DNA testing in low-resource settings: A mixed methods approach. *BMC Public Health, 14*(1), 596.

Barthel, E. R., et al. (2011). Availability of a pediatric trauma center in a disaster surge decreases triage time of the pediatric surge population: A population kinetics model. *Theoretical Biology and Medical Modeling, 8*(38), 1–32.

Bernardin, F., Maheut-Bosser, A., & Paille, F. (2014). Cognitive impairments in alcohol dependent subjects. *Frontiers in Psychiatry, 5*(78), 1–6.

Bhandarwar, A. H., et al. (2012). Surgical response to the 2008 Mumbai terror attack. *British Journal of Surgery, 99*(3), 368–372.

Boscarino, J. A. (2011). Introduction to special issue commemorating the 10th anniversary of September 11, 2001. *International Journal of Emergency Mental Health, 13*(2), 65–67.

Boscarino, J. A., & Adams, R. E. (2008). Overview of findings from the World Trade Center disaster outcome study: Recommendations for future research after exposure to psychological trauma. *International Journal of Emergency Mental Health, 10*(4), 275–290.

Braithwaite, A. (2013). The logic of public fear in terrorism and counter-terrorism. *Journal of Police and Criminal Psychology, 28*(2), 95–101.

Bread, K. (2014). Long-term health problems after natural disasters strike. http://www.usnews.com/news/articles/2014/01/06/long-term-health-problems-after-natural-disasters-strike.

Bryant, R. A., et al. (2011). A randomized controlled effectiveness trial of cognitive behavior therapy for post-traumatic stress disorder in terrorist-affected people in Thailand. *World Psychiatry, 10*, 205–209.

Cameron, L., & Shah, M. (2015). Risk-taking behavior in the wake of natural disasters. *Journal of Human Resources, 50*(2), 484–515.

Centers for Disease Control and Prevention (CDC). (2006). Strategies for clinical management of MRSA in the community: Summary of an experts' meeting convened by the Centers for Disease Control and Prevention. http://www.cdc.gov/mrsa/pdf/MRSA-Strategies-ExpMtgSummary-2006.pdf.

Centers for Disease Control and Prevention (CDC). (2010). MRSA. https://www.cdc.gov/mrsa/.

Centers for Disease Control and Prevention (CDC). (2011). MRSA and the workplace. http://www.cdc.gov/niosh/topics/mrsa/.

Centers for Disease Control and Prevention (CDC). (2012a). Global health programs: International Micronutrient Malnutrition Prevention and Control Program (IMMPaCT). http://www.cdc.gov/globalhealth/programs/IMMPaCT.htm.

Centers for Disease Control and Prevention (CDC). (2012b). Precautions to prevent spread of MRSA. https://www.cdc.gov/mrsa/healthcare/clinicians/precautions.html.

Centers for Disease Control and Prevention (CDC). (2012c). Violence prevention. http://www.cdc.gov/violenceprevention/.

Centers for Disease Control and Prevention (CDC). (2012d). Emergency preparedness and response. https://emergency.cdc.gov/.

Centers for Disease Control and Prevention (CDC). (2014). The public health system and the 10 essential public health services. http://www.cdc.gov/nphpsp/essentialservices.html.

Center for Disease Control and Prevention (CDC). (2015a). Intimate partner violence: Risk and protective factors. http://www.cdc.gov/violenceprevention/intimatepartnerviolence/riskprotectivefactors.html.

Centers for Disease Control and Prevention (CDC). (2015b). HPV-associated cancers and precancers. http://www.cdc.gov/std/tg2015/hpv-cancer.htm.

Centers for Disease Control and Prevention (CDC). (2016a). Ebola (Ebola virus disease). http://www.cdc.gov/vhf/ebola.

Centers for Disease Control and Prevention (CDC). (2016b). Zika and pregnancy. http://www.cdc.gov/zika/about/index.html.

Centers for Disease Control and Prevention (CDC). (2016c). Zika virus. Tools for health care providers. https://www.cdc.gov/zika/hc-providers/.

Centers for Disease Control and Prevention (CDC). (2016d). Zika virus and sexual transmission. http://www.cdc.gov/zika/transmission/sexual-transmission.html.

Centers for Disease Control and Prevention (CDC). (2016e). Bioterrorism overview. https://www.emergency.cdc.gov/bioterrorism/pdf/bioterrorism_overview.pdf.

Centers for Disease Control and Prevention (CDC). (2016f). Syndrome definitions for diseases associated with critical bioterrorism-associated agents. http://emergency.cdc.gov/bioterrorism/surveillance.asp.

Centers for Disease Control and Prevention (CDC). (2016g). The threat. http://www.cdc.gov/anthrax/bioterrorism/threat.html.

Centers for Disease Control and Prevention (CDC). (2016h). Symptoms. http://www.cdc.gov/anthrax/basics/symptoms.html.

Centers for Disease Control and Prevention (CDC). (2016i). Prevention. http://www.cdc.gov/anthrax/medical-care/prevention.html.

Centers for Disease Control and Prevention (CDC). (2016j). Smallpox fact sheet. Smallpox overview. The disease. https://stacks.cdc.gov/view/cdc/26503/Share.

Centers for Disease Control and Prevention (CDC). (2016k). Side effects of smallpox vaccination. https://www.cdc.gov/smallpox/vaccine-basics/vaccination-effects.html.

Centers for Disease Control and Prevention (CDC). (2016l). Diagnosis and evaluation. https://www.cdc.gov/smallpox/clinicians/diagnosis-evaluation.html.

Centers for Disease Control and Prevention (CDC). (2016m). Emergency preparedness and response. http://emergency.cdc.gov/disasters/.

Centers for Disease Control and Prevention (CDC). (2016n). Human papillomavirus. http://www.cdc.gov/hpv.

Centers for Disease Control and Prevention (CDC). (2016o). US Zika Pregnancy Registry. http://www.cdc.gov/zika/hc-providers/registry.html.

Centers for Disease Control and Prevention (CDC). (2016p). Living with HIV. http://www.cdc.gov/hiv/basics/livingwithhiv.

Centers for Disease Control and Prevention (CDC). (2016q). Evaluating patients for smallpox: Acute, generalized vesicular or pustular rash illness protocol. https://www.cdc.gov/smallpox/clinicians/algorithm-protocol.html.

Central Intelligence Agency (CIA). (2015a). Life expectancy at birth. https://www.cia.gov/library/publications/the-world-factbook/rankorder/2102rank.html.

Central Intelligence Agency (CIA). (2015b). HIV/AIDS adult prevalence rates. https://www.cia.gov/library/publications/the-world-factbook/rankorder/2155rank.html.

Coelho, F. C., et al. (2016). Higher incidence of Zika in adult women than adult men in Rio de Janeiro suggests a significant contribution of sexual transmission from men to women. *International Journal of Infectious Diseases, 51*, 128–132.

Compaore, S., et al. (2015). Barriers to cervical cancer screening in Burkina Faso: Needs for patient and professional education. *Journal of Cancer Education*, 1–7.

De Vuyst, H., et al. (2013). The burden of human papillomavirus infections and related diseases in sub-Saharan Africa. *Vaccine, 31*, F32–F46.

Dickenson-Jones, G., Hyslop, D., & Vaira-Lucero, M. (2014). Estimating the global costs of violence. *Business, Peace and Sustainable Development, 2014*(2), 6–27.

Dunne, E. F., et al. (2015). Reduction in HPV vaccine type prevalence among young women screened for cervical cancer in an integrated health care delivery system, United States 2007 and 2012-2013. *Journal of Infectious Diseases, 212*(12), 1970–1975.

Falconier, M. K., et al. (2013). Interpartner violence among Latinos: Community perceptions on help seeking and needed programs. *Partner Abuse, 4*(3), 356–379.

Fan, F., et al. (2015). Longitudinal trajectories of post-traumatic stress disorder symptoms among adolescents after the Wenchuan earthquake in China. *Psychological Medicine, 45*(13), 2885–2896.

Fekete, T. (2007). Emerging infections: What you need to know, part 1. *Consultant, 47*(12), 1013–1016.

Ferrer, H. B., et al. (2014). Barriers and facilitators to HPV vaccination of young women in high-income countries: A qualitative systematic review and evidence synthesis. *BMC Public Health, 14*, 700.

Fischer, W. A., & Wohl, D. A. (2016). Confronting Ebola as a sexually transmitted infection. *Clinical Infectious Diseases : an Official Publication of the Infectious Diseases Society of America*, doi:10.1093/cid/ciw123.

Food and Agriculture Organization of the United Nations. (2016). Malnutrition. http://www.fao.org/3/a-i4646e.pdf.

Food and Agriculture Organization of the United Nations, International Fund for Agricultural Development, & World Food Programme (2015). *The state of food insecurity in the World 2015. Meeting the 2015 international hunger targets: taking stock of uneven progress.* Rome: Food and Agriculture Organization.

Fulu, E., et al. (2013). Prevalence of and factors associated with male perpetration of intimate partner violence: Findings from the UN multi-country cross-sectional study on men and violence in Asia and the Pacific. *The Lancet Global Health, 1*(4), e187–e207.

GAVI Alliance. (2014). 1.5 million girls set to benefit from vaccine against cervical cancer. http://www.gavi.org/library/news/press-releases/2014/1-5-million-girls-set-to-benefit-from-vaccine-against-cervical-cancer.

Gelting, R., et al. (2013). Water, sanitation and hygiene in Haiti: Past, present, and future. *The American Journal of Tropical Medicine and Hygiene, 89*(4), 665–670.

Gilbert, L., et al. (2012). Substance use and partner violence among urban women seeking emergency care. *Psychology of Addictive Behaviors, 26*(2), 226–235.

Glass, N., et al. (2015). A safety app to respond to dating violence for college women and their friends: The MyPlan study randomized controlled trial protocol. *BMC Public Health, 15*(1), 871.

Gouws, E., & Guchi, P. (2015). Focusing on HIV response through estimating the major modes of HIV transmission: A multi-country analysis. *Sexually Transmitted Infections, 88*, i76–i85.

Gribble, K. D., & Berry, N. (2011). Emergency preparedness for those who care for infants in developed country contexts. *International Breastfeeding Journal, 6*(16), http://www.internationalbreastfeedingjournal.com/content/pdf/1746-4358-6-16.pdf.

Griebeler, M., et al. (2012). Parental beliefs and knowledge about male human papillomavirus vaccination in the U.S.: A survey of a pediatric clinic population. *International Journal of Adolescent Medicine & Health, 24*(4), 315–320.

Hendricks, K. A., et al. (2014). Centers for Disease Control and Prevention Expert Panel meetings on prevention and treatment of anthrax in adults. *Emerging Infectious Diseases, 20*(2), http://wwwnc.cdc.gov/eid/article/20/2/13-0687_article.

Hu, S. H., et al. (2015). Recovery from post-traumatic stress disorder after a flood in China: A 13-year follow-up and its prediction by degree of collective action. *BMC Public Health, 15*(615), 2–7.

Inter-Agency Standing Committee Gender Sub-Working Group (2009). *Sex and age disaggregated data in humanitarian action: SADD project.* New York: Inter-Agency Standing Committee Gender Sub-Working Group.

International Agency for Research on Cancer. (2013). Latest world cancer statistics. Global cancer burden rises to 14.1 million new cases in 2012. Marked increases in breast cancer must be addressed. Press release no.223. https://www.iarc.fr/en/media-centre/pr/2013/pdfs/pr223_E.pdf.

International Federation of Red Cross and Red Crescent Societies. (2015). World disaster report 2015. https://ifrc-media.org/interactive/wp-content/uploads/2015/09/1293600-World-Disasters-Report-2015_en.pdf.

Jeronimo, J., et al. (2014). A multicountry evaluation of careHPV testing, visual inspection with acetic acid, and Papanicolaou testing for the detection of cervical cancer. *International Journal of Gynecological Cancer, 24*(3), 576–585.

Joint United Nations Programme on HIV/AIDS (UNAIDS). (2007). NGO/Civil Society Participation in PCB. http://www.unaids.org/en/aboutunaids/unaidsprogrammecoordinatingboard/ngocivilsocietyparticipationinpcb.

Joint United Nations Programme on HIV/AIDS (UNAIDS). (2011). Getting to zero: UNAIDS strategies 2011–2015. http://www.unaids.org/en/media/unaids/contentassets/documents/unaidspublication/2010/JC2034_UNAIDS_Strategy_en.pdf.

Joint United Nations Programme on HIV/AIDS. (UNAIDS). (2014). HIV and AIDS estimates. http://www.unaids.org/en/regionscountries/countries/afghanistan.

Joint United Nations Programme on HIV/AIDS (UNAIDS). (2017). Getting to zero: How will we fast track the aids response? Discussion paper for consultations on UNAIDS strategy 2016-2021. http://www.icad-cisd.com/pdf/UNAIDS/Strategy-Consultations/1-UNAIDS-Discussion-Paper_2016-2021-Strategy-Consultations.

Kallen, A. J., et al. (2010). Health care-associated invasive MRSA infections, 2005-2008. *Journal of the American Medical Association, 304*(6), 641–648.

Khoury, N. M., et al. (2012). Explanatory models and mental health treatment: Is vodou an obstacle to psychiatric treatment in rural Haiti? *Culture, Medicine and Psychiatry, 36*(3), 514–534.

Kirkland, E. B., & Adams, B. B. (2008). Methicillin-resistant *Staphylococcus aureus* and athletes. *Journal of the American Academy of Dermatology, 59*(3), 494–502.

Koistinen, I., & Holma, J. (2015). Finnish health care professionals' views of patients who experience family violence. *Sage Open, 5*(1), 2158244015570392.

Kouadio, I. K., et al. (2012). Infectious diseases following natural disasters: Prevention and control measures. *Expert Review of Anti-infective Therapy, 10*(1), 95–104.

Lau, M., Lin, H., & Flores, G. (2012). Factors associated with human papillomavirus vaccine-series initiation and healthcare provider recommendation in US adolescent females: 2007 National Survey of Children's Health. *Vaccine, 30*(20), 3112–3118. doi:10.1016/j.vaccine.2012.02.034.

Learmonth, D., van Vuuren, A. J., & De Abreu, C. (2015). The influence of gender roles and traditional healing on cervical screening adherence amongst women in a Cape Town peri-urban settlement. *South African Family Practice, 57*(2), 62–63.

Lim, J. N. W., & Ojo, A. A. (2016). Barriers to utilisation of cervical cancer screening in sub-Saharan Africa: A systematic review. *European Journal of Cancer Care,* doi:10.1111/ecc.12444.

Liu, C., et al. (2011). Clinical practice guidelines by the Infectious Diseases Society of America for the treatment of methicillin-resistant *Staphylococcus aureus* infections in adults and children. *Clinical Infectious Diseases: An Official Publication of the Infectious Diseases Society of America, 52*(3), e18–e55.

Loke, A. Y., & Fung, O. W. M. (2014). Nurses' competencies in disaster nursing: Implications for curriculum development and public health. *International Journal of Environmental Research and Public Health, 11*(3), 3289–3303.

Lupton, K. (2015). Preparing nurses to work in Ebola treatment centres in Sierra Leone. *British Journal of Nursing, 24*(3), 168–172.

Marion, D., Charlebois, P. B., & Kao, R. (2016). The healthcare workers' clinical skill set requirements for a uniformed international response to the Ebola virus disease outbreak in West Africa: The Canadian perspective. *Journal of the Royal Army Medical Corps, 162*(3), 207–211.

Mazurana, D., et al. (2011). *Sex and age matter: Improving humanitarian response in emergencies.* Medford, MA: Feinstein International Center, Tufts University.

McAlister, E. A. (2016). Vodou: Haitian religion. http://www.britannica.com/topic/Vodou.

McFarlane, J., et al. (2014). Maternal-child dyads of functioning: The intergenerational impact of violence against women on children. *Maternal and Child Health Journal, 18*(9), 2236–2243.

Modibbo, F. I., et al. (2016). Qualitative study of barriers to cervical cancer screening among Nigerian women. *BMJ Open, 6*(1), e008533.

Nanyonga, M., et al. (2016). Sequelae of Ebola virus disease, Kenema District, Sierra Leone. *Clinical Infectious Diseases: An Official Publication of the Infectious Diseases Society of America, 62*(1), 125–126.

National Council on Alcoholism and Drug Dependence. (2015). Alcohol, drugs and crime. https://www.ncadd.org/about-addiction/addiction-update/alcohol-drugs-and-crime.

Pandey, A., et al. (2014). Strategies for containing Ebola in West Africa. *Science, 346*(6212), 991–995.

Perencevich, E. N., & Diekema, D. J. (2010). Decline in invasive MRSA infection: Where to go from here? *Journal of the American Medical Association, 304*(6), 687–689.

Purnell, L. D. (2008). Transcultural diversity and health care. In L. D. Purnell & B. J. Paulanka (Eds.), *Transcultural health care: A culturally competent approach* (pp. 1–18). Philadelphia: F.A. Davis.

Rogstad, K. E., & Tunbridge, A. (2015). Ebola virus as a sexually transmitted infection. *Current Opinion in Infectious Diseases, 28*(1), 83–85.

Ross, R., et al. (2009). The Satellite sexual violence assessment and care guide. *Women's Health Care, 8*(11), 25–31.

Ross, R., et al. (2010). The bridge: Providing nursing care for survivors of sexual violence. *Journal of the American Academy of Nurse Practitioner, 22,* 1–8.

Ross, R., et al. (2015). Intimate partner violence, emotional support, and health outcomes among Thai women: A mixed methods study. *Journal of the Royal Thai Army Nurses, 16*(1), 14–24.

Sawangchareon, K., et al. (2013). Developing nurses' competency on screening and helping women who had experienced intimate partner violence. *Journal of Nursing Science & Health, 36*(3), 95–105.

Schlievert, P. M., et al. (2010). *Staphylococcus aureus* exotoxins are present in vivo in tampons. *Clinical and Vaccine Immunology: CVI, 17*(5), 722–727.

Sedighi, I., Moez, H. J., & Alikhani, M. Y. (2011). Nasal carriage of methicillin resistant *Staphylococcus aureus* and their antibiotic susceptibility patterns in children attending day-care centers. *Acta Microbiologica et Immunologica Hungarica, 58*(3), 227–234.

Sullivan, T. P. (2013). Think outside: Advancing risk and protective factor research beyond the intimate-partner-violence box. *Psychology of Violence, 3*(2), 121.

Thomson Reuters Foundation. (2015). Haiti earthquake. http://news.trust.org//spotlight/Haiti-earthquake-2010/?tab=background.

Tiffany, A., et al. (2016). Ebola virus disease complications as experienced by survivors in Sierra Leone. *Clinical Infectious Diseases: An Official Publication of the Infectious Diseases Society of America, 62*(11), 1360–1366.

United Nations Children's Fund (UNICEF). (2012). The Baby-Friendly Hospital Initiative. http://www.unicef.org/programme/breastfeeding/baby.htm.

Warsini, S., et al. (2015). Post-traumatic stress disorder among survivors two years after the 2010 Mount Merapi volcano eruption: A survey study. *Nursing & health sciences, 17*(2), 173–180.

Waxman, D. (2011). Living with terror, not living in terror: The impact of chronic terrorism on Israeli society. *Perspectives on Terrorism, 5*(5-6), 4–26.

White, L., Waldrop, J., & Waldrop, C. (2016). Human papillomavirus and vaccination of males: Knowledge and attitudes of registered nurses. *Pediatric Nursing, 42*(1), 21–35.

William, M., et al. (2014). Assessment of psychological barriers to cervical cancer screening among women in Kumasi, Ghana using a mixed methods approach. *African Health Sciences, 13*(4), 1054–1061.

World Health Organization (WHO) (2000). *Turning the tide of malnutrition: Responding to the challenge of the 21st century. WHO/NHD/00.7.* Geneva: World Health Organization.

World Health Organization (WHO) (2004). *Serious childhood problems in countries with limited resources: Background book on management of the child with a serious infection or severe malnutrition.* Geneva: World Health Organization.

World Health Organization (WHO). (2011). The WHO child growth standards. http://www.who.int/childgrowth/standards/en/.

World Health Organization (WHO). (2012a). Obesity and overweight. http://www.who.int/mediacentre/factsheets/fs311/en/.

World Health Organization (WHO). (2012b). Violence. http://www.who.int/topics/violence/en/.

World Health Organization (WHO). (2012c). Suicide prevention (SUPRE). http://www.who.int/mental_health/prevention/suicide/suicideprevent/en/.

World Health Organization (WHO). (2012d). Mental health. http://www.who.int/topics/suicide/en/.

World Health Organization (WHO). (2014). New WHO guide to prevent and control cervical cancer. http://www.who.int/mediacentre/news/releases/2014/preventing-cervical-cancer/en/.

World Health Organization (WHO). (2015a). Global health observatory data. http://www.who.int/gho/ncd/mortality_morbidity/en/.

World Health Organization (WHO). (2015b). The top 10 causes of death. http://www.who.int/mediacentre/factsheets/fs310/en/index1.html.

World Health Organization (WHO). (2015c). Human papillomavirus (HPV) and cervical cancer. http://www.who.int/mediacentre/factsheets/fs380/en/.

World Health Organization (WHO). (2016a). Ebola virus disease. http://www.who.int/mediacentre/factsheets/fs103/en/.

World Health Organization (WHO). (2016b). Zika virus. http://www.who.int/topics/zika/en/.

World Health Organization (WHO). (2016c). Definition and typology of violence. http://www.who.int/violenceprevention/approach/definition/en/.

World Health Organization (WHO). (2016d). Epidemic intelligence—systematic event detection. http://www.who.int/csr/alertresponse/epidemicintelligence/en/.

World Health Organization (WHO). (2016e). Alert, response, and capacity building under the International Health Regulations (IHR). http://www.who.int/features/qa/39/en/index.html.

World Health Organization (WHO). (2016f). Mental health atlas 2011. Haiti. http://www.who.int/mental_health/evidence/atlas/profiles/hti_mh_profile.pdf?ua=1.

World Health Organization (WHO). (2016g). IASC guidelines on mental health and psychosocial support in emergency settings. http://www.who.int/mental_health/emergencies/IASC_guidelines.pdf.

World Health Organization (WHO). (2016h). What is malnutrition? http://www.who.int/features/qa/malnutrition/en/.

World Health Organization (WHO), & United Nations Children's Fund (UNICEF). (2009). Child growth standards and the identification of severe acute malnutrition in infants and children. http://www.who.int/nutrition/publications/severemalnutrition/9789241598163_eng.pdf.

World Hunger Education Service. (2012). 2011 world hunger and poverty facts and statistics. http://www.worldhunger.org/articles/Learn/world%20hunger%20facts%202002.htm.

Wosu, A. C., Gelaye, B., & Williams, M. A. (2015). History of childhood sexual abuse and risk of prenatal and postpartum depression or depressive symptoms: An epidemiologic review. *Archives of Women's Mental Health*, 18(5), 659–671.

Wright, J. G., et al. (2014). Effect of reduced dose schedules and intramuscular injection of anthrax vaccine adsorbed on immunological response and safety profile: A randomized trial. *Vaccine*, 32(8), 1019–1028.

Zhong, S., et al. (2014). Progress and challenges of disaster health management in China: A scoping review. *Global Health Action*, 7, 24986. doi:10.3402/gha.v7.24986.

# INDEX

Page numbers followed by *f* indicates figures; *t*, indicates tables; *b*, indicates boxes.